# TISSUE ENGINEERING
## PRINCIPLES AND PRACTICES

# TISSUE ENGINEERING
## PRINCIPLES AND PRACTICES

Edited by
John P. Fisher
Antonios G. Mikos
Joseph D. Bronzino
Donald R. Peterson

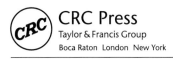

CRC Press
Taylor & Francis Group
Boca Raton   London   New York

CRC Press is an imprint of the
Taylor & Francis Group, an **informa** business

CRC Press
Taylor & Francis Group
6000 Broken Sound Parkway NW, Suite 300
Boca Raton, FL 33487-2742

First issued in paperback 2017

© 2013 by Taylor & Francis Group, LLC
CRC Press is an imprint of Taylor & Francis Group, an Informa business

No claim to original U.S. Government works

Version Date: 20120730

ISBN 13: 978-1-138-07786-7 (pbk)
ISBN 13: 978-1-4398-7400-4 (hbk)

---

**Library of Congress Cataloging-in-Publication Data**

---

Tissue engineering : principles and practices / edited by John P. Fisher [et al.].
    p. ; cm.
  Includes bibliographical references and index.
  ISBN 978-1-4398-7400-4 (hardcover : alk. paper)
  I. Fisher, John P.
  [DNLM: 1. Tissue Engineering. 2. Biocompatible Materials--therapeutic use. QT 37]

610.28--dc23

2012029517

---

**Visit the Taylor & Francis Web site at**
**http://www.taylorandfrancis.com**

**and the CRC Press Web site at**
**http://www.crcpress.com**

# Contents

Preface.................................................................................................................. ix

Editors ................................................................................................................ xi

Contributors ...................................................................................................... xv

## SECTION I  Fundamentals

1  Strategic Directions................................................................................**1**-1
   *Peter C. Johnson*

2  Silks .......................................................................................................**2**-1
   *Monica A. Serban and David L. Kaplan*

3  Calcium Phosphates ..............................................................................**3**-1
   *Kemal Sariibrahimoglu, Joop G.C. Wolke, Sander C.G. Leeuwenburgh,
   and John A. Jansen*

4  Engineered Protein Biomaterials..........................................................**4**-1
   *Andreina Parisi-Amon and Sarah C. Heilshorn*

5  Synthetic Biomaterials .........................................................................**5**-1
   *Joshua S. Katz and Jason A. Burdick*

6  Growth Factors and Morphogens: Signals for Tissue Engineering.............**6**-1
   *A. Hari Reddi*

7  Signal Expression in Engineered Tissues .............................................**7**-1
   *Martha O. Wang and John P. Fisher*

8  Pluripotent Stem Cells .........................................................................**8**-1
   *Todd C. McDevitt and Melissa A. Kinney*

9  Hematopoietic Stem Cells.....................................................................**9**-1
   *Ian M. Kaplan, Sebastien Morisot, and Curt I. Civin*

10  Mesenchymal Stem Cells.....................................................................**10**-1
   *Pamela C. Yelick and Weibo Zhang*

# SECTION II  Enabling Technologies

11  Nanobiomaterials for Tissue Engineering ..................................................... **11**-1
    *Pramod K. Avti, Sunny C. Patel, Pushpinder Uppal, Grace O'Malley, Joseph Garlow,
    and Balaji Sitharaman*

12  Biomimetic Approaches in Tissue Engineering .......................................... **12**-1
    *Indong Jun, Min Sup Kim, Ji-Hye Lee, Young Min Shin, and Heungsoo Shin*

13  Molecular Biology Techniques ..................................................................... **13**-1
    *X.G. Chen, Y.L. Fang, and W.T. Godbey*

14  Biomaterial Mechanics .................................................................................. **14**-1
    *Kimberly M. Stroka, Leann L. Norman, and Helim Aranda-Espinoza*

15  Mechanical Conditioning .............................................................................. **15**-1
    *Elaine L. Lee and Horst A. von Recum*

16  Micropatterned Biomaterials for Cell and Tissue Engineering .................. **16**-1
    *Murugan Ramalingam and Ali Khademhosseini*

17  Drug Delivery ................................................................................................ **17**-1
    *Prinda Wanakule and Krishnendu Roy*

18  Gene Therapy ................................................................................................. **18**-1
    *C. Holladay, M. Kulkarni, W. Minor, and Abhay Pandit*

19  Nanotechnology-Based Cell Engineering Strategies for Tissue
    Engineering and Regenerative Medicine Applications ............................... **19**-1
    *Joaquim Miguel Oliveira, João Filipe Mano, and Rui Luís Reis*

20  Cell Encapsulation ........................................................................................ **20**-1
    *Stephanie J. Bryant*

21  Coculture Systems for Mesenchymal Stem Cells ....................................... **21**-1
    *Song P. Seto and Johnna S. Temenoff*

22  Tissue Engineering Bioreactors ................................................................... **22**-1
    *Sarindr Bhumiratana, Elisa Cimetta, Nina Tandon, Warren Grayson, Milica Radisic,
    and Gordana Vunjak-Novakovic*

23  Shear Forces .................................................................................................. **23**-1
    *Jose F. Alvarez-Barreto, Samuel B. VanGordon, Brandon W. Engebretson,
    and Vasilios I. Sikavitsas*

24  Vascularization of Engineered Tissues ........................................................ **24**-1
    *Monica L. Moya and Eric M. Brey*

25  Biomedical Imaging of Engineered Tissues ................................................ **25**-1
    *Nicholas E. Simpson and Athanassios Sambanis*

26  Multiscale Modeling of *In Vitro* Tissue Cultivation ................................... **26**-1
    *Kyriacos Zygourakis*

# SECTION III    Applications

27  Bone Engineering ........................................................................ 27-1
    *Lucas A. Kinard, Antonios G. Mikos, and F. Kurtis Kasper*

28  Dental and Craniofacial Bioengineering .................................... 28-1
    *Hemin Nie and Jeremy J. Mao*

29  Tendon and Ligament Engineering ............................................ 29-1
    *Nicholas Sears, Tyler Touchet, Hugh Benhardt, and Elizabeth Cosgriff-Hernández*

30  Cartilage Tissue Engineering .................................................... 30-1
    *Emily E. Coates and John P. Fisher*

31  TMJ Engineering ...................................................................... 31-1
    *Michael S. Detamore*

32  Interface Tissue Engineering ..................................................... 32-1
    *Helen H. Lu, Nora Khanarian, Kristen Moffat, and Siddarth Subramony*

33  The Bioengineering of Dental Tissues ....................................... 33-1
    *Rena N. D'Souza, Katherine R. Regan, Kerstin M. Galler, and Songtao Shi*

34  Tissue Engineering of the Urogenital System ............................ 34-1
    *In Kap Ko, Anthony Atala, and James J. Yoo*

35  Vascular Tissue Engineering ..................................................... 35-1
    *Laura J. Suggs*

36  Neural Engineering ................................................................... 36-1
    *Yen-Chih Lin and Kacey G. Marra*

37  Tumor Engineering: Applications for Cancer Biology and
    Drug Development ..................................................................... 37-1
    *Joseph A. Ludwig and Emily Burdett*

Index ............................................................................................. Index-1

# Preface

Tissue engineering research continues to captivate the interest of researchers and the general public. Popular media outlets like the *New York Times*, *Time*, and *Wired* continue to engage a wide audience and foster excitement for the field as regenerative medicine inches toward becoming a clinical reality. The availability of tissue engineering knowledge and research is astounding. From the time the concept of "tissue engineering" and its terminology first originated in 1985, the field has continued to expand and evolve. A September 2012 PubMed database search through the National Library of Medicine for the term "tissue engineering" yields almost 26,000 literature citations and abstracts, with near 7,700 free, full-text journal articles. Ongoing research incorporates a diverse array of technologies from other fields, including nanotechnology, polymer sciences, and cell and molecular biology, contributing to the exponential growth of the vast body of literature surrounding the subject.

In an effort to put the numerous advances in the field into a broad context, this collection is devoted to the dissemination of current thoughts on the development of engineered tissues. To this end, the work has been divided into three sections: Fundamentals, Enabling Technologies, and Applications. The Fundamentals section examines the properties of stem cells, primary cells, growth factors, and extracellular matrix as well as their impact on the development of tissue-engineered devices. The Enabling Technologies section focuses upon those strategies typically incorporated into tissue-engineered devices or utilized in their development, including scaffolds, nanocomposites, bioreactors, drug delivery systems, and gene therapy techniques. Finally, the Applications section presents synthetic tissues and organs that are currently under development for regenerative medicine applications.

The contributing authors are a diverse group with backgrounds in academia, clinical medicine, and industry. Furthermore, this book includes contributions from Europe, Asia, and North America, helping to broaden the views on the development and application of tissue-engineered devices.

The format of this book is derived from the Advances in Tissue Engineering short course, which has been held at Rice University since 1993. This short course has educated researchers, students, clinicians, and engineers on both the fundamentals of tissue engineering and recent advances in many of the most prominent tissue engineering laboratories around the world. For many of the contributors, their chapter included in this book presents findings that have been recently discussed at the Advances in Tissue Engineering short course.

The target audience for this book includes not only researchers but also advanced students and industrial investigators. This book should be a useful reference for courses devoted to tissue engineering fundamentals and those laboratories developing tissue-engineered devices for regenerative medicine therapy.

**John P. Fisher**

**Antonios G. Mikos**

**Joseph D. Bronzino**

**Donald R. Peterson**

# Editors

**John P. Fisher** is professor and associate chair for undergraduate studies in the Fischell Department of Bioengineering at the University of Maryland. He completed a BS in chemical engineering at the Johns Hopkins University (1995), an MS in chemical engineering at the University of Cincinnati (1998), a PhD in bioengineering at Rice University (2003), and a postdoctoral fellowship in cartilage biology and engineering at the University of California, Davis (2003).

Dr. Fisher, the director of the Tissue Engineering and Biomaterials Laboratory, investigates biomaterials, stem cells, and bioreactors for the regeneration of lost tissues, particularly bone, cartilage, vasculature, and skeletal muscle. His research focuses on the development of novel, implantable, biocompatible materials that can support the development of both adult progenitor and adult stem cells, and he particularly examines how biomaterials affect endogenous molecular signaling among embedded cell populations. He is the author of over 65 publications, 120 scientific presentations, and 4 patents. Fisher has mentored 3 MS students and 10 PhD students. In addition, Fisher has mentored over 40 undergraduate researchers in his own lab, including 2 who were named University of Maryland Outstanding Undergraduate Researchers, 4 who have received Howard Hughes Medical Institute Undergraduate Research Fellowships, and 18 supported by Maryland Technology Enterprise Institute ASPIRE Awards.

In 2012, Dr. Fisher was elected Fellow of the American Institute for Medical and Biological Engineering. In addition, he has received an NSF (National Science Foundation) CAREER Award (2005), the Arthritis Foundation's Investigator Award (2006), the University of Maryland Invention of the Year Award (2006), the Outstanding Graduate Alumnus Award from the Department of Bioengineering at Rice University (2007), the Engalitcheff Award from the Arthritis Foundation (2008), the University of Maryland Professor Venture Fair Competition (2009), and the Teaching Excellence Award from the Fischell Department of Bioengineering at the University of Maryland (2011).

Since 2007, Dr. Fisher has directed the NSF-supported Molecular and Cellular Bioengineering Research Experiences for Undergraduates Site. He has served as editor of several works, and he is currently the editor-in-chief of the journal *Tissue Engineering, Part B: Reviews*. He has edited two books, and he was the tissue engineering editor for the third edition of *The Biomedical Engineering Handbook* (2006).

**Antonios G. Mikos** is the Louis Calder Professor of Bioengineering and Chemical and Biomolecular Engineering at Rice University. He is the director of the J.W. Cox Laboratory for Biomedical Engineering and the director of the Center for Excellence in Tissue Engineering at Rice University. He received the Dipl.Eng. (1983) from the Aristotle University of Thessaloniki, Greece, and a PhD (1988) in chemical engineering from Purdue University. He was a postdoctoral researcher at the Massachusetts Institute of Technology and the Harvard Medical School before joining the Rice Faculty in 1992 as an assistant professor.

Dr. Mikos' research focuses on the synthesis, processing, and evaluation of new biomaterials for use as scaffolds for tissue engineering, as carriers for controlled drug delivery, and as nonviral vectors for gene therapy. His work has led to the development of novel orthopedic, dental, cardiovascular, neurological, and ophthalmological biomaterials. He is the author of over 450 publications and 25 patents. He is the editor of 14 books and the author of one textbook (*Biomaterials: The Intersection of Biology and Materials Science*, Pearson Prentice Hall, 2008). He has been cited over 30,000 times and has an h-index of 96.

Dr. Mikos is a member of the National Academy of Engineering and a member of the Academy of Medicine, Engineering and Science of Texas. He is a fellow of the American Institute for Medical and Biological Engineering, a fellow of the International Union of Societies for Biomaterials Science and Engineering, a fellow of the Biomedical Engineering Society, a fellow of the Controlled Release Society, and a fellow of the American Association for the Advancement of Science. He has been recognized by various awards, including the *Founders Award* and the *Clemson Award for Contributions to the Literature* of the Society for Biomaterials, the *Robert A. Pritzker Distinguished Lecturer Award* of the Biomedical Engineering Society, the *Alpha Chi Sigma Award for Chemical Engineering Research* and the *Food, Pharmaceutical and Bioengineering Award in Chemical Engineering* of the American Institute of Chemical Engineers, the *Meriam/Wiley Distinguished Author Award* and the *Chemstations Lectureship Award* of the American Society for Engineering Education, the *Edith* and *Peter O'Donnell Award in Engineering* of the Academy of Medicine, Engineering and Science of Texas, the *Marshall R. Urist Award for Excellence in Tissue Regeneration Research* of the Orthopaedic Research Society, the *Distinguished Scientist Award—Isaac Schour Memorial Award* of the International Association for Dental Research, and the *Outstanding Chemical Engineer Award* of Purdue University.

Dr. Mikos has mentored 52 graduate students on their way to completing their doctoral studies, as well as 36 postdoctoral fellows, 22 of whom remain in academia at institutions, including Georgia Tech, Hanyang University, Mayo Clinic, Texas A&M University, Tulane University, University of Maryland, University of New Mexico, University of Oklahoma, University of Texas at Austin, Virginia Tech, and Rice University. He is the organizer of the continuing education course *Advances in Tissue Engineering* offered annually at Rice University since 1993.

Dr. Mikos is a founding editor and editor-in-chief of the journals *Tissue Engineering, Part A, Tissue Engineering, Part B: Reviews,* and *Tissue Engineering, Part C: Methods* and a member of the editorial boards of the journals *Advanced Drug Delivery Reviews, Cell Transplantation, Journal of Biomaterials Science Polymer Edition, Journal of Biomedical Materials Research (Parts A and B),* and *Journal of Controlled Release.*

**Joseph D. Bronzino** earned a BSEE from Worcester Polytechnic Institute, Worcester, Massachusetts, in 1959, an MSEE from the Naval Postgraduate School, Monterey, California, in 1961, and a PhD in electrical engineering from Worcester Polytechnic Institute in 1968. He is presently the Vernon Roosa Professor of Applied Science, an endowed chair at Trinity College, Hartford, Connecticut, and president of the Biomedical Engineering Alliance and Consortium (BEACON), a nonprofit organization consisting of academic and medical institutions as well as corporations dedicated to the development and commercialization of new medical technologies (www.beaconalliance.org).

Dr. Bronzino is the author of over 200 articles and 11 books, including *Technology for Patient Care* (C.V. Mosby, 1977), *Computer Applications for Patient Care* (Addison-Wesley, 1982), *Biomedical Engineering: Basic Concepts and Instrumentation* (PWS Publishing Co., 1986), *Expert Systems: Basic Concepts* (Research Foundation of State University of New York, 1989), *Medical Technology and Society: An Interdisciplinary Perspective* (MIT Press and McGraw-Hill, 1990), *Management of Medical Technology* (Butterworth/Heinemann, 1992), *The Biomedical Engineering Handbook* (CRC Press, 1st Ed., 1995; 2nd Ed., 2000; 3rd Ed., 2005 ), and *Introduction to Biomedical Engineering* (Academic Press 1st Ed., 1999; 2nd Ed., 2005),

Dr. Bronzino is a fellow of IEEE and the American Institute of Medical and Biological Engineering (AIMBE), an honorary member of the Italian Society of Experimental Biology, past chairman of the Biomedical Engineering Division of the American Society for Engineering Education (ASEE), a charter member and former vice president of the Connecticut Academy of Science and Engineering (CASE), and a charter member of the American College of Clinical Engineering (ACCE), the Association for the

Advancement of Medical Instrumentation (AAMI), past president of the IEEE-Engineering in Medicine and Biology Society (EMBS), past chairman of the IEEE Health Care Engineering Policy Committee (HCEPC), past chairman of the IEEE Technical Policy Council in Washington, DC, and presently editor-in-chief of Elsevier's BME Book Series and CRC Press's *The Biomedical Engineering Handbook*.

Dr. Bronzino received the Millennium Award from IEEE/EMBS in 2000 and the Goddard Award from Worcester Polytechnic Institute for Professional Achievement in June 2004.

**Donald R. Peterson** is an associate professor of medicine and the director of the biodynamics laboratory in the School of Medicine at the University of Connecticut (UConn). He serves jointly as the director of the biomedical engineering undergraduate program in the School of Engineering and recently served as the director of the graduate program and as the BME Program chair. He earned a PhD in biomedical engineering and an MS in mechanical engineering at UConn and a BS in aerospace engineering and a BS in biomechanical engineering from Worcester Polytechnic Institute. Dr. Peterson has 16 years of experience in biomedical engineering education and offers graduate-level and undergraduate-level courses in BME in the areas of biomechanics, biodynamics, biofluid mechanics, and ergonomics, and he teaches in medicine in the subjects of gross anatomy, occupational biomechanics, and occupational exposure and response. Dr. Peterson's scholarly activities include over 50 published journal articles, 3 textbook chapters, and 12 textbooks, including his new appointment as co-editor-in-chief for *The Biomedical Engineering Handbook* by CRC Press.

Dr. Peterson has over 21 years of experience in biomedical engineering research and has been recently focused on measuring and modeling human, organ, and/or cell performance, including exposures to various physical stimuli and the subsequent biological responses. This work also involves the investigation of human–device interaction and has led to applications on the design and development of tools and various medical devices. Dr. Peterson is faculty within the occupational and environmental medicine group at the UConn Health Center, where his work has been directed toward the objective analysis of the anatomic and physiological processes involved in the onset of musculoskeletal and neuromuscular diseases, including strategies of disease mitigation. Recent applications of his research include human interactions with existing and developmental devices such as powered and non-powered tools, spacesuits and space tools for NASA, surgical and dental instruments, musical instruments, sports equipment, and computer-input devices. Other overlapping research initiatives focus on cell mechanics and cellular responses to fluid shear stress, the acoustics of hearing protection and communication, human exposure and response to vibration, and the development of computational models of biomechanical performance.

Dr. Peterson is also the co-executive director of the Biomedical Engineering Alliance and Consortium (BEACON; www.beaconalliance.org), which is a nonprofit entity dedicated to the promotion of collaborative research, translation, and partnership among academic, medical, and industry people in the field of biomedical engineering to develop new medical technologies and devices.

# Contributors

**Jose F. Alvarez-Barreto**
Human Tissue Engineering Laboratory
Ciencia y Tecnología para la Salud
Instituto de Estudios Avanzados
Caracas, Venezuela

**Helim Aranda-Espinoza**
Fischell Department of
    Bioengineering
University of Maryland
College Park, Maryland

**Anthony Atala**
Wake Forest Institute for
    Regenerative Medicine
Wake Forest University School of
    Medicine
Winston-Salem, North Carolina

**Pramod K. Avti**
Department of Biomedical
    Engineering
Stony Brook University
Stony Brook, New York

**Hugh Benhardt**
Department of Biomedical
    Engineering
Texas A&M University
College Station, Texas

**Sarindr Bhumiratana**
Department of Biomedical
    Engineering
Columbia University
New York, New York

**Eric M. Brey**
Pritzker Institute of Biomedical Science and
    Engineering
Department of Biomedical Engineering
Illinois Institute of Technology
and
Research Service
Edward Hines Jr. Veterans Hospital
Chicago, Illinois

**Stephanie J. Bryant**
Department of Chemical and Biological
    Engineering
University of Colorado
Boulder, Colorado

**Emily Burdett**
Department of Bioengineering
BioScience Research Collaborative
Houston, Texas

**Jason A. Burdick**
Department of Bioengineering
University of Pennsylvania
Philadelphia, Pennsylvania

**X.G. Chen**
Department of Chemical and Biomolecular
    Engineering
Tulane University
New Orleans, Louisiana

**Elisa Cimetta**
Department of Biomedical Engineering
Columbia University
New York, New York

**Curt I. Civin**
Center for Stem Cell Biology and
    Regenerative Medicine
University of Maryland School of
    Medicine
Baltimore, Maryland

**Emily E. Coates**
Fischell Department of
    Bioengineering
University of Maryland
College Park, Maryland

**Elizabeth Cosgriff-Hernández**
Department of Biomedical
    Engineering
Texas A&M University
College Station, Texas

**Michael S. Detamore**
Department of Chemical and Petroleum
    Engineering
University of Kansas
Lawrence, Kansas

**Rena N. D'Souza**
Department of Biomedical
    Sciences
Texas A&M Health Science Center—Baylor
    College of Dentistry
Dallas, Texas

**Brandon W. Engebretson**
Department of Bioengineering
University of Oklahoma
Norman, Oklahoma

**Y.L. Fang**
Department of Chemical and Biomolecular
    Engineering
Tulane University
New Orleans, Louisiana

**John P. Fisher**
Fischell Department of
    Bioengineering
University of Maryland
College Park, Maryland

**Kerstin M. Galler**
Department of Restorative Dentistry and
    Periodontology
University of Regensburg
Regensburg, Germany

**Joseph Garlow**
Department of Biomedical Engineering
Stony Brook University
Stony Brook, New York

**W.T. Godbey**
Department of Chemical and Biomolecular
    Engineering
Tulane University
New Orleans, Louisiana

**Warren Grayson**
Department of Biomedical Engineering
Johns Hopkins University
Baltimore, Maryland

**Sarah C. Heilshorn**
Department of Materials Science and Engineering
Stanford University
Stanford, California

**C. Holladay**
Network of Excellence for Functional
    Biomaterials
National University of Ireland, Galway
Galway, Ireland

**John A. Jansen**
Department of Biomaterials
Radboud University Nijmegen Medical Center
Nijmegen, The Netherlands

**Peter C. Johnson**
Research and Development
Avery-Dennison Medical Solutions
Chicago, Illinois

and

Scintellix, LLC
Raleigh, North Carolina

**Indong Jun**
Department of Bioengineering
Hanyang University
Seoul, Korea

**David L. Kaplan**
Department of Biomedical Engineering
Tufts University
Medford, Massachusetts

**Ian M. Kaplan**
Program in Cellular and Molecular Medicine
Johns Hopkins School of Medicine
and
Center for Stem Cell Biology and
    Regenerative Medicine
University of Maryland School of Medicine
Baltimore, Maryland

**F. Kurtis Kasper**
Department of Bioengineering
Rice University
Houston, Texas

**Joshua S. Katz**
Dow Chemical Company
Spring House, Pennsylvania

**Ali Khademhosseini**
WPI Advanced Institute for Materials Research
Tohoku University
Sendai, Japan
and
Department of Medicine
Brigham and Women's Hospital
Harvard Medical School
and
Harvard-MIT Division of Health Sciences
    and Technology
Massachusetts Institute of Technology
Cambridge, Massachusetts

**Nora Khanarian**
Columbia University
New York, New York

**Min Sup Kim**
Department of Bioengineering
Hanyang University
Seoul, Korea

**Lucas A. Kinard**
Department of Bioengineering
Rice University
Houston, Texas

**Melissa A. Kinney**
Georgia Institute of Technology
Atlanta, Georgia

**In Kap Ko**
Wake Forest Institute for
    Regenerative Medicine
Wake Forest University School of
    Medicine
Winston-Salem, North Carolina

**M. Kulkarni**
Network of Excellence for Functional
    Biomaterials
National University of Ireland,
    Galway
Galway, Ireland

**Elaine L. Lee**
Department of Biomedical
    Engineering
Case Western Reserve University
Cleveland, Ohio

**Ji-Hye Lee**
Department of Bioengineering
Hanyang University
Seoul, Korea

**Sander C.G. Leeuwenburgh**
Department of Biomaterials
Radboud University Nijmegen
    Medical Center
Nijmegen, The Netherlands

**Yen-Chih Lin**
Department of Plastic Surgery
University of Pittsburgh
Pittsburgh, Pennsylvania

**Helen H. Lu**
Columbia University
New York, New York

**Joseph A. Ludwig**
Department of Sarcoma Medical Oncology
MD Anderson Cancer Center
University of Texas, Houston
Houston, Texas

**João Filipe Mano**
3B's Research Group—Biomaterials,
    Biodegradables, and Biomimetics
University of Minho
and
ICVS/3B's
PT Government Associated Laboratory
Guimarães, Portugal

**Jeremy J. Mao**
Tissue Engineering and Regenerative Medicine
    Laboratory
Center for Craniofacial Regeneration
Columbia University Medical Center
New York, New York

**Kacey G. Marra**
Departments of Plastic Surgery and Bioengineering
University of Pittsburgh
Pittsburgh, Pennsylvania

**Todd C. McDevitt**
Georgia Institute of Technology
Atlanta, Georgia

**Antonios G. Mikos**
Department of Bioengineering
Rice University
Houston, Texas

**W. Minor**
Network of Excellence for Functional Biomaterials
National University of Ireland, Galway
Galway, Ireland

**Kristen Moffat**
Columbia University
New York, New York

**Sebastien Morisot**
Center for Stem Cell Biology and Regenerative
    Medicine
University of Maryland School
    of Medicine
Baltimore, Maryland

**Monica L. Moya**
Department of Biomedical Engineering
University of California, Irvine
Irvine, California

**Hemin Nie**
Tissue Engineering and Regenerative
    Medicine Laboratory
Center for Craniofacial Regeneration
Columbia University Medical Center
New York, New York

**Leann L. Norman**
Fischell Department of Bioengineering
University of Maryland
College Park, Maryland

**Joaquim Miguel Oliveira**
3B's Research Group—Biomaterials,
    Biodegradables, and Biomimetics
University of Minho
and
ICVS/3B's
PT Government Associated
    Laboratory
Guimarães, Portugal

**Grace O'Malley**
Department of Biomedical Engineering
Stony Brook University
Stony Brook, New York

**Abhay Pandit**
Network of Excellence Functional
    Biomaterials
National University of Ireland,
    Galway
Galway, Ireland

**Andreina Parisi-Amon**
Department of Bioengineering
Stanford University
Stanford, California

**Sunny C. Patel**
Department of Biomedical Engineering
Stony Brook University
Stony Brook, New York

**Milica Radisic**
Department of Chemical Engineering and
    Applied Chemistry
University of Toronto
Toronto, Ontario, Canada

**Murugan Ramalingam**
WPI Advanced Institute for Materials
    Research
Tohoku University
Sendai, Japan

**A. Hari Reddi**
University of California, Davis
Davis, California

**Katherine R. Regan**
Department of Biomedical Sciences
Texas A&M Health Science Center—Baylor
    College of Dentistry
Dallas, Texas

**Rui Luís Reis**
3B's Research Group—Biomaterials,
    Biodegradables, and Biomimetics
University of Minho
and
ICVS/3B's
PT Government Associated Laboratory
Guimarães, Portugal

**Krishnendu Roy**
Department of Biomedical Engineering
University of Texas, Austin
Austin, Texas

**Athanassios Sambanis**
School of Chemical and Biomolecular
    Engineering
Georgia Institute of Technology
Atlanta, Georgia

**Kemal Sariibrahimoglu**
Department of Biomaterials
Radboud University Nijmegen
    Medical Center
Nijmegen, The Netherlands

**Nicholas Sears**
Department of Biomedical Engineering
Texas A&M University
College Station, Texas

**Monica A. Serban**
Department of Biomedical Engineering
Tufts University
Medford, Massachusetts

**Song P. Seto**
Department of Biomedical Engineering
Georgia Institute of Technology
and
Emory University
Atlanta, Georgia

**Songtao Shi**
Center for Craniofacial Biology
University of Southern California School of
    Dentistry
Los Angeles, California

**Heungsoo Shin**
Department of Bioengineering
Hanyang University
Seoul, Korea

**Young Min Shin**
Department of Bioengineering
Hanyang University
Seoul, Korea

**Vasillios I. Sikavitsas**
Department of Bioengineering
University of Oklahoma
Norman, Oklahoma

**Nicholas E. Simpson**
Department of Medicine
University of Florida
Gainesville, Florida

**Balaji Sitharaman**
Department of Biomedical Engineering
Stony Brook University
Stony Brook, New York

**Kimberly M. Stroka**
Fischell Department of Bioengineering
University of Maryland
College Park, Maryland

**Siddarth Subramony**
Columbia University
New York, New York

**Laura J. Suggs**
Department of Biomedical
    Engineering
University of Texas, Austin
Austin, Texas

**Nina Tandon**
Department of Biomedical Engineering
Columbia University
New York, New York

**Johnna S. Temenoff**
Department of Biomedical Engineering
Georgia Institute of Technology
and
Emory University
Atlanta, Georgia

**Tyler Touchet**
Department of Biomedical Engineering
Texas A&M University
College Station, Texas

**Pushpinder Uppal**
Department of Biomedical Engineering
Stony Brook University
Stony Brook, New York

**Samuel B. VanGordon**
Department of Bioengineering
University of Oklahoma
Norman, Oklahoma

**Horst A. von Recum**
Department of Biomedical Engineering
Case Western Reserve University
Cleveland, Ohio

**Gordana Vunjak-Novakovic**
Department of Biomedical Engineering
Columbia University
New York, New York

**Prinda Wanakule**
Department of Biomedical Engineering
University of Texas, Austin
Austin, Texas

**Martha O. Wang**
Fischell Department of Bioengineering
University of Maryland
College Park, Maryland

**Joop G.C. Wolke**
Department of Biomaterials
Radboud University Nijmegen Medical Center
Nijmegen, The Netherlands

**Pamela C. Yelick**
Tufts University School of Dental Medicine
Boston, Massachusetts

**James J. Yoo**
Wake Forest Institute for Regenerative
  Medicine
Wake Forest University School of Medicine
Winston-Salem, North Carolina

**Weibo Zhang**
Tufts University School of Dental Medicine
Boston, Massachusetts

**Kyriacos Zygourakis**
Department of Chemical and Biomolecular
  Engineering
Rice University
Houston, Texas

# I

# Fundamentals

1 **Strategic Directions** *Peter C. Johnson* ............................................................1-1
Introduction • Previous Approaches to the Assignment of Strategic
Directions in Tissue Engineering • Tools in the Identification of Strategic
Directions • Summary • References

2 **Silks** *Monica A. Serban and David L. Kaplan*............................................................2-1
Introduction to Silks • Tissue Engineering Applications of Silks • Concluding
Remarks • References

3 **Calcium Phosphates** *Kemal Sariibrahimoglu, Joop G.C. Wolke,
Sander C.G. Leeuwenburgh, and John A. Jansen* ................................................3-1
Introduction • Physicochemical Properties of CaP Compounds • CaP Blocks/
Granules • CaP Cements • Conclusion • References

4 **Engineered Protein Biomaterials** *Andreina Parisi-Amon and Sarah C. Heilshorn* ....... 4-1
Engineered Protein Biomaterials as an Alternative to "Traditional"
Biomaterials • Synthesis of Engineered Protein Biomaterials • Design of Engineered
Protein Biomaterials • Applications of Engineered Protein Biomaterials • References

5 **Synthetic Biomaterials** *Joshua S. Katz and Jason A. Burdick*...........................................5-1
Introduction • Choice of Monomer • Polymerization Mechanisms • Biomaterial
Degradation • Poly(ethylene glycol) • Poly(esters) • Poly(anhydrides) • Poly(ortho
esters) • Poly(urethanes) • Pseudo Poly(amino acids) • Poly(acrylates) and
Poly(methacrylates) • Non-Polymeric Synthetic Biomaterials • Conclusions • References

6 **Growth Factors and Morphogens: Signals for Tissue Engineering** *A. Hari Reddi*........ 6-1
Introduction • Tissue Engineering and Morphogenesis • The Bone Morphogenetic
Proteins • Growth Factors • BMPs Bind to Extracellular Matrix • Clinical
Applications • Challenges and Opportunities • Acknowledgments • References

7 **Signal Expression in Engineered Tissues** *Martha O. Wang and John P. Fisher* ...........7-1
Introduction • Biology of Osteoblasts • Biology of Chondrocytes • Signaling
Pathway Overview • Anabolic Growth Factors/Cytokines • Catabolic Growth
Factors/Cytokines • Hormones • Mechanotransduction • Dual Growth Factor
Studies • Conclusion • References

8 **Pluripotent Stem Cells** *Todd C. McDevitt and Melissa A. Kinney*.................................. 8-1
Origin and Derivation of Embryonic Stem Cells • Characteristics • Alternate
Derivation Methods • Propagation • Differentiation • Clinical
Outlook • Conclusion • References

**9   Hematopoietic Stem Cells**  *Ian M. Kaplan, Sebastien Morisot, and Curt I. Civin*......... **9**-1
Introduction: The Hematopoietic Hierarchy • The Hematopoietic Lineage Commitment
Process • Hematopoietic Stem Cells • Sources of Hematopoietic Stem Cells for Clinical
Transplantation • *Ex Vivo* Expansion of HSCs • Conclusion • References

**10   Mesenchymal Stem Cells**  *Pamela C. Yelick and Weibo Zhang*...................................... **10**-1
Definition • Cell Characteristics • Potential Therapeutic Applications •
Potential Concerns • Conclusion • References

# 1

# Strategic Directions

| | | |
|---|---|---|
| 1.1 | Introduction | 1-1 |
| 1.2 | Previous Approaches to the Assignment of Strategic Directions in Tissue Engineering | 1-2 |
| 1.3 | Tools in the Identification of Strategic Directions | 1-3 |
| | Identification of Concepts Having General Criticality • Cohesive Technology Opportunity Stratification • Modulators of Strategy | |
| 1.4 | Summary | 1-8 |
| | References | 1-9 |

Peter C. Johnson
*Avery-Dennison*
*Medical Solutions*
*Scintellix, LLC*

## 1.1 Introduction

Properly identified strategic directions for technology development optimize our ability to bring robustly engineered tissues to humanity. They guide our work within the dual envelopes of technical possibility and social/commercial acceptability. As we have learned, the effective engineering of human tissues represents a challenge of the highest order (Table 1.1). In order to make effective progress, some marshalling of resources and establishment of common directions are becoming ever more essential. A reasoned declaration of strategy is now more necessary for our field than ever.

Strategy implies the efficient application of resources toward a common end. It begins with the end in sight and works backwards to define tactics, boundary conditions and a temporal sequence that together, enable the end to be reached. What is this "end" in the field of tissue engineering? Simply stated, it is the creation of reproducible tissue replacement/augmentation technologies that are safe, effective, and economically attractive for use in day-to-day healthcare across the entire population.

Strategy, although forward-looking, is limited by what is known at the point in time when it is crafted. It is axiomatic that "best laid plans" are commonly thwarted by either a misappreciation of challenges or by the emergence of previously unknown accelerators of development. Nonetheless, what is important about strategy is its capacity—when well designed—to bring key stakeholders together into a common understanding of goals, tactics, and limitations. The set of stakeholders who have a vested interest in tissue engineering success is quite broad—and their interests are diverse (Table 1.2). The development of a comprehensive strategy for the field requires that their needs as a group be carefully considered.

The complete aggregation of these stakeholders in a robust strategic planning exercise has never been achieved, though such processes are now being designed. In harmony with the nature of a *Bioengineering Handbook*, this piece will therefore not provide a specific set of strategic directions for the field but rather, a system through which strategic directions can be defined. The techniques presented here can be used not only to support pan-stakeholder strategy development but also the strategic directions of individual investigators and their laboratory teams.

**TABLE 1.1**   Components of the Overall Challenge Facing the Field of Tissue Engineering

| Challenge Component | Concern |
| --- | --- |
| Intellectual | Can we attract and retain sufficient multidisciplinary talent having the imagination and tenacity to overcome present technical limitations? Can we sufficiently unify the focus of tissue engineers to meet technical goals? |
| Technical | Can cells be reproducibly sourced and tissues be manufactured to specification? Can we master the requirements for both 2D and 3D tissues, the latter as perfusable systems? |
| Regulatory | Can engineered tissues exhibit safety and efficacy thresholds that will trigger FDA clearance for marketing? |
| Commercial | Can engineered tissues replace existing technologies with enhanced function and lower cost? |
| Social | Will caregivers and patients embrace engineered tissues as solutions to multiple health care problems? |

**TABLE 1.2**   Stakeholders

| Stakeholders | Primary Concerns |
| --- | --- |
| Patients | Safety, efficacy, cost |
| Caregivers | Safety, efficacy, cost, ease of use, improvement upon other technology |
| Payers | Safety, efficacy, cost-effectiveness |
| Scientists/engineers | Technically possible |
| Research funding agencies | Probability of technical success and successful application in humans |
| Regulatory bodies | Safety and efficacy |
| Investors/companies/employees | Commercial profitability |
| General public | Understandability and acceptability as a technology; nonthreatening |

*Note:* The stakeholders in the field of tissue engineering represent a complex set of capabilities and interests, all of which must be considered in the assignment of strategic directions for the field.

## 1.2 Previous Approaches to the Assignment of Strategic Directions in Tissue Engineering

While there have been several scholarly assessments of the state of technical and commercial development in tissue engineering, formal, pan-stakeholder strategic directions have seldom been a focus of such work.[1–9] In a 2007 publication,[3] Johnson et al. reviewed a general, primarily technical strategy for the field. Using Hoshin strategic assessment methodology, the authors surveyed the worldwide editorial board of the journal, *Tissue Engineering*. By putting forth a goal of strong clinical penetration of tissue engineering technologies by the year 2021, they were able to elicit those steps that the editors felt were required to achieve the goal. They then compared the relative dominance of the identified steps (Table 1.3) and incorporated an assessment of present progress (Table 1.4) to further stratify the steps by priority. The result is shown in Table 1.5.

This study had the advantage of inclusion of international participants but was limited to a single component of the stakeholder pool—scientists and engineers. Although certainly not causal, the article presaged the recent explosion of literature in the angiogenesis,[10] stem cell,[11] and systems biology categories. Since these were deemed the most critical positive influencers of the other steps, it remains to be seen how technical accomplishments in the field will accelerate as a consequence. The article also identifies technology development funding as a critical element but perhaps surprisingly, only as a follower to the other strategic steps. A cohesive story and preliminary data, after all, are always requirements for

**TABLE 1.3** Relative Dominance of Strategic Steps

| Strategic Step | Relative Dominance |
| --- | --- |
| Stem cell science | 12 |
| Molecular biology/systems biology | 11 |
| Clinical understanding/interaction | 10 |
| Cell sourcing and cell/tissue interaction | 10 |
| Angiogenic control | 9 |
| Immunologic understanding and control | 7 |
| Standardized models | 5 |
| Regulatory transparency | 5 |
| Multidisciplinary understanding/cooperation | 5 |
| Manufacturing/scale up | 4 |
| Enhanced biomaterial functionality | 4 |
| Expectation management/communication | 2 |
| Pharmacoeconomic/commercial pathway | 1 |
| Multilevel funding | 0 |

*Note:* All of the strategic steps listed are considered to be critical to the achievement of the goal. However, their relative dominance is shown on the right as the number of other steps over which they are felt to be stronger in a pairwise comparison.[3]

**TABLE 1.4** Strategic Steps: Progress to Date (2007)

| Strategic Step | Progress to Date (2007) |
| --- | --- |
| Multidisciplinary understanding/cooperation | 6.5 |
| Expectation management/communication | 5.5 |
| Multilevel funding | 4.8 |
| Enhanced biomaterial functionality | 4.8 |
| Standardized models | 4.8 |
| Clinical understanding/Interaction | 4.5 |
| Regulatory transparency | 4.5 |
| Molecular biology/systems biology | 4.0 |
| Cell sourcing and cell/tissue characterization | 3.8 |
| Stem cell science | 3.8 |
| Pharmacoeconomic/commercial pathway | 3.8 |
| Manufacturing/scale up | 3.5 |
| Immunologic understanding and control | 3.5 |
| Angiogenic control | 2.8 |

*Note:* Progress was semi quantitatively assigned using a continuous scale from 1 = No Progress to 10 = Fully Complete.[3]

funding to occur. Future articles of this type would do well to enhance inclusion of the stakeholder pool along the lines outlined in Table 1.1.

## 1.3 Tools in the Identification of Strategic Directions

### 1.3.1 Identification of Concepts Having General Criticality

It is often difficult to physically assemble a significant number of representatives of the stakeholder pools shown in Table 1.1 in order to gain their feedback on the elements of strategic direction for a field.

**TABLE 1.5**   Normalized Dominance of Strategic Steps

| Normalized Dominance of Strategic Steps | Ratio of Dominance/ Progress |
|---|---|
| Angiogenic control | 3.3 |
| Stem cell science | 3.2 |
| Molecular biology/systems biology | 2.8 |
| Cell sourcing and cell/tissue characterization | 2.7 |
| Clinical understanding/interaction | 2.2 |
| Immunologic understanding and control | 2.0 |
| Manufacturing/scale up | 1.1 |
| Regulatory transparency | 1.1 |
| Standardized models | 1.1 |
| Enhanced biomaterial functionality | 0.8 |
| Multidisciplinary understanding/cooperation | 0.8 |
| Expectation management/communication | 0.4 |
| Pharmacoeconomic/commercial pathway | 0.3 |
| Multilevel funding | 0.0 |

*Note:* When the Relative Dominance number in Table 1.3 is divided by the Progress number in Table 1.4, a normalization of strategic step priority is achieved. This approach enables the identification of the sequence of steps that will be the most efficient in the achievement of the goal.[3]

**TABLE 1.6**   Generally Critical Concepts for Tissue Engineering

| Concepts Having General Criticality for Tissue Engineering |
|---|
| Clinical need |
| Degree of improvement over alternative therapy |
| Technical feasibility |
| Cost effectiveness |
| Likeliness to pass the regulatory process |
| Likeliness to be reimbursed |
| Manufacturability |
| Ease of distribution |
| Potential for general use |
| Likeliness of caregiver adoption |
| Degree to which free of biological risk |

As previously discussed, online or mailed survey instruments may be effectively used to gain information from these groups. Table 1.6 depicts an example set of Generally Critical Concepts (GCC) that might be gleaned from a comprehensive survey of all stakeholder groups (in the author's estimation).

While good general directions can be gleaned in this fashion, it is difficult to determine specific technology development directions from them, such as which tissue or which clinical indication would be best to focus on at any point in time.

## 1.3.2 Cohesive Technology Opportunity Stratification

A follow-on methodology known as Cohesive Technology Opportunity Stratification (CTOS) can be used to leverage agreed-upon concepts having General Criticality in order to provide this functionality.

Briefly described, CTOS assembles GCC, weights them by their importance relative to one another and incorporates these weights into an algorithm-driven technology stratification spreadsheet. In the latter, intensity of fit scales are developed under each Generally Critical Concept to allow assignment of a value to any technology being assessed. In addition, the weight of the GCC is multiplied by the scalar assignment in each column and these are summed for all GCCs as shown in Figure 1.1. Weights and scales are ideally assigned/developed together by representatives of all stakeholder groups. An example of how weights are assigned is shown in Table 1.7 (author's impressions are only shown).

While the assignment of weights in this example are the author's alone, they were assigned with a general appreciation for the points of view of the stakeholder groups in Table 1.1. If these values were to be ratified in a formal pan-stakeholder survey and assignment, the relative criticality of concepts would be illuminating. For example, the likeliness of reimbursement, the ability to pass regulatory review, cost-effectiveness and absence of biological risk loom large in the assessment of any technology. Conversely, technical feasibility weighs in only weakly as a deciding element. This is because tissue engineering, to be successful as an applied medical discipline, must begin any assessment of its strategic direction at the "end." That is, any tissue engineering technology must pass through the same hurdles (reimbursement, regulation, cost-effectiveness, risk) as do present, nontissue engineering technologies. Another way to put this is that the most technically feasible tissue engineering technology is of little worth to humanity if it cannot pass through these critical hurdles that enable commercialization.

Figure 1.1 shows the aforementioned Technology Stratification Spreadsheet. Note that the spreadsheet has both "Perfect" and "Threshold" entries. The Perfect technology would achieve the highest scalar scores for each of the GCCs. The Threshold technology values (numerics assigned by the author only) represent the minimum that would be acceptable for a tissue engineering technology to reach human use. Note that both the weighting and stratification mechanisms are time and progress-sensitive. Should there be changes in reimbursement or regulatory systems or if technology advanced rapidly to reduce risk and enhance cost-effectiveness, scalar and weight values could change, perhaps also changing the Threshold value for acceptable technology. These tools are simply provided as examples of ways in which the processing of strategic directions can be made more objective.

Also to be noted in Figure 1.1 is that assigning scalar values for each GCC assesses several tissue targets for development. These are then processed according to the multiplication (by weight) and summation algorithm. Note the tissues that fall above and below the Threshold level at this point in time (author's numeric assignments only). A general assessment of the stakeholder pools in tissue engineering is presently underway and will be the topic of a future report. Until then, any stratification of this type must be considered tentative.

An analysis of this type takes into consideration the circumstances of the time of the analysis and perhaps a short look into the future only. As such, the tissue targets deemed most worthy of development today can change over time, as factors such as technical feasibility, reimbursability, regulatory clearance potential and the like change. The numbers shown in this analysis represent the best guess of the author only. In a formal strategic planning session, all stakeholder groups would agree upon these. In this analysis, there is no surprise that the tissues deemed most readily developable in today's timeframe have almost all demonstrated some degree of commercial momentum. Also, the temporal progression from 1D (cell) to 2D (planar sheets of cells and matrix) and 3D (vascularized organs or organoids) tissue development appears to hold up as a function of construct complexity.

## 1.3.3 Modulators of Strategy

As previously alluded, strategic direction represents a best guess as to the optimal course a field of endeavor can pursue, given present and immediate future restraints. However, what if these restraints are underestimated? Or better, what if new discoveries are made that bypass present restraints? Under these circumstances, a revisitation of strategy will be called for immediately, as the game will have changed. Modulators of strategy can come in many forms. Table 1.8 illustrates several such unexpected modulators, both inhibitors and accelerators. It is important to watch for these, since they can have a major impact on the timing of development of the essential technology bases of the field.

Strategic Selection of Tissue Engineering Solutions

| Criteria | Clinical Need | Degree of Improvement Upon Alternate Therapy | Technical Feasibility | Cost Effectiveness | Likeliness to Pass the Regulatory Process | Likeliness to Be Reimbursed | Manufactur-ability | Ease of Distribution | Potential for General Use | Likeliness of Caregiver Adoption | Degree To Which Free of Biological Risk | Total |
|---|---|---|---|---|---|---|---|---|---|---|---|---|
| Scale | 0 = None<br>1 = Minimal<br>2 = Clear<br>3 = Extensive | 0 = None<br>1 = Minimal<br>2 = Clear<br>3 = Extensive | 0 = Not Feasible<br>1 = Possible<br>2 = Probable<br>3 = Certain | 0 = Not Cost Effective<br>1 = Possible<br>2 = Probable<br>3 = Certain | 0 = Impossible<br>1 = Possible<br>2 = Probable<br>3 = Certain | 0 = Impossible<br>1 = Possible<br>2 = Probable<br>3 = Certain | 0 = Impossible<br>1 = Possible<br>2 = Probable<br>3 = Certain | 0 = Impossible<br>1 = Possible<br>2 = Probable<br>3 = Certain | 0 = None<br>1 = Minimal<br>2 = Clear<br>3 = Extensive | 0 = Impossible<br>1 = Possible<br>2 = Probable<br>3 = Certain | 0 = High Risk<br>1 = Medium<br>2 = Low<br>3 = None | |
| *Weight* | 3 | 6 | 1 | 7 | 9 | 10 | 3 | 2 | 3 | 4 | 7 | |
| **Solutions** | | | | | | | | | | | | |
| Perfect | 3 | 3 | 3 | 3 | 3 | 3 | 3 | 3 | 3 | 3 | 3 | 165.0 |
| Skin Equivalents | 2.5 | 1.8 | 3 | 1.8 | 3 | 3 | 3 | 2.5 | 1.7 | 1.8 | 2 | 131.2 |
| Ligament | 3 | 2.5 | 2.5 | 1.8 | 2 | 2.3 | 2.5 | 3 | 3 | 2.7 | 2 | 127.4 |
| Cartilage | 3 | 2.5 | 2.5 | 1.5 | 2.3 | 2 | 2 | 3 | 3 | 2.7 | 2 | 123.5 |
| Bladder | 2.5 | 3 | 2.7 | 2 | 2 | 2 | 2 | 2 | 1.8 | 2.5 | 2 | 119.6 |
| Vessels | 3 | 3 | 2 | 1.8 | 1.8 | 1.8 | 2 | 2 | 2 | 2 | 2 | 113.8 |
| Bone (Long) | 3 | 2.3 | 2 | 1.8 | 2 | 2 | 2 | 2 | 2 | 2 | 2 | 113.4 |
| Myocardial Stem Cells | 3 | 2.5 | 0.8 | 1.7 | 1.8 | 2.2 | 2 | 2 | 2.5 | 2.5 | 1 | 109.4 |
| Stem Cells (Tendon) | 2 | 2 | 2.3 | 2 | 2 | 2 | 2.5 | 2.5 | 2.5 | 2.5 | 2 | 109.3 |
| **Threshold** | 2 | 2 | 2 | 2 | 2 | 2 | 2 | 1 | 1.5 | 2 | 2 | 106.5 |
| Bone (Craniofacial) | 1.6 | 2 | 0.5 | 1 | 1.5 | 1.5 | 2 | 2 | 2 | 2.5 | 2 | 94.3 |
| Kidney | 3 | 3 | 2.3 | 1 | 1 | 1 | 1.5 | 1 | 2 | 2 | 2 | 93.0 |
| Heart Valve | 2.5 | 1.8 | 1.5 | 1 | 1 | 1 | 2 | 2 | 2 | 2 | 2 | 84.6 |
| Skeletal Muscle | 1.3 | 1.5 | 0.5 | 1 | 1 | 1 | 1 | 1 | 2 | 2 | 2 | 73.4 |
| Liver (Whole or Segment) | 2.5 | 2 | 1 | 1 | 0.8 | 1 | 0.8 | 0.8 | 2 | 2 | 1.5 | 72.7 |
| Neural Tissue | 1.5 | 1.8 | 1 | 1 | 1 | 1 | 0.8 | 1 | 1.5 | 1.5 | 1.5 | 68.3 |

**FIGURE 1.1** Example of comprehensive technology opportunity stratification, taking into consideration weighted General Critical Concepts and scalars. Each assigned scalar for each GCC is multiplied by the weight of that GCC and these are summed across all GCCs to provide the total. (Numbers assigned here are by the author only as an example.)

**TABLE 1.7** Assignment of Weights to Generally Critical Concepts

| | Clinical Need | Degree of Improvement upon Alternate Therapy | Technical Feasibility | Cost Effectiveness | Likeliness to Pass the Regulatory Process | Likeliness to Be Reimbursed | Manufactur- ability | Ease of Distribution | Potential for General Use | Likeliness of Care- giver Adoption | Degree to Which Free of Biological Risk | Weight |
|---|---|---|---|---|---|---|---|---|---|---|---|---|
| Clinical need | | | | | | | | 1 | 1 | 1 | | 3 |
| Degree of improvement upon alternate therapy | 1 | | 1 | | | | 1 | 1 | 1 | 1 | | 6 |
| Technical feasibility | 1 | | | | | | | | | | | 1 |
| Cost effectiveness | | 1 | 1 | | | | 1 | 1 | 1 | 1 | 1 | 7 |
| Likeliness to pass the regulatory process | 1 | 1 | 1 | 1 | | | 1 | 1 | 1 | 1 | 1 | 9 |
| Likeliness to be reimbursed | 1 | 1 | 1 | 1 | 1 | | 1 | 1 | 1 | 1 | 1 | 10 |
| Manufacturability | 1 | | 1 | | | | | 1 | | | | 3 |
| Ease of distribution | 1 | | 1 | | | | | | | | | 2 |
| Potential for general use | | | 1 | | | | 1 | 1 | | | | 3 |
| Likeliness of caregiver adoption | | | 1 | 1 | | | 1 | | 1 | | | 4 |
| Degree to which free of biological risk | 1 | 1 | 1 | | | | 1 | 1 | 1 | 1 | | 7 |

*Note:* The GCCs in the leftmost column are compared to all other GCCs in the topmost column. If the leftmost column GCC is more critical than the topmost row GCC, a "1" is placed in the cell. If the reverse, the cell is left blank. The rightmost column depicts the summed weight of relative criticality of leftmost column GCCs.

**TABLE 1.8**   Modulators of Strategy

| Inhibitors | Accelerators |
| --- | --- |
| Enhanced risk aversion of regulatory bodies | New evidence supporting the safety and efficacy of engineered tissues |
| Federal restrictions on stem cell research | New, enhanced federal financial and legal support for stem cell research |
| New evidence that tissue vascularization cannot be maintained in vitro | Identification of genes responsible for the modular vascularization of tissues in any environment |
| Limited interdisciplinary understanding and cooperation | New educational methodologies that enable standardized cross-disciplinary understanding |

*Note:* Example inhibitors and accelerators of strategy are shown. Each type can substantially alter the verity of previously described strategic directions. In the event that any such modulator is material, a new assessment of strategic directions should be undertaken.

In Table 1.8, one of the identified Inhibitors of strategy is "Limited Interdisciplinary Understanding and Cooperation." This has recently been formally investigated in a survey of the membership of the Tissue Engineering and Regenerative Medicine Society, North American chapter (TERMIS-NA)[12] that was carried out by that organization's Industry Committee. In an attempt to understand the hurdles to commercialization of tissue engineering technologies, members were asked to assign themselves to one of the following groups, based upon their present employment:

- Academia
- A Start-Up Company (i.e., having products in early development)
- A Development Stage Company (i.e., having products in late development or early sales)
- An Established Company (i.e., ongoing, predictable product sales and growth)

In an online survey, sets of group-specific feasible hurdles were presented to participants. They were asked to identify the most difficult hurdles not only for their group *but for all other groups, as well.* This enabled the authors to determine what each group identified as its critical hurdles to product commercialization. In addition, it enabled the authors to determine the degree to which cross-disciplinary understanding (or its lack) might contribute to the modulation of strategy.

The authors also asked survey participants to characterize the intensity of the difficulties of their hurdles, relative to the perceived hurdles of other groups.

The results are interesting. Not only did all groups assess their own hurdles as significantly more difficult than those of other groups but there was an approximately 40% error in the assessment of the specific difficult hurdles of other groups. In other words, in a field such as ours that needs technology to be handed off to ever better structured commercial entities in order to reach the marketplace, there are multiple barriers to understanding—probably a clearly Inhibitory modulator. The Industry Committee of TERMIS-NA is using these data to structure its educational programs to rectify this situation—an example of action that may provide an Acceleratory modulation of strategy. Clearly, of all the Inhibitors and Accelerators of strategy, the human element looms largest.

## 1.4 Summary

The development of strategic directions is not a rote exercise though it can be approached objectively. Reduced to its essentials, it is very similar to the way in which design engineers clarify the nuanced elements of successful products. They do this by first asking any and every person who may be impacted by the technology to offer their opinion regarding form and function. They then stratify features by priority for inclusion in the ultimate product.

Tissue engineering products have the potential to deeply impact the future of medicine. However, not all potential tissue engineering products have the same probability of technical or commercial success. Leveraging stakeholder understanding to identify GCCs that serve as success filters sets the stage for the rational stratification of potential products. Any such analysis represents only the reality of a point in time and certainly should not inhibit creative endeavor among investigators. However, the exercise creates a sense of inclusion for stakeholders, enhances mutual understanding by all parties and creates a mechanism for structured information sharing among investigators and others. Through greater and more structured information sharing, new and more rapid permutations of ideas may ensue. Ironically, the greatest benefit of this process may be the enhancement of the potential for *serendipity* in both technical and commercial development.

# References

1. Advancing Tissue Science and Engineering: A Multi-Agency Strategic Plan, U.S. Government Multi-Agency Tissue Engineering Science (MATES) Interagency Working Group, National Science and Technology Council, 2007. Web site: http://tissueengineering.gov/welcome-s.htm.
2. McIntire, LV, Ed. *WTEC Panel on Tissue Engineering Research*, Academic Press, San Diego, 2003.
3. Johnson, PC, Mikos, AG, Fisher, JP, and Jansen, JA. Strategic directions in tissue engineering, *Tissue Eng.* 2007 Dec; 13(12):2827–37.
4. Lysaght, MJ, Jaklenec, A, and Deweerd, E. Great expectations: Private sector activity in tissue engineering, regenerative medicine, and stem cell therapeutics, *Tissue Eng. Part A* 2008 Feb; 14(2):305–15.
5. Lysaght, MJ and Hazlehurst, AL. Tissue engineering: The end of the beginning, *Tissue Eng.* 2004 Jan–Feb; 10(1–2):309–20.
6. Lysaght, MJ and Hazlehurst, AL. Private sector development of stem cell technology and therapeutic cloning, *Tissue Eng.* 2003 June; 9(3):555–61.
7. Lysaght, MJ and Reyes, J. The growth of tissue engineering, *Tissue Eng.* 2001 Oct; 7(5):485–93. Review.
8. Lysaght, MJ, Nguy, NA, and Sullivan, K. An economic survey of the emerging tissue engineering industry, *Tissue Eng.* 1998 Fall; 4(3):231–8.
9. Lysaght, MJ. Product development in tissue engineering, *Tissue Eng.* 1995 Summer; 1(2):221–8.
10. Johnson, PC and Mikos, AG. *Advances in Tissue Engineering: Volume 1—Angiogenesis*, Mary Ann Liebert, Inc., Publishers, New Rochelle, NY, 2010.
11. Johnson, PC and Mikos, AG. *Advances in Tissue Engineering: Volume 2—Stem Cells*, Mary Ann Liebert, Inc., Publishers, New Rochelle, NY, 2010.
12. Johnson, PC, Bertram, TA, Tawil, B, and Hellman, KB. Hurdles in tissue engineering/regenerative medicine product commercialization: A survey of North American academia and industry, *Tissue Eng., Part A* 2011 Jan; 17(1–2):5–15.

# 2

# Silks

Monica A. Serban
*Tufts University*

David L. Kaplan
*Tufts University*

2.1  Introduction to Silks ........................................................ 2-1
  Origin • Overview
2.2  Tissue Engineering Applications of Silks ...................... 2-5
  Silk-Based Biomaterials • Target Tissue Engineering Applications
2.3  Concluding Remarks .......................................................... 2-11
References ................................................................................ 2-11

## 2.1 Introduction to Silks

Historically silks were known to the ancient Chinese since 3000 B.C. To the Western world, the art of silk production and processing was largely unknown for centuries as the process of sericulture was kept secret. Over time, migration, commerce, and wars led to the birth of the Silk Road, and the loss of the monopoly on silk production. Later, silks transitioned from textile-targeted materials into surgical sutures. Subsequently, silk stirred the interest of the scientific community and in 1913 the capacity of silk to diffract x-rays was reported (Lucas et al., 1958).

### 2.1.1 Origin

The original, ancient silk source is believed to be *Bombyx Mandarina Moore* or the wild silk moth/ worm, a species living on white mulberry trees and specific to China. For a very long time silk worms constituted the main silk source. Because of the increasing demand of silk, with time, these insects were domesticated to the point where they are now blind, flightless and depend entirely on human care for feeding and protection (Hyde, 1984). The resulting, highly inbred silk moth/worm strains (*Bombyx mori*), are however "optimized" for the number of generations produced per year, larval growth rates, disease resistance, environmental tolerance, and most importantly silk yield.

In addition to silk moths/worms, silks are produced by many other species of insects and spiders (Kaplan et al., 1992, 1993, 1998). Unlike silk moth-derived silk, spider silks are not widely used in the textile industry because of their limited availability. Spiders naturally produce less silk than a silk worm cocoon (~137 m of fiber can be obtained from the ampullate gland of a spider while one silkworm cocoon yields 600–900 m of fiber) (Lewis, 1996) and, spiders being solitary and predatory in nature, cannot be raised in large numbers. However, it was documented that spider silks are just as suitable for textile production as their insect counterparts (Kaplan et al., 1993). Consequentially, for biomaterial development, silk moths/worms and spiders are the main silk sources.

## 2.1.2 Overview

### 2.1.2.1 Structure

Silk fibers are comprised of two filaments of fibroin protein and a glue-like sericin protein-based coating that keeps the filaments together. Evolutionarily, silks evolved to fulfill vital functions such as prey capture or construction of cocoon-like habitats for the offsprings (spiders, moths). As a result, the amino acid sequence of these natural polymers is tightly correlated with their function. Although often divergent in function, fibroins do exhibit common hallmarks. At the primary structure level, all fibroins contain regions with highly repetitive peptide sequences. While the exact nature of the repeats is species specific (Table 2.1), all primary sequences contain glycine, alanine, or other uncharged amino acids. These hydrophobic repeating blocks are interspersed with more hydrophilic amino acid clusters, and are flanked at both ends of the protein chain with conserved domains, consisting of standard amino acids. At the three-dimensional (3D) level, the hydrophobic blocks interact physically and organize the macromolecules into beta-sheet rich structures (Craig and Riekel, 2002). The extent of the 3D packing correlates with the mechanical properties of fibroins. Aside the aforementioned commonalities, silk fibroins diverge in their "shape and form" from species to species. The most comprehensive compositional and structural information is available for silkworm and spider silks.

In *B. mori*, the fibroin consists of a heavy chain and a light chain linked together through a single disulfide bond (Tanaka et al., 1999). The heavy chain was extensively studied and consists of 5263 amino acids and has a molecular weight of 391 kDa (Zhou et al., 2001). The first 22 amino acids are thought to be involved in signaling and cleaved post-translationally to yield the mature protein (Wang et al., 2006a). The polypeptide chain is structured into antiparallel beta-sheets and confers the fibroin with the characteristic mechanical and biological properties (discussed below). The light chain consists of 262 amino acids that include a short cleavable signal peptide. The mature chain consists of 244 amino acids with a molecular weight of 25.8 kDa (Yamaguchi et al., 1989). In contrast to the heavy chain, its function is not fully elucidated; however, the impairment of the heavy and light assembly led to defective intracellular transport and secretion of the protein (Takei et al., 1984, 1987).

In contrast to silk worms, spiders secrete more than one type of silk—known as spidroins, each with unique function-tailored properties. Moreover, only a few have been characterized and the available structural information is often contradictory (Vollrath and Knight, 2001). One of the most studied web is that of the European garden spider (*Araneus diadematus*), consisting of several types of spidroins, each with different properties. Two different types of proteins constitute the frame and radii of the web for strong, rigid fibers. The same type of fiber is used for the lifeline (dragline). The capture spiral, located at the center of the web, consists of a different type of spidroin with highly elastic properties. Two other proteins are synthesized to complete the web. All the spidroins display the architectural fibroin hallmarks, with 90% of protein consisting of repetitive sequences and nonrepetitive regions located at the protein termini.

**TABLE 2.1**  Repetitive Amino Acid Sequences Found in Silkworm and Spider Fibroins

| Species | Repeating Peptide Sequences |
| --- | --- |
| Silkworms (Zhou et al., 2001) | GAGAGS |
| | GAGAGY |
| | GAGAGA |
| | GAGYGA |
| Spiders (Romer and Scheibel, 2008) | GPGQQ |
| | GPGGX |

**TABLE 2.2**   Summary of the Mechanical Properties of Some Silk Fibers and Other Materials

| Material | Density (g/cm³) | Strength (GPa) | Elasticity (%) | Toughness (MJ/m³) |
|---|---|---|---|---|
| Silkworm silk | 1.3 | 0.6 | 18 | 70 |
| Spider silk | 1.3 | 0.5–1.1 | 27–270 | 150–180 |
| Kevlar 49 | 1.4 | 3.6 | 2.78 | 50 |
| Steel | 7.8 | 1.5 | 0.8 | 6 |

*Source:* Adapted from Romer, L. and Scheibel, T. 2008. *Prion*, 2, 154–61.

### 2.1.2.2 Mechanical Properties

The mechanical properties of fibroins reflect their 3D structural organization (Vollrath, 2000, 2005). The ability of these proteins to compact into various degrees of beta structures endows them with light weight, high strength, and remarkable toughness (Table 2.2) (Romer and Scheibel, 2008). Kevlar 49 is a high-tenacity synthetic polymer from the para-aramid family commonly used in plastic reinforcement for boat hulls, airplanes, and bicycles. In comparison, the elasticity of silks is 6–100 times higher and 1.4–3.6 times tougher. Compared to steel, silks have half the strength, but they are 6-times lighter, 22.5-times more elastic and 11–30 times harder to break. As illustrated in Table 2.2, the mechanical properties of silks are species-dependent. Insect silks are generally weaker and less extensible than spider silks (Vollrath et al., 2001). Intriguingly, depending on protein folding conditions, the mechanics of silk worm silk can be shifted between elastic and strong, while spider silks naturally combine both characteristics (Shao and Vollrath, 2002). Spider silks elicit additional features, such as torsional shape memory (Emile et al., 2006, 2007) (prevents uncontrolled twisting and turning during the spider's descent), and supercontraction (ensures web durability by tightening fibers through water absorption) (Liu et al., 2005). Overall, all the aforementioned properties rank silks as the toughest natural fibers.

### 2.1.2.3 Biocompatibility

Silks have been used as sutures for centuries (Moy et al., 1991). As biomaterials, silks were initially tested in two-dimensional (2D) cell culture systems. Silk films cast from fibroin, collected from silk worm glands, were found to promote fibroblast attachment and proliferation and were comparable to collagen films in terms of cytocompatibility (Minoura et al., 1995a,b). The same group showed that silk films prepared from the wild-type silk worm supported better cell attachment. This difference was explained by the presence of RGD-like attachment sequences in the native sequence (Minoura et al., 1995b). Additional reports confirmed these findings and demonstrated that silks, prepared from regenerated native (Inouye et al., 1998) or RGD-modified silk worm fibroin, sustain the attachment and proliferation of both animal and human cell lines (Gotoh et al., 1998, Sofia et al., 2001).

Insect silks are secreted in combination with sericin, a glue-like protein that holds the fibers together. Sericin was also showed to promote cell attachment (Minoura et al., 1995a, Tsubouchi et al., 2005) and proliferation (Ogawa et al., 2004, Terada et al., 2005). Intriguingly, in *in vivo* applications, silks caused allergic responses, sometimes months after the initial exposure (Kurosaki et al., 1999, Rossitch et al., 1987). However, when sericin and silk fibroin were separated and their individual immunogenicity tested, it was found that sericin was the main allergen (Dewair et al., 1985, Wen et al., 1990, Zaoming et al., 1996).

The biocompatibility of spider silk has also been investigated. In one report, human primary Schwann cells were adherent and elongated along dragline silk fibers (Allmeling et al., 2006). Another group found that spider silks isolated from the dragline and egg sacks of garden spiders supported primary chondrocyte attachment and growth for up to 3 weeks (Gellynck et al., 2008b). Interestingly, the same group showed that egg sack silk induced a severe acute response when subcutaneously implanted into rats (Gellynck et al., 2008a). However, the extent of the reaction could be significantly diminished by enzymatically treating the fibers. The *in vivo* biocompatibility of spider silks was further supported by data on subcutaneous implantation in pigs, with reported tolerance levels comparable to polyurethane or collagen (Vollrath et al., 2002). Recombinant spider silks, developed in recent years to address the scarce availability are not as extensively characterized in terms of biocompatibility. However, there are a few studies that demonstrated the in-growth and proliferation of mouse fibroblasts in 3D recombinant silk scaffolds (Bini et al., 2006) or osteogenic differentiation of human mesenchymal cells (hMSC) on recombinant silk films (Agapov et al., 2009). In terms of *in vivo* compatibility of these recombinant materials, reported adverse effects were correlated with the presence of expression host-derived contaminants (Bini et al., 2006). The development of an advanced purification and endotoxin removal method was reported to overcome the aforementioned issues and yielded spidroins that were well tolerated in rat subcutaneous implants (Hedhammar et al., 2008).

### 2.1.2.4 Biodegradability

The biodegradability of silks is largely dictated by their processing and beta sheet content. Early *in vitro* studies showed that fibroin, specifically the amorphous domains of the protein, is susceptible to chymotrypsin degradation (Zahn et al., 1967). The list of silk-degrading enzymes has since expanded and currently, various proteases capable of also digesting the beta-sheet crystals are employed to evaluate the *in vitro* durability of silk-based biomaterials (Horan et al., 2005, Minoura et al., 1990). Interestingly, it was assumed that there are no specific mammalian enzymes that degrade silk. However, new data indicate that pancreatic elastase, a serine protease that hydrolyses peptide bonds adjacent to the carboxyl groups of alanines, is capable of digesting silk worm derived silk with high specificity (Serban et al., 2010). Elastins also have a high number of GAG repeats in their primary structure, therefore structure similarities between the two proteins might account for the enzymatic specificity.

The *in vivo* degradation of silks is largely dependent on the biomaterial formulation/morphology (film, gel, sponge, fiber) and on the local enzymatic activity. In a comparative study of 10 types of sutures, silk lost 55% of strength and 16% elasticity within 6 weeks, indicative of degradation (Greenwald et al., 1994). In a subcutaneous implantation rat model, significant loss of silk fiber mechanical properties was reported within 10 days (Bucknall et al., 1983). In a rat muscle pouch defect model, 3D porous silk scaffolds were still present after 4 weeks (Mauney et al., 2007). To date, the biodegradability and biocompatibility of silk films have not yet been fully characterized (Wang et al., 2006c). One study addressed the *in vivo* degradation rate dependence on 3D scaffold processing method (aqueous versus hexafluoro-isopropanol) and pore size (Wang et al., 2008). It was found that aqueous processed scaffolds implanted into rats completely degraded between 2 and 6 months postimplantation. In contrast, the organic solvent-processed equivalents were still detectable after one year. The scaffold pore size also impacted the scaffold degradation rates. Smaller pore sizes were found to sustain less tissue in-growth and therefore less degradation. A similar correlation was found between the overall silk concentration of the scaffold and the degradation rate—highly concentrated (~17% silk) scaffolds elicited slow degradation rates. In conclusion, based on the data available, silks classify as biodegradable materials but their degradation rates is highly dependent on the structural features and the local enzymatic pool.

A debatable subject related to silk degradation is the potential for generation of amyloid-like, predominantly parallel beta-sheet containing structures, despite any evidence for such correlations and despite long history of silk sutures. Beta sheets, specifically amyloid structures, are associated with serious pathological conditions such as Alzheimer's disease or spongiform encephalitis, yet it is important to note that silk worm and spider silks elicit antiparallel beta pleated sheet structures, very different in chemistry and structure. Recent data demonstrated that proteolytic silk fibroin degradation (protease XIV) occurred through a different mechanism than that associated with amyloid formation. This mechanism implies the full degradation of beta-sheet structures to noncytotoxic nanofibrils, nanofilaments, and soluble fractions (Numata et al., 2010).

# 2.2 Tissue Engineering Applications of Silks

Tissue engineering applications rely on a well orchestrated interplay between biomaterials/scaffolds, cells, and biological cues commonly provided by growth factors. According to the consensus definition set at the *1st Biomaterials Consensus Conference* in 1986, a biomaterial is defined as "a nonviable material used in a medical device, intended to interact with biological systems." Despite the plethora of biomaterials reported in the scientific literature, it is clear that due to the complexity of the systems/tissues targeted for regeneration no one material will be able to satisfy all the demands. Silk-based biomaterials emerged as a natural alternative for tissue regeneration scaffolds, based on their previously discussed attractive characteristics—mechanics, biocompatibility and slow degradability among others. Imposed by availability, silks from *B. mori* are currently the hallmark for silk-based biomaterials. Commonly, silk worm fibroin is generated by dissolving silkworm cocoons in concentrated lithium bromide solution and then exchanging the solvent to water. Other methods involve the use of highly concentrated sulfuric acid, formic acid, hexafluoro-isopropanol (HFIP) or calcium nitrate to resolubilize the fibers. Once in solution, the fibroin can be processed into a multitude of morphologies that include films, gels, sponges, fibers, coatings, adhesives, and other formats. Based on their final format, which intimately correlates with crystallinity and beta-sheet content, the biomaterials are targeted to various regenerative applications.

## 2.2.1 Silk-Based Biomaterials

### 2.2.1.1 Native Silks

Native silks are obtained by collection directly from the glands of the producing organisms, spider webs or by extraction from silk worm cocoons or spider egg sacks. As previously mentioned, the domestication of silk worms provides a convenient and abundant source of silk fibroin, easily extractable in just a few steps (Wang et al., 2006c). Specifically, silk cocoons are boiled in sodium carbonate containing water to remove sericin and extract the insoluble fibroin fibers. Fibers are subsequently solubilized typically in concentrated lithium bromide solution and then dialyzed against water. The clear, yellowish silk fibroin solution obtained can then be processed or stored at 4°C for months. As already mentioned, the majority of silk-based biomaterials involve *B. mori* derived silks. Conversely, the mechanical properties of spider silks are superior to that of insects and constitute attractive biomaterial building blocks, if adequate supplies can be generated. Spidroins are characteristically obtained from webs or egg sacs through mechanical processing (Blackledge and Hayashi, 2006). Another method of spidroin isolation involves the direct collection of the protein from silk-producing glands. This method commonly involves the drawing of a single fiber from the spinnerets of the spider (Xu and Lewis, 1990). However, to generate a pound of silk several hundred thousand spiders would be needed (Kaplan et al., 1993). To overcome this hurdle, biotechnological alternatives are currently being explored, such as recombinant spidroin or spidroin-like protein expression in bacterial hosts and transgenic animals and plants.

### 2.2.1.2 Genetically Engineered Silks

In an effort to increase spider silk availability, various recombinant DNA techniques have been developed. This approach is not without major challenges, considering the long, repetitive sequences that cause toxicity to hosts systems, truncations, rearrangements, and translational pauses. Codon usage and growth media optimization, along with screening an array of host systems were needed to successfully clone spidroins. The variety of expression hosts and general information about the cloned proteins are summarized in Table 2.3 (Rising et al., 2005). *Escherichia coli (E. coli)* is the most common expression system utilized due to its well characterized genetics and fermentation process (Rising et al., 2005). This system also led to the successful expression of fairly large, native-sized (~285 kDa) recombinant constructs (Xia et al., 2010). To date, spider silk expression in plants and mammalian cell expression systems have provided low yields (Menassa et al., 2004, Williams, 2003, Xu et al., 2007). Transgenic

**TABLE 2.3**   Summary of Expression Hosts for Recombinant Silk Expression and Length Range of Recombinant Constructs Obtained

| Host System | Protein Description | Protein Size (kDa) |
|---|---|---|
| | Prokaryotes | |
| *Escherichia coli* | Synthetic repeats | 76–89 |
| | Repeats (spider) | 11–163 |
| | C-terminal (spider) | 10–43 |
| | Glycine-rich domains (spider) | 9–36 |
| *Salmonella typhimurium* | Repeats (spider) | 30–56 |
| | Eukaryotes | |
| *Pichia pastoris* | Synthetic repeats | 28–32 |
| | Repeats (spider) | 65–113 |
| *Nicotiana tobaccum (tobacco)* | Repeats (spider) | 13–100 |
| *Solanum tuberosum (potato)* | Repeats (spider) | 13–100 |
| *Arabidopsis thaliana* | Repeats (spider) | 64 |
| | Cells | |
| Mammalian (immortalized ephitelian mammary cell line MAC-T; baby hamster kidney cells—BHK; monkey kidney cells–COS-1) | C-terminal (spider) | 60–140 |
| | Repeats (spider) | 22 |
| Insect (*Spodoptera fruiperda*) | C-terminal (spider) | 28–60 |
| | Transgenic Animals | |
| Mice (*Mus musculus*) | Repeats (spider) | 31–66 |
| Silkworms (*Bombyx mori*) | Repeats (spider) | 70 |
| Goats (*Capra hircus*) | Repeats (spider) | N/A |

*Source:* Adapted from Rising, A. et al., 2005. *Zoolog Sci*, 22, 273–81.

silk worms led to spider silks with improved mechanical properties, but recombinant spidroin ratios in the final blend were unsatisfactory (Wen et al., 2010, Zhu et al., 2010). Purification of the cloned repeats posed additional challenges as the proteins tended to aggregate. The aggregate resolubilization commonly requires harsh solvents that later need to be removed for physiological applications (Bini et al., 2006, Fukushima, 1998, Slotta et al., 2008). The removal process, however, often results in re-aggregation of the protein. In the case of successful resolubilization, subsequent techniques, such as wet spinning, hand drawing or electrospinning are needed to form fibers from recombinant spidroins (Bogush et al., 2009, Lazaris et al., 2002, Lewis et al., 1996, Yang et al., 2005). Other material morphologies (i.e., films, beads, microspheres, 3D porous scaffolds) could be successfully obtained through beta-sheet inductive processes such as dehydration or salting out with solvents (Agapov et al., 2009, Bini et al., 2006, Lammel et al., 2008, Liebmann et al., 2008). With all the current advances in the recombinant silk area and processing methods, to date none of these materials fully recapitulates the extraordinary mechanical properties of their native counterparts.

Chimeric recombinant systems have also been developed, in an effort to combine the mechanical properties of silks with the biological features of other macromolecules. In one study, the consensus sequence of the major component of the dragline silk from *Nephila clavipes* was bioengineered into protein variants that incorporated RGD domains and expressed in *E. coli*. These recombinant proteins were able to maintain their beta-sheet forming abilities and were processable into films and fibers. Both RGD recombinant and recombinant silk without RGD supported human mesenchymal stem cell (hMSC) attachment and osteogenic differentiation. A separate study reported the fusion of domains from the major amplullate spidroin 1 protein from *N. clavipes* with silica precipitating peptide (R5) from *Cylindrotheca fusiformis*. The recombinant protein yielded unique biomaterials with the ability to regulate and induce silica precipitation in aqueous, physiological environments at low temperatures. Silica particles precipitated on recombinant substrates had diameters of 0.5–2 μm compared to 0.5–10 μm obtained on R5 peptide-only substrates. Moreover, the morphologies and structures of the precipitated silica could be modulated by the processing conditions of the recombinant protein (Wong Po Foo et al., 2006).

Silk-elastin-like protein polymers were also developed biotechnologically (Cappello et al., 1990). These systems consisted of tandemly repeated silk-like (GAGAGS) and elastin-like (GVGVP) blocks. The polymers retained their self assembling properties, stimuli-sensitivity, biodegradability and biocompatibility. These features, along with the ability to respond to various external stimuli (i.e., temperature, pH, ionic strength), targeted the chimeric constructs for applications in drug delivery devices, tissue engineering, and biosensors.

### 2.2.1.3 Chemically Modified Silks

The tuning of silk properties can be achieved through molecular biology techniques as previously described, or by chemical approaches. As already stated, the primary sequence of silk consists mainly of chemically inert amino acids. Spider silks have a more chemistry-friendly sequence, with a higher number of charged amino acids. However, as discussed, there is the problem of low spidroin availability for biomaterials-related needs. Chemical modifications of silks are generally aimed at improving the material interactions with cells (i.e., RGD attachment) or to expand other functional features (Murphy and Kaplan, 2009). To this end, conjugation of silks to poly(D,L-lactic acid) by a zero-degree carbodiimide crosslinker, promoted osteoblast attachment and proliferation (Cai et al., 2002). Diazonium coupling of silk with functionalities that altered the protein hydrophilicity and hydrophobicity led to materials that promoted human mesenchymal stem cell attachment and proliferation (Murphy et al., 2008). Covalent attachment of lactose to silk by using cyanuric chloride as a coupling spacer increased the adherence of hepatocytes to the surface, but did not promote cell spreading (Gotoh et al., 2004). Incorporation of RGD peptides via carbodiimide coupling led to materials with increased cell adherence and differentiation capacity when studied with osteoblasts, fibroblasts, and bone marrow-derived stem cells (Chen et al., 2003, Sofia et al., 2001). In a more recent study, fibroblasts attached better to a silk-lactose biomaterial than myofibroblasts (Acharya et al., 2008). Moreover, fibroblasts lost their differentiation capacity into myofibroblasts when cultured on these substrates. This observation would indicate that lactose derivatization would render silk-lactose based biomaterials suitable for scar-free wound-healing applications.

Sulfonation of silk through the reaction of fibroin with chlorosulfonic acid yielded heparin-mimetic materials with anticoagulant activity while maintaining characteristic silk properties (Ma et al., 2006). Conjugation of insulin (Zhang et al., 2006) or L-asparaginase (Zhang et al., 2004, 2005, Nazarov et al., 2004) to silks prolonged the biological stability of the molecules and established silk as a drug delivery vehicle. All these reports indicate that chemical alternatives are a reliable method for fine tuning the biological properties of silk-based biomaterials.

### 2.2.1.4 Silk Blends

Silk blends represent an alternative for modulating silk-based material properties in a simplistic manner. Various components have been used to yield novel biomaterial formulations with diverse mechanical and biological properties.

Silk-keratin blends were used in an abdominal wall musculo-fascial defect model in guinea pigs (Gobin et al., 2006). The blended materials sustained deposition of new extracellular matrix, uniform vascularization and cellular infiltration. Moreover, the mechanical parameters at the repair site were comparable to that of the native tissue. In a separate study, porous scaffolds prepared by blending hyaluronan and silk were evaluated in a 3-week *in vitro* culture of human mesenchymal stem cells (Garcia-Fuentes et al., 2009). Histological evaluation of the constructs showed enhanced cellular in-growth into silk fibroin/hyaluronan scaffolds when compared to plain silk fibroin scaffolds. Moreover, in the presence of tissue-inductive stimuli, more efficient tissue formation, measured by glycosaminoglycan and type I and type III collagen gene expression, were observed on silk fibroin/hyaluronan scaffolds compared to plain silk fibroin scaffolds. In a different approach, *in vitro* disease models (kidney) were generated by infusing 3D porous silk scaffolds with matrix proteins (collagen, Matrigel) (Subramanian et al., 2010). The results indicated collagen–Matrigel-mediated morphogenesis for both (normal and disease) cell types, supported coculturing with fibroblasts and led to kidney-like tissue formation.

The studies discussed here touch on the array of tissue engineering applications that involve silks, the available alternatives for fine-tuning their properties and highlight the multifaceted nature of these proteins. The following section will focus on a few examples of specific, engineered organs and tissues with silk-based biomaterials.

## 2.2.2 Target Tissue Engineering Applications

This section will focus on tissue engineering and regenerative applications with the diverse set of silk-based biomaterial formats. Cases, illustrating recent advances toward the regeneration of commonly targeted organs will be discussed below.

### 2.2.2.1 Bone

Bones are mineralized, highly organized tissues with essential functions in support, motility, protection, hematopoiesis and calcium homeostasis. Structurally, compact (cortical) bones have supportive functions, while spongy (cancellous) bones fulfill metabolic functions (Sandy et al., 2002). Bone engineering poses challenges because of the morphological, structural, and functional complexity. Bone repair however is a frequent procedure in the medical world. Tissue engineering offers alternatives that could avoid repeated surgery and reduce second site morbidity.

Processing techniques currently used to yield silk based biomaterials allow for the generation of scaffolds that mechanically match or compare to those of the native tissue. Porous 3D silk fibroin scaffolds emerged as optimal candidates for bone regeneration (Kim et al., 2005a, Meinel et al., 2004, 2005). These scaffolds are commonly obtained by either all aqueous or HFIP processing followed by salt leaching, gas foaming, and freeze-drying, to generate the porous structures (Kim et al., 2005a). Depending on the processing path, different porosities could be obtained which translate into different mechanical properties and degradation rates. Typically aqueous processing yields rougher scaffolds, with interconnected pores and higher mechanical parameters (Kim et al., 2005b). Nevertheless, both *in vitro* and *in vivo*, these aqueous-based scaffolds degrade at a faster rate than their HFIP processed counterparts (Kim et al., 2005b, Wang et al., 2008). This correlates with the extent of beta-sheet content formed during processing, which is a major determinant of different degradation rates (Kim et al., 2005b, Nazarov et al., 2004).

The relationship between scaffold degradability and human mesenchymal stem cell (hMSC) osteogenesis in *in vitro* dynamic cultures has been investigated (Park et al., 2010). Scaffolds with different degradation rates were obtained by the aforementioned processing methods. Scanning electron microscopy, von Kossa, type I collagen staining and calcium content determination showed extensively mineralized extracellular matrices (ECM) formed in the scaffolds designed to degrade more rapidly. Levels of ECM osteogenic markers were also significantly higher in the more rapidly degrading scaffolds than in the more slowly degrading scaffolds over 56 days of study *in vitro*. Metabolic glucose and lactate levels were also scaffold-dependent, with the more rapidly degrading scaffolds supporting higher levels of glucose consumption and lactate synthesis by the differentiated cells, in comparison to the more slowly degrading scaffolds.

Dynamic culturing conditions of hMSCs were also used to engineer bone implants for critical sized calvarial bone repair in nude mice (Meinel et al., 2004, 2005). The engineered bone implants displayed trabecular-like bone networks with ECM similar to the native tissue. Good integration was observed after 5-weeks postimplantation, and constructs stained positive for osteogenic markers (sialoprotein, osteocalcin, and osteopontin). The controls (scaffolds alone, unfilled defects) did not support regeneration or were less substantial in terms of bone formation, as was the case for freshly cell-seeded scaffolds.

In a critical size femoral defect study organic solvent-based silk scaffolds infused with bone morphogenetic protein (BMP-2) and seeded with hMSCs, with or without prior osteogenic differentiation, induced significant bone morphogenesis compared to the untreated controls (Kirker-Head et al., 2007). BMP-2 addition induced more bone formation than observed in the noninfused scaffolds. Moderately good bridging between the native and regenerated bone was attained.

These few examples are illustrative of the advances made toward recreating functional bone and also pinpoint the issues that still need to be address. Scaffold preparation methods, scaffold mechanical, physico-chemical and biological properties, cell culture conditions, and the addition of growth factors are all parameters that interplay in the tissue engineering process of bones in order to recapitulate the properties of native tissues.

### 2.2.2.2 Cartilage

Cartilage is a stiff, inelastic tissue comprised of chondrocytes that secrete abundant collagen type II rich matrices. This system is avascular, with nutrient influx and efflux dictated by diffusion and facilitated by tissue mechanics (compression, elongation). The lack of an abundant nutrient supply translates into a system with low and slow regenerative capacity. Cartilage damage caused by developmental abnormalities or immunological disorders, trauma or aging, is associated with chronic pain and gradual loss of mobility. Current treatment options are aimed at reducing pain and decreasing cartilage degradation rates, but they fail to restore normal cartilage function.

Tissue engineering approaches using both stem and primary cells have been employed on this direction. Porous, aqueous-based silk scaffolds seeded with hMSCs and primary chondrocytes were studied *in vitro* for cartilage regeneration (Wang et al., 2005, 2006b). Stem cells cultured on silk scaffolds under static conditions underwent chondrogenesis as evaluated by real-time RT-PCR analysis for cartilage-specific ECM gene markers, histological and immunohistochemical evaluations of cartilage-specific ECM components (Wang et al., 2005). Upon 3 weeks in culture, most cells acquired a spherical morphology (essential for the synthesis of cartilage-specific ECM components), and were embedded in scaffold-specific lacunae-like niches resembling the native tissue architecture. Moreover, collagen type II distribution in the hMSC-silk scaffold constructs resembled those in native articular cartilage tissue. No calcium deposition was detected by von Kossa staining indicating the lack of osteogenesis. However, dexamethasone and transforming growth factor (TGF)-beta3 were supplemented in the culture media of these constructs, while they were absent in the controls. This fact encumbers the interpretation of the data and the separation of scaffold-cell versus additive effects on chondrogenesis.

Aqueous-based porous silk fibroin scaffolds were also studied when seeded with adult human chondrocytes (hCHs) (Wang et al., 2006b). The attachment, proliferation and re-differentiation of hCHs in the scaffolds in serum-free chemically defined medium with TGF-beta1 was evaluated based on cell morphology, levels of cartilage-related gene transcripts, and the presence of cartilage-specific ECM. Compared to hMSC attachment, primary cells attached more slowly and cell density appeared critical for the re-differentiation of culture-expanded hCHs in the silk fibroin scaffolds. Moreover, there was an upregulation in the level of cartilage-related transcripts (aggrecan core protein, collagen type II, transcription factor Sox 9 and collagen type II/collagen type I ratio) and deposition of cartilage-specific ECM in constructs initiated with higher seeding density compared to their hMSC seeded counterparts. In contrast to hMSCs, all hCH cells adopted spherical morphologies after a 3-week culture period. This study indicates that primary chondrocytes might be competitive for tissue regenerative applications, but these results will need to be further confirmed in *in vivo* models.

### 2.2.2.3 Tendon/Ligament

Tendons and ligaments are both fibrous tissues comprised of fibroblasts arranged in parallel that secrete a collagen type I and proteoglycan-rich matrix. Tendons connect muscles to bones, ligaments link bones to bones and both tissues need to sustain significant mechanical stress. This is achieved by a strict hierarchical organization starting with collagen fibers assembled into microfibrils, microfibrils into subfibrils, subfibrils into fibrils interspersed with fibroblasts to form fascicles. Fascicles are then clustered together to form the tendon or ligaments.

Tendon and ligament repair is especially prevalent in sports medicine. Challenges arise in the ability to recreate a mechanically functional tissue. Classical treatment options imply lengthy recovery time, arthritis, donor site morbidity, and degenerative joint disease. Lack of mechanical stimulation after reconstructive procedures frequently leads to undesired inter-hierarchical structural adhesions that result in impairment or loss of function. Tissue engineering approaches in this area are still in their infancy, due to the complexity of the tissue. To date, attempts were made to recapitulate the native tissue architecture by employing fiber-like biomaterials. An initial effort in this direction used a wire-rope model designed silk-fiber matrix to engineer anterior cruciate ligaments (ACL)-like structures (Altman et al., 2002). The matrix matched the mechanical requirements of native human ACL including the fatigue performance. In addition, scanning electron microscopy, DNA quantitation and detection of collagen types I and III and tenascin-C marker expression indicated hMSC attachment, expansion and differentiation. A different approach used RGD-modified silk sutures cultured with human tenocytes (Kardestuncer et al., 2006). These substrates supported increased cell adhesion after 3 days when compared with unmodified silk fibers and tissue cultured plastic. Collagen type I and decorin transcript levels were also higher on the RGD-modified sutures compared with unmodified silk and tissue culture plastic at 6 weeks. These studies indicate the compatibility of silks for tendon and ligament regeneration and repair.

### 2.2.2.4 Skin/Wound Healing

Since skin covers the entire surface of the body, it is highly prone to injury. Skin regeneration can be less challenging compared to other organs and tissues, with an architecture that is fairly uncomplicated, and achievable mechanical properties, such as an elastic modulus of ~120 kPa (Diridollou et al., 2000). A myriad of synthetic and natural biomaterials have been employed as wound dressings and regenerative scaffolds, each with its merits and pitfalls. Silk-based scaffolds have also been employed for this purpose in various forms, including epidermal growth factor (EGF)-releasing silk mats (Schneider et al., 2009). A human skin-equivalent wound model, displaying similar architecture and molecular and cellular healing mechanisms as the native organ, was used to evaluate the silk-based constructs. Silk mats maintained their structure and biocompatibility, slowly released EGF and increased wound closure time by 90% compared to no treatment. These results establish silks as potential candidates for skin regeneration and wound repair and open avenues for testing novel silk-based biomaterial formulations.

### 2.2.2.5 Cornea

The cornea—the transparent structure covering the anterior part of the eye—is responsible for approximately two-thirds of the eye's total optical power. Corneal blindness represents a major issue worldwide. Therapeutic approaches utilize corneal grafting, commonly from cadaveric donors. However, by 4–5 years post implantation the immunological rejection rate is ~25% and continues to increase over the life of the patient (George and Larkin, 2004, Nishida et al., 2004). Synthetic keratoprostheses, constructed of poly-2-hydroxyethylmethacrylate, are currently available yet they also exhibit a relatively high host rejection rate (Ilhan-Sarac and Akpek, 2005, Myung et al., 2007). Corneal tissue engineering builds on the native tissue architecture. The corneal transparency is a reflection of its stromal organization, with an extracellular matrix consisting of hybrid type I/V collagen fibrils, extraordinarily uniform in diameter and regularly arranged into a pseudolattice. Moreover, the fibrils are kept at defined distances by proteoglycans (Knupp et al., 2009).

Silk film biomaterials were used to recreate the stacked architecture of the cornea (Lawrence et al., 2009). Films were 2 μm thick mimicking corneal collagen lamellae dimensions and porous to permit nutrient trans-lamellar diffusion and promote cell–cell interactions. In addition, film surfaces were patterned to guide human and rabbit corneal fibroblast cell alignment. The final constructs sustained cell proliferation, alignment and corneal extracellular matrix expression, were optically clear and had good mechanical integrity indicating the suitability of silks for such applications.

### 2.2.2.6 Peripheral Nerves

The peripheral nervous system consists of cord-like structures containing bundles of nerve fibers that carry information from limbs and organs to the spinal cord and back. In contrast to the brain and spinal cord that have very limited healing capacity, peripheral nerves can regenerate, even when completely severed, resulting in complete or nearly complete recovery of the patient. However, in some cases, the process is slow enough to cause the affected organ to be paralyzed or to atrophy. Autologous grafts are typically used in peripheral nerve reconstructive surgery (Subramanian et al., 2009). However, autografts have drawbacks such as limited availability, mismatch of donor-site nerve size with the recipient site, neuroma formation and lack of functional recovery. As an alternative, allogenic grafts from cadavers address the availability issue, but often cause immune rejection.

A silk fibroin conduit loaded with neurotrophic factors was recently evaluated in a small nerve gap repair model (Madduri et al., 2010). This system was functionalized with aligned and nonaligned silk fibers to aid axon orientation. Both sensory and spinal cord motor neurons from chick embryos exhibited increased length and rate of axonal outgrowth parallel to the aligned nanofibers. Glial cells from dorsal root ganglions proliferated and migrated in close association and even slightly ahead of the outgrowing axon while on nonaligned fibers both axonal and glial growth was slower and randomly oriented. These data suggest that silk fibroin-based conduits have the potential to enhance functional recovery of injured peripheral nerves and may offer a viable treatment option for rapid recovery.

## 2.3 Concluding Remarks

Key features of silks, their extraordinary potential as biomaterials, along with a few organ-specific tissue engineering applications have been described. Despite silk as a well-known fiber for eons, the unraveling of the novel characteristics of these fibers has recently led to a new generation of tissue-related applications. Further, the novel properties identified for medical devices and regenerative medicine have also spilled over into parallel technologies in fields like photonics, nanotechnology, electronics, optics, and microfluidics, increasing the high-technology web of silk applications. As technology progresses, silks tailored for specific needs should continue to lead to new applications. As silk-based devices proceed through the FDA and into more common use, the impact of this novel protein in many areas of human health and wellness are expected to continue to grow, all originating from the astonishing properties of this protein fiber from nature.

## References

Acharya, C., Hinz, B., and Kundu, S. C. 2008. The effect of lactose-conjugated silk biomaterials on the development of fibrogenic fibroblasts. *Biomaterials*, 29, 4665–75.

Agapov, II, Pustovalova, O. L., Moisenovich, M. M., Bogush, V. G., Sokolova, O. S., Sevastyanov, V. I., Debabov, V. G., and Kirpichnikov, M. P. 2009. Three-dimensional scaffold made from recombinant spider Silk protein for tissue engineering. *Dokl Biochem Biophys*, 426, 127–30.

Allmeling, C., Jokuszies, A., Reimers, K., Kall, S., and Vogt, P. M. 2006. Use of spider silk fibres as an innovative material in a biocompatible artificial nerve conduit. *J Cell Mol Med*, 10, 770–7.

Altman, G. H., Horan, R. L., Lu, H. H., Moreau, J., Martin, I., Richmond, J. C., and Kaplan, D. L. 2002. Silk matrix for tissue engineered anterior cruciate ligaments. *Biomaterials*, 23, 4131–41.

Bini, E., Foo, C. W., Huang, J., Karageorgiou, V., Kitchel, B., and Kaplan, D. L. 2006. Rgd-functionalized bioengineered spider dragline silk biomaterial. *Biomacromolecules*, 7, 3139–45.

Blackledge, T. A. and Hayashi, C. Y. 2006. Silken toolkits: Biomechanics of silk fibers spun by the orb web spider *Argiope argentata* (Fabricius 1775). *J Exp Biol*, 209, 2452–61.

Bogush, V. G. et al. 2009. A novel model system for design of biomaterials based on recombinant analogs of spider silk proteins. *J Neuroimmune Pharmacol*, 4, 17–27.

Bucknall, T. E., Teare, L., and Ellis, H. 1983. The choice of a suture to close abdominal incisions. *Eur Surg Res*, 15, 59–66.

Cai, K., Yao, K., Cui, Y., Yang, Z., Li, X., Xie, H., Qing, T., and Gao, L. 2002. Influence of different surface modification treatments on poly(D,L-lactic acid) with silk fibroin and their effects on the culture of osteoblast in vitro. *Biomaterials*, 23, 1603–11.

Cappello, J., Crissman, J., Dorman, M., Mikolajczak, M., Textor, G., Marquet, M., and Ferrari, F. 1990. Genetic engineering of structural protein polymers. *Biotechnol Prog*, 6, 198–202.

Chen, J., Altman, G. H., Karageorgiou, V., Horan, R., Collette, A., Volloch, V., Colabro, T., and Kaplan, D. L. 2003. Human bone marrow stromal cell and ligament fibroblast responses on Rgd-modified silk fibers. *J Biomed Mater Res A*, 67, 559–70.

Craig, C. L. and Riekel, C. 2002. Comparative architecture of silks, fibrous proteins and their encoding genes in insects and spiders. *Comp Biochem Physiol B Biochem Mol Biol*, 133, 493–507.

Dewair, M., Baur, X., and Ziegler, K. 1985. Use of immunoblot technique for detection of human IgE and IgG antibodies to individual silk proteins. *J Allergy Clin Immunol*, 76, 537–42.

Diridollou, S., Patat, F., Gens, F., Vaillant, L., Black, D., Lagarde, J. M., Gall, Y., and Berson, M. 2000. *In vivo* model of the mechanical properties of the human skin under suction. *Skin Res Technol*, 6, 214–21.

Emile, O., Le Floch, A., and Vollrath, F. 2006. Biopolymers: Shape memory in spider draglines. *Nature*, 440, 621.

Emile, O., Le Floch, A., and Vollrath, F. 2007. Time-resolved torsional relaxation of spider draglines by an optical technique. *Phys Rev Lett*, 98, 167402.

Fukushima, Y. 1998. Genetically engineered syntheses of tandem repetitive polypeptides consisting of glycine-rich sequence of spider dragline silk. *Biopolymers*, 45, 269–79.

Garcia-Fuentes, M., Meinel, A. J., Hilbe, M., Meinel, L., and Merkle, H. P. 2009. Silk fibroin/hyaluronan scaffolds for human mesenchymal stem cell culture in tissue engineering. *Biomaterials*, 30, 5068–76.

Gellynck, K., Verdonk, P., Forsyth, R., Almqvist, K. F., Van Nimmen, E., Gheysens, T., Mertens, J., Van Langenhove, L., Kiekens, P., and Verbruggen, G. 2008a. Biocompatibility and biodegradability of spider egg sac silk. *J Mater Sci Mater Med*, 19, 2963–70.

Gellynck, K., Verdonk, P. C., Van Nimmen, E., Almqvist, K. F., Gheysens, T., Schoukens, G., Van Langenhove, L., Kiekens, P., Mertens, J., and Verbruggen, G. 2008b. Silkworm and spider silk scaffolds for chondrocyte support. *J Mater Sci Mater Med*, 19, 3399–409.

George, A. J. and Larkin, D. F. 2004. Corneal transplantation: The forgotten graft. *Am J Transplant*, 4, 678–85.

Gobin, A. S., Butler, C. E., and Mathur, A. B. 2006. Repair and regeneration of the abdominal wall musculofascial defect using silk fibroin-chitosan blend. *Tissue Eng*, 12, 3383–94.

Gotoh, Y., Niimi, S., Hayakawa, T., and Miyashita, T. 2004. Preparation of lactose-silk fibroin conjugates and their application as a scaffold for hepatocyte attachment. *Biomaterials*, 25, 1131–40.

Gotoh, Y., Tsukada, M., and Minoura, N. 1998. Effect of the chemical modification of the arginyl residue in *Bombyx mori* silk fibroin on the attachment and growth of fibroblast cells. *J Biomed Mater Res*, 39, 351–7.

Greenwald, D., Shumway, S., Albear, P., and Gottlieb, L. 1994. Mechanical comparison of 10 suture materials before and after *in vivo* incubation. *J Surg Res*, 56, 372–7.

Hedhammar, M., Rising, A., Grip, S., Martinez, A. S., Nordling, K., Casals, C., Stark, M., and Johansson, J. 2008. Structural properties of recombinant nonrepetitive and repetitive parts of major ampullate spidroin 1 from *Euprosthenops australis*: Implications for fiber formation. *Biochemistry*, 47, 3407–17.

Horan, R. L., Antle, K., Collette, A. L., Wang, Y., Huang, J., Moreau, J. E., Volloch, V., Kaplan, D. L., and Altman, G. H. 2005. *In vitro* degradation of silk fibroin. *Biomaterials*, 26, 3385–93.

Hyde, N. 1984. Silk, the queen of textiles. *National Geographic*, 165, 2–49.

Ilhan-Sarac, O. and Akpek, E. K. 2005. Current concepts and techniques in keratoprosthesis. *Curr Opin Ophthalmol,* 16, 246–50.

Inouye, K., Kurokawa, M., Nishikawa, S., and Tsukada, M. 1998. Use of *Bombyx mori* silk fibroin as a substratum for cultivation of animal cells. *J Biochem Biophys Methods,* 37, 159–64.

Kaplan, D. L., Adams, W. W., Farmer, B., and Viney, C. 1993. Silk: Biology, structure, properties, and genetics. *Silk Polymers.* Washington, DC: ACS Symposium Series.

Kaplan, D. L., Fossey, S., Viney, C., and Muller, W. 1992. Self-organization (assembly) in biosynthesis of silk fibers—A hierarchical problem. *In*: Aksay, I. A., Baer, E., Sarikaya, M., and Tirrell, D. A. (eds.) Hierarchically structured materials. *Materials Res Symp Proc.* 255, 19–29.

Kaplan, D. L., Mello, S. M., Arcidiacono, S., Fossey, S., Senecal, K., and Muller, W. 1998. Silk. *In*: McGrath, K. and Kaplan, D. L. (eds.) *Protein Based Materials.* Boston: Birkhauser, pp. 103–31.

Kardestuncer, T., Mccarthy, M. B., Karageorgiou, V., Kaplan, D., and Gronowicz, G. 2006. RGD-tethered silk substrate stimulates the differentiation of human tendon cells. *Clin Orthop Relat Res,* 448, 234–9.

Kim, H. J., Kim, U. J., Vunjak-Novakovic, G., Min, B. H., and Kaplan, D. L. 2005a. Influence of macroporous protein scaffolds on bone tissue engineering from bone marrow stem cells. *Biomaterials,* 26, 4442–52.

Kim, U. J., Park, J., Kim, H. J., Wada, M., and Kaplan, D. L. 2005b. Three-dimensional aqueous-derived biomaterial scaffolds from silk fibroin. *Biomaterials,* 26, 2775–85.

Kirker-Head, C. et al. 2007. BMP-silk composite matrices heal critically sized femoral defects. *Bone,* 41, 247–55.

Knupp, C., Pinali, C., Lewis, P. N., Parfitt, G. J., Young, R. D., Meek, K. M., and Quantock, A. J. 2009. The architecture of the cornea and structural basis of its transparency. *Adv Protein Chem Struct Biol,* 78, 25–49.

Kurosaki, S., Otsuka, H., Kunitomo, M., Koyama, M., Pawankar, R., and Matumoto, K. 1999. Fibroin allergy. IgE mediated hypersensitivity to silk suture materials. *Nippon Ika Daigaku Zasshi,* 66, 41–4.

Lammel, A., Schwab, M., Slotta, U., Winter, G., and Scheibel, T. 2008. Processing conditions for the formation of spider silk microspheres. *ChemSusChem,* 1, 413–6.

Lawrence, B. D., Marchant, J. K., Pindrus, M. A., Omenetto, F. G., and Kaplan, D. L. 2009. Silk film biomaterials for cornea tissue engineering. *Biomaterials,* 30, 1299–308.

Lazaris, A., Arcidiacono, S., Huang, Y., Zhou, J. F., Duguay, F., Chretien, N., Welsh, E. A., Soares, J. W., and Karatzas, C. N. 2002. Spider silk fibers spun from soluble recombinant silk produced in mammalian cells. *Science,* 295, 472–6.

Lewis, R. 1996. *Bioscience,* 46, 636–8.

Lewis, R. V., Hinman, M., Kothakota, S., and Fournier, M. J. 1996. Expression and purification of a spider silk protein: a new strategy for producing repetitive proteins. *Protein Expr Purif,* 7, 400–6.

Liebmann, B., Hummerich, D., Scheibel, T., and Fehr, M. 2008. Formulation of poorly water soluble substances using self-assembling spider silk protein. *Colloids Surf. A Physicochem. Eng. Aspects,* 331, 126–132.

Liu, Y., Shao, Z. and Vollrath, F. 2005. Relationships between supercontraction and mechanical properties of spider silk. *Nat Mater,* 4, 901–5.

Lucas, F., Shaw, J. T., and Smith, S. G. 1958. The silk fibroins. *Adv Protein Chem,* 13, 107–242.

Ma, X., Cao, C., and Zhu, H. 2006. The biocompatibility of silk fibroin films containing sulfonated silk fibroin. *J Biomed Mater Res B Appl Biomater,* 78, 89–96.

Madduri, S., Papaloizos, M., and Gander, B. 2010. Trophically and topographically functionalized silk fibroin nerve conduits for guided peripheral nerve regeneration. *Biomaterials,* 31, 2323–34.

Mauney, J. R., Nguyen, T., Gillen, K., Kirker-Head, C., Gimble, J. M., and Kaplan, D. L. 2007. Engineering adipose-like tissue *in vitro* and *in vivo* utilizing human bone marrow and adipose-derived mesenchymal stem cells with silk fibroin 3D scaffolds. *Biomaterials,* 28, 5280–90.

Meinel, L., Fajardo, R., Hofmann, S., Langer, R., Chen, J., Snyder, B., Vunjak-Novakovic, G., and Kaplan, D. 2005. Silk implants for the healing of critical size bone defects. *Bone,* 37, 688–98.

Meinel, L., Karageorgiou, V., Fajardo, R., Snyder, B., Shinde-Patil, V., Zichner, L., Kaplan, D., Langer, R., and Vunjak-Novakovic, G. 2004. Bone tissue engineering using human mesenchymal stem cells: Effects of scaffold material and medium flow. *Ann Biomed Eng, 32,* 112–22.

Menassa, R., Zhu, H., Karatzas, C. N., Lazaris, A., Richman, A., and Brandle, J. 2004. Spider dragline silk proteins in transgenic tobacco leaves: Accumulation and field production. *Plant Biotechnol J, 2,* 431–8.

Minoura, N., Aiba, S., Gotoh, Y., Tsukada, M., and Imai, Y. 1995a. Attachment and growth of cultured fibroblast cells on silk protein matrices. *J Biomed Mater Res, 29,* 1215–21.

Minoura, N., Aiba, S., Higuchi, M., Gotoh, Y., Tsukada, M., and Imai, Y. 1995b. Attachment and growth of fibroblast cells on silk fibroin. *Biochem Biophys Res Commun, 208,* 511–6.

Minoura, N., Tsukada, M., and Nagura, M. 1990. Physico-chemical properties of silk fibroin membrane as a biomaterial. *Biomaterials, 11,* 430–4.

Moy, R. L., Lee, A., and Zalka, A. 1991. Commonly used suture materials in skin surgery. *Am Fam Phys, 44,* 2123–8.

Murphy, A. R. and Kaplan, D. L. 2009. Biomedical applications of chemically-modified silk fibroin. *J Mater Chem, 19,* 6443–6450.

Murphy, A. R., St John, P., and Kaplan, D. L. 2008. Modification of silk fibroin using diazonium coupling chemistry and the effects on HMSC proliferation and differentiation. *Biomaterials, 29,* 2829–38.

Myung, D., Koh, W., Bakri, A., Zhang, F., Marshall, A., Ko, J., Noolandi, J., Carrasco, M., Cochran, J. R., Frank, C. W., and Ta, C. N. 2007. Design and fabrication of an artificial cornea based on a photolithographically patterned hydrogel construct. *Biomed Microdevices, 9,* 911–22.

Nazarov, R., Jin, H. J., and Kaplan, D. L. 2004. Porous 3-D scaffolds from regenerated silk fibroin. *Biomacromolecules, 5,* 718–26.

Nishida, K., Yamato, M., Hayashida, Y., Watanabe, K., Yamamoto, K., Adachi, E., Nagai, S., Kikuchi, A., Maeda, N., Watanabe, H., Okano, T., and Tano, Y. 2004. Corneal reconstruction with tissue-engineered cell sheets composed of autologous oral mucosal epithelium. *N Engl J Med, 351,* 1187–96.

Numata, K., Cebe, P., and Kaplan, D. L. 2010. Mechanism of enzymatic degradation of beta-sheet crystals. *Biomaterials, 31,* 2926–33.

Ogawa, A., Terada, S., Kanayama, T., Miki, M., Morikawa, M., Kimura, T., Yamaguchi, A., Sasaki, M., and Yamada, H. 2004. Improvement of islet culture with sericin. *J Biosci Bioeng, 98,* 217–9.

Park, S. H., Gil, E. S., Kim, H. J., Lee, K., and Kaplan, D. L. 2010. Relationships between degradability of silk scaffolds and osteogenesis. *Biomaterials, 31,* 6162–72.

Rising, A., Nimmervoll, H., Grip, S., Fernandez-Arias, A., Storckenfeldt, E., Knight, D. P., Vollrath, F., and Engstrom, W. 2005. Spider silk proteins—Mechanical property and gene sequence. *Zoolog Sci, 22,* 273–81.

Romer, L. and Scheibel, T. 2008. The elaborate structure of spider silk: Structure and function of a natural high performance fiber. *Prion, 2,* 154–61.

Rossitch, E., Jr., Bullard, D. E., and Oakes, W. J. 1987. Delayed foreign-body reaction to silk sutures in pediatric neurosurgical patients. *Childs Nerv Syst, 3,* 375–8.

Sandy, C., Marks, J., and Odgren, P. R. 2002. Structure and developmant of the skeleton. *In:* John, P. B., Lawrence, G. R., and Gideon, A. R. (eds.) *Principles of Bone Biology.* 2nd ed. New York, USA: Academic Press.

Schneider, A., Wang, X. Y., Kaplan, D. L., Garlick, J. A., and Egles, C. 2009. Biofunctionalized electrospun silk mats as a topical bioactive dressing for accelerated wound healing. *Acta Biomater, 5,* 2570–8.

Serban, M. A., Kluge, J. A., Laha, M. M., and Kaplan, D. L. 2010. Modular elastic patches: Mechanical and biological effects. *Biomacromolecules, 11,* 2230–7.

Shao, Z. and Vollrath, F. 2002. Surprising strength of silkworm silk. *Nature, 418,* 741.

Slotta, U. K., Rammensee, S., Gorb, S., and Scheibel, T. 2008. An engineered spider silk protein forms microspheres. *Angew Chem Int Ed Engl, 47,* 4592–4.

Sofia, S., Mccarthy, M. B., Gronowicz, G., and Kaplan, D. L. 2001. Functionalized silk-based biomaterials for bone formation. *J Biomed Mater Res, 54,* 139–48.

Subramanian, A., Krishnan, U. M., and Sethuraman, S. 2009. Development of biomaterial scaffold for nerve tissue engineering: Biomaterial mediated neural regeneration. *J Biomed Sci,* 16, 108.

Subramanian, B., Rudym, D., Cannizzaro, C., Perrone, R., Zhou, J., and Kaplan, D. L. 2010. Tissue-engineered three-dimensional *in vitro* models for normal and diseased kidney. *Tissue Eng Part A,* 16, 2821–31.

Takei, F., Kikuchi, Y., Kikuchi, A., Mizuno, S., and Shimura, K. 1987. Further evidence for importance of the subunit combination of silk fibroin in its efficient secretion from the posterior silk gland cells. *J Cell Biol,* 105, 175–80.

Takei, F., Oyama, F., Kimura, K., Hyodo, A., Mizuno, S., and Shimura, K. 1984. Reduced level of secretion and absence of subunit combination for the fibroin synthesized by a mutant silkworm, Nd(2). *J Cell Biol,* 99, 2005–10.

Tanaka, K., Kajiyama, N., Ishikura, K., Waga, S., Kikuchi, A., Ohtomo, K., Takagi, T., and Mizuno, S. 1999. Determination of the site of disulfide linkage between heavy and light chains of silk fibroin produced by *Bombyx mori. Biochim Biophys Acta,* 1432, 92–103.

Terada, S., Sasaki, M., Yanagihara, K., and Yamada, H. 2005. Preparation of silk protein sericin as mitogenic factor for better mammalian cell culture. *J Biosci Bioeng,* 100, 667–71.

Tsubouchi, K., Igarashi, Y., Takasu, Y., and Yamada, H. 2005. Sericin enhances attachment of cultured human skin fibroblasts. *Biosci Biotechnol Biochem,* 69, 403–5.

Vollrath, F. 2000. Strength and structure of spiders' silks. *J Biotechnol,* 74, 67–83.

Vollrath, F. 2005. Spiders' webs. *Curr Biol,* 15, R364–5.

Vollrath, F., Barth, P., Basedow, A., Engstrom, W., and List, H. 2002. Local tolerance to spider silks and protein polymers in vivo. *In Vivo,* 16, 229–34.

Vollrath, F. and Knight, D. P. 2001. Liquid crystalline spinning of spider silk. *Nature,* 410, 541–8.

Vollrath, F., Madsen, B., and Shao, Z. 2001. The effect of spinning conditions on the mechanics of a spider's dragline silk. *Proc Biol Sci,* 268, 2339–46.

Wang, S. P., Guo, T. Q., Guo, X. Y., Huang, J. T., and Lu, C. D. 2006a. *In vivo* analysis of fibroin heavy chain signal peptide of silkworm *Bombyx mori* using recombinant baculovirus as vector. *Biochem Biophys Res Commun,* 341, 1203–10.

Wang, Y., Blasioli, D. J., Kim, H. J., Kim, H. S., and Kaplan, D. L. 2006b. Cartilage tissue engineering with silk scaffolds and human articular chondrocytes. *Biomaterials,* 27, 4434–42.

Wang, Y., Kim, H. J., Vunjak-Novakovic, G., and Kaplan, D. L. 2006c. Stem cell-based tissue engineering with silk biomaterials. *Biomaterials,* 27, 6064–82.

Wang, Y., Kim, U. J., Blasioli, D. J., Kim, H. J., and Kaplan, D. L. 2005. *In vitro* cartilage tissue engineering with 3D porous aqueous-derived silk scaffolds and mesenchymal stem cells. *Biomaterials,* 26, 7082–94.

Wang, Y., Rudym, D. D., Walsh, A., Abrahamsen, L., Kim, H. J., Kim, H. S., Kirker-Head, C., and Kaplan, D. L. 2008. *In vivo* degradation of three-dimensional silk fibroin scaffolds. *Biomaterials,* 29, 3415–28.

Wen, C. M., Ye, S. T., Zhou, L. X., and Yu, Y. 1990. Silk-induced asthma in children: a report of 64 cases. *Ann Allergy,* 65, 375–8.

Wen, H., Lan, X., Zhang, Y., Zhao, T., Wang, Y., Kajiura, Z., and Nakagaki, M. 2010. Transgenic silkworms (*Bombyx mori*) produce recombinant spider dragline silk in cocoons. *Mol Biol Rep,* 37, 1815–21.

Williams, D. 2003. Sows' ears, silk purses and goats' milk: New production methods and medical applications for silk. *Med Device Technol,* 14, 9–11.

Wong Po Foo, C., Patwardhan, S. V., Belton, D. J., Kitchel, B., Anastasiades, D., Huang, J., Naik, R. R., Perry, C. C., and Kaplan, D. L. 2006. Novel nanocomposites from spider silk-silica fusion (chimeric) proteins. *Proc Natl Acad Sci USA,* 103, 9428–33.

Xia, X. X., Qian, Z. G., Ki, C. S., Park, Y. H., Kaplan, D. L., and Lee, S. Y. 2010. Native-sized recombinant spider silk protein produced in metabolically engineered *Escherichia coli* results in a strong fiber. *Proc Natl Acad Sci USA,* 107, 14059–63.

Xu, H. T., Fan, B. L., Yu, S. Y., Huang, Y. H., Zhao, Z. H., Lian, Z. X., Dai, Y. P., Wang, L. L., Liu, Z. L., Fei, J., and Li, N. 2007. Construct synthetic gene encoding artificial spider dragline silk protein and its expression in milk of transgenic mice. *Anim Biotechnol,* 18, 1–12.

Xu, M. and Lewis, R. V. 1990. Structure of a protein superfiber: Spider dragline silk. *Proc Natl Acad Sci USA,* 87, 7120–4.

Yamaguchi, K., Kikuchi, Y., Takagi, T., Kikuchi, A., Oyama, F., Shimura, K., and Mizuno, S. 1989. Primary structure of the silk fibroin light chain determined by cDNA sequencing and peptide analysis. *J Mol Biol,* 210, 127–39.

Yang, J., Barr, L. A., Fahnestock, S. R., and Liu, Z. B. 2005. High yield recombinant silk-like protein production in transgenic plants through protein targeting. *Transgenic Res,* 14, 313–24.

Zahn, H., Schade, W., and Ziegler, K. 1967. Fractionation of the chymotryptic precipitate of *Bombyx mori* silk fibroin. *Biochem J,* 104, 1019–26.

Zaoming, W., Codina, R., Fernandez-Caldas, E., and Lockey, R. F. 1996. Partial characterization of the silk allergens in mulberry silk extract. *J Investig Allergol Clin Immunol,* 6, 237–41.

Zhang, Y. Q., Ma, Y., Xia, Y. Y., Shen, W. D., Mao, J. P., Zha, X. M., Shirai, K., and Kiguchi, K. 2006. Synthesis of silk fibroin-insulin bioconjugates and their characterization and activities in vivo. *J Biomed Mater Res B Appl Biomater,* 79, 275–83.

Zhang, Y. Q., Tao, M. L., Shen, W. D., Zhou, Y. Z., Ding, Y., Ma, Y., and Zhou, W. L. 2004. Immobilization of L-asparaginase on the microparticles of the natural silk sericin protein and its characters. *Biomaterials,* 25, 3751–9.

Zhang, Y. Q., Zhou, W. L., Shen, W. D., Chen, Y. H., Zha, X. M., Shirai, K., and Kiguchi, K. 2005. Synthesis, characterization and immunogenicity of silk fibroin-L-asparaginase bioconjugates. *J Biotechnol,* 120, 315–26.

Zhou, C. Z., Confalonieri, F., Jacquet, M., Perasso, R., Li, Z. G., and Janin, J. 2001. Silk fibroin: structural implications of a remarkable amino acid sequence. *Proteins,* 44, 119–22.

Zhu, Z., Kikuchi, Y., Kojima, K., Tamura, T., Kuwabara, N., Nakamura, T., and Asakura, T. 2010. Mechanical properties of regenerated Bombyx mori silk fibers and recombinant silk fibers produced by transgenic silkworms. *J Biomater Sci Polym Ed,* 21, 395–411.

# 3

# Calcium Phosphates

Kemal
Sariibrahimoglu
*Radboud University
Nijmegen Medical Center*

Joop G.C. Wolke
*Radboud University
Nijmegen Medical Center*

Sander C.G.
Leeuwenburgh
*Radboud University
Nijmegen Medical Center*

John A. Jansen
*Radboud University
Nijmegen Medical Center*

3.1 Introduction ........................................................................ 3-1
3.2 Physicochemical Properties of CaP Compounds ...................... 3-1
    Dicalcium Phosphate • Tricalcium Phosphate • Tetracalcium
    Phosphate • Octacalcium Phosphate • Apatites
3.3 CaP Blocks/Granules............................................................ 3-5
    Production Methods • Structure–Property Relationships
3.4 CaP Cements ..................................................................... 3-11
    Setting of Cement • Structure–Property Relationships
3.5 Conclusion ....................................................................... 3-15
References............................................................................... 3-15

## 3.1 Introduction

Tissue engineering is a combination of materials engineering and biology and involves the application of materials to induce tissue regeneration (Langer and Vacanti 1993). The overall goal of tissue engineering is to manipulate cellular interaction with synthetic advanced materials for the treatment of structurally degenerated organs in the human body. In view of this, various types of scaffold materials have already been developed to cure musculoskeletal disorders. Engineering materials that can be used for bone tissue engineering are metals, polymers, and ceramics. Both metals and polymers are used since decennia to replace bone defects in the body, but they are usually separated from the adjacent bone by a nonphysiological capsule causing a mismatch in functional properties between bone tissue and artificial implant. Frequently, the implantation of these materials is also accompanied by wound infection, mobility, and resorption of the adjacent bone (Frame and Brady 1987). An approach to overcome this problem is to use calcium phosphate (CaP) based ceramic materials.

The main interest in CaP materials for bone regeneration relates to the fact that the inorganic phase of bone mainly consists of CaP (70%). CaP ceramics are considered to be bioactive, which implies that they possess the capacity to form a strong chemical bond with adjacent bone (Daculsi et al. 1990; Frayssinet et al. 1993). Despite the fact that CaP ceramics generally exhibit favorable properties for bone tissue engineering, the biological response depends strongly on their physicochemical properties, which will be discussed in the following paragraph.

## 3.2 Physicochemical Properties of CaP Compounds

Many attempts have been made to synthesize CaP ceramics with optimal properties for bone reconstruction. An overview of these different CaP compounds and their Ca/P ratios are given in Table 3.1. The thermodynamic stabilities in aqueous solution as a function of pH are also cited.

**TABLE 3.1** Abbreviations of the CaP Compounds with Corresponding Formulas and Ca/P Ratios

| Ca/P | Formula | Abbreviation | Name | Remarks |
|---|---|---|---|---|
| 0.50 | $Ca(H_2PO_4)\cdot H_2O$ | MCPM | Monocalcium phosphate monohydrate | Stability: <pH 2 |
| 1.00 | $CaHPO_4\cdot 2H_2O$ | DCPD | Dicalcium phosphate dihydrate | Stability: 2 < pH < 4 |
| 1.00 | $CaHPO_4$ | DCPA | Dicalcium phosphate anhydrous (monetite) | Stability: 2 < pH < 4 |
| 1.33 | $Ca_8(HPO_4)_2(PO_4)_4\cdot 5H_2O$ | OCP | Octacalcium phosphate | Stability: 6.5 < pH < 8 |
| 1.50 | $Ca_3(PO_4)_2\cdot xH_2O$ | ACP | Amorphous calcium phosphate | Stability: 4 < pH < 8 |
| 1.50 | $Ca_9(HPO_4)(PO_4)_5\cdot OH$ | CDHA (ns-HA) | Calcium deficient hydroxyapatite | Stability: 5 < pH < 10 |
| 1.50 | $Ca_3(PO_4)_2$ | α-TCP | Alpha-tricalcium phosphate | Stability: 6 < pH < 8, more stable than DCPD but less than CDHA |
| 1.50 | $Ca_3(PO_4)_2$ | β-TCP | Beta-tricalcium phosphate | Stability: 6 < pH < 8, more stable than α-TCP |
| 1.67 | $Ca_{10}(PO_4)_6(OH)_2$ | s-HA | Stoichiometric hydroxyapatite | Stability: 4 < pH |
| 2.00 | $Ca_4(PO_4)_2O$ | TTCP | Tetracalcium phosphate | Less stable than CDHA, DCPD or OCP in water at pH 7.4 |

## 3.2.1 Dicalcium Phosphate

Two different crystalline dicalcium phosphates (DCP) are known at ambient conditions: (i) brushite (dicalcium phosphate dihydrate (DCPD), $CaHPO_4\cdot 2H_2O$) and (ii) monetite (dicalcium phosphate anhydrous (DCPA), $CaHPO_4$). The hydrated DCPD has a monoclinic (*Ia*) structure. $OH^-$ molecules in the unit cell occupy an interlayer between $Ca^{2+}$ and $PO_4^{3-}$ chains, which are arranged parallel to each other (Wang and Nancollas 2008). Absence of $OH^-$ molecules in the structure is referred to as monetite (DCPA). DCPA has a triclinic structure with a Ca/P ratio of 1.5 (Elliott 1994). DCPA can be prepared by the precipitation reaction of $Ca(OH)_2$ or $CaCO_3$ slurry with $H_3PO_4$ solution at a pH of 3.5 around 90°C or by evaporation of a $Ca(NO_3)_2\cdot 4H_2O$ and $NH_4H_2PO_4$ mixture in water at room temperature (Louati et al. 2005; Tas 2009).

At all pH values, DCPA is less soluble than the DCPD structure (Elliott 1994; Fernandez et al. 1999a), but both types of DCP's are stable at a pH lower than 4.2 (Table 3.1). Under biological conditions, DCPA is thermodynamically more stable than DCPD (Lilley et al. 2005). Both phases have been proposed as a precursor in bone mineralization (Boanini et al. 2010).

DCPA and DCPD are widely used as an initial precursor component of self-setting CaP bone cements (Barrere et al. 2006; Hofmann et al. 2009). It is reported that cells are able to rapidly resorb DCP ceramics (Gilardino et al. 2009). However, this structure is metastable under physiological conditions and transforms towards a more stable apatitic structure (Elliott 1994). Many attempts have been made to maintain its structure under conditions where the apatite formation is favored thermodynamically. It is reported that the presence of magnesium ions strongly reduces the transformation rate (Boanini et al. 2010). Absorbance of magnesium ions into DCPD crystal nuclei prevents crystallization and gradually decreases the mechanical properties (Lilley et al. 2005). However, maximally 0.3 wt.% $Mg^{2+}$ can be replaced with $Ca^{2+}$ atomic sites (Elliott 1994).

## 3.2.2 Tricalcium Phosphate

Two polymorphous forms of tricalcium phosphates (TCPs) are beta-tricalcium phosphate (β-TCP) and alpha-tricalcium phosphate (α-TCP). α-TCP is stable between 1120°C and 1470°C and β-TCP is stable below 1120°C (Mathew and Takagi 2001).

β-TCP crystallizes into the R3*c* rhombohedral space group (Yashima et al. 2003). The structure is less stable than apatite under physiological conditions. β-TCP is more soluble than hydroxyapatite (HA), which is formed by sintering at high temperatures (Yang et al. 2008).

Thermodynamically, the most stable structure of β-TCP is whitlockite, where 15% calcium ion vacancies can be occupied by magnesium ions ($Ca_9(Mg)(PO_4)6(PO_3OH)$). Substitution with $Mg^{2+}$ ions decreases its solubility to a lower extent. Moreover, $Mg^{2+}$ plays an important role in the control of the degradation as well as osteoinductivity of β-TCP ceramics (Qi et al. 2008; Pina et al. 2009).

A-TCP crystallizes into the monoclinic ($P2_1/a$) space group (Elliott 1994). The major difference with β-TCP is its strong degree of lattice misfit and the presence of atomic vacancies, which creates a higher internal energy. Thus, the solubility and the biodegradability of α-TCP is higher than β-TCP ceramics (Mathew et al. 1977). Therefore, the main application area of α-TCP is as constituent of CaP cements (CPC), because α-TCP powders easily hydrolyze toward stable HA phases under physiological conditions (Ginebra et al. 2004).

A-TCP can also be sintered as a dense or porous ceramic. The main drawback of this ceramic form is its high reactivity owing to its high solubility (Yuan et al. 2001). In an attempt to counteract excessive degradation, α-TCP/β-TCP biphasic porous ceramics have been produced. The degradation rate of biphasic α-TCP/β-TCP ceramics was reported to be more effective for bone regeneration than α-TCP or β-TCP alone (Kamitakahara 2008).

## 3.2.3 Tetracalcium Phosphate

Tetracalcium phosphate ($Ca_4(PO_4)_2$, TTCP) crystallizes into the monoclinic unit cell. TTCP is prepared by heating an equimolar mixture of DCPA and $CaCO_3$ at higher temperatures (>1300°C) (Fukase et al. 1990).

Generally, TTCP is highly basic and its Ca/P ratio is higher than stoichiometric apatite. The main application of TTCP is as constituent of self-setting CaP cement (Fukase et al. 1990). It can be combined with other CaP cement compounds with lower Ca/P ratios (Chow and Takagi 2001; Mathew and Takagi 2001). More acidic DCP is frequently used to dissolve TTCP with TTCP/DCP molar ratios of 1:1, 1:2, 1:3 (Hirayama et al. 2008). Under physiological conditions, it is easily hydrolyzed toward large rod-like or plate-like HA crystals (calcium deficient hydroxyapatite, CDHA or s-HA) (Fukase et al. 1990). The solubility of the final compound increases with the use of low TTCP/DCP ratios. Consequently, fast bioresorbable CaP cements can be prepared with low TTCP/DCP ratios (Chow and Takagi 2001; Hirayama et al. 2008).

## 3.2.4 Octacalcium Phosphate

Synthetic octacalcium phosphate (OCP) materials are crystallized into the triclinic structure (P1) (Mathew and Takagi 2001). OCP ($Ca_8(HPO_4)_2(PO_4)_4 \cdot 5H_2O$) has a Ca/P ratio of 1.33. Its unit cell consists of CaP apatitic layers with hydrated interlayers (Brown 1962). OCP contains less water molecules than DCPD, which explains its lower solubility (Elliott 1994). Weakly bonded water molecules near the center of hydrated layer allow incorporation of other ions (Brown 1962; Johnsson and Nancollas 1992). OCP is instable in physiological conditions and it tends to convert into the HA structure (Suzuki 2010).

## 3.2.5 Apatites

The CaP phase as present in the inorganic mineral component of calcified tissue is referred to as apatite (Biltz and Pellegrino 1983). The general formula of synthetic CaP apatite is $Ca_5(PO_4)_3X$. When the X position is occupied by $OH^-$ groups, the apatite is referred to as HA. HAs can be grouped into two categories: (i) stoichiometric apatite (s-HA) or (ii) nonstoichiometric apatite (ns-HA) (Elliott 1994).

Stoichiometric apatite has a hexagonal structure (P63/$m$) with a Ca/P ratio of 1.67 (Elliott 1994; Yubao et al. 1996). Sintered s-HA has generally large crystallite sizes and thus a low solubility. As a result, the biodegradation rate of s-HA is generally low (Driessens et al. 1995).

**TABLE 3.2** Chemical and Crystallographic Characteristics of Biologic Apatites

| Composition (wt.%) | Bone | Dentin | Enamel |
|---|---|---|---|
| Calcium[a] | 36.6 | 40.3 | 37.6 |
| Phosphorus[a] | 17.1 | 18.6 | 18.3 |
| Sodium[b] | 1.0 | 0.6 | 0.5 |
| Magnesium[b] | 0.7 | 1.2 | 0.4 |
| Potassium[b] | 0.07 | 0.07 | 0.05 |
| Carbonate[b] | 7.4 | 5.6 | 3.5 |
| Fluoride[c] | 0.03 | 0.06 | 0.01 |
| Chloride[a,d] | 0.33 | 0.01 | 0.30 |
| Ca/P[a] | 1.65 | 1.67 | 1.59 |
| Lattice Parameters (±003 Å) | | | |
| $a$-axis (Å) | 9.41[c] | 9.42[c] | 9.44[e] |
| $c$-axis (Å) | 6.89[c] | 6.88[c] | 6.87[e] |

[a] Elliott (1994). The composition is relative to the ash content of whole dentin (73 wt%) and enamel (96%). Bone is from bovine cortical bone (taken as 73 wt% of fat-free dry bone).

[b] Boanini et al. (2010).

[c] Dorozhkin (2009).

[d] Handschin and Stern (1995).

[e] Elliott et al. (1985).

Nonstoichiometric apatite (CDHA) has a formula of $Ca_{10-x}(OH)_{2-x}(HPO_4)_x(PO_4)_{6-x}$ $0 < x \leq 1$). The lack of $Ca^{2+}$ and $OH^-$ ions in nonstoichiometric apatite creates atomic vacancies, which increase the susceptibility to acidic dissolution (Yubao et al. 1996). As a consequence, they are structurally and physically more reactive than s-HA.

Chemical analysis of biological apatites, on the other hand, indicated that bone apatite structure also contains trace elements such as Mg, Na, Si, Cl, and F (Table 3.2).

### 3.2.5.1 Fluorapatite

The ionic radii of the $OH^-$ lattice positions as located in the apatite structure, allow for substitution by fluoride ions (FAp: $Ca_{10}(PO_4)_6(OH)_{2-x}F_x$) (Lin et al. 1981). Incorporation of fluoride ions into the apatite structure results into stabilization of the lattice and correspondingly a decreased solubility (Little and Rowley 1961). Clinical studies on dental caries have revealed that fluoride inhibits acidic etching (Lin et al. 1981). FAp's resistance to acid etching is higher than all other CaP compounds (Budz et al. 1987).

### 3.2.5.2 Carbonated Apatite

As shown in Table 3.2, bone mineral contains a high amount of carbonate. Biological apatites as present in human bone can therefore be referred to as carbonated apatite (CHA). Carbonate in biological apatites primarily substitutes for phosphate groups (B-type substitution). This type of substitution in synthetic $CO_3$-Aps can be obtained by synthesis at lower temperatures (60–100°C) (LeGeros 1965). On the other hand, when the reaction is performed at high temperatures (800–1000°C) for several hours in dry $CO_2$, the substitution preferentially takes place on $OH^-$ molecular sites (A-type substitution) (Elliott 1994).

Both A-type and B-type carbonated apatite structure are chemically unstable yielding a HA structure that is more reactive than synthetic HA under physiological conditions (Habibovic et al. 2010).

### 3.2.5.3 Silicon-Substituted Apatite

Silicon-substituted CaPs have received much attention because of their supposed positive effect on bone healing (Bohner 2009). Apatites having 1.5–4.6 wt% of Si incorporated into the lattice have been suggested to display improved bone formation (Gasqueres et al. 2007; Boanini et al. 2010). The incorporation of Si in HA is suggested to enhance its bioactivity by increasing the number of defect sites, which are responsible for partial dissolution of the apatite structure (Regi and Arcos 2005). Moreover, released Si ions are claimed to stimulate cellular activity by affecting the adsorption of proteins onto silicon-substituted apatites (Gasqueres et al. 2007). Nevertheless, final evidence for the supposed effect of silicon substitution has not been found in animal studies (Bohner 2009).

## 3.3 CaP Blocks/Granules

The CaP compounds as mentioned in the previous chapter have been primarily fabricated in the form of blocks/granules. They have been used in dental and orthopedic applications (Bucholz et al. 1989; Navarro et al. 2008). The majority of CaP blocks/granules are chemically based on HA, β-TCP, and biphasic CaPs (HA/β-TCP, BCP). Commercially available CaP blocks/granules as being currently marketed are listed in Table 3.3.

### 3.3.1 Production Methods

CaP blocks/granulate powder can be fabricated by precipitation, sol–gel and hydrothermal synthesis (Orlovskii et al. 2002; Tanaja and Yamashite 2008). The precipitation route is a widely used technique to obtain CaP powders. In this method, powders are prepared by the reaction of diammonium hydrogen phosphate with calcium nitrate (Zhang and Gonsalves 1997) or orthophosphoric acid with calcium hydroxide (lime: $Ca(OH)_2$) at pH 10 (Bernard et al. 1999; Kweh et al. 1999). Parameters such as stirring rate and temperature have an influence on chemical composition, crystallinity, morphology, size, shape, and specific surface area (Bernard et al. 1999). The sol–gel method involves the calcination of ammonium, urea, and calcium nitrate tetradihydrate solution to produce s-HA powders (Ca/P = 1.67) (Sopyan et al. 2008). During hydrothermal processing; monetite, brushite, or amorphous calcium phosphate (ACP) compounds can be used to obtain more homogeneous and 30–50 nm in length needle-like HA particles under steam pressure at high temperature (Mahabole et al. 2005).

The processing of powders into block-form can be done by solid-state high-temperature sintering (<1500°C) and hot isostatic pressing (10–300 MPa) (Orlovskii et al. 2002). The sintering temperatures depend on the powder characteristics. For instance, sintering of β-TCP powders at high temperature (>1250°C) leads to the composition transformation toward the α-TCP form, which slows down the sintering process. Therefore, this process is usually performed under water vapor in order to be able to increase the temperature while preserving the crystal phase (Tanaja and Yamashite 2008). The sintering process under water vapor increases the crystallite size, removes impurities, and facilitates the production of dense blocks.

Another limitation related to high temperature sintering is excessive grain growth, high density, loss of porosity, and correspondingly low-specific surface area (Komlev and Barinov 2002; Hsu et al. 2007). For example, densification of HA above 700°C decreases the specific area from 50–200 to 1 m²/g. In contrast, the specific area of bone is around 80 m²/g (Muralithran and Ramesh 2000; Bohner 2001; Kasten et al. 2003; Bailliez and Nzihou 2004).

In order to improve the biological success of CaP ceramics, interconnected macroporous CaP blocks or granules have been developed. Macroporosity within the ceramic increases the success of the implant by enabling vascularization and bone ingrowth throughout the ceramic material. Macroporosity in CaP ceramics can be introduced by polymeric substances or production of gas bubbles ($CO_2$). Although

**TABLE 3.3**   Commercially Available Calcium Phosphate Blocks/Granules Substitutes

| Company | Commercially Available Product | Available Forms | Macro Porosity (µm) | Resorption | Comp. Strength (MPa) | Target Area | Reference |
|---|---|---|---|---|---|---|---|
| Biomet OsteoBiologics, US | ProOsteon 500R | CHA • Blocks | 500 | 9–18 months | 6 | Distal radius for internal-external fixation, cervical fusion, oral and maxillofacial surgery, orthognathic applications, posttraumatic metaphyseal defects | Wolfe 1999; Thalgott et al. 2001; Korovessis et al. 2005 |
| | Endobon | HA • Blocks • Granules | 100–1.500 | >5 years | 2.5–16 | Blocks: Tibial plateau fractures, pelvis, and femur, acetabulum, pseudarthrosis defects Granules: bone cysts in hand, feet, knee, and spine | Gierse and Donath 1999; Baer et al. 2002 |
| | ProOsteon 200R | CHA • Granules | 200 | 6–13 months | — | Anterior/posterior iliac crest corticocancellous bone graft | Shord 1999; Stubbsa et al. 2004 |
| DePuy Spine US | Conduit | β-TCP • Granules | 1–600 | 64% 6–7 months | — | Femoral neck fractures, vertebral body compression fractures | Bodde et al. 2006 |
| Ceraver, France | Cerapatite | HA • Granules | 100–400 | Several years | 40–45 | — | Henno et al. 2003 |
| | Calciresorb | β-TCP • Granules | 100–400 500–1000 | — | 40–45 | Sinus augmentation | Gruber et al. 2008 |
| FH Orthopedics, France | Eurocer 400 | BCP 55%HA/45%β-TCP • Granules | 300–500 | 6–12 months | No mech. resistance | Femoral systems, metaphyseal fractures | Schwartz et al. 1999; Schwartz and Bordei 2005 |
| | Eurocer 200+ | BCP 65%/35%β-TCP • Blocks | 150–300 | >15 months | 10 | Femoral systems, arthrodeses, ankle fractures | Schwartz et al. 1999 |
| Medtronic, US | BCP | BCP 60%HA/40%β-TCP • Granules | 200–500 | — | 1–2 | Iliac crest | Krijnen et al. 2008 |
| Sybron Implant Solutions, Germany | Bioresorb | β-TCP • Granules | 200–500 500–1000 1000–2000 1400–3200 | 2 years | 15 | Osteochondritis, mandibular cysts, ankle-foot fracture, calcaneus cystic lipoma, acetabular revision, tumoral cavities | Galois et al. 2001; Knežević et al. 2007 |

| Wright Medical Technology, U.S. | Cellplex TCP | BCP • α-TCP/β-TCP/ HA Granules | — | 62% 8 weeks | 1.4 | Metadiaphyseal fracture of tibia | Fredericks et al. 2004 |
|---|---|---|---|---|---|---|---|
| Mitsubishi Materials Corp. Japan | Bonfil | HA • Blocks • Granules | 90–200 | >160 weeks | Blocks: 15 granules: 2–3 | Distal radius for internal, external fixation, hip arthroplasty, ilium, dental applications | Yaszemski et al. 2004; Ogose et al. 2006 |
| Sumitomo Osaka Cement Co. Japan | Boneceram | HA • Blocks • Granules | 50–300 | — | 44–68.6 | Spinal surgery: cervical laminoplasty | Kokubun et al. 1994; Yoshikawa et al. 2009 |
| Pentax Corp. Japan | Apaceram | HA • Dense granules • Porous granules | 100–400 | >20 months | Dense: 210 Porous: 66 (40%) | Maxillofacial reconstruction: buccal, inferior mandibular, and posterior margins | Li et al. 1997; Saijo et al. 2008; Yamasaki et al. 2009 |
| Olympus Terumo Biomaterials, Japan | Osferion | β-TCP • Granules | 100–500 | 24 weeks | 2 | Acetabulum, distal femur, proximal femur | Ogose et al. 2006 |
| Curasan, CryoLife and Spinal Con., Germany | Cerosorb | β-TCP • Blocks • Granules | 50–2000 | 80–90% within 12 months | — | Sinus floor augmentation, periodontal applications | Horch et al. 2006 |

macroporosity enhances the resorption and cellular interaction, the reduced mechanical resistance of the material does not allow its use in load-bearing applications (Habraken et al. 2007).

## 3.3.2 Structure–Property Relationships

### 3.3.2.1 Mechanical Properties

The stiffness of a biomaterial should be comparable to that of cortical and trabecular bone to support loading at the fracture site (Nilsson 2003). Therefore, bone substitutes have to be designed in order to withstand long-term or short-term compressive and bending forces. The main drawback of CaPs materials is their brittleness and poor strength, limiting their use as implants in loaded situations.

Porous CaPs are attractive for a wide variety of applications. However, deterioration of mechanical properties is the main disadvantage of these structures. It is reported that high macroporosity (>40%) induces bone growth, but decreases the elastic modulus and compressive strength more than 10-fold (Zheltonoga and Gabriwlov 1979; Chevalier et al. 2008). Therefore, a remarkable increase in mechanical properties and biological performance can be achieved by controlling the preparation conditions.

### 3.3.2.2 Bioresorption

Bioresorption is a biological erosion process by which a material is resorbed and replaced by tissue over a period of time. Bioresorption of CaP ceramics is divided into two main categories: (i) active resorption, and (ii) passive resorption (Frayssinet et al. 1993; Blokhuis et al. 2000; Ooms et al. 2003).

Passive resorption is a solution-mediated process (extracellular liquid of the body) and predominantly initiates at potential stress accumulated regions in the structure. Porosities, grain boundaries, dislocations, cracks, irregularities, substitution ion sites, and atomic vacancies are known to be potential dissolution sites in ceramic apatites because of their higher sensitivity to acidic etching (Koerten and van der Meulen 1999; Ambard and Museninghoff 2006).

Active resorption takes place by osteoclasts. Upon implantation of CaP ceramics, the activity of the osteoclasts determines the dissolution and remodeling characteristics of the CaP ceramic.

Remodeling of the CaP material is strongly influenced by the presence of porosity. Microporosity (<10 μm) allows the influx of body liquids. The material serves then as a nutrition provider for osteoprogenitor cells. Macroporosity (>100 μm) enables the penetration of fibrovascular tissue and the development of mature osteons (Afonso et al. 1996; Smith et al. 2006). It is reported that the ideal pore size for CaP ceramics is between 100 and 400 μm in order to act as a convenient template for rapid bone growth (Tsuruga et al. 1997). Interconnections between pores are also favorable for nourishment and colonization of the material with blood vessels.

### 3.3.2.3 Biological Properties

#### *3.3.2.3.1 In Vivo Animal Studies*

The bone-healing capacity of various CaP ceramics has been tested in different animal models (Figure 3.1). CaP biomaterials with various amounts of HA and TCP (BCP) blocks were reported to have high bone-forming capacity (Yuan et al. 2001).

Compared to high-temperature sintered β-TCP, α-TCP, and HA ceramics that showed low amount of bone formation in a dog implantation study due to an unbalanced passive resorption (Yuan et al. 1998), high biodegradability and bone regeneration was observed for low-temperature sintered (1150°C) BCP ceramics (80/20, 60/40 wt% HA/β-TCP) in goat and sheep experiments (Le Nihouannena et al. 2005; Wilson et al. 2006). In another study, the optimum bone formation rate of six different CaP ceramic implants (HA/β-TCP: 100/0, 76/24, 63/37, 56/44, 20/80) was determined in a femoral gap defect as created in rats. More bone formation within 12 weeks was determined in the BCP group, which consisted of 56/44 and 20/80 wt% HA/β-TCP. The high amount of bone formation in the BCP group was attributed to a low activity of osteoclast induced by $Ca^{2+}$ release (Livinston et al. 2003).

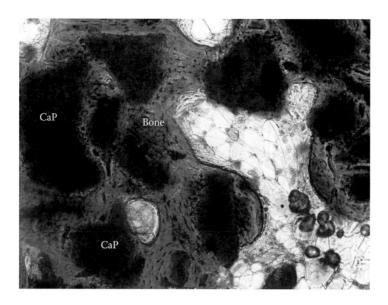

**FIGURE 3.1** Photomicrographs showing the tissue response of CaP granules after 12 weeks of implantation in sheep. A close contact between the newly formed bone and the CaP granules supporting the osteoconductive properties of the CaP ceramic materials.

### 3.3.2.3.2 Clinical Applications

*3.3.2.3.2.1 Hydroxyapatite*  HA granules can be used as filler of bone defects and blocks can be used to prevent, for example, dorsal displacement of the distal fragments in orthopedic fractures (Figure 3.2). However, many clinical results demonstrated a lower quantity of bone growth on HA granules when used in human craniofacial and maxillofacial bone defects in long-term follow-up studies (Sakano et al. 2001; Fortunato et al. 1997; Bonucci et al. 2007).

The main problem with the granules is their migration in the defect site and the unpredictable bone growth. On the other hand, HA blocks overcome these problems by producing a stable augmentation. HA blocks can successfully support teeth and bone segments in their replaced positions

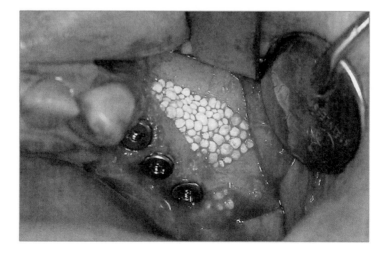

**FIGURE 3.2** Placement of HA granules into pockets created between the soft tissues and the alveolar bone.

and they are convenient materials for alveolar ridge augmentation procedures (Frame 1987; Frame and Brady 1987). Histological studies showed good bony healing and early host bone attachment with no evidence of any foreign body reaction. However, it is difficult to shape the solid-dense HA blocks during surgery. This may result into implant migration through the cavity (Quayle et al. 1990).

*3.3.2.3.2.2 Coral-Derived Apatites*   In an attempt to enhance the osteoconductivity and osteoinductivity of apatites, thermochemically treated marine coral apatites ($CaCO_3$, Porites, Goniopora) have been developed. When corals are treated with ammonium phosphate solution under hydrothermal conditions at pH 7 for 3 days, their structure is converted into resorbable osteoconductive coralline hydroxyapatite (Sivakumar et al. 1996; Zaffe 2005).

Currently, the most commonly used commercial coral-derived carbonated apatite blocks/granules are Biocoral®, ProOsteon®500, and Interpore®200 (ProOsteon®200). They have been reported to be bioresorbable and osteoinductive (Damien and Revell 2004). They can be used for alveolar ridge augmentation, periodontal, and orthognathic reconstructions (White and Shors 1986). It is reported that when coralline blocks are used for the repair of lumbar discogenic pain surgery in 40 patients with an anterior lumbar interbody fusion technique, a success rate of 82.5% with a fusion rate of 92.5% can be achieved in patients. Histological analysis after 24 months confirmed conclusive evidence of bone ingrowth (Thalgott et al. 2001). Another histological study showed a 93.5% implant success rate when coralline apatite granules were used in the posterior maxilla and mandible for the placement of dental implants during a 3–8 year follow-up period in 21 patients (Sandor et al. 2003).

*3.3.2.3.2.3 β-Tricalcium Phosphate*   Biodegradable CaP materials are used to replace a defect sites with newly formed bone. In many bone reconstruction surgeries, bioresorbable β-TCP blocks/granules attract more attention for tissue engineering applications because of their osteoinductivity. Although β-TCP has almost the same chemical composition ($Ca_3(PO_4)_2$) as HA, the crystallographic difference strongly influences its dissolution and resorption activity.

β-TCP granules such as Conduit™, RTR®, or Osferion® alone, possess a fast resorption rate and superior osteoconductivity (Dong et al. 2002; Ogose et al. 2006; Bodde et al. 2007). *In vivo* studies have revealed that β-TCP resorption depending on passive erosion due to its reactivity at biologic conditions (Kotani et al. 1991).

*3.3.2.3.2.4 Biphasic Calcium Phosphate*   As implants made of dense pure HA are maintained in the defect area for many years because of their thermodynamic stability and β-TCP implants can degrade too fast before bone formation can occur, the soluble HA/TCP (BCP) composite calcium biomaterials have been developed for biomedical applications. Notably, the use of two CaP phases has gained in importance due to its high bone growth rate at physiological conditions (Chena et al. 2004).

Clinical application of BCPs is shown in a study of Mailac et al. 2008, who used 21% microporous and 49% macroporous (macropores: >300 µm) 60/40 wt% HA/TCP granules in a sinus lift augmentation procedure in human. After 6 months of implantation, 53% of the granules were resorbed and almost completely replaced by newly formed bone (Mailac and Daculsi 2008). Vascularization and hematopoietic cells around the residual HA material confirmed the high osteoconduction properties of BCP granules. Besides their biological activity, a broad pore size range production stimulates infiltration of large osteoclast and small leukocytes, which enhance cellular interactions and bone regeneration (Le Nihouannena et al. 2005).

The bioactivity of BCPs is also ascribed to the HA/β-TCP ratio. When 50/50 wt% BCP granules (pore size: 90–100 µm) were used in the anterior maxilla, gradual resorption, and new bone substitution is observed with no evidence of inflammatory response (Piattelli et al. 1996). High bone remodeling of low HA/β-TCP ratio occurs by (i) partial dissolution of β-TCP, (ii) carbonated HA transformation associated with an organic matrix, (iii) mineralization of the collagen fibrils, and (iv) a rapid remodeling process (Daculsi 1998).

Although the bone-repairing ceramics based on HA or β-TCP become more and more applied, biphasic structure grafts provide a significant alternative to autogenous bone for orthopedic and dental applications.

## 3.4 CaP Cements

In contrast to premade CaP blocks or granules, which are difficult to handle from a clinical point of view, self-setting CPC have been developed. These materials are injectable, which allows for optimal defect filling.

Injectable CaP cements for the use as a bone graft were first described by Chow and Brown in 1985. Their cement is based on at least two sparingly soluble CaP mixtures that are precipitated apatite crystals in an aqueous environment. Under physiological conditions, the end product is an apatite structure, which is remarkably biocompatible (Brown and Chow 1985). So far, a large number of CPC have been developed as a potential grafting material for use in orthopedics and dentistry (Table 3.4). For each formulation, *in vivo* tests have been performed to prove the success of CaP cements. Cements having identical chemical compositions display large differences in physicochemical and biological properties due to several factors such as the presence of impurities, the particle size distribution, and correspondingly specific surface area resulting into differences in solubility of the precursor phases (Fernandez et al. 1999b; Vanderschot et al. 2007).

**TABLE 3.4**  List of Commercially Available Calcium Phosphate Cements

| Company | Cement Type | Components | Solution Mixture | End Product | Compressive Strength (MPa) |
|---|---|---|---|---|---|
| Teknimed | Cementek® | α-TCP<br>TTCP<br>Ca(OH)$_2$ | H$_2$O + Ca(OH)$_2$, H$_3$PO$_4$ | HA Ca/P = 1.64 | 20 |
| Biomed | Calcibon® | α-TCP (61%)<br>DCPA (26%)<br>CaCO$_3$ (10%)<br>pHA (3%) | H$_2$O + Na$_2$HPO$_4$ | Carbonated apatite (CHA) | 60–70 |
|  | Mimix™ | α-TCP<br>TTCP<br>C$_6$H$_5$O$_7$Na$_3$ · 2H$_2$O | H$_2$O + C$_6$H$_8$O$_7$ | HA | 22 |
| ETEX | Biobon® | ACP(50%)<br>DCPD (50%) | H$_2$O | HA Ca/P = 1.45 | 12 |
| Stryker-Leibinger | BoneSource® | TTCP (73%)<br>DCPD (27%) | H$_2$O + Na$_2$HPO$_4$ + NaH$_2$PO$_4$ | HA Ca/P = 1.67 | 36 |
| Synthes-Norian | Norian®SRS | α-TCP (85%)<br>CaCO$_3$ (12%)<br>MCPM (3%) | H$_2$O + Na$_2$HPO$_4$ | Brushite Ca/P = 1.67 | 28–55 |
|  | chronOS™ | β-TCP (42%)<br>MCPM (21%)<br>MgHPO$_4$ · 3H$_2$O (5%) | H$_2$O + Sodium hyaluronate (0.5%) | Brushite | 3 |
| Mitsubishi materials | Biopex® | α-TCP (75%)<br>TTCP (18%)<br>DCPD (5%)<br>HA (2%) | H$_2$O, sodium succinate (12%), sodium chondroitin sulfate | HA | 80 |

*Source:*  Adapted from Habraken, W. J., Wolke, J. G., and Jansen, J. A. 2007. *Advances in Drug Delivery Reviews* 59: 234–48.

### 3.4.1 Setting of Cement

CaP cements are formulated as a solid–liquid mixture. The general principle of mixing more than one CaP compound is to balance the precipitation reaction of CaP compounds with respect to solubility. Dry CaP sources may include: $Ca_3(PO_4)_2$ (TCP), $CaHPO_4$ (DCP), $Ca_4(PO_4)_2O$ (TTCP), $Ca_3(PO_4)_2H_2O$ (ACP). Alternatively, calcium sources include: $CaCO_3$ (calcite), CaO (calcium oxide), $Ca(OH)_2$ (calcium hydroxide), while phosphate sources can be: $H_3PO_4$ (phosphoric acid), $Na_2HPO_4$ (disodium hydro-phosphate), or $NaH_2PO_4$ (sodium dihydrophosphate) (Constantz et al. 2007). When mixed in aque-ous solvents that often contain buffers based on, for example, phosphate or acetate, these dry powders convert into a self-setting paste that can be injected into bone cavities and subsequently harden within 10–20 min (Figure 3.3).

The setting behavior of the paste is an important property that strongly affects its clinical per-formance. The setting time should not be too fast or too long because it can only be shaped before it hardens, whereas the wound area can only be closed after hardening. Generally, the final setting time of the cement should be below 15 min for optimal clinical handling (Khairoun et al. 1997). In order to accelerate the setting time of the paste, $Na_2HPO_4$ (pH > 7) and/or $NaH_2PO_4$ (pH < 6) liquid addi-tives can be used (Fernandez et al. 1994). These additives not only modify the pH of the medium for dissolution reaction, but also supply $PO_4^{3-}$ sources to accelerate the precipitation reaction (Fernandez et al. 1999b).

The liquid/powder ratio (L/P) is an important aspect of the cement that affects the workability and the injectability of the paste. Generally, low L/P ratio's cause flowable and viscous pastes, while liquid deprivation reduces the injectability of the paste. On the other hand, excess aqueous solution is often associated with the phenomenon of filter-pressing, which implies that the liquid flows faster than the ceramic particles (Bohner et al. 2010). Although liquid films surrounding the particles keep the particles separated, improve the fluidity and allow injection by minimally invasive techniques, the final setting time of the cement increases due to delayed crystallization, which causes a weaker structure due to a high micro and nanoporosity in the final cement (Ginebra et al. 2004; Espanol et al. 2009).

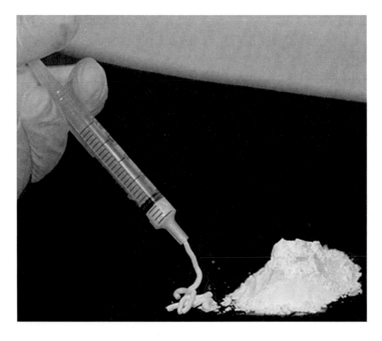

**FIGURE 3.3**  Injection of CaP cement from syringe.

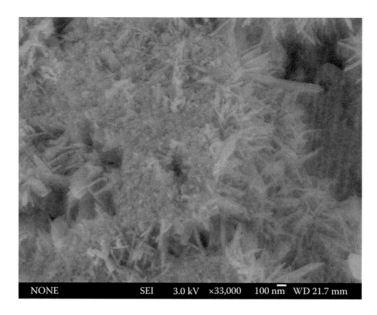

**FIGURE 3.4** SEM pictures of the acicular microcrystalline HA structure (×33.000).

The cohesion is the ability of the paste to maintain its shape upon contact with body liquid. Washout of the cement may result in inflammatory reactions at the defect site (Ishikawa 2008). Small particle sizes, low L/P ratios or addition of gelling agents (0.2–2% sodium alginate, 0.4–1.5% chitosan, 2–4% hydroxypropylmethyl or carboxymethyl cellulose) can be used to prevent disintegration of the paste (Takechi et al. 1996; Cherng et al. 1997; Ishikawa et al. 1997).

The evolution of the crystal structure is governed by the dissolution/precipitation, crystallization, and crystal growth mechanism (Figure 3.4). In relatively high supersaturations, an ACP is the phase that forms first.

Incorporation of carbonate and other impurities occurs during irreversible hydrolysis reactions of ceramic precursors towards precipitation of HA. These ions decrease the transformation rate and crystal size of precipitated HA (LeGeros 2008).

## 3.4.2 Structure–Property Relationships

### 3.4.2.1 Mechanical Properties

A critical limitation for long-term performance of CPCs is their relatively low mechanical strength. Because of the self-setting reaction and the absence of high sintering temperatures, compressive strengths of CPC are up to 10 times lower than sintered CaP compounds (Komath and Varma 2003). However, the compressive strength of CPCs is still comparable to that of cortical bone (88–164 MPa) (Nissan et al. 2008).

CaP cements exhibit a high amount of nano- and microporosity. Porosity that develops between entangled crystals is the main reason for the weak mechanical structure of cements. For example, a decrease in microporosity from 50% to 31% in the end product of TTCP/DCPA cements, increased the wet compressive strength from 4 to 37 MPa, respectively (Barralet et al. 2002). Additionally, an addition of 10 wt% silica or titanium oxide in TTCP/DCPA cements significantly increased the compressive strength (80–100 MPa) due to the more dense structure (Gbureck et al. 2003). On the other hand, for α-TCP cement, which sets into CDHA as end product, a compressive strength of 40 MPa was obtained by using fine particles of about 2–3 μm to obtain a structure with a low porosity (Ginebra et al. 2004).

### 3.4.2.2 Bioresorption

CaP cements consisting of α-TCP/DCP, TTCP/DCP, or β-TCP/MCPM (monocalcium phosphate mono-hydrate) powders set into highly osteoconductive and osteoinductive HA, CDHA, or DCPD final products (Table 3.4) (Ohura et al. 1996; Lew et al. 1997; Ooms et al. 2003). Their resorption rate and bone formation rate has been reported to be higher than sintered HA-based ceramics (Fujikawa et al. 1995). Due to the low density of the final HA structure, these cements can be resorbed by osteoclasts (Sugawara et al. 2008). Moreover, because of the uniform distribution of the paste throughout the bone defect, new bone formation can occur more rapidly and uniformly in the entire defect area due to calcium release into the surrounding medium by active and passive resorption of the cement (Sugawara et al. 1993).

### 3.4.2.3 Biological Properties

#### 3.4.2.3.1 In Vivo Animal Studies

CaP cements have been proven to be effective as bone substitutes because of their high biocompatibility and osteoconductive structure (Figure 3.5).

Several histological and histomorphometrical examinations confirmed the excellent bone biocompatibility, osteoconductivity, and bone-healing capacity of apatite and brushite cements in various animal models (Lew et al. 1997; Theiss et al. 2005; Sugawara et al. 2008). Apatite cements have been reported to be able to enhance osteoblast and osteoclast activity and increased mesenchymal cell differentiation when implanted in rabbits and goats (Ooms et al. 2002; Camiré et al. 2006). Upon implantation, fully osseointegration of the apatitic cement to the rim of the acetabulum in 22 sheep was also reported (Timperley et al. 2010). For brushite cements, on the other hand, the resorption occurred through body liquid dissolution with cement disintegration, which is accompanied with new bone formation when implanted in sheep femur defects for a period of 8 weeks (Theiss et al. 2005). However, the osteoinduction rate for brushite cements is higher when vascular endothelial growth factor and platelet derived growth factor (VEGF/PDGF) are loaded into this material (De la Riva et al. 2010).

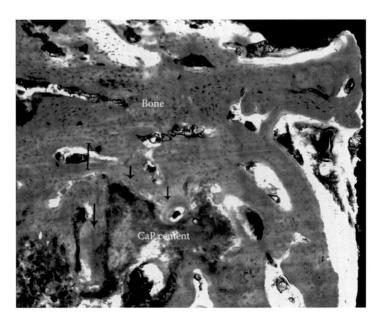

**FIGURE 3.5** Low magnification photomicrograph of a transversal section of the CaP cement after 24 weeks of sinus implantation in goat model. Parts of the cement mass is resorbed and followed by bone ingrowth (arrow-heads). A close contact between the newly formed bone and the CaP cement, (end product: CDHA, Ca/P: 1.54) supporting the osteoconductive properties of the cement (original magnification 2.5×, bar = 400 μm).

### *3.4.2.3.2 Clinical Applications*

Various bone cement materials are currently being commercialized for various clinical indications. The most important are discussed below.

The first commercially available injectable cement, Norian Skeletal Repair System (SRS), (Norian/ Synthes USA, Paoli, PA), was marketed in the 1990s (Ilan and Ladd 2003). Norian Skeletal is a CaP cement consisting of MCPM, α-TCP, and $CaCO_3$, while the liquid phase contains phosphate source. Within 10 min, the cement begins to crystallize into carbonated apatite with a molar calcium–phosphate ratio of 1.67. The hardening reaction is almost completed after 12 h. The final compressive strength equals 55 MPa which is higher than cancellous bone (Constantz et al. 1995). The end product of the cement setting reaction is biocompatible, osteoconductive, and stimulates osteogenesis (Manzotti et al. 2006). The cement is approved for more general orthopedic use in tibial and femoral metaphyseal bone defects and displaced tibial plateau fractures (Frankenburg et al. 1998). Bioresorption of SRS in cancellous bone defect is completed as early as 16 weeks after implantation (Constantz et al. 1995). Long-term follow up (1 year) with Norian cements in cranial defects and bony deformities showed that the main complications were related to sterile seroma and infection due to cement fragmentation. However, problems related to infections could be solved with antibiotic therapy. The complication rate was observed to increase in patients who received more than 25 g of Norian (Gilardino et al. 2009).

BoneSource® (Stryker-Howmedica-Osteonics, Rutherford, NJ) is another CaP cement, which consists of TTCP and DCPD with a powder–liquid ratio of 4:1. Hardening of the paste is reached between 10 and 15 min resulting into complete conversion towards HA (Ca/P: 1.65–1.67) as an end product (Fukase et al. 1990). BoneSource® has been approved for use in metaphyseal fractures. High success rates are reported for craniofacial defects for time periods between 24 months to 6 years (Friedman et al. 1998). Effectiveness and healing of metaphyseal bone voids, translabyrinthine, middle cranial fossa, and suboccipital craniectoy have also been reported, but long-term stability of final product is the main disadvantage of this cement type when high amounts of the cement are used at the defect site (Kneton et al. 1995; Kveton et al. 1995; Dickson et al. 2002).

## 3.5 Conclusion

The osteoconductivity and in some cases osteoinductivity of CaP ceramics render these materials highly suitable as scaffold material for the engineering of bone tissue. Still, the biological performance of these ceramics in terms of biodegradation and the amount of new bone formation is strongly dependent on their physicochemical properties, which stresses the fact that proper characterization of CaP scaffolds is of utmost importance. Although CaP based blocks/granules have been safely and effectively used in a wide range of orthopedic and dental applications, recent evidence indicates that self-hardening cements can be as effective as sintered CaP granules to regenerate bone tissue. In combination with their superior clinical handling, it can be concluded that CPC with controlled injectability, porosity, and degradation can become the preferred material of choice for hard tissue engineering applications.

## References

Afonso, A., Santos, J. D., Vasconcelos, M., Branco, R., and Cavalheiro, J. 1996. Granules of osteoapatite and glass-reinforced hydroxyapatite implanted in rabbit tibiae. *Journal of Materials Science: Materials in Medicine* 7: 507–10.

Ambard, J. A. and Museninghoff, L. 2006. Calcium phosphate cement: Reviews of mechanical and biological properties. *Journal of Prosthondontics* 15: 321–28.

Baer, W., Schaller, P., and Carl, H. D. 2002. Spongy hydroxyapatite in hand surgery—A five year follow up. *Journal of Hand Surgery* 27B: 101–03.

Bailliez, S. and Nzihou, A. 2004. The kinetics of surface area reduction during isothermal sintering of hydroxyapatite adsorbent. *Chemical Engineering Journal* 98: 141–52.

Barralet, J. E., Gaunt, T., Wright, A. J., Gibson, I. R., and Knowles, J. C. 2002. Effect of porosity reduction by compaction on compressive strength and microstructure of calcium phosphate cement. *Journal of Biomedical Materials Research* 63: 1–9.

Barrere, F., van Blitterswijk, C. A., and de Groot, K. 2006. Bone regeneration: Molecular and cellular interactions with calcium phosphate ceramics. *International Journal of Nanomedicine* 1: 317–32.

Bernard, L., Freche, M., Lacout, J. L., and Biscans, B. 1999. Preparation of hydroxyapatite by neutralization at low temperature-influence of purity of raw material. *Powder Technology* 103: 19–25.

Biltz, R. M. and Pellegrino, E. D. 1983. The composition of recrystallized bone mineral. *Journal of Dental Research* 62: 1190–95.

Blokhuis, T. J., Termaat, M. F., den Boer, F. C., Patka, P., Bakker, F. C., and Haarman, H. J. 2000. Properties of calcium phosphate ceramics in relation to their *in vivo* behavior. *The Journal of Trauma: Injury, Infection, and Critical Care* 48: 179–86.

Boanini, E., Gazzano, M., and Bigi, A. 2010. Ionic substitutions in calcium phosphates synthezed at low temperature. *Acta Biomaterialia* 6: 1882–94.

Bodde, E. W. H., Wolke, J. G. C., Kowalski, R. S. Z., and Jansen, J. A. 2007. Bone regeneration of porous-tricalcium phosphate (conduit-tcp) and of biphasic calcium phosphate ceramic (biosel) in trabecular defects in sheep. *Journal of Biomedical Materials Research Part A* 82A: 711–22.

Bohner, M. 2001. Physical and chemical aspects of calcium phosphates used in spinal surgery. *European Spine Journal* 10: 114–21.

Bohner, M. 2009. Silicon-substituted calcium phosphates—A critical view. *Biomaterials* 30: 6403–06.

Bohner, M., Barroud, G., and Gasser, B. 2010. Critical aspects in the use of injectable calcium phosphates in spinal surgery. *Biomaterials* 31: 4609–11.

Bonucci, E., Marini, E., Valdinucci, F., and Fortunate, G. 2007. Osteogenic response to hydroxyapatite-fibrin implants in maxillofacial bone defects. *European Journal of Oral Sciences* 105: 557–61.

Brown, E. W. 1962. Octacalcium phosphate and hydroxyapatite: Crystal structure of octacalcium phosphate. *Nature* 196: 1048–50.

Brown, W. E., and Chow, L. C. 1985. Dental restorative cement paste. US Patent: 4,518,430.

Bucholz, R. W., Carlton, A., and Holmes, R. 1989. Interporous hydroxyapatite as a bone graft substitute in tibial plateau fractures. *Clinical Orthopaedics and Related Research* 240: 53–62.

Budz, J. A., Lore, M., and Nancollas, G. H. 1987. Hydroxyapatite and carbonated apatite as models for the dissolution behaviour of human dental enamel. *Advances in Dental Research* 1: 314–21.

Camiré, C. L., Saint-Jean, S. J., Mochales, C., Nevsten, P., Wang, J. S., Lidgren, L., McCarthy, I., and Ginebra, M. P. 2006. Material characterization and *in vivo* behavior of silicon substituted alpha-tricalcium phosphate cement. 76B: 424–31.

Chena, T. M., Shihb, C., Linc, F. T., and Lin, F. H. 2004. Reconstruction of calvarial bone defects using an osteoconductive material and post-implantation hyperbaric oxygen treatment. *Materials Science and Engineering C* 24: 855–60.

Cherng, A., Takagi, S., and Chow, L. C. 1997. Effects of hydroxypropyl methylcellulose and other gelling agents on the handling properties of calcium phosphate cement. *Journal of Biomedical Materials Research Part A* 35: 273–77.

Chevalier, E., Chulia, D., Pouget, C., and Viana, M. 2008. Fabrication of porous substrates: A review of processes using pore forming agents in the biomaterial field. *Journal of Pharmaceutical Sciences* 97: 1135–54.

Chow, C. L. and Takagi, S. 2001. A natural bone cement—A laboratory novelty led to the development of revolutionary new biomaterials. *Journal of Research of the National Institute of Standards and Technology* 106: 1029–33.

Constantz, B. R., Delaney, D., and Yetkinler, D. 2007. Rapid setting calcium phosphate cements. US Patents: 7,252,841 B2.

Constantz, B. R., Ison, I. C., Fulmer, M. T., Poser, R. D., Smith, S. T., VanWagoner, M., Ross, J., Goldstein, S. A., Jupiter, J. B., and Rosenthal, D. I. 1995. Skeletal repair by *in situ* formation of the mineral phase of bone. *Science* 267: 1796–99.

Daculsi, G. 1998. Biphasic calcium phosphate concept applied to artificial bone, implant coating and injectable bone substitute. *Biomaterials* 19: 1473–78.

Daculsi, G., LeGeros, R. Z., Heughebaert, M., and Barbieux, I. 1990. Formation of carbonate-apatite crystals after implantation of calcium phosphate cermics. *Calcified Tissue International* 46: 20–27.

Damien, E. and Revell, P. A. 2004. Coralline hydroxyapatite bone graft substitute: A review of experimental studies and biomedical applications. *Journal of Applied Biomaterials and Biomechanics* 2: 65–73.

De la Riva, B., Sánchez, E., Hernández, A., Reyes, R., Tamimi, F., López-Cabarcos, E., Delgado, A., and Évora, C. 2010. Local controlled release of VEGF and PDGF from a combined brushite-chitosan system enhances bone regeneration. *Journal of Controlled Release* 143: 45–52.

Dickson, K. F., Friedman, J., Buchholz, J. G., and Flandry, F. D. 2002. The use of bonesource hydroxyapatite cement for traumatic metaphyseal bone void filling. *The Journal of Trauma: Injury, Infection, and Critical Care* 53: 1103–08.

Dong, J., Uemura, T., Shirasaki, Y., and Tateishi, T. 2002. Promotion of bone formation using highly pure porous b-TCP combined with bone marrow-derived osteoprogenitor cells. *Biomaterials* 23: 4493–502.

Dorozhkin, S. V. 2009. Calcium orthophosphates in nature, biology and medicine. *Materials* 2: 399–498.

Driessens, F. C. M., Boltong, M. G., Zapatero, M. I., Verbeeck, R. M. H., Bonfield, W., Bermudez, O., Fernandez, E., Ginebra, M. P., and Planell, J. A. 1995. *In vivo* behaviour of three calcium phosphate cements and magnesium phosphate cement. *Journal of Materials Science: Materials in Medicine* 6: 272–78.

Elliott, J. C. 1994. *Structure and Chemistry of the Apatites and other Calcium Orthophosphates*. Amsterdam: Elsevier Science.

Elliott, J. C., Holcomb, D. W., and Young, R. A. 1985. Infrared determination of the degree of substitution of hydroxyl by carbonate ions in human enamel. *Calcified Tissue International* 37: 372–75.

Espanol, M., Perez, R. A., Montufar, E. B., Marichal, C., Sacco, A., and Ginebra, M. P. 2009. Intrinsic porosity of calcium phosphate cements and its significance for drug delivery and tissue engineering applications. *Acta Biomaterialia* 5: 2752–62.

Fernandez, E., Boltong, M. G., Ginebra, M. P., Bermudez, O., Driessens, F. C. M., and Planell, J. A. 1994. Common ion effect on some calcium phosphate cements. *Clinical Materials* 16: 99–103.

Fernandez, E., Gil, F. J., Ginebra, M. P., Driessens, F. C. M., Planell, J. A., and Best, S. M. 1999a. Calcium phosphate bone cements for clinical applications, Part 1: Solution chemistry. *Material Science: Material in Medicine* 10: 169–76.

Fernandez, E., Gil, F. J., Ginebra, M. P., Driessens, F. C. M., Planell, J. A., and Best, S. M. 1999b. Production and characterization of new calcium phosphate bone cements in the $CaHPO_4$-TCP system: pH, workability and setting times. *Journal of Materials Science: Materials in Medicine* 10: 223–30.

Fortunato, G., Marini, E., Valdinucci, F., and Bonucci, E. 1997. Long-term results of hydroxyapatite-fibrin sealant implantation in plastic and reconstructive craniofacial surgery. *Journal of Cranio-Maxillofacial Surgery* 25: 124–35.

Frame, J. W. 1987. Hydroxyapatite as a biomaterial for alveolar ridge augmentation. *International Journal of Oral and Maxillofacial Surgery* 16: 642–55.

Frame, J. W. and Brady, C. L. 1987. The versatility of hydroxyapatite blocks in maxillofacial surgery. *British Journal of Oral and Maxillofacial Surgery* 25: 452–64.

Frankenburg, E. P., Goldstein, S. A., Bauer, T. W., Harris, S. A., and Poser, R. D. 1998. Biomechanical and histological evaluation of a calcium phosphate cement. *The Journal of Bone and Joint Surgery* 80: 1112–24.

Frayssinet, P., Trouillet, J. L., Rouquet, N., Azimus, E., and Autefage, A. 1993. Osseointegration of macroporous calcium phosphate ceramics having a different chemical composition. *Biomaterials* 14: 423–29.

Fredericks, D. C., Bobst, J. A., Petersen, E. B., Nepola, J. V., Dennis, J. E., Caplan, A. I., Burgess, A. V., Overby, R. J., and Schulz, O. H. 2004. Cellular interactions and bone healing responses to a novel porous tricalcium phosphate bone graft material. *Orthophedics* 27: 167–73.

Friedman, C. D., Costantino, P. D., Takagi, S., and Chow, L. C. 1998. BoneSource™ hydroxyapatite cement: A novel biomaterial for craniofacial skeletal tissue engineering and reconstruction. *Journal Biomedical Materials Research Part B: Applied Biomaterials* 43: 428–32.

Fujikawa, K., Sugawara, A., Murai, S., Nishiyama, M., Takagi, S., and Chow, C. L. 1995. Histopathological reaction of calcium phosphate cement in periodontal bone defect. *Dental Materials Journal* 14: 45–57.

Fukase, Y., Eanes, E. D., Takagi, S., Chow, L. C., and Brown, W. E. 1990. Setting reactions and compressive strenghts of calcium phosphate cements. *Journal of Dental Research* 69: 1852–56.

Galois, L., Mainard, D., Pfeffer, F., Traversari, R., and Delagoutte, J. P. 2001. Use of [beta]-tricalcium phosphate in foot and ankle surgery: A report of 20 cases. *Foot and Ankle Surgery* 7: 217–27.

Gasqueres, G., Bonhomme, C., Maquet, J., Babonneau, F., Hayakawa, S., Kanaya, T., and Osaka, A. 2007. Revisiting silicate substituted hydroxyapatite by solid-state NMR. *Magnetic Resonance in Chemistry* 46: 342–46.

Gbureck, U., Spatz, K., and Thull, R. 2003. Improvement of mechanical properties of self setting calcium phosphate bone cements mixed with different metal oxides. *Materialswissenschaff und Werkstofftechnik* 34: 1036–40.

Gierse, H. and Donath, K. 1999. Reactions and complications after the implantation of Endobon including morphological examination of explants. *Archives of Orthopaedic and Trauma Surgery* 119: 349–55.

Gilardino, S. M., Cabiling, S. D., and Bartlett, P. S. 2009. Long-term follow-up experience with carbonated calcium phosphate cement (Norian) for cranioplasty in children and adults. *Plastic Reconstruction Surgery* 123: 983–94.

Ginebra, M. P., Driessens, F. C. M., and Planell, J. A. 2004. Effect of the particle size on the micro and nanostructural features of a calcium phosphate cement: A kinetic analysis. *Biomaterials* 25: 3453–62.

Gruber, R. M., Ludwig, A., Merten, H. A., Achilles, M., Poehling, S., and Schliephake, H. 2008. Sinus floor augmentation with recombinant human growth and differentiation factor-5 (rhGDF-5): A histological and histomorphometric study in the Goettingen miniature pig. *Clinical Oral Implants Research* 19: 522–29.

Habibovic, P., Juhl, V. M., Clyens, S., Martinetti, R., Dolcini, L., Theilgaard, N., and van Blitterswijk, C. A. 2010. Comparison of two apatite ceramics *in vivo*. *Acta Biomaterialia* 6: 2219–26.

Habraken, W. J., Wolke, J. G., and Jansen, J. A. 2007. Ceramic composites as matrices and scaffolds for drug delivery in tissue engineering. *Advances in Drug Delivery Reviews* 59: 234–48.

Handschin, R. G. and Stern, W. B. 1995. X-ray diffraction studies on the lattice perfection of human bone apatite (Crista Iliaca). *Bone* 16: S355–63.

Henno, S., Lambotte, J. C., Glez, D., Guigand, M., Lancien, G., and Cathelineau, G. 2003. Characterisation and quantification of angiogenesis in [beta]-tricalcium phosphate implants by immunohistochemistry and transmission electron microscopy. *Biomaterials* 24: 3173–81.

Hirayama, S., Takagi, S., Marcovic, M., and Chow, C. L. 2008. Properties of calcium phosphate cements with different tetracalcium phosphate and dicalcium phosphate anhydrous molar ratios. *Journal of Research of the National Institute of Standards and Technology* 113: 311–20.

Hofmann, M. P., Mohammed, A. R., Perrie, Y., Gbureck, U., and Barralet, J. E. 2009. High-strength resorbable brushite bone cement with controlled drug-releasing capabilities. *Acta Biomaterialia* 5: 43–49.

Horch, H. H., Sader, R., Pautke, C., Neff, A., Deppe, H., and Kolk, A. 2006. Synthetic, pure-phase betatricalcium phosphate ceramic granules (Cerasorb) for bone regeneration in the reconstructive surgery of the jaws. *International Journal of Oral Maxillofacial Surgery* 35: 708–13.

Hsu, H. Y., Turner, G. I., and Miles, W. A. 2007. Fabrication and mechanical testing of porous calcium phosphate bioceramic granules. *Journal Material Science: Materials in Medicine* 18: 1931–37.

Ilan, D. I. and Ladd, A. L. 2003. Bone Graft Substitutes. *Operative Techniques in Plastic and Reconstructive Surgery* 9: 151–60.

Ishikawa, K. 2008. Calcium phosphate cement. In: *Bioceramics and their Clinical Applications*, ed. T. Kokubo. Boca Raton: CRC Press, pp. 438–63.

Ishikawa, K., Miyamoto, M., Takechi, M., Toh, T., Kon, M., Nagayama, M., and Asaoka, K. 1997. Non-decay type fast-setting calcium phosphate cement: Hydroxyapatite putty containing an increased amount of sodium alginate. *Journal of Biomedical Materials Research Part A* 36: 393–99.

Johnsson, M. S. and Nancollas, G. H. 1992. The role of brushite and octacalcium phosphate in apatite formation. *Critical Reviews in Oral Biology & Medicine* 3: 61–82.

Kamitakahara, M. 2008. Review paper: Behavior of ceramic biomaterials derived from tricalcium phosphate in physiological condition. *Journal of Biomaterials Applications* 23: 197–12.

Kasten, P., Luginbuhl, R., van Griensven, M., Barkhausen, T., Krettek, C., Bohner, M., and Bosch, U. 2003. Comparison of human bone marrow stromal cells seeded on calcium-deficient hydroxyapatite, β-tricalcium phosphate and demineralized bone matrix. *Biomaterials* 24: 2593–603.

Khairoun, I., Boltong, M. G., Driessens, F. C. M., and Planell, J. A. 1997. Effect of calcium carbonate on the compliance of an apatitic calcium phosphate bone cement. *Biomaterials* 18: 1535–39.

Kneton, J. F., Friedman, C. D., and Costantino, P. D. 1995. Indications for hydroxyapatite cement reconstraction in lateral skull base surgery. *American Journal of Otolaryngology* 16: 465–69.

Knežević, G., Rinčić, M., and Knežević, D. 2007. Radiological evaluation of the healing of bone defects filled with tricalcium phosphate (bioresorb) after cystectomy of the mandible. *Acta Stomatologica* 41: 66–73.

Koerten, H. K. and van der Meulen, J. 1999. Degradation of calcium phosphate ceramics. *Journal of Biomedical Materials Research Part A* 44: 78–86.

Kokubun, S., Kashimoto, O., and Tanaka, Y. 1994. Histological verification of bone bonding and ingrowth into porous hydroxyapatite pinous process spacer for cervical aminoplasty. *The Tohoku Journal of Experimental Medicine* 173: 337–44.

Komath, M. and Varma, H. K. 2003. Development of a fully injectable calcium phosphate cement for orthopedic and dental applications. *Bulletin of Material Science* 26: 415–22.

Komlev, V. S. and Barinov, S. M. 2002. Porous hydroxyapatite ceramics of bi-modal pore size distribution. *Journal of Materials Science: Materials in Medicine* 13: 295–99.

Korovessis, P., Koureas, G., Zacharatos, S., Papazisis, Z., and Lambiris, E. 2005. Correlative radiological, self-assessment and clinical analysis of evolution in instrumented dorsal and lateral fusion for degenerative lumbar spine disease. Autograft versus coralline hydroxyapatite. *European Spine Journal* 14: 630–38.

Kotani, S., Fujita, Y., Kitsugi, T., Nakamura, T., Yamamuro, T., Ohtsuki, C., and Kukubo, T. 1991. Bone bonding mechanism of beta-tricalcium phosphate. *Journal Biomedical Materials Research* 1: 1303–15.

Krijnen, M. R., Smit, T. H., Everts, V., and Wuisman, P. I. J. M. 2008. PLDLA mesh and 60/40 biphasic calcium phosphate in iliac crest regeneration in the goat. *Journal of Biomedical Materials Research Part B: Applied Biomaterials* 89B: 9–17.

Kveton, J. F., Friedman, C. D., Piepmeier, J. M., and Costantino, P. D. 1995. Reconstruction of suboccipital craniectomy defects with hydroxyapatite cement: A preliminary report. *Laryngoscope* 105: 156–59.

Kweh, S. W. K., Khor, K. A., and Cheang, P. 1999. The production and characterization of hydroxyapatite (HA) powders. *Journal of Materials Processing Technology* 89–90: 373–77.

Langer, R. and Vacanti, J. P. 1993. Tissue engineering. *Science* 260: 920–26.

Le Nihouannena, D., Daculsi, G., Saffarzadeh, A., Gauthier, O., Delplace, S., Pilet, P., and Layrolle, P. 2005. Ectopic bone formation by microporous calcium phosphate ceramic particles in sheep muscles. *Bone* 36: 1086–93.

LeGeros, R. Z. 1965. Effect of carbonate on the lattice parameters of apatite. *Nature* 4982: 403–04.

LeGeros, R. Z. 2008. Calcium phosphate-based osteoinductive materials. *Chemical Rewievs* 108: 4742–53.

Lew, D., Farrell, B., Bardach, J., and Keller, J. 1997. Repair of craniofacial defects with hydroxyapatite cement. *Journal of Oral and Maxillofacial Surgery* 55: 1441–49.

Li, D. J., Ohsa, K., Li, K., Ye, Q., Nobuto, Y., Tenshin, S., and Yamamoto, T. T. 1997. Long-term observation of subcutaneous tissue reaction to synthetic auditory ossicle (Apaceram®) in rats. *The Journal of Laryngology and Otology* 111: 702–06.

Lilley, K. J., Gbureck, U., Knowles, J. C., Farrar, D. F., and Barralet, J. E. 2005. Cement from magnesium substituted hydroxyapatite. *Journal of Materials Science: Materials in Medicine* 16: 455–60.

Lin, J., Raghavan, S., and Fuerstenau, D. W. 1981. The adsorption of fluoride ions by hydroxyapatite from aqueous solution. *Colloids and Surfaces* 3: 357–70.

Little, F. M. and Rowley, J. 1961. Studies on the carbon dioxide component of human enamel III. The effect of neutral and acid fluoride. *Journal of Dental Research* 40: 915–20.

Livinston, T. L., Gordon, S., Archambault, M., Kadiyala, S., McIntosh, K., Smith, A., and Peter, S. J. 2003. Mesenchymal stem cells combined with biphasic calcium phosphate ceramics promote bone regeneration *Journal of Materials Science: Materials in Medicine* 14: 211–18.

Louati, B., Hlel, F., Guidara, K., and Gargouri, M. 2005. Analysis of the effects of thermal treatments on $CaHPO_4$ by 31P NMR spectroscopy. *Journal of Alloys and Compounds* 394: 13–18.

Mahabole, M. P., Aiyer, R. C., Ramakrishna, C. V., Sreedhar, B., and Khairnar, R. S. 2005. Synthesis, characterization and gas sensing property of hydroxyapatite ceramic. *Bulletin of Material Science* 28: 535–45.

Mailac, N. and Daculsi, G. 2008. Bone ingrowth for sinus lift augmentation with micro macroporous biphasic calcium human cases evaluation using microct and histomorphometry. *Key Engineering Materials* 361: 1347–50.

Manzotti, A., Confalonieri, N., and Pullen, C. 2006. Grafting of tibial bone defects in knee replacement using norian skeletal repair system. *Archives of Orthopaedic and Trauma Surgery* 126: 594–98.

Mathew, M., Schroeder, L. W., Dickens, B., and Brown, W. E. 1977. The crystal structure of a-$Ca_3(PO_4)_2$. *Acta Cryst* B33: 1325–33.

Mathew, M. and Takagi, S. 2001. Structures of biological minerals in dental research. *Journal of Research of the National Institute of Standards and Technology* 106: 1035–44.

Muralithran, G. and Ramesh, S. 2000. The effects of sintering temperature on the properties of hydroxyapatite. *Ceramics International* 26: 221–30.

Navarro, M., Michiardi, A., Castano, O., and Planell, J. A. 2008. Biomaterials in orthopaedics. *Journal of Royal Society Interface* 5: 1137–58.

Nilsson, M. 2003. Injectable calcium sulphate and calcium phosphate bone substitutes. PhD thesis. Lund University.

Nissan, B. B., Choi, A. H., and Cordingley, R. 2008. Alumina ceramics. In: *Bioceramics and their Clinical Applications*, ed. T. Kokubo. Boca Raton, FL: Woodhead Publishing, CRC Press, pp. 223–42.

Ogose, A., Kondo, N., Umezu, H., Hotta, T., Kawashima, H., Tokunaga, K., Ito, T., Kudo, N., Hoshino, M., Gu, W., and Endo, N. 2006. Histological assessment in grafts of highly purified beta-tricalcium phosphate (OSferion) in human bones. *Biomaterials* 27: 1542–49.

Ohura, K., Bohner, M., Hardouin, P., Lemaitre, J., Pasquier, G., and Flautre, B. 1996. Resorption of, and bone formation from, new beta-tricalcium phosphate-monocalcium phosphate cements: An *in vivo* study. *Journal Biomedical Materials Research* 30: 193–200.

Ooms, E. M., Wolke, J. G. C., van de Heuvel, R., Jeschke, B., and Jansen, J. A. 2003. Histological evaluation of the bone response to calcium phosphate cement implanted in cortical bone. *Biomaterials* 24: 989–1000.

Ooms, E. M., Wolke, J. G. C., van der Waerden, J. P. C. M., and Jansen, J. A. 2002. Trabecular bone response to injectable calcium phosphate (Ca-P) cement. *Journal Biomedical Materials Research* 61: 9–18.

Orlovskii, P. V., Komlev, V. S., and Barinov, S. M. 2002. Hydroxyapatite and hydroxyapatite based ceramics. *Inorganic Materials* 38: 1159–72.

Piattelli, A., Scarano, A., and Mangano, C. 1996. Clinical and histologic aspects of biphasic calcium phosphate (bcp) ceramic used in connection with implant placement. *Biomaterials* 17: 1767–70.

Pina, S., Olhero, S. M., Gheduzzi, S., Miles, A. Q., and Ferreira, J. M. F. 2009. Influence of setting liquid composition and liquid-to-powder ratio on properties of a Mg-substituted calcium phosphate cement. *Acta Biomaterialia* 5: 1233–40.

Qi, G., Zhang, S., Khor, K. A., Lye, S. W., Zeng, X., Weng, W., Liu, C., Venkatraman, S. S., and Ma, L. L. 2008. Osteoblastic cell response on magnesium-incorporated apatite coatings. *Applied Surface Science* 255: 304–07.

Quayle, A. A., Marouf, H., and Holland, I. 1990. Alveolar ridge augmentation using a new design of inflatable tissue expander: Surgical technique and preliminary results. *British Journal of Oral and Maxillofacial Surgery* 28: 375–82.

Regi, V. M. and Arcos, D. 2005. Silicon substituted hydroxyapatites: A method to upgrate calcium phosphate based implants. *Journal of Materials Chemistry* 15: 1509–16.

Saijo, H., Chung, I., Igawa, K., Mori, Y., Chikazu, D., Iino, M., and Takato, T. 2008. Clinical application of artificial bone in the maxillofacial region. *Journal of Artificial Organs* 11: 171–76.

Sakano, H., Koshino, T., Takeuchi, R., Sakai, N., and Saito, T. 2001. Treatment of the unstable distal radius fracture with external fixation and a hydroxyapatite spacer. *The Journal of Hand Surgery* 26: 923–930.

Sandor, G. K. B., Kainulainen, V. T., Queiroz, J. O., Carmichael, R. P., and Oikarinen, K. S. 2003. Preservation of ridge dimensions following grafting with coral granules of 48 post-traumatic and post-extraction dento-alveolar defects. *Dental Traumatology* 19: 221–27.

Schwartz, C., and Bordei, R. 2005. Biphasic phospho-calcium ceramics used as bone substitutes are efficient in the management of severe acetabular bone loss in revision total hip arthroplasties. *European Journal of Orthopaedic Surgery and Traumatology* 15: 191–96.

Schwartz, C., Liss, P., Jacquemaire, B., Lecestre, P., and Frayssinet, P. 1999. Biphasic synthetic bone substitute use in orthopaedic and trauma surgery: Clinical, radiological and histological results. *Journal of Materials Science: Materials in Medicine* 10: 821–25.

Shord, E. C. 1999. Coralline bone graft substitutes. *Orthopedic Clinics of North America* 30: 599–13.

Sivakumar, M., Kumar, T. S., Shanta, K. L., and Rao, K. P. 1996. Development of hydroxyapatite derived from Indian coral. *Biomaterials* 17: 1709–14.

Smith, I. A., McCabe, L. R., and Baumann, M. J. 2006. MC3T3-E1 osteoblast attachment and proliferation on porous hydroxyapatite scaffolds fabricated with nanophase powder. *International Journal of Nanomedicine* 1: 189–94.

Sopyan, I., Singh, R., and Hamdi, M. 2008. Synthesis of nano sized hydroxyapatite powder using sol-gel technique and its conversion to dense and porous bodies. *Indian Journal of Chemistry* 47A: 1626–31.

Stubbsa, D., Deakina, M., Sheatha, P. C., Bruceb, W., Debesc, J., Gillies, R. M., and Walsh, W. R. 2004. *In vivo* evaluation of resorbable bone graft substitutes in a rabbit tibial defect mode. *Biomaterials* 25: 5037–44.

Sugawara, A., Fujikawa, K., Takagi, S., and Chow, L. C. 2008. Histological analysis of calcium phosphate bone grafts for surgically created periodontal bone defects in dogs. *Dentistry Materials Journal* 27: 787–94.

Sugawara, A., Kusama, K., Nishimura, S., Nishiyama, M., Moro, I., Kudo, I., Takagi, S., and Chow, C. L. 1993. Histopathological reactions to calcium phosphate cement for bone filling. *Dental Materials Journal* 12: 691–98.

Suzuki, O. 2010. Octacalcium phosphate: Osteoconductivity and crystal chemistry. *Acta Biomaterialia* 6: 3379–87.

Takechi, M., Miyamoto, Y., Ishikawa, K., Yuasa, M., Nagayama, M., Kon, M., and Asaoka, K. 1996. Non-decay type fast-setting calcium phosphate cement using chitosan. *Journal of Materials Science: Materials in Medicine* 7: 317–22.

Tanaja, Y. and Yamashite, K. 2008. Fabrication processes for bioceramics. In: *Bioceramics and Their Clinical Applications*, ed. T. Kokubo. Woodhead Publishing in Materials. Boca Raton, FL: CRC Press, pp. 30–40.

Tas, A. C. 2009. Monetite synthesis in ethanol at room temperature. *Journal of the American Ceramic Society* 92: 2907–12.

Thalgott, J. S., Giuffre, J. M., Fritts, K., Timlin, M., and Klezl, Z. 2001. Instrumented posterolateral lumbar fusion using coralline hydroxyapatite with or without demineralized bone matrix, as an adjunct to autologous bone. *The Spine Journal* 1: 131–37.

Theiss, F., Apelt, D., Brand, B., Kutter, A., Zlinszky, K., Bohner, M., Matter, S., Frei, C., Auer, J. A., and von Rechenberg, B. 2005. Biocompatibility and resorption of a brushite calcium phosphate cement. *Biomaterials* 26: 4383–94.

Timperley, A. J., Nusem, I., Wilson, K., Whitehouse, S. L., Buma, P., and Crawford, R. W. 2010. A modified cementing technique using BoneSource to augment fixation of the acetabulum in a sheep model. *Acta Orthopaedica* 81: 503–07.

Tsuruga, E., Takita, H., Itoh, H., Wakisaka, Y., and Kuboki, Y. 1997. Pore size of porous hydoxyapatite as the cell-substratum controls BMP-induced osteogenesis. *Journal of Biochemistry* 121: 317–24.

Vanderschot, P., Muylaert, D., and Schepers, E. 2007. CaP-cement as a bone substitute in defect areas: An animal study. *Injury Extra* 38: 102–03.

Wang, L. and Nancollas, H. G. 2008. Calcium orthophosphates: Crystallization and dissolution. *Chemical Reviews* 108: 4628–69.

White, E. and Shors, E. 1986. Biomaterial aspects of Interpore-200 porous hydroxyapatite. *Dental Clinics of North America* 30: 49–67.

Wilson, C. E., Kruyt, M. C., De Bruijn, J. D., Van Blitterswijk, C. A., Oner, C. F., Verbout, A. J., and Dhert, W. J. A. 2006. A new *in vivo* screening model for posterior spinal bone formation: Comparison of ten calcium phosphate ceramic material treatments. *Biomaterials* 27: 302–14.

Wolfe, S. W. 1999. Augmentation of distal radius fracture fixation with coralline HA bone graft substitutes. *Journal of Hand Surgery* 24A: 816–27.

Yamasaki, N., Hirao, M., Nanno, K., Sugiyasu, K., Tamai, N., Hashimoto, N., Yoshikawa, H., and Myoui, A. 2009. A comparative assessment of synthetic ceramic bone substitutes with different composition and microstructure in rabbit femoral condyle model. *Journal of Biomedical Materials Research Part B: Applied Biomaterials* 91: 788–98.

Yang, H., Thompson, I., Yang, S., Chi, X., Evans, J., and Cook, R. 2008. Dissolution characteristics of extrusion freeformed hydroxyapatite–tricalcium phosphate scaffolds. *Journal of Materials Science: Materials in Medicine* 19: 3345–53.

Yashima, M., Sakai, A., Kamiyama, T., and Hoshikawa, A. 2003. Crystal structure analysis of $\beta$-tricalcium phosphate $Ca_3(PO_4)_2$ by neutron powder diffraction. *Journal of Solid State Chemistry* 175: 272–77.

Yaszemski, M. J., Trantolo, D. J., Lewandrowski, K. U., Hasirci, V., Altobelli, D. E., and Donald, L. W. 2004. *Biomaterials in Orthopedics*. New York: Northeastern University Press.

Yoshikawa, H., Tamai, N., Murase, T., and Myoui, A. 2009. Interconnected porous hydroxyapatite ceramics for bone tissue engineering. *Journal of the Royal Society Interface* 6: 341–48.

Yuan, H., Yang, Z., de Bruijn, J. D., de Groot, K., and Zhang, X. 2001. Material-dependent bone induction by calcium phosphate ceramics: A 2.5-year study in dog. *Biomaterials* 22: 2617–23.

Yuan, H., Yang, Z., Li, Y., Zhang, X., De Bruijn, J. D., and De Groot, K. 1998. Osteoinduction by calcium phosphate biomaterials. *Journal of Materials Science: Materials in Medicine* 9: 723–26.

Yubao, L., Xıngdongo, Z., and de Groot, K. 1996. Hydroxlysis and phase transition of alpha-tricalcium phosphate. *Biomaterials* 18: 737–41.

Zaffe, D. 2005. Some considerations on biomaterials and bone. *Micron* 36: 583–92.

Zhang, S. and Gonsalves, K. E. 1997. Preparation and characterization of thermally stable nanohydroxyapatite. *Journal of Materials Science: Materials in Medicine* 8: 25–28.

Zheltonoga, L. A. and Gabriwlov, I. P. 1979. Characteristics of crack growth in sintered materials *Powder Metallurgy and Metal Ceramics* 18: 744–48.

# 4

# Engineered Protein Biomaterials

Andreina
Parisi-Amon
*Stanford University*

Sarah C.
Heilshorn
*Stanford University*

4.1 Engineered Protein Biomaterials as an Alternative to
    "Traditional" Biomaterials ................................................................. 4-1
4.2 Synthesis of Engineered Protein Biomaterials ........................... 4-3
4.3 Design of Engineered Protein Biomaterials ............................... 4-5
    Crosslinking Domains • Structural Domains • Degradation
    Domains • ECM Cell-Binding Domains • Cell–Cell Adhesion
    Domains • Cell-Directive Domains
4.4 Applications of Engineered Protein Biomaterials .................... 4-11
References ................................................................................................ 4-11

## 4.1 Engineered Protein Biomaterials as an Alternative to "Traditional" Biomaterials

Materials that are ideal for *in vitro* cell studies and *in vivo* transplantation studies, en route to clinical translation, aim to mimic the complex milieu of biochemical and biomechanical signals found in the extracellular matrix (ECM) while remaining biocompatible and biodegradable. Protein engineering of biomaterials relies on the designer to dictate precise protein polymer sequences using amino acid building blocks, which in turn dictate the material's structure and functionality. Coupled with recombinant technology, which permits direct genetic fusion of multiple peptide functionalities into a single protein, protein engineering aims to produce modular biomaterials that meet the goals of biocompatibility and biodegradability while enabling predictable cell–material interactions that dictate cell responses.

Deriving inspiration from nature, scientists have designed protein-engineered biomaterials that include specific peptide domains to direct crosslinking, material structure, degradation, cell-binding, growth factor-binding, and cell-signaling. The fusion of these various peptide domains to create a full-length, protein-engineered biomaterial results in an inherently modular design strategy. Combinatorial variation in domain choices and sequences creates a family of scaffolds with properties customized for different cell types and tissue engineering applications (Figure 4.1). The DNA sequence of the designed protein is then encoded in a recombinant DNA plasmid that is transformed into a host organism, which translates and transcribes the protein. The engineered protein is then harvested and purified for use as a biomaterial.

As seen in Figure 4.1, many peptide domains used in protein-engineered biomaterials are derived from amino acid sequences found in the natural ECM. Naturally existing biomaterials such as collagen and Matrigel (a complex mixture of biomacromolecules primarily consisting of laminin) clearly have physiologically relevant biofunctionalities, as they are harvested directly from mammalian sources. However,

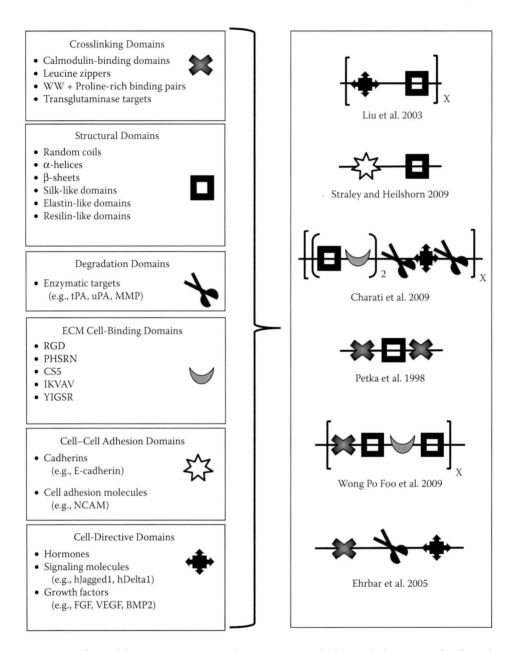

**FIGURE 4.1** In the modular protein engineering design strategy, multiple peptide domains are fused together to design novel, multifunctional, recombinant protein polymers with specific properties.

while the complex biochemical compositions of these materials are valued for their ability to initiate multiple cellular signaling pathways, their compositions also make naturally derived materials nonideal, as their properties cannot be easily tailored. Moreover, harvesting and processing of these materials may destroy their higher-order structures (such as fibers) while also producing undesirable batch-to-batch variability. In addition, some natural materials are known to cause high levels of immunogenic response and can have additional clinical translation difficulties due to their mammalian origins. Borrowing biofunctional peptide domains from natural ECM proteins and including them within engineered proteins enables the creation of multifunctional biomaterials that address many of these concerns.

An alternative approach to create tailorable biomaterials is the use of synthetic polymers such as PEG (polyethlyene glycol), PMMA (poly(methyl methacrylate)), PHEMA (poly(2-hydroxyethyl methacrylate)), and PLGA (poly(lactic-*co*-glycolic acid)) derivatives. While these materials are easily tailored, they are usually bio-inert without further modification. As such, these materials can only achieve biofunctionality with the incorporation of additional components such as ECM-derived peptides and proteins. Often however, these functional peptides play a role in the mechanical structure, making it difficult to independently tune the biofunctionality and mechanical properties of the biomaterial (Thompson et al. 2006). In addition, the synthetic chemistries inherent to these materials may carry the risk of toxic crosslinkers, activating agents, and degradation fragments (Williams et al. 2005, Seymour et al. 1987).

While protein-engineered biomaterials overcome some of the concerns associated with natural and synthetic biomaterials, they also have their own limitations. Before these materials can be considered for clinical translation, the laboratory-scale synthesis and purification processes typically used during the biomaterial design phase must be optimized to achieve efficient scale-up of production. Although the materials are generally made from protein building blocks native to the human body, rendering them cytocompatible and bioresorbable, they may nonetheless trigger an immunogenic response, particularly due to their synthesis in a foreign host organism. For example, proteins made in Gram-negative bacteria, such as *Escherichia coli* (*E. coli*), must be sufficiently purified to remove endotoxin, a lipopolysaccharide that can trigger an innate immune response (Rietschel et al. 1994). Even with these challenges, protein-engineered materials constitute an exciting area of biomaterials research given their exquisite design control that enables the creation of novel biomimetic cell scaffolds. In this chapter, we will focus on recent developments in the field of engineered protein biomaterials and highlight opportunities for future advances.

## 4.2 Synthesis of Engineered Protein Biomaterials

Following the design of a specific protein polymer (which is discussed in the following section), a variety of methods can be used to synthesize and purify the protein. Solid-phase synthesis is the process by which novel proteins are manually created through the sequential addition of individual amino acids (Kates and Albericio 2000). While this process has become more optimized and commonplace over the past several years, the resulting proteins are limited in length and the process is too time consuming and expensive to scale-up to the high levels of production needed for potential therapies. Instead, with the discovery of molecular cloning in the 1970s, scientists have been able to harness the protein factories that exist in nature—cells (Porro et al. 2005). Mammalian (Nagaoka et al. 2002), insect (Tomita et al. 1999), plant (Karg and Kallio 2009), fungal (yeast) (Graf et al. 2009), and bacterial (Zerbs et al. 2009) cells have all been used for recombinant protein synthesis, each with their advantages and disadvantages. Irrespective of the host, the creation of a protein through the cellular processes of transcription and translation is inherently advantageous, as it provides efficient molecular-level control of the protein synthesis. Furthermore, built-in accuracy and error-checking mechanisms by the ribosome ensure that the desired protein sequence is being produced (Zaher and Green 2009).

Choosing which host to use is a key step in recombinant protein synthesis, as it determines the complexity of the protein sequence that can be produced, as well as the efficiency with which the production can take place. Microorganisms such as *E. coli* and *Saccharomyces cerevisiae* (yeast), with their relative ease of genetic modification, low cost of culture, and high growth rates compared to mammalian cells, are often chosen as the host. In fact, for simple protein structures, prokaryotic *E. coli* is often the first host of choice due to its simplicity and versatility. However, for more complex proteins that require post-transcriptional possessing for correct structure and resulting function, eukaryotic yeast, such as *S. cerevisiae* and *Pichia pastoris* are more often chosen, as they combine the high growth rate and simplicity of a single-celled microorganism with the organelles needed for specialized folding and modification.

Once the host is chosen, the exact nucleotide sequence must be designed, while keeping in mind that various hosts may have different tolerances to specific sequences. While some basic tenets are known, such as the fact that highly repetitive sequences have an increased susceptibility of resulting in unwanted recombination events (Bzymek and Lovett 2001), it is difficult to predict *a priori* which sequences will have high translational efficiency and yield, therefore making sequence design an iterative process. To that end, scientists are working to create sequence design programs that use host-specific algorithms to improve expression (Gao et al. 2004). Once designed, the completed sequence is synthesized and introduced into the host cell for production. Culture conditions, such as pH, temperature, and oxygen abundance also play a complex role in the yield of protein production.

After protein production, the product must be collected from the cell, either through secretion or cell lysis, and then purified such that only the protein of interest remains. Purification can be achieved through various chromatographic methods, in which the product-containing solution is run through a resin-packed column that takes advantage of specific properties of the target protein, such as size, charge, hydrophobicity, or ligand binding. The basic process includes binding or capturing the protein of interest to the resin, allowing all impurities to run through, and then releasing the purified product for collection (Nilsson et al. 1997). Often multiple iterations are required to isolate the target protein with the desired level of purity. To scale up the process for larger yields, chromatographic methods are often deemed too expensive and time-intensive; therefore, alternative techniques utilizing differential target protein solubility are often developed. For example, target proteins that include an elastin-like sequence typically exhibit lower critical solution temperature behavior, whereby the protein forms a highly concentrated coacervate at elevated temperatures while most other contaminating proteins remain in solution (McPherson et al. 1996). This thermodynamic phenomenon can be exploited to purify the target protein through a simple sequence of centrifugations at alternating temperatures above and below the target protein's lower critical solution temperature (Meyer and Chilkoti 1999). Finally, additional purification may be needed to make the product cytocompatible for proteins expressed in Gram-negative bacteria such as *E. coli*. These target proteins are often contaminated with residual amounts of endotoxin (i.e., lipopolysaccharide), a component of the bacterial cell wall that can activate an innate immune

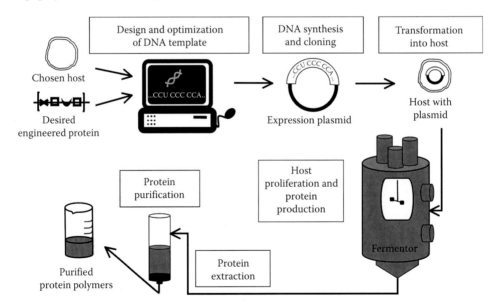

**FIGURE 4.2** Design and synthesis of recombinantly engineered protein polymers. First, an expression host and target amino acid sequence are chosen. This information is used to design a DNA template that encodes the engineered protein polymer. After synthesis and cloning of the DNA template into a recombinant expression plasmid, the plasmid is introduced into the host organism. A fermentor is used to control environmental parameters during host proliferation and protein expression. Following protein extraction and purification, a pure sample of engineered protein polymer remains.

response. Several techniques have been developed for efficient endotoxin purification, with the most commonly used being an affinity-based column (Petsch and Anspach 2000).

Through iterative optimization, the use of microorganism hosts for recombinant protein engineering provides an economical and efficient method to synthesize engineered proteins in therapeutic quantities (Figure 4.2). Optimized protocols and laboratory-scale fermentors enable the growth of high-density cultures in volumes from 1 to 200 L, enabling the production of multigram protein yields (Heilshorn et al. 2003, Chow et al. 2006, Welsh and Tirrell 2000, Shiloach and Fass 2005).

## 4.3 Design of Engineered Protein Biomaterials

The inherent modularity of the peptide building-block design strategy of protein-engineered biomaterials provides the ability not only to design materials emulating a specific biological niche, but also to create a versatile family of materials simply through the inclusion or removal of singular peptide domains. The domains that are fused together to create full-length proteins can be classified by the functionalities they convey to the final product (Figure 4.1). For example, many biologically inspired domains can interact directly with cells through the promotion of cell–ligand interactions, cell–cell adhesion mimicry, or behavioral instruction (i.e., regulation of proliferation, differentiation, etc.). Alternatively, other domains can affect material properties, such as degradability and elastic modulus (i.e., the stiffness of a material), which may further direct cell behavior (Discher et al. 2005). Other selected domains can impart specific structural motifs, such as random coils (Davis et al. 2009), coiled-coils (Stevens et al. 2004), β-sheets (Marini et al. 2002), and hierarchical self-assembling domains (Chung et al. 2010) to the protein polymers, which affect the material's microstructure.

Historically, these peptides were identified by isolating domains of interest from naturally evolved proteins. The tripeptide RGD sequence (arginine–glycine–aspartic acid), a commonly used cell-adhesion domain, is a prime example of this. RGD was isolated in 1983 from the extracellular and plasma protein fibronectin and was identified as the minimal sequence necessary to promote cell-attachment properties (Pierschbacher and Ruoslahti 1984). Other commonly used domains include elastin-like sequences, which are derived from the protein elastin found in connective tissue (Meyer and Chilkoti 2002), and recombinant-silks (Prince et al. 1995). Both of these peptide domains are used to confer their unique mechanical properties (i.e., resilience, elasticity, and strength) to the resulting biomaterial.

More recently, the design of protein-engineered biomaterials has not been limited to domains found in nature. As computational design (Hin Yan Tong et al. 2002) and high-throughput screens (Sidhu et al. 2003) are increasingly being used in peptide development, the variety and specificity of domains available for biomaterials design are rapidly expanding. The design process, however, is not always straightforward. For example, the functionality of a given peptide can be affected by the context of the fully assembled protein, that is, the identity of the flanking peptide domains (Heilshorn et al. 2005). As such, the activity of the domains in each protein composition must be evaluated after the initial design phase. Another complication in peptide selection is the lack of clarity surrounding exactly which properties are imperative for specific niches. Because protein-engineered biomaterials are synthesized to include rationally chosen domains, this design strategy enables iterative testing and optimization of cell–material interactions to overcome both of the limitations discussed above. To illustrate this inherent design flexibility, the sections below give several specific examples of peptide domains identified from naturally evolved proteins, through computational design, or by high-throughput screening to confer specific biomaterial functionalities.

### 4.3.1 Crosslinking Domains

The inclusion of crosslinking domains enables the formation of a network from the individual designed protein polymer chains, forming two- and three-dimensional material structures with the desired mechanical integrity for supporting cells. Because many cellular behaviors, including spreading, signaling, and gene transcription, are known to be responsive to the stiffness of the biomaterial, it is critical to exert control over this design variable in order to direct cell growth and differentiation (Discher et al. 2005). The monodispersity of recombinant proteins, resulting in polymers with identical composition, allows for the tight regulation of the frequency and distance between crosslinking sites, with higher crosslinking densities generating stiffer materials (Welsh and Tirrell 2000). Several crosslinking strategies exist for protein-engineered biomaterials, including enzymatic covalent crosslinking, chemical covalent crosslinking, and physical (i.e., noncovalent) crosslinking via peptide domains that associate through electrostatic or hydrophobic/hydrophilic interactions.

An example of enzymatic covalent crosslinking is the use of the enzyme transglutaminase (TGase). TGase is found naturally in the processes of wound healing and ECM stabilization, where it catalyzes covalent bond formation between lysine (K) and glutamine (Q) residues through a calcium-dependent reaction (Greenberg et al. 1991). Through a process of rational peptide design and screening, several amino acid sequences were identified to have high specificity and tight binding to TGase (Hu and Messersmith 2003). In one example, these optimized TGase crosslinking peptides were included as domains within a family of engineered proteins with varying molecular weights between the lysine-containing domains, resulting in a family of biomaterials with a fourfold range in modulus, from 4 to 16 kPa (Davis et al. 2010).

The binding of calmodulin protein to calmodulin-binding domains (CBDs) is another calcium-dependent crosslinking reaction, although this strategy results in physical (rather than covalent) crosslinks. Upon binding four calcium ions, calmodulin undergoes a conformational change, allowing it to bind to the hundreds CBDs found in other proteins. This binding is reversible upon the depletion of calcium ions. The myriad of both natural and engineered CBDs improves the versatility of this binding method, as calmodulin–CBD pairs can be chosen with binding affinities that range over five-orders of magnitude and with differing calcium dependencies, ultimately enabling control over the material's modulus and the reversibility of network formation (Topp et al. 2006).

Leucine zippers comprise another interesting crosslinking domain that allows for reversible self-assembly, in this case through the noncovalent association of coiled-coil domains (Petka et al. 1998). Naturally evolved leucine zippers function as DNA-binding domains in various transcriptional regulatory proteins. The motif has been well characterized and is known for its heptad amino acid repeat with hydrophobic amino acids at positions one and four and charged amino acids at positions five and seven (Landschulz et al. 1988). At specific pH and temperature conditions, the zipper peptide folds into a helical structure with both hydrophobic residues on one face, promoting interhelical interactions between multiple folded zippers and leading to association. Connecting concatenated zipper motifs by a hydrophilic amino acid sequence creates a triblock co-polymer that utilizes the natural protein–protein interactions for the formation of a hydrogel, where the zipper domains provide the physical crosslinks (Petka et al. 1998). This system lends itself to independent tuning of both the hydrophilic domain (length, composition, and charge density) as well as the zipper domain (electrostatic charge), thereby fine-tuning the overall properties of the gelation phase diagram. Recently, additional functionality has been imparted into leucine zipper hydrogels through the incorporation of folded globular proteins. For example, the inclusion of an alcohol dehydrogenase with aldo–keto reductase activity (AdhD) into a leucine zipper protein polymer led to a thermostable, self-assembling hydrogel with enzymatic activity (Wheeldon et al. 2008).

WW and proline-rich domains represent another example of associating peptides that have been used to design protein-engineered hydrogels. Numerous WW domains, so named for their conserved tryptophan (W) residues, have been identified in intracellular proteins and also derived computationally (Russ et al. 2005). WW domains bind to proline-rich sequences, which are divided into several different classes with varying dissociation constants. The design of protein block copolymers containing multiple WW or proline-rich domains connected by hydrophilic peptide spacers enabled the formation of a mixing-induced, two-component hydrogel (Wong Po Foo et al. 2009). The large library of various WW and proline-rich domains allowed for modulation of the crosslinking strength, and hence hydrogel viscoelastic properties, based on the binding affinity of the chosen domains. In addition, the use of transient physical crosslinks to form the protein hydrogel resulted in a shear-thinning and self-healing biomaterial, which is required for injectable theraputic applications.

## 4.3.2 Structural Domains

In addition to the density of crosslinking sites, the mechanical properties of a protein-engineered biomaterial can also be controlled by including various structural peptide domains in the primary sequence. Elastomeric proteins contain domains that cause them to exhibit rubber-like elasticity, enabling them to undergo high levels of reversible deformation under high stress (Tamburro et al. 2010). Elastin and silk are elastomeric proteins that have been extensively studied and whose desirable mechanical properties have been incorporated into many different biomaterials. In addition to their structural properties, elastin-inspired polymers have been explored for use as injectable biomaterials and implantable scaffolds due to their biocompatibility and thermal sensitivity (Cappello et al. 1990). Through a combination of protein sequence selection and spinning conditions, silk fibers have an outstanding combination of mechanical properties—high strength, elasticity, and resistance to compression failure—that is highly desirable for biomaterials (Gosline et al. 1999). In addition, they have been found to have tunable degradation rates and to be biocompatible (Park et al. 2010). Attempting to harness these properties, researchers have succeeded in designing multiple versions of recombinant silk through expression in host systems, such as yeast, *E. coli*, and mammalian cells (Fahnestock and Bedzyk 1997, Asakura et al. 2003).

A recent addition to the library of structural domains included in protein-engineered biomaterials is resilin. This protein enables many insects to fly, jump, and vocalize, both by storing energy in sound-producing organs and by constraining vibrations during flight. Natural resilin from locusts and dragonflies has demonstrated a remarkable fatigue lifetime and up to 92% resilience (ability to recover after deforming under applied stress) (Tamburro et al. 2010, Elvin et al. 2005). Resilin-derived peptide sequences were observed to have no stable secondary structure and instead underwent continuous interconversion between extended (poly-L-proline II) and folded (β-turn) conformations, allowing resilin to act as an entropic spring. The structural resilin domain has been incorporated into engineered protein biomaterials combining multiple biofunctional domains, including the RGD ligand for cell binding, a matrix metalloproteinase-sensitive sequence for proteolytic degradation, and a heparin-binding domain for the binding and controlled release of growth factors (Charati et al. 2009). The crosslinked material was found to be both highly elastic and to promote cell attachment and proliferation, making it an ideal candidate for mechanically demanding tissue engineering applications.

Another way to use proteins as structural domains is to harness their self-associative interactions to create specifically shaped nanostructures. For example, structures such as hollow cages may be used as drug or gene delivery materials (Uchida et al. 2007), while self-assembled compact structures, such as M13 bacteriophages, can be used to display a high density of a cell-binding peptide (Chung et al. 2010). While the above examples utilized protein self-assembly to form naturally evolved structures, scientists can also mix and match various peptide domains to form novel self-assembling nanostructures. As an example, several rigid α-helical peptide domains that either dimerize or trimerize were fused together at specific angles to create a family of engineered proteins that self-assembled into both cage-like and filamentous nanostructures (Padilla et al. 2001).

## 4.3.3 Degradation Domains

For many tissue engineering applications, the ideal biomaterial will eventually fully degrade, thereby promoting cell invasion and allowing the injured site to be completely replaced by new host tissue. The ability to degrade can be incorporated into protein-engineered biomaterials by incorporating peptide domains that undergo proteolytic degradation in response to cell-secreted protease enzymes. Matrix metalloproteinases (MMPs), such as collagenase, are proteases that have been recognized as key in cell migration (Moses 1997, Gailit and Clark 1994). Seminal work proving the concept of engineered biodegradation was preformed using synthetic PEG polymers crosslinked by synthesized peptides that served as proteolytic MMP-target sites (West and Hubbell 1999). Building on this work, the use of proteolytic target peptides to enable biodegradation has been extended to a wide range of synthetic polymeric biomaterials and recombinant protein-engineered biomaterials.

The designed biomaterial degradation rate can be tailored by controlling the concentration of protease degradation sites within the engineered protein or by altering the amino acid sequence of the protease target site. As an example, elastin-like domains were alternated with proteolytic target sites that degrade in response to tissue plasminogen activator (tPA) or urokinase plasminogin activator (uPA), enzymes produced by endothelial and neuronal cells (Straley and Heilshorn 2009b). Altering the three flanking residues upstream of the proteolytic target site resulted in a family of engineered proteins with 97% sequence homology, identical mechanical properties, and a 200-fold range in protease degradation rate. Engineered proteins with differing degradation kinetics were patterned to form composite biomaterials that sequentially degraded to reveal internally patterned three-dimensional structures. The engineered proteins were further modified to enable the release of two encapsulated small molecules with distinct spatial and temporal delivery profiles (Straley and Heilshorn 2009b).

The well-planned placement of proteolytic degradation sites has also been utilized to control the release of tethered growth factors such as vascular endothelial growth factor (VEGF) (Ehrbar et al. 2005). In this example, a plasmin cleavage site was placed between the VEGF and a crosslinking domain that enabled tethering of the recombinant engineered protein to a fibrin biomaterial. This design enabled slow, plasmin-induced release of the VEGF that could be predictably tuned through implementation of a simple mathematical model. Clearly there are a multitude of variations that can be conceived from this framework, using different degradation sites and various growth factors, cytokines, or other signaling molecules. An especially interesting scenario would be one in which multiple growth factors are tethered into a single biomaterial and released in a timed manner to emulate a specific developmental pathway. These examples show great promise for the advent of biomaterials that not only degrade in response to cell-secreted proteases, but also undergo three-dimensional pattern formation or biochemical release to further direct cell behavior.

### 4.3.4 ECM Cell-Binding Domains

A central role of the ECM is to mediate cellular adhesion through peptide ligands that are recognized by various cell-surface receptors, most notably integrins. Integrins are a class of heterodimeric, transmembrane receptors that exist in a variety of sub-unit combinations. Many cell types present several different integrin receptor combinations on their cell surfaces at different times (Plow et al. 2000). Integrin–ligand binding induces multiple intracellular signaling cascades that can influence cell morphology, migration, gene expression, and differentiation. To recreate these cell-binding events in engineered materials, peptides identified as cell-binding domains from ECM proteins are commonly incorporated into synthetic polymeric and protein-engineered biomaterials. Exemplifying the complexity often found in natural systems, certain peptide ligands are substrates for multiple integrins, certain integrins are receptors for multiple peptide ligands, and certain peptide ligands are present in multiple ECM proteins (Ruoslahti and Pierschbacher 1987, Ruoslahti 1988). Given this complexity, the presentation of peptide ligands within engineered biomaterials offers an opportunity to mechanistically study integrin signaling responses. By presenting various cell-binding domains within an engineered protein biomaterial, scientists often can control the identity and concentration of peptide ligands without altering other material properties such as mechanical stiffness. For example, two different fibronectin-derived peptide ligands, RGD and REDV, were included as cell-binding domains interspersed with elastin-like domains to form two different protein-engineered biomaterials with different integrin specificities. In a direct comparison, human umbilical vein endothelial cells were observed to spread more rapidly and adhere more strongly to the RGD-containing proteins (Liu et al. 2004).

In a second example, the activity of the RGD domain was studied in combination with the so-called "synergy site" of fibronectin, PHSRN. Each cell-binding domain was fused to a serine esterase to enable covalent linkage of the engineered protein to a self-assembled monolayer (Eisenberg et al. 2009). While both domains were observed to independently mediate adhesion, RGD presented a much higher binding affinity. However, at relatively low ligand densities, the co-presentation of PSHRN with RGD led to more efficient cell adhesion than the presentation of RGD alone, confirming the synergistic interaction of these two binding domains.

In addition to exerting control over cell adhesion, ECM cell-binding domains can also be employed to influence cell morphology and phenotype. For example, the cell-binding domain IKVAV, naturally found at the end of the α1 chain of laminin, has been utilized to promote neurite outgrowth from neuronal cells on protein-engineered biomaterials (Nakamura et al. 2009). Similarly, the IKVAV domain has also been implicated in promoting endothelial cell migration and angiogenic behavior (Nakamura et al. 2008). In a direct comparison of RGD and IKVAV cell-binding domains incorporated within self-assembling β-sheet hydrogels, the RGD domain promoted firm endothelial cell adhesion and a traditional cobblestone-like cell morphology, while the IKVAV domain promoted minimal cell adhesion and a spindle-shaped, elongated cell morphology (Jung et al. 2009). These results corroborate previous findings that suggest the IKVAV domain may promote a more migratory endothelial cell phenotype (Schnaper et al. 1993).

Often, the minimal amino acid sequence known to induce integrin binding may have a slightly altered functionality compared to the exact same sequence presented within the context of the full-length, naturally evolved protein. Similarly, when ECM cell-binding domains are incorporated into protein-engineered biomaterials, the context of the flanking amino acid residues can greatly impact the functionality. Often, the minimal amino acid sequence is flanked by spacer sequences to enhance conformational flexibility or a larger amino acid sequence derived from the natural ECM protein. Even in these cases, amino acid choice quite distal to the ECM cell-binding domain can alter cellular response, as observed by differential strengths of cell adhesion to two engineered proteins containing identical REDV domains and different elastin-like domains (Heilshorn et al. 2005). Recently, this ability to alter peptide ligand conformational stability has been utilized to modulate integrin specificity and ultimately differentiation of mesenchymal stem cells (Martino et al. 2009).

These few examples demonstrate how optimization of ligand identity, ligand concentration, and ligand stability can be used to impart cell-instructive properties to protein-engineered biomaterials. As additional mechanistic insight is gained into the actions of integrin signaling (both in response to single ligands or combinations of ligands), the development of cell-instructive biomaterials is expected to increase.

## 4.3.5 Cell–Cell Adhesion Domains

Cell–cell interactions mediate many aspects of cell behavior, including proliferation, migration, and differentiation. These interactions range from stable cell–cell junctions formed within epithelial linings to the transient influence of immune cells on white blood cells during infection. These cell–cell interactions are generally mediated through cell–cell adhesion proteins presented on the cell surface such as selectins, cadherins, and members of the immunoglobulin (Ig) superfamily (Cooper 2000). Similar to the integrin-binding domains described above, cell–cell binding domains can be incorporated into protein-engineered biomaterials to mimic the action of cell–cell interactions and exert control over cell behavior.

As an example, E-cadherin forms calcium-dependent cell–cell adhesion homophilic interactions that are needed for tissue morphogenesis and the maintenance of organized solid tissues (Nagaoka et al. 2010). The E-cadherin extracellular domain was fused to the heavy chain, crystallizable fragment (Fc) of the IgG antibody to form an engineered protein that could be easily tethered to tissue-culture plastic surfaces through adsorption of the Fc region, resulting in presentation of the E-cadherin domain. Hepatocyte culture on this substrate induced cellular responses typical of increased cell–cell interactions, including decreased proliferation and promotion of the differentiated phenotype (Nagaoka et al.

2002). Embryonic stem cells cultured on these E-cadherin-mimetic surfaces did not form colonies, retained their pluripotency, displayed increased proliferation, and had higher transfection efficiency than cells in colony-forming cultures (Nagaoka et al. 2006).

The Ig superfamily includes both cell surface and soluble proteins involved in many roles of cell recognition, binding, and adhesion, all linked by the common "Ig fold" structure of immunoglobulins. Some members of the superfamily, such as the Neural Cell Adhesion Molecule (NCAM), fall in the cell–cell adhesion domain category. NCAM is found on the surfaces of most neural cells and is involved in cell–cell interactions during brain development, synaptic plasticity, and regeneration (Cambon et al. 2004). Peptides encompassing different portions of NCAM have been identified and found to influence neurite growth (Soroka et al. 2002). These peptides are promising for use in biomaterials focused on neural regeneration; for example, recently a fusion protein was created that combines an elastin-like sequence and the P2 peptide of NCAM (Straley and Heilshorn 2009a).

## 4.3.6 Cell-Directive Domains

The category of cell-directive domains includes hormones, growth factors, cytokines, and other signaling molecules. These molecules generally act in a cell-type specific and context-dependent manner to modulate many cell processes, including proliferation, differentiation, migration, adhesion, and gene expression (Silva et al. 2009).

For example, growth factors such as VEGF, fibroblast growth factor (FGF), and bone morphogenetic protein-2 (BMP2) have been studied extensively for their important roles in wound healing, angiogenesis, and bone formation, respectively. While growth factors often have been blended with or tethered to synthetic materials to impart biofunctionality, the recombinant synthesis strategy of producing protein-engineered biomaterials enables the direction incorporation of growth factor domains within the primary polymeric backbone. One such example was discussed previously in Section 4.3.3, where a VEGF domain was fused to a proteolytic target domain and a crosslinking domain (Ehrbar et al. 2005). A second example is the linking of FGF to the RGD cell-binding domain of fibronectin, resulting in a fusion protein with enhanced angiogenic activity (Hashi et al. 1994). Another family of cell-directive molecules includes the hDelta1 and hJagged1 domains, which make up part of the Notch signaling pathway that is key in cell developmental fate decision-making (Beckstead et al. 2006). Both of these functional domains have been interspersed within elastin-like structural domains to create a family of covalently crosslinkable proteins for Notch activity modulation (Liu et al. 2003).

An interesting example within this category is the p21 peptide, which induces cell cycle arrest by interfering with proliferating cell nuclear antigen function and inhibiting cyclin-dependent-kinase activity (Mutoh et al. 1999). This peptide is being investigated for potential cancer therapeutics to target tumor cells and prevent their continued proliferation. The p21 peptide was fused to the C-terminus of an elastin-like domain to render the engineered protein thermally responsive (Massodi et al. 2010). At temperatures below the critical solution temperature, the engineered protein remains soluble, while at higher temperature a reversible aggregate is formed. Thermal induction of aggregation may enable specific targeting of the p21 peptide to a heated solid tumor. In addition, a cell penetrating peptide was fused to the N-terminus of the engineered protein, resulting in increased cellular uptake by cancerous cells (Massodi et al. 2010).

The six peptide domain categories described above are the functionalities most commonly incorporated into protein-engineered biomaterials. Despite the large library of potential peptide domains that are included in these categories, the immense diversity of other potential peptide functionalities has only begun to be realized. Recently, a wide variety of other peptide functionalities, such as inorganic precipitation domains (Wong Po Foo et al. 2006), enzymatic domains (Lu et al. 2010), and enzymatic inhibitor domains (Roberge et al. 2002) have been successfully designed into protein-engineered biomaterials. As the protein-engineered biomaterials field continues to mature, it is expected that an increasing diversity of multifunctional, cell-responsive biomaterials will continue to be developed for a variety of applications.

# 4.4 Applications of Engineered Protein Biomaterials

The two most common applications of protein-engineered biomaterials are (i) use as an ECM-mimetic for studies of cell–environment interactions and (ii) various potential clinical uses. Due to their modular design and exact biosynthesis, protein-engineered biomaterials are ideal platforms for reductionist biological studies. Protein-engineered biomaterials are highly reproducible, engineered matrices that may represent a more physiologically relevant *in vitro* environment compared to traditional cell culture on rigid tissue-culture polystyrene. Because matrix biochemistry, biophysics, and dimensionality (i.e., two- versus three-dimensional environments) are all known to impact cell behavior, utilizing a reproducible cell culture platform that attempts to recreate key aspects of the *in vivo* ECM may lead to more physiologically relevant results. In addition, insights gained from these fundamental investigations of cell response will lead to enhanced understanding of cell–peptide domain interactions, thereby informing the design of future protein-engineered biomaterials.

Protein-engineered biomaterials aimed for use in the clinic include space-filling and structural implants for tissue engineering, as well as injectable materials that function as cell carriers, endogenous cell recruiters, or delivery systems for drugs, growth factors, and other signaling molecules. While many exciting and promising research projects are underway, the barrier to entering clinical trials is high, as the final product must prove to be efficacious and safe, as well as cost-effective with scalable production. As with all biomaterials, a panel of preclinical and clinical safety studies, including potential negative immune system responses, must be performed prior to potential commercialization. Another critical consideration is the ease of use of the material in a clinical setting and the roles of the physician and the patient in deploying the biomaterial. For example, an implant whose use requires a more invasive and time consuming surgery, a disadvantage for both the patient's health and the physician's time, is much less likely to be adopted than a material that can be implanted through a comparatively less invasive injection.

A current example of a protein-engineered biomaterial entering the clinical landscape is that of NuCore® Injectable Nucleus, which is being investigated as a replacement for disc tissue lost due to herniation or surgery to reduce disc degeneration, with the goal of easing the associated back and leg pain. The material is a fusion protein combining silk-like and elastin-like domains, one of which is altered to allow enable chemical crosslinking (Boyd and Carter 2006). The properties of the material have been designed to closely emulate the pH, complex modulus, and protein and water content of natural disc tissue (Boyd and Carter 2006). Initially developed by Protein Polymer Technologies, Inc., NuCore was approved by the United States Food and Drug Administration (FDA) for Investigational Device Exemption (IDE) feasibility studies in 2006 under the direction of Spine Wave, Inc. Results of a 2-year follow-up pilot clinical study were promising, showing NuCore to be biocompatible and effective in reducing the back and leg pain that accompanies herniated lumbar discs requiring surgery (Berlemann and Schwarzenbach 2009).

The continued progress of protein-engineered biomaterials, such as NuCore, toward clinical approval is very encouraging and exciting for the entire field. With the wide-variety of multi-functional, protein-engineered biomaterials that are currently the subject of intense research and preclinical trials and the immense future potential to include new biofunctionalities into these materials, it seems imminent that this class of materials will bring forward a new realm of therapies as they enter clinical use in the near future.

# References

Asakura, T., Nitta, K., Yang, M. et al. 2003. Synthesis and characterization of chimeric silkworm silk. *Biomacromolecules,* 4: 815–20.

Beckstead, B. L., Santosa, D. M., and Giachelli, C. M. 2006. Mimicking cell-cell interactions at the biomaterial-cell interface for control of stem cell differentiation. *J Biomed Mater Res A,* 79: 94–103.

Berlemann, U. and Schwarzenbach, O. 2009. An injectable nucleus replacement as an adjunct to microd-iscectomy: 2 year follow-up in a pilot clinical study. *Eur Spine J,* 18: 1706–12.

Boyd, L. M. and Carter, A. J. 2006. Injectable biomaterials and vertebral endplate treatment for repair and regeneration of the intervertebral disc. *Eur Spine J,* 15 Suppl 3: S414–21.

Bzymek, M. and Lovett, S. T. 2001. Instability of repetitive DNA sequences: The role of replication in mul-tiple mechanisms. *Proc Natl Acad Sci USA,* 98: 8319–25.

Cambon, K., Hansen, S. M., Venero, C. et al. 2004. A synthetic neural cell adhesion molecule mimetic pep-tide promotes synaptogenesis, enhances presynaptic function, and facilitates memory consolidation. *J Neurosci,* 24: 4197–204.

Cappello, J., Crissman, J., Dorman, M. et al. 1990. Genetic engineering of structural protein polymers. *Biotechnol Prog,* 6: 198–202.

Charati, M. B., Ifkovits, J. L., Burdick, J. A., Linhardt, J. G., and Kiick, K. L. 2009. Hydrophilic elastomeric biomaterials based on resilin-like polypeptides. *Soft Matter,* 5: 3412–6.

Chow, D. C., Dreher, M. R., Trabbic-Carlson, K., and Chilkoti, A. 2006. Ultra-high expression of a thermally responsive recombinant fusion protein in *E. coli. Biotechnol Prog,* 22: 638–46.

Chung, W.-J., Merzlyak, A., and Lee, S. 2010. Fabrication of engineered M13 bacteriophages into liquid crys-talline films and fibers for directional growth and encapsulation of fibroblasts. *Soft Matter,* 6: 4454–9.

Cooper, G. M. 2000. The cell surface: Cell–cell interactions. *The Cell: A Molecular Approach.* 2nd Edition ed. Sunderland, MA: Sinaur Assosiates.

Davis, N. E., Ding, S., Forster, R. E., Pinkas, D. M., and Barron, A. E. 2010. Modular enzymatically cross-linked protein polymer hydrogels for *in situ* gelation. *Biomaterials,* 31: 7288–97.

Davis, N. E., Karfeld-Sulzer, L. S., Ding, S., and Barron, A. E. 2009. Synthesis and characterization of a new class of cationic protein polymers for multivalent display and biomaterial applications. *Biomacromolecules,* 10: 1125–34.

Discher, D. E., Janmey, P., and Wang, Y. L. 2005. Tissue cells feel and respond to the stiffness of their sub-strate. *Science,* 310: 1139–43.

Ehrbar, M., Metters, A., Zammaretti, P., Hubbell, J. A., and Zisch, A. H. 2005. Endothelial cell proliferation and progenitor maturation by fibrin-bound VEGF variants with differential susceptibilities to local cellular activity. *J Control Release,* 101: 93–109.

Eisenberg, J. L., Piper, J. L., and Mrksich, M. 2009. Using self-assembled monolayers to model cell adhesion to the 9th and 10th type III domains of fibronectin. *Langmuir,* 25: 13942–51.

Elvin, C. M., Carr, A. G., Huson, M. G. et al. 2005. Synthesis and properties of crosslinked recombinant pro-resilin. *Nature,* 437: 999–1002.

Fahnestock, S. R. and Bedzyk, L. A. 1997. Production of synthetic spider dragline silk protein in *Pichia pastoris. Appl Microbiol Biotechnol,* 47: 33–9.

Gailit, J. and Clark, R. A. F. 1994. Wound repair in the context of extracellular matrix. *Current Opinion in Cell Biology,* 6: 717–25.

Gao, W., Rzewski, A., Sun, H., Robbins, P. D., and Gambotto, A. 2004. UpGene: Application of a web-based DNA codon optimization algorithm. *Biotechnol Prog,* 20: 443–8.

Gosline, J. M., Guerette, P. A., Ortlepp, C. S., and Savage, K. N. 1999. The mechanical design of spider silks: From fibroin sequence to mechanical function. *Journal of Experimental Biology,* 202: 3295–303.

Graf, A., Dragosits, M., Gasser, B., and Mattanovich, D. 2009. Yeast systems biotechnology for the produc-tion of heterologous proteins. *FEMS Yeast Research,* 9: 335–48.

Greenberg, C. S., Birckbichler, P. J., and Rice, R. H. 1991. Transglutaminases: Multifunctional cross-linking enzymes that stabilize tissues. *FASEB J,* 5: 3071–7.

Hashi, H., Hatai, M., Kimizuka, F., Kato, I., and Yaoi, Y. 1994. Angiogenetic activity of a fusion protein of the cell-binding domain of fibronectin and the basic fibroblast growth-factor. *Cell Structure and Function,* 19: 37–47.

Heilshorn, S. C., Dizio, K. A., Welsh, E. R., and Tirrell, D. A. 2003. Endothelial cell adhesion to the fibronec-tin CS5 domain in artificial extracellular matrix proteins. *Biomaterials,* 24: 4245–52.

Heilshorn, S. C., Liu, J. C., and Tirrell, D. A. 2005. Cell-binding domain context affects cell behavior on engineered proteins. *Biomacromolecules,* 6: 318–23.

Hin Yan Tong, A., Drees, B., Nardelli, G. et al. 2002. A combined experimental and computational strategy to define protein interaction networks for peptide recognition modules. *Science,* 295: 321–4.

Hu, B. H. and Messersmith, P. B. 2003. Rational design of transglutaminase substrate peptides for rapid enzymatic formation of hydrogels. *J Am Chem Soc,* 125: 14298–9.

Jung, J. P., Nagaraj, A. K., Fox, E. K. et al. 2009. Co-assembling peptides as defined matrices for endothelial cells. *Biomaterials,* 30: 2400–10.

Karg, S. R. and Kallio, P. T. 2009. The production of biopharmaceuticals in plant systems. *Biotechnology Advances,* 27: 879–94.

Kates, S. A. and Albericio, F. 2000. *Solid-Phase Synthesis: A Practical Guide,* New York, Marcel Dekker, Inc.

Landschulz, W. H., Johnson, P. F., and Mcknight, S. L. 1988. The leucine zipper: A hypothetical structure common to a new class of DNA binding proteins. *Science,* 240: 1759–64.

Liu, C. Y., Apuzzo, M. L. J., and Tirrell, D. A. 2003. Engineering of the extracellular matrix: Working toward neural stem cell programming and neurorestoration—Concept and progress report. *Neurosurgery,* 52: 1154–65.

Liu, J. C., Heilshorn, S. C., and Tirrell, D. A. 2004. Comparative cell response to artificial extracellular matrix proteins containing the RGD and CS5 cell-binding domains. *Biomacromolecules,* 5: 497–504.

Lu, H. D., Wheeldon, I. R., and Banta, S. 2010. Catalytic biomaterials: Engineering organophosphate hydrolase to form self-assembling enzymatic hydrogels. *Protein Eng Des Sel,* 23: 559–66.

Marini, D. M., Hwang, W., Lauffenburger, D. A., Zhang, S. G., and Kamm, R. D. 2002. Left-handed helical ribbon intermediates in the self-assembly of a beta-sheet peptide. *Nano Lett,* 2: 295–9.

Martino, M. M., Mochizuki, M., Rothenfluh, D. A. et al. 2009. Controlling integrin specificity and stem cell differentiation in 2D and 3D environments through regulation of fibronectin domain stability. *Biomaterials,* 30: 1089–97.

Massodi, I., Moktan, S., Rawat, A., Bidwell, G. L., 3rd and Raucher, D. 2010. Inhibition of ovarian cancer cell proliferation by a cell cycle inhibitory peptide fused to a thermally responsive polypeptide carrier. *Int J Cancer,* 126: 533–44.

McPherson, D. T., Xu, J., and Urry, D. W. 1996. Product purification by reversible phase transition following *Escherichia coli* expression of genes encoding up to 251 repeats of the elastomeric pentapeptide GVGVP. *Protein Expr Purif,* 7: 51–7.

Meyer, D. E. and Chilkoti, A. 1999. Purification of recombinant proteins by fusion with thermally-responsive polypeptides. *Nat Biotechnol,* 17: 1112–5.

Meyer, D. E. and Chilkoti, A. 2002. Genetically encoded synthesis of protein-based polymers with precisely specified molecular weight and sequence by recursive directional ligation: Examples from the elastin-like polypeptide system. *Biomacromolecules,* 3: 357–67.

Moses, M. A. 1997. The regulation of neovascularization by matrix metalloproteinases and their inhibitors. *Stem Cells,* 15: 180–9.

Mutoh, M., Lung, F. D., Long, Y. Q. et al. 1999. A p21(Waf1/Cip1)carboxyl-terminal peptide exhibited cyclin-dependent kinase-inhibitory activity and cytotoxicity when introduced into human cells. *Cancer Res,* 59: 3480–8.

Nagaoka, M., Ise, H., and Akaike, T. 2002. Immobilized E-cadherin model can enhance cell attachment and differentiation of primary hepatocytes but not proliferation. *Biotechnol Lett,* 24: 6.

Nagaoka, M., Jiang, H. L., Hoshiba, T., Akaike, T., and Cho, C. S. 2010. Application of recombinant fusion proteins for tissue engineering. *Ann Biomed Eng,* 38: 683–93.

Nagaoka, M., Koshimizu, U., Yuasa, S. et al. 2006. E-cadherin-coated plates maintain pluripotent ES cells without colony formation. *PLoS One,* 1: e15.

Nakamura, M., Mie, M., Mihara, H., and Kobatake, E. 2009. Construction of a multi-functional extracellular matrix protein that increases number of N1E-115 neuroblast cells having neurites. *J Biomed Mater Res B Appl Biomater,* 91: 425–32.

Nakamura, M., Mie, M., Mihara, H., Nakamura, M., and Kobatake, E. 2008. Construction of multi-functional extracellular matrix proteins that promote tube formation of endothelial cells. *Biomaterials,* 29: 2977–86.

Nilsson, J., Stahl, S., Lundeberg, J., Uhlen, M., and Nygren, P. A. 1997. Affinity fusion strategies for detection, purification, and immobilization of recombinant proteins. *Protein Expr Purif,* 11: 1–16.

Padilla, J. E., Colovos, C., and Yeates, T. O. 2001. Nanohedra: Using symmetry to design self assembling protein cages, layers, crystals, and filaments. *Proc Natl Acad Sci USA,* 98: 2217–21.

Park, S. H., Gil, E. S., Shi, H. et al. 2010. Relationships between degradability of silk scaffolds and osteogenesis. *Biomaterials,* 31: 6162–72.

Petka, W. A., Harden, J. L., Mcgrath, K. P., Wirtz, D., and Tirrell, D. A. 1998. Reversible hydrogels from self-assembling artificial proteins. *Science,* 281: 389–92.

Petsch, D. and Anspach, F. B. 2000. Endotoxin removal from protein solutions. *J Biotechnol,* 76: 97–119.

Pierschbacher, M. D. and Ruoslahti, E. 1984. Cell attachment activity of fibronectin can be duplicated by small synthetic fragments of the molecule. *Nature,* 309: 30–3.

Plow, E. F., Haas, T. A., Zhang, L., Loftus, J., and Smith, J. W. 2000. Ligand binding to integrins. *J Biol Chem,* 275: 21785–8.

Porro, D., Sauer, M., Branduardi, P., and Mattanovich, D. 2005. Recombinant protein production in yeasts. *Mol Biotechnol,* 31: 245–59.

Prince, J. T., Mcgrath, K. P., Digirolamo, C. M., and Kaplan, D. L. 1995. Construction, cloning, and expression of synthetic genes encoding spider dragline silk. *Biochemistry,* 34: 10879–85.

Rietschel, E. T., Kirikae, T., Schade, F. U. et al. 1994. Bacterial endotoxin: Molecular relationships of structure to activity and function. *FASEB J,* 8: 217–25.

Roberge, M., Peek, M., Kirchhofer, D., Dennis, M. S., and Lazarus, R. A. 2002. Fusion of two distinct peptide exosite inhibitors of Factor VIIa. *Biochem J,* 363: 387–93.

Ruoslahti, E. 1988. Fibronectin and its receptors. *Annu Rev Biochem,* 57: 375–413.

Ruoslahti, E. and Pierschbacher, M. D. 1987. New perspectives in cell adhesion: RGD and integrins. *Science,* 238: 491–7.

Russ, W. P., Lowery, D. M., Mishra, P., Yaffe, M. B., and Ranganathan, R. 2005. Natural-like function in artificial WW domains. *Nature,* 437: 579–83.

Schnaper, H. W., Kleinman, H. K., and Grant, D. S. 1993. Role of laminin in endothelial cell recognition and differentiation. *Kidney Int,* 43: 20–5.

Seymour, L. W., Duncan, R., Strohalm, J., and Kopecek, J. 1987. Effect of molecular weight (Mw) of N-(2-hydroxypropyl) methacrylamide copolymers on body distribution and rate of excretion after subcutaneous, intraperitoneal, and intravenous administration to rats. *J Biomed Mater Res,* 21: 1341–58.

Shiloach, J. and FASS, R. 2005. Growing E. coli to high cell density—A historical perspective on method development. *Biotechnol Adv,* 23: 345–57.

Sidhu, S. S., Bader, G. D., and Boone, C. 2003. Functional genomics of intracellular peptide recognition domains with combinatorial biology methods. *Curr Opin Chem Biol,* 7: 97–102.

Silva, A. K., Richard, C., Bessodes, M., Scherman, D., and Merten, O. W. 2009. Growth factor delivery approaches in hydrogels. *Biomacromolecules,* 10: 9–18.

Soroka, V., Kiryushko, D., Novitskaya, V. et al. 2002. Induction of neuronal differentiation by a peptide corresponding to the homophilic binding site of the second Ig module of the neural cell adhesion molecule. *J Biol Chem,* 277: 24676–83.

Stevens, M. M., Allen, S., Sakata, J. K. et al. 2004. pH-dependent behavior of surface-immobilized artificial leucine zipper proteins. *Langmuir,* 20: 7747–52.

Straley, K. S. and Heilshorn, S. C. 2009a. Design and adsorption of modular engineered proteins to prepare customized, neuron-compatible coatings. *Front Neuroeng,* 2: 9.

Straley, K. S. and Heilshorn, S. C. 2009b. Dynamic, 3D-pattern formation within enzyme-responsive hydrogels. *Adv Mater,* 21: 4148.

Tamburro, A. M., Panariello, S., Santopietro, V. et al. 2010. Molecular and supramolecular structural studies on significant repetitive sequences of resilin. *Chembiochem,* 11: 83–93.

Thompson, M. T., Berg, M. C., Tobias, I. S. et al. 2006. Biochemical functionalization of polymeric cell substrata can alter mechanical compliance. *Biomacromolecules,* 7: 1990–5.

Tomita, M., Yoshizato, K., Nagata, K., and Kitajima, T. 1999. Enhancement of secretion of human procollagen I in mouse HSP47-expressing insect cells. *J Biochem,* 126: 1118–26.

Topp, S., Prasad, V., Cianci, G. C., Weeks, E. R., and Gallivan, J. P. 2006. A genetic toolbox for creating reversible Ca2+-sensitive materials. *J Am Chem Soc,* 128: 13994–5.

Uchida, M., Klem, M. T., Allen, M. et al. 2007. Biological containers: Protein cages as multifunctional nanoplatforms. *Adv Mater,* 19: 1025–1042.

Welsh, E. R. and Tirrell, D. A. 2000. Engineering the extracellular matrix: A novel approach to polymeric biomaterials. I. Control of the physical properties of artificial protein matrices designed to support adhesion of vascular endothelial cells. *Biomacromolecules,* 1: 23–30.

West, J. L. and Hubbell, J. A. 1999. Polymeric biomaterials with degradation sites for proteases involved in cell migration. *Macromolecules,* 32: 241–244.

Wheeldon, I. R., Gallaway, J. W., Barton, S. C., and Banta, S. 2008. Bioelectrocatalytic hydrogels from electron-conducting metallopolypeptides coassembled with bifunctional enzymatic building blocks. *Proc Natl Acad Sci USA,* 105: 15275–80.

Williams, C. G., Malik, A. N., Kim, T. K., Manson, P. N., and Elisseeff, J. H. 2005. Variable cytocompatibility of six cell lines with photoinitiators used for polymerizing hydrogels and cell encapsulation. *Biomaterials,* 26: 1211–8.

Wong Po Foo, C., Patwardhan, S. V., Belton, D. J. et al. 2006. Novel nanocomposites from spider silk-silica fusion (chimeric) proteins. *Proc Natl Acad Sci USA,* 103: 9428–33.

Wong Po Foo, C. T., Lee, J. S., Mulyasasmita, W., Parisi-Amon, A., and Heilshorn, S. C. 2009. Two-component protein-engineered physical hydrogels for cell encapsulation. *Proc Natl Acad Sci USA,* 106: 22067–72.

Zaher, H. S. and Green, R. 2009. Quality control by the ribosome following peptide bond formation. *Nature,* 457: 161–6.

Zerbs, S., Frank, A. M., and Collart, F. R. 2009. Bacterial systems for production of heterologous proteins. *Methods Enzymol,* 463: 149–68.

# 5

# Synthetic Biomaterials

5.1   Introduction ........................................................................... 5-1
5.2   Choice of Monomer................................................................ 5-2
5.3   Polymerization Mechanisms ................................................ 5-2
5.4   Biomaterial Degradation ......................................................5-4
      Hydrolytic Degradation • Enzymatic Degradation •
      Stimuli-Responsive Degradation • Degradation By-Products
5.5   Poly(ethylene glycol) ........................................................... 5-6
5.6   Poly(esters)............................................................................ 5-7
      Poly(α-esters) • Poly(propylene fumarate) • Other Poly(esters)
5.7   Poly(anhydrides) ................................................................. 5-10
5.8   Poly(ortho esters) ............................................................... 5-11
5.9   Poly(urethanes) ................................................................... 5-11
5.10  Pseudo Poly(amino acids) .................................................. 5-12
5.11  Poly(acrylates) and Poly(methacrylates) ......................... 5-13
5.12  Non-Polymeric Synthetic Biomaterials............................ 5-14
5.13  Conclusions.......................................................................... 5-16
References............................................................................................. 5-16

**Joshua S. Katz**
*Dow Chemical Company*

**Jason A. Burdick**
*University of Pennsylvania*

## 5.1 Introduction

Synthetic biomaterials have been developed over the last century for a range of applications, including for dental fillings, bone cements, prosthetics, and contact lenses (Griffith 2000, Langer and Tirrell 2004, Ratner and Bryant 2004). In recent years, synthetic biomaterials have evolved to address problems in the field of tissue engineering, namely as three-dimensional scaffolding material to provide structure during tissue formation. This chapter will begin with an overview of the development and properties of synthetic biomaterials for tissue engineering and then focus on the various classes of materials that have been developed. The specific focus will be on synthetic polymers and primarily those that undergo degradation.

When designing and using synthetic biomaterials for tissue engineering applications, it is important to consider many criteria (Drury and Mooney 2003, Lutolf and Hubbell 2005, Shin et al. 2003). This includes the specific tissue of interest (e.g., cartilage versus liver) with respect to the healing potential, cell sources for repair, and vascularization. The scaffold should degrade in accordance with tissue healing (to facilitate, but not impede tissue growth) and into non-toxic by-products. The processing of the polymer must be possible into the desired structure, including as hydrogels, fibrous scaffolds, or macroporous materials. It may also be desirable to incorporate cells, growth factors, and other molecules to aid in the healing response. The bulk mechanical properties are also of concern depending on the local tissue loading and the influence of mechanical properties on cell behavior. With these criteria in mind, nearly endless compositions have been investigated for many tissue types. This chapter will cover materials that exhibit a range of properties and cell and tissue interactions.

The evolution of materials for use in tissue engineering began with various natural materials (e.g., collagen, fibrin), then turned to synthetic materials used for other biomedical applications (e.g., sutures), and now to more complex materials and scaffolds. Added complexity may include control over materials in both time and space, as well as the inclusion of biological components that can lead to optimal cellular signaling. However, the development of new materials opens up questions related to bulk properties, as well as the *in vivo* tissue response and cellular interactions. The overall goal is to better understand the materials toward their use in clinical applications for tissue repair.

## 5.2 Choice of Monomer

The most significant factor in determining the material properties of a polymer is the structure of the monomer(s) selected for polymerization. Monomer choice dictates both side chain and backbone structure, the latter which determines the polymer classification. Even minor changes to the chemical modification of a monomer (and the resulting polymer) can have drastic effects on polymer solubility, mechanical strength, crystallinity, and sensitivity to degradation. Consequently, the choice of monomer also often dictates the manner in which the material can be processed for biomedical applications.

As a general rule, hydrophilic polymers are processed into hydrogels whereas hydrophobic polymers are processed into solid, porous scaffolds (e.g., foams or fibrous structures). Hydrogels are water-swollen networks held together by cross-links (either chemical or physical, depending on the material) between the polymers. In the absence of cross-links, the polymers typically would simply dissolve. Because water is ubiquitous in these materials, it is important that hydrolysis be controlled to better manipulate degradation timing with tissue formation. Hydrogels are generally soft materials because of their high water content and are therefore generally more suitable for soft tissue applications.

In contrast, hydrophobic polymers must be processed into three-dimensional porous scaffolds to support cell and tissue population, as well as nutrient and waste transport. This topic will be discussed in more detail in other chapters. Water does not penetrate hydrophobic materials extensively, so swelling is generally negligible. As hydrophobic materials can span a large range of material properties, they have potential for applications in both hard and soft tissue engineering. Generally, poly(ethylene glycols) (PEGs) and some of the poly(acrylates) and poly(methacrylates) are used as hydrophilic materials, while there are many examples of hydrophobic materials, which will be discussed in more detail below.

## 5.3 Polymerization Mechanisms

In addition to monomer selection determining polymer behavior, the ultimate structure of the polymer, such as its molecular weight, polydispersity, and degree of branching can also have profound effects on the material properties. These characteristics can be controlled through the polymerization mechanism and corresponding choice of initiators, terminating molecules, and reaction conditions. Polymers are generally synthesized through one of two mechanisms: step growth or chain growth polymerization (Odian 2004).

The vast majority of polymers produced are synthesized using a step growth mechanism. In step growth polymerizations, all monomeric species are equally able to react with other monomers in a stepwise manner, slowly building dimers, trimers, tetramers, etc. In addition, small oligomers can react with each other (e.g., dimer + trimer → pentamer). Because all monomers are able to react at the beginning of polymerization, at early time points, while conversion is high, the molecular weights remain low. Only at very high conversion it is possible to obtain high molecular weight species. For polymerization to proceed, monomers must contain at least two reactive groups (where the presence of more than two reactive groups enables branching and/or cross-linking). Monofunctional monomers cause chain termination and can be used to control the molecular weight of the final polymer. In addition, for copolymer systems in which multiple monomers react with each other (e.g., "A" only reacts with "B" and "B"

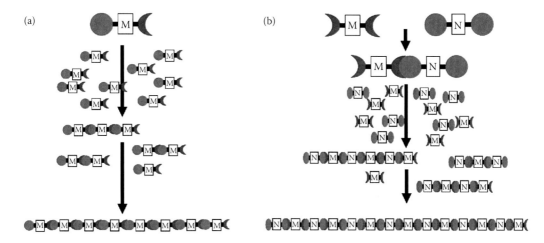

**FIGURE 5.1** Step growth polymerization. In step growth polymerization, monomers slowly react with each other until ultimately a high molecular weight species is formed. Monomers can react with themselves (a), or with a complementary monomer (b), forming an alternating copolymer.

only reacts with "A"), molecular weight can be controlled through the monomer feed ratio. Schematics of both types of step-growth polymerization can be found in Figure 5.1.

In contrast to step growth polymerizations, chain growth polymerizations require activation of monomer by an initiator species. The active initiator reacts with a monomer, forming a bond and transferring the reactive point to the end of the monomer, allowing it to react with another, quickly forming a chain (Figure 5.2). Consequently, unlike with step growth polymerizations, even at very low conversions, the polymers present may be of high molecular weight. The most common chain growth polymerization is free radical polymerization. In free radical polymerizations, a radical is introduced to the system through an initiator that activates in the presence of light or heat, or through reductive/oxidative mechanisms. As free radicals are very unstable, the active initiator quickly reacts with monomer (usually a vinyl monomer), transferring the radical to the monomer, which can then react with another monomer, growing the chain. Growth is halted by the reaction of the free radical with another species present in solution to quench the radical such as inhibitors, oxygen, other free radicals, or scission of another polymer's backbone. Free radical polymerization is used to produce both linear polymers that can be further processed into structural materials or to cross-link materials directly into a structure, such as a hydrogel.

In more recent years, a significant amount of research has involved the development of catalysts for controlling chain growth polymerizations such that high molecular weights and narrow polydispersities can be obtained. In these reactions, known as "living polymerizations" the catalysts stabilize the growing reactive chain end, enabling slow and uniform growth of the polymers. Consequently, the

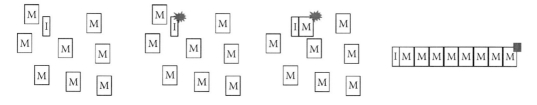

**FIGURE 5.2** Chain growth polymerization. In chain growth polymerization, an initiator molecule is activated and rapidly transfers its activity to a monomer, which continues to react with more monomers in succession until a termination reaction occurs.

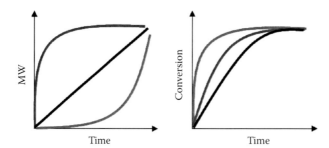

**FIGURE 5.3** (**See color insert.**) Progression of polymer molecular weight and monomer conversion with time for step growth (red), chain growth (blue), and living (black) polymerizations.

molecular weight changes are linear with time and conversion. In addition, due to the high stability of the growing chain ends, living polymerizations allow for the synthesis of high-fidelity diblock copolymers. Figure 5.3 demonstrates the molecular weight and monomer conversion profiles for all three typical polymerization mechanisms.

## 5.4 Biomaterial Degradation

To facilitate the replacement of synthetic scaffold materials with natural tissue, many materials are now being processed and designed to degrade under physiological conditions. Degradation can also be used as a tool to deliver molecules (e.g., growth factors) or cells to aid in the tissue healing and to manipulate material properties with time. This section explores the various routes of degradation that have been used in synthetic materials for tissue engineering.

### 5.4.1 Hydrolytic Degradation

The vast majority of degradable synthetic materials degrade *in vivo* through water hydrolysis of polymer bonds. Classically, degradation and erosion of a biomaterial have been described in one of two ways, namely surface erosion or bulk erosion. Which mode of erosion a material undergoes is dictated by both the ability of water to penetrate the material (hydrophobicity) and the rate of bond hydrolysis (lability). Materials that are highly hydrophobic but also exhibit relatively labile bonds undergo surface erosion because the fast degradation at the surface is more rapid than water penetration into the material. Consequently, surface eroding materials exhibit a relatively linear decrease in mass with time (depending on the sample geometry), as the hydrolyzed portion of the material, located solely at the water–material interface, becomes free to dissolve into the surrounding solution. In contrast, materials that undergo slow hydrolysis and are more hydrophilic are more susceptible to bulk degradation. In bulk-degrading materials, little mass loss is observed at (relatively) early time points until enough of the material has degraded throughout, leading to nearly complete dissolution of the polymer. The slow degradation rate enables penetration of water throughout the material, allowing uniform hydrolysis. However, at early times, as the majority of the material remains intact, even those portions that have been hydrolyzed remain with the material, trapped from escape, and hence the minimal mass loss. However, practically all materials exhibit some combination of bulk and surface erosion, leading to hybrid degradation profiles (Figure 5.4).

### 5.4.2 Enzymatic Degradation

Few synthetic materials are susceptible to recognition and degradation by endogenous enzymes found in human tissues. Consequently, several groups have recently begun to incorporate synthetic peptides

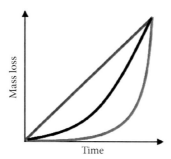

**FIGURE 5.4**  (**See color insert.**) Mass loss profile for idealized bulk eroding (red) and surface eroding (blue) polymeric materials. The actual mass loss profile is a hybrid of the two profiles, shown in black.

containing consensus sequences sensitive to proteolytic enzymes, such as matrix metalloproteinases (MMP) (Lutolf et al. 2003). Using solid phase peptide synthesis, these specialty peptides are designed to cross-link hydrogels. Most of this work has focused on natural materials or PEG-based hydrogels. Several approaches have been taken to fabricate these gels, including the use of multi-arm PEGs with bifunctional peptides cross-linking them or building large repeating PEG-peptide-PEG macromers that then crosslink using UV light (Lutolf and Hubbell 2005, Miller et al. 2010). The MMP peptides were coupled to the PEG using a Michael-type addition through terminal cysteines on the peptide and vinyl groups on the PEGs. Once the gels have been formed, surrounding cells (either encapsulated or at the surface) produce MMPs as they migrate into and through the gel, slowly degrading the synthetic network and allowing it to be replaced by new tissue.

### 5.4.3  Stimuli-Responsive Degradation

Another potential route to inducing degradation is through the cleavage of reduction-sensitive linkages, such as disulfide bonds (Cerritelli et al. 2007, Lee and Park 1998). The vast majority of research in this field has focused on nano-sized drug delivery vehicles, as most reduction occurs inside endosomal and lysosomal compartments of cells. As the extracellular environment is generally non-reductive in nature, reductive degradation is unlikely to find significant use as a degradation route for materials being developed for tissue engineering applications, as in such applications, the materials are not taken up by cells. Alternatively, light is now being used as a trigger for polymer degradation, where ultraviolet light exposure of incorporated *o*-nitrobenzyl moieties can lead to polymer cleavage (Katz and Burdick 2010, Kloxin et al. 2009). This provides precise spatial and temporal control over material properties and user-dictated degradation.

### 5.4.4  Degradation By-Products

When designing a biodegradable implant, it is important to keep in mind the products of the material's degradation (Nair and Laurencin 2007). Most materials undergoing hydrolysis liberate large amounts of acid as the degradation products. For rapidly degrading materials, such a large local concentration of acid could prove to be toxic, interfering with the intended application of the material while inducing inflammation. In addition, as many materials' degradation profiles are affected by pH, the generation of acids (or bases) locally could significantly alter the continued degradation of the material. The choice of monomer must be considered when designing synthetic polymers as it will be a component of the degradation products and care should be taken to understand the resulting cell and tissue interactions with degradation. Generally, the quantity and timing of degradation product release, as well as monomer toxicity, correlates to cytotoxicity and the *in vivo* inflammatory response.

## 5.5 Poly(ethylene glycol)

PEG (also known as poly(ethylene oxide)) is one of the most widely used materials in tissue engineering (Drury and Mooney 2003). As a result of its extreme hydrophilicity, PEG is highly resistant to protein adsorption and therefore works well as a non-fouling, non-immunogenic surface in a biological environment. This makes PEG materials a "blank slate" so that cellular interactions can be precisely controlled through added features (e.g., peptides). Furthermore, because it is one of the few synthetic hydrophilic materials available, it has become a prime candidate for use in many soft tissue applications, where hydrogels are preferable to hard materials.

PEG is synthesized by the ring-opening polymerization of ethylene oxide and very narrow molecular weight distributions can be obtained through the use of living catalysts (Figure 5.5). The choice of initiator determines the end group chemistry, which is important for enabling post-functionalization of the polymer to allow for cross-linking into networks and chemical functionalization of the resulting material. The use of a multifunctional initiator allows for multi-branched PEGs. Many PEGs are commercially available with alcohol termini, ranging in molecular weight from a few hundred Daltons to several million. The most common functionality added to PEG to process it into a three-dimensional biomaterial is the acrylate group which enables polymerization and (if more than one acrylate per polymer) cross-linking through free radical routes. Hydrogels of PEG diacrylate are non-degradable under physiological conditions on time scales of interest for tissue engineering. To address this issue, several groups have added short polyesters to the PEG termini prior to acrylation (Metters et al. 2000, Sawhney et al. 1993). These short polyester chains provide a route to hydrolytic degradation, the kinetics of which can be tuned by the choice of polyester and number of groups incorporated.

Although beneficial in that it resists nearly all non-specific binding, PEG materials are limited because of the inability of cells to attach to these gels and grow. To address this issue, multi-functional PEGs are now being developed and used that incorporate a route to present a biologically relevant ligand to enhance cell interactions (Burdick and Anseth 2002, Hern and Hubbell 1998). PEG hydrogels have also been investigated that degrade via enzymes or through light (as discussed above) and have found utility for a wide range of tissue engineering applications.

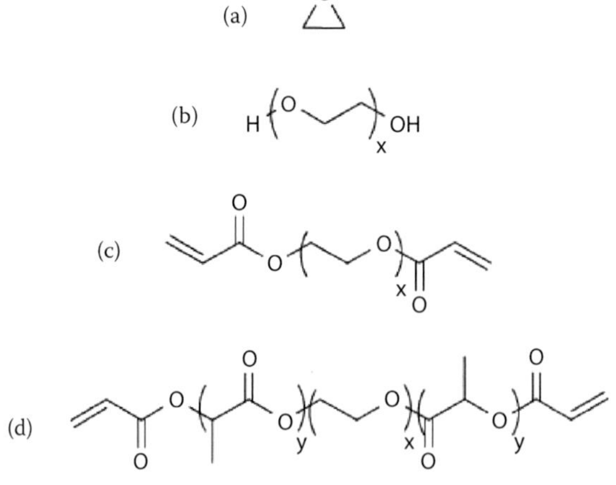

**FIGURE 5.5**    Poly(ethylene glycol) is synthesized by the ring-opening polymerization of ethylene oxide (a) and has the structure shown in (b). PEG can be modified with acrylate groups for cross-linking (c) or with short poly(ester) chains and acrylate groups for crosslinking and degradability (d).

# 5.6 Poly(esters)

## 5.6.1 Poly(α-esters)

The poly(α-esters) are a class of thermoplastic polymers that are widely used in surgical implant materials (Nair and Laurencin 2007) and are likely the most investigated hydrophobic polymer class used in tissue engineering applications. The properties of this class of material vary widely depending on the polymer molecular weight, hydrophobicity of the monomer, and the degree of crystallinity of the resulting polymer. Poly(α-esters) can be synthesized through either step or living chain growth polymerizations. Step growth polymers are formed by the condensation of alcohols and carboxylic acids (or activated esters). To produce robust polymers, high temperature and vacuum are required to remove the water by-product. Even with such extreme conditions, however, the synthesis of high molecular weight species is fairly limited. In contrast, living polymerization can be achieved through the ring opening polymerization of lactones (Labet and Thielemans 2009). These reactions proceed at relatively low temperatures (as low as room temperature has been achieved) and monodisperse, high molecular weight polymers can be obtained. The most common catalyst for chain growth polymerization of lactones is stannous octoate, though many other electron rich catalysts such as alkyl aluminums and heterocyclic carbenes have been employed to provide further control over the reaction progression and to produce multi-block polymers. Figure 5.6 shows the structures of the monomers and polymers to be discussed in the next section.

The glycolide monomer is the smallest unit in the poly(α-ester) series. The resulting polymer, poly(glycolic acid) is crystalline with a $T_g$ in the range of 40°C and melting temperature over 200°C. As a result of its high crystallinity, it has a very strong tensile modulus, making it a promising candidate for many tissue engineering applications. Its ability to form fibers has also made it a strong candidate for bioresorbable sutures. Poly(glycolic acid) is a bulk degrading polymer, breaking down into naturally occurring glycine. However, owing to the rapidly produced acidic degradation products, poly(glycolic acid) may be limited to only a few *in vivo* applications (Li 1999, Nair and Laurencin 2007).

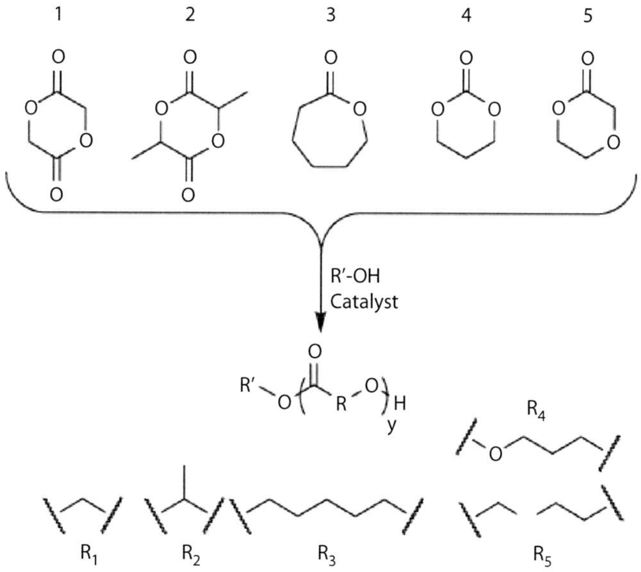

**FIGURE 5.6** Cyclic lactones undergo ring-opening polymerization to form the poly(α-esters). Monomers shown are (1) glycolide, (2) lactide, (3) caprolactone, (4) trimethylene carbonate, and (5) dioxanone.

Lactic acid is a naturally occurring chiral molecule whose polymer properties vary significantly based on the chirality of the monomer feed. Enantiomerically pure monomer feeds (all D-lactide or L-lactide) produce highly crystalline polymers. As L-lactide is the naturally occurring species, poly(L-lactic acid) (PLLA) is more often used for medical applications. These polymers have a $T_g$ around 60°C and melt at temperatures slightly lower than poly(glycolic acid), around 175°C. As a result of the crystalline nature of the polymer—and that it is more hydrophobic than poly(glycolic acid)—degradation is relatively slower, with resorption taking several years. In contrast to PLLA, polymers made from a racemic mixture of monomer are amorphous in nature, with a $T_g$ approximately 5°C less than the optically pure polymers. Owing to the amorphous nature, these polymers are significantly softer than PLLA and hydrolyze in a manner of months. In all cases, these polymers undergo primarily bulk degradation and produce lactic acid as their degradation product (Li 1999).

Significant research has also been conducted on copolymers of lactic and glycolic acid (PLGA), an FDA-approved biomaterial. These polymers degrade relatively rapidly (weeks to months), as they do not benefit from the crystalline stability afforded materials of the homopolymers and have the added hydrophilicity from the glycolide. The degradation rate depends on the actual polymer composition, molecular weight, and how the material has been processed. Applications of PLGA range from tissue engineering scaffolds, to fast-degrading sutures, to drug-delivery vehicles (Li 1999).

Several larger cyclic monomers have also been used for the production of more hydrophobic polyesters. Poly(dioxanone) (PDN) and poly(caprolactone) (PCL) are polyesters with significantly reduced glass transition temperatures, PDN being around −5°C and PCL being as low as −60°C. PDN has a melting temperature of around 110°C, whereas the melting temperature of PCL is closer to 60°C. Both polymers undergo bulk degradation over very long periods of time, their rates limited by their hydrophobicity and crystallinity. Consequently, these polymers are potentially useful for applications requiring the long-term presence of the material, such as long-term releasing drug-delivery devices or slow-growth tissue regeneration (Nair and Laurencin 2007).

Similar to the poly(α-esters), both in structure and route of preparation, is poly(trimethylene carbonate) (PTMC). PTMC is a soft amorphous polymer that is highly elastic. Unlike the poly(α-esters), PTMC does not undergo bulk degradation, but rather is subject to surface-erosion. Interestingly, the rate of surface erosion is significantly higher in an *in vivo* setting compared with *in vitro* (Zhang et al. 2006). This enhanced rate of degradation is caused by the ability of PTMC to undergo enzymatic degradation in addition to simple hydrolysis. PTMC is one of the very few completely synthetic materials that can be subject to enzymatic hydrolysis, making it a particularly interesting candidate for materials development.

## 5.6.2 Poly(propylene fumarate)

Poly(propylene fumarate) (PPF) is a classical example of a degradable poly(ester) synthesized by step-growth polymerization. There are several methods for synthesis of the polymer including transesterification of a fumaric ester or direct esterification of 1,2-propanediol and fumaric acid using an acidic catalyst (Gresser et al. 1995, Suggs et al. 1997). Both fumaric acid and 1,2-propanediol are known to be biocompatible, translating to minimal adverse responses to the material *in vivo* (Nair and Laurencin 2007). An advantage of the PPF structure is an unsaturated double bond in each repeat unit of the polymer (Figure 5.7). This double bond enables further polymerization and cross-linking of PPF polymers following casting into a desired shape (i.e., a tissue defect). PPF can also be used as a biodegradable cross-linker for other vinyl monomers, such as *N*-vinyl pyrrolidone or methyl methacrylate (Frazier et al. 1997, Gresser et al. 1995). These two added benefits—cross-linking and copolymerization—have enabled a broad spectrum of material properties accessible to PPF materials. However, research with PPF has mainly been centered on applications in bone tissue engineering, and as a result, in order to better mimic bone, it is often combined in a composite with beta-tricalcium phosphate (Temenoff and Mikos 2000, Wolfe et al. 2002).

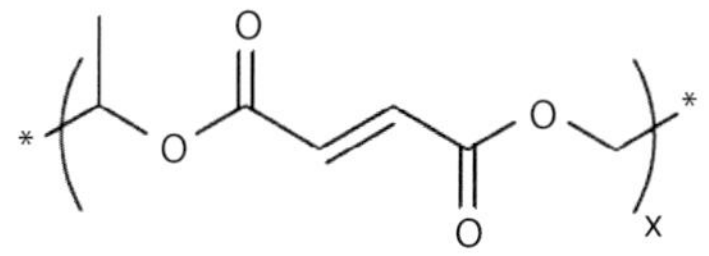

**FIGURE 5.7** Structure of poly(propylene fumarate). The unsaturated double bond enables further polymerization and cross-linking of the polymer.

## 5.6.3 Other Poly(esters)

In addition to ring-opening polymerization and transesterification reactions, condensation reactions can also afford polyesters, though with less control over the molecular weight and polydispersity of the resulting polymers. These materials are obtained by the condensation of alcohols and carboxylic acids or activated esters. One such example material that has been explored for tissue engineering is a copolymer of sebacic acid and glycerol, shown in Figure 5.8 (Wang et al. 2003). Synthesized in the melt, high temperature, and vacuum facilitates condensation and removal of water. If allowed to proceed to completion, the material cures owing to the three alcohols on glycerol providing a route to cross-linking. Others have stopped the reaction prior to curing and in a second step, acrylated the polymer, which could then be cross-linked following radical initiation (Ifkovits et al. 2008). Poly(glycerol-co-sebacate) is an elastomeric material, making it a suitable candidate for tissue engineering of soft flexible tissues such as muscle.

Recently, a new class of poly(esters), poly(β-amino esters) (PBAEs), has been developed (Anderson et al. 2006). Originally designed as a potential gene-delivery vehicle, PBAEs have demonstrated promise in the field of tissue engineering as scaffold materials (Brey et al. 2010). PBAEs are synthesized through step-growth polymerization via Michael-type addition of an amine across the vinyl bond of an acrylate (Figure 5.9). The use of diacrylate monomers allows for polymerization (each amine can add to two double bonds, linking the monomers). These polymers are synthesized in the bulk without the production of by-products. The monomer (diacrylate and amine) ratios are set to ensure that the polymer end-groups are acrylates, allowing for radical cross-linking of the material. A large combinatorial library of PBAEs was screened for mechanical and degradation properties, and the choice of monomers can have a significant effect on both. Although all formulations were found to bulk degrade, the most hydrophilic polymers were found to degrade too quickly for applications in tissue engineering, indicating the need for at least a moderate hydrophobicity to the material to have applicability in tissue engineering.

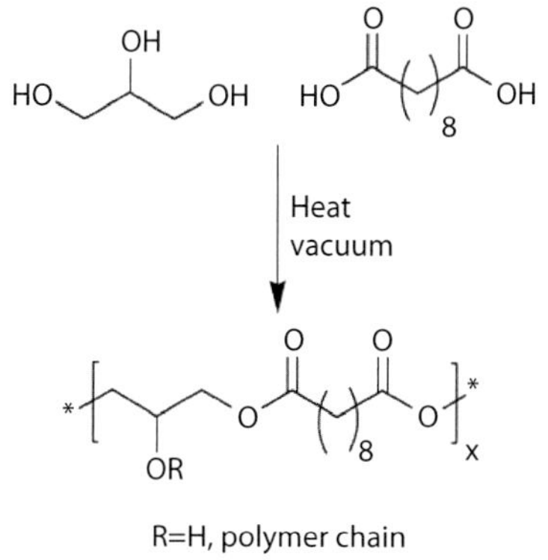

**FIGURE 5.8** Glycerol and sebacic acid esterify to form poly(glycerol sebacate), an elastomeric material.

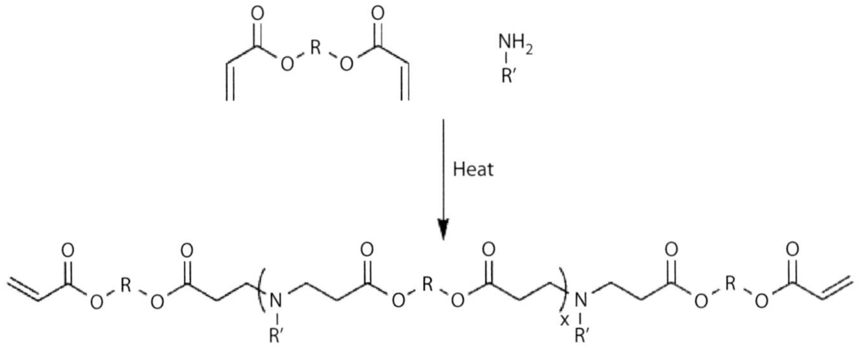

**FIGURE 5.9**   Acrylates and primary amines react by Michael addition to form poly(β-amino esters). The mechanical and degradation properties of the PBAEs vary greatly based on the R and R′ groups.

## 5.7 Poly(anhydrides)

The major class of surface-eroding polymers is poly(anhydrides) (Kumar et al. 2002). More sensitive to hydrolytic cleavage than esters, the anhydride backbone is able to degrade relatively quickly, allowing less time for water penetration into the material and, therefore, the resulting surface-eroding profile. The use of hydrophobic moieties surrounding the anhydride linkage further limits water penetration into the bulk. Poly(anhydrides) are synthesized predominantly by condensation reactions of carboxylic acids or their activated derivatives—activated esters or acyl chlorides, though ring opening polymerization of adipic anhydride has also been achieved (Albertsson and Lundmark 1988, Kumar et al. 2002). Various catalysts that coordinate the carbonyl have been introduced that accelerate the synthesis and also afford higher molecular weight polymers. The range of monomers that have been investigated for poly(anhydride) synthesis and applications is vast, ranging from simple aliphatic diacids (i.e., sebacic acid or adipic acid) which degrade in a matter of weeks to bulky aromatic diacids such as 1,3-bis(*p*-carboxyphenoxy) propane which must be used as copolymers to reduce brittleness (Kumar et al. 2002). Such a copolymer is shown in Figure 5.10. Others have made poly(anhydrides) from fatty acids and amino acids or with branches (Domb 1990, Domb et al. 1995, Maniar et al. 1990). In one particularly interesting example, poly(anhydrides) were synthesized with a salicylic acid-based monomer, degrading into the common analgesic drug (Erdmann and Uhrich 2000).

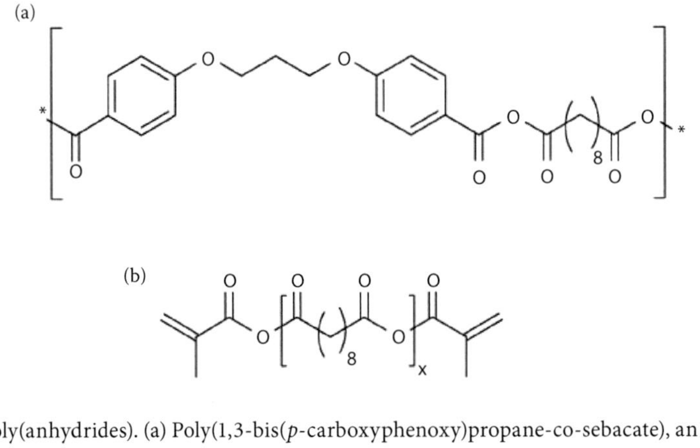

**FIGURE 5.10**   Poly(anhydrides). (a) Poly(1,3-bis(*p*-carboxyphenoxy)propane-co-sebacate), an aliphatic-aromatic copoly(anhydride). (b) Methacrylated poly(sebacate), which can undergo cross-linking through the methacrylate groups.

Poly(anhydrides) made inroads in the field of biomaterials through their use in drug-delivery applications (Kumar et al. 2002). Because they surface erode, a linear release of encapsulated drugs could be achieved, allowing for constant, sustained drug concentrations *in vivo*. Poly(anhydrides), however, are somewhat limited in their applications as their processing can be difficult owing to high degrees of crystallinity, leading to poor solubility in most solvents, and any hydrophilic candidate would hydrolyze at a rate too fast for any practical application. To address this concern, methacrylated poly(anhydrides), which begin soft and moldable and can then be cross-linked into a defect, have also been developed and investigated for tissue engineering applications (Muggli et al. 1999).

## 5.8 Poly(ortho esters)

Another major class of surface-eroding polymers is the poly(ortho esters) (POE; Figure 5.11) (Heller et al. 2002). Four classes of POEs have been developed for applications in controlled drug delivery, as they exhibit linear release profiles of encapsulated contents. The POE structure is a carbon bonded to three oxygens, two of which are part of the backbone of the polymer. They exhibit pH-dependent hydrolysis, cleaving to yield alcohols and esters, though the esters often further hydrolyze to the corresponding alcohol and acid. POE I was the first POE developed, a copolymer of tetrahydrofuran and a diol. However, because POE I degrades into hydroxybutyric acid (from butyrolactone), which further catalyzes (and accelerates) degradation, focus was turned to other POEs. POE II is a far more stable POE than POE I, and through the choice of diol, the material properties of the polymer can be tuned from glassy to semi solid. However, because of the extreme hydrophobicity of this POE II, there was little control over the very slow degradation rate, limiting their applicability. POE III is a semi-solid polymer; however, it was limited in development by difficulties in obtaining reproducible synthetic results. The most advanced POE is POE IV, a modified version of POE II to address the slow hydrolysis. POE IV is a copolymer of POE II and short PLA or PGA segments. The PLA or PGA offers a route to facile hydrolysis and the production of either lactic or glycolic acid further catalyzes the decay of the POE. By controlling the amount of PLA or PGA added, the degradation rate can be easily tuned.

## 5.9 Poly(urethanes)

Poly(urethanes) are a class of polymer that have been explored for many applications in the materials science field (Santerre et al. 2005). As a result of their ability to form segmented block copolymers, a wide range of material properties is accessible, making them a particularly attractive class of polymers. Polyurethanes are synthesized by the polycondensation of diols and diisocyanates. To form segmented diblock copolymers, polymeric diols (e.g., PEG or a polyester) are used as a small percentage of the diol feed (with the remainder being a low molecular weight diol or diamine called a chain extender). Figure 5.12 shows a poly(urethane) with a poly(ester) segment. Upon condensation, the polymeric diol forms

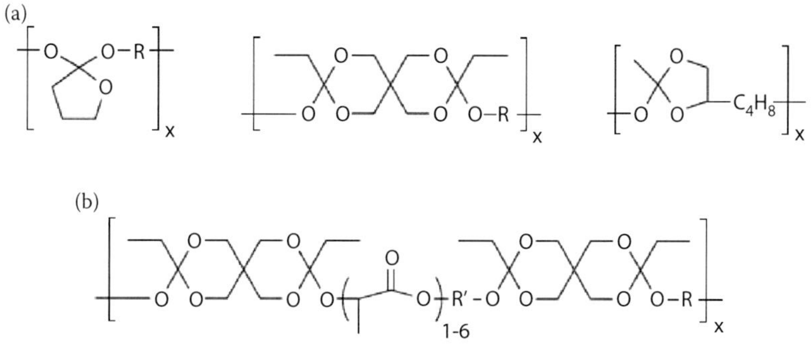

**FIGURE 5.11** The poly(orthoesters). (a) left to right: POE-I, POE-II, and POE-III. (b) POE-IV.

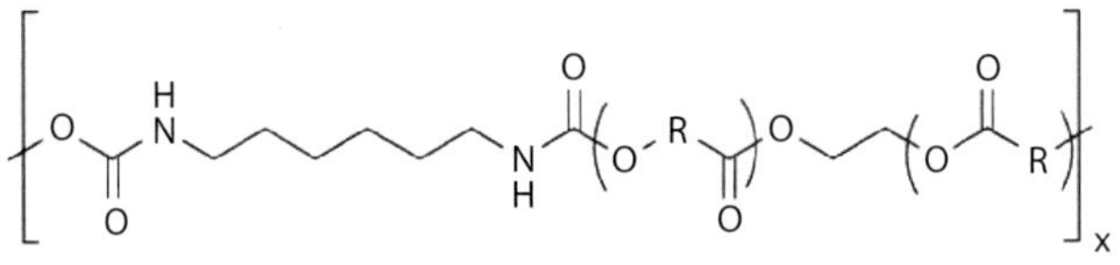

**FIGURE 5.12** The general structure of a poly(urethane), synthesized from hexamethylene diisocyanate and a poly(ester) diol.

one block (soft segment), while the small diol/diamine in conjunction with the diisocyanate forms the other (hard segment). One limitation to the use of poly(urethanes) for tissue engineering applications, however, has been the severe toxicity associated with the degradation products of the most common diisocyanate monomers. To address these concerns about toxicity, more recently, several biocompatible diisocyanates have been developed, including lysine diisocyanate, based on the natural amino acid and hexamethylene diisocyanate. Used in conjunction with biocompatible soft segments such as PCL or PEG, these materials hold much promise for the engineering of many tissues (Loh et al. 2008). Specific functionalities have also been explored for incorporation in poly(urethanes) through the use of sugars (i.e., sucrose), amino acids or even drugs as part of the hard segment or the polymer (Santerre et al. 2005).

## 5.10 Pseudo Poly(amino acids)

To better mimic natural materials, tyrosine has been used as a base for the development of a series of polymers that offer much promise for tissue engineering applications (Bourke and Kohn 2003). Desaminotyrosyl-tyrosine alkyl esters can be processed into a variety of polymers including poly(carbonates) and poly(arylates). The backbone structure contains an amide bond (linking the tyrosine and desaminotyrosine) and the carbonate or arylate (ester) bond (Figure 5.13). The polymers are produced by step growth polymerization and usually have a polydispersity between 1.4 and 1.8. Having a biphenolic monomer structure lends the polymer the ability to have the robust mechanical properties that are accessible for other commercial plastics, whereas the use of tyrosine as the base for the monomer enables biocompatibility. Varying the side chain alkyl length and diacid linkage (for arylates) further enhances the mechanical properties. Indeed, different versions of these polymers can range from amorphous to liquid crystalline. As a result of the hydrophobicity of the backbone, the water content of

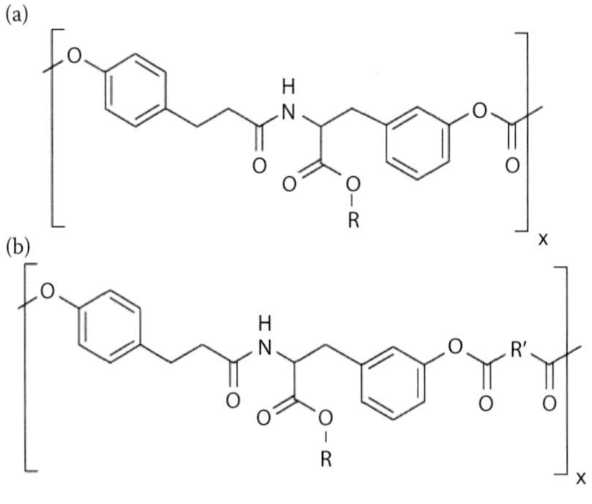

**FIGURE 5.13** Pseudo poly(amino acids). Poly(carbonate) (a) and poly(arylate) (b) desaminotyrosyl-tyrosine copolymers. The R group is usually an alkyl chain.

the polymers is also quite low, remaining at only a few percent, leading to very slow degradation times. In addition, because the monomers themselves are relatively water insoluble, mass loss is also very slow, even though there is some bulk degradation. The degradation products also have fewer equivalents of acid compared with the poly(α-esters), which should lead to less inflammation at a site of implantation. To increase the water content, PEG has been incorporated into the backbone of the polymer through the ether or carbonate linkages. In addition, the inclusion of PEG increased the degradation rate of the polymer and decreased the mechanical stiffness. These PEGylated materials are being further explored for self-assembly for drug delivery and soft tissue engineering applications and in medical devices (Johnson et al. 2010, Sheihet et al. 2007, Yu and Kohn 1999).

## 5.11 Poly(acrylates) and Poly(methacrylates)

In addition to the use of acrylates as a route to cross-linking PEG as described above, small molecule acrylates can also be polymerized to form materials useful for tissue engineering. Poly(methacrylates) were first developed for use as bone cements and dental sealants, forming hard, hydrophobic, insoluble materials upon cross-linking (Anseth et al. 1995, Mousa et al. 2000). More recently, (meth)acrylates have been developed for more advanced tissue engineering applications. The properties of poly(acrylates) and poly(methacrylates) are highly influenced by the pendant side group (Figure 5.14). When the side chains are hydrophilic, such as hydroxyethyl, short chains of PEG or the free acid, the resulting materials are highly hydrophilic and form hydrogels upon cross-linking (Guvendiren et al. 2009). Conversely, saturated hydrocarbon or aromatic ring (i.e., butyl methacrylate or benzyl methacrylate) side chains lend the polymer a hydrophobic character, insolubility in water, and depending on the exact side chain, the polymer can also be quite crystalline. As the backbone of poly(acrylates) and poly(methacrylates) are saturated hydrocarbons, there is no route for degradation of the backbone polymer in a physiological environment. Consequently, hydrophobic materials are very slowly degrading *in vivo*. Hydrophilic poly(acrylates) and poly(methacrylates) are generally water soluble unless cross-linked, and cross-linked versions can only degrade when degradable units are included in the cross-linker.

Responsive (meth)acrylates have also been developed, offering responses to light and pH. 2-Nitrobenzyl (meth)acrylate is a light-sensitive, protected form of (meth)acrylic acid (Doh and Irvine

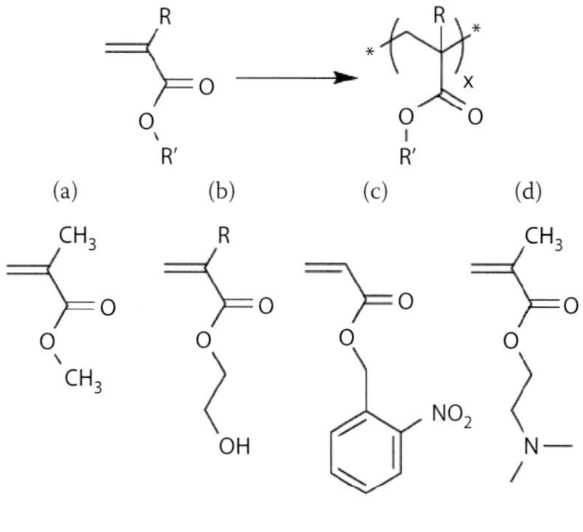

**FIGURE 5.14** (Top) Acrylates (R=H) and methacrylates (R=CH₃) polymerize to form poly(acrylates) and poly(methacrylates), which have saturated hydrocarbon backbones. (Bottom) Four common (meth)acrylate monomers. (a) Methyl methacrylate is a hydrophobic monomer commonly used in bone cements. (b) 2-Hydroxyethyl(meth) acrylate is a hydrophilic monomer used in soft tissue engineering. (c) 2-Nitrobenzyl acrylate is a protected form of acrylic acid and deprotects upon exposure to UV light. (d) 2-Dimethylaminoethyl methacrylate is a pH-sensitive monomer.

2004). When polymerized, due to the presence of the 2-nitrobenzyl group, the polymer is highly hydrophobic. However, on exposure to UV light, the 2-nitrobenzyl moiety is cleaved, producing (meth)acrylic acid, which is highly hydrophilic. This polymer (or copolymers of it) has been useful for producing materials where UV light can be used to spatially and temporally alter the hydrophilicity of the material. Poly(methacrylates) containing secondary and tertiary amines in their side chains offer pH responsiveness (Lee et al. 1999). At elevated (and neutral) pH, the amines are uncharged, lending a hydrophobic character to the polymer. However, on dropping the pH, the polymer quickly becomes charged through protonation of the amines, making the material hydrophilic. These materials offer a route to enhanced cellular delivery of drugs and proteins, as only in the lower pH of the endosome does the polymer become charged, making the delivery vehicle dissolve or swell and release its contents (Hu et al. 2007).

Poly(acrylates) and poly(methacrylates) are synthesized through chain growth or living mechanisms. The most common route to their preparation is free radical polymerization. However, to obtain higher molecular weights with more narrow dispersities, living routes (either living radical or anionic) must be used, which stabilize the reactive, growing species. There are several well-established living radical polymerization routes. Atom transfer radical polymerization uses a transition metal catalyst (usually copper) that sits in equilibrium between two oxidation states to coordinate and stabilize the growing radical (Coessens et al. 2001). As the non-radical oxidation state is preferred in the equilibrium, the progression of the reaction is stabilized, leading to fewer side and termination reactions compared with normal free radical polymerization. Homeolytic scission of an alkyl-halide bond by the catalyst initiates the reaction, and the halide is carried throughout the polymerization, remaining present even at termination. Two other living radical polymerization routes are reversible addition-fragmentation chain transfer (RAFT) and nitroxide-mediated polymerizations (NMP). RAFT stabilizes growing radicals through the reversible addition and fragmentation of the radical across the C–S double bond of a chain transfer agent, a di- or tri-thiocarbonyl compound (Moad et al. 2005). The reduction in number of actively growing species (compared with temporarily dormant species) allows for the reaction to proceed in a living manner. NMP stabilizes the reaction by temporarily deactivating the growing polymer chain and a nitroxide scavenger reversibly accepting the free radical (Sciannamea et al. 2008). As nitroxide radicals are very stable, side reactions are diminished and the number of growing chains at any given time is reduced. However, NMP is somewhat limited by the number of commercially available initiators. The full details of these mechanisms are beyond the scope of this chapter, but several excellent reviews, referenced above, have been written on atom transfer radical polymerization, RAFT, and NMP.

## 5.12 Non-Polymeric Synthetic Biomaterials

Although the majority of synthetic materials explored for applications in tissue engineering are polymers, several research groups have explored the use of non-polymeric synthetic materials that can be processed into materials conducive to tissue engineering applications.

As a greater class, poly(peptides) are generally considered to be natural materials. However, with the advent and optimization of solid phase synthesis techniques, many peptides now being explored for tissue engineering can be considered synthetic. In addition, while in the natural sphere peptides are usually confined to containing only the canonical 20 L-amino acids, solid phase synthesis has allowed for the facile introduction of many other unnatural amino acids, further increasing the possible sequences available. Synthetic peptides have generally been explored in two arenas: in conjunction with other materials to enhance their properties or as stand-alone self-assembling materials. Many biologically relevant proteins have short consensus sequences that can be synthesized to modify non-bioactive materials. The most common sequence is the RGD (arginine-glycine-aspartic acid), an integrin-binding domain from the extracellular matrix protein fibronectin (Hersel et al. 2003, Hubbell 1995). Many variations of this three-amino acid sequence have been explored to couple the peptide to various materials and to enhance its binding properties. Cysteine residues can be used to couple the peptide to synthetic materials containing maleiimide, vinyl sulfone, or acrylate groups through Michael addition. Multiple cysteine residues have also been used to lock the RGD into a specific conformation through introduction of a disulfide bridge in the peptide. Many other peptides have been explored as well to enhance specific functionality of a biomaterial, including IKVAV and YIGSR (laminin peptides). In addition to introducing side functionality to materials, short peptides have also been used to cross-link synthetic and natural materials, providing a route for cellular remodeling of scaffolds. For example, many groups have explored the use of MMP-sensitive peptides to cross-link hydrogels, where cross-links are cleaved by cellular produced MMPs (Khetan et al. 2009, Lutolf et al. 2003).

Non-naturally occurring peptides have also been developed that self-assemble into hydrogels through non-covalent interactions within the peptides (Charati et al. 2009). Such peptides have been engineered on multiple length scales, ranging from short oligomers that can interact and assemble through pi-stacking of aromatic residues to large peptides containing helical domains that interact, providing a route to physical cross-linking. Many of these larger peptides are too large to produce using solid phase routes and therefore require synthesis using molecular biology techniques, limiting the choice of amino acids and sequences to those that are naturally occurring. Recently there have been several advances in improving molecular biology to enable the addition of unnatural amino acids through directed evolution of tRNA–tRNA synthetase pairs toward the desired unnatural amino acid (Wang and Schultz 2005). However, such advances still do not offer the same variety that can be obtained through solid phase techniques.

In addition to synthesizing self-assembling peptides, several groups have begun to look at peptide derivatives for applications in medicine, for example a class of materials known as peptide amphiphiles (Cui et al. 2010, Hartgerink et al. 2002). An example peptide amphiphile is shown in Figure 5.15. These materials are surfactant hybrids of peptides and lipids. Under physiological conditions, the peptide amphiphiles self assemble, undergoing a hydrophobic condensation of the lipid tail and hydrophobic amino acid residues while being stabilized in solution by the hydrophilic peptide residues at the terminus of the amphiphile. Most often the peptide amphiphiles assemble to form long fibers in solution, where entanglement of the fibers causes gelation of the material. Use of consensus sequences (such as those described above) in the peptide portion of the material allows for the creation of bioactive hydrogels that promote cell infiltration and growth.

Moving still a little further away from basic poly(peptide) structure are poly(peptoids), developed by the Barron group at Stanford University (Kirshenbaum et al. 1998, Patch and Barron 2002). Unlike typical peptides, poly(peptoids) have a structure in which rather than being on the α-carbon, the amino acid side chain is attached to the amine itself, forming a tertiary amine (Figure 5.16). Similar to synthetic peptides, they can be synthesized in a facile manner on a solid phase peptide synthesizer. The Barron group has found that these materials can be good mimics for naturally occurring peptides while avoiding significant recognition by the immune system and offering enhanced biostability. This is an example

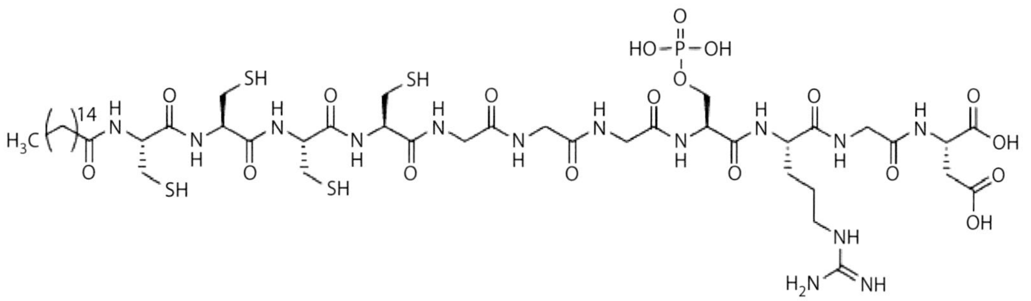

**FIGURE 5.15** A self-assembling peptide amphiphile. Upon exposure to salts, the amphiphile self-assembles into fibers, entangling to form a gel. The fibers can be stabilized by oxidation of the SH groups on the cysteines. The RGD head of the amphiphile encourages cell binding and the phosphate encourages mineralization. (Adapted from Hartgerink, J. D., E. Beniash, and S. I. Stupp 2002. *Proceedings of the National Academy of Sciences of the United States of America.* 99: 5133–38.)

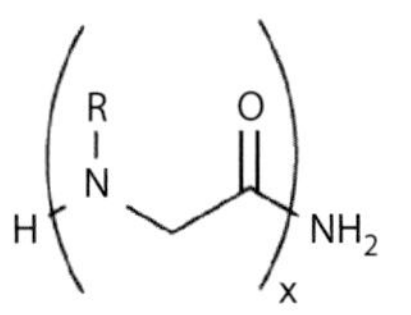

**FIGURE 5.16** The basic structure of a poly(peptoid), in which the R group of the peptide is attached to the amine rather than the α-carbon.

of materials that have enhanced complexity and may lead to more improved structures for tissue engineering applications in the future.

## 5.13 Conclusions

As chemistry advances our ability to design novel monomers and routes to polymerization, the quality and quantity of materials available for research in tissue engineering will continue to increase. Early, classical polymers and polymeric materials have pushed open the door for the development of and advances in tissue engineering as a field. However, while these classical polymers have been utilized for early applications in the field, as research progresses, it appears as though further advances in the smart design of polymers and their resulting materials will better enhance our ability to improve, restore, and replace damaged tissue function.

## References

Albertsson, A. C. and S. Lundmark 1988. Synthesis of poly(adipic anhydride) by use of ketene. *Journal of Macromolecular Science-Chemistry.* A25: 247–58.

Anderson, D. G., C. A. Tweedie, N. Hossain et al. 2006. A combinatorial library of photocrosslinkable and degradable materials. *Advanced Materials.* 18: 2614–18.

Anseth, K. S., S. M. Newman, and C. N. Bowman 1995. Polymeric dental composites: Properties and reaction behavior of multimethacrylate dental restorations. *Advances in Polymer Science.* 122: 177–217.

Bourke, S. L. and J. Kohn 2003. Polymers derived from the amino acid L-tyrosine: Polycarbonates, polyarylates and copolymers with poly(ethylene glycol). *Advanced Drug Delivery Reviews.* 55: 447–66.

Brey, D. M., C. Chung, K. D. Hankenson, J. P. Garino, and J. A. Burdick 2010. Identification of osteoconductive and biodegradable polymers from a combinatorial polymer library. *Journal of Biomedical Materials Research Part A.* 93A: 807–16.

Burdick, J. A. and K. S. Anseth 2002. Photoencapsulation of osteoblasts in injectable RGD-modified PEG hydrogels for bone tissue engineering. *Biomaterials.* 23: 4315–23.

Cerritelli, S., D. Velluto, and J. A. Hubbell 2007. PEG-SS-PPS: Reduction-sensitive disulfide block copolymer vesicles for intracellular drug delivery. *Biomacromolecules.* 8: 1966–72.

Charati, M. B., J. L. Ifkovits, J. A. Burdick, J. G. Linhardt, and K. L. Kiick 2009. Hydrophilic elastomeric biomaterials based on resilin-like polypeptides. *Soft Matter.* 5: 3412–16.

Coessens, V., T. Pintauer, and K. Matyjaszewski 2001. Functional polymers by atom transfer radical polymerization. *Progress in Polymer Science.* 26: 337–77.

Cui, H. G., M. J. Webber, and S. I. Stupp 2010. Self-assembly of peptide amphiphiles: From molecules to nanostructures to biomaterials. *Biopolymers.* 94: 1–18.

Doh, J. and D. J. Irvine 2004. Photogenerated polyelectrolyte bilayers from an aqueous-processible photoresist for multicomponent protein patterning. *Journal of the American Chemical Society.* 126: 9170–71.

Domb, A. J. 1990. Biodegradable polymers derived from amino-acids. *Biomaterials.* 11: 686–89.

Domb, A. J. and R. Nudelman 1995. Biodegradable polymers derived from natural fatty-acids. *Journal of Polymer Science Part A-Polymer Chemistry.* 33: 717–25.

Drury, J. L. and D. J. Mooney 2003. Hydrogels for tissue engineering: Scaffold design variables and applications. *Biomaterials.* 24: 4337–51.

Erdmann, L. and K. E. Uhrich 2000. Synthesis and degradation characteristics of salicylic acid-derived poly(anhydride-esters). *Biomaterials.* 21: 1941–46.

Frazier, D. D., V. K. Lathi, T. N. Gerhart, and W. C. Hayes 1997. Ex vivo degradation of a poly(propylene glycol-fumarate) biodegradable particulate composite bone cement. *Journal of Biomedical Materials Research.* 35: 383–89.

Gresser, J. D., S. H. Hsu, H. Nagaoka et al. 1995. Analysis of a vinyl pyrrolidone poly(propylene fumarate) resorbable bone-cement. *Journal of Biomedical Materials Research.* 29: 1241–47.

Griffith, L. G. 2000. Polymeric biomaterials. *Acta Materialia.* 48: 263–77.

Guvendiren, M., S. Yang, and J. A. Burdick 2009. Swelling-induced surface patterns in hydrogels with gradient crosslinking density. *Advanced Functional Materials.* 19: 3038–45.

Hartgerink, J. D., E. Beniash, and S. I. Stupp 2002. Peptide-amphiphile nanofibers: A versatile scaffold for the preparation of self-assembling materials. *Proceedings of the National Academy of Sciences of the United States of America.* 99: 5133–38.

Heller, J., J. Barr, S. Y. Ng, K. S. Abdellauoi, and R. Gurny 2002. Poly(ortho esters): Synthesis, characterization, properties and uses. *Advanced Drug Delivery Reviews.* 54: 1015–39.

Hern, D. L. and J. A. Hubbell 1998. Incorporation of adhesion peptides into nonadhesive hydrogels useful for tissue resurfacing. *Journal of Biomedical Materials Research.* 39: 266–76.

Hersel, U., C. Dahmen, and H. Kessler 2003. RGD modified polymers: Biomaterials for stimulated cell adhesion and beyond. *Biomaterials.* 24: 4385–415.

Hu, Y., T. Litwin, A. R. Nagaraja et al. 2007. Cytosolic delivery of membrane-impermeable molecules in dendritic cells using PH-responsive core-shell nanoparticles. *Nano Letters.* 7: 3056–64.

Hubbell, J. A. 1995. Biomaterials in tissue engineering. *Bio-Technology.* 13: 565–76.

Ifkovits, J. L., R. F. Padera, and J. A. Burdick 2008. Biodegradable and radically polymerized elastomers with enhanced processing capabilities. *Biomedical Materials.* 3: 034104.

Johnson, P. A., A. Luk, A. Demtchouk et al. 2010. Interplay of anionic charge, poly(ethylene glycol), and iodinated tyrosine incorporation within tyrosine-derived polycarbonates: Effects on vascular smooth muscle cell adhesion, proliferation, and motility. *Journal of Biomedical Materials Research Part A.* 93A: 505–14.

Katz, J. S. and J. A. Burdick 2010. Light-responsive biomaterials: Development and applications. *Macromolecular Bioscience.* 10: 339–48.

Khetan, S., J. S. Katz, and J. A. Burdick 2009. Sequential crosslinking to control cellular spreading in 3-dimensional hydrogels. *Soft Matter.* 5: 1601–06.

Kirshenbaum, K., A. E. Barron, R. A. Goldsmith et al. 1998. Sequence-specific polypeptoids: A diverse family of heteropolymers with stable secondary structure. *Proceedings of the National Academy of Sciences of the United States of America.* 95: 4303–08.

Kloxin, A. M., A. M. Kasko, C. N. Salinas, and K. S. Anseth 2009. Photodegradable hydrogels for dynamic tuning of physical and chemical properties. *Science.* 324: 59–63.

Kumar, N., R. S. Langer, and A. J. Domb 2002. Polyanhydrides: An overview. *Advanced Drug Delivery Reviews.* 54: 889–910.

Labet, M. and W. Thielemans 2009. Synthesis of polycaprolactone: A review. *Chemical Society Reviews.* 38: 3484–504.

Langer, R. and D. A. Tirrell 2004. Designing materials for biology and medicine. *Nature.* 428: 487–92.

Lee, A. S., A. P. Gast, V. Butun, and S. P. Armes 1999. Characterizing the structure of PH dependent polyelectrolyte block copolymer micelles. *Macromolecules.* 32: 4302–10.

Lee, H. and T. G. Park 1998. Reduction/oxidation induced cleavable/crosslinkable temperature-sensitive hydrogel network containing disulfide linkages. *Polymer Journal.* 30: 976–80.

Li, S. M. 1999. Hydrolytic degradation characteristics of aliphatic polyesters derived from lactic and glycolic acids. *Journal of Biomedical Materials Research.* 48: 342–53.

Loh, X. J., K. B. C. Sng, and J. Li 2008. Synthesis and water-swelling of thermo-responsive poly(ester urethane)s containing poly(epsilon-caprolactone), poly(ethylene glycol) and poly(propylene glycol). *Biomaterials.* 29: 3185–94.

Lutolf, M. P. and J. A. Hubbell 2005. Synthetic biomaterials as instructive extracellular microenvironments for morphogenesis in tissue engineering. *Nature Biotechnology.* 23: 47–55.

Lutolf, M. P., J. L. Lauer-Fields, H. G. Schmoekel et al. 2003. Synthetic matrix metalloproteinase-sensitive hydrogels for the conduction of tissue regeneration: Engineering cell-invasion characteristics. *Proceedings of the National Academy of Sciences of the United States of America.* 100: 5413–18.

Maniar, M., X. D. Xie, and A. J. Domb 1990. Polyanhydrides. 5. Branched polyanhydrides. *Biomaterials.* 11: 690–94.

Metters, A. T., K. S. Anseth, and C. N. Bowman 2000. Fundamental studies of a novel, biodegradable PEG-b-PLA hydrogel. *Polymer.* 41: 3993–4004.

Miller, J. S., C. J. Shen, W. R. Legant et al. 2010. Bioactive hydrogels made from step-growth derived PEG-peptide macromers. *Biomaterials.* 31: 3736–43.

Moad, G., E. Rizzardo, and S. H. Thang 2005. Living radical polymerization by the raft process. *Australian Journal of Chemistry.* 58: 379–410.

Mousa, W. F., M. Kobayashi, S. Shinzato et al. 2000. Biological and mechanical properties of PMMA-based bioactive bone cements. *Biomaterials.* 21: 2137–46.

Muggli, D. S., A. K. Burkoth, and K. S. Anseth 1999. Crosslinked polyanhydrides for use in orthopedic applications: Degradation behavior and mechanics. *Journal of Biomedical Materials Research.* 46: 271–78.

Nair, L. S. and C. T. Laurencin 2007. Biodegradable polymers as biomaterials. *Progress in Polymer Science.* 32: 762–98.

Odian, G. 2004. *Principles of polymerization.* Hoboken, NJ: John Wiley & Sons, Inc.

Patch, J. A. and A. E. Barron 2002. Mimicry of bioactive peptides via non-natural, sequence-specific peptidomimetic oligomers. *Current Opinion in Chemical Biology.* 6: 872–77.

Ratner, B. D. and S. J. Bryant 2004. Biomaterials: Where we have been and where we are going. *Annual Review of Biomedical Engineering.* 6: 41–75.

Santerre, J. P., K. Woodhouse, G. Laroche, and R. S. Labow 2005. Understanding the biodegradation of polyurethanes: From classical implants to tissue engineering materials. *Biomaterials.* 26: 7457–70.

Sawhney, A. S., C. P. Pathak, and J. A. Hubbell 1993. Bioerodible hydrogels based on photopolymerized poly(ethylene glycol)-co-poly(alpha-hydroxy acid) diacrylate macromers. *Macromolecules.* 26: 581–87.

Sciannamea, V., R. Jerome, and C. Detrembleur 2008. In-situ nitroxide-mediated radical polymerization (NMP) processes: Their understanding and optimization. *Chemical Reviews.* 108: 1104–26.

Sheihet, L., K. Piotrowska, R. A. Dubin, J. Kohn and D. Devore 2007. Effect of tyrosine-derived triblock copolymer compositions on nanosphere self-assembly and drug delivery. *Biomacromolecules.* 8: 998–1003.

Shin, H., S. Jo, and A. G. Mikos 2003. Biomimetic materials for tissue engineering. *Biomaterials.* 24: 4353–64.

Suggs, L. J., R. G. Payne, M. J. Yaszemski, L. B. Alemany, and A. G. Mikos 1997. Synthesis and characterization of a block copolymer consisting of poly(propylene fumarate) and poly(ethylene glycol). *Macromolecules.* 30: 4318–23.

Temenoff, J. S. and A. G. Mikos 2000. Injectable biodegradable materials for orthopedic tissue engineering. *Biomaterials.* 21: 2405–12.

Wang, L. and P. G. Schultz 2005. Expanding the genetic code. *Angewandte Chemie-International Edition.* 44: 34–66.

Wang, Y. D., Y. M. Kim, and R. Langer 2003. In vivo degradation characteristics of poly(glycerol sebacate). *Journal of Biomedical Materials Research Part A.* 66A: 192–97.

Wolfe, M. S., D. Dean, J. E. Chen et al. 2002. In vitro degradation and fracture toughness of multilayered porous poly(propylene fumarate)/beta-tricalcium phosphate scaffolds. *Journal of Biomedical Materials Research.* 61: 159–64.

Yu, C. and J. Kohn 1999. Tyrosine-PEG-derived poly(ether carbonate)s as new biomaterials—Part I: Synthesis and evaluation. *Biomaterials.* 20: 253–64.

Zhang, Z., R. Kuijer, S. K. Bulstra, D. W. Grijpma, and J. Feijen 2006. The in vivo and in vitro degradation behavior of poly(trimethylene carbonate). *Biomaterials.* 27: 1741–48.

# 6

# Growth Factors and Morphogens: Signals for Tissue Engineering

6.1 Introduction ................................................................. 6-1
6.2 Tissue Engineering and Morphogenesis ...................................... 6-1
6.3 The Bone Morphogenetic Proteins............................................ 6-2
6.4 Growth Factors.............................................................. 6-3
6.5 BMPs Bind to Extracellular Matrix ......................................... 6-3
6.6 Clinical Applications....................................................... 6-4
6.7 Challenges and Opportunities................................................ 6-4
Acknowledgments................................................................. 6-4
References...................................................................... 6-4

A. Hari Reddi
*University of
California, Davis*

## 6.1 Introduction

Tissue engineering is the exciting discipline of design and construction of spare parts for the human body to restore function based on biology and biomedical engineering. The basis of tissue engineering is the triad of signals for tissue induction, responding stem cells, and the scaffolding of extracellular matrix. Among the many tissues in the human body, bone has the highest power of regeneration and therefore is a prototype model for tissue engineering based on morphogenesis. Morphogenesis is the developmental cascade of pattern formation, body plan establishment, and culmination of the adult body form. The cascade of bone morphogenesis in the embryo is recapitulated by demineralized bone matrix-induced bone formation. The inductive signals for bone morphogenesis, the bone morphogenetic proteins (BMPs) were isolated from demineralized bone matrix. BMPs and related cartilage-derived morphogenetic proteins (CDMPs) initiate cartilage and bone formation. The promotion and maintenance of the initiated skeleton is regulated by several growth factors. Tissue engineering is the symbiosis of signals (growth factors and morphogens), stem cells, and scaffolds (extracellular matrix). The rules of architecture for tissue engineering are a true imitation of principles of developmental biology and morphogenesis.

## 6.2 Tissue Engineering and Morphogenesis

An understanding of the molecular principles of development and morphogenesis, is a prerequisite for tissue engineering. We define tissue engineering as the science of design and manufacture of new tissues for functional restoration of the impaired organs and replacement of lost parts due to disease, trauma, and tumors [1]. Tissue engineering is based on principles of developmental biology and morphogenesis, biomedical engineering, and biomechanics.

Morphogenesis is initiated by morphogens. The promotion and maintenance of morphogenesis is achieved by a variety of growth factors. Generally, morphogens are first identified in fly and frog embryos by genetic approaches, differential displays, and subtractive hybridization expression cloning. An alternate biochemical approach of "grind and find" from adult mammalian bone led to the isolation of BMPs, the premier signals for bone morphogenesis. We now discuss the identification, isolation, and molecular cloning of BMPs from a natural biomaterial, the demineralized bone matrix.

## 6.3 The Bone Morphogenetic Proteins

Bone grafts have been used to aid the healing of recalcitrant fractures. Demineralized bone matrix induced new bone formation. Bone induction by demineralized bone matrix is a sequential cascade [2–4]. The key steps in this cascade are chemotaxis of progenitor cells, proliferation of progenitor cells, and finally differentiation first into cartilage and then bone. The demineralized bone matrix is devoid of any living cells and is a biomaterial that elicits new bone formation. The insoluble collagenous bone matrix binds plasma fibronectin [3] and promotes the proliferation of cells. Proliferation was maximal on day 3, chondroblast differentiation was evident on day 5, and chondrocytes were abundant on day 7. The cartilage hypotrophied on day 9 with concominant vascular invasion and osteogenesis. On days 10–12 maximal alkaline phosphatase activity, a marker of bone formation, was observed. Hematopoietic differentiation was observed in the ossicle on day 21. The sequential bone development cascade is reminiscent of bone morphogenesis in limb.

A systematic study of the biochemical basis of bone induction was initiated. A bioassay for bone induction was established *in vivo* in rats. The insoluble demineralized bone matrix was extracted in 4-M guanidine hydrochloride, a dissociative extractant. About 3% of the proteins were solubilized and the rest was the insoluble residue. The extract and the residue alone were unable to induce bone formation. However, reconstitution of the extract to residue yielded new bone morphogenesis. Thus, there is collaboration between soluble signals and the insoluble matrix scaffold to yield new bone formation [5,6]. This key experiment predates the term tissue engineering and demonstrates the collaboration of soluble signals and insoluble scaffolding as a critical concept in practical tissue engineering. Collagen appears to be an optimal scaffold [7]. The bone induction is dependent on the hormonal status including vitamin D [8,9]. Irradiation of the recipient blocked the cellular cascade of osteogenesis [10].

This bioassay was a critical development in the quest for the purification of the bioactive bone morphogens, the BMPs [11–15]. There are nearly 15 members of BMPs in the human genome (Table 6.1). BMPs are dimeric molecules with a single disulfide bond. The mature monomer consists of seven canonical cysteines contributing to three interchain disulfides and one interchain disulfide bond.

BMPs stimulate chondrogenesis in limb bud mesodermal cells [16]. BMP 2 stimulates osteoblast maturation [17]. BMPs are chemotactic for human monocytes [18]. In addition to initiating chondrogenesis, BMPs maintain proteoglycan biosynthesis in bovine articular cartilage explants [19,20]. Recombinant human growth/differentiation factors (GDF-5) stimulate chondrogenesis during limb development [21].

BMPs interact with BMP receptors I and II on the cell surface/membrane [1,22]. BMP receptors are serine/threonine kinases. The intracellular substrates for these kinases called Smads function as relays to activate the transcriptional machinery [23]. The three functional classes are (1) receptor-regulated Smads, namely, Smads 1, 5, and 8; (2) the common partner Smad—4; and (3) the inhibitory Smads 6 and 7. There are Smad-dependent and independent pathways for activation of BMP signaling including new bone formation.

**TABLE 6.1**  The BMP Family in Mammals[a]

| BMP Subfamily | Generic Name | BMP Designation |
|---|---|---|
| BMP 2/4 | BMP-2A | BMP-2 |
| | BMP-2B | BMP-4 |
| BMP-3 | Osteogenin | BMP-3 |
| | GDF-10 | BMP-3B |
| OP-1/BMP-7 | BMP-5 | BMP-5 |
| | Vegetal related-1 (Vgr-1) | BMP-6 |
| | Osteogenic protein-1 (OP-1) | BMP-7 |
| | Osteogenic protein-1 (OP-2) | BMP-8 |
| | Osteogenic protein-1 (OP-3) | BMP-8B |
| | GDF-2 | BMP-9 |
| | BMP-10 | BMP-10 |
| | GDF-11 | BMP-11 |
| GDF-5,6,7 | GDF-7 or cartilage-derived morphogenetic protein-3 (CDMP-3) | BMP-12 |
| | GDF-6 or cartilage-derived morphogenetic protein-2 (CDMP-2) | BMP-13 |
| | GDF-5 or cartilage-derived morphogenetic protein-1 (CDMP-1) | BMP-14 |
| | BMP-15 | BMP-15 |

[a] BMP-1 is not a BMP family member with seven canonical cysteines. It is a procollagen-C proteinase related to *Drosophila* tolloid.

# 6.4 Growth Factors

Growth factors are proteins with profound influence on proliferation and growth of cells. Growth factors stimulate the differentiation of progenitor/stem cells. The growth factors include many subgroups and such as insulin-like growth factors (IGFs), fibroblast growth factors (FGFs), and platelet-derived growth factors (PDGFs).

IGFs are polypeptides related to insulin. There are two members, IGF-I and IGF-II. The liver is the predominant site of IGF-I synthesis, and is stimulated by pituitary growth hormone. IGF biological activity is modulated by IGF-binding proteins. There are six different IGF-binding proteins. IGFs promote extracellular matrix biosynthesis by osteoblasts.

FGFs are proteins with multiple members. FGFs are mitogens for endothelial cells. Along with vascular endothelial growth factors, FGFs are critical for bone formation. It is well known that vascular invasion is a prerequisite for endochodral bone formation.

PDGFs come in three isoforms, namely, AA, AB, and BB. They are primarily produced by platelets in blood. Various isoforms stimulate bone formation.

# 6.5 BMPs Bind to Extracellular Matrix

The critical role of extracellular matrix in morphogenesis of many tissues during development is well known. The extracellular matrix is a supramolecular assembly of collagens, proteoglycans, and glycoproteins. The collagens are tissue specific and the proteoglycans include chondroitin sulfate, dermatan sulfate, heparan sulfate/heparin, and keratan sufate. Recombinant BMP 4 and BMP 7 bind to heparan sulfate/heparin, collagen IV of the basement membrane [24]. The binding of a soluble morphogen to insoluble extracellular matrix renders the morphogen to act locally and protects it from proteolytic degradation and therefore extends its biological half-life. Thus, extracellular matrix scaffolding is an efficient delivery system for tissue engineering. Growth factors such as FGFs bind to heparan sulfate. An emerging concept for tissue engineering is the tethering of signals to scaffolds to restrict their diffusion.

## 6.6 Clinical Applications

Recombinant BMP 2 has been approved by the Food and Drug Administration for spine fusion and open fractures of tibia due to orthopedic trauma. There have been several clinical applications of BMPs in orthopedic surgery [25–29]. The developing experience of BMPs will be of immense utility to the nascent field of tissue engineering, the science of design-based manufacture of spare parts for human skeleton based on signals, stem cells, and scaffolding [1,30] in medicine and dentistry. A prototype paradigm has validated the proof of principle for tissue engineering based on tissue transformation by BMPs and scaffolding [31,32].

## 6.7 Challenges and Opportunities

Despite the exciting advances in clinical applications of BMPs, there remain many challenges. Foremost among them is the need for developing synthetic scaffolds to deliver recombinant BMPs for skeletal tissue engineering. The development of synthetic scaffolds with an ability to respond to biomechanical influences that are known to be critical for musculoskeletal structures will lead to a quantum improvement of current tissue engineering approaches to bone, cartilage, and meniscus. The remaining challenges make the field of morphogen-based tissue engineering an exciting frontier with unlimited opportunities.

## Acknowledgments

The research in the Center for Tissue Regeneration is supported by the Lawrence Ellision Chair in Musculoskeletal Molecular Biology and grants from the NIH and DOD. I thank Danielle Neff for the outstanding help in completion of this article.

## References

1. Reddi, A.H., 1998. Role of morphogenetic proteins in skeletal tissue engineering and regeneration, *Nat. Biotechnol.*, 16, 247.
2. Reddi, A.H. and Anderson, W.A. 1976. Collagenous bone matrix-induced endochondral ossification hemopoiesis, *J. Cell Biol.*, 69, 557.
3. Weiss, R.E. and Reddi, A.H. 1980. Synthesis and localization of fibronectin during collagenous matrix-mesenchymal cell interaction and differentiation of cartilage and bone *in vivo*, *Proc. Natl. Acad. Sci. USA*, 77, 2074.
4. Reddi, A.H. 1981. Cell biology and biochemistry of endochondral bone development, *Coll. Relat. Res.*, 1, 209.
5. Sampath, T.K. and Reddi, A.H. 1981. Dissociative extraction and reconstitution of extracellular matrix components involved in local bone differentiation, *Proc. Natl. Acad. Sci. USA*, 78, 7599.
6. Sampath, T.K. and Reddi, A.H. 1983. Homology of bone-inductive proteins from human, monkey, bovine, and rat extracellular matrix, *Proc. Natl. Acad. Sci. USA*, 80, 6591.
7. Ma, S., Chen, G., and Reddi, A.H. 1990. Collaboration between collagenous matrix and osteogenin is required for bone induction, *Ann. NY Acad. Sci.,* 580, 524.
8. Reddi, A.H. 1984. Extracellular matrix and development, in *Extracellular Matrix Biochemistry*, Piez, K.A. and Reddi, A.H. Eds., Elsevier, New York, p. 247.
9. Sampath, T.K., Wientroub, S., and Reddi, A.H. 1984. Extracellular matrix proteins involved in bone induction are vitamin D dependent, *Biochem. Biophys. Res. Commun.*, 124, 829.
10. Wientroub, S. and Reddi, A.H. 1988. Influence of irradiation on the osteoinductive potential of demineralized bone matrix, *Calcif. Tissue Int.*, 42, 255.
11. Wozney, J.M. et al. 1988. Novel regulators of bone formation: Molecular clones and activities, *Science*, 242, 1528.

12. Luyten, F.P. et al. 1989. Purification and partial amino acid sequence of osteogenin, a protein initiating bone differentiation, *J. Biol. Chem.,* 264, 13377.

13. Celeste A.J. et al. 1990. Identification of transforming growth factor beta family members present in bone-inductive protein purified from bovine bone, *Proc. Natl. Acad. Sci. USA,* 87, 9843.

14. Ozkaynak, E. et al. 1990. OP-1 cDNA encodes an osteogenic protein in the TGF-beta family, *EMBO J.,* 9, 2085.

15. Wang, E.A. et al. 1990. Recombinant human bone morphogenetic protein induces bone formation, *Proc. Natl Acad. Sci. USA*, 87, 2220.

16. Chen, P. et al. 1991. Stimulation of chondrogenesis in limb bud mesoderm cells by recombinant human bone morphogenetic protein 2B (BMP-2B) and modulation by transforming growth factor beta 1 and beta 2, *Exp. Cell Res.*, 195, 509.

17. Yamaguchi, A. et al. 1991. Recombinant human bone morphogenetic protein-2 stimulates osteoblastic maturation and inhibits myogenic differentiation *in vitro, J. Cell Biol.,* 113, 681.

18. Cunningham, N.S., Paralkar, V., and Reddi, A.H. 1992. Osteogenin and recombinant bone morphogenetic protein 2B are chemotactic for human monocytes and stimulate transforming growth factor beta 1 mRNA expression, *Proc. Natl. Acad. Sci. USA,* 89, 11740.

19. Luyten, F.P. et al. 1992. Natural bovine osteogenin and recombinant human bone morphogenetic protein-2B are equipotent in the maintenance of proteoglycans in bovine articular cartilage explant cultures, *J. Biol. Chem.,* 267, 3691.

20. Lietman, S.A. et al. 1997. Stimulation of proteoglycan synthesis in explants of porcine articular cartilage by recombinant osteogenic protein-1 (bone morphogenetic protein-7), *J. Bone Joint Surg. Am.,* 79, 1132.

21. Khouri, R.K., Koudsi, B., and Reddi, A.H. 1991. *M* Tissue transformation into bone *in vivo* a potential practical application, *JAMA,* 266, 1953.

22. ten Dijke, P. et al. 1994. Identification of type I receptors for osteogenic protein-1 and bone morphogenetic protein-4, *J. Biol. Chem.,* 269, 16985.

23. Imamura T. et al. 1997. Smad6 inhibits signalling by the TGF-beta superfamily (see comments), *Nature,* 389, 622.

24. Paralkar, V.M. et al. 1990. Interaction of osteogenin, a heparin binding bone morphogenetic protein, with type IV collagen, *J. Biol. Chem.,* 265, 17281.

25. Einhorn, T.A. 2003. Clinical applications of recombinant BMPs: Early experience and future development, *J. Bone Joint Surg.,* 85A, 82.

26. Li, R.H. and Wozney, J.M. 2001. Delivering on the promise of bone morphogenetic proteins, *Trends Biotechnol.,* 19, 255.

27. Ripamonti, U., Ma, S., and Reddi A.H. 1992. The critical role of geometry of porous hydroxyapatite delivery system in induction of bone by osteogenin, a bone morphogenetic protein, *Matrix,* 12, 202.

28. Geesink, R.G., Hoefnagels, N.H., and Bulstra, S.K. 1999. Osteogenic activity of OP1, bone morphogenetic protein 7 (BMP 7) in a human fibular defect, *J. Bone Joint Surg.,* 81, 710.

29. Friedlaender, G.E. et al. 2001. Osteogenic protein 1 (bone morphogenic protein 7) in the treatment of tibial non-unions, *J. Bone Joint Surg. Am.,* 83A, S151.

30. Govender et al. 2002. Recombinant human bone morphogenetic protein 2 for treatment of open tibiol fractures: A prospective, controlled, randomized study of four hundred and fifty patients. *J. Bone Joint Surg. Am.*, 84A, 2123.

31. Nakashima, M. and Reddi, A.H. 2003. The application of bone morphogenetic protein to dental tissue engineering, *Nat. Biotechnol.*, 21, 1025.

32. Khouri, R.K., Koudsi, B., and Reddi, A.H. 1991. Tissue transformation into bone *in vivo*: A potential practical application. *JAMA,* 266, 1953.

# 7

# Signal Expression in Engineered Tissues

7.1  Introduction ..................................................................................7-1
7.2  Biology of Osteoblasts.................................................................7-1
      Bone Extracellular Matrix
7.3  Biology of Chondrocytes ............................................................ 7-4
      Cartilage ECM
7.4  Signaling Pathway Overview ...................................................... 7-4
7.5  Anabolic Growth Factors/Cytokines........................................... 7-5
      Insulin-Like Growth Factor • TGF-β Superfamily • VEGF,
      Platelet-Derived Growth Factor, and Fibroblastic Growth Factor
7.6  Catabolic Growth Factors/Cytokines.........................................7-10
      Interleukin-1 • Interleukin-6 • Tumor Necrosis Factor
7.7  Hormones.................................................................................. 7-13
      Growth Hormone and Parathyroid Hormone • Adiponectin
7.8  Mechanotransduction................................................................7-14
      Osteoblasts • Chondrocytes
7.9  Dual Growth Factor Studies ......................................................7-16
7.10 Conclusion ...............................................................................7-17
References....................................................................................7-17

**Martha O. Wang**
*University of Maryland*

**John P. Fisher**
*University of Maryland*

## 7.1 Introduction

Current trends in tissue engineering focus on the impact of exogenous and endogenous signals on cells seeded in scaffolds. To fully understand the potential impact of these signaling molecules we must first review their signal expression pathways. In this chapter we focus on two of the most common cells used in skeletal tissue engineering, osteoblasts and chondrocytes. We will discuss the basic biology of the skeletal system and investigate the impact of the different signaling molecules such as hormones, cytokines, growth factors, and the mechanotransduction signaling pathway on cell phenotype and gene expression.

In tissue engineering the implementation of a successful tissue scaffold is dependent on three factors: an appropriate cell type, developing a scaffold to mimic the surrounding tissue, and then using cell signaling to drive cells to express the correct phenotype and genes. Through understanding of the signals that impact osteoblast and chondrocyte functions we can improve *in vivo* use of engineered tissue scaffolds (Table 7.1).

## 7.2 Biology of Osteoblasts

### 7.2.1 Bone Extracellular Matrix

The skeleton's primary purpose is to provide structural support: however, its secondary purpose is metabolic (Rubin et al., 2006). These purposes are accomplished through maintenance of a rigid skeletal

**TABLE 7.1** List of Abbreviations

| | |
|---|---|
| Akt | v-akt murine thymoma viral oncogene homolog |
| ALP | Alkaline phosphatase |
| BAD | BCL2-associated agonist of cell death |
| BAX | BCL2-associated X protein |
| BCL-2 | B-cell chronic lymphocytic leukemia/lymphoma 2 |
| BMP | Bone morphogenic protein |
| CD44 | CD44 molecule (Indian blood group) |
| c-fos | FBJ osteosarcoma oncogene |
| ECM | Extracellular matrix |
| ERK | Extracellular signal-regulated kinase |
| FAC | Focaladhesion complex |
| FADD | Fas-activated death domain protein |
| FAK | Focal adhesion kinase |
| Fas | TNF receptor superfamily, member 6 |
| FGF | Fibroblastic growth factor |
| GAGs | Glycosaminoglycan |
| GH | Growth hormone |
| gp130 | Interleukin 6 signal transducer (gp130, oncostatin M receptor) |
| Grb2 | Growth factor receptor-binding protein 2 |
| Herp2 | Homocysteine-responsive endoplasmic reticulum-resident ubiquitin-like domain member 2 protein |
| HesR-1 | Hairy and enhancer of split related 1 |
| HeyI | Hairy/enhancer of split related with YRPW motif 1 |
| IGF | Insulin-like growth factor |
| IGF-1R | Insulin-like growth factor-1 receptor |
| IGFBP | Insulin-like growth factor binding protein |
| IL | Interleukin |
| IL-1RA | Interleukin-1 receptor antagonist |
| IL-1RAP | Interleukin-1 receptor associated protein |
| IL-6R | Interleukin-6 receptor |
| IL-R | Interleukin receptor |
| IRAK | Interleukin-1 receptor activate kinase |
| IRS | Insulin receptor substrate |
| JNK | c-Jun N-terminal kinases |
| JunB | Jun B proto-oncogene |
| Lrp-5 | Low-density lipoprotein receptor-related protein 5 |
| MAPK | Mitogen-activated protein (MAP) kinases |
| M-CSF | Macrophage colony-stimulating factor |
| MEK | Map erk kinase |
| MGP | Matrix Gla protein |
| MMP | Matrix metalloproteinase |
| NF-κB | Nuclear transcription factor-kappaB |
| NO | Nitric oxide |
| NOS2 | Nitric oxide synthase type II |
| OCN | Osteonectin |
| PDGFR | Platelet-derived growth factor receptor |
| PGDF | Platelet-derived growth factor |
| PGE2 | Prostaglandin E2 |
| PI3K | Phosphatidylinositol 3-kinases |

**TABLE 7.1**   (continued) List of Abbreviations

| | |
|---|---|
| PK | Protein kinase |
| PKA | Protein kinase A |
| PKC | Protein kinase C |
| PTH | Parathyroid hormone |
| Raf | Proto-oncogene serine/threonine-protein kinase |
| Ras | Rat sarcoma guanine triphosphatase |
| Rel | C-Rel proto-oncogene protein |
| Runx2 | Runt-related transcription factor 2 |
| Shc | Src homology 2 domain containing transforming protein 1 |
| sIL-6R | Soluble interleukin-6 receptor |
| Smad | Mothers against decapentaplegic homolog |
| Smurfs | Smad ubiquitin regulatory factors |
| Sox9 | Sex-determining region Y-related gene |
| Src | Sarcoma |
| STAT | Signal transducer and activator of transcription |
| Tcf7 | Transcription factor 7 |
| TGF | Transforming growth factor |
| TIMP | Tissue inhibitor of metalloproteinase |
| TNF | Tumor necrosis factor |
| TRADD | Tumor necrosis factor receptor-associated death domain protein |
| TRAF | Tumor necrosis factor receptor-associated factor |
| VEGF | Vascular endothelial growth factor |
| Vg1 | Vegetalising factor 1 |
| Wnt | Wingless-type MMTV (mouse mammary tumor virus) integration site family |

extracellular matrix (ECM) regulated for the release of ions through hormones. Bone is made of three cells, osteoblasts, osteocytes, and osteoclasts, and the ECM. Osteoblasts are responsible for the secretion and mineralization of ECM. Osteocytes are mature osteoblasts encased within the ECM. Osteoclasts are responsible for ECM resorption allowing for the remodeling of bone.

The ECM consists mainly, >90%, of type 1 collagen (Allori et al., 2008a). The noncollagenous components of the ECM include γ-carboxyglutamic acid-containing proteins, glycoproteins, enzymes, and sialoproteins (Allori et al., 2008a). The γ-carboxyglutamic acid-containing proteins in the ECM are osteonectin (OCN) and matrix Gla protein (MGP). OCN is only found in mineralized tissues and is one of the most abundant noncollagen proteins in the ECM (Allori et al., 2008b). MGP is structurally similar to OCN but is found in many tissues throughout the body (Allori et al., 2008a). The sialoproteins osteopontin and bone sialoprotein are RGD-containing (Arg-Gly-Asp peptide sequence-containing) matrix proteins within the SIBLING family. The enzymes in bone ECM are alkaline phosphatase (ALP) and matrix metalloproteinases (MMP). MMP all have the ability to digest ECM facilitating the movement of cells and therefore moderating the resorption and remodeling of bone. MMPs are used as a metric of bone homeostasis. Fibronectin, OCN, thrombospondin, and proteoglycans are the glycoproteins found in the ECM (Allori et al., 2008a).

Osteoblasts are responsible for the secretion and mineralization of the ECM. Osteoblasts differentiate from pluripotent mesenchymal cells through four stages. Each stage has a distinct phenotype with the expression of different bone matrix proteins. The first stage consists of the differentiation into an osteoprogenitor cell. In this stage bone morphogenic protein (BMP)-2 and wingless-type MMTV integration site family (Wnt) signaling is upregulated for the commitment to the osteoblastic cell line. The second stage is the transition from an osteoprogenitor to a preosteoblast cell. Parathyroid hormone (PTH) helps to commit the osteoprogenitor to this process; this stage is identified by the upregulation of ALP, runt-related transcription factor 2 (Runx2), and collagen Ia gene expression (Zhang et al., 2010, Westendorf et al., 2004). The third stage, the mature osteoblast is identified by the upregulation of ALP, collagen Ia, OCN, Runx2, Osterix, and other genes (Lian et al., 2004). We will focus on the signaling impact of mature osteoblasts, the main producer of ECM proteins and the subsequent mineralization of the ECM (Westendorf et al., 2004, Lian et al., 2004). The fourth stage occurs with the terminal differentiation of the mature osteoblast into an osteocyte and elevated levels of apoptosis (Westendorf et al., 2004, Lian et al., 2004). OCN, Runx2, and low density lipoprotein receptor-related protein 5 (Lrp-5) are the main genes expressed in this stage (Westendorf et al., 2004).

## 7.3 Biology of Chondrocytes

### 7.3.1 Cartilage ECM

Articular cartilage is a heterogenous avascular, aneural, and alymphatic tissue consisting of chondrocytes and its surrounding ECM (Yoon and Fisher, 2007, Leipzig et al., 2006, Davies et al., 2008). Its purpose is to act as a low-friction material that is resistant to compressive loading. The ECM is divided into four zones: superficial, middle, deep, and calcified (Leipzig et al., 2006, Almarza and Athanasiou, 2004). The ECM consists mainly of collagen, proteoglycans, and noncollagenous proteins (Shakibaei et al., 2008). Unlike bone ECM, chondrocyte ECM is composed of 90% type II collagen. Other collagen types present are collagen types VI, IX, X, and XI (Mollenhauer, 2008, Shakibaei et al., 2008). The remaining ECM is composed of proteoglycans, aggrecan, glycosaminoglycan (GAGs), hyaluronic acid, decorin, biglycan, and perlecan (Otero and Goldring, 2007). Proteoglycans are heavily glycosylated, consisting of a long linear chain of carbohydrate polymers that are covalently bonded to GAG chains (Allori et al., 2008a). GAGs are negatively charged allowing them to swell with water so when depressed they are able to dispel the water, compress and reform when the compression subsides (Burrage et al., 2006). Collagen fibers create a mesh of these molecules by binding decorin and biglycan to collagen fibers and then trapping proteoglycans and GAGs within the network (Almarza and Athanasiou, 2004, Millward-Sadler and Salter, 2004). This collagen meshwork works to provide great tensile strength and the ability to remain intact under compressive forces (Millward-Sadler and Salter, 2004, Almarza and Athanasiou, 2004, Shakibaei et al., 2008).

Though chondrocytes only compose ~5% of the total volume and are sparsely distributed throughout the tissue they are responsible for synthesizing and maintaining cartilage homeostasis (Van der Kraan et al., 2002, Yoon and Fisher, 2007, Mollenhauer, 2008). Chondrocytes are spherical in morphology and contained within a pericellular matrix, made of type VI collagen and biglycan (Shakibaei et al., 2008, Otero and Goldring, 2007). Type VI collagen fibers interact with hyaluronic acid, biglycan, and decorin to provide the framework for ECM attachment and the transmission of mechanical stimuli to the cell (Shakibaei et al., 2008, Otero and Goldring, 2007).

Chondrocytes also differentiate from pluripotent mesenchymal cells to either hypertrophic chondrocytes (transient cartilage) or to chondrocytes (permanent articular cartilage) (Woods et al., 2007, Zuscik et al., 2008). Transient cartilage refers to the cartilage that is found during chondrogenesis in endochondral ossification and growth plate development (Woods et al., 2007, Zuscik et al., 2008). We will focus on the terminal differentiation into chondrocytes located in permanent articular cartilage. The differentiation of the mesenchymal cell into a chondrocyte is marked by the upregulation of sex-determining region Y-related gene (Sox9) and the secretion of ECM components type IIb collagen and aggrecan and is upregulated by the addition of transforming growth factor (TGF)-$\beta$1 and BMP-7 (Yamane and Reddi, 2008, Woods et al., 2007, Zuscik et al., 2008).

## 7.4 Signaling Pathway Overview

Intracellular cell signaling occurs through the translation of extracellular mechanical or chemical stimuli into a cellular response. The signaling pathways from these translations occur through the same general process. An extracellular signal, such as a cytokine, growth factor or hormone, is transmitted through the cellular membrane into the cytoplasm. Once inside the cell it may either continue to the nucleus via second messengers, or interact within the intracellular region with other cell components (e.g., the cytoskeleton) leading to the desired cellular effect whether it is a change in gene expression, phenotype, or metabolism. The cell signaling pathway studies referenced in this chapter used bovine, murine, human, and other mammalian derived cells. Since this is an overview of the major cell signaling pathways we have not differentiated between each mammalian cell type.

Autocrine signaling occurs when signaling molecules released from a cell bind to receptors located on the same cell. Similarly paracrine signaling refers to signaling molecules that bind to receptors located on neighboring cells. Endocrine signal occurs when systemically circulating signaling molecules (e.g., hormones) bind to receptors located in cells external to their place of production.

Cytokines, growth factors and hormones are some of the extracellular signaling molecules that initiate signaling pathways. Cytokines (e.g., interleukins, interferons) are primarily used for maintaining cell homeostasis and the body's defensive pathways. Growth factors, closely related to cytokines, are primarily used in the regulation of cell growth and proliferation such as TGF-$\beta$ superfamily and insulin-like growth factor (IGF). Hormones (e.g., PTH, growth hormone [GH]) interact with cells through endocrine signaling.

Signaling pathways occur through the attachment of an extracellular signal, a ligand, to a cell receptor protein either spanning or extending from the plasma membrane of the cell. Receptor proteins are most commonly transmembrane, structurally consisting of three segments: extracellular, intracellular, and a hydrophobic segment located within the plasma membrane. One notable exception is for hormone signaling which mainly occurs through intracellular receptors. Once the ligand binds to the receptor the intracellular protein has a conformational change initiating the signal cascade through activation of proteins or other second messengers (e.g., kinase, phosphatase, calcium). Since multiple signals may lead to the same phenotypic response or to different outcomes it can cause a whole tissue response from the same signaling molecules interacting with different receptors and cells.

Once the desired cellular effect has occurred the ligand may be released from the receptor, then either degrade or bind with another receptor. Receptor and ligand complexes may also be internalized through clathrin-mediated endocytosis. Once internalized the complexes may be recycled back to the cell surface via early endosomes or degraded in late stage endosomes. Alternatively complexes may be degraded through endocytosis and transportation to the proteasome by calveolin-positive vesicles. For example, TGF-$\beta$ receptors are internalized through both the clathrin-mediated and caveolar pathways (Di Guglielmo et al., 2003, Le Roy and Wrana, 2005). Intracellularly, after second messengers complete their role in the signaling cascade they may be degraded through ubiquitination and observe a conformational change to become inactive permanently or inactive until later activation.

Cell homeostasis is maintained through complex feedback loops and the balance of anabolic and catabolic growth factors and cytokines (Pujol et al., 2008). Anabolic growth factors and cytokines work to maintain homeostasis by increasing the expression of gene for increased cell proliferation and for the proteins that make up the ECM. In contrast, catabolic growth factors and cytokines work to change gene expression levels to produce proteins that work to degrade the proteins that are components of the ECM.

Since osteoblasts and chondrocytes share much of the same environment, the skeletal system, they are exposed to some of the same signaling molecules. However, the same signaling molecules may impact osteoblasts and chondrocytes differently. We will look in depth at some shared cytokines and growth factors such as TGF-$\beta$1, IGF-1, BMP-2, BMP-7, tissue necrosis factor (TNF)-$\alpha$, and interleukin (IL)-1.

# 7.5 Anabolic Growth Factors/Cytokines

## 7.5.1 Insulin-Like Growth Factor

IGF-1 is considered to be the main anabolic factor for chondrocyte growth, proliferation, and survival (Van der Kraan et al., 2002, Davies et al., 2008, Starkman et al., 2005). It is structurally similar to insulin and consists of a single chain of 70 amino acids, with a molecular weight of ~7.5 kDa (Baserga et al., 1997). IGF functions as an endocrine, autocrine, and paracrine growth factor (Starkman et al., 2005,

Giustina et al., 2008). As an endocrine growth factor it is circulated systemically after production in liver but it also may act through autocrine or paracrine signaling as in osteoblasts and chondrocytes when it is synthesized and incorporated into the ECM (Davies et al., 2008, Govoni et al., 2005). To maintain stability in the ECM IGF-1 is bound to an antagonist, the insulin-like growth factor binding protein (IGFBP) (Govoni et al., 2005).

### 7.5.1.1 IGF Signaling Pathway

IGF-1 signaling is initiated through the ligand binding of insulin-like growth factor-1 receptor (IGF-1R), a transmembrane glycoprotein tetramer. IGF-1R is a tyrosine kinase receptor with its two α and two β subunits connect by disulfide bonds (Yoon and Fisher, 2007, Giustina et al., 2008). For IGF-1 to bind to its receptor it must first cleave the antagonist IGFBP. There are six known IGFBPs that may bind to both IGF-1 and IGF-2 (Conover, 2008, Baserga et al., 1997). IGFBPs are used for IGF transport and increasing IGF stability and therefore their half lives (Govoni et al., 2005). After cleavage ligand binding occurs with the extracellular α subunit IGF-1R then the β subunit, which spans the membrane and autophosphorylates its intracellular tyrosine phosphorylation site (Samani et al., 2007). Once phosphorylated, the major substrates, insulin receptor substrate (IRS)-1, IRS-2, and src homology 2 domain containing transforming protein 1 (Shc) may bind, become phosphorylated, and then begin the signaling pathways (Baserga et al., 1997, Perrini et al., 2010, Humbel, 1990) (Figure 7.1). IRS-1 initiates the phosphatidylinositol 3-kinases/v-akt murine thymoma viral oncogene homolog (PI3K/Akt) pathway mediating the antiapoptotic effects of IGF-1R by phosphorylating and therefore inactivating BCL2-associated agonist of cell death (BAD) (Perrini et al., 2010). Concomitantly the rat sarcoma guanine triphosphatase/ mitogen-activated protein kinases (Ras/MAPK) pathway is initiated by the IRS-2 pathway and by the

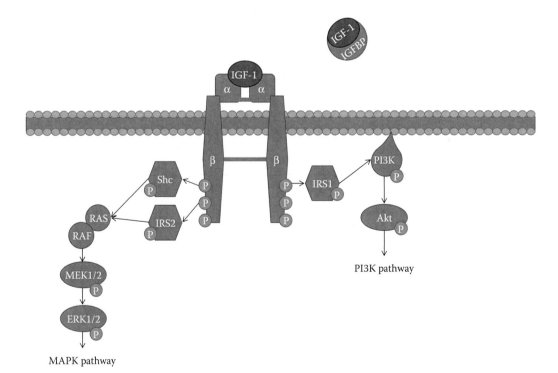

**FIGURE 7.1** IGF-1 signaling pathway. To initiate the IGF-1 signaling pathway first the antagonist IGFBR must be cleaved from the ligand. After proteolysis, the IGF-1 ligand may bind with its receptor, IGF-1R to initiate auto phosphorylation. Once IGF-1R is phosphorylated it subsequently initiates a phosphorylation chain of Shc and IRS1/2 to activate the MAPK and PI3K pathways. (Adapted from Perrini, S. et al. 2010. *Journal of Endocrinology*, 205, 201–210.)

phosphorylation of Shc. The Ras/MAPK pathway leads to increased cell proliferation, and possibly the mediation of oxidative stress cell damage and apoptosis (Perrini et al., 2010, Yoon and Fisher, 2007).

### 7.5.1.2 IGF-1 in Osteoblast and Chondrocytes

Of all the growth factors osteoblasts produce, IGF-1 and IGF-II are the most abundant (Govoni et al., 2005). Although osteoblasts are capable of producing all six IGFBR, in osteoblasts IGF primarily binds with IGFBP-3, -4, -5 (Conover, 2008, Giustina et al., 2008). Of which IGFBPs-4 and -5 are the most abundant within the ECM (Govoni et al., 2005). Of the six, IGFBP-1, -2, -4, -6 are known to inhibit osteoblast function while IGFBP-3 stimulates (Govoni et al., 2005). IGFBP-5 is the most controversial as it both inhibits and stimulates IGF interaction with osteoblasts (Conover, 2008, Govoni et al., 2005). IGFBR concentrations may differ depending on the levels of IGF-1 through autocrine and paracrine signaling (Giustina et al., 2008). In order to access IGF-1 osteoblasts secrete MMP and serine proteases which cleave IGFBPs (Giustina et al., 2008) to free IGF-1 for ligand binding. Osteoblast apoptosis is mediated through the IGF-1 activation of the PI3K/Akt pathway (Perrini et al., 2010). Additionally osteoblast proliferation is regulated through the activation of the extracellular signal-regulated kinase/mitogen-activated protein (MAP) kinases (ERK/MAPK) pathway (Perrini et al., 2010). In osteoblasts IGF-1 is known to be under the control of PTH, where exposure to PTH causes osteoblasts to express IGF-1 (Giustina et al., 2008). In turn, IGF-1 has shown to stimulate osteoblast proliferation and ECM production (Bernstein et al., 2010).

In chondrocytes IGF-1 stimulates an increase of proteoglycans, aggrecan, hyaluronan, and collagen synthesis (Davies et al., 2008, Starkman et al., 2005). IGF-1 initiates proteoglycan production by activating both the PI3K and ERK/MAPK pathways; however, only the PI3K pathway is required for the synthesis (Starkman et al., 2005, Zhang et al., 2009). Also through the activation of the PI3K pathway chondrocytes have been shown to express type II collagen (Yoon and Fisher, 2007). IGF-1 has been shown to inhibit ECM degradation by decreasing the production of MMP-13, one of the major factors in ECM degradation (Zhang et al., 2009, Burrage et al., 2006). Reduction of MMP production occurs through the activation of the ERK/MAPK pathway (Zhang et al., 2009, Malemud, 2004). Also, IGF-1 in chondrocytes upregulates IL-1RII, a decoy receptor for the cytokine IL-1, protecting the cell from the catabolic IL-1 signaling pathway (Wang et al., 2003). Interestingly, IGF-1 in chondrocytes has shown to not activate either the c-Jun N-terminal kinases (JNK) or p38 proteins as seen in other cell types (Malemud, 2004). IGF-1 also is able to inhibit apoptosis that is normally caused through the TNF receptor superfamily, member 6 (Fas) antibody activation creating an imbalance in BCL2-associated X protein/B-cell CCL/lymphoma 2 (BAX/BCL-2) concentration levels, as well as a decrease of focal adhesion kinase (FAK) and integrin expression (Wang et al., 2006). As discussed previously IGF-1 increases integrin expression and therefore increases the number of mechanoreceptors available which may increase MAPK pathway activation (Perrini et al., 2010, Yoon and Fisher, 2007).

## 7.5.2 TGF-β Superfamily

Among the many signaling molecules that effect osteoblasts and chondrocytes, the TGF-β superfamily has the largest range of impact. The TGF-β superfamily can regulate cell differentiation, proliferation, maintenance, and apoptosis (Hay et al., 2004, Massague, 1990, 1998, Westendorf et al., 2004). The TGF-β superfamily consists of a set of structurally conserved dimeric proteins held in place through hydrophobic interactions. TGF-β1, TGF-β2, TGF-β3 isoforms, bone morphogenetic proteins (BMPs), vegetalising factor-1 (Vg1), and Activin are some of the proteins within the superfamily (Massague, 1990, 1998).

### 7.5.2.1 TGF-β Signaling Pathway

The TGF-β superfamily cell signaling pathways are well characterized (Figure 7.2). Cell signaling occurs through association with two transmembrane serine/threonine glycoprotein kinase receptors, type I

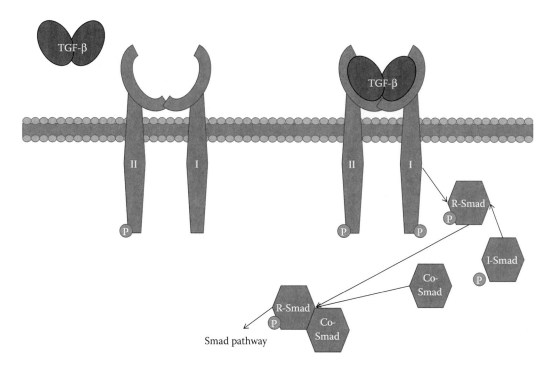

**FIGURE 7.2**  TGF-β signaling pathway. When the ligand, TGF-β, binds to its receptor the signaling pathway is activated. Once ligand binding occurs the constitutively phosphorylated TβR-II receptor phosphorylates TβR-I. This initiates the phosphorylation of R-Smads, and the subsequent binding with Co-Smads to activate the Smad pathway. (Adapted from Izzi, L. and Attisano, L. 2004. *Oncogene*, 23, 2071–2078.)

(TβR-I) and type II (TβR-II) (Janssens et al., 2005). Both receptors are dimers; upon ligand binding to the TβR-II, TβR-I is recruited to make a heterotrimeric complex. The dormant TβR-I is activated through phosphorylation by the constitutively phosphorylated active TβR-II. After phosphorylation TβR-I most commonly initiates the signaling pathway by phosphorylating the mothers against decapentaplegic homolog (Smad) receptor protein, or less commonly via the Non-Smad pathway (Janssens et al., 2005, Selvamurugan et al., 2004, Massagué and Gomis, 2006, Moustakas and Heldin, 2005).

Smads, or mothers against decapentaplegic homologs, are made of three subclasses: receptor regulated (R)-, inhibitory (I)-, and common mediator (Co)-Smads. R-Smads, Smad1, Smad2, Smad3, Smad5, Smad8, bind with the activated TβR-I. Once phosphorylated R-Smads bind with Co-Smad, Smad4, and enter the nucleus to regulate gene transcription. I-Smads, Smad-6, and Smad-7, regulate gene expression through inhibiting the interaction of TβR-I and R-Smads (Canalis et al., 2003, Massagué et al., 2005).

The Smad pathway regulates the transcription of specific genes through three methods. First is the direct binding of a R-Smad–Smad4 complex to the DNA. The second method occurs through the interaction with other protein receptors to activate transcription. Additionally R-Smad–Smad4 complexes may effect gene transcription through binding with either genes co-activators or co-repressors (Miyazono, 2000).

### 7.5.2.2  Transforming Growth Factor β1

TGF-β1, is the most abundant member of the TGF-β superfamily (Janssens et al., 2005). It impacts cell proliferation, differentiation, and apoptosis of both chondrocytes and osteoblasts (Selvamurugan et al., 2004). TGF-β1 signaling pathway occurs through Smad activation as well as through non-Smad pathways including activation of the ERK, JNK, and p38 MAPK pathways (Moustakas and Heldin, 2005, Blaney Davidson et al., 2007). TGF-β is found in the ECM surrounding osteoblasts as well as in chondrocytes.

In osteoblasts TGF-β1 blocks apoptosis and allows for the transdifferentiation into osteocytes. TGF-β1 impacts osteoblasts during early differentiation by increasing the expression of Runx2, along with BMP; however, during late differentiation and osteoblast maturation it suppresses Runx2, collagen 1, ALP, and osteocalcin production. Additionally as the osteoblasts mature it has been demonstrated that all receptors are down regulated therefore it is hypothesized that mature osteoblasts are less sensitive to TGF-β1 and its inhibition of matrix mineralization (Janssens et al., 2005). During late-differentiation osteoblasts express collagen 3 (MMP13) which leads to the degradation of ECM, signaling the transition for osteoclast resorption (Selvamurugan et al., 2004). Studies have shown that the increased collagen 3 expression caused by TGF-β1 signaling occurs optimally through activation of both the MAPK and the Smad pathways (Selvamurugan et al., 2004). TGF-β1 also down regulates ALP, osteocalcin, collagen I, and BMP-2 mRNA expression (Sykaras and Opperman, 2003).

In chondrocytes the impact of TGF-β1 on ECM production has conflicting reviews (Davies et al., 2008, Darling and Athanasiou, 2005, Li and O'Keefe, 2005). It has been shown to both stimulate the synthesis of ECM and decrease proteoglycan production (Blaney Davidson et al., 2007, Davies et al., 2008). Specifically chondrocytes in the presence of TGF-β expresses increased levels of aggrecan (Roman-Blas et al., 2007). Additionally TGF-β1 has been shown to prevent chondrocyte apoptosis when stimulated with TNF-α (Lires-Deán et al., 2008). TGF-β1 plays a main role in ECM maintenance by reducing ECM degrading enzymes such as collagenase and MMP inhibitors (Edwards et al., 1987, 1996). Owing to the success of prior individual studies using TGF-β1 or IGF-1 to improve chondrocyte growth, proliferation, and ECM production, current work focuses on combining these growth factors and has shown increased collagen and proteoglycan synthesis (Leipzig et al., 2006, Davies et al., 2008, Koay et al., 2008).

### 7.5.2.3 Bone Morphogenic Protein

One of the best characterized growth factor of the TGF-β superfamily for use with osteoblasts is BMP. Since their identification in the 1960s there have been over 30 BMP family members identified and 20 of which have been well characterized (Urist, 1965, Xiao et al., 2007, Balemans and Van Hul, 2002). Structurally BMPs are a dimeric protein with seven cystine amino acid residues, six of which form an intrachain disulfide bonds and the seventh is used to form dimers through an interchain disulfide bond (Bessa et al., 2008).

Since BMPs are part of the TGF-β superfamily they follow the same cell signaling pathway, through binding of serine/threonine kinase receptors which initiate the Smad and non-Smad pathways (Bessa et al., 2008). Whereas the TGF-βs use Smad2 and Smad3 for signal transduction, the BMP family uses Smad1, Smad5, and Smad8 as R-Smads. As in TGF-β signaling, Smad4 is the Co-Smad and Smad6/7 are I-Smads. BMP signaling may be inhibited in five ways, the nonsignaling of pseudoreceptors, intracellularly through I-Smads, ubiquitination caused by Smad ubiquitin regulatory factors (Smurfs), and antagonist binding of R-Smads, and extracellularly through antagonist binding of BMP (Gazzerro and Minetti, 2007, Canalis et al., 2003). Some of the BMP antagonists are noggin, gremlin, sclerostin (Gazzerro and Minetti, 2007, Cao and Chen, 2005).

#### 7.5.2.3.1 BMP-2 and BMP-7

The effects of BMP-2 and BMP-7 on osteoblast differentiation, growth, proliferation, and apoptosis are well documented, and currently are used for clinical applications in the healing bone defects (Hay et al., 2004, Bessa et al., 2008). Of the BMP family, BMP-2, is known as a main factor in osteoblast homeostasis and BMP-7, is regarded as a main factor in chondrocyte function (Yoon and Fisher, 2007).

BMP-2 can be a positive or a negative factor in osteoblast homeostasis. BMP-2 has been shown to promote osteoblast apoptosis as well as impact Notch and Wnt signaling through the regulation of hairy/enhancer-of-split related with YRPW motif 1 (*Hey1*) also known as hairy and enhancer of split related-1 (HesR-1) or homocysteine-responsive endoplasmic reticulum-resident ubiquitin-like domain member 2 protein (Herp2) and transcription factor 7 (Tcf7) transcription factors (Hay et al., 2004, Haÿ et al., 2001, Miyazono et al., 2005). BMP-2 promotion of apoptosis occurs through the BMP-1 receptor

(Hay et al., 2004). It also has been shown to promote apoptosis through a non-Smad protein kinase (PK) C-dependent pathway (Haÿ et al., 2001). The non-Smad PKC-dependant path increases BAX/BCL-2 and increases the amount of cytochrome *c* released from the mitochondria therefore which activates caspase-9 and the other effector caspases to initiate osteoblast apoptosis (Haÿ et al., 2001). TGF-β1 exerts a negative regulation of BMP-2 at transcription (Sykaras and Opperman, 2003).

For chondrocytes BMP-2 has been shown to increase the expression of some ECM proteins, such as aggrecan and type II collagen (Gründer et al., 2004, Yoon and Fisher, 2007). However, it was also shown to have negative impacts as well such as ECM degradation (Yoon and Fisher, 2007). BMP-2 has also been shown to upregulate vascular endothelial growth factor (VEGF) transcription and translation in chondrocytes (Bluteau et al., 2007).

BMP-7 is known to have a positive effect on cartilage homeostasis, maintaining levels of collagen II and ECM (Klooster and Bernier, 2005, Khalafi et al., 2007). Chondrocytes incubated with BMP-7 had increased levels of proteoglycan synthesis even in the presence of the catabolic cytokine, IL-1 (Chubinskaya et al., 2007). Additionally BMP-7 is known to improve chondrocyte survival as well as inhibit proinflammatory responses initiated by exposure to IL-1 or IL-6 (Chubinskaya et al., 2007).

### 7.5.3  VEGF, Platelet-Derived Growth Factor, and Fibroblastic Growth Factor

Other major growth factors in osteoblast and chondrocyte functioning are VEGF, platelet-derived growth factor (PDGF), and fibroblastic growth factor (FGF). VEGF, made of seven members, VEGF-A—VEGF-F is constitutively expressed by chondrocytes and osteoblasts (Saadeh et al., 2000, Ferrara, 2004). In osteoblasts VEGF synthesis is believed to be upregulated by BMP-2 and by TGF-β1 through the MAPK pathway (Dai and Rabie, 2007, Ferrara, 2004). VEGF interacts with osteoblast cell receptors for the regulation of cell migration and ECM mineralization (Tombran-Tink and Barnstable, 2004, Dai and Rabie, 2007). On chondrocytes VEGF interacts with cell receptors that regulate cell survival (Dai and Rabie, 2007). VEGF levels are low in mature chondrocytes in articular cartilage but are higher in the growth phase, leading to the idea that increased expression of VEGF could lead to increased matrix synthesis (Murata et al., 2008). Additionally VEGF is thought to regulate chondrocyte apoptosis through regulating the BCL-2/BAD concentration levels (Murata et al., 2008).

PDGF binds to the platelet-derived growth factor receptor (PDGFR) on osteoblasts to increase gene expression for osteoblast proliferation through tenascin-C (Hofmann et al., 2008). Studies evaluating the effect of PDGF, or platelet-derived growth factor, on chondrocytes concluded that PDGF had a stimulatory effect on chondrocytes. However, for differentiating chondrocytes PDGF has been shown to be an antagonist, causing a decrease in the amount of proteoglycan produced (Van der Kraan et al., 2002).

FGF-2 is a highly conserved heparin-binding growth factor. In osteoblasts and chondrocytes it is produced and then stored in the ECM (Vincent et al., 2007, Takai et al., 2007). FGF-2 induces increased osteoblastic proliferation and TGF-β1 production (Saadeh et al., 2000). FGF-2 also is known to improve cell survival in osteoblasts through PI3K/Akt pathway and through the inhibition of caspase-3 (Xing and Boyce, 2005, Takai et al., 2007). Additionally FGF-2 activates the MAPK pathway in osteoblasts (Takai et al., 2007). In chondrocytes, FGF-2 is known to increase cell proliferation and upregulate GAG synthesis (Veilleux and Spector, 2005). Also with mechanical loading chondrocytes use FGF-2 to activate the ERK1/2 pathway (Vincent et al., 2007).

## 7.6  Catabolic Growth Factors/Cytokines

To maintain tissue homeostasis catabolic growth factors must provide ECM degradation at the same rate of the anabolic growth factor ECM expression. The main catabolic cytokines are interleukins, interferons, lymphokines, and prostaglandins. We will focus on IL-1, IL-6, and TNF-α, proinflammatory cytokines associated with the degradation of both bone and cartilage ECM (Burrage et al., 2006, Yoon and Fisher, 2007).

## 7.6.1 Interleukin-1

IL-1 is a family of more than nine polypeptides, originally discovered as IL-1β, IL-1α, and interleukin-1 receptor antagonist (IL-1Ra). It is one of the best understood proinflammatory cytokine (Boch et al., 2001, Saklatvala, 2007). It is believed to be a main factor in the development of osteoarthritis is diarthrodial joints (Malemud, 2004, Fan et al., 2004, Wang et al., 2003). IL-1 is synthesized in its inactive form and is activated by a protease cleavage to begin the signaling cascade.

The expression of IL-1 is controlled by two antagonists IL-1RI and IL-1RII (Wang et al., 2003) (Figure 7.3). Signaling is only initiated with the ligand binding of IL-1 to IL-1RI because IL-1RII is a decoy receptor and will not initiate the IL-1 signaling pathway (Boch et al., 2001, Wang et al., 2003). Once IL-1RI binding occurs, IL-1RI recruits and binds with IL1RAP (Saklatvala, 2007). Interleukin-1 receptor activate kinase-1/interleukin-1 receptor activate kinase-2 (IRAK1/2) and the adaptor protein MyD88 then activate tumor necrosis factor receptor-associated factor (TRAF)-6 (Boch et al., 2001, Saklatvala, 2007). TRAF6 then initiates the ERK, MAPK, JNK, p38, and NF-κB pathways (Roman-Blas and Jimenez, 2008, Saklatvala, 2007, Bankers-Fulbright et al., 1996).

NF-κB is regarded as the "master switch" of the inflammation cascade (Otero and Goldring, 2007). It is a member of the C-Rel proto-oncogene protein (Rel) family (Wang et al., 2007). As an inactive protein it is bound to I-κB, if I-κB is phosphorylated the NF-κB subunits, (commonly 50 and p65), reform into a dimer and initiate the NF-κB signaling pathway (Bonizzi and Karin, 2004, Wang et al., 2007).

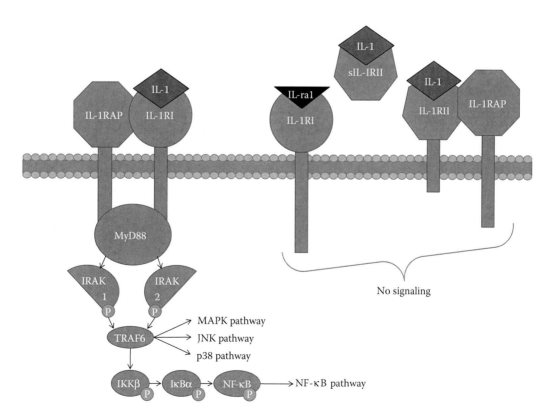

**FIGURE 7.3** IL-1 signaling pathway. IL-1 signaling is controlled by IL-1RI and IL-1RII. IL-1RII is a decoy receptor and signaling is only initiated when IL-1 binds with IL1-RI. Once bound, IL-1RAP is recruited and along with the adaptor protein, MYD88, IRAK1/2 are phosphorylated to initiate the NF-κB pathway. (Adapted from Boch, J. A., Wara-Aswapati, N., and Auron, P. E. 2001. *Journal of Dental Research,* 80, 400; Blanchard, F. et al. 2009. *Cytokine and Growth Factor Reviews,* 20, 19–28.)

NF-κB translocates to the nucleus and mediates gene transcription through binding to DNA at κB sites (Saklatvala, 2007, Fan et al., 2004).

### 7.6.1.1 IL-1 in Osteoblasts and Chondrocytes

IL-1 has been identified as the main cytokine for the resorption of bone while inhibiting new bone formation since the discovery of its role in 1983 (Gowen et al., 1983, Fujisaki et al., 2006). IL-1α inhibits ECM mineralization, decreases type I collagen synthesis, and decreases ALP (Tanabe et al., 2004). IL-1α also increases bone resorption by stimulating osteoblast expression of macrophage colony-stimulating factor (M-CSF) and prostaglandin E2 (PGE$_2$) while decreasing expression of OPG, all known factors in the recruitment and differentiation of osteoclasts (Tanabe et al., 2005). IL-1β is also known to increase osteoblast apoptosis through the increased expression of Fas (Tsuboi et al., 1999).

The impact of IL-1 on chondrocytes in osteoarthritic cartilage has been well studied. In response to IL-1 and lipopolysaccharide stimulation chondrocytes have been shown to use nitric oxide (NO) to inhibit proteoglycan synthesis and cell proliferation (Lee et al., 2000). Additionally IL-1 increases NO production by activating nitric oxide synthase type II (NOS2) (Otero and Goldring, 2007). Chondrocytes cultured with IL-1 had inhibited levels of collagen type II synthesis known to occur through the down regulation of one component of type II collagen (Pujol et al., 2008, Malemud, 2004). Not only does IL-1 reduce collagen II production but it also upregulates the production of MMPs and aggrecanases to degrade the ECM (Pujol et al., 2008). IL-1 moderates the impact of TGF-β by initiating the nuclear transcription factor—kappaB (NF-κB) pathway to synthesize a transcription factor that competes with the transcription factors for TGF-β and in turn causes the down regulation of TGF-β (Pujol et al., 2008). IL-1 also accomplishes this through the increased expression of Smad7 to inhibit TGF-β signaling (Pujol et al., 2008).

## 7.6.2 Interleukin-6

There are 10 identified members of the IL-6 family however, IL-6 has been shown to be the most influential on bone resorption and formation (Blanchard et al., 2009). It has been shown to be anabolic by increasing ECM mineralization, ALP expression, and inhibiting apoptosis but also has catabolic effects through the inhibition of osteoblast proliferation and stimulating osteoclastic resorption (Mundy, 2007, Blanchard et al., 2009). Since osteoblasts express low levels of interleukin-6 receptor (IL-6R), soluble interleukin-6 receptor sIL-6R is necessary for IL-6 to have a significant impact at physiological levels.

IL-6 signaling is initiated with ligand binding to IL-6R and interleukin 6 signal transducer (gp130) (Steeve et al., 2004). IL-6 binding causes the activation of tyrosine kinases on JNK to activate the SHP2/SCH and signal transducer and activator of transcription (STAT) 1/3/5 pathways. STAT1/3/5 leads to the catabolic phenotypes through p21, RANKL, BAX/BCL2 pathways (Blanchard et al., 2009, Franchimont et al., 2005). The activation of SHP2/SHC leads to the anabolic pathways of IRS1/2, PI3K, and Ras/proto-oncogene serine/threonine-protein kinase (Raf). These anabolic phenotypes are seen through the expression of IL-6, tissue inhibitor of metalloproteinase (TIMP)-1, Mcl-1, FBJ osteosarcoma oncogene (c-fos), and jun B proto-oncogene (JunB) (Blanchard et al., 2009). Additionally culturing osteoblasts with IL-6 increased the transcription of IGF-1 and BMP-6, both growth factors known to increase osteoblast proliferation (Franchimont et al., 2005). However, IL-6 also acts catabolically though the stimulation of osteoblasts to release paracrine factors to activate osteoclasts (Steeve et al., 2004).

The effects of IL-6 on chondrocytes are also in debate. Chondrocytes cultured with IL-6 showed catabolic effects including reduced proteoglycan synthesis and increased MMP production (Malemud, 2004, Otero and Goldring, 2007). Other studies showed that IL-6 had anabolic effects with chondrocytes increasing TIMP production and activation of collagen synthesis (Malemud, 2004). This difference seems to be dependent on the availability of sIL-6R (Otero and Goldring, 2007). If sIL-6R is present then the catabolic inhibition of proteoglycan synthesis and MMP stimulation occurs (Otero and Goldring, 2007).

## 7.6.3 Tumor Necrosis Factor

TNF-$\alpha$ is a membrane-bound protein that once cleaved may act as a cytokine similar in function to IL-1 (Malemud, 2004). TNF-$\alpha$ is proteolytically cleaved by MMPs then binds with TNF-R1 or TNF-R2, both found on osteoblasts and chondrocytes (Malemud, 2004) Once bound the TNF receptor and ligand complex form a trimer and begins the signaling pathway. TNF receptors associate with tumor necrosis factor receptor-associated death domain protein (TRADD) to initiate the signaling pathways through FADD and TRAF2/5 (Yoon and Fisher, 2007, Nanes, 2003). TRAF 2/5 lead to the activation of the NF-$\kappa$B and MAPK pathways (Yoon and Fisher, 2007, Malemud, 2004, Nanes, 2003). The FADD pathway initiates apoptosis through the activation of the caspase pathway.

TNF-$\alpha$ inhibits osteoblastic mineralization of the ECM by decreasing gene expression of collagen Ia, IGF-1, ALP, and osteocalcin (Nanes, 2003). Additionally in osteoblasts TNF-$\alpha$ is able to inhibit anabolic BMP signaling through the activation of NF-$\kappa$B and the degradation of Runx2 by upregulation of Smurf1/2 (Yamazaki et al., 2009, Kaneki et al., 2006). TNF-$\alpha$ also inhibits ALP activity, preventing bone growth after remodeling (Yamazaki et al., 2009). Apoptosis of osteoblasts is also promoted through the NF-$\kappa$B pathway (Kaneki et al., 2006). In osteoblasts and in chondrocytes TNF-$\alpha$ increases catabolic activity by stimulating gene expression of MMPs (Klooster and Bernier, 2005, Nanes, 2003).

Increased levels of TNF-$\alpha$ is known to be a marker of damaged cartilage (Yoon and Fisher, 2007). TNF-$\alpha$ regulates a number of chondrocyte factors including ECM degradation, apoptosis, and MMP synthesis (Lehmann et al., 2005, Djouad et al., 2009). TNF-$\alpha$ controls the synthesis of ECM components through multiple pathways. It inhibits the synthesis of collagen II through the NF-$\kappa$B pathway and decreases the mRNA production of aggrecan through the MAPK pathway (Klooster and Bernier, 2005). TNF-$\alpha$ also initiates ECM degradation through the upregulation of MMPs and aggrecanase through the MAPK pathway (Sondergaard et al., 2009, Djouad et al., 2009). Like IL-1, TNF-$\alpha$ also increases the production of NO through the activation of NOS2 (Otero and Goldring, 2007).

## 7.7 Hormones

### 7.7.1 Growth Hormone and Parathyroid Hormone

Endocrine signaling is an important regulator of osteoblast and chondrocyte signaling (Perrini et al., 2010, Qin et al., 2004). GH and PTH are two of the most dynamic regulators of cell growth, proliferation, ECM synthesis, and survival (Lian et al., 2004, Perrini et al., 2008, 2010, Giustina et al., 2008). GH is a key regulator of IGF-1 through the activation of IRS-1 by JNK within the GH pathway. GH can also activate ERK1/2 and MAPK signaling pathway in osteoblasts. Similarly PTH works to regulate both osteoblast proliferation and apoptosis (Qin et al., 2004). PTH activates both the PKA and PKC pathways to regulate the expression of gene for the production of collagenase III, osteocalcin (Qin et al., 2004). PTH inhibits osteoblast apoptosis through both the regulation of BCL-2/BAD ratio and the increased expression of Runx2 to maintain survival genes (Bellido et al., 2003). PTH has also been shown to increase the production of IL-6, which may activate osteoclast functions (Allori et al., 2008a).

### 7.7.2 Adiponectin

Adiponectin is a hormone that is more present in women than in men, similar in structure to TNF-$\alpha$ (Ehling et al., 2006). Recent studies have linked increased levels of adiponectin to cartilage degeneration (Lago et al., 2008). Culture of chondrocytes with adiponectin showed an increased production of IL-6, MMP-3, and MMP-9. It also increased the production of NOS2 (Lago et al., 2008). In osteoblasts adiponectin has an alternate effect. It has shown to upregulate mRNA expression of ALP along with causing an increase in matrix mineralization (Oshima et al., 2005).

# 7.8 Mechanotransduction

In addition to initiating intracellular signal expression through the binding of signaling molecules to receptors, changes in the physical environment also initiate cell signaling through a process called mechanotransduction. Physical stimuli is transferred from the ECM to receptors on the cell surface then through the cell membrane and transmitted to the nucleus to make changes in gene expression (Liedert et al., 2006). Mechanotransduction occurs through three steps: (1) ECM-coupling, where the mechanically stimulated ECM interacts with the transmembrane protein, (2) coupling, where the forces are transmitted from the transmembrane protein to biochemical signals within the cell, and (3) gene expression change, biochemical signals are regulated by nuclear transcription changing gene expression levels (Millward-Sadler and Salter, 2004).

For both chondrocytes and osteoblasts mechanotransduction occurs through integrins, cadherins, and $Ca^{2+}$ channels (Liedert et al., 2006, Damsky, 1999). Integrins are the main mode of mechanotransduction as they connect the ECM to the cytoskeleton and other intracellular signaling molecules (Katsumi et al., 2004, Rubin et al., 2006, Millward-Sadler and Salter, 2004). Integrins are a $\alpha\beta$ heterodimeric transmembrane receptors (Millward-Sadler and Salter, 2004). Each integrin domain consists of an extracellular segment, a transmembrane region and an intracellular region (Millward-Sadler and Salter, 2004, Rubin et al., 2006, Shakibaei et al., 2008). There are 18 known $\alpha$ and 8 known $\beta$ subunits in mammals (Woods et al., 2007, Millward-Sadler and Salter, 2004). Principally, in the cytoplasm the $\beta$ subunit is for binding where as the $\alpha$ subunit functions in a for regulatory manner (Shakibaei et al., 2008). Integrin ligand binding can occur with collagen, fibronectin, vitronectin, and laminin (Millward-Sadler and Salter, 2004) depending on the domain structure.

Integrin signal pathways are initiated by ligand binding to either an extracellular or intracellular subunit domain. For this chapter we will focus on the integrin pathway for extracellular mechanotransduction as it is the most common transmission of physical stimuli. Once the extracellular domain binds with a ligand, multiple actions occur, including the clustering of multiple integrins, the recruitment of FAKs and adapter proteins (Millward-Sadler and Salter, 2004) (Figure 7.4). Adapter proteins (paxillin, tensin, talin, $\alpha$-actin) bind, along with FAK to form a complex allowing the binding of the cytoplasmic tail to the actin cytoskeleton forming actin stress fibers (Millward-Sadler and Salter, 2004, Rubin et al., 2006, Westendorf et al., 2004, Giancotti and Ruoslahti, 1999). FAK is one of the main components of the integrin mechanotransduction pathway (Rubin et al., 2006, Shakibaei et al., 2008). Once associated with the focal adhesion complex (FAC), FAK is subsequently activated, autophosphorylates and then binds with sarcoma (Src) to form a Src-homology-2 binding domain (Millward-Sadler and Salter, 2004, Yoon and Fisher, 2007). As an SHC-2 it is able to phosphorylate other proteins such as paxillin and tensin (Millward-Sadler and Salter, 2004, Giancotti and Ruoslahti, 1999).

This process is additive as the concomitant phosphorylation activates additional paxillin and tensin, forming more FACs. The recruitment of these enzymes, proteins, and other necessary substrates to a concentrated area improve reaction kinetics by reducing any spatial dependence on substrates necessary for signal transduction. Activated FAK also initiates the PI3K, p38, and JNK pathways, as well as ERK1/2 to concomitantly initiate the MAPK pathway. The MAPK pathway may control cell proliferation, survival, and differentiation, as it can function in an anabolic or catabolic manner (Takai et al., 2007, Saklatvala, 2007, Shakibaei et al., 2008).

Integrin binding and subsequent clustering may activate other mechanosensing cell components such as stretch activated ion channels and growth factor receptors and cell-surface associated proteoglycans (Millward-Sadler and Salter, 2004). This allows for other signal transduction through other mechanoreceptors such as lipid raft domains, caveolins, and adherens junctions (Rubin et al., 2006, Liedert et al., 2006).

Growth factors such as TGF-$\beta$1 and IGF-1 have shown to increase the expression of integrins as well as the production of Shc, Erk1/2, and other second messengers seen in the integrin pathway therefore there is an interaction between growth factor and integrin signaling pathways (Van der Kraan et al.,

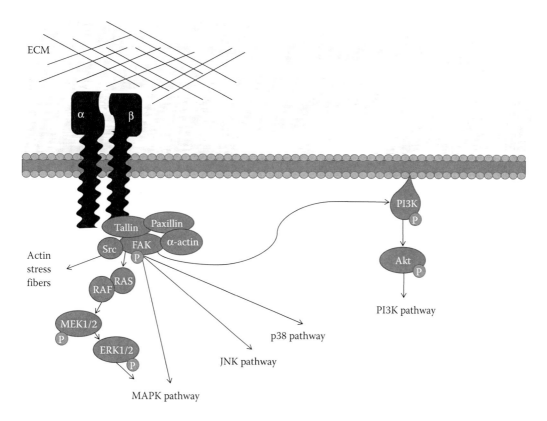

**FIGURE 7.4** Integrin mechanotransduction signaling. Ligand binding initiates mechanotransduction. Once ligand binding occurs, additional integrins, FAK, and adapter proteins are recruited to create FACs. With the subsequent activation and autophosphorylation of FAK the MAPK, JNK, p38, and PI3K pathways are initiated. (Adapted from Guo, W. and Giancotti, F. G. 2004. *Nature Reviews Molecular Cell Biology*, 5, 816–826.)

2002, Loeser, 2000, Shakibaei et al., 2008, Perrini et al., 2008, Loeser, 2002). This is especially seen by the activation of the MAPK pathway by both growth factors and integrins to regulate cell proliferation and survival (Perrini et al., 2010).

## 7.8.1 Osteoblasts

Bone is known to be sensitive to loading and shear stresses and may be anabolic depending the rate, degree, and frequency of loading (Rubin et al., 2006, Liedert et al., 2006, 2010). For osteoblasts ion channels, integrins, connexins, and plasmid membrane components play a role in transmitting mechanical stimuli into chemical signals (Rubin et al., 2006, Liedert et al., 2006). Integrins are a primary method of mechanotransduction in osteoblasts (Rubin et al., 2006). These integrins transmit signals mainly through the β1 subunit (Rubin et al., 2006). Specifically osteoblasts have been demonstrated to activate integrin αvβ1 and integrin β1 during periods of mechanical stress (Rubin et al., 2006). FAK is phosphorylated at tyrosine during osteoblast mechanical stimulation which then concomitantly activates the MAPK pathway through interactions with c-src, Ras, and growth factor receptor-binding protein 2 (Grb2) (Rubin et al., 2006). Specifically the MAPK pathway is activated through ERK1/2 which has shown to increase the production of collagen III and collagen I as well as increase proliferation (Rubin et al., 2006, Sanchez et al., 2008). Loading has also been shown to activate osteoblasts to increase matrix production, upregulate IGF-1, VEGF, TGF-β1, BMP-2, and

BMP-4 (Liedert et al., 2006). Mechanical stress through shear stress also impacts osteoblast function causing the tyrosine phosphorylation in FAK which may regulate cell growth and survival in osteoblasts (Rubin et al., 2006). The upregulation of these growth factors leads to the conclusion that there is likely crosstalk between the anabolic growth factors and integrin signaling to upregulate bone's response to physical stimuli (Liedert et al., 2006).

### 7.8.2 Chondrocytes

Understanding mechanotransduction in chondrocytes is integral in developing an optimal tissue engineered cartilage replacement because of the wide range of mechanical stresses that cartilage endures. Without this understanding of the impact of tensile, shear, or compressive forces on chondrocytes *in vivo* one cannot develop a tissue replacement robust enough to ensure cell survival and proliferation (Millward-Sadler and Salter, 2004). Mechanical cyclical stimulation from the ECM impacts chondrocyte development, morphology, phenotype, function, and even survival (Lee et al., 1998, Shakibaei et al., 2008).

Chondrocytes receive mechanical stimuli through multiple receptors including stretch-activated ion channels, CD44 molecule (Indian blood group) (CD44), anchorin II, and integrins. As in chondrocytes the main mechanotransduction receptors are integrins. The main integrins expressed in chondrocytes are: α1, α3, αv, and α5β1, with α1β5 as the primary integrin (Shakibaei et al., 2008, Loeser, 2002). The α1β5 integrins transmit mechanical changes to the ECM through its interactions with fibronectin (Villanueva et al., 2009). Integrin transduction of mechanical stimuli can regulate differentiation, matrix remodeling, and cell survival for chondrocytes (Loeser, 2000, Shakibaei et al., 2008). In chondrocyte ligand binding of collagen II to the integrin β1 subunit causes the activation of Shc and subsequently the Ras–MAPK signaling pathway (Shakibaei et al., 2008). The Ras–MAPK pathway is known to regulate chondrocyte growth, differentiation, and apoptosis (Saklatvala, 2007, Shakibaei et al., 2008). The Ras–MAPK pathway may induce apoptosis through multiple pathways: activating caspase 3 and subsequent PARP cleavage; inhibiting map erk kinase (MEK), and by activating JNK pathway (Shakibaei et al., 2008).

Chondrocytes cultured under cyclical loading show an increase in GAG production (Preiss-Bloom et al., 2009). Even in the presence of catabolic cytokines, IL-1β, mechanical loading of chondrocytes caused an upregulation of both proteoglycan synthesis and cell proliferation (Lee et al., 2000, Chowdhury et al., 2006). Oscillatory loading of superficial zone chondrocytes increased proteoglycan synthesis but not in middle or deep zone chondrocytes (Vanderploeg et al., 2008). Not all stress is anabolic to chondrocytes, chondrocytes in monolayer express higher levels of NO in response to increasing fluid flow shear stresses (Lee et al., 2000). NO may contribute to chondrocyte loss of phenotype, apoptosis, and ECM degradation (Wang et al., 2007, Lago et al., 2008, Blanco et al., 1995).

## 7.9 Dual Growth Factor Studies

With the success of many anabolic growth factors increasing cell proliferation and ECM synthesis current studies are interested in elucidating any positive impact by combining multiple growth factors in tissue engineering scaffolds. Exogenous delivery of multiple growth factors works to recapitulate the complex *in vivo* environment. See Table 7.2 for a list of different biomaterials, delivery of growth factors and their impact on cell proliferation and ECM synthesis. Newer studies have begun to elucidate the role of sequentially adding growth factors to best recapitulate the *in vivo* milieu. This is the next logical step in growth factor studies to develop/design an optimal tissue engineering scaffold. However, there are currently not enough studies to be able to conclusively determine which combination of anabolic growth factors provide the optimal signaling for cell proliferation and ECM synthesis.

**TABLE 7.2**    Impact of Dual Growth Factor Delivery

| Growth Factors | Targeted Cell Type | Growth Factor Delivery Material | ECM Synthesis | Cell Proliferation | Reference(s) |
|---|---|---|---|---|---|
| BMP-2, IGF-1 | Chondrocyte | Agarose Gel | + + | | Elder and Athanasiou (2009) |
| BMP-2, IGF-I, TGF-β1 | Chondrocyte | Agarose Gel | | + | Elder and Athanasiou (2009) |
| IGF-1, TGF-β | Chondrocyte | Oligo (poly(ethylene glycol) fumarate), gelatin | – | – | Holland et al. (2005, 2007) |
| IGF-1, TGF-β | Chondrocyte | Poly(lactic acid-*co*-glycolic acid) | + | | Elisseeff et al. (2001) |
| IGF-1, TGF-β1 | Chondrocyte | Poly(ethylene oxide) hydrogels in poly(lactic acid-*co*-glycolic acid) (PLGA) | + | | Elisseeff et al. (2001) |
| IGF-1, TGF-β1 | Osteoblast | Poly(D,L-lactide) | + | | Wildemann et al. (2004) |
| IGF-1, TGF-β1 | Chondrocyte | Polyglycolic acid | – | + | Blunk et al. (2002) |
| VEGF, BMP-2 | Osteoblast (Bone) | PLGA microspheres in PPF rod surrounded by gelatin hydrogel | + + | | Kempen et al. (2009) |
| VEGF, BMP-2 | (Osteoblast) Bone | Gelatin microsphere in PPF scaffold | + + | | Patel et al. (2008) |

## 7.10  Conclusion

Understanding the wide range of impact from cytokines, growth factors, and hormones on osteoblasts and chondrocytes allows for their combination and use in designing an optimal tissue engineering scaffold for the skeletal system. Growth factors such as TGF-β and IGF-1 are anabolic for both osteoblasts and chondrocytes; whereas cytokines such as IL-1 and TNF-α are catabolic. In addition to the growth factors and cytokines that act as autocrine and paracrine signaling molecules one must take into account the impact of hormones such as PTH, GH, and adiponectin when developing bone and cartilage replacements. With further studies as to the additive effects of dual delivery of growth factors one will be able to determine the optimal factors in developing a tissue engineering replacement for either bone or cartilage.

## References

Allori, A. C., Sailon, A. M., and Warren, S. M. 2008a. Biological basis of bone formation, remodeling, and repair—Part I: Biochemical signaling molecules. *Tissue Engineering Part B-Reviews,* 14, 259–273.

Allori, A. C., Sailon, A. M., and Warren, S. M. 2008b. Biological basis of bone formation, remodeling, and repair—Part II: Extracellular matrix. *Tissue Engineering Part B-Reviews,* 14, 275–283.

Almarza, A. J. and Athanasiou, K. A. 2004. Design characteristics for the tissue engineering of cartilaginous tissues. *Annals of Biomedical Engineering,* 32, 2–17.

Balemans, W. and Van Hul, W. 2002. Extracellular regulation of BMP signaling in vertebrates: A cocktail of modulators. *Developmental Biology,* 250, 231–250.

Bankers-Fulbright, J. L., Kalli, K. R., and Mckean, D. J. 1996. Interleukin-1 signal transduction. *Life Sciences,* 59, 61–83.

Baserga, R., Hongo, A., Rubini, M., Prisco, M., and Valentinis, B. 1997. The IGF-I receptor in cell growth, transformation and apoptosis. *Biochimica et Biophysica Acta (BBA)—Reviews on Cancer,* 1332, F105–F126.

Bellido, T., Ali, A. A., Plotkin, L. I. et al. 2003. Proteasomal degradation of Runx2 shortens parathyroid hormone-induced anti-apoptotic signaling in osteoblasts. *Journal of Biological Chemistry*, 278, 50259.

Bernstein, A., Mayr, H. O., and Hube, R. 2010. Can bone healing in distraction osteogenesis be accelerated by local application of IGF-1 and TGF- 1? *Journal of Biomedical Materials Research Part B: Applied Biomaterials*, 92, 215–225.

Bessa, P. C., Casal, M., and Reis, R. L. 2008. Bone morphogenetic proteins in tissue engineering: The road from the laboratory to the clinic, part I (basic concepts). *Journal of Tissue Engineering and Regenerative Medicine*, 2, 1–13.

Blanchard, F., Duplomb, L., Baud'Huin, M., and Brounais, B. 2009. The dual role of IL-6-type cytokines on bone remodeling and bone tumors. *Cytokine and Growth Factor Reviews*, 20, 19–28.

Blanco, F. J., Ochs, R. L., Schwarz, H., and Lotz, M. 1995. Chondrocyte apoptosis induced by nitric oxide. *The American Journal of Pathology*, 146, 75.

Blaney Davidson, E. N., Van der Kraan, P. M., and Van Den Berg, W. B. 2007. TGF-[beta] and osteoarthritis. *Osteoarthritis and Cartilage*, 15, 597–604.

Blunk, T., Sieminski, A. L., Gooch, K. J., Courter, D. L., Hollander, A. P., Nahir, A. M., Langer, R., Vunjak-Novakovic, G., and Freed, L. E. 2002. Differential effects of growth factors on tissue-engineered cartilage. *Tissue Engineering*, 8, 73–84.

Bluteau, G., Julien, M., Magne, D. et al. 2007. VEGF and VEGF receptors are differentially expressed in chondrocytes. *Bone*, 40, 568–576.

Boch, J. A., Wara-Aswapati, N., and Auron, P. E. 2001. Concise review biological: Interleukin 1 signal transduction—Current concepts and relevance to periodontitis. *Journal of Dental Research*, 80, 400.

Bonizzi, G. and Karin, M. 2004 The two NF-[kappa]B activation pathways and their role in innate and adaptive immunity. *Trends in Immunology*, 25, 280–288.

Burrage, P. S., Mix, K. S., and Brinckerhoff, C. E. 2006. Matrix metalloproteinases: Role in arthritis. *Frontiers in Bioscience*, 11, 529–543.

Canalis, E., Economides, A. N., and Gazzerro, E. 2003. Bone morphogenetic proteins, their antagonists, and the skeleton. *Endocrine Reviews*, 24, 218–235.

Cao, X. and Chen, D. 2005. The BMP signaling and *in vivo* bone formation. *Gene*, 357, 1–8.

Chowdhury, T. T., Appleby, R. N., Salter, D. M., Bader, D. A., and Lee, D. A. 2006. Integrin-mediated mechanotransduction in IL-1 stimulated chondrocytes. *Biomechanics and Modeling in Mechanobiology*, 5, 192–201.

Chubinskaya, S., Hurtig, M., and Rueger, D. C. 2007. OP-1/BMP-7 in cartilage repair. *International Orthopaedics*, 31, 773–781.

Conover, C. A. 2008. Insulin-like growth factor-binding proteins and bone metabolism. *American Journal of Physiology—Endocrinology and Metabolism*, 294, E10–14.

Dai, J. and Rabie, A. B. M. 2007. VEGF: An essential mediator of both angiogenesis and endochondral ossification. *Journal of Dental Research*, 86, 937.

Damsky, C. H. 1999. Extracellular matrix–integrin interactions in osteoblast function and tissue remodeling. *Bone*, 25, 95–96.

Darling, E. M. and Athanasiou, K. A. 2005. Growth factor impact on articular cartilage subpopulations. *Cell and Tissue Research*, 322, 463–473.

Davies, L. C., Blain, E. J., Gilbert, S. J., Caterson, B., and Duance, V. C. 2008. The potential of IGF-1 and TGF 1 for promoting adult" articular cartilage repair: An *in vitro* study. *Tissue Engineering Part A*, 14, 1251–1261.

Di Guglielmo, G. M., Le Roy, C., Goodfellow, A. F., and Wrana, J. L. 2003. Distinct endocytic pathways regulate TGF-[beta] receptor signalling and turnover. *Nature Cell Biology*, 5, 410–421.

Djouad, F., Rackwitz, L., Song, Y., Janjanin, S., and Tuan, R. S. 2009. ERK1/2 Activation induced by inflammatory cytokines compromises effective host tissue integration of engineered cartilage. *Tissue Engineering Part A*, 15, 2825.

Edwards, D. R., Leco, K. J., Beaudry, P. P. et al. 1996. Differential effects of transforming growth factor-[beta] 1 on the expression of matrix metalloproteinases and tissue inhibitors of metalloproteinases in young and old human fibroblasts. *Experimental Gerontology,* 31, 207–223.

Edwards, D. R., Murphy, G., Reynolds, J. J. et al. 1987. Transforming growth factor beta modulates the expression of collagenase and metalloproteinase inhibitor. *The EMBO Journal,* 6, 1899.

Ehling, A., Schaffler, A., Herfarth, H. et al. 2006. The potential of adiponectin in driving arthritis. *The Journal of Immunology,* 176, 4468.

Elder, B. D. and Athanasiou, K. A. 2009. Systematic assessment of growth factor treatment on biochemical and biomechanical properties of engineered articular cartilage constructs. *Osteoarthritis and Cartilage,* 17, 114–123.

Elisseeff, J., McIntosh, W., Fu, K., Blunk, T., and Langer, R. 2001. Controlled-release of IGF-I and TGF-β1 in a photopolymerizing hydrogel for cartilage tissue engineering. *Journal of Orthopaedic Research,* 19, 6.

Fan, Z. Y., Bau, B., Yang, H. Q., and Aigner, T. 2004. IL-1 beta induction of IL-6 and LIF in normal articular human chondrocytes involves the ERK, p38 and NF kappa B signaling pathways. *Cytokine,* 28, 17–24.

Ferrara, N. 2004. Vascular endothelial growth factor: Basic science and clinical progress. *Endocrine Reviews,* 25, 581–611.

Franchimont, N., Wertz, S., and Malaise, M. 2005. Interleukin-6: An osteotropic factor influencing bone formation? *Bone,* 37, 601–606.

Fujisaki, K., Tanabe, N., Suzuki, N. et al. 2006. The effect of IL-1[alpha] on the expression of matrix metalloproteinases, plasminogen activators, and their inhibitors in osteoblastic ROS 17/2.8 cells. *Life Sciences,* 78, 1975–1982.

Gazzerro, E. and Minetti, C. 2007. Potential drug targets within bone morphogenetic protein signaling pathways. *Current Opinion in Pharmacology,* 7, 325–333.

Giancotti, F. G. and Ruoslahti, E. 1999. Integrin signaling. *Science,* 285, 1028.

Giustina, A., Mazziotti, G., and Canalis, E. 2008. Growth hormone, insulin-like growth factors, and the skeleton. *Endocrine Reviews,* 29, 535–559.

Govoni, K., Baylink, D. J., and Mohan, S. 2005. The multi-functional role of insulin-like growth factor binding proteins in bone. *Pediatric Nephrology,* 20, 261–268.

Gowen, M., Wood, D. D., Ihrie, E. J., Mcguire, M. K. B., and Russell, R. G. G. 1983. An interleukin 1 like factor stimulates bone resorption *in vitro. Nature,* 306, 378–380.

Gründer, T., Gaissmaier, C., Fritz, J. et al. 2004. Bone morphogenetic protein (BMP)-2 enhances the expression of type II collagen and aggrecan in chondrocytes embedded in alginate beads. *Osteoarthritis and Cartilage,* 12, 559–567.

Guo, W. and Giancotti, F. G. 2004. Integrin signalling during tumour progression. *Nature Reviews Molecular Cell Biology,* 5, 816–826.

Haÿ, E., Lemonnier, J., Fromigué, O., and Marie, P. J. 2001. Bone morphogenetic protein-2 promotes osteoblast apoptosis through a Smad-independent, protein kinase C-dependent signaling pathway. *Journal of Biological Chemistry,* 276, 29028.

Hay, E., Lemonnier, J., Fromigue, O., Guenou, H., and Marie, P. J. 2004. Bone morphogenetic protein receptor IB signaling mediates apoptosis independently of differentiation in osteoblastic cells. *Journal of Biological Chemistry,* 279, 1650–1658.

Hofmann, A., Ritz, U., Hessmann, M. H. et al. 2008. Cell viability, osteoblast differentiation, and gene expression are altered in human osteoblasts from hypertrophic fracture non-unions. *Bone,* 42, 894–906.

Holland, T. A., Tabata, Y., and Mikos, A. G. 2005. Dual growth factor delivery from degradable oligo(poly(ethylene glycol) fumarate) hydrogel scaffolds for cartilage tissue engineering. *Journal of Controlled Release,* 101, 111–125.

Holland, T. A., Bodde, E. W. H., Cuijpers, V. M. J. I., Baggett, L. S., Tabata, Y., Mikos, A. G., and Jansen, J. A. 2007. Degradable hydrogel scaffolds for in vivo delivery of single and dual growth factors in cartilage repair. *Osteoarthritis and Cartilage,* 15, 187–197.

Humbel, R. E. 1990. Insulin-like growth factors I and II. *European Journal of Biochemistry,* 190, 445–462.

Izzi, L. and Attisano, L. 2004. Regulation of the TGF signalling pathway by ubiquitin-mediated degradation. *Oncogene,* 23, 2071–2078.

Janssens, K., Ten Dijke, P., Janssens, S., and Van Hul, W. 2005. Transforming growth factor-beta 1 to the bone. *Endocrine Reviews,* 26, 743–774.

Kaneki, H., Guo, R., Chen, D. et al. 2006. Tumor necrosis factor promotes Runx2 degradation through up-regulation of Smurf1 and Smurf2 in osteoblasts. *Journal of Biological Chemistry,* 281, 4326–4333.

Katsumi, A., Orr, A. W., Tzima, E., and Schwartz, M. A. 2004. Integrins in mechanotransduction. *Journal of Biological Chemistry,* 279, 12001–12004.

Kempen, D. H. R., Lu, L., Heijink, A., Hefferan, T. E., Creemers, L. B., Maran, A., Yaszemski, M. J., and Dhert, W. J. A. 2009. Effect of local sequential VEGF and BMP-2 delivery on ectopic and orthotopic bone regeneration. *Biomaterials,* 30, 2816–2825.

Khalafi, A., Schmid, T. M., Neu, C., and Reddi, A. H. 2007. Increased accumulation of superficial zone protein (SZP) in articular cartilage in response to bone morphogenetic protein-7 and growth factors. *Journal of Orthopaedic Research,* 25, 293–303.

Klooster, A. R. and Bernier, S. M. 2005. Tumor necrosis factor alpha and epidermal growth factor act additively to inhibit matrix gene expression by chondrocyte. *Arthritis Research & Therapy,* 7, R127–R138.

Koay, E. J., Ofek, G., and Athanasiou, K. A. 2008. Effects of TGF-1 and IGF-I on the compressibility, biomechanics, and strain-dependent recovery behavior of single chondrocytes. *Journal of Biomechanics,* 41, 1044–1052.

Lago, R., Gomez, R., Otero, M. et al. 2008. A new player in cartilage homeostasis: Adiponectin induces nitric oxide synthase type II and pro-inflammatory cytokines in chondrocytes. *Osteoarthritis and Cartilage,* 16, 1101–1109.

Le Roy, C. and Wrana, J. L. 2005. Clathrin-and non-clathrin-mediated endocytic regulation of cell signalling. *Nature Reviews Molecular Cell Biology,* 6, 112–126.

Lee, D. A., Noguchi, T., Frean, S. P., Lees, P., and Bader, D. L. 2000. The influence of mechanical loading on isolated chondrocytes seeded in agarose constructs. *Biorheology,* 37, 149–161.

Lee, D. A., Noguchi, T., Knight, M. M. et al. 1998. Response of chondrocyte subpopulations cultured within unloaded and loaded agarose. *Journal of Orthopaedic Research,* 16, 726–733.

Lehmann, W., Edgar, C. M., Wang, K. et al. 2005. Tumor necrosis factor alpha (TNF-alpha) coordinately regulates the expression of specific matrix metalloproteinases (MMPS) and angiogenic factors during fracture healing. *Bone,* 36, 300–310.

Leipzig, N. D., Eleswarapu, S. V., and Athanasiou, K. A. 2006. The effects of TGF-[beta] 1 and IGF-I on the biomechanics and cytoskeleton of single chondrocytes. *Osteoarthritis and Cartilage,* 14, 1227–1236.

Li, T. F. and O'Keefe, R. J. 2005. TGF- signaling in chondrocytes. *Frontiers in Bioscience: A Journal and Virtual Library,* 10, 681.

Lian, J. B., Javed, A., Zaidi, S. K. et al. 2004. Regulatory controls for osteoblast growth and differentiation: Role of Runx/Cbfa/Aml factors. *Critical Reviews in Eukaryotic Gene Expression,* 14, 1–41.

Liedert, A., Kaspar, D., Blakytny, R., Claes, L., and Ignatius, A. 2006. Signal transduction pathways involved in mechanotransduction in bone cells. *Biochemical and Biophysical Research Communications,* 349, 1–5.

Liedert, A., Wagner, L., Seefried, L. et al. 2010. Estrogen receptor and Wnt signaling interact to regulate early gene expression in response to mechanical strain in osteoblastic cells. *Biochemical and Biophysical Research Communications,* 394, 755–759.

Lires-Deán, M., Caramés, B., Cillero-Pastor, B. et al. 2008. Anti-apoptotic effect of transforming growth factor-[beta]1 on human articular chondrocytes: Role of protein phosphatase 2A. *Osteoarthritis and Cartilage,* 16, 1370–1378.

Loeser, R. F. 2000. Chondrocyte integrin expression and function. *Biorheology,* 37, 109–116.

Loeser, R. F. 2002. Integrins and cell signaling in chondrocytes. *Biorheology,* 39, 119–124.

Malemud, C. J. 2004. Cytokines as therapeutic targets for osteoarthritis. *BioDrugs,* 18, 23–35.

Massague, J. 1990. The transforming growth-factor-beta family. *Annual Review of Cell Biology,* 6, 597–641.

Massague, J. 1998. TGF-beta signal transduction. *Annual Review of Biochemistry,* 67, 753–791.

Massagué, J. and Gomis, R. R. 2006. The logic of TGF [beta] signaling. *FEBS Letters,* 580, 2811–2820.

Massagué, J., Seoane, J., and Wotton, D. 2005. Smad transcription factors. *Genes and Development,* 19, 2783.

Millward-Sadler, S. J. and Salter, D. M. 2004. Integrin-dependent signal cascades in chondrocyte mechano-transduction. *Annals of Biomedical Engineering,* 32, 435–446.

Miyazono, K. 2000. TGF-[beta] signaling by Smad proteins. *Cytokine & Growth Factor Reviews,* 11, 15–22.

Miyazono, K., Maeda, S., and Imamura, T. 2005. BMP receptor signaling: Transcriptional targets, regulation of signals, and signaling cross-talk. *Cytokine & Growth Factor Reviews,* 16, 251–263.

Mollenhauer, J. A. 2008. Perspectives on articular cartilage biology and osteoarthritis. *Injury,* 39, 5–12.

Moustakas, A. and Heldin, C. H. 2005. Non-Smad TGF-beta signals. *Journal of Cell Science,* 118, 3573–3584.

Mundy, G. R. 2007. Osteoporosis and Inflammation. *Nutrition Reviews,* 65, S147-S151.

Murata, M., Yudoh, K., and Masuko, K. 2008. The potential role of vascular endothelial growth factor (VEGF) in cartilage: How the angiogenic factor could be involved in the pathogenesis of osteoarthritis? *Osteoarthritis and Cartilage,* 16, 279–286.

Nanes, M. S. 2003. Tumor necrosis factor-alpha: molecular and cellular mechanisms in skeletal pathology. *Gene,* 321, 1–15.

Oshima, K., Nampei, A., Matsuda, M. et al. 2005. Adiponectin increases bone mass by suppressing osteoclast and activating osteoblast. *Biochemical and Biophysical Research Communications,* 331, 520–526.

Otero, M. and Goldring, M. B. 2007. Cells of the synovium in rheumatoid arthritis. Chondrocytes. *Arthritis Research and Therapy,* 9, 220.

Patel, Z. S., Yamamoto, M., Yasuhiko, H., Tabata, U., and Mikos, A. G. 2008. Biodegradable gelatin microparticles as delivery systems for the controlled release of bone morphogenetic protein-2. *Acta Biomaterialia,* 4, 1126–1138.

Perrini, S., Laviola, L., Carreira, M. C. et al. 2010. The GH/IGF1 axis and signaling pathways in the muscle and bone: mechanisms underlying age-related skeletal muscle wasting and osteoporosis. *Journal of Endocrinology,* 205, 201–210.

Perrini, S., Natalicchio, A., Laviola, L. et al. 2008. Abnormalities of insulin-like growth factor-I signaling and impaired cell proliferation in osteoblasts from subjects with osteoporosis. *Endocrinology,* 149, 1302.

Preiss-Bloom, O., Mizrahi, J., Elisseeff, J., and Seliktar, D. 2009. Real-time monitoring of force response measured in mechanically stimulated tissue-engineered cartilage. *Artificial Organs,* 33, 318–327.

Pujol, J.-P., Chadjichristos, C., Legendre, F. et al. 2008. Interleukin-1 and transforming growth factor-ss 1 as crucial factors in osteoarthritic cartilage metabolism. *Connective Tissue Research,* 49, 293–297.

Qin, L., Raggatt, L. J., and Partridge, N. C. 2004. Parathyroid hormone: a double-edged sword for bone metabolism. *Trends in Endocrinology and Metabolism,* 15, 60–65.

Roman-Blas, J. A. and Jimenez, S. A. 2008. Targeting NF-kappa B: A promising molecular therapy in inflammatory arthritis. *International Reviews of Immunology,* 27, 351–374.

Roman-Blas, J. A., Stokes, D. G., and Jimenez, S. A. 2007. Modulation of TGF-[beta] signaling by proinflammatory cytokines in articular chondrocytes. *Osteoarthritis and Cartilage,* 15, 1367–1377.

Rubin, J., Rubin, C., and Jacobs, C. R. 2006. Molecular pathways mediating mechanical signaling in bone. *Gene,* 367, 1–16.

Saadeh, P. B., Mehrara, B. J., Steinbrech, D. S. et al. 2000. Mechanisms of fibroblast growth factor-2 modulation of vascular endothelial growth factor expression by osteoblastic cells. *Endocrinology,* 141, 2075.

Saklatvala, J. 2007. Inflammatory signaling in cartilage: MAPK and NF-B pathways in chondrocytes and the use of inhibitors for research into pathogenesis and therapy of osteoarthritis. *Current Drug Targets,* 8, 305–313.

Samani, A. A., Yakar, S., Leroith, D., and Brodt, P. 2007. The role of the IGF system in cancer growth and metastasis: Overview and recent insights. *Endocrine Reviews,* 28, 20.

Sanchez, C., Gabay, O., Henrotin, Y. E., and Berenbaum, F. 2008. Osteoblast: A cell under compression. *Bio-Medical Materials & Engineering,* 18, 221–224.

Selvamurugan, N., Kwok, S., Alliston, T., Reiss, M., and Partridge, N. C. 2004. Transforming growth factor-1 regulation of collagenase-3 expression in osteoblastic cells by cross-talk between the Smad and MAPK signaling pathways and their components, Smad2 and Runx2. *Journal of Biological Chemistry,* 279, 19327.

Shakibaei, M., Csaki, C., and Mobasheri, A. 2008. *Diverse Roles of Integrin Receptors in Articular Cartilage,* Springer Verlag, Berlin.

Sondergaard, B. C., Schultz, N., Madsen, S. H. et al. 2009. MAPKs are essential upstream signaling pathways in proteolytic cartilage degradation—Divergence in pathways leading to aggrecanase and MMP-mediated articular cartilage degradation. *Osteoarthritis and Cartilage,* 18, 279–288.

Starkman, B. G., Cravero, J. D., Delcarlo Jr, M., and Loeser, R. F. 2005. IGF-I stimulation of proteoglycan synthesis by chondrocytes requires activation of the PI 3-kinase pathway but not ERK MAPK. *Biochemical Journal,* 389, 723.

Steeve, K. T., Marc, P., Sandrine, T., Dominique, H., and Yannick, F. 2004. IL-6, RANKL, TNF-alpha/IL-1: Interrelations in bone resorption pathophysiology. *Cytokine and Growth Factor Reviews,* 15, 49–60.

Sykaras, N. and Opperman, L. A. 2003. Bone morphogenetic proteins (BMPs): How do they function and what can they offer the clinician? *Journal of Oral Science,* 45, 57–74.

Takai, S., Tokuda, H., Hanai, Y., and Kozawa, O. 2007. Activation of phosphatidylinositol 3-kinase/Akt limits FGF-2-induced VEGF release in osteoblasts. *Molecular and Cellular Endocrinology,* 267, 46–54.

Tanabe, N., Ito-Kato, E., Suzuki, N. et al. 2004. IL-1[alpha] affects mineralized nodule formation by rat osteoblasts. *Life Sciences,* 75, 2317–2327.

Tanabe, N., Maeno, M., Suzuki, N. et al. 2005. IL-1[alpha] stimulates the formation of osteoclast-like cells by increasing M-CSF and Pge2 production and decreasing OPG production by osteoblasts. *Life Sciences,* 77, 615–626.

Tombran-Tink, J. and Barnstable, C. J. 2004. Osteoblasts and osteoclasts express PEDF, VEGF-A isoforms, and VEGF receptors: possible mediators of angiogenesis and matrix remodeling in the bone. *Biochemical and Biophysical Research Communications,* 316, 573–579.

Tsuboi, M., Kawakami, A., Nakashima, T. et al. 1999. Tumor necrosis factor-[alpha] and interleukin-1 [beta] increase the Fas-mediated apoptosis of human osteoblasts. *Journal of Laboratory and Clinical Medicine,* 134, 222–231.

Urist, M. R. 1965. Bone: Formation by autoinduction. *Science,* 150, 893–899.

Van der Kraan, P. M., Buma, P., Van Kuppevelt, T., and Van Den Berg, W. B. 2002. Interaction of chondrocytes, extracellular matrix and growth factors: relevance for articular cartilage tissue engineering. *Osteoarthritis and Cartilage,* 10, 631–637.

Vanderploeg, E. J., Wilson, C. G., and Levenston, M. E. 2008. Articular chondrocytes derived from distinct tissue zones differentially respond to *in vitro* oscillatory tensile loading. *Osteoarthritis and Cartilage,* 16, 1228–1236.

Veilleux, N. and Spector, M. 2005. Effects of FGF-2 and IGF-1 on adult canine articular chondrocytes in Type II collagen-glycosaminoglycan scaffolds in vitro. *Osteoarthritis and Cartilage,* 13, 278–286.

Villanueva, I., Weigel, C. A., and Bryant, S. J. 2009. Cell-matrix interactions and dynamic mechanical loading influence chondrocyte gene expression and bioactivity in PEG-RGD hydrogels. *Acta Biomaterialia,* 5, 2832–2846.

Vincent, T. L., Mclean, C. J., Full, L. E., Peston, D., and Saklatvala, J. 2007. FGF-2 is bound to perlecan in the pericellular matrix of articular cartilage, where it acts as a chondrocyte mechanotransducer. *Osteoarthritis and Cartilage,* 15, 752–763.

Wang, H., Wang, Z., Chen, J., and Wu, J. 2007. Apoptosis induced by NO via phosphorylation of p38 MAPK that stimulates NF-[kappa] B, p53 and caspase-3 activation in rabbit articular chondrocytes. *Cell Biology International,* 31, 1027–1035.

Wang, J., Elewaut, D., Veys, E. M., and Verbruggen, G. 2003. Insulin-like growth factor 1-induced interleukin-1 receptor II overrides the activity of interleukin-1 and controls the homeostasis of the extracellular matrix of cartilage. *Arthritis and Rheumatism,* 48, 1281–1291.

Wang, Y.-J., Shi, Q., Sun, P. et al. 2006. Insulin-like growth factor-1 treatment prevents anti-fas antibody-induced apoptosis in endplate chondrocytes. *Spine*, 31, 736–741 10.1097/01.brs.0000208128.49912.64.

Westendorf, J. J., Kahler, R. A., and Schroeder, T. M. 2004. Wnt signaling in osteoblasts and bone diseases. *Gene*, 341, 19–39.

Wildemann, B., Bamdad, P., Holmer, C., Haas, N. P., Raschke, M., and Schmidmaier, G. 2004. Local delivery of growth factors from coated titanium plates increases osteotomy healing in rats. *Bone*, 34, 862–868.

Woods, A., Wang, G., and Beier, F. 2007. Regulation of chondrocyte differentiation by the actin cytoskeleton and adhesive interactions. *Journal of Cellular Physiology*, 213, 1–8.

Xiao, Y.-T., Xiang, L.-X., and Shao, J.-Z. 2007. Bone morphogenetic protein. *Biochemical and Biophysical Research Communications*, 362, 550–553.

Xing, L. and Boyce, B. F. 2005. Regulation of apoptosis in osteoclasts and osteoblastic cells. *Biochemical and Biophysical Research Communications*, 328, 709–720.

Yamane, S. and Reddi, A. H. 2008. Induction of chondrogenesis and superficial zone protein accumulation in synovial side population cells by Bmp-7 and TGF- 1. *Journal of Orthopaedic Research*, 26, 485–492.

Yamazaki, M., Fukushima, H., Shin, M. et al. 2009. Tumor necrosis factor alpha represses Bone Morphogenetic Protein (BMP) Signaling by interfering with the DNA binding of Smads through the activation of NF-kappa B. *Journal of Biological Chemistry*, 284, 35987–35995.

Yoon, D. M. and Fisher, J. P. 2007. Chondrocyte signaling and artificial matrices for articular cartilage engineering. *Tissue Engineering*, 67–86.

Zhang, M., Zhou, Q., Liang, Q. Q. et al. 2009. Igf-1 regulation of type II collagen and MMP-13 expression in rat endplate chondrocytes via distinct signaling pathways. *Osteoarthritis and cartilage/OARS, Osteoarthritis Research Society*, 17, 100–106.

Zhang, Y., Deng, X., Scheller, E. L. et al. 2010. The effects of Runx2 immobilization on poly (caprolactone) on osteoblast differentiation of bone marrow stromal cells *in vitro*. *Biomaterials*, 31, 3231–3236.

Zuscik, M. J., Hilton, M. J., Zhang, X., Chen, D., and O'keefe, R. J. 2008. Regulation of chondrogenesis and chondrocyte differentiation by stress. *The Journal of Clinical Investigation*, 118, 429–438.

# 8

# Pluripotent Stem Cells

8.1  Origin and Derivation of Embryonic Stem Cells ........................ 8-1
History of Embryonic Stem Cell Research • Derivation of
ESCs • Early Embryonic Development
8.2  Characteristics................................................................................. 8-5
Self-Renewal and Pluripotency • *In Vivo* Differentiation Capacity:
Teratoma Formation and Chimerism • Genetic Markers of
Pluripotency
8.3  Alternate Derivation Methods....................................................... 8-7
Blastomere Derivation • Somatic Cell Nuclear Transfer • Induced
Pluripotent Stem Cells
8.4  Propagation...................................................................................... 8-9
Culture Conditions for Undifferentiated ESCs • Epiblast Stem Cells
8.5  Differentiation .............................................................................. 8-11
Late Embryonic Development • ESC Differentiation in
Monolayer • Embryoid Body Differentiation
8.6  Clinical Outlook ........................................................................... 8-15
8.7  Conclusion .................................................................................... 8-15
References................................................................................................ 8-15

Todd C. McDevitt
*Georgia Institute of
Technology*

Melissa A. Kinney
*Georgia Institute of
Technology*

## 8.1 Origin and Derivation of Embryonic Stem Cells

### 8.1.1 History of Embryonic Stem Cell Research

Embryonic stem cells (ESCs) possess the unique capacity to proliferate indefinitely in culture and differentiate into all somatic cells, thereby serving as a promising cell source for tissue engineering applications, including the treatment of degenerative diseases, traumatic injuries and chronic wounds. ESCs have garnered much public attention, largely via media coverage, due to frequent discussions and changes in legislative regulations at the state and federal levels. Much of the controversy surrounding ESCs stems from the methods used to harvest stem cells, which traditionally results in the destruction of blastocysts during the stages of development prior to implantation.

Opposition to biomedical research involving the use of embryos has its origins in the beginning of the anti-abortion movement following the 1973 Supreme Court case of Roe v. Wade, which stated that decisions about abortion are between a woman and her doctor and cannot be regulated by individual states. Although ESCs had not yet been successfully derived from mammalian species, research interest in cells from embryonic sources was growing due to the derivation of pluripotent embryonic carcinoma (EC) cells in the early 1970s. The public outcry in response to the legislation led to concerns regarding the lack of regulation and possible exploitation of aborted fetuses for research purposes. Subsequently, the Department of Health and Human Services placed an indefinite federal funding ban on research using human embryos, embryonic or fetal tissue, or cells from *in vitro* fertilization (IVF), with the rationalization that such research could potentially increase the number of abortions; however, research using embryonic tissues remained unregulated in the private sector, and federal funding was available for the use of ESCs derived from non-human sources. In response to limited federal funding, several states, including most notably California, Maryland, and New York, took steps in the past decade to start up funding programs for human ESC research. Legislative bills that were intended to expand federal funding of human ESC research were passed by the US Senate and Congress in 2006 and 2007, but were subsequently vetoed by President George W. Bush on each occasion. In 2009, an executive order was passed by President Barack Obama, and stipulates that only cells obtained from left over IVF treatments could be used for the derivation of ESCs. In response to this change in policy, the National Institute of Health developed a registry, which enumerates hESC lines that are eligible for funding through the government organization.

Despite the ongoing public debate and legal barriers to human ESC research, there has been an exponential increase in the number of publications related to ESCs from the 1980s until the present day (Figure 8.1, source: Pubmed). Much of the work during the past decades has focused on the use of mouse ESCs, initially derived in 1981, as a model system for studying cell differentiation and understanding the therapeutic potential of ESCs. In addition, federal funding barriers prompted the development of several promising alternative derivation methods for human ESCs. The growth of ESC research is paralleled by a similar expansion of tissue engineering publications, indicating a general interest in functional tissue replacement technologies. However, beginning in the late 1990s, the two fields began to coalesce, which is demonstrated by a steady increase in the percentage of tissue engineering publications that mention ESCs. The increasing discussion of ESCs in the context of tissue engineering is likely due to the derivation of ESCs from primate and human sources in 1995 and 1998, respectively, which helped to fully realize the clinical potential of ESCs. The interest in stem cells in recent years has also been apparent through the establishment of scientific journals dedicated to stem cell research, as well as the increasing impact factors of existing journals, such as a 40% increase in the impact factor of *Cell Stem Cell* between 2008 and 2009 (from 16.826 to 23.563).

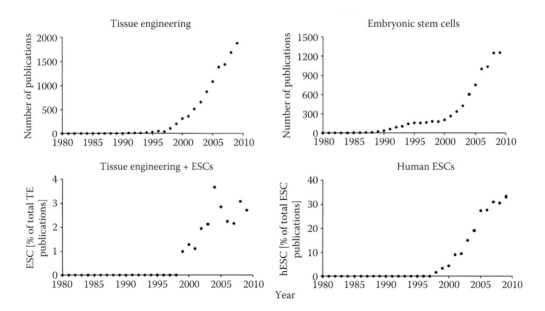

**FIGURE 8.1**  Publication records depicting the prevalence of embryonic stem cells and tissue engineering. On the basis of publication records, tissue engineering and ESC research have experienced exponential growth from the late 1990s until present, with an increasing number of ESC publications relating to both tissue engineering and human ESC research.

## 8.1.2 Derivation of ESCs

Prior to the isolation of pluripotent cells from embryonic sources, carcinomas were the most widely understood source of highly proliferative cells. Teratocarcinomas, or germ cell tumors, were known to consist of many cell types at various stages of differentiation (Stevens and Little 1954, Pierce and Dixon 1959). Investigators postulated that the differentiated cell types found within the tumors were all derived from a common source, which they termed EC cells (Pierce et al. 1960). Isolation of EC cells, based on morphological appearance and proliferative capacity, validated this hypothesis, as aggregates of EC cells, termed embryoid bodies (EBs), as well as single EC cells produced similar tumors when injected subcutaneously or intraperitoneally in animals (Pierce and Verney 1961, Kleinsmith and Pierce 1964). When cultured *in vitro*, EC cells differentiated into derivatives of all three embryonic germ layers (Kahan and Ephrussi 1970, Rosenthal et al. 1970, Lehman et al. 1974, Martin and Evans 1974). EC cells also incorporated into all somatic tissues when injected into a blastocyst; however, tumor induction was also commonly observed (Illmensee and Mintz 1976). EC cells have been derived and characterized from both mouse and human (Andrews et al. 1984, Pera et al. 1989) sources, permitting studies of differentiation and mammalian embryogenesis. However, due to their derivation from tumor sources, EC cells are often aneuploid (Roach et al. 1993), harbor genetic variability and exhibit varied capacities depending on the cell line, including the potential to differentiate and form EBs (Jacob 1977, Pera et al. 1987).

Many of the advances in the establishment of *in vitro* cell culture methods and phenotyping of EC cells (Jacob 1977) led to the successful derivation of pluripotent stem cells from blastocyst-stage embryos (Evans and Kaufman 1981, Martin 1981). Comparison of surface antigens present on EC cells led to the derivation of epiblast cells from post-implantation mouse embryos, based on similar markers. Changing hormonal conditions through the process of ovariectomy resulted in the embryos entering a state of diapause, in which the process of implantation was disrupted to ease the isolation of epiblast cells. Individual blastocysts were isolated and cultured in drops of tissue culture media, and after about 48 h attached to the dish and began to exhibit trophoblast propagation. The trophoblast was then removed and the resulting inner cell mass (ICM) cells were separated by enzymatic trypsin treatment. Cells with similar morphology to EC cells were then individually selected and propagated for over 30 passages *in vitro* using previously established feeder-dependent or conditioned media culture conditions (Evans and Kaufman 1981). ESCs derived from the ICM exhibited similar growth characteristics to ECs, as well as the capacity to differentiate into derivatives of all three germ lineages as EBs *in vitro* and form teratomas *in vivo* (Martin 1981). Karyotypically normal cells have been isolated from murine (Evans and Kaufman 1981, Martin 1981), primate (Thomson et al. 1995), and human (Thomson et al. 1998, Reubinoff et al. 2000) sources. Human ESCs were derived from fresh or frozen morula stage embryos obtained from IVF.

## 8.1.3 Early Embryonic Development

ESCs derived from the ICM of pre-implantation embryos exhibit unique properties that have been useful to understanding the events associated with early stages of development and the genetic regulation of pluripotent tissues. Many established culture conditions for the maintenance of undifferentiated cells, as well as for directing differentiation into desired somatic cells and tissues rely on signaling pathways active during embryogenesis.

At the time of fertilization, the resultant zygote is responsible for all of the cellular programming required for the specification and patterning of tissues within the embryo. The cells of the zygote initially undergo several rapid divisions, referred to as "cleavages," in which the resulting cells, or blastomeres, become increasingly smaller with each division and the overall cell cluster, referred to as the morula, remains approximately the same size as the original zygote. At the eight-cell stage, the morula undergoes compaction, in which cell–cell adhesions are initiated via adherens and tight junctions (Vestweber et al. 1987). Compaction is largely mediated by the adhesion molecule E-cadherin (Hyafil et al. 1980); inhibition of the binding capabilities of E-cadherin prevents the embryo from undergoing compaction (Vestweber and Kemler 1984). The mechanisms through which the compaction processes is initiated, however, are unclear. Studies have indicated that both E-cadherin and its binding partners, such as β-catenin, are present during earlier stages prior to compaction (Ohsugi et al. 1999). It is therefore hypothesized that post-translational protein modifications may be responsible for the initiation of embryonic compaction (Kidder and Mclachlin 1985, Levy et al. 1986). Prior to compaction, the cells do not exhibit polarity; however, after the establishment of cell–cell adhesions, the apical and basolateral sides of cells become well-defined (Ziomek and Johnson 1980, Johnson and Ziomek 1981). Many of the cytoplasmic components are reorganized, including the basolateral localization of the nuclei (Reeve and Kelly 1983) and the movement of actin filaments (Johnson and Maro 1984) and endosomes (Fleming and Pickering 1985) near the apical side of the cells. In subsequent cleavages, the polarity is retained, resulting in two distinct populations comprising the interior and exterior of the developing embryo.

Owing to the changes during compaction, specification of distinct cell types occurs during the 32-cell stage. The specification of cells is likely mediated by cell polarity and adhesions, as changing the location of cells within the blastocyst can influence the cell fate during subsequent stages of differentiation (Handyside 1978, Rossant and Lis 1979). Specification yields a 70–100-cell blastocyst, containing spatially distinct structures, including an outer layer of epithelial trophoblast cells, which envelops a tightly packed ICM, from which ESCs are derived (Figure 8.2). One of the functions of the trophoblast is to pump sodium into the structure, simultaneously increasing water content, thereby forming the fluid-filled blastocoel cavity within the blastocyst (Barcroft et al. 2003). The blastocyst typically implants into the uterine wall about 4.5 days *post coitum* in mice and a week in humans (Edwards et al. 1981). At the time of implantation, the cell types within the blastocyst are transcriptionally and epigenetically distinct, and will ultimately give rise to divergent cells and tissues (Santos et al. 2002, Rossant et al. 2003). Specification of the trophoblast leads to generation of extraembryonic supporting tissues, including

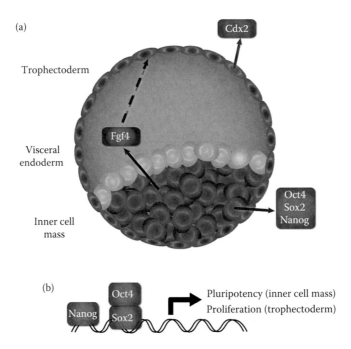

**FIGURE 8.2** Blastocyst (a) structure and (b) signaling. Blastocyst structure comprises three distinct cell types, including the ICM, visceral endoderm, and the trophoblast. Distinct signaling patterns within the ICM (Fgf4) and trophoblast (Cdx2) are responsible maintenance of the divergent cell types. Several factors produced by the ICM (Oct4, Nanog, Sox2) are transcriptional regulators of both trophectoderm proliferation and ICM pluripotency.

components of the placenta, whereas the ICM segregates into extraembryonic primitive endoderm and epiblast, which is responsible for development of the embryo proper.

Events leading to early specification of trophoblast and ICM remain largely unknown; however, there are several key genes that are likely responsible for initiating and maintaining distinct cell phenotypes. Cdx2 and Eomes are both found in trophectoderm cells, and are thought to regulate the specification of early trophoblast and ICM cells (Albert and Peters 2009). As early as the eight-cell stage, Cdx2 is found at the apical domain of blastomeres (Jedrusik et al. 2008). In contrast, several genes that are highly expressed in the ICM, including octamer-binding transcription factor 4 (Oct4), Nanog and Sox2 are found at very low levels in the trophoblast (Palmieri et al. 1994). The downregulation of ICM genes, however, occurs after Cdx2 becomes restricted to the exterior cells, indicating the possible role of Cdx2 in the downregulation of ICM genes (Beck et al. 1995). Within Cdx2-deficient ($Cdx2^{-/-}$) embryos, the spatial patterning of genes within the ICM does not occur, resulting in failure of the outer cells to differentiate into trophoblast, and leading to eventual cell death (Strumpf et al. 2005).

High levels of expression of several key genes are responsible for maintaining pluripotency within the ICM. Oct4 is a maternally derived transcription factor, which is present from unfertilized oocytes through the blastocyst (Schöler et al. 1989). Embryos deficient in Oct4 ($Oct4^{-/-}$) develop to the blastocyst stage, but the cells of the ICM are not pluripotent, and instead differentiate similarly to trophoblast cells (Nichols et al. 1998). Oct4 is known to regulate two promoters: E1A-like activity (Schöler et al. 1991) and Fgf4 (Yuan et al. 1995). Dimerization of Sox2 and Oct4 can result in transcriptional activation of the gene Fgf4 (Yuan et al. 1995, Avilion et al. 2003), a signaling molecule responsible for trophectoderm proliferation (Nichols et al. 1998). Nanog, another transcription factor, which has been implicated in the maintenance of pluripotency, associates with many of the same target sites as Sox2 and Oct4, indicating cooperative activation and repression of many genes by Sox2, Oct4, and Nanog (Boyer et al. 2005, Loh et al. 2006, Masui et al. 2007). Therefore, the reciprocal expression of genes in the ICM and trophoblast is responsible for maintaining pluripotency, as well as for paracrine signaling to direct divergent lineages (Chew et al. 2005, Okumura-Nakanishi et al. 2005).

# 8.2 Characteristics

## 8.2.1 Self-Renewal and Pluripotency

Owing to their derivation from the ICM, ESCs retain unique properties, which distinguish them from adult cells. ESCs are defined by the ability to self-renew indefinitely, producing more stem cells, as well as the capacity to differentiate into other cell types. Self-renewal is accomplished via both symmetric divisions, which produce two daughter cells of the same fate, as well as through asymmetric divisions, which result in one daughter ESC and one destined to differentiate. Asymmetric divisions of ESCs are similar to divisions near the exterior of the morula during embryonic cell cleavages, which produce one polar and one apolar cell (Johnson and Ziomek 1981, Sutherland et al. 1990). Owing to their capacities to divide asymmetrically and increase telomerase activity, ESCs are capable of indefinite self-renewal in an undifferentiated state under defined culture conditions (Thomson et al. 1998). The highly proliferative nature of undifferentiated ESCs, therefore, affords derivation of a population of cells from a single-cell clone. Similar to the cells of the ICM, ESCs are considered pluripotent because they can give rise to all three primary germ lineages simultaneously—endoderm, ectoderm, and mesoderm—as well as germ cells (Evans and Kaufman 1981, Martin 1981, Thomson et al. 1998). In contrast, many adult stem and progenitor cells, such as mesenchymal stem cells, are considered multipotent due to the limited capacity to differentiate, often along a single germ lineage of related cell types (Baum et al. 1992, Pittenger et al. 1999). Many progenitor and somatic cells are not capable of differentiating, and are therefore unipotent. One of the unique traits of pluripotent ESCs is the capacity to generate any cell type, including cells which cannot be easily isolated from primary sources, such as pancreatic β-cells (Shi et al. 2005, Bernardo et al. 2009, Champeris Tsaniras and Jones 2010), neurons (Strübing et al. 1995, Sasai 2002,

Nakayama and Inoue 2006), and cardiomyocytes (Wobus et al. 1991, Maltsev et al. 1994, Boheler et al. 2002, Fijnvandraat et al. 2003). Although more differentiated cells, such as multipotent adult stem cells, are already partially committed to a certain lineage and therefore may be easier to coax toward a desired phenotype, the proliferative capacity also generally decreases rather dramatically as cells differentiate. In addition, more differentiated cells often do not survive when transplanted *in vivo*, and necessitate tissue-specific stromal cells. Although current methods for ESC differentiation often result in heterogeneous populations, there is promise for the creation of complex tissues comprising multiple cell types.

## 8.2.2 *In Vivo* Differentiation Capacity: Teratoma Formation and Chimerism

Similar to teratocarcinomas formed by EC cells, the hyperproliferative capacity of ESCs can result in the generation of benign tumors (i.e., teratomas) when injected subcutaneously. Teratoma formation *in vivo* is a relatively straightforward assay to test the pluripotency of ESCs. The resultant teratomas comprise a heterogeneous, disorganized mass of tissue consisting of cells from all three germ layers, and histological analysis often reveals organization into discernable somatic structures (Figure 8.3). Although the formation of teratomas from ESCs is a useful qualitative analytical technique to establish differentiation potential along divergent lineages, the binary output of tumor formation does not conclusively establish the ability of ESCs to generate all somatic cells.

To examine the full pluripotency of ESCs, chimeras can be formed by injection of ESCs into blastocyst stage embryos (Eggan et al. 2002). The resultant animals contain two populations of genetically distinct cells derived from the original embryonic cells, and from the artificially introduced ESCs. Analysis of the genetic profile of cells within different tissues can indicate the pluripotency of ESCs by the ability to contribute to all somatic tissues. Tetraploid complementation is a more specialized form of chimerism, which is used to determine the potential of the ESCs to form a complete embryo. Tetraploid cells are created by electrically fusing the two cells of an embryo after the first cleavage, resulting in a single cell that is considered tetraploid because it has four chromosomes, twice as many as somatic cells. Tetraploid embryos will develop to the blastocyst stage and are capable of implanting in the uterine wall, but tetraploid cells often form the extraembryonic supporting tissues, such as the trophoblast and rarely contribute to the embryo itself. The formation of a tetraploid embryo can, therefore, be used to combine with ESCs in the morula or blastula stage. The diploid ESCs progress to form the somatic tissues, resulting in an embryo derived entirely from the ESCs, and conclusively indicating that the ESCs are pluripotent. Although the formation of chimeras from ESCs has been useful as a method for establishing pluripotency of mouse ESCs, such chimera studies have not been conducted with human cells due to biological and ethical concerns related to inter-species mixing. Therefore, characterization techniques for human ESC research have relied largely upon the establishment of molecular markers of pluripotency.

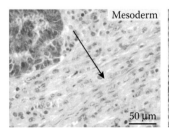 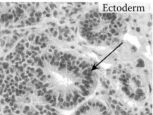 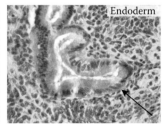

**FIGURE 8.3** Teratoma formation demonstrating differentiation into cells from each of the three germ lineages. Hematoxylin and eosin-stained histological sections of a single teratoma from injection of mESCs *in vivo* result in the development of structures resembling mesoderm, ectoderm, and endoderm.

### 8.2.3 Genetic Markers of Pluripotency

Owing to the inability to functionally test hESCs in the same manner as mouse ESCs, the genetic profile of both mouse and human ESCs has been extensively studied. Many of the markers for pluripotency have been established from expression patterns in the embryo. For example, Oct-4, Sox2, and Nanog are commonly expressed in the ICM and used as markers of the undifferentiated pluripotent state. However, gene and protein expression alone may not be sufficient to unequivocally determine functional pluripotency. For example, the specific levels of Oct-4 expression govern cell fate, with a narrow range of expression leading to pluripotency, and increases and decreases in Oct-4 resulting in mesoderm/endoderm and trophectoderm differentiation, respectively (Niwa et al. 2000). Nanog was first described as a critical factor for maintaining pluripotency and self-renewal of ESCs (Chambers et al. 2003, Mitsui et al. 2003), and is believed to work in concert with other important pluripotency factors such as Oct-4 and Sox2; however, recent evidence suggests that the loss of Nanog results in a reversibly uncommitted, yet primed state for differentiation (Chambers et al. 2007). Although commonly associated with ESCs, Nanog may not be strictly required for the maintenance of pluripotency. Other established indicators of pluripotency include the enzymatic activity of alkaline phosphatase and the expression of stage-specific embryonic antigens (SSEAs), with SSEA-1 expressed in mESCs and SSEA-3,4 in hESCs, as well as TRA1-60 and TRA1-81 in hESCs (Beck et al. 1995, Vallier et al. 2005). The sum of recent investigations suggests that no single unequivocal marker for the pluripotency of ESCs exists; therefore, multiple functional and genetic analyses may be necessary to rigorously characterize the establishment of new cell lines.

## 8.3 Alternate Derivation Methods

### 8.3.1 Blastomere Derivation

One of ethical concerns regarding ESC research is that dissociation of blastocysts to extract ICM cells deprives embryos of the potential to develop into viable animals if they were successfully implanted (Figure 8.4, ICM). Thus, in attempts to address ethical concerns, it was discovered that a

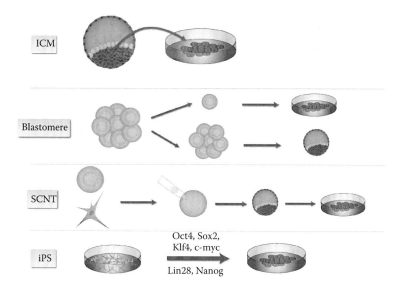

**FIGURE 8.4** Alternate methods for deriving pluripotent stem cells. In addition to conventional derivation of ESCs from the ICM of blastocyst stage embryos, ESCs have also been derived from a single blastomere derived from eight-cell morulas, by injection of a somatic cell nucleus into an enucleated egg, or by treating somatic cells with defined factors for reprogramming the differentiation state.

single blastomere could be propagated *in vitro* for the isolation of ESCs. Seven-cell morulas continue to undergo cleavage events and develop into morphologically and functionally normal blastocysts in several species, including mice (Rossant 1976), sheep (Moore et al. 1968), rabbits (Willadsen 1981), and primates (Chan et al. 2000). The method of deriving single blastomeres (Figure 8.4, blastomere) is regularly used in IVF clinics for pre-implantation genetic diagnosis and employs the use of piezo-pulse drilling to create a hole in the zona pellucida to obtain a single-cell biopsy. Early attempts to culture blastomeres *in vitro* resulted in the derivation of cells that were morphologically similar to trophoblast and failed to form a pluripotent population (Tarkowski and Wróblewska 1967). However, coculture of the isolated blastomere as aggregates with ESCs from the same species led to the derivation of pluripotent stem cells. Studies also established propagation methods utilizing mouse embryonic fibroblasts (MEFs) rather than coculture with other ESCs (Chung et al. 2008) and determined that the efficiency of derivation was increased using blastomeres at earlier stages (two to four cells) of the morula (Wakayama et al. 2007). Subsequent analysis confirmed the functional, morphological, genetic, and karyotypic similarities to ICM-derived ESCs in both mouse and human (Klimanskaya et al. 2006) species.

## 8.3.2  Somatic Cell Nuclear Transfer

Somatic cell nuclear transfer (SCNT), or the insertion of a nucleus into an enucleated egg, is a widely publicized technique that is often associated with ESCs (Figure 8.4, SCNT). SCNT was first conducted to establish the difference between nuclei from embryonic and fully differentiated cell sources. Although early work had established that the nuclei of individual blastomeres are identical, the nuclear mechanisms behind differentiation were still unclear. The method was first established by inserting the nuclei from blastula cells into enucleated frog eggs (Briggs and King 1952). The resultant cells were capable of developing into full embryos. Subsequent studies utilized the nuclei from terminally differentiated cells to establish that the somatic nuclei were capable of deriving functional embryos, albeit with much lower efficiency compared with the nuclei of less differentiated cells (Gurdon 1962). SCNT has become publicized due to the controversial ability to create genetically identical animals (genetic clones), as was demonstrated with the example of "Dolly" the sheep in 1996 (Campbell et al. 1996). However, SCNT has also provided a means of studying genetic and epigenetic changes in development and disease through the isolation of ESCs from blastocyst stage SCNT embryos. The efficient derivation of pluripotent cells with somatic nuclei first introduced the concept of "reprogramming," in which epigenetic changes can radically reverse the differentiation potential of somatic cells.

The ability to reprogram somatic cells highlighted the possibility of deriving autologous ESCs for clinical applications. It was originally thought that ICM-derived ESCs would not incite an immune response, based on the limited expression of major histocompatibility complex proteins (Drukker et al. 2002, Swijnenburg et al. 2005, Nussbaum et al. 2007). However, it has since been demonstrated that differentiation is accompanied by increases in the expression of immunogenic molecules that could provoke inflammatory and immune responses *in vivo* (Nussbaum et al. 2007). SCNT, therefore, was originally identified as a promising method for the derivation of autologous ESCs. However, studies indicate that some propensities cannot be completely reversed by SCNT. For example, ESCs derived from transfer of EC cell nuclei retain the same tumorigenic potential when induced to form chimeras (Blelloch et al. 2004, Hochedlinger et al. 2004). The retained susceptibility to forming cancerous cells demonstrates that some genetic changes are not reversible. Several groups have also discovered abnormal methylation patterns in SCNT-derived cells and found that the epigenetic regulation is more closely related to the donor cell compared with embryonic cells (Dean et al. 1998, Bourc'his et al. 2001, Dean et al. 2001, Koo et al. 2001, Ohgane et al. 2001). Despite the possibility of incomplete reprogramming, SCNT represents the first route to derivation of "autologous" ESCs that would avoid the rejection issues associated with allogeneic transplantation.

### 8.3.3 Induced Pluripotent Stem Cells

In 2006, Takahashi and Yamanaka reported the ability to reprogram differentiated somatic cells (Figure 8.4, "induced" pluripotent stem [iPS] cell) by retroviral transduction of several embryonic genes (Takahashi and Yamanaka 2006). The iPS cells exhibit similar characteristics of ESCs, including self-renewal and differentiation capacities (Narazaki et al. 2008, Schenke-Layland et al. 2008, Zhang et al. 2009). iPS cells, therefore, are a promising alternative source of autologous pluripotent cells for regenerative and therapeutic applications. Studies indicate that iPS cells are epigenetically similar to hESCs, including re-activation of the silent X-chromosome in female cells, as well as methylation patterns and histone modifications (Maherali et al. 2007). In subsequent studies, iPS cells have been derived independently by several groups introducing a variety of combinations of factors including Oct3/4, Sox2, Klf4, c-myc (termed the "Yamanaka factors"), as well as Nanog and Lin28 (Takahashi and Yamanaka 2006, Okita et al. 2007, Takahashi et al. 2007, Yu et al. 2007, Nakagawa et al. 2008) in both mouse and human somatic cells. Reprogramming has also been accomplished by transient expression of the same factors using adenoviral or plasmid delivery methods *in lieu* of viral vectors, which can permanently insert into the genome of cells and increase the potential for tumor formation (Okita et al. 2008, Stadtfeld et al. 2008). Therefore, the transient expression of many factors found in the ICM is sufficient for induction of pluripotency in somatic cells. As was found with SCNT, the efficiency of reprogramming is related to the differentiation state of the somatic cell; however, the inhibition of epigenetic modifying enzymes such as histone deacetylase (Huangfu et al. 2008a,b) and DNA methylation (Mikkelsen et al. 2008) can increase the efficiency of reprogramming.

iPS cells offer several advantages compared with ESCs, including the abilities to derive autologous cells for therapeutic applications and create disease-specific cell lines. Thus far, iPS cells from autologous sources have been used to treat sickle cell disease (Hanna et al. 2007) and Parkinson's (Wernig et al. 2008) in animal models. Diseased somatic cells may also be amenable to integration with other technologies, such as gene therapy, for the correction of genetic anomalies prior to replacement (Rideout et al. 2002). Alternatively, iPS cells also provide a means of deriving diseased cell lines from somatic cells, to understand the sequence of changes as the disease progresses from immature cells (Park et al. 2008, Soldner et al. 2009). However, for the realization of therapeutic applications, further examination is necessary to directly compare the molecular and functional similarities and differences between iPS cells and ESCs, as well as to establish standardized protocols for efficient reprogramming with regard to specific transcription factors and delivery methods (Kaichi et al. 2010, Kulkeaw et al. 2010, Tokumoto et al. 2010).

## 8.4 Propagation

### 8.4.1 Culture Conditions for Undifferentiated ESCs

The standard culture conditions for mESC growth were largely adapted from established EC cells culture techniques (Martin 1981). When maintained as a monolayer in coculture with stromal cells, such as mitotically inactivated MEFs, mESCs can be maintained in an undifferentiated state (Park et al. 2003). Subsequent analysis of the paracrine factors that contribute to the maintenance of pluripotency revealed the key roles of leukemia inhibitory factor (LIF) and bone morphogenetic proteins (BMPs) (Williams et al. 1988, Qi et al. 2004, Xu et al. 2005b). LIF acts via activation of the Stat3 pathway to maintain the self-renewal potential of mESCs (Niwa et al. 1998, Ernst et al. 1999, Matsuda et al. 1999). More recent work has established feeder-free culture methods for mESCs, which employ defined substrates, such as gelatin, to promote mESC attachment and media supplemented with exogenous LIF ($10^3$ U/mL) and BMP-containing serum. However, hESCs are not responsive to LIF and require different factors such as basic fibroblast growth factor (Xu et al. 2005a,b). hESCs, therefore, require slightly different culture techniques, and have been instead maintained with MEFs or on ECM-derived Matrigel™ substrates

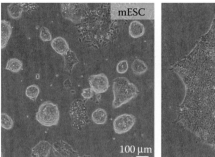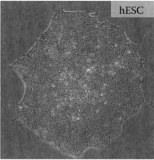

**FIGURE 8.5**   Phase images of undifferentiated mESC and hESC colonies. ESCs derived from mouse and human sources exhibit several differences, including the colony morphology, with mESCs growing in a more tightly packed dome-like colonies, whereas hESCs exhibit more flattened and spread out morphology.

(Xu et al. 2001, Eiselleova et al. 2008). However, paracrine signaling from MEFs is complex and the composition of Matrigel™ is variable between lots, which does not afford uniformity between hESC cultures. Thus, recent work has also utilized chemical screening techniques to establish individual factors necessary for maintaining pluripotency (Beattie et al. 2005, James et al. 2005, Vallier et al. 2005, Wang et al. 2005). For example, inhibition of the mitogen-activated protein kinase (Erk) pathway, which is known to induce differentiation of ESCs, by small molecule inhibitors of glycogen synthase kinase-3, effectively sustains pluripotency in hESCs (Silva and Smith 2008, Ying et al. 2008). Future work in the formulation of defined media conditions will assist in standardization of ESC culture (Ludwig et al. 2006). For clinical purposes, completely xenogenic-free methods for the propagation of human cells in the absence of animal products are thought to be necessary to meet anticipated safety and regulatory standards (Ellerström et al. 2006, Skottman et al. 2006).

In addition to morphogenic cues required for pluripotency, mESCs and hESCs exhibit distinct differences in morphology, culture conditions, and genetic signatures (Sato et al. 2003, Ginis et al. 2004, Wei et al. 2005). For example, mESCs grow in colonies that are compact and dome-like in morphology, whereas hESC colonies are more flattened and spread out in two-dimensional culture (Figure 8.5). Additionally, mESCs exhibit activation of the X chromosome, consistent with the epigenetic state of pre-implantation embryos, whereas the chromosome is silenced in hESCs. Spontaneous differentiation of mESCs and hESCs can occur due to confluence; however, methods of passaging the cells vary between species. mESCs are regularly passaged by enzymatic dissociation using trypsin into single cells when the culture reaches approximately 70% confluence, whereas hESCs are resistant to passaging as single cells and therefore are typically either passaged by physical removal of entire colonies or by enzymatic passaging into single cells in the presence of rho-associated kinase (ROCK) inhibitors. Inhibition of the ROCK pathway using direct inhibitors Y-27632 and 2,4-disubstituted thiazole (Thiazovivin/Tzv) decreases dissociation-induced apoptosis by stabilization of cadherins required for adhesion (Watanabe et al. 2007, Harb et al. 2008, Xu et al. 2010). The discrepancies between culture conditions for mouse and human ESCs warrant further studies to identify the underlying differences between the cells derived from different species.

## 8.4.2  Epiblast Stem Cells

Differences between mouse and human culture conditions have prompted questions regarding the pluripotent state of cell lines derived from different species. Some groups argue the existence of multiple pluripotent states (Chou et al. 2008). The states have been designated as naive and primed pluripotent states, and can be compared to distinct stem cells derived from post-implantation embryos, termed epiblast stem cells (EpiSCs). Although EpiSCs express all of the markers of pluripotency and can give rise to teratomas, EpiSCs of murine origins cannot contribute to chimeras (Tesar et al. 2007, Guo et al. 2009). EpiSCs also exhibit inactivation of an X chromosome, consistent with the more mature post-implantation blastocyst state. hESCs, likewise, exhibit a silenced X chromosome; however, as noted previously, chimerism cannot be tested in humans. Differences in culture conditions and morphology between rodent EpiSCs and mESCs has led investigators to hypothesize that hESCs may be more similar to EpiSCs, possibly due to continued development of IVF embryos in culture prior to ESC derivation (Brons et al. 2007, Tesar et al. 2007, Rossant and Auguste 2008). Investigators have successfully reprogrammed mEpiSCs using only the factor Klf4, which results in X chromosome reactivation and all of the other hallmarks of ESCs, including chimerism (Guo et al. 2009). Furthermore, reprogrammed hESCs can exhibit similar genetic profiles and culture conditions compared with mESCs (Hanna et al. 2010). Therefore, it is likely that currently established cultures of hESCs are in a primed pluripotent state, similar to cells of the epiblast. Alternative derivation methods or reversal of the primed state by reprogramming will likely yield a population of hESCs that can be maintained through methods similar to those established for mESCs.

## 8.5  Differentiation

### 8.5.1  Late Embryonic Development

After the formation of the blastocyst, embryogenesis progresses through the specification of the ICM in a process known as gastrulation. The ICM is initially composed of a visceral endoderm layer at the interface between the blastocoel cavity and the epiblast. The anterior visceral endoderm (AVE) is responsible for much of the signaling that results in spatial patterning of the epiblast (Thomas and Beddington 1996, Bielinska et al. 1999). Gastrulation progresses through axis formation, which establishes the posterior side of the embryo, where the transient structure known as the primitive streak (PS) is formed. Spatial patterning occurs within the epiblast by secretion of inhibitory signals from the PS and AVE (Lawson et al. 1991). The PS is associated with expression of transforming growth factor β (TGFβ) (Lefty 1, Nodal) and Wnt, whereas the AVE secretes Nodal and Wnt repressors (Dkk-1, Sfrp1, and Sfrp5) (Finley et al. 2003, Kemp et al. 2005, Rivera-Pérez and Magnuson 2005). Cells traverse the PS to form the mesoderm and definitive endoderm lineages in a spatially and temporally controlled manner within the embryo (Lawson et al. 1991). For example, cells of the extraembryonic mesoderm are the first mobilized within the PS and localize within the posterior end of the embryo, whereas cardiac mesoderm and definitive endoderm migrate toward the anterior (Burdsal et al. 1993). Cells of the ectoderm lineage arise from epiblast cells that do not enter the PS. Expression patterns of agonists and inhibitors, which lead to PS formation and cell specification during embryogenesis, highlight several key genetic pathways which are likely responsible for the temporal and spatial regulation of various differentiation events in ESCs.

### 8.5.2  ESC Differentiation in Monolayer

The ability of ESCs to form teratomas and incorporate within chimeras indicates the exquisite sensitivity of the cells to environmental cues. Therefore, many differentiation approaches have relied heavily on understanding the changes during embryogenesis to define environmental parameters for the differentiation of ESCs. Many protocols rely on soluble delivery of factors in monolayer and exploit pathways known to be important in the context of early development (Figure 8.6).

In the absence of anti-differentiation factors such as LIF, mESCs spontaneously differentiate. Early specification of ESCs proceeds similarly to gastrulation, with the commitment of either neuroectoderm or a PS-like population. Neuroectoderm specification is often referred to as the "default" pathway, because ESCs differentiate into neural precursors with high fidelity without the supplementation of serum of other exogenous growth factors (Ying et al. 2003). Cells have been induced to enter the PS lineage by

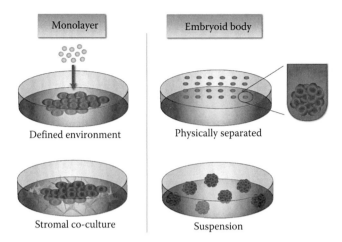

**FIGURE 8.6**  ESC differentiation formats. ESCs have been induced to differentiate in several formats, including monolayer culture with defined soluble factors or as a coculture, and as three-dimensional EBs, which can be formed by spontaneous aggregation, either in physically separated or mass suspension environments.

BMP4, which requires active signaling of the FGF and TGFβ/Nodal/activin pathways (Wiles and Keller 1991, Ng et al. 2005a, Nostro et al. 2008, Zhang et al. 2008). Addition of PS-inducing morphogens results in inhibition of neuroectoderm differentiation, which is consistent with the active signaling pathways during gastrulation (Aubert et al. 2002, Kubo et al. 2004). PS induction was initially accomplished by the addition of serum; however, the components of serum are highly variable between lots and the identification of factors that actively promote differentiation has led to the creation of serum-free defined media. The levels of various factors are also important, which is exemplified by the differential induction of mesoderm or endoderm, depending on the concentration of exogenous activin A (Kubo et al. 2004).

Delivery of exogenous small molecules and growth factors is most often accomplished via monolayer culture of ESCs in the absence of anti-differentiation factors. Monolayer format affords uniform application of external stimuli, including biochemical factors and mechanical forces, resulting in increased efficiency of directed differentiation compared with other formats (Zweigerdt et al. 2003). Monolayer culture of ESCs also permits coculture with stromal cells, as a method of directing differentiation via paracrine signaling (Nakano et al. 1994). For example, ESCs have been induced to differentiate into hematopoietic precursors by coculture with OP9 bone marrow-derived stromal cells (Nakano et al. 1994, Cho et al. 1999, Schmitt et al. 2004), thereby elucidating possible mechanisms of hematopoietic differentiation *in vivo*. Coculture methods do not require supplementation with exogenous growth factors; however, the signaling from stromal cells is often complex and poorly defined. Monolayer culture is also amenable to high throughput screening methods using various morphogens and substrate properties (Anderson et al. 2004). Substrate elasticity has been demonstrated as an important parameter with respect to ESC spreading, migration, and differentiation, likely due to signaling from changes in cadherin and integrin adhesions (Engler et al. 2006). Substrate parameters have be modulated by the seeding of cells on various artificial and natural substrates, including polyacrylamide, collagen, laminin, and Matrigel™ (Levenberg et al. 2003, Flaim et al. 2005). Control of defined substrates and delivery of exogenous factors in monolayer affords systematic studies of *in vitro* differentiation of ESCs, without the complexity of adhesions and signaling *in vivo*.

### 8.5.3  Embryoid Body Differentiation

The term "EB" (Figure 8.6) is broadly used to define aggregates of differentiating pluripotent cells, which are thought to more accurately recapitulate the complex cellular adhesions and signaling of native tissue

(Akins et al. 2010, Chang and Hughes-Fulford 2009). EBs are formed by enzymatically dissociating ESC colonies to obtain a single-cell suspension, whereby ESCs spontaneously aggregate to form spheroids (Larue et al. 1996, Dasgupta et al. 2005). When cultured as EBs, the differentiation of ESCs is similar to many of the events during early embryogenesis, including simultaneous differentiation into endoderm, mesoderm, and ectoderm lineages (Coucouvanis and Martin 1995, Keller 1995, Doevendans et al. 2000, Itskovitz-Eldor et al. 2000, Höpfl et al. 2004). The complexity of the three-dimensional structure, however, leads to transport limitations stemming from size of aggregates and the formation of a nonpermissive "shell" of epithelial cells at the exterior of the EB (Sachlos and Auguste 2008, Carpenedo et al. 2009). Transport properties underscore the inability to efficiently deliver morphogens to EBs for directing ESC differentiation, which contributes to the heterogeneity in resulting cell types.

Spontaneous aggregation of ESCs is mediated by E-cadherin, a $Ca^{2+}$-dependent homophilic adhesion molecule, which is also expressed in the morula and blastocyst stage of embryogenesis (Larue et al. 1996). As aggregates of ESCs begin to differentiate, the first specification leads to a layer of primitive endoderm cells at the exterior of the EB. The formation of primitive endoderm is thought to be mediated largely by FGF signaling and the downstream PI 3-kinase pathway (Chen et al. 2000, Esner et al. 2002). The primitive endoderm then differentiates to form the visceral and parietal endoderm, which deposit a basement membrane-like layer of ECM comprised largely of laminin and collagen IV (Wan et al. 1984, Li et al. 2001). It is thought that cell survival within the EB is dependent on contact with the basement membrane layer, and death of interior cells often results in the formation of cystic cavities within EBs (Coucouvanis and Martin 1995, Smyth et al. 1999, Murray and Edgar 2000). After specification of the exterior endoderm cells, differentiation of the remaining cells within the EB proceeds to form the three germ lineages. The genetic regulation during differentiation demonstrates a temporal sequence of events similar to the processes of embryonic gastrulation and specification (Itskovitz-Eldor et al. 2000, Dvash et al. 2004). For example, in both embryonic cardiogenesis and ESC differentiation, Wnt signaling, which is important in initial PS formation, exhibits biphasic regulation, in which the pathway must be inhibited at later stages of differentiation to form committed cardiac cells (Kwon et al. 2007, Lin et al. 2007, Qyang et al. 2007, Ueno et al. 2007). Morphologically, germ layer differentiation can be visualized through the formation of blood islands, contractile foci, and neurite extensions when plated on adhesive substrates (Doetschman et al. 1985).

Initiation of EB formation can be accomplished by the creation of hanging drops, in which ESCs are forced to aggregate within small volumes (20–30 μL) of media suspended from the lid of a Petri dish (Yoon et al. 2006). The number of cells incorporated into each EB can be easily manipulated by controlling the concentration of cells and the volume of drops. The size of EBs formed using the hanging drop method typically varies from approximately 200 to 1000 cells per drop. Larger EBs cannot be easily formed because the media volume is usually limited to less than approximately 50 μL, due to the surface tension needed to keep the inverted drops suspended from lid surface. The hanging drop method is not readily amenable to frequent media exchanges (due to the small volume) and the technique is not convenient for the larger-scale production of EBs. After approximately 2–3 days of aggregate formation, EBs formed using hanging drops are typically transferred into suspension culture to facilitate media exchanges and monitor the progression of differentiation. One of the caveats of culturing EBs in suspension is the agglomeration of individual EBs, leading to increased heterogeneity in the overall population of cell aggregates. Although the hanging drop method of EB formation affords reproducible control of EB size and yields an initially uniform population of EBs, the method is also labor intensive, produces relatively few EBs and is not suitable for sustained EB culture for days to weeks.

Alternatively, larger yields of EBs (i.e., 1000s) can be produced simply by inoculation of a single-cell population of ESCs into suspension culture in bacteriological grade dishes or dishes coated with non-adhesive materials such as agar or hydrophilic polymers (Doetschman et al. 1985). Because hESCs are sensitive to enzymatic digestion and single-cell culture, EBs are formed through physical separation of colonies from the culture surface, or by using ROCK inhibitors to obtain single-cell populations (Watanabe et al. 2007). Typical inoculation densities range from approximately $10^4$ to $10^6$ cells/mL. The

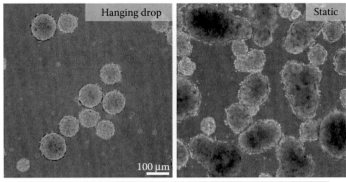

| | Hanging drop | Semi-solid media | Suspension |
|---|---|---|---|
| Uniformity (size/shape) | + | + | − |
| Throughput | − | + | + |
| Control of formation | + | + | − |
| Ease of media exchange | − | − | + |

**FIGURE 8.7**   EB formation methods. EBs formed by physical separation in hanging drop culture result in controlled formation, with increased homogeneity of size and shape. In contrast, EBs from suspension cultures are more heterogeneous, but can be produced easily in higher throughput and enable media exchange. Culture in semisolid media demonstrates an intermediate method, which is higher throughput than hanging drop, but can physically separate individual ESCs.

EBs form via random aggregation of cells and are largely dependent on inoculation concentrations and local interactions between cells. After initial aggregation, individual spheroids often agglomerate to form larger masses, resulting in large, irregularly shaped EBs that are widely variable in size and shape. When comparing different EB formation and culture methods, it is apparent that there is an inherent tradeoff between the ability to control EB formation and the yield of cells produced (Figure 8.7) (Dang et al. 2002, Kurosawa et al. 2003, Carpenedo et al. 2007).

A compromise between the two previously discussed methods is the use of a semi-solid media, such as methylcellulose, to physically isolate single-cell populations. The high viscosity of methylcellulose prevents movement of cells, and thus limits the spontaneous aggregation of cells and spheroids. Within a 1% methylcellulose medium, ESCs are typically inoculated at concentrations of approximately 1000–3000 cells/mL. The mass transfer properties within methylcellulose create a different culture environment compared with liquid suspension cultures because there is likely accumulation of paracrine factors, as well as limited transport of oxygen, nutrients, and waste. Therefore, EB formation within semi-solid media is more amenable to understanding endogenous differentiation without the supplementation of morphogens. The semi-solid cultures have been used for efficiently deriving hematopoietic and endothelial cells (Wiles and Keller 1991), likely due to the low-oxygen environment within the methylcellulose (Potocnik et al. 1994). Alternatively, naturally derived matrices, such as fibrin (Liu et al. 2006) and hyaluronic acid (Gerecht et al. 2007), have been used to encapsulate ESCs. As the hydrogels are derived from natural ECM components, the ESCs are capable of binding through integrin and other adhesion receptors, which may influence the spreading, migration, and differentiation of ESCs.

Recently, new methods have been established which provide increased control of EB size and homogeneity, yet are amenable to higher throughput production. Such methods rely on physical separation of EBs to promote controlled formation (Ng et al. 2005b, Mohr et al. 2006, Torisawa et al. 2007, Moeller et al. 2008, Ungrin et al. 2008). Control of EB size has been accomplished using encapsulation of ESCs within beads, physical separation using microwells and growth of ESC colonies on adhesive micropatterned substrates. Controlled formation methods permit more systematic analysis of the effects of EB size, with initial analyses demonstrating that differentiation is related to EB size, and may contribute to heterogeneity in uncontrolled suspension cultures (Bauwens et al. 2008, Mohr et al. 2010). Therefore, the uniformity of the resulting EB populations, both in terms of size and aggregation kinetics, enables more systematic analysis of environmental perturbations without confounding factors stemming from EB heterogeneity.

## 8.6 Clinical Outlook

For the purposes of functional tissue replacement, it has been estimated that upwards of $10^9$ cells will be necessary for regenerative therapies (Tzanakakis et al. 2000, Lock and Tzanakakis 2007, Jing et al. 2008). Therefore, the development of methods for increasing the scale of ESC culture is important to produce clinically relevant yields. In their pluripotent state, ESCs are typically cultured in monolayer, which restricts the number of cells produced, dependent on the culture surface area. Some groups have established methods for using beads made of alginate or other adhesive materials, to increase the surface area for growth (Fernandes et al. 2007, Lock and Tzanakakis 2009). Alternatively, when cultured as small aggregates in the presence of LIF or fibroblast conditioned media, ESCs maintain pluripotency (Cormier et al. 2006, Ouyang et al. 2007).

Suspension culture is amenable to scale-up for larger volume cultures, such as bioreactors (Gerecht-Nir et al. 2004, Bauwens et al. 2005, Fok and Zandstra 2005, Cameron et al. 2006, Wang et al. 2006, Zur Nieden et al. 2007, Niebruegge et al. 2008, Krawetz et al. 2010). Common formats include spinner flasks, rotating wall vessels (high aspect rotating vessel, slow turning lateral vessel) and large-scale bioreactors. Large-volume culture systems are also amenable to modifications for increased monitoring and control of the culture environment, which is important for uniformity between culture environments (Côme et al. 2008, Gerlach et al. 2010). Large-scale culture systems, however, all necessitate mixing to prevent gradients of nutrients and waste within the culture (Bilgen et al. 2005, 2006, Sargent et al. 2010). Hydrodynamic mixing within cultures may impact EB homogeneity, viability, and differentiation (Carpenedo et al. 2007, Sargent et al. 2010). Therefore, it is important to consider the impact of the environmental changes necessary for increasing the scale of cultures for clinical settings.

## 8.7 Conclusion

Although hESCs are a promising cell source for many translational applications, much remains to be determined regarding the proteomic, genetic, and epigenetic mechanisms that regulate pluripotency and differentiation. ESCs, therefore, may provide a useful platform to understand embryonic developmental events that cannot be perturbed *in vivo* due to lethality of genetic knockouts. For example, cell lines transduced with reporter constructs allow real-time monitoring of genetic changes during differentiation and are amenable to high-throughput screening approaches. iPS may, additionally, provide insight into regulatory mechanisms, specifically with respect to the epigenetic changes during reprogramming of somatic cells. The derivation of individualized iPS lines provides methods for understanding the pathophysiology of disease-specific cell lines, and as platforms for drug testing and autologous transplantation. From an engineering perspective, understanding the interactions of ESCs with their environment will enable the development of modified culture approaches to modulate cell potential through cell–cell adhesions, morphogen delivery, and mechanical factors. Understanding the ESC microenvironment may also enable alternative therapeutic approaches, including harnessing the paracrine potential of secreted growth factors and ECM for directing somatic cell functions *in vivo*.

## References

Akins, R. E., Rockwood, D., Robinson, K. G. et al. 2010. Three-dimensional culture alters primary cardiac cell phenotype. *Tissue Eng Part A* 16(2): 629–41.

Albert, M. and Peters, A. H. F. M. 2009. Genetic and epigenetic control of early mouse development. *Curr Opin Genet Dev* 19(2): 113–21.

Anderson, D., Levenberg, S., and Langer, R. 2004. Nanoliter-scale synthesis of arrayed biomaterials and application to human embryonic stem cells. *Nat Biotechnol* 22(7): 863–66.

Andrews, P. W., Damjanov, I., Simon, D. et al. 1984. Pluripotent embryonal carcinoma clones derived from the human teratocarcinoma cell line tera-2. Differentiation *in vivo* and in vitro. *Lab Invest* 50(2): 147–62.

Aubert, J., Dunstan, H., Chambers, I., and Smith, A. 2002. Functional gene screening in embryonic stem cells implicates wnt antagonism in neural differentiation. *Nat Biotechnol* 20(12): 1240–5.

Avilion, A. A., Nicolis, S. K., Pevny, L. H. et al. 2003. Multipotent cell lineages in early mouse development depend on sox2 function. *Genes Dev* 17(1): 126–40.

Barcroft, L. C., Offenberg, H., Thomsen, P., and Watson, A. J. 2003. Aquaporin proteins in murine trophectoderm mediate transepithelial water movements during cavitation. *Dev Biol* 256(2): 342–54.

Baum, C. M., Weissman, I. L., Tsukamoto, A. S., Buckle, A. M., and Peault, B. 1992. Isolation of a candidate human hematopoietic stem-cell population. *Proc Natl Acad Sci U S A* 89(7): 2804–8.

Bauwens, C., Yin, T., Dang, S., Peerani, R., and Zandstra, P. W. 2005. Development of a perfusion fed bioreactor for embryonic stem cell-derived cardiomyocyte generation: Oxygen-mediated enhancement of cardiomyocyte output. *Biotechnol Bioeng* 90(4): 452–61.

Bauwens, C. L., Peerani, R., Niebruegge, S. et al. 2008. Control of human embryonic stem cell colony and aggregate size heterogeneity influences differentiation trajectories. *Stem Cells* 26(9): 2300–10.

Beattie, G. M., Lopez, A. D., Bucay, N. et al. 2005. Activin a maintains pluripotency of human embryonic stem cells in the absence of feeder layers. *Stem Cells* 23(4): 489–95.

Beck, F., Erler, T., Russell, A., and James, R. 1995. Expression of cdx-2 in the mouse embryo and placenta: Possible role in patterning of the extra-embryonic membranes. *Dev Dyn* 204(3): 219–27.

Bernardo, A. S., Cho, C. H.-H., Mason, S. et al. 2009. Biphasic induction of pdx1 in mouse and human embryonic stem cells can mimic development of pancreatic beta-cells. *Stem Cells* 27(2): 341–51.

Bielinska, M., Narita, N., and Wilson, D. B. 1999. Distinct roles for visceral endoderm during embryonic mouse development. *Int J Dev Biol* 43(3): 183–205.

Bilgen, B., Chang-Mateu, I. M., and Barabino, G. A. 2005. Characterization of mixing in a novel wavy-walled bioreactor for tissue engineering. *Biotechnol Bioeng* 92(7): 907–19.

Bilgen, B., Sucosky, P., Neitzel, G. P., and Barabino, G. A. 2006. Flow characterization of a wavy-walled bioreactor for cartilage tissue engineering. *Biotechnol Bioeng* 95(6): 1009–22.

Blelloch, R. H., Hochedlinger, K., Yamada, Y. et al. 2004. Nuclear cloning of embryonal carcinoma cells. *Proc Natl Acad Sci USA* 101(39): 13985–90.

Boheler, K. R., Czyz, J., Tweedie, D. et al. 2002. Differentiation of pluripotent embryonic stem cells into cardiomyocytes. *Circ Res* 91(3): 189–201.

Bourc'his, D., Le Bourhis, D., Patin, D. et al. 2001. Delayed and incomplete reprogramming of chromosome methylation patterns in bovine cloned embryos. *Curr Biol* 11(19): 1542–6.

Boyer, L. A., Lee, T. I., Cole, M. F. et al. 2005. Core transcriptional regulatory circuitry in human embryonic stem cells. *Cell* 122(6): 947–56.

Briggs, R. and King, T. J. 1952. Transplantation of living nuclei from blastula cells into enucleated frogs' eggs. *Proc Natl Acad Sci USA* 38(5): 455–63.

Brons, I. G. M., Smithers, L. E., Trotter, M. W. B. et al. 2007. Derivation of pluripotent epiblast stem cells from mammalian embryos. *Nature* 448(7150): 191–5.

Burdsal, C. A., Damsky, C. H., and Pedersen, R. A. 1993. The role of e-cadherin and integrins in mesoderm differentiation and migration at the mammalian primitive streak. *Development* 118(3): 829–44.

Cameron, C. M., Hu, W.-S., and Kaufman, D. S. 2006. Improved development of human embryonic stem cell-derived embryoid bodies by stirred vessel cultivation. *Biotechnol Bioeng* 94(5): 938–48.

Campbell, K. H., Mcwhir, J., Ritchie, W. A., and Wilmut, I. 1996. Sheep cloned by nuclear transfer from a cultured cell line. *Nature* 380(6569): 64–6.

Carpenedo, R. L., Sargent, C. Y., and Mcdevitt, T. C. 2007. Rotary suspension culture enhances the efficiency, yield, and homogeneity of embryoid body differentiation. *Stem Cells* 25(9): 2224–34.

Carpenedo, R. L., Bratt-Leal, A. M., Marklein, R. A. et al. 2009. Homogeneous and organized differentiation within embryoid bodies induced by microsphere-mediated delivery of small molecules. *Biomaterials* 30(13): 2507–15.

Chambers, I., Colby, D., Robertson, M. et al. 2003. Functional expression cloning of nanog, a pluripotency sustaining factor in embryonic stem cells. *Cell* 113(5): 643–55.

Chambers, I., Silva, J., Colby, D. et al. 2007. Nanog safeguards pluripotency and mediates germline development. *Nature* 450(7173): 1230–4.

Champeris Tsaniras, S. and Jones, P. M. 2010. Generating pancreatic beta-cells from embryonic stem cells by manipulating signaling pathways. *J Endocrinol* 206(1): 13–26.

Chan, A. W., Dominko, T., Luetjens, C. M. et al. 2000. Clonal propagation of primate offspring by embryo splitting. *Science* 287(5451): 317–9.

Chang, T. T. and Hughes-Fulford, M. 2009. Monolayer and spheroid culture of human liver hepatocellular carcinoma cell line cells demonstrate distinct global gene expression patterns and functional phenotypes. *Tissue Eng Part A* 15(3): 559–67.

Chen, Y., Li, X., Eswarakumar, V. P., Seger, R., and Lonai, P. 2000. Fibroblast growth factor (fgf) signaling through pi 3-kinase and akt/pkb is required for embryoid body differentiation. *Oncogene* 19(33): 3750–6.

Chew, J.-L., Loh, Y.-H., Zhang, W. et al. 2005. Reciprocal transcriptional regulation of pou5f1 and sox2 via the oct4/sox2 complex in embryonic stem cells. *Mol Cell Biol* 25(14): 6031–46.

Cho, S. K., Webber, T. D., Carlyle, J. R. et al. 1999. Functional characterization of b lymphocytes generated *in vitro* from embryonic stem cells. *Proc Natl Acad Sci USA* 96(17): 9797–802.

Chou, Y.-F., Chen, H.-H., Eijpe, M. et al. 2008. The growth factor environment defines distinct pluripotent ground states in novel blastocyst-derived stem cells. *Cell* 135(3): 449–61.

Chung, Y., Klimanskaya, I., Becker, S. et al. 2008. Human embryonic stem cell lines generated without embryo destruction. *Cell Stem Cell* 2(2): 113–7.

Côme, J., Nissan, X., Aubry, L. et al. 2008. Improvement of culture conditions of human embryoid bodies using a controlled perfused and dialyzed bioreactor system. *Tissue Eng C, Methods* 14(4): 289–98.

Cormier, J. T., Zur Nieden, N. I., Rancourt, D. E., and Kallos, M. S. 2006. Expansion of undifferentiated murine embryonic stem cells as aggregates in suspension culture bioreactors. *Tissue Eng* 12(11): 3233–45.

Coucouvanis, E. and Martin, G. R. 1995. Signals for death and survival: A two-step mechanism for cavitation in the vertebrate embryo. *Cell* 83(2): 279–87.

Dang, S. M., Kyba, M., Perlingeiro, R., Daley, G. Q., and Zandstra, P. W. 2002. Efficiency of embryoid body formation and hematopoietic development from embryonic stem cells in different culture systems. *Biotechnol Bioeng* 78(4): 442–53.

Dasgupta, A., Hughey, R., Lancin, P., Larue, L., and Moghe, P. V. 2005. E-cadherin synergistically induces hepatospecific phenotype and maturation of embryonic stem cells in conjunction with hepatotrophic factors. *Biotechnol Bioeng* 92(3): 257–66.

Dean, W., Bowden, L., Aitchison, A. et al. 1998. Altered imprinted gene methylation and expression in completely es cell-derived mouse fetuses: Association with aberrant phenotypes. *Development* 125(12): 2273–82.

Dean, W., Santos, F., Stojkovic, M. et al. 2001. Conservation of methylation reprogramming in mammalian development: Aberrant reprogramming in cloned embryos. *Proc Natl Acad Sci USA* 98(24): 13734–8.

Doetschman, T., Eistetter, H., Katz, M., Schmidt, W., and Kemler, R. 1985. The *in vitro* development of blastocyst-derived embryonic stem cell lines: Formation of visceral yolk sac, blood islands and myocardium. *J Embryol Exp Morphol* 87: 27–45.

Doevendans, P. A., Kubalak, S. W., An, R. H. et al. 2000. Differentiation of cardiomyocytes in floating embryoid bodies is comparable to fetal cardiomyocytes. *J Mol Cell Cardiol* 32(5): 839–51.

Drukker, M., Katz, G., Urbach, A. et al. 2002. Characterization of the expression of mhc proteins in human embryonic stem cells. *Proc Natl Acad Sci USA* 99(15): 9864–9.

Dvash, T., Mayshar, Y., Darr, H. et al. 2004. Temporal gene expression during differentiation of human embryonic stem cells and embryoid bodies. *Hum Reprod* 19(12): 2875–83.

Edwards, R. G., Purdy, J. M., Steptoe, P. C., and Walters, D. E. 1981. The growth of human preimplantation embryos in vitro. *Am J Obstet Gynecol* 141(4): 408–16.

Eggan, K., Rode, A., Jentsch, I. et al. 2002. Male and female mice derived from the same embryonic stem cell clone by tetraploid embryo complementation. *Nat Biotechnol* 20(5): 455–9.

Eiselleova, L., Peterkova, I., Neradil, J. et al. 2008. Comparative study of mouse and human feeder cells for human embryonic stem cells. *Int J Dev Biol* 52(4): 353–63.

Ellerström, C., Strehl, R., Moya, K. et al. 2006. Derivation of a xeno-free human embryonic stem cell line. *Stem Cells* 24(10): 2170–6.

Engler, A. J., Sen, S., Sweeney, H. L., and Discher, D. E. 2006. Matrix elasticity directs stem cell lineage specification. *Cell* 126(4): 677–89.

Ernst, M., Novak, U., Nicholson, S. E., Layton, J. E., and Dunn, A. R. 1999. The carboxyl-terminal domains of gp130-related cytokine receptors are necessary for suppressing embryonic stem cell differentiation. Involvement of stat3. *J Biol Chem* 274(14): 9729–37.

Esner, M., Pachernik, J., Hampl, A., and Dvorak, P. 2002. Targeted disruption of fibroblast growth factor receptor-1 blocks maturation of visceral endoderm and cavitation in mouse embryoid bodies. *Int J Dev Biol* 46(6): 817–25.

Evans, M. J. and Kaufman, M. H. 1981. Establishment in culture of pluripotential cells from mouse embryos. *Nature* 292(5819): 154–6.

Fernandes, A. M., Fernandes, T. G., Diogo, M. M. et al. 2007. Mouse embryonic stem cell expansion in a microcarrier-based stirred culture system. *J Biotechnol* 132(2): 227–36.

Fijnvandraat, A. C., Van Ginneken, A. C. G., De Boer, P. A. J. et al. 2003. Cardiomyocytes derived from embryonic stem cells resemble cardiomyocytes of the embryonic heart tube. *Cardiovasc Res* 58(2): 399–409.

Finley, K. R., Tennessen, J., and Shawlot, W. 2003. The mouse secreted frizzled-related protein 5 gene is expressed in the anterior visceral endoderm and foregut endoderm during early post-implantation development. *Gene Expr Patterns* 3(5): 681–4.

Flaim, C. J., Chien, S., and Bhatia, S. N. 2005. An extracellular matrix microarray for probing cellular differentiation. *Nat Methods* 2(2): 119–25.

Fleming, T. P. and Pickering, S. J. 1985. Maturation and polarization of the endocytotic system in outside blastomeres during mouse preimplantation development. *J Embryol Exp Morphol* 89: 175–208.

Fok, E. Y. L. and Zandstra, P. W. 2005. Shear-controlled single-step mouse embryonic stem cell expansion and embryoid body-based differentiation. *Stem Cells* 23(9): 1333–42.

Gerecht, S., Burdick, J. A., Ferreira, L. S. et al. 2007. Hyaluronic acid hydrogel for controlled self-renewal and differentiation of human embryonic stem cells. *Proc Natl Acad Sci USA* 104(27): 11298–303.

Gerecht-Nir, S., Cohen, S., and Itskovitz-Eldor, J. 2004. Bioreactor cultivation enhances the efficiency of human embryoid body (heb) formation and differentiation. *Biotechnol Bioeng* 86(5): 493–502.

Gerlach, J. C., Hout, M., Edsbagge, J. et al. 2010. Dynamic 3d culture promotes spontaneous embryonic stem cell differentiation in vitro. *Tissue Eng Part C, Methods* 16(1): 115–21.

Ginis, I., Luo, Y., Miura, T. et al. 2004. Differences between human and mouse embryonic stem cells. *Dev Biol* 269(2): 360–80.

Guo, G., Yang, J., Nichols, J. et al. 2009. Klf4 reverts developmentally programmed restriction of ground state pluripotency. *Development* 136(7): 1063–9.

Gurdon, J. B. 1962. The developmental capacity of nuclei taken from intestinal epithelium cells of feeding tadpoles. *J Embryol Exp Morphol* 10: 622–40.

Handyside, A. H. 1978. Time of commitment of inside cells isolated from preimplantation mouse embryos. *J Embryol Exp Morphol* 45: 37–53.

Hanna, J., Cheng, A. W., Saha, K. et al. 2010. Human embryonic stem cells with biological and epigenetic characteristics similar to those of mouse escs. *Proc Natl Acad Sci USA* 107(20): 9222–7.

Hanna, J., Wernig, M., Markoulaki, S. et al. 2007. Treatment of sickle cell anemia mouse model with ips cells generated from autologous skin. *Science* 318(5858): 1920–3.

Harb, N., Archer, T. K., and Sato, N. 2008. The rho-rock-myosin signaling axis determines cell-cell integrity of self-renewing pluripotent stem cells. *PLoS ONE* 3(8): e3001.

Hochedlinger, K., Rideout, W. M., Kyba, M. et al. 2004. Nuclear transplantation, embryonic stem cells and the potential for cell therapy. *Hematol J* 5 Suppl 3: S114–7.

Höpfl, G., Gassmann, M., and Desbaillets, I. 2004. Differentiating embryonic stem cells into embryoid bodies. *Methods Mol Biol* 254: 79–98.

Huangfu, D., Maehr, R., Guo, W. et al. 2008a. Induction of pluripotent stem cells by defined factors is greatly improved by small-molecule compounds. *Nat Biotechnol* 26(7): 795–7.

Huangfu, D., Osafune, K., Maehr, R. et al. 2008b. Induction of pluripotent stem cells from primary human fibroblasts with only oct4 and sox2. *Nat Biotechnol* 26(11): 1269–75.

Hyafil, F., Morello, D., Babinet, C., and Jacob, F. 1980. A cell surface glycoprotein involved in the compaction of embryonal carcinoma cells and cleavage stage embryos. *Cell* 21(3): 927–34.

Illmensee, K. and Mintz, B. 1976. Totipotency and normal differentiation of single teratocarcinoma cells cloned by injection into blastocysts. *Proc Natl Acad Sci USA* 73(2): 549–53.

Itskovitz-Eldor, J., Schuldiner, M., Karsenti, D. et al. 2000. Differentiation of human embryonic stem cells into embryoid bodies compromising the three embryonic germ layers. *Mol Med* 6(2): 88–95.

Jacob, F. 1977. Mouse teratocarcinoma and embryonic antigens. *Immunol Rev* 33: 3–32.

James, D., Levine, A. J., Besser, D., and Hemmati-Brivanlou, A. 2005. Tgfbeta/activin/nodal signaling is necessary for the maintenance of pluripotency in human embryonic stem cells. *Development* 132(6): 1273–82.

Jedrusik, A., Parfitt, D.-E., Guo, G. et al. 2008. Role of cdx2 and cell polarity in cell allocation and specification of trophectoderm and inner cell mass in the mouse embryo. *Genes Dev* 22(19): 2692–706.

Jing, D., Parikh, A., Canty, J. M., and Tzanakakis, E. S. 2008. Stem cells for heart cell therapies. *Tissue Eng B, Rev* 14(4): 393–406.

Johnson, M. H. and Ziomek, C. A. 1981. Induction of polarity in mouse 8-cell blastomeres: Specificity, geometry, and stability. *J Cell Biol* 91(1): 303–8.

Johnson, M. H. and Maro, B. 1984. The distribution of cytoplasmic actin in mouse 8-cell blastomeres. *J Embryol Exp Morphol* 82: 97–117.

Kahan, B. W. and Ephrussi, B. 1970. Developmental potentialities of clonal *in vitro* cultures of mouse testicular teratoma. *J Natl Cancer Inst* 44(5): 1015–36.

Kaichi, S., Hasegawa, K., Takaya, T. et al. 2010. Cell line-dependent differentiation of induced pluripotent stem cells into cardiomyocytes in mice. *Cardiovasc Res* 88(2): 314–23.

Keller, G. M. 1995. *In vitro* differentiation of embryonic stem cells. *Curr Opin Cell Biol* 7(6): 862–9.

Kemp, C., Willems, E., Abdo, S., Lambiv, L., and Leyns, L. 2005. Expression of all wnt genes and their secreted antagonists during mouse blastocyst and postimplantation development. *Dev Dyn* 233(3): 1064–75.

Kidder, G. M. and Mclachlin, J. R. 1985. Timing of transcription and protein synthesis underlying morphogenesis in preimplantation mouse embryos. *Dev Biol* 112(2): 265–75.

Kleinsmith, L. J. and Pierce, G. B. 1964. Multipotentiality of single embryonal carcinoma cells. *Cancer Research* 24: 1544–51.

Klimanskaya, I., Chung, Y., Becker, S., Lu, S.-J., and Lanza, R. 2006. Human embryonic stem cell lines derived from single blastomeres. *Nature* 444(7118): 481–5.

Koo, D. B., Kang, Y. K., Choi, Y. H. et al. 2001. Developmental potential and transgene expression of porcine nuclear transfer embryos using somatic cells. *Mol Reprod Dev* 58(1): 15–21.

Krawetz, R., Taiani, J., Liu, S. et al. 2010. Large-scale expansion of pluripotent human embryonic stem cells in stirred suspension bioreactors. *Tissue Eng Part C, Methods* 16(4): 573–82.

Kubo, A., Shinozaki, K., Shannon, J. M. et al. 2004. Development of definitive endoderm from embryonic stem cells in culture. *Development* 131(7): 1651–62.

Kulkeaw, K., Horio, Y., Mizuochi, C., Ogawa, M., and Sugiyama, D. 2010. Variation in hematopoietic potential of induced pluripotent stem cell lines. *Stem Cell Rev Rep* 6(3): 381–89.

Kurosawa, H., Imamura, T., Koike, M., Sasaki, K., and Amano, Y. 2003. A simple method for forming embryoid body from mouse embryonic stem cells. *J Biosci Bioeng* 96(4): 409–11.

Kwon, C., Arnold, J., Hsiao, E. C. et al. 2007. Canonical wnt signaling is a positive regulator of mammalian cardiac progenitors. *Proc Natl Acad Sci USA* 104(26): 10894–9.

Larue, L., Antos, C., Butz, S. et al. 1996. A role for cadherins in tissue formation. *Development* 122(10): 3185–94.

Lawson, K. A., Meneses, J. J., and Pedersen, R. A. 1991. Clonal analysis of epiblast fate during germ layer formation in the mouse embryo. *Development* 113(3): 891–911.

Lehman, J. M., Speers, W. C., Swartzendruber, D. E., and Pierce, G. B. 1974. Neoplastic differentiation: Characteristics of cell lines derived from a murine teratocarcinoma. *J Cell Physiol* 84(1): 13–27.

Levenberg, S., Huang, N. F., Lavik, E. et al. 2003. Differentiation of human embryonic stem cells on three-dimensional polymer scaffolds. *Proc Natl Acad Sci USA* 100(22): 12741–6.

Levy, J. B., Johnson, M. H., Goodall, H., and Maro, B. 1986. The timing of compaction: Control of a major developmental transition in mouse early embryogenesis. *J Embryol Exp Morphol* 95: 213–37.

Li, X., Talts, U., Talts, J. F. et al. 2001. Akt/pkb regulates laminin and collagen iv isotypes of the basement membrane. *Proc Natl Acad Sci USA* 98(25): 14416–21.

Lin, L., Cui, L., Zhou, W. et al. 2007. Beta-catenin directly regulates islet1 expression in cardiovascular progenitors and is required for multiple aspects of cardiogenesis. *Proc Natl Acad Sci USA* 104(22): 9313–8.

Liu, H., Collins, S. F., and Suggs, L. J. 2006. Three-dimensional culture for expansion and differentiation of mouse embryonic stem cells. *Biomaterials* 27(36): 6004–14.

Lock, L. T. and Tzanakakis, E. S. 2007. Stem/progenitor cell sources of insulin-producing cells for the treatment of diabetes. *Tissue Eng* 13(7): 1399–412.

Lock, L. T. and Tzanakakis, E. S. 2009. Expansion and differentiation of human embryonic stem cells to endoderm progeny in a microcarrier stirred-suspension culture. *Tissue Eng A* 15(8): 2051–63.

Loh, Y.-H., Wu, Q., Chew, J.-L. et al. 2006. The oct4 and nanog transcription network regulates pluripotency in mouse embryonic stem cells. *Nat Genet* 38(4): 431–40.

Ludwig, T. E., Levenstein, M. E., Jones, J. M. et al. 2006. Derivation of human embryonic stem cells in defined conditions. *Nat Biotechnol* 24(2): 185–7.

Maherali, N., Sridharan, R., Xie, W. et al. 2007. Directly reprogrammed fibroblasts show global epigenetic remodeling and widespread tissue contribution. *Cell Stem Cell* 1(1): 55–70.

Maltsev, V. A., Wobus, A. M., Rohwedel, J., Bader, M., and Hescheler, J. 1994. Cardiomyocytes differentiated *in vitro* from embryonic stem cells developmentaly express cardiac-specific genes and ionic currents. *Circ Res* 75(2): 233–44.

Martin, G. R. 1981. Isolation of a pluripotent cell line from early mouse embryos cultured in medium conditioned by teratocarcinoma stem cells. *Proc Natl Acad Sci USA* 78(12): 7634–8.

Martin, G. R. and Evans, M. J. 1974. The morphology and growth of a pluripotent teratocarcinoma cell line and its derivatives in tissue culture. *Cell* 2(3): 163–72.

Masui, S., Nakatake, Y., Toyooka, Y. et al. 2007. Pluripotency governed by sox2 via regulation of Oct3/4 expression in mouse embryonic stem cells. *Nat Cell Biol* 9(6): 625–35.

Matsuda, T., Nakamura, T., Nakao, K. et al. 1999. Stat3 activation is sufficient to maintain an undifferentiated state of mouse embryonic stem cells. *EMBO J* 18(15): 4261–9.

Mikkelsen, T. S., Hanna, J., Zhang, X. et al. 2008. Dissecting direct reprogramming through integrative genomic analysis. *Nature* 454(7200): 49–55.

Mitsui, K., Tokuzawa, Y., Itoh, H. et al. 2003. The homeoprotein nanog is required for maintenance of pluripotency in mouse epiblast and es cells. *Cell* 113(5): 631–42.

Moeller, H.-C., Mian, M. K., Shrivastava, S., Chung, B. G., and Khademhosseini, A. 2008. A microwell array system for stem cell culture. *Biomaterials* 29(6): 752–63.

Mohr, J. C., De Pablo, J. J., and Palecek, S. P. 2006. 3-d microwell culture of human embryonic stem cells. *Biomaterials* 27(36): 6032–42.

Mohr, J. C., Zhang, J., Azarin, S. M. et al. 2010. The microwell control of embryoid body size in order to regulate cardiac differentiation of human embryonic stem cells. *Biomaterials* 31(7): 1885–93.

Moore, N. W., Adams, C. E., and Rowson, L. E. 1968. Developmental potential of single blastomeres of the rabbit egg. *J Reprod Fertil* 17(3): 527–31.

Murray, P. and Edgar, D. 2000. Regulation of programmed cell death by basement membranes in embryonic development. *J Cell Biol* 150(5): 1215–21.

Nakagawa, M., Koyanagi, M., Tanabe, K. et al. 2008. Generation of induced pluripotent stem cells without myc from mouse and human fibroblasts. *Nat Biotechnol* 26(1): 101–6.

Nakano, T., Kodama, H., and Honjo, T. 1994. Generation of lymphohematopoietic cells from embryonic stem cells in culture. *Science* 265(5175): 1098–101.

Nakayama, T. and Inoue, N. 2006. Neural stem sphere method: Induction of neural stem cells and neurons by astrocyte-derived factors in embryonic stem cells in vitro. *Methods Mol Biol* 330: 1–13.

Narazaki, G., Uosaki, H., Teranishi, M. et al. 2008. Directed and systematic differentiation of cardiovascular cells from mouse induced pluripotent stem cells. *Circulation* 118(5): 498–506.

Ng, E. S., Azzola, L., Sourris, K. et al. 2005a. The primitive streak gene mixl1 is required for efficient haematopoiesis and bmp4-induced ventral mesoderm patterning in differentiating es cells. *Development* 132(5): 873–84.

Ng, E. S., Davis, R. P., Azzola, L., Stanley, E. G., and Elefanty, A. G. 2005b. Forced aggregation of defined numbers of human embryonic stem cells into embryoid bodies fosters robust, reproducible hematopoietic differentiation. *Blood* 106(5): 1601–3.

Nichols, J., Zevnik, B., Anastassiadis, K. et al. 1998. Formation of pluripotent stem cells in the mammalian embryo depends on the pou transcription factor oct4. *Cell* 95(3): 379–91.

Niebruegge, S., Nehring, A., Bär, H. et al. 2008. Cardiomyocyte production in mass suspension culture: Embryonic stem cells as a source for great amounts of functional cardiomyocytes. *Tissue Eng A* 14(10): 1591–601.

Niwa, H., Burdon, T., Chambers, I., and Smith, A. 1998. Self-renewal of pluripotent embryonic stem cells is mediated via activation of stat3. *Genes Dev* 12(13): 2048–60.

Niwa, H., Miyazaki, J., and Smith, A. G. 2000. Quantitative expression of oct-3/4 defines differentiation, dedifferentiation or self-renewal of es cells. *Nat Genet* 24(4): 372–6.

Nostro, M. C., Cheng, X., Keller, G. M., and Gadue, P. 2008. Wnt, activin, and bmp signaling regulate distinct stages in the developmental pathway from embryonic stem cells to blood. *Cell Stem Cell* 2(1): 60–71.

Nussbaum, J., Minami, E., Laflamme, M. A. et al. 2007. Transplantation of undifferentiated murine embryonic stem cells in the heart: Teratoma formation and immune response. *FASEB J* 21(7): 1345–57.

Ohgane, J., Wakayama, T., Kogo, Y. et al. 2001. DNA methylation variation in cloned mice. *Genesis* 30(2): 45–50.

Ohsugi, M., Butz, S., and Kemler, R. 1999. Beta-catenin is a major tyrosine-phosphorylated protein during mouse oocyte maturation and preimplantation development. *Dev Dyn* 216(2): 168–76.

Okita, K., Ichisaka, T., and Yamanaka, S. 2007. Generation of germline-competent induced pluripotent stem cells. *Nature* 448(7151): 313–7.

Okita, K., Nakagawa, M., Hyenjong, H., Ichisaka, T., and Yamanaka, S. 2008. Generation of mouse induced pluripotent stem cells without viral vectors. *Science* 322(5903): 949–53.

Okumura-Nakanishi, S., Saito, M., Niwa, H., and Ishikawa, F. 2005. Oct-3/4 and sox2 regulate oct-3/4 gene in embryonic stem cells. *J Biol Chem* 280(7): 5307–17.

Ouyang, A., Ng, R., and Yang, S.-T. 2007. Long-term culturing of undifferentiated embryonic stem cells in conditioned media and three-dimensional fibrous matrices without extracellular matrix coating. *Stem Cells* 25(2): 447–54.

Palmieri, S. L., Peter, W., Hess, H., and Schöler, H. R. 1994. Oct-4 transcription factor is differentially expressed in the mouse embryo during establishment of the first two extraembryonic cell lineages involved in implantation. *Dev Biol* 166(1): 259–67.

Park, I.-H., Arora, N., Huo, H. et al. 2008. Disease-specific induced pluripotent stem cells. *Cell* 134(5): 877–86.

Park, J. H., Kim, S. J., Oh, E. J. et al. 2003. Establishment and maintenance of human embryonic stem cells on sto, a permanently growing cell line. *Biol Reprod* 69(6): 2007–14.

Pera, M. F., Blasco Lafita, M. J., and Mills, J. 1987. Cultured stem-cells from human testicular teratomas: The nature of human embryonal carcinoma, and its comparison with two types of yolk-sac carcinoma. *Int J Cancer* 40(3): 334–43.

Pera, M. F., Cooper, S., Mills, J., and Parrington, J. M. 1989. Isolation and characterization of a multipotent clone of human embryonal carcinoma cells. *Differentiation* 42(1): 10–23.

Pierce, G. B. and Dixon, F. J. 1959. Testicular teratomas. I. Demonstration of teratogenesis by metamorphosis of multipotential cells. *Cancer* 12(3): 573–83.

Pierce, G. B., Dixon, F. J., and Verney, E. L. 1960. An ovarian teratocarcinoma as an ascitic tumor. *Cancer Res* 20: 106–11.

Pierce, G. B. and Verney, E. L. 1961. An *in vitro* and *in vivo* study of differentiation in teratocarcinomas. *Cancer* 14: 1017–29.

Pittenger, M. F., Mackay, A. M., Beck, S. C. et al. 1999. Multilineage potential of adult human mesenchymal stem cells. *Science* 284(5411): 143–7.

Potocnik, A. J., Nielsen, P. J., and Eichmann, K. 1994. *In vitro* generation of lymphoid precursors from embryonic stem cells. *EMBO J* 13(22): 5274–83.

Qi, X., Li, T.-G., Hao, J. et al. 2004. Bmp4 supports self-renewal of embryonic stem cells by inhibiting mitogen-activated protein kinase pathways. *Proc Natl Acad Sci USA* 101(16): 6027–32.

Qyang, Y., Martin-Puig, S., Chiravuri, M. et al. 2007. The renewal and differentiation of isl1+ cardiovascular progenitors are controlled by a wnt/beta-catenin pathway. *Cell Stem Cell* 1(2): 165–79.

Reeve, W. J. and Kelly, F. P. 1983. Nuclear position in the cells of the mouse early embryo. *J Embryol Exp Morphol* 75: 117–39.

Reubinoff, B. E., Pera, M. F., Fong, C. Y., Trounson, A., and Bongso, A. 2000. Embryonic stem cell lines from human blastocysts: Somatic differentiation in vitro. *Nat Biotechnol* 18(4): 399–404.

Rideout, W. M., Hochedlinger, K., Kyba, M., Daley, G. Q., and Jaenisch, R. 2002. Correction of a genetic defect by nuclear transplantation and combined cell and gene therapy. *Cell* 109(1): 17–27.

Rivera-Pérez, J. A. and Magnuson, T. 2005. Primitive streak formation in mice is preceded by localized activation of brachyury and wnt3. *Dev Biol* 288(2): 363–71.

Roach, S., Cooper, S., Bennett, W., and Pera, M. F. 1993. Cultured cell lines from human teratomas: Windows into tumour growth and differentiation and early human development. *Eur Urol* 23(1): 82–7; discussion 87–8.

Rosenthal, M. D., Wishnow, R. M., and Sato, G. H. 1970. *In vitro* growth and differetiation of clonal populations of multipotential mouse clls derived from a transplantable testicular teratocarcinoma. *J Natl Cancer Inst* 44(5): 1001–14.

Rossant, J. 1976. Postimplantation development of blastomeres isolated from 4- and 8-cell mouse eggs. *J Embryol Exp Morphol* 36(2): 283–90.

Rossant, J. and Lis, W. T. 1979. Potential of isolated mouse inner cell masses to form trophectoderm derivatives in vivo. *Dev Biol* 70(1): 255–61.

Rossant, J., Chazaud, C., and Yamanaka, Y. 2003. Lineage allocation and asymmetries in the early mouse embryo. *Philos Trans R Soc Lond, B, Biol Sci* 358(1436): 1341–8; discussion 49.

Rossant, J. 2008. Stem cells and early lineage development. *Cell* 132(4): 527–31.

Sachlos, E. and Auguste, D. T. 2008. Embryoid body morphology influences diffusive transport of inductive biochemicals: A strategy for stem cell differentiation. *Biomaterials* 29(34): 4471–80.

Santos, F., Hendrich, B., Reik, W., and Dean, W. 2002. Dynamic reprogramming of DNA methylation in the early mouse embryo. *Dev Biol* 241(1): 172–82.

Sargent, C. Y., Berguig, G. Y., Kinney, M. A. et al. 2010. Hydrodynamic modulation of embryonic stem cell differentiation by rotary orbital suspension culture. *Biotechnol Bioeng* 105(3): 611–26.

Sasai, Y. 2002. Generation of dopaminergic neurons from embryonic stem cells. *J Neurol* 249 Suppl 2: II41–4.

Sato, N., Sanjuan, I. M., Heke, M. et al. 2003. Molecular signature of human embryonic stem cells and its comparison with the mouse. *Dev Biol* 260(2): 404–13.

Schenke-Layland, K., Rhodes, K. E., Angelis, E. et al. 2008. Reprogrammed mouse fibroblasts differentiate into cells of the cardiovascular and hematopoietic lineages. *Stem Cells* 26(6): 1537–46.

Schmitt, T. M., De Pooter, R. F., Gronski, M. A. et al. 2004. Induction of t cell development and establishment of t cell competence from embryonic stem cells differentiated in vitro. *Nat Immunol* 5(4): 410–7.

Schöler, H. R., Ciesiolka, T., and Gruss, P. 1991. A nexus between oct-4 and e1a: Implications for gene regulation in embryonic stem cells. *Cell* 66(2): 291–304.

Schöler, H. R., Hatzopoulos, A. K., Balling, R., Suzuki, N., and Gruss, P. 1989. A family of octamer-specific proteins present during mouse embryogenesis: Evidence for germline-specific expression of an oct factor. *EMBO J* 8(9): 2543–50.

Shi, Y., Hou, L., Tang, F. et al. 2005. Inducing embryonic stem cells to differentiate into pancreatic beta cells by a novel three-step approach with activin a and all-trans retinoic acid. *Stem Cells* 23(5): 656–62.

Silva, J. and Smith, A. 2008. Capturing pluripotency. *Cell* 132(4): 532–6.

Skottman, H., Dilber, M. S., and Hovatta, O. 2006. The derivation of clinical-grade human embryonic stem cell lines. *FEBS Lett* 580(12): 2875–8.

Smyth, N., Vatansever, H. S., Murray, P. et al. 1999. Absence of basement membranes after targeting the lamc1 gene results in embryonic lethality due to failure of endoderm differentiation. *J Cell Biol* 144(1): 151–60.

Soldner, F., Hockemeyer, D., Beard, C. et al. 2009. Parkinson's disease patient-derived induced pluripotent stem cells free of viral reprogramming factors. *Cell* 136(5): 964–77.

Stadtfeld, M., Nagaya, M., Utikal, J., Weir, G., and Hochedlinger, K. 2008. Induced pluripotent stem cells generated without viral integration. *Science* 322(5903): 945–9.

Stevens, L. C. and Little, C. C. 1954. Spontaneous testicular teratomas in an inbred strain of mice. *Proc Natl Acad Sci USA* 40(11): 1080–7.

Strübing, C., Ahnert-Hilger, G., Shan, J. et al. 1995. Differentiation of pluripotent embryonic stem cells into the neuronal lineage *in vitro* gives rise to mature inhibitory and excitatory neurons. *Mech Dev* 53(2): 275–87.

Strumpf, D., Mao, C.-A., Yamanaka, Y. et al. 2005. Cdx2 is required for correct cell fate specification and differentiation of trophectoderm in the mouse blastocyst. *Development* 132(9): 2093–102.

Sutherland, A. E., Speed, T. P., and Calarco, P. G. 1990. Inner cell allocation in the mouse morula: The role of oriented division during fourth cleavage. *Dev Biol* 137(1): 13–25.

Swijnenburg, R.-J., Tanaka, M., Vogel, H. et al. 2005. Embryonic stem cell immunogenicity increases upon differentiation after transplantation into ischemic myocardium. *Circulation* 112(9 Suppl): I166–72.

Takahashi, K. and Yamanaka, S. 2006. Induction of pluripotent stem cells from mouse embryonic and adult fibroblast cultures by defined factors. *Cell* 126(4): 663–76.

Takahashi, K., Tanabe, K., Ohnuki, M. et al. 2007. Induction of pluripotent stem cells from adult human fibroblasts by defined factors. *Cell* 131(5): 861–72.

Tarkowski, A. K. and Wróblewska, J. 1967. Development of blastomeres of mouse eggs isolated at the 4- and 8-cell stage. *J Embryol Exp Morphol* 18(1): 155–80.

Tesar, P. J., Chenoweth, J. G., Brook, F. A. et al. 2007. New cell lines from mouse epiblast share defining features with human embryonic stem cells. *Nature* 448(7150): 196–9.

Thomas, P. and Beddington, R. 1996. Anterior primitive endoderm may be responsible for patterning the anterior neural plate in the mouse embryo. *Curr Biol* 6(11): 1487–96.

Thomson, J. A., Itskovitz-Eldor, J., Shapiro, S. S. et al. 1998. Embryonic stem cell lines derived from human blastocysts. *Science* 282(5391): 1145–7.

Thomson, J. A., Kalishman, J., Golos, T. G. et al. 1995. Isolation of a primate embryonic stem cell line. *Proc Natl Acad Sci USA* 92(17): 7844–8.

Tokumoto, Y., Ogawa, S., Nagamune, T., and Miyake, J. 2010. Comparison of efficiency of terminal differentiation of oligodendrocytes from induced pluripotent stem cells versus embryonic stem cells in vitro. *J Biosci Bioeng* 109(6): 622–8.

Torisawa, Y.-S., Chueh, B.-H., Huh, D. et al. 2007. Efficient formation of uniform-sized embryoid bodies using a compartmentalized microchannel device. *Lab Chip* 7(6): 770–6.

Tzanakakis, E. S., Hess, D. J., Sielaff, T. D., and Hu, W. S. 2000. Extracorporeal tissue engineered liver-assist devices. *Annu Rev Biomed Eng* 2: 607–32.

Ueno, S., Weidinger, G., Osugi, T. et al. 2007. Biphasic role for wnt/beta-catenin signaling in cardiac specification in zebrafish and embryonic stem cells. *Proc Natl Acad Sci USA* 104(23): 9685–90.

Ungrin, M. D., Joshi, C., Nica, A., Bauwens, C., and Zandstra, P. W. 2008. Reproducible, ultra high-throughput formation of multicellular organization from single cell suspension-derived human embryonic stem cell aggregates. *PLoS ONE* 3(2): e1565.

Vallier, L., Alexander, M., and Pedersen, R. A. 2005. Activin/nodal and fgf pathways cooperate to maintain pluripotency of human embryonic stem cells. *J Cell Sci* 118(Pt 19): 4495–509.

Vestweber, D. and Kemler, R. 1984. Some structural and functional aspects of the cell adhesion molecule uvomorulin. *Cell Differ* 15(2–4): 269–73.

Vestweber, D., Gossler, A., Boller, K., and Kemler, R. 1987. Expression and distribution of cell adhesion molecule uvomorulin in mouse preimplantation embryos. *Dev Biol* 124(2): 451–6.

Wakayama, S., Hikichi, T., Suetsugu, R. et al. 2007. Efficient establishment of mouse embryonic stem cell lines from single blastomeres and polar bodies. *Stem Cells* 25(4): 986–93.

Wan, Y. J., Wu, T. C., Chung, A. E., and Damjanov, I. 1984. Monoclonal antibodies to laminin reveal the heterogeneity of basement membranes in the developing and adult mouse tissues. *Journal of Cell Biology* 98(3): 971–9.

Wang, G., Zhang, H., Zhao, Y. et al. 2005. Noggin and bfgf cooperate to maintain the pluripotency of human embryonic stem cells in the absence of feeder layers. *Biochem Biophys Res Commun* 330(3): 934–42.

Wang, X., Wei, G., Yu, W. et al. 2006. Scalable producing embryoid bodies by rotary cell culture system and constructing engineered cardiac tissue with ES-derived cardiomyocytes in vitro. *Biotechnol Prog* 22(3): 811–8.

Watanabe, K., Ueno, M., Kamiya, D. et al. 2007. A rock inhibitor permits survival of dissociated human embryonic stem cells. *Nat Biotechnol* 25(6): 681–6.

Wei, C. L., Miura, T., Robson, P. et al. 2005. Transcriptome profiling of human and murine escs identifies divergent paths required to maintain the stem cell state. *Stem Cells* 23(2): 166–85.

Wernig, M., Zhao, J.-P., Pruszak, J. et al. 2008. Neurons derived from reprogrammed fibroblasts functionally integrate into the fetal brain and improve symptoms of rats with parkinson's disease. *Proc Natl Acad Sci USA* 105(15): 5856–61.

Wiles, M. V. and Keller, G. 1991. Multiple hematopoietic lineages develop from embryonic stem (es) cells in culture. *Development* 111(2): 259–67.

Willadsen, S. M. 1981. The development capacity of blastomeres from 4- and 8-cell sheep embryos. *J Embryol Exp Morphol* 65: 165–72.

Williams, R. L., Hilton, D. J., Pease, S. et al. 1988. Myeloid leukaemia inhibitory factor maintains the developmental potential of embryonic stem cells. *Nature* 336(6200): 684–7.

Wobus, A. M., Wallukat, G., and Hescheler, J. 1991. Pluripotent mouse embryonic stem cells are able to differentiate into cardiomyocytes expressing chronotropic responses to adrenergic and cholinergic agents and ca2+ channel blockers. *Differentiation* 48(3): 173–82.

Xu, C., Inokuma, M. S., Denham, J. et al. 2001. Feeder-free growth of undifferentiated human embryonic stem cells. *Nat Biotechnol* 19(10): 971–4.

Xu, C., Rosler, E., Jiang, J. et al. 2005a. Basic fibroblast growth factor supports undifferentiated human embryonic stem cell growth without conditioned medium. *Stem Cells* 23(3): 315–23.

Xu, R.-H., Peck, R. M., Li, D. S. et al. 2005b. Basic fgf and suppression of bmp signaling sustain undifferentiated proliferation of human es cells. *Nat Methods* 2(3): 185–90.

Xu, Y., Zhu, X., Hahm, H. S. et al. 2010. Revealing a core signaling regulatory mechanism for pluripotent stem cell survival and self-renewal by small molecules. *Proc Natl Acad Sci USA* 107(18): 8129–34.

Ying, Q.-L., Stavridis, M., Griffiths, D., Li, M., and Smith, A. 2003. Conversion of embryonic stem cells into neuroectodermal precursors in adherent monoculture. *Nat Biotechnol* 21(2): 183–6.

Ying, Q.-L., Wray, J., Nichols, J. et al. 2008. The ground state of embryonic stem cell self-renewal. *Nature* 453(7194): 519–23.

Yoon, B. S., Yoo, S. J., Lee, J. E. et al. 2006. Enhanced differentiation of human embryonic stem cells into cardiomyocytes by combining hanging drop culture and 5-azacytidine treatment. *Differentiation* 74(4): 149–59.

Yu, J., Vodyanik, M. A., Smuga-Otto, K. et al. 2007. Induced pluripotent stem cell lines derived from human somatic cells. *Science* 318(5858): 1917–20.

Yuan, H., Corbi, N., Basilico, C., and Dailey, L. 1995. Developmental-specific activity of the fgf-4 enhancer requires the synergistic action of sox2 and oct-3. *Genes Dev* 9(21): 2635–45.

Zhang, D., Jiang, W., Liu, M. et al. 2009. Highly efficient differentiation of human es cells and ips cells into mature pancreatic insulin-producing cells. *Cell Res* 19(4): 429–38.

Zhang, P., Li, J., Tan, Z. et al. 2008. Short-term bmp-4 treatment initiates mesoderm induction in human embryonic stem cells. *Blood* 111(4): 1933–41.

Ziomek, C. A. and Johnson, M. H. 1980. Cell surface interaction induces polarization of mouse 8-cell blastomeres at compaction. *Cell* 21(3): 935–42.

Zur Nieden, N. I., Cormier, J. T., Rancourt, D. E., and Kallos, M. S. 2007. Embryonic stem cells remain highly pluripotent following long term expansion as aggregates in suspension bioreactors. *J Biotechnol* 129(3): 421–32.

Zweigerdt, R., Burg, M., Willbold, E., Abts, H., and Ruediger, M. 2003. Generation of confluent cardiomyocyte monolayers derived from embryonic stem cells in suspension: A cell source for new therapies and screening strategies. *Cytotherapy* 5(5): 399–413.

# 9

# Hematopoietic Stem Cells

9.1 Introduction: The Hematopoietic Hierarchy................................**9**-1
Mature Blood Cells • Precursor Cells • Progenitor
Cells • Hematopoietic Stem Cells (HSC)

9.2 The Hematopoietic Lineage Commitment Process....................**9**-3
Common Myeloid Progenitors and Their Progeny • Common
Lymphoid Progenitors and Their Progeny • Multipotent Cells

9.3 Hematopoietic Stem Cells ..............................................................**9**-7
Identification Strategies • Quiescence and Cell Fate
Decisions • Transplant Assays • The Hematopoietic Niche

9.4 Sources of Hematopoietic Stem Cells for Clinical
Transplantation................................................................................**9**-11
Bone Marrow • G-CSF Mobilized Peripheral Blood • Umbilical
Cord Blood

9.5 *Ex Vivo* Expansion of HSCs ..........................................................**9**-12

9.6 Conclusion ........................................................................................**9**-12

References................................................................................................**9**-13

Ian M. Kaplan
*Johns Hopkins School
of Medicine*
*University of Maryland
School of Medicine*

Sebastien
Morisot
*University of Maryland
School of Medicine*

Curt I. Civin
*University of Maryland
School of Medicine*

## 9.1 Introduction: The Hematopoietic Hierarchy

The cellular components of the blood are essential for the survival of complex multicellular organisms. The human hematopoietic system produces billions of mature blood cells every day for a lifetime in order to replace the constantly turning-over pool of mature cells. This tour de force of multilineage cell output, on the order of $200 \times 10^9$ red blood cells and $100 \times 10^8$ white blood cells per day in the average human (Metcalf 1988), is accomplished via a highly orchestrated hierarchy of stem cells, progenitors, precursors, and mature cells (Figure 9.1).

### 9.1.1 Mature Blood Cells

The major types of mature blood cells are relatively short-lived and postmitotic, meaning they are no longer dividing. These mature blood cells are responsible for the functions of the hematopoietic system and include red blood cells (erythrocytes) that carry oxygen, granulocytes and monocytes that fight infections, and platelets that help clot the blood and aid wound healing.

B and T cells, two types of lymphocytes, comprise a special class of mature cell. Upon activation, B and T cells can expand clonally to give rise to both effector and memory cells. Unstimulated memory lymphocytes have very long half-lives, on the order of years to decades. These memory cells can be reactivated at a later time, upon recurrence of an infection, and expand clonally, repeatedly. Although memory B and T lymphocytes are unipotent (i.e., they cannot differentiate into a different cell type) their maintenance requires self-renewal capability, an essential property of stem cells. Thus, memory B and T lymphocytes have been called "honorary" stem cells (Jones and Armstrong 2008).

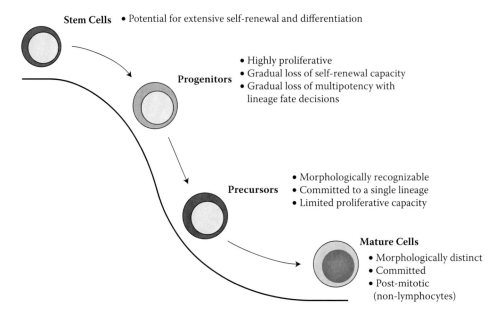

**FIGURE 9.1**  A simplified hierarchy of blood cell differentiation. Hematopoietic cells are arranged in a hierarchy of stem, progenitor, precursor and mature cells. Differentiation is a down-hill process, in that the progeny of a stem cell that has committed to differentiation cannot regain stem cell properties of extensive self-renewal and differentiation capacity.

The major mature blood and immune cell types (erythrocytes, granulocytes, monocytes, and lymphocytes) are easily identifiable by microscopic observation of histochemically stained cell preparations, but distinguishing between mature cell subclasses such as B and T lymphocytes requires the use of monoclonal antibody staining for cell surface proteins in combination with multicolor flow cytometry (discussed later).

### 9.1.2  Precursor Cells

Every mature cell is the product of a precursor cell, a cell that is completely lineage restricted but not fully differentiated. Precursor cells can be identified morphologically, as each precursor type shares histochemical characteristics with the relevant mature cell type.

### 9.1.3  Progenitor Cells

The massive numbers of hematopoietic cells produced daily are due largely to the proliferative capacity of progenitor cells. A progenitor cell type is named based on the lineages to which it gives rise *in vivo* or the type of colony that it produces in semi-solid (most commonly, methylcellulose-containing) medium. These *in vitro* colony-forming cells are termed CFU for colony-forming units or CFC for colony-forming cells, and are also designated for the types of mature cells they produce (e.g., CFC-G for unipotential progenitor cells that generate only granulocytes; CFC-GM for bipotential progenitors that produce granulocytes and monocytes; CFC-Mix for progenitors that produce multiple blood cell types including erythrocytes, granulocytes, monocytes, and megakaryocytes/platelets; note that lymphocytes do not survive *in vitro* and so "CFC-L" cannot be enumerated in standard *in vitro* hematopoietic colony-forming assays).

The earlier multipotent or bipotent progenitor cells have not yet committed to a single lineage. Beginning with multipotent progenitors, capable of producing every blood cell type, these cells expand exponentially as their lineage spectrum becomes restricted. Progenitors cannot be distinguished from each other morphologically; however, the advent of monoclonal antibodies (Kohler and Milstein 1975) and multicolor flow cytometry (Herzenberg et al. 2002) has provided hematologists with the means to identify and subclassify these progenitors based on cell surface markers (immunophenotyping).

### 9.1.4 Hematopoietic Stem Cells (HSCs)

At the pinnacle of the hematopoietic hierarchy are the hematopoietic stem cells, which give rise to all of the lympho-hematopoietic cells for the lifetime of the organism. A long-term HSC (LT-HSC) has two fundamental properties; it has the capacity for extensive self-renewal and the ability to differentiate into every blood and immune cell. These two cardinal properties can only be assessed *in vivo* and, as of today, transplant into an irradiated recipient animal remains the gold standard assay for LT-HSCs (discussed later).

## 9.2 The Hematopoietic Lineage Commitment Process

The generation of a fully functional lympho-hematopoietic system is a gradual yet dynamic process. As the differentiation-committed progeny of LT-HSCs expand, they undergo progressive gene-expression changes that ultimately result in the development of mature cells with a range of very different functional capacities. In hematopoiesis, the process of differentiation is tightly coupled with proliferation.

Progenitor cell subtypes and HSCs are morphologically indistinguishable, unlike precursors and mature cells. Therefore, we rely on immunophenotyping schemes to identify and purify cell subsets enriched in each population specified by hematopoietic models. Characterization of distinct cell populations by stage and lineage is achieved best by cell surface marker stains, using monoclonal antibodies, and/or dye efflux capacity (discussed later in detail) and assessed by fluorescence-activated cell sorting (FACS), followed by assays to assess their functional capacity. However, given the fluid, gradual nature of differentiation, a cell population that we might define operationally as representative of a particular stem-progenitor subtype, actually is a snapshot of cells at approximately that stage and lineage of hematopoietic differentiation. In addition, an immunophenotypically defined population has a high probability of containing slightly varied types of cells with respect to proliferative state, as well as stage and lineage. Thus, we must emphasize that a cell type of interest can rarely be "purified" to complete homogeneity; instead, the term "enriched" better describes the limited heterogeneity of any FACS-sorted population.

Currently, the accepted model of hematopoiesis (Figure 9.2) is a schematic representation of a fluid process. Each hematopoietic stem or progenitor cell (HSPC) subtype is an ancestral cell that is defined by the types of mature cells that it can produce and the duration of time over which it can sustain mature cell production. The dynamic nature of the differentiation process implies the "Heisenberg"-type impossibility of simultaneously isolating a single cell for some novel analysis and functionally defining the same cell and its progeny in a functional assay. These progenitor populations should therefore be treated as our best approximation or model of the process of hematopoiesis, rather than as actual cells. Therefore, we should remain open to the possibility, for example, that an enriched subset of "myeloid" or "lymphoid" progenitors might have the capacity to give rise to other lineages under appropriate conditions. A recent study illustrates the ability of human monocytes and dendritic cells to arise from a population previously believed to be lymphoid-restricted (Doulatov et al. 2010).

The following section will describe the process of lineage commitment in hematopoiesis, according to established models.

### 9.2.1 Common Myeloid Progenitors and Their Progeny

The current model of hematopoiesis proposes the existence of a CMP, a myelo-erythroid restricted progenitor. The CMP proliferates and gives rise to two bi-potent progenitors, the granulocyte–monocyte progenitor (GMP) and the megakaryocyte–erythroid progenitor (MEP).

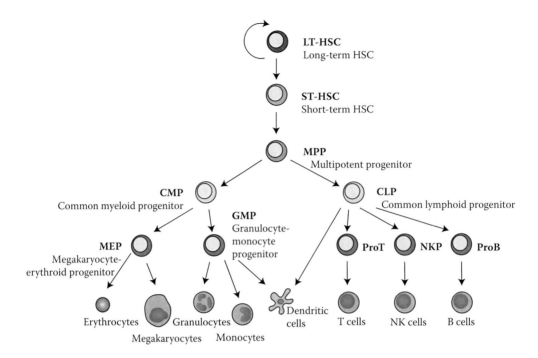

**FIGURE 9.2** Tree diagram of hematopoiesis. Hematopoiesis is organized in a hierarchy that is sustained by a very small population of quiescent, LT-HSCs that persist for the lifetime of the organism. These cells are capable of differentiating sequentially into ST-HSCs and MPPs that have reduced self-renewal capacity but greater proliferation. The progeny of MPPs become lineage-restricted CLPs or CMPs. Their progeny gradually expand and differentiate into vast numbers of morphologically-recognizable precursors and then mature functional blood and immune cells, many of which are non-proliferative and have short half-lives. An exquisitely regulated balance between the self-renewal and the differentiation of HSCs allows for a lifetime of blood cell production, without exhausting the small pool of HSCs.

### 9.2.1.1 Red Blood Cells (Erythrocytes)

Mature red blood cells, or erythrocytes, deliver oxygen to the tissues. They are rich in cytoplasmic hemoglobin, an iron-containing protein responsible for their red color, which binds oxygen with a high affinity. Erythrocytes develop from erythroid-committed progenitors within the bone marrow in a process termed erythropoiesis. In semisolid cultures containing erythropoietin (EPO), early and late erythroid progenitors are characterized functionally as BFU-E (burst-forming units erythroid) and CFU-E (colony-forming units erythroid), respectively; the names of erythroid colonies have been preserved over their long history. Erythroid-committed progenitors express glycophorin A (CD235a) and high levels of transferrin receptor (CD71) (Loken et al. 1987, Socolovsky et al. 2001). Expression of glycophorin A is erythroid-specific. Although essentially every mitotic cell type expresses transferrin receptor, because iron is required for cell division, erythroid progenitors can be distinguished by their very high CD71 expression, consistent with the high levels of hemoglobin being synthesized. As they differentiate, erythroid precursors undergo sequential morphological changes before extruding their nuclei and becoming reticulocytes, which in turn develop into mature erythrocytes that circulate for 3 months in humans. Senescent erythrocytes are endocytosed by macrophages which recycle their iron back into the circulation (Koury et al. 2002).

### 9.2.1.2 Platelets

Platelets are anucleate cell fragments that bind to damaged tissues where they are instrumental in the blood clotting and wound-healing processes. Megakaryoblasts and megakaryocytes are multinucleated platelet precursors that develop from MEPs. Megakaryocytic progenitors will form CFC-Mk in methylcellulose in the presence of thrombopoietin (TPO). Platelets and megakaryocytes can be immunophenotyped based on their expression of cell surface CD41, CD42a, CD42b, CD42c, CD42d, and CD61— receptors for the clotting factors fibrinogen, fibronectin, and von Willebrand factor (Kaushansky 2008). Mature megakaryocytes migrate to capillary sinusoids where they shed mature platelets into the circulation. A single megakaryocyte can produce over 1000 mature platelets (Kaushansky 2008) which circulate for around 10 days in the human body (Mason et al. 2007).

### 9.2.1.3 Granulocytic and Monocytic Cells

Precursors of granulocytes and monocytes arise from GMPs. The close developmental relationship between granulocytes and monocytes can be demonstrated simply in a colony-forming assay. Whole bone marrow plated in semisolid medium containing IL-3, IL-6, and SCF for mouse or IL-3, SCF, G-CSF and GM-CSF for human, readily forms bipotent CFC-GM, which contain both granulocytes and monocytes, as well as unipotent CFC-G and CFC-M, which form only granulocytes or monocytes, respectively. CD33 is a pan myeloid marker. Human monocytes and granulocytes can be distinguished by their expression of CD14 (Goyert et al. 1988) and CD15 (Skubitz et al. 1988), respectively. In the mouse, monocytes can be identified with CD115 (the M-CSF receptor) and granulocytes by their high Gr1 expression (Alder et al. 2008). Developing granulocytes can be identified morphologically at the promyelocyte stage when their cytoplasmic granules become evident in microscopic evaluation of Wright's stained histologic bone marrow cell smears. Mature granulocytes are easily identifiable morphologically due to their highly compacted nuclei that become multilobed, in human, or ring shaped, in mouse (Friedman 2002). Neutrophils, the major type of granulocytes, are the shortest-lived mature cell type in the hematopoietic system with a half-life on the order of days (Pillay et al. 2010). Neutrophil granules are loaded with potent enzymes and reactive oxygen species (ROS) that function as a first line of defense against invading pathogens. Each day, about $10^9$ neutrophils/kg of body weight, in the human, die via apoptosis and are efficiently phagocytosed by monocytes and macrophages (Luo and Loison 2008), which prevents the potentially harmful release of their enzymes and ROS. Monocytes are phagocytic cells that engulf pathogens and cellular debris that they encounter. Monocytes develop into tissue macrophages and antigen-presenting dendritic cells.

## 9.2.2 Common Lymphoid Progenitors and Their Progeny

The current hematopoietic model also proposes the existence of a lymphoid-restricted CLP, which can be separated from the CMP based on expression of the IL-7 receptor. The progeny of the CLP develop into B cell precursors that remain in the bone marrow or T cell precursors that migrate to the thymus. Although mature lymphocytes are generally quiescent, specific memory T and B cells can be reactivated by their cognate antigen to proliferate, expand, and fight infection.

### 9.2.2.1 B Cells

B cells are effector cells of the adaptive immune system producing surface bound immunoglobulins (antibodies) that can be secreted upon B cell activation and differentiation into plasma cells. B cells acquired their name because their development in birds takes place in a specialized organ called the bursa of Fabricius. The bursa of Fabricius is absent in mammals, and B cell development proceeds in the bone marrow, in close proximity with specialized stromal cells, where each cell rearranges the genetic regions responsible for antibody-binding specificity, called variable regions. This process occurs by randomly joining gene segments, in a process called V-D-J rearrangement, and introducing mutations at the junction regions to produce a repertoire of B cell clones with a vast variety of different variable regions. Those B cells that make productive rearrangements, such that their entire immunoglobulin proteins are intact, are positively selected for and survive; those that do not make productive rearrangements do not receive positive signals and undergo apoptosis. Finally, B cells with productive rearrangements that have high affinity for self-proteins are eliminated by a process called negative selection, which provides protection against deleterious autoimmune reactions (LeBien and Tedder 2008).

B cells that encounter a molecule (usually a protein) that binds to their specific immunoglobulin, called an antigen, can undergo further affinity maturation in secondary lymphoid organs such as the spleen or lymph nodes. In this process, activated B cells proliferate and acquire additional genetic changes in their immunoglobulin variable regions, a process called somatic hypermutation, to give rise to subclones producing antibodies with even greater affinity for that antigen. The expansion of activated B cell clones and their affinity maturation is the basis for the accelerated secondary response to infections that an individual has previously encountered. B cells have extremely long half-lives and can persist in the circulation or tissues for years to decades (Matthias and Rolink 2005). Early developing B cells express CD19 and CD10. Mature B cells can be distinguished by their expression of CD21 and CD22 and the lack of CD10 (Loken et al. 1988).

### 9.2.2.2 T Cells

The process of T cell development is analogous to B cell development, although T cell development takes place in the thymus. Developing thymocytes rearrange the genetic regions that encode their T cell receptors. There are two major differences between B cell receptors—surface bound antibodies—and T cell receptors. B cell receptors can be surface bound and then secreted, following activation, whereas T cell receptors are always surface bound. B cell receptors bind directly to antigens while T cell receptors can only recognize peptide antigens expressed by MHC molecules. There are two classes of MHC proteins. MHC class I molecules are expressed by all nucleated cells, and present peptides from within the cell. Thus, the peptides expressed on MHC class I represent a random sampling of the proteins within a given cell. These peptides can be nonimmunogenic portions of self-proteins or degraded from an invading pathogen or altered self-protein (e.g., in a viral infection or cancer, respectively). MHC class II molecules are expressed only by professional antigen-presenting cells (APCs)—dendritic cells, activated B cells or activated macrophages—and are "loaded" with MHC-bound peptides from proteins that have been phagocytosed by these APCs.

Early thymic progenitors (ETP) have migrated from the bone marrow and retain the ability to differentiate into monocytes, NK cells, and dendritic cells. ETPs begin at the double negative (DN) stage, as they do not express CD4 or CD8, co-receptors for the TCR. DN progenitors gradually rearrange their TCR genes. A productive rearrangement results in positive selection and progression to the double positive (DP) stage, where both CD4 and CD8 are expressed. DP progenitors successively undergo negative selection, in order to eliminate any T cell clones with high affinity for self-peptides expressed by MHC molecules on thymic stromal cells, followed by the fate decision to either CD4+ or CD8+ expression.

T cell clones will also expand upon activation by binding to an MHC molecule and peptide combination for which their TCR and co-receptor will bind. CD8+ "cytotoxic" T cells eliminate host cells that express a peptide–MHCI combination that a given T cell clone recognizes as foreign. CD4+ "helper" T cells play an instrumental role in activating B cells that express a peptide–MHCII combination that they recognize. Similarly to B cells, T cells are extremely long-lived (Rothenberg et al. 2008). Mature T cells can be identified by their expression of CD3, CD4 or CD8, and TCR (Toribio et al. 1988).

### 9.2.2.3 Dendritic Cells

Dendritic cells (DCs) are the most potent (therefore, called "professional") APCs: their role in the immune system is to constantly phagocytose antigens and display their peptides on MHC molecules. DCs can be found in the spleen, skin, lymph nodes, lung, liver, and kidney. Tissue-resident DCs can have very long half-lives.

There are a variety of tissue resident DC types, each with specific cell surface markers and gene-expression profiles. For example, in the spleen there are both CD8+CD205+ and CD8-33D1+ DC sub-types. The CD8+ DCs in the spleen are more efficient at phagocytosing apoptotic bodies and "cross-priming" the antigens onto MHC class I molecules, for the detection of viral and tumor antigens. The CD8- subtype presents phagocytosed antigens on MHC class II molecules in the more classical method.

The origin of DCs is somewhat promiscuous, and both highly purified CMPs and CLPs have the capacity to generate DCs. In the bone marrow, DCs can be traced back to a bipotent monocyte-DC progenitor (MDP). ETPs and early DN T cell precursors also have the capacity to generate DCs (Liu and Nussenzweig 2010, Rothenberg et al. 2008).

#### 9.2.2.4 Natural Killer Cells

Natural killer (NK) cells are lymphocytes that are instrumental in the cellular response against tumors and pathogen-infected cells. Mature NK cells express cell surface receptors that bind to MHC class I molecules on the surface of host cells. Viral infections and tumor initiation are often accompanied by aberrant expression of MHC class I molecules, which can be recognized by these receptors, and thereby trigger NK cells to release cytotoxic proteins (perforins and granzymes) from their granules. Additionally, NK cells can be activated to release the contents of their granules upon recognition of antibodies bound to the surface of a pathogen infected cell, in a process called antibody-dependent cellular cytotoxicity (ADCC).

NK cell development proceeds from the CLP stage in the bone marrow and from ETPs in the thymus, but these two populations of NK cells may be functionally distinct. Unlike other lymphocyte types, NK cell development does not require the rearrangement of any specialized receptors. NK precursors in the bone marrow express CD122, the common β chain of the IL-2 and IL-15 receptors. As NK precursors differentiate, they gradually acquire the expression of cell surface molecules required for their function including CD56, CD94 (MHCI binding protein) and CD16/CD32 (FcRγ) (Boos et al. 2008).

### 9.2.3 Multipotent Cells

The most primitive hematopoietic cells—long-term HSCs (LT-HSCs), short-term HSCs (ST-HSCs), and multipotent progenitors (MPPs)—are categorized functionally based on the duration for which they can support multilineage blood production. MPPs and ST-HSCs provide short-term reconstitution to a transplant recipient for up to 4–6 weeks and 3–4 months (Yang et al. 2005), respectively. A true LT-HSC, at the apex of the hematopoietic hierarchy, is capable of providing an entire lympho-hematopoietic system to a transplant recipient for a lifetime (Osawa et al. 1996) and can do this repeatedly as can be revealed by serial transplantation into secondary, tertiary, and subsequent recipients. While, all of these multipotent cell types satisfy one requirement for defining stem cells, the capacity for multilineage differentiation, only the LT-HSC has the capacity for such extensive self-renewal. Thus, the most rigorous test for a stem cell is self-renewal, as assessed by the serial transplant assay. For the purpose of this chapter, we will refer to human LT-HSCs simply as HSCs, since they have not been fractionated to the same purity as mouse LT-HSCs, mainly due to both the paucity of markers available to characterize human HSCs, and suboptimal immunodeficient mouse models (discussed below in detail).

## 9.3 Hematopoietic Stem Cells

LT-HSCs are extremely rare, comprising <0.005% (based on our own observations and Kiel et al. 2005, Yang et al. 2005) of nucleated cells in adult mouse bone marrow. The remaining > 99.99% of the marrow is comprised of the progeny of LT-HSCs.

### 9.3.1 Identification Strategies

It is important to remember that there is no single marker or characteristic that perfectly identifies HSCs. Obtaining HSC preparations of absolute purity proves to be challenging, and as mentioned above, most studies achieve "enrichment" rather than "isolation" of HSCs or other rare hematopoietic subsets. In addition, HSCs and other hematopoietic subsets must be defined by function. Morphologically, HSCs are virtually indistinguishable from lymphocytes. Indeed, the first enrichment strategies relied on the observation that HSCs are small cells. Using the CFU-S assay, which was believed to be an HSC assay at the time, fractions of small cells that had been separated by density-gradient sedimentation were found to be enriched in CFU-S (Worton et al. 1969). Later it was shown that HSCs could be fractionated away from CFU-S by elutriation, which separates cells based on their size and density (Jones et al. 1990). Currently, more sensitive methods are available to identify HSCs.

### 9.3.1.1 Immunophenotype

Using FACS, subsets of cells can be prospectively enriched, based on their light scattering characteristics and cell surface marker expression then probed for their ability to reconstitute the hematopoietic system. Simple immunophenotypic cell purifications can also be performed utilizing magnetic beads instead of FACS. Magnetic separations are robust and cost effective, and therefore can be used clinically (in the case of CD34 for human hematopoietic stem-progenitor cells (HSPCs) (Civin et al. 1996)) or to partially purify cell subsets prior to cell sorting for definitive cell purification.

#### 9.3.1.1.1 Enriching for Mouse HSCs

HSPCs in the mouse are found within the $Kit^+Sca^+Lin^-$ (KSL) population (Orlic et al. 1993, Spangrude et al. 1988) which comprises ~0.25% of whole bone marrow cells. This population includes LT-HSCs, ST-HSCs and MPPs. One in 30 KSL cells generates long-term engraftment in an irradiated recipient mouse. The KSL population can be further subdivided using either of two marker schemes, either the $KSLCD34^{lo}Flt3^-$ LT-HSC definition (Yang et al. 2005), the $KSLCD150^+CD48^-$ definition (Kiel et al. 2005), or a combination of the two to achieve extremely high purity (requiring seven-color flow cytometry) (Wilson et al. 2008).

#### 9.3.3.1.2 Enriching for Human HSPCs

Human HSPCs can be isolated from bone marrow, umbilical cord blood or mobilized peripheral blood (see sources of HSCs below). *In vivo* repopulating HSCs are enriched in the $CD34^+CD38^-$ population (Civin et al. 1984, 1987, Terstappen et al. 1991). This population is approximately equivalent in purity to the mouse KSL population—it is enriched for HSCs but ~95% are progenitors and will not provide long-term hematopoiesis. Somewhat enhanced purity can be achieved using CD90 (Thy1) and CD45RA; LT-HSCs are enriched in the $CD34^+CD38^-CD90^+CD45RA^-$ cell population (Baum et al. 1992, Majeti et al. 2007).

### 9.3.1.2 Functional Characteristics

#### 9.3.1.2.1 Side Population

Goodell and colleagues first demonstrated that HSCs could be enriched based on efflux of the DNA staining dye Hoechst 33342 (Goodell et al. 1996). Mouse bone marrow stained with Hoechst 33342 at 37°C displays a curious staining pattern when visualized on a flow cytometer. A small subset of cells, known as the side-population (SP), can be observed with low blue and red fluorescence. The SP subset can be abolished by incubating the cells with Verapamil or other MDR (multidrug resistance) pump inhibitors. The SP technique can be combined with immunophenotypic markers to more highly enrich for HSCs (Weksberg et al. 2008).

#### 9.3.1.2.2 Aldefluor

Aldehyde dehydrogenase (ALDH) enzymes are a family of enzymes that oxidize and thereby detoxify a variety of aldehydes, including retinaldehyde. The high expression of ALDHs in stem and progenitor cells can be exploited using fluorogenic aldehyde substrates that differentially label cells with high levels of ALDH expression (Jones et al. 1995, Storms et al. 1999). Like SP labeling, Aldefluor staining enriches for both human (Hess et al. 2004) and mouse (Jones et al. 1996) HSCs, although the mouse data are somewhat controversial (Pearce and Bonnet 2007). Also as with SP, Aldefluor can be used in combination with cell surface markers (Pearce and Bonnet 2007).

### 9.3.1.2.3 Day 2 Homing Assay

The Sharkis lab purified quiescent, marrow-homed mouse HSPCs and showed they are highly enriched in *in vivo* engrafting HSCs (Juopperi et al. 2007, Juopperi and Sharkis 2008). Briefly, cells collected at the 1.081/1.087 g/mL density-gradient interface are collected, depleted for lineage antigen-positive cells, and stained with the membrane dye PKH26 that will be diluted with every cell division. The stained cells are then injected into irradiated recipient mice. Any cell that does not divide extensively will retain bright PKH staining. Two days posttransplant, the bone marrow from the recipient mice is collected and PKH[bright] cells, which represent relatively quiescent cells with homing capability, are sorted by FACS.

## 9.3.2 Quiescence and Cell Fate Decisions

The ability of HSCs to constantly support hematopoiesis is dependent on their relative quiescence. At any given time, the majority of HSCs are in the $G_0$, quiescent or inactive, phase of the cell cycle, and the hematopoietic content of the marrow and the periphery is the product of only a small percent of the individual's LT-HSCs. A single quiescent HSC becomes active, produces highly proliferative progeny (that in turn produce blood for several months), and then returns to quiescence. While the activation of HSCs appears to be a stochastic process at the single cell level, it is an exquisitely well-orchestrated process at the systems level (Mangel and Bonsall 2008). Label retention studies of mouse HSCs have shown that a bone marrow LT-HSC divides only about 5 times over the course of the mouse's lifetime (Trumpp et al. 2010). Quiescence helps ensure the integrity of the genome, since every round of replication can potentially introduce mutations. Although, the kinetics of human HSCs could be different, since human bone marrow produces the same number of cells in a day that a typical mouse produces in a lifetime (Metcalf 1988), mice do nonetheless provide a valuable model for the study of most aspects of HSC biology.

An actively dividing HSC has three distinct fate decisions (Figure 9.3): a symmetrical division producing two identical daughter cells with the same stem cell capacities as the parent cell, a symmetrical division producing two differentiating daughter cells, or an asymmetrical division producing an HSC and a daughter cell destined for differentiation. Any HSC division—symmetrical or asymmetrical—that gives rise to a daughter HSC identical to the parent HSC is called self-renewal. A symmetrical division that produces two daughter HSCs leads to HSC expansion, whereas an asymmetrical division that produces both an HSC and a differentiation daughter cell leads to HSC maintenance during steady-state hematopoieis.

The ability of HSCs to switch from steady-state (maintenance) divisions to expansion is apparent in the bone marrow transplant assay. There are approximately $2 \times 10^4$ HSCs in an adult C57Bl/6 mouse. A lethally irradiated mouse can be transplanted with $2.5 \times 10^5$ bone marrow mononuclear cells—containing

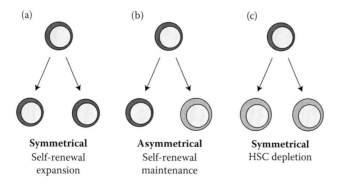

| (a) | (b) | (c) |
|---|---|---|
| **Symmetrical** | **Asymmetrical** | **Symmetrical** |
| Self-renewal | Self-renewal | HSC depletion |
| expansion | maintenance | |

**FIGURE 9.3** HSC fate decisions. An actively dividing HSC has three possible fates. (a) Symmetrical cell division that produces two identical, daughter HSCs by self-renewal. (b) An asymmetrical self-renewal division that produces one daughter HSC and one daughter cell destined for differentiation. (c) A symmetrical division that produces two daughter cells destined for differentiation.

only ~30 HSCs—which will home to the host bone marrow, expand, and fully repopulate the hematopoietic system before returning to a relatively quiescent state. The capacity for extensive self-renewal can be assessed only by the *in vivo* transplant assay; there is currently no *in vitro* assay that measures HSC function. Primary transplanted marrow can be serially transplanted to secondary or tertiary recipients to assess self-renewal capacity even more rigorously.

### 9.3.3 Transplant Assays

#### 9.3.3.1 CD45 Isoforms as Valuable Tools for Studying Mouse HSCs

The CD45 congenic system has proven to be a most useful toolkit for studying murine HSCs. Congenic strains of C57Bl/6 mice express either of two isoforms of the CD45 receptor, which is present on all nucleated hematopoietic cells. These isoforms were originally designated Ly-5a and Ly5-b (Shen et al. 1985) but their current standard designation is CD45.2 and CD45.1, respectively; the isoforms can be clearly discriminated using commercially available antibodies. The CD45 isoforms do not elicit an immune response (rejection) when transplanted into a congenic mouse expressing the other isoform. Therefore, CD45.1 cells can be transplanted into a CD45.2 recipient mouse, or vice versa, and both donor and host cells can be quantitated using monoclonal antibodies and flow cytometry.

Transgenic and knock-out mice generally must be backcrossed onto the C57Bl/6 background to enable use of the CD45 isoforms in transplantation experiments. The CD45 congenic system and the above described immunophenotyping paradigms can then be used for prospective identification of phenotypic HSCs and for assessing the role of specific genes on HSC function. For example, deletion of the cell cycle regulator p21 has no apparent affect on HSCs. However, serial transplantation of $p21^{-/-}$ marrow reveals a severe defect in HSC fitness (Cheng et al. 2000). In addition, using the CD45 system along with HSC immunophenotypes, investigators have been able to demonstrate that as few as 1 Lin⁻ $Kit^+Sca^+CD34^{lo}$ donor cell can engraft a recipient mouse (Osawa et al. 1996).

#### 9.3.3.2 Immunodeficient Animal Models for Studying Human HSCs

The study of human HSC function also requires *in vivo* models. Quantitative models for human engraftment have been slower to develop since the immune system in the recipient recognizes donor human cells as foreign. Fetal sheep (Civin et al. 1996) or myeloablated mice were first used to study human hematopoiesis *in vivo*. The low levels of engraftment observed in these models spurred a need for more sensitive, genetically engineered, immunocompromised mice, to prevent graft rejection. Various immunocompromised mouse strains have been discovered and improved upon over time to minimize immune rejection of the xenogeneic human stem cells (Shultz et al. 2007).

NOD-*scid* IL-2Rγ$^{-/-}$ mice (NSG) are arguably the most immunocompromised mouse strain currently available and have been shown to be the most sensitive mouse strain to assess low numbers of HSCs (Ishikawa et al. 2005). Similar to transplant of mouse HSCs, the transplant of human HSCs into an immunodeficient animal, will give rise to all blood lineages, and serial transplant into a secondary recipient will reveal the self-renewal capacity of HSCs (Ishikawa et al. 2005). Most human lineages successfully develop in the NSG mouse, including T cells. However, the absence of HLA expression on thymic stromal cells and lymph nodes (e.g., for positive and negative selection) still constrains the full modeling of development of a human immune system in the NSG mouse. In addition, there is a paucity of mature human blood cell types, due to the absence of human hematopoietic growth factors. Finally, there is still a need to develop more sensitive mouse models that can support the growth of single human HSCs and mimic the human marrow microenvironment.

### 9.3.4 The Hematopoietic Niche

The function and fate of HSCs is inextricably linked to microenvironmental cues: although HSCs are partially maintained by cell-intrinsic molecules, such as Bmi-1 (Akala and Clarke 2006), the extracellular hematopoietic microenvironment, or niche, provides extrinsic signals that are necessary for the maintenance of HSCs and their functional capacity. HSCs removed from their niche and cultured *ex vivo* rapidly lose their engrafting capacity (Antonchuk et al. 2002). The extrinsic signals involved in maintaining HSC identity are a complex, and not fully understood, combination of soluble factors, cell–cell contact signals and oxygen gradients. Unlike the intestinal stem cell niche, where intestinal stem cells and transit-amplifying cells reside in distinct locations in the intestinal crypts, the HSC niche is not an absolute location within the bone marrow.

The HSC niche in adult bone marrow is located at the endosteum, a vascularized region at the junction between bone and marrow, and is lined by osteoblasts, osteoclasts and stromal cells. These cells provide a complex milieu, which directs HSCs to remain quiescent and pluripotent through signals such as Wnt, Notch, SDF-1, TPO, and Cadherin binding. Within the endosteal niche, HSCs are subjected to a relatively hypoxic environment, which has the benefit of reduced concentrations of DNA-damaging oxygen free radicals (Trumpp et al. 2010). In one model of hematopoiesis, active HSCs migrate out of the endosteal niche and into perivascular regions in close proximity to capillaries and the nutrients they provide, in order to proliferate and differentiate. However, this observation that HSCs are found in close proximity to vasculature may also be altered by the fact that HSCs regularly egress from the niche into the circulation and return to their niche (Trumpp et al. 2010).

# 9.4 Sources of Hematopoietic Stem Cells for Clinical Transplantation

For clinical and research applications, there are three main sources of human HSCs: bone marrow, G-CSF mobilized peripheral blood, and umbilical cord blood (UCB). For clinical purposes, harvests of marrow, mobilized blood, or UCB may be enriched for HSPCs by CD34 (Civin et al. 1996). Such clinical HSPC preparations are a heterogeneous population composed mainly of progenitor cells along with <1% HSCs.

## 9.4.1 Bone Marrow

Bone marrow has been harvested as a source of HSPCs for over 50 years. Whole bone marrow is extracted from donors under general anesthesia, from the iliac crest of the pelvic bone, by puncturing the bone with a syringe followed by aspiration. Harvested bone marrow includes HSPCs (~5% of whole marrow), mature cells, stromal cells and adipocytes. Since bone marrow harvesting is painful (requiring the marrow donor to receive general or regional anesthesia in an operating room), the majority of HSPC harvests are now mobilized blood (Peters et al. 2010).

## 9.4.2 G-CSF Mobilized Peripheral Blood

HSPC egress from the marrow is a naturally occurring process. At any given time, very small numbers of HSPCs can be found circulating in the bloodstream before they return to the bone marrow (Wright et al. 2001). HSPC egress can be exaggerated by administration of G-CSF (granulocyte colony-stimulating factor), which causes large numbers of HSPCs to "mobilize" into the circulation, where they can be collected from a donor's blood (Arslan and Moog 2007, Sica et al. 1992). Leukocytes are then harvested by a minimally invasive procedure called leukaphaeresis, with erythrocytes subsequently returned to the donor. Harvested cells can then be enriched for HSPCs, as described above. Mobilized blood leads to more rapid hematopoietic repopulation than marrow, thus reducing the risk of infections and bleeding, a major advantage for the recipient (Bonig et al. 2007). The collection of HSPCs directly from the blood does not require anesthesia, another advantage for the donor, although G-CSF administration has certain, usually minor side effects (Arslan and Moog 2007). Bone marrow and mobilized peripheral blood harvests run the risk of being harmful to the transplant recipient if any T cells are left in the HSPC prep.

T cells are the major mediator of graft versus host disease (GVHD) a potentially fatal side effect of any HSPC transplant (Couriel et al. 2004).

### 9.4.3 Umbilical Cord Blood

The placenta is a site of ongoing hematopoiesis during fetal development. Immediately after the birth of a newborn, the placenta and the umbilical cord still contain relatively high concentrations of HSPCs that would otherwise be discarded. UCB can be drawn out of the placenta and umbilical cord and cryopreserved, therefore converting a waste product into a valuable clinical resource (Gluckman 2009). However, the numbers of HSCs in a UCB harvest are limiting because the amount of blood in the placenta contains ~10–100-fold fewer total cells than the typical bone marrow harvest. Therefore, UCB harvests are optimally sufficient only for transplant of smaller children, not larger children or adults (Kelly et al. 2009). UCB has the major advantage of containing few mature T cells. Therefore, the occurrence and severity of GVHD is lower in patients transplanted with UCB than in those transplanted with bone marrow or mobilized blood.

## 9.5 *Ex Vivo* Expansion of HSCs

The ability to expand HSPCs *in vitro* has numerous potential clinical applications. For instance, if the number of HSCs from a single donor could be augmented, the need for large-scale harvesting of HSPC sources could be reduced (Kelly et al. 2009). However, most investigators agree that current *ex vivo* HSPC culture strategies are accompanied by loss of *in vivo* engrafting capacity (Sorrentino 2004). Although progenitor cells can be readily expanded, optimal conditions to induce HSC self-renewal *in vitro* remains a technical challenge, despite use of many combinations of cytokines, stromal cells, and continuous perfusion systems. Possibly, an optimal combination of growth factors (Zhang et al. 2006), some provided by stromal cells in 3-dimensional matrices mimicking the bone marrow microenvironment, will eventually support expansion of self-renewing HSCs. Alternatively, it might be possible to develop techniques to generate large numbers of HSCs from human embryonic stem cells or induced pluripotent stem cells (Kaufman 2009) in the future.

## 9.6 Conclusion

The hematopoietic system is a tightly regulated cellular hierarchy, with astonishing potential. Remarkably, a single self-renewing HSC, if placed in the appropriate conditions and environment, is able to reconstitute an entire fully functional lympho-hematopoietic system. Historically, the hematopoietic system is arguably the most characterized stem cell hierarchical model. The lessons of stem cell biology learned from hematopoiesis have been applied to all stem cell systems including, but not limited to, neural stem cells, intestinal stem cells and even cancer stem cells. The hematopoietic system is also a wonderful example of the ability of science to be translated from bench to bedside. The thorough identification and characterization of stem and progenitors cells, at a fundamental level, has been successfully translated to the clinic with the advent of bone marrow transplantations for several blood disorders and hematologic malignancies.

The dysregulation of such a complex system can lead to the transformation of stem or progenitors cells into leukemia stem cells, that harbor a stem-cell like self-renewal property, and can sustainably generate leukemia cell subtypes. Often, the same genes so fundamental for normal HSC biology are the ones that drive leukemogenesis when altered. Therefore, by studying HSCs we hope to better understand and fight leukemia. Reflexively, studying leukemia has helped us unravel HSC regulation. Additionally, the improvement of *ex vivo* expansion techniques, and the generation of iPS cells capable of differentiating into HSCs, although at very preliminary stages, holds great promise for the treatment of blood disorders and cancers.

# References

Akala, O. O. and Clarke, M. F. 2006. Hematopoietic stem cell self-renewal. *Curr Opin Genet Dev.* 16:496–501.

Alder, J. K., Georgantas, R. W., 3rd, Hildreth, R. L. et al. 2008. Kruppel-like factor 4 is essential for inflammatory monocyte differentiation in vivo. *J Immunol.* 180:5645–52.

Antonchuk, J., Sauvageau, G., and Humphries, R. K. 2002. HOXB4-induced expansion of adult hematopoietic stem cells ex vivo. *Cell.* 109:39–45.

Arslan, O. and Moog, R. 2007. Mobilization of peripheral blood stem cells. *Transfus Apher Sci.* 37:179–85.

Baum, C. M., Weissman, I. L., Tsukamoto, A. S., Buckle, A. M., and Peault, B. 1992. Isolation of a candidate human hematopoietic stem-cell population. *PNAS.* 89:2804–8.

Bonig, H., Priestley, G. V., Oehler, V., and Papayannopoulou, T. 2007. Hematopoietic progenitor cells (HPC) from mobilized peripheral blood display enhanced migration and marrow homing compared to steady-state bone marrow HPC. *Exp Hematol.* 35:326–34.

Boos, M. D., Ramirez, K., and Kee, B. L. 2008. Extrinsic and intrinsic regulation of early natural killer cell development. *Immunol Res.* 40:193–207.

Cheng, T., Rodrigues, N., Shen, H. et al. 2000. Hematopoietic stem cell quiescence maintained by p21cip1/waf1. *Science.* 287:1804–8.

Civin, C., Strauss, L., Brovall, C. et al. 1984. Antigenic analysis of hematopoiesis. III. A hematopoietic progenitor cell surface antigen defined by a monoclonal antibody raised against KG-1a cells. *J Immunol.* 133:157–65.

Civin, C. I., Almeida-Porada, G., Lee, M. J. et al. 1996. Sustained, retransplantable, multilineage engraftment of highly purified adult human bone marrow stem cells in vivo. *Blood.* 88:4102–9.

Civin, C. I., Banquerigo, M. L., Strauss, L. C., and Loken, M. R. 1987. Antigenic analysis of hematopoiesis. VI. Flow cytometric characterization of My-10-positive progenitor cells in normal human bone marrow.

Civin, C. I., Trischmann, T., Kadan, N. S. et al. 1996. Highly purified CD34-positive cells reconstitute hematopoiesis. *J Clin Oncol.* 14:2224–33.

Couriel, D., Caldera, H., Champlin, R., and Komanduri, K. 2004. Acute graft-versus-host disease: Pathophysiology, clinical manifestations, and management. *Cancer.* 101:1936–46.

Doulatov, S., Notta, F., Eppert, K. et al. 2010. Revised map of the human progenitor hierarchy shows the origin of macrophages and dendritic cells in early lymphoid development. *Nat Immunol.* 11:585–93.

Friedman, A. D. 2002. Transcriptional regulation of granulocyte and monocyte development. *Oncogene.* 21:3377–90.

Gluckman, E. 2009. History of cord blood transplantation. *Bone Marrow Transplant.* 44:621–6.

Goodell, M. A., Brose, K., Paradis, G., Conner, A. S., and Mulligan, R. C. 1996. Isolation and functional properties of murine hematopoietic stem cells that are replicating in vivo. *J Exp Med.* 183:1797–806.

Goyert, S. M., Ferrero, E., Rettig, W. J. et al. 1988. The CD14 monocyte differentiation antigen maps to a region encoding growth factors and receptors. *Science.* 239:497–500.

Herzenberg, L. A., Parks, D., Sahaf, B., Perez, O., and Roederer, M. 2002. The history and future of the fluorescence activated cell sorter and flow cytometry: A view from Stanford. *Clin Chem.* 48:1819–27.

Hess, D. A., Meyerrose, T. E., Wirthlin, L. et al. 2004. Functional characterization of highly purified human hematopoietic repopulating cells isolated according to aldehyde dehydrogenase activity. *Blood.* 104:1648–55.

Ishikawa, F., Yasukawa, M., Lyons, B. et al. 2005. Development of functional human blood and immune systems in NOD/SCID/IL2 receptor {gamma} chain(null) mice. *Blood.* 106:1565–73.

Jones, R., Barber, J., Vala, M. et al. 1995. Assessment of aldehyde dehydrogenase in viable cells. *Blood.* 85:2742–6.

Jones, R., Collector, M., Barber, J. et al. 1996. Characterization of mouse lymphohematopoietic stem cells lacking spleen colony-forming activity. *Blood.* 88:487–91.

Jones, R. J. and Armstrong, S. A. 2008. Cancer stem cells in hematopoietic malignancies. *Biol Blood Marrow Transplant.* 14:12–6.

Jones, R. J., Wagner, J. E., Celano, P., Zicha, M. S., and Sharkis, S. J. 1990. Separation of pluripotent haematopoietic stem cells from spleen colony-forming cells. *Nature*. 347:188–9.

Juopperi, T. A., Schuler, W., Yuan, X. et al. 2007. Isolation of bone marrow-derived stem cells using density-gradient separation. *Exp Hematol*. 35:335–41.

Juopperi, T. A. and Sharkis, S. J. 2008. Isolation of quiescent murine hematopoietic stem cells by homing properties. *Methods Mol Biol*. 430:21–30.

Kaufman, D. S. 2009. Toward clinical therapies using hematopoietic cells derived from human pluripotent stem cells. *Blood*. 114:3513–23.

Kaushansky, K. 2008. Historical review: Megakaryopoiesis and thrombopoiesis. *Blood*. 111:981–6.

Kelly, S. S., Sola, C. B., de Lima, M., and Shpall, E. 2009. ex vivo expansion of cord blood. *Bone Marrow Transplant*. 44:673–81.

Kiel, M. J., Yilmaz, M. H., Iwashita, T. et al. 2005. SLAM family receptors distinguish hematopoietic stem and progenitor cells and reveal endothelial niches for stem cells. *Cell*. 121:1109–21.

Kohler, G. and Milstein, C. 1975. Continuous cultures of fused cells secreting antibody of predefined specificity. *Nature*. 256:495–7.

Koury, M. J., Sawyer, S. T., and Brandt, S. J. 2002. New insights into erythropoiesis. *Curr Opin Hematol*. 9:93–100.

LeBien, T. W. and Tedder, T. F. 2008. B lymphocytes: How they develop and function. *Blood*. 112:1570–1580.

Liu, K. and Nussenzweig, M. C. 2010. Origin and development of dendritic cells. *Immunological Reviews*. 234:45–54.

Loken, M. R., Shah, V. O., Dattilio, K. L., and Civin, C. I. 1987. Flow cytometric analysis of human bone marrow: I. Normal erythroid development. *Blood*. 69:255–63.

Loken, M. R., Shah, V. O., Hollander, Z., and Civin, C. I. 1988. Flow cytometric analysis of normal B lymphoid development. *Pathol Immunopathol Res*. 7:357–70.

Luo, H. R. and Loison, F. 2008. Constitutive neutrophil apoptosis: Mechanisms and regulation. *Am J Hematol*. 83:288–95.

Majeti, R., Park, C. Y., and Weissman, I. L. 2007. Identification of a hierarchy of multipotent hematopoietic progenitors in human cord blood. *Cell Stem Cell*. 1:635–45.

Mangel, M. and Bonsall, M. B. 2008. Phenotypic evolutionary models in stem cell biology: Replacement, quiescence, and variability. *PLoS ONE*. 3:e1591.

Mason, K. D., Carpinelli, M. R., Fletcher, J. I. et al. 2007. Programmed anuclear cell death delimits platelet life span. *Cell*. 128:1173–86.

Matthias, P. and Rolink, A. G. 2005. Transcriptional networks in developing and mature B cells. *Nat Rev Immunol*. 5:497–508.

Metcalf, D. 1988. *The Molecular Control of Blood Cells*. Cambridge, MA: Harvard University Press.

Orlic, D., Fischer, R., Nishikawa, S., Nienhuis, A., and Bodine, D. 1993. Purification and characterization of heterogeneous pluripotent hematopoietic stem cell populations expressing high levels of c-kit receptor. *Blood*. 82:762–70.

Osawa, M., Hanada, K.-I., Hamada, H. and Nakauchi, H. 1996. Long-term lymphohematopoietic reconstitution by a single CD34-low/negative hematopoietic stem cell. *Science*. 273:242–5.

Pearce, D. J. and Bonnet, D. 2007. The combined use of Hoechst efflux ability and aldehyde dehydrogenase activity to identify murine and human hematopoietic stem cells. *Exp Hematol*. 35:1437–46.

Pearce, D. J. and Bonnet, D. 2007. The combined use of Hoechst efflux ability and aldehyde dehydrogenase activity to identify murine and human hematopoietic stem cells. *Exp. Hematol*. 35:1437–46.

Peters, C., Cornish, J. M., Parikh, S. H., and Kurtzberg, J. 2010. Stem cell source and outcome after hematopoietic stem cell transplantation (HSCT) in children and adolescents with acute leukemia. *Pediatr Clin North Am*. 57:27–46.

Pillay, J., den Braber, I., Vrisekoop, N. et al. 2010. *In vivo* labeling with $2H_2O$ reveals a human neutrophil lifespan of 5.4 days. *Blood*. 116:625–7.

Rothenberg, E. V., Moore, J. E., and Yui, M. A. 2008. Launching the T-cell-lineage developmental programme. *Nat Rev Immunol.* 8:9–21.

Shen, F. W., Saga, Y., Litman, G. et al. 1985. Cloning of Ly-5 cDNA. *Proc Natl Acad Sci USA.* 82:7360–3.

Shultz, L. D., Ishikawa, F., and Greiner, D. L. 2007. Humanized mice in translational biomedical research. *Nat Rev Immunol.* 7:118–30.

Sica, S., Salutari, P., Teofili, L., Menichella, G., and Leone, G. 1992. G-CSF and peripheral blood progenitor cells. *Lancet.* 339:1411.

Skubitz, K. M., Mendiola, J. R., and Collett, M. S. 1988. CD15 monoclonal antibodies react with a phosphotyrosine-containing protein on the surface of human neutrophils. *J Immunol.* 141:4318–23.

Socolovsky, M., Nam, H.-S., Fleming, M. D. et al. 2001. Ineffective erythropoiesis in Stat5a-/-5b-/mice due to decreased survival of early erythroblasts. *Blood.* 98:3261–73.

Sorrentino, B. P. 2004. Clinical strategies for expansion of haematopoietic stem cells. *Nat Rev Immunol.* 4:878–88.

Spangrude, G. J., Heimfeld, S., and Weissman, I. L. 1988. Purification and characterization of mouse hematopoietic stem cells. *Science.* 241:58–62.

Storms, R. W., Trujillo, A. P., Springer, J. B. et al. 1999. Isolation of primitive human hematopoietic progenitors on the basis of aldehyde dehydrogenase activity. *PNAS.* 96:9118–23.

Terstappen, L., Huang, S., Safford, M., Lansdorp, P., and Loken, M. 1991. Sequential generations of hematopoietic colonies derived from single nonlineage-committed CD34 + CD38- progenitor cells. *Blood.* 77:1218–27.

Toribio, M. L., de la Hera, A., Regueiro, J. R. et al. 1988. Alpha/beta heterodimeric T-cell receptor expression early in thymocyte differentiation. *J Mol Cell Immunol.* 3:347–62.

Trumpp, A., Essers, M., and Wilson, A. 2010. Awakening dormant haematopoietic stem cells. *Nat Rev Immunol.* 10:201–9.

Weksberg, D. C., Chambers, S. M., Boles, N. C., and Goodell, M. A. 2008. CD150- side population cells represent a functionally distinct population of long-term hematopoietic stem cells. *Blood.* 111:2444–51.

Wilson, A., Laurenti, E., Oser, G. et al. 2008. Hematopoietic stem cells reversibly switch from dormancy to self-renewal during homeostasis and repair. *Cell.* 135:1118–29.

Worton, R. G., McCulloch, E. A., and Till, J. E. 1969. Physical separation of hemopoietic stem cells differing in their capacity for self-renewal. *J Exp Med.* 130:91–103.

Wright, D. E., Wagers, A. J., Gulati, A. P., Johnson, F. L., and Weissman, I. L. 2001. Physiological migration of hematopoietic stem and progenitor cells. *Science.* 294:1933–6.

Yang, L., Bryder, D., Adolfsson, J. et al. 2005. Identification of Lin-Sca1 + kit + CD34 + Flt3- short-term hematopoietic stem cells capable of rapidly reconstituting and rescuing myeloablated transplant recipients. *Blood.* 105:2717–23.

Zhang, C. C., Kaba, M., Ge, G. et al. 2006. Angiopoietin-like proteins stimulate ex vivo expansion of hematopoietic stem cells. *Nat Med.* 12:240–5.

# 10

# Mesenchymal Stem Cells

| | | |
|---|---|---|
| 10.1 | Definition | 10-1 |
| 10.2 | Cell Characteristics | 10-2 |
| | Cell Isolation • Colony Forming Unit Assay • Cell Surface Marker and Flow Cytometry • Self-Renewal Capacity • Cell Differentiation Capacity • The MSC Niche | |
| 10.3 | Potential Therapeutic Applications | 10-5 |
| 10.4 | Potential Concerns | 10-6 |
| 10.5 | Conclusion | 10-7 |
| References | | 10-7 |

Pamela C. Yelick
*Tufts University School of Dental Medicine*

Weibo Zhang
*Tufts University School of Dental Medicine*

## 10.1 Definition

The term "mesenchymal stem cells" (MSCs) was originally used to refer to the non-hematopoietic stem cells derived from the bone marrow, which can differentiate into a variety of cell types (Prockop, 1997). These cells are also referred to as bone marrow stromal cells (BMSCs) as they are derived from the complex supporting tissues present in the bone marrow.

Research on BMSCs can be traced back to more than 130 years ago (Cohnheim, 1867), when Cohnheim injected an analine dye into the veins and found dye-labeled fibroblast-like cells in a distal wound site (Prockop, 1997). This observation suggested the presence of non-hematopoietic stem cells in the bone marrow. In the 1970s, Friedenstein noticed that a small population of cells obtained from bone marrow aspirates were able to attach to the bottom of plastic culture dish. The attached cells were heterogenous in appearance, but mainly consisted of spindle-shaped. Most importantly, they were capable of differentiating to form small mineralized deposits resembling bone or cartilage (Friedenstein et al., 1976). Later, the same group demonstrated that these cells retained their potential to differentiate into bone, cartilage, and fibrous tissue *in vivo,* even after 20 or 30 cell doublings in culture (Friedenstein et al., 1987). Further studies confirmed this observation and proved that BMSCs were able to differentiate into osteoblasts, chondroblasts, adipocytes, and myoblasts (Wakitani et al., 1995, Clark and Keating, 1995). Caplan was the first to coin the term MSCs to describe these cells with multilineage differentiation potential (Caplan, 1991). Other terms have also been used to describe the bone marrow-derived pluripotent cells, such as marrow-isolated adult multilineage inducible cells (D'Ippolito et al., 2004), very small embryonic-like cells (Kucia et al., 2006), multipotent adult progenitor cells (Belema-Bedada et al., 2008), and pre-MSC (Anjos-Afonso and Bonnet, 2007).

Adult stem cells, also known as postnatal stem cells, have been isolated from other mesenchymal tissues, such as umbilical cord blood (Mareschi et al., 2001), fat (Zuk et al., 2001), muscle (Collins et al., 2005), synovium (De Bari et al., 2001), and dental pulp (Gronthos et al., 2000, Miura et al., 2003). Although the cell characteristics of stem cells derived from different tissues are not identical, they all share the two basic properties of stem cells, self-renewal and pluripotency, like the BMSC populations.

Currently, the term MSCs is used to indicate multipotent stem cells derived from mesenchymal tissues, which can differentiate into a variety of cell types (Kirschstein and Skirboll, 2001). Various protocols have been used for MSC isolation and purification, making experimental results from different groups somewhat difficult to compare. In order to diminish this confusion, in 2006 the Mesenchymal and Tissue Stem Cell Committee of the International Society for Cellular Therapy proposed four minimal criteria to define human MSCs: (1) MSCs must be plastic-adherent when maintained in standard culture conditions; (2) MSCs must have the potential for osteogenic, adipogenic, and chondrogenic differentiation; (3) MSCs must express CD73, CD90, and CD105; and (4) MSCs must lack the expression of CD45, CD34, CD14, or CD11b, CD79alpha or CD19 and human leukocyte antigen (HLA)-DR (Dominici et al., 2006). As MSCs derived from the bone marrow are best characterized and most advanced in clinical use, in this chapter we will review progress in research pertaining to bone marrow-derived MSCs.

## 10.2  Cell Characteristics

### 10.2.1  Cell Isolation

MSCs isolation is fairly easy, because they can be obtained from a small amount of tissue. For instance, BMSCs are usually cultured from 25 to 50 mL of bone marrow aspirate. The traditional method used to harvest BMSCs is density gradient centrifugation, in which BMSCs concentrated at the high-density interface are collected and seeded onto tissue culture plates and cultured in medium with 10% fetal calf serum. Most of the attached mononuclear cells are MSCs. Some hematopoietic cells can also adhere, but will be washed away over time. Gradually, the morphology of the cells with heterogeneous appearance becomes more and more uniform after serial passages. The typical morphology of MSCs is a spindle-shaped cell body, with a large, round nucleus containing a prominent nucleolus. Some MSCs are polygonal in shape, exhibit a few long cell processes, and are characterized by small numbers of Golgi apparati, rough endoplasmic reticulum, mitochondria, and polyribosomes present in cytoplasm.

MSCs from tissues other than the bone marrow can be isolated via enzymatic digestion and selected by their adherence to plastic tissue culture plates. They all show phenotypic heterogeneity initially, and become homogenous after a few passages in culture (Huang et al., 2008, Katz et al., 2005, Nomura et al., 2007). Alternative protocols for MSCs isolation have been tested to achieve more purified stem cell populations (Smith et al., 2004). However, plastic attachment is still considered to be the most reliable method.

### 10.2.2  Colony Forming Unit Assay

When MSCs were plated at low cell seeding density, individual precursor can proliferate to form a colony. The number of colony forming units (CFUs) reflects the number of progenitor cells present in the cell population, and in turn the mesenchymal tissue potential. For human MSCs, each colony is generated by a single cell. Although more than one colony can be generated by a single mouse or rat MSCs because they can detach and reseed in the plate (Javazon et al., 2001). CFU of fibroblasts measuring assay is considered to be a gold standard *in vitro* assay to identify MSCs (Friedenstein et al., 1970). A refined method for colony-forming ability of MSCs is single-cell colony forming unit assay. That is the method to seed the cells into individual wells of a microtiter plate to ensure that each observed colony was generated by a single cell, which showed a smaller variation than the standard CFU assay (Pochampally, 2008). Several groups estimated that 0.01% to 0.0001% of nucleated marrow cells are MSCs in the bone marrow (Castro-Malaspina et al., 1980, Perkins and Fleischman, 1990). Most of the MSCs derived from tissues other than bone marrow can form colonies *in vitro*. However, CFU assay has not been routinely successful for the detection of MSCs in peripheral blood and cord blood (Deans and Moseley, 2000).

## 10.2.3 Cell Surface Marker and Flow Cytometry

Recently, significant increase in knowledge on MSC surface markers has been gathered using microarray and cell-sorting methods, including fluorescence activated cell sorting and magnetic bead sorting. However, additional data still need to be accumulated in order to complete the cell surface antigenic profile. To date, no specific single marker of MSCs has been identified. Reasons for this include the fact that current protocols for MSCs isolation result in highly heterogeneous cell populations, and also that MSCs isolated from different tissues represent highly variable cell populations.

It is generally accepted that MSCs lack typical hematopoietic cell surface antigens, such as CD14, CD31, CD34, and CD45. However, CD34 expression was observed in MCSs harvested from some mice strains (Peister et al., 2004). MSCs also lack the expression of CD 11b (Integrin alpha M), CD79alpha or CD19, and HLA-DR. BMSCs also do not express the co-stimulatory molecules CD80, CD86, CD40, the adhesion molecules CD31 (platelet/endothelial cell adhesion molecule [PECAM]-1), CD18 (leukocyte function-associated antigen-1 [LFA-1]), or CD56 (neuronal cell adhesion molecule-1). Other than the three markers, CD73, CD90, and CD105, identified by the Mesenchymal and Tissue Stem Cell Committee of the International Society, BMSCs also express STRO-1, CD105 (SH2), CD73 (SH3/4), CD44, CD71, and CD90 (Thy-1), as well as the adhesion molecules CD106 (vascular cell adhesion molecule [VCAM]-1), CD166 (activated leukocyte cell adhesion molecule [ALCAM]), intercellular adhesion molecule (ICAM)-1, and CD29 (Pittenger et al., 1999). Mesenchymal stem cells are also known to express numerous receptors important for cell adhesion with hematopoietic cells. Eleven common genes were identified as stemness genes because there are highly expressed in undifferentiated and de-differentiated MSCs by comparing the gene profiles of undifferentiated and de-differentiated MSCs to differentiated osteoblasts, chondrocyte, and adipocytes (Song et al., 2006).

## 10.2.4 Self-Renewal Capacity

One of the two main characteristics of stem cells is their capacity of self-renewal. There are two types of stem cell division, symmetric and asymmetric (Morrison and Kimble, 2006). Asymmetric replication is a defining characteristic of stem cells, where each stem cell divides into one daughter cell with a stem cell fate, and one daughter cell with a differentiated cell fate. Symmetric division of one stem cell will produce two identical daughter cells, both of which can retain their stem cell characteristics (Knoblich, 2008). In this way, MSCs can maintain the cell number and keep their self-renewal potential though symmetric and asymmetric division (Ramasamy et al., 2007). It has been shown that embryonic stem cells (ESCs) have unlimited self-renewal capacity, but there is no evidence that the self-renewal capacity of MSCs is comparable to that of ESCs, the pluripotent stem cells derived from the inner cell mass of the blastocyst from an early-stage embryo (Thomson et al., 1998). Self-renewal potential of bone marrow-derived MSCs has been confirmed by numerous research groups, but with highly variable results (Bruder et al., 1997, Colter et al., 2000).

## 10.2.5 Cell Differentiation Capacity

Multilineage differentiation potential is another specific property of MSCs. MSCs can differentiate into all of the cell types of the tissues or organ that they were originally harvested from. More recently, reports indicate that MSCs can cross lineage boundary and differentiate into a variety of tissue-specific cell types, a capacity termed "plasticity" (Herzog et al., 2003, Zipori, 2005). MSCs can give rise to all somatic cells in variety of tissues and organs, such as the brain, lung, liver, spleen, kidney, blood, and skin when injected into blastocysts (Jiang et al., 2002). The *in vitro* and *in vivo* differentiation potential of bone marrow-derived MSCs has been studied most extensively. Other than the identical tri-differentiation (osteo/adipo/chondro) potentials, many studies also demonstrate that bone marrow-derived MSCs can differentiate into various functional cell types in all three germ layers, including mesoderm, ectoderm, and endoderm, both *in vitro* and *in vivo*. The specific cell types into which BMSCs have differentiated included, but not limited to, cardiomyocytes (Makino et al., 1999, Psaltis et al., 2008, Valarmathi et al., 2010), lung epithelial cells (Popov et al., 2007), endothelial cells (Oswald et al., 2004), hepatocytes (Kang et al., 2005, Ke et al., 2008), pancreatic islets (Eberhardt et al., 2006), bladder cells (Tian et al., 2010), and neurons (Cho et al., 2005). Recent reports also suggest the potential of BMSCs for hematopoietic cell differentiation (Zhao et al., 2008, Rafii and Lyden, 2003). Human BMSCs were able to differentiate into site-specific cells after intraperitoneal injection (Liechty et al., 2000). After intravenous infusion, MSCs can be detected in a variety of tissues (Devine et al., 2003), especially at sites of inflammation or injury (Mouiseddine et al., 2007). The mechanism behind this BMSC localization remains unclear, although one theories is that MSCs migrate via the stromal cell-derived factor 1/chemokine CSC receptor 4 pathway (Shi et al., 2007, Dar et al., 2006).

The differentiation capabilities of MSCs derived from tissues other than bone has been verified by various studies. However, no report indicates that the differentiation potential of MSCs is as strong as ESCs. Moreover, debate of the differentiation potential of MSCs continues, due to the heterogeneous nature of these cells.

A number of possible mechanisms could explain the plasticity of MSCs. One possibility is transdifferentiation, by which a cell directly differentiates into another cell type, under the influence of environmental cues. Another theory is de-differentiation, where a differentiated cell can revert back to a more primitive differentiation stage, and then can be induced to form another differentiated cell lineage (Song et al., 2006). For example, Song and Tuan (2004) have proved that cloned osteoblasts can differentiate into chondrocytes or adipocytes. Delorme et al. (2009) reported that cloned MSCs that were differentiated into vascular smooth muscle cells, can in turn form adipocytes, osteoblasts, or chondrocytes. However, no definitive evidence for either theory has been found, and the molecular basis for plasticity remains poorly understood. Plasticity may be related to lineage priming, as differentiation in the primed lineages would not entail resetting the entire molecular program, but rather the up-regulation of only a few of the differentiation program components (Delorme et al., 2009).

## 10.2.6 The MSC Niche

It is well known that MSCs can be released from their local resident and participate in the tissue repair or regeneration under the stimulation of specific signals. *In vivo*, BMSCs are widely dispersed and the adjacent extracellular matrix is populated by a few reticular fibrils but is devoid of the other types of collagen fibrils (Brighton and Hunt, 1997). However, the exact anatomical location of MSCs remains uncertain because there is no identified single marker for stem cells. Current evidences suggest that those MSCs are resident in a common stem cell microenvironment within different tissues, which is termed niche (Bianco and Robey, 2001, Gronthos et al., 2003, da Silva Meirelles et al., 2006). MSCs can maintain their stem cell properties in those niches. More and more evidences indicated that those stem cell niches are situated in close proximity within the vascular wall (Covas et al., 2008).

MSCs in the bone marrow form the niches which can support hematopoietic stem cell maintenance and differentiation in the bone marrow by producing matrix to provide physical support and secreting growth factors to offer signals.

The origin of the MSCs is under debate. One of the theories is all the MSCs from different tissue actually circulating cells derived from the bone marrow. Because tissue-specific MSCs display many common characteristics attributed to bone marrow-derived MSCs although they are vary in phenotype, proliferation rate and differentiation potentials, which suggest all those cells share a similar ontogeny.

Another argument is that the tissue-specific MSCs are actually pericytes (Crisan et al., 2008b). Pericytes is also referred as Rouget or mural cells, mesangial cells in the kidney, or Ito cells in the liver (Kuhn and Tuan, 2010). Pericytes reside in close proximity to endothelial cells in capillaries (Andreeva et al., 1998), and similar to MSCs, have the multilineage capacity to differentiate into adipogenic, osteogenic, and chondrogenic cell lineages (Doherty et al., 1998, Crisan et al., 2008a, Farrington-Rock et al., 2004).

Furthermore, both types of cells express similar markers, such as STRO-1, CD146, and α-smooth muscle actin (Shi and Gronthos, 2003).

# 10.3 Potential Therapeutic Applications

The major function of MSCs reside in the body is to migrate and repair the injured tissue in response of systemic signals. However, the efficiency is fairly low only with the natural stimulation. Increasing the local concentration of MSCs can help to achieve better outcome. It has been demonstrated that MSCs can help the new tissue formation when being injected peripherally or directly into the injured organ, especially in soft tissues (Dumont et al., 2002, Plotnikov et al., 2007). For hard tissue engineering, seeding MSCs onto scaffolds will help the cell maintenance and differentiation, and benefit the new tissue regeneration sequentially. MSCs have been widely tested for tissue engineering and other cell-based therapies. Some of them have reached the clinical trial level, including osteogenesis imperfect (Horwitz et al., 2002), heart stroke (Guhathakurta et al., 2009), graft-versus-host disease (Le Blanc et al., 2004), and severe inflammatory disease (Iyer et al., 2009). The endothelial (CD34[+]) fraction of BMSCs was able to benefit cardiac repair though improving the vascular growth and regeneration (Sekiguchi et al., 2009).

Other than the fact that MSCs have the potential to differentiate into specific cell types at the site with injury or inflammation, MSCs can also stimulate proliferation and differentiation of the local progenitor cells. Furthermore, MSCs can also secrete cytokines and growth factors to promote the recovery of injured cells (Uccelli et al., 2007).

Previous report suggested that MSCs are able to migrate specifically to tumors, under the continuous stimulation of the inflammatory mediators produce in those regions (Loebinger and Janes, 2010, Dvorak, 1986). Recent *in vitro* transwell migration assays and *in vivo* animal tumor models both supported this observation (Menon et al., 2007, Studeny et al., 2002, Komarova et al., 2006). This tumor-homing property advocates the possibility of tumor treatment by MSCs. Furthermore, MSCs express high levels of amphotropic receptors that makes MSCs can be easily transduced by integrating vectors (Marx et al., 1999). Other reports proved that MSCs are capable of long-term gene expression after gene transduction without affecting their basic phenotype (Chan et al., 2005, Van Damme et al., 2006). Genetic modification of MSCs can turn the cells into drug-delivery vehicle and enhance the anti-tumor effect (Ren et al., 2008, Kallifatidis et al., 2008). Furthermore, the secretory nature of MSCs suggests the possibility to treat the protein deficiency with gene-corrected MSCs from patient (Koc et al., 2002).

As result of their self-renewal capacity and multilineage differential ability to functional cell types, MSCs are considered as an essential cell source for tissue engineering and regenerative medicine. It is possible to achieve autologous MSCs and transplanted back to the individual themselves, eliminating the complications associated with immune rejection. Furthermore, MSCs do not target the foreign cytotoxic T cells or NK cells (Ramasamy et al., 2007, Spaggiari et al., 2006). Human MSCs are major histocompatibility class (MHC) I positive and MHC II negative, which obviates the need for HLA matching and allogeneic transplant not require immunosuppression (Le Blanc et al., 2005, Weiss et al., 2008). Therefore, allogenic MSCs can be obtained and used for different patients, without the need for severe immunosupression or causing immune-rejection.

Most of the publications of MSCs are focused on bone marrow-derived MSCs, and they are considered as the "gold standard." Adipose tissue-derived MSCs is another cell source which reaches clinical trial (Fang et al., 2007, Garcia-Olmo et al., 2005).

ESCs is another widely used cell source. ESCs can replicate indefinitely while the self-renewal capacity of MSCs is limited. It is also widely accepted that the differentiation potential of MSCs is incomparable with ESCs. ESCs are pluripotent, which means they are able to differentiation into all derivatives of the three primary germ layers (Ying et al., 2003). However, MSCs are still considered as a potential alternative cell source to ESCs. Unlike MSCs, it is impossible to perform autologous transplantation of ESCs. Allogenic ESCs may arouse immunologic incompatibility reaction. Furthermore, it is possible that ESCs develop malignant neoplasms or teratomas (Wakitani et al., 2003, Gerecht-Nir et al., 2004). The use of MSCs also arouses less ethical debate than that of ESCs.

Recently, another type of stem cells with great differentiation potency, induced pluripotent stem (iPS) cells, have been created (Takahashi et al., 2007, Yu et al., 2007, Takahashi and Yamanaka, 2006). The iPS cells were generated from somatic cells by overexpress key factors via viral modification. That method offered the possibility of producing autologous stem cell. Furthermore, the differentiation potential of iPS cells is comparable with ESC. Even though, most commonly used technique to generate iPS cells is through retroviruses transfection, which may increase the possibility of tumor formation (Okita et al., 2007). Also, the modified genetic information of iPS cells makes their fates more unpredictable.

## 10.4 Potential Concerns

Despite the increasing knowledge and characterizations of MSCs, and the mounting enthusiasm for the use of MSCs in regenerative therapies in humans, the mechanisms of MSCs proliferation and differentiation are still not fully understood. The current lack of reliable methods to control MSC cell fate, especially in the *in vivo* condition, is one of the main problems that needs to be addressed.

MSCs selection is another issue, due to the lack of a single definitive stem cell marker. Current isolation methods can only achieve heterogeneous cell populations, and the proportions of MSC progenitors in enriched MSC populations can vary even when the samples are obtained from the same donor at the same time (Digirolamo et al., 1999). Individual MSC clones derived from the same source showed completely differently cell characteristics, including size, morphology, proliferation, and differentiation potentials (Friedenstein et al., 1987, Owen and Friedenstein, 1988). Gronthos et al. (1994) revealed that only 48% of the CFU of fibroblasts clones derived from STRO-1$^+$ hBMSCs showed the capacity to differentiate into adipocytes *in vitro*. Previous research also indicated that only one-third of the initial adherent bone marrow-derived MSCs clones showed tri-lineage (osteo/adipo/chondro) differentiation potential (Pittenger et al., 1999). A later report demonstrated that only 30% of the BMSC clones had tri-lineage differentiation potential, while the rest exhibited a bi-linage (osteo/chondro) or a uni-lineage (osteo) potential (Muraglia et al., 2000). Even highly purified BMSC populations contained clones with differential capacity to form bone *in vivo* (Gronthos et al., 2003). Further confounding this issue is the fact that the cell properties of clones generated from a single clone are also variable. Kuznetsove et al. (1997) reported that bone formation was observed in only 58.8% of the single colony-derived clones transplanted with hydroxyapatite-tricalcium phosphate ceramic scaffolds *in vivo*. Even the results of current clinical trials proved that the purified cell population is unnecessary to get positive result (Prockop, 2007), obtain the more purified MSCs will help to achieve more reliable result.

Moreover, MSCs tend to spontaneously differentiate into osteoblastic cell, adipocytes, and stromal cells under the current culturing condition (Banfi et al., 2000, Izadpanah et al., 2008). Attempts to maintain the "stemness" of MSCs showed higher possible population doublings. One of the methods is to culture the cells in a condition similar to the *in vivo* circumstance of stem cell niche, such as culturing cells on fibronectin matrices under low oxygen tension (3%) (Chow et al., 2001a,b). Another method is to cultured the MSCs at low seeding density in low serum (Sekiya et al., 2002). However, no differentiation potential report was included in any of those publications.

Most of the published research of MSCs was performed on heterogeneous cell populations, making it difficult, if not impossible, to determine whether multilineage differentiation potential is a property of a single MSC, versus a variety of progenitor cells. To solve the inconsistencies of MSCs researches, it is necessary to develop standardized protocols for MSCs isolation and expansion. Identified the unique gene will benefit the purification and enrichment of homogenous MSC populations.

Although fetal bovine serum (FBS) is a common supplement for culture medium used to achieve high cell proliferation, the use of FBS and other animal products increases the potential risk of transmitting animal diseases. Currently, alternative media for human MSC culture has generated a great deal of enthusiasm, and a variety of serum-free media have been reported (Muller et al., 2006, Lindroos et al., 2009, Agata et al., 2009). Various substitutes for FBS, such as autologous serum, fresh frozen plasma, and human platelet lysates, have also been tested (Lange et al., 2007, Le Blanc et al., 2007).

The low frequency of MSCs in harvested tissue is another problem. *In vivo* cell therapy requires large numbers of cells, and insufficient cell numbers will not provide positive outcome (Habisch et al., 2007). For most of the cases, *in vitro* expansion is necessary to achieve adequate cells. Previous study proved that BMSCs express telomerase, which maintained telomere length many cell doublings but not thought to be immortal (Morrison et al., 1996). Moreover, some publications indicated that MSCs may lose their multipotentiality after six or seven passages *in vitro* culture (Colter et al., 2000, Sekiya et al., 2002). Increase the lifespan of MSCs by viral transduction of human telomerase reverse transcriptase may help to solve the problem.

Tumorigenesis potential of MSCs is much less than ESCs. However, MSCs still show the possibility of cancer initiation. Because those self-renewable stem cells can spontaneously transform *in vitro* (Rubio et al., 2005), which may cause the formation of malignant cells under the *in vivo* environment.

## 10.5 Conclusion

The mechanism behind the special cell properties of these multifunctional cells remains unclear. The therapeutic potential of MSCs is not fully predictable, especially under the *in vivo* environment. However, the self-renewal capacity, plasticity, and tumor-homing ability still make MSCs one of the most promising cell sources for tissue engineering and cell-based therapies. Further studies are necessary for better understanding and control of MSCs.

## References

Agata, H., Watanabe, N., Ishii, Y., Kubo, N., Ohshima, S., Yamazaki, M., Tojo, A., and Kagami, H. 2009. Feasibility and efficacy of bone tissue engineering using human bone marrow stromal cells cultivated in serum-free conditions. *Biochem Biophys Res Commun*, 382, 353–8.

Andreeva, E. R., Pugach, I. M., Gordon, D., and Orekhov, A. N. 1998. Continuous subendothelial network formed by pericyte-like cells in human vascular bed. *Tissue Cell*, 30, 127–35.

Anjos-Afonso, F. and Bonnet, D. 2007. Nonhematopoietic/endothelial SSEA-1+ cells define the most primitive progenitors in the adult murine bone marrow mesenchymal compartment. *Blood*, 109, 1298–306.

Banfi, A., Muraglia, A., Dozin, B., Mastrogiacomo, M., Cancedda, R., and Quarto, R. 2000. Proliferation kinetics and differentiation potential of ex vivo expanded human bone marrow stromal cells: Implications for their use in cell therapy. *Exp Hematol*, 28, 707–15.

Belema-Bedada, F., Uchida, S., Martire, A., Kostin, S., and Braun, T. 2008. Efficient homing of multipotent adult mesenchymal stem cells depends on FROUNT-mediated clustering of CCR2. *Cell Stem Cell*, 2, 566–75.

Bianco, P. and Robey, P. G. 2001. Stem cells in tissue engineering. *Nature*, 414, 118–21.

Brighton, C. T. and Hunt, R. M. 1997. Early histologic and ultrastructural changes in microvessels of periosteal callus. *J Orthop Trauma*, 11, 244–53.

Bruder, S. P., Jaiswal, N., and Haynesworth, S. E. 1997. Growth kinetics, self-renewal, and the osteogenic potential of purified human mesenchymal stem cells during extensive subcultivation and following cryopreservation. *J Cell Biochem*, 64, 278–94.

Caplan, A. I. 1991. Mesenchymal stem cells. *J Orthop Res*, 9, 641–50.

Castro-Malaspina, H., Gay, R. E., Resnick, G., Kapoor, N., Meyers, P., Chiarieri, D., Mckenzie, S., Broxmeyer, H. E., and Moore, M. A. 1980. Characterization of human bone marrow fibroblast colony-forming cells (CFU-F) and their progeny. *Blood*, 56, 289–301.

Chan, J., O'donoghue, K., De La Fuente, J., Roberts, I. A., Kumar, S., Morgan, J. E., and Fisk, N. M. 2005. Human fetal mesenchymal stem cells as vehicles for gene delivery. *Stem Cells*, 23, 93–102.

Cho, K. J., Trzaska, K. A., Greco, S. J., Mcardle, J., Wang, F. S., Ye, J. H., and Rameshwar, P. 2005. Neurons derived from human mesenchymal stem cells show synaptic transmission and can be induced to produce the neurotransmitter substance P by interleukin-1 alpha. *Stem Cells,* 23, 383–91.

Chow, D. C., Wenning, L. A., Miller, W. M., and Papoutsakis, E. T. 2001a. Modeling pO(2) distributions in the bone marrow hematopoietic compartment. I. Krogh's model. *Biophys J,* 81, 675–84.

Chow, D. C., Wenning, L. A., Miller, W. M., and Papoutsakis, E. T. 2001b. Modeling pO(2) distributions in the bone marrow hematopoietic compartment. II. Modified Kroghian models. *Biophys J,* 81, 685–96.

Clark, B. R. and Keating, A. 1995. Biology of bone marrow stroma. *Ann N Y Acad Sci,* 770, 70–8.

Cohnheim, J. 1867. Ueber entzündung und eiterung. *Path Anat Physiol Klin Med,* 40, 1.

Collins, C. A., Olsen, I., Zammit, P. S., Heslop, L., Petrie, A., Partridge, T. A., and Morgan, J. E. 2005. Stem cell function, self-renewal, and behavioral heterogeneity of cells from the adult muscle satellite cell niche. *Cell,* 122, 289–301.

Colter, D. C., Class, R., Digirolamo, C. M., and Prockop, D. J. 2000. Rapid expansion of recycling stem cells in cultures of plastic-adherent cells from human bone marrow. *Proc Natl Acad Sci USA,* 97, 3213–8.

Covas, D. T., Panepucci, R. A., Fontes, A. M., Silva, W. A., Jr., Orellana, M. D., Freitas, M. C., Neder, L., Santos, A. R., Peres, L. C., Jamur, M. C., and Zago, M. A. 2008. Multipotent mesenchymal stromal cells obtained from diverse human tissues share functional properties and gene-expression profile with CD146+ perivascular cells and fibroblasts. *Exp Hematol,* 36, 642–54.

Crisan, M., Deasy, B., Gavina, M., Zheng, B., Huard, J., Lazzari, L., and Peault, B. 2008a. Purification and long-term culture of multipotent progenitor cells affiliated with the walls of human blood vessels: Myoendothelial cells and pericytes. *Methods Cell Biol,* 86, 295–309.

Crisan, M. et al. 2008b. A perivascular origin for mesenchymal stem cells in multiple human organs. *Cell Stem Cell,* 3, 301–13.

D'ippolito, G., Diabira, S., Howard, G. A., Menei, P., Roos, B. A., and Schiller, P. C. 2004. Marrow-isolated adult multilineage inducible (MIAMI) cells, a unique population of postnatal young and old human cells with extensive expansion and differentiation potential. *J Cell Sci,* 117, 2971–81.

da Silva Meirelles, L., Chagastelles, P. C., and Nardi, N. B. 2006. Mesenchymal stem cells reside in virtually all post-natal organs and tissues. *J Cell Sci,* 119, 2204–13.

Dar, A., Kollet, O., and Lapidot, T. 2006. Mutual, reciprocal SDF-1/CXCR4 interactions between hematopoietic and bone marrow stromal cells regulate human stem cell migration and development in NOD/SCID chimeric mice. *Exp Hematol,* 34, 967–75.

De Bari, C., Dell'accio, F., Tylzanowski, P., and Luyten, F. P. 2001. Multipotent mesenchymal stem cells from adult human synovial membrane. *Arthritis Rheum,* 44, 1928–42.

Deans, R. J. and Moseley, A. B. 2000. Mesenchymal stem cells: Biology and potential clinical uses. *Exp Hematol,* 28, 875–84.

Delorme, B., Ringe, J., Pontikoglou, C., Gaillard, J., Langonne, A., Sensebe, L., Noel, D., Jorgensen, C., Haupl, T., and Charbord, P. 2009. Specific lineage-priming of bone marrow mesenchymal stem cells provides the molecular framework for their plasticity. *Stem Cells,* 27, 1142–51.

Devine, S. M., Cobbs, C., Jennings, M., Bartholomew, A., and Hoffman, R. 2003. Mesenchymal stem cells distribute to a wide range of tissues following systemic infusion into nonhuman primates. *Blood,* 101, 2999–3001.

Digirolamo, C. M., Stokes, D., Colter, D., Phinney, D. G., Class, R., and Prockop, D. J. 1999. Propagation and senescence of human marrow stromal cells in culture: A simple colony-forming assay identifies samples with the greatest potential to propagate and differentiate. *Br J Haematol,* 107, 275–81.

Doherty, M. J., Ashton, B. A., Walsh, S., Beresford, J. N., Grant, M. E., and Canfield, A. E. 1998. Vascular pericytes express osteogenic potential *in vitro* and in vivo. *J Bone Miner Res,* 13, 828–38.

Dominici, M., Le Blanc, K., Mueller, I., Slaper-Cortenbach, I., Marini, F., Krause, D., Deans, R., Keating, A., Prockop, D., and Horwitz, E. 2006. Minimal criteria for defining multipotent mesenchymal stromal cells. The International Society for Cellular Therapy position statement. *Cytotherapy,* 8, 315–7.

Dumont, R. J., Dayoub, H., Li, J. Z., Dumont, A. S., Kallmes, D. F., Hankins, G. R., and Helm, G. A. 2002. ex vivo bone morphogenetic protein-9 gene therapy using human mesenchymal stem cells induces spinal fusion in rodents. *Neurosurgery,* 51, 1239–44; discussion 1244–5.

Dvorak, H. F. 1986. Tumors: Wounds that do not heal. Similarities between tumor stroma generation and wound healing. *N Engl J Med,* 315, 1650–9.

Eberhardt, M., Salmon, P., Von Mach, M. A., Hengstler, J. G., Brulport, M., Linscheid, P., Seboek, D., Oberholzer, J., Barbero, A., Martin, I., Muller, B., Trono, D., and Zulewski, H. 2006. Multipotential nestin and Isl-1 positive mesenchymal stem cells isolated from human pancreatic islets. *Biochem Biophys Res Commun,* 345, 1167–76.

Fang, B., Song, Y., Zhao, R. C., Han, Q., and Lin, Q. 2007. Using human adipose tissue-derived mesenchymal stem cells as salvage therapy for hepatic graft-versus-host disease resembling acute hepatitis. *Transplant Proc,* 39, 1710–3.

Farrington-Rock, C., Crofts, N. J., Doherty, M. J., Ashton, B. A., Griffin-Jones, C., and Canfield, A. E. 2004. Chondrogenic and adipogenic potential of microvascular pericytes. *Circulation,* 110, 2226–32.

Friedenstein, A. J., Chailakhjan, R. K., and Lalykina, K. S. 1970. The development of fibroblast colonies in monolayer cultures of guinea-pig bone marrow and spleen cells. *Cell Tissue Kinet,* 3, 393–403.

Friedenstein, A. J., Chailakhyan, R. K., and Gerasimov, U. V. 1987. Bone marrow osteogenic stem cells: *In vitro* cultivation and transplantation in diffusion chambers. *Cell Tissue Kinet,* 20, 263–72.

Friedenstein, A. J., Gorskaja, J. F., and Kulagina, N. N. 1976. Fibroblast precursors in normal and irradiated mouse hematopoietic organs. *Exp Hematol,* 4, 267–74.

Garcia-Olmo, D., Garcia-Arranz, M., Herreros, D., Pascual, I., Peiro, C., and Rodriguez-Montes, J. A. 2005. A phase I clinical trial of the treatment of Crohn's fistula by adipose mesenchymal stem cell transplantation. *Dis Colon Rectum,* 48, 1416–23.

Gerecht-Nir, S., Osenberg, S., Nevo, O., Ziskind, A., Coleman, R., and Itskovitz-Eldor, J. 2004. Vascular development in early human embryos and in teratomas derived from human embryonic stem cells. *Biol Reprod,* 71, 2029–36.

Gronthos, S., Graves, S. E., Ohta, S., and Simmons, P. J. 1994. The STRO-1+ fraction of adult human bone marrow contains the osteogenic precursors. *Blood,* 84, 4164–73.

Gronthos, S., Mankani, M., Brahim, J., Robey, P. G., and Shi, S. 2000. Postnatal human dental pulp stem cells (DPSCs) *in vitro* and in vivo. *Proc Natl Acad Sci USA,* 97, 13625–30.

Gronthos, S., Zannettino, A. C., Hay, S. J., Shi, S., Graves, S. E., Kortesidis, A., and Simmons, P. J. 2003. Molecular and cellular characterisation of highly purified stromal stem cells derived from human bone marrow. *J Cell Sci,* 116, 1827–35.

Guhathakurta, S., Subramanyan, U. R., Balasundari, R., Das, C. K., Madhusankar, N., and Cherian, K. M. 2009. Stem cell experiments and initial clinical trial of cellular cardiomyoplasty. *Asian Cardiovasc Thorac Ann,* 17, 581–6.

Habisch, H. J. et al. 2007. Intrathecal application of neuroectodermally converted stem cells into a mouse model of ALS: Limited intraparenchymal migration and survival narrows therapeutic effects. *J Neural Transm,* 114, 1395–406.

Herzog, E. L., Chai, L., and Krause, D. S. 2003. Plasticity of marrow-derived stem cells. *Blood,* 102, 3483–93.

Horwitz, E. M., Gordon, P. L., Koo, W. K., Marx, J. C., Neel, M. D., Mcnall, R. Y., Muul, L., and Hofmann, T. 2002. Isolated allogeneic bone marrow-derived mesenchymal cells engraft and stimulate growth in children with osteogenesis imperfecta: Implications for cell therapy of bone. *Proc Natl Acad Sci USA,* 99, 8932–7.

Huang, T. F., Chen, Y. T., Yang, T. H., Chen, L. L., Chiou, S. H., Tsai, T. H., Tsai, C. C., Chen, M. H., MA, H. L., and Hung, S. C. 2008. Isolation and characterization of mesenchymal stromal cells from human anterior cruciate ligament. *Cytotherapy,* 10, 806–14.

Iyer, S. S., Co, C., and Rojas, M. 2009. Mesenchymal stem cells and inflammatory lung diseases. *Panminerva Med,* 51, 5–16.

Izadpanah, R., Kaushal, D., Kriedt, C., Tsien, F., Patel, B., Dufour, J., and Bunnell, B. A. 2008. Long-term *in vitro* expansion alters the biology of adult mesenchymal stem cells. *Cancer Res,* 68, 4229–38.

Javazon, E. H., Colter, D. C., Schwarz, E. J., and Prockop, D. J. 2001. Rat marrow stromal cells are more sensitive to plating density and expand more rapidly from single-cell-derived colonies than human marrow stromal cells. *Stem Cells,* 19, 219–25.

Jiang, Y. et al. 2002. Pluripotency of mesenchymal stem cells derived from adult marrow. *Nature,* 418, 41–9.

Kallifatidis, G. et al. 2008. Improved lentiviral transduction of human mesenchymal stem cells for therapeutic intervention in pancreatic cancer. *Cancer Gene Ther,* 15, 231–40.

Kang, X. Q., Zang, W. J., Song, T. S., Xu, X. L., Yu, X. J., Li, D. L., Meng, K. W., Wu, S. L., and Zhao, Z. Y. 2005. Rat bone marrow mesenchymal stem cells differentiate into hepatocytes in vitro. *World J Gastroenterol,* 11, 3479–84.

Katz, A. J., Tholpady, A., Tholpady, S. S., Shang, H., and Ogle, R. C. 2005. Cell surface and transcriptional characterization of human adipose-derived adherent stromal (hADAS) cells. *Stem Cells,* 23, 412–23.

Ke, Z., Zhou, F., Wang, L., Chen, S., Liu, F., Fan, X., Tang, F., Liu, D., and Zhao, G. 2008. Down-regulation of Wnt signaling could promote bone marrow-derived mesenchymal stem cells to differentiate into hepatocytes. *Biochem Biophys Res Commun,* 367, 342–8.

Kirschstein, R. and Skirboll, L. R. 2001. Stem Cells: Scientific Progress and Future Research Directions. National Institutes of Health, Department of Health and Human Services. Accessed May 17, 2005, http://stemcells.nih.gov/info/basics/.

Knoblich, J. A. 2008. Mechanisms of asymmetric stem cell division. *Cell,* 132, 583–97.

Koc, O. N., Day, J., Nieder, M., Gerson, S. L., Lazarus, H. M., and Krivit, W. 2002. Allogeneic mesenchymal stem cell infusion for treatment of metachromatic leukodystrophy (MLD) and Hurler syndrome (MPS-IH). *Bone Marrow Transplant,* 30, 215–22.

Komarova, S., Kawakami, Y., Stoff-Khalili, M. A., Curiel, D. T., and Pereboeva, L. 2006. Mesenchymal progenitor cells as cellular vehicles for delivery of oncolytic adenoviruses. *Mol Cancer Ther,* 5, 755–66.

Kucia, M., Reca, R., Campbell, F. R., Zuba-Surma, E., Majka, M., Ratajczak, J., and Ratajczak, M. Z. 2006. A population of very small embryonic-like (VSEL) CXCR4(+)SSEA-1(+)Oct-4+ stem cells identified in adult bone marrow. *Leukemia,* 20, 857–69.

Kuhn, N. Z. and Tuan, R. S. 2010. Regulation of stemness and stem cell niche of mesenchymal stem cells: Implications in tumorigenesis and metastasis. *J Cell Physiol,* 222, 268–77.

Kuznetsov, S. A., Krebsbach, P. H., Satomura, K., Kerr, J., Riminucci, M., Benayahu, D., and Robey, P. G. 1997. Single-colony derived strains of human marrow stromal fibroblasts form bone after transplantation in vivo. *J Bone Miner Res,* 12, 1335–47.

Lange, C., Cakiroglu, F., Spiess, A. N., Cappallo-Obermann, H., Dierlamm, J., and Zander, A. R. 2007. Accelerated and safe expansion of human mesenchymal stromal cells in animal serum-free medium for transplantation and regenerative medicine. *J Cell Physiol,* 213, 18–26.

Le Blanc, K. et al. 2005. Fetal mesenchymal stem-cell engraftment in bone after in utero transplantation in a patient with severe osteogenesis imperfecta. *Transplantation,* 79, 1607–14.

Le Blanc, K., Rasmusson, I., Sundberg, B., Gotherstrom, C., Hassan, M., Uzunel, M., and Ringden, O. 2004. Treatment of severe acute graft-versus-host disease with third party haploidentical mesenchymal stem cells. *Lancet,* 363, 1439–41.

Le Blanc, K., Samuelsson, H., Lonnies, L., Sundin, M., and Ringden, O. 2007. Generation of immunosuppressive mesenchymal stem cells in allogeneic human serum. *Transplantation,* 84, 1055–9.

Liechty, K. W., Mackenzie, T. C., Shaaban, A. F., Radu, A., Moseley, A. M., Deans, R., Marshak, D. R., and Flake, A. W. 2000. Human mesenchymal stem cells engraft and demonstrate site-specific differentiation after in utero transplantation in sheep. *Nat Med,* 6, 1282–6.

Lindroos, B., Boucher, S., Chase, L., Kuokkanen, H., Huhtala, H., Haataja, R., Vemuri, M., Suuronen, R., and Miettinen, S. 2009. Serum-free, xeno-free culture media maintain the proliferation rate and multipotentiality of adipose stem cells in vitro. *Cytotherapy,* 11, 958–72.

Loebinger, M. R. and Janes, S. M. 2010. Stem cells as vectors for antitumour therapy. *Thorax,* 65, 362–9.

Makino, S., Fukuda, K., Miyoshi, S., Konishi, F., Kodama, H., Pan, J., Sano, M., Takahashi, T., Hori, S., Abe, H., Hata, J., Umezawa, A., and Ogawa, S. 1999. Cardiomyocytes can be generated from marrow stromal cells in vitro. *J Clin Invest,* 103, 697–705.

Mareschi, K., Biasin, E., Piacibello, W., Aglietta, M., Madon, E., and Fagioli, F. 2001. Isolation of human mesenchymal stem cells: Bone marrow versus umbilical cord blood. *Haematologica,* 86, 1099–100.

Marx, J. C., Allay, J. A., Persons, D. A., Nooner, S. A., Hargrove, P. W., Kelly, P. F., Vanin, E. F., and Horwitz, E. M. 1999. High-efficiency transduction and long-term gene expression with a murine stem cell retroviral vector encoding the green fluorescent protein in human marrow stromal cells. *Hum Gene Ther,* 10, 1163–73.

Menon, L. G., Picinich, S., Koneru, R., Gao, H., Lin, S. Y., Koneru, M., Mayer-Kuckuk, P., Glod, J., and Banerjee, D. 2007. Differential gene expression associated with migration of mesenchymal stem cells to conditioned medium from tumor cells or bone marrow cells. *Stem Cells,* 25, 520–8.

Miura, M., Gronthos, S., Zhao, M., Lu, B., Fisher, L. W., Robey, P. G., and Shi, S. 2003. Shed: Stem cells from human exfoliated deciduous teeth. *Proc Natl Acad Sci USA,* 100, 5807–12.

Morrison, S. J. and Kimble, J. 2006. Asymmetric and symmetric stem-cell divisions in development and cancer. *Nature,* 441, 1068–74.

Morrison, S. J., Prowse, K. R., Ho, P., and Weissman, I. L. 1996. Telomerase activity in hematopoietic cells is associated with self-renewal potential. *Immunity,* 5, 207–16.

Mouiseddine, M., Francois, S., Semont, A., Sache, A., Allenet, B., Mathieu, N., Frick, J., Thierry, D., and Chapel, A. 2007. Human mesenchymal stem cells home specifically to radiation-injured tissues in a non-obese diabetes/severe combined immunodeficiency mouse model. *Br J Radiol,* 80 Spec No 1, S49–55.

Muller, I., Kordowich, S., Holzwarth, C., Spano, C., Isensee, G., Staiber, A., Viebahn, S., Gieseke, F., Langer, H., Gawaz, M. P., Horwitz, E. M., Conte, P., Handgretinger, R., and Dominici, M. 2006. Animal serum-free culture conditions for isolation and expansion of multipotent mesenchymal stromal cells from human BM. *Cytotherapy,* 8, 437–44.

Muraglia, A., Cancedda, R., and Quarto, R. 2000. Clonal mesenchymal progenitors from human bone marrow differentiate *in vitro* according to a hierarchical model. *J Cell Sci,* 113(Pt 7), 1161–6.

Nomura, T., Ashihara, E., Tateishi, K., Ueyama, T., Takahas-Hi, T., Yamagishi, M., Kubo, T., Yaku, H., Matsubara, H., and Oh, H. 2007. Therapeutic potential of stem/progenitor cells in human skeletal muscle for cardiovascular regeneration. *Curr Stem Cell Res Ther,* 2, 293–300.

Okita, K., Ichisaka, T., and Yamanaka, S. 2007. Generation of germline-competent induced pluripotent stem cells. *Nature,* 448, 313–7.

Oswald, J., Boxberger, S., Jorgensen, B., Feldmann, S., Ehninger, G., Bornhauser, M., and Werner, C. 2004. Mesenchymal stem cells can be differentiated into endothelial cells in vitro. *Stem Cells,* 22, 377–84.

Owen, M. and Friedenstein, A. J. 1988. Stromal stem cells: Marrow-derived osteogenic precursors. *Ciba Found Symp,* 136, 42–60.

Peister, A., Mellad, J. A., Larson, B. L., Hall, B. M., Gibson, L. F., and Prockop, D. J. 2004. Adult stem cells from bone marrow (MSCs) isolated from different strains of inbred mice vary in surface epitopes, rates of proliferation, and differentiation potential. *Blood,* 103, 1662–8.

Perkins, S. and Fleischman, R. A. 1990. Stromal cell progeny of murine bone marrow fibroblast colony-forming units are clonal endothelial-like cells that express collagen IV and laminin. *Blood,* 75, 620–5.

Pittenger, M. F., Mackay, A. M., Beck, S. C., Jaiswal, R. K., Douglas, R., Mosca, J. D., Moorman, M. A., Simonetti, D. W., Craig, S., and Marshak, D. R. 1999. Multilineage potential of adult human mesenchymal stem cells. *Science,* 284, 143–7.

Plotnikov, A. N. et al. 2007. Xenografted adult human mesenchymal stem cells provide a platform for sustained biological pacemaker function in canine heart. *Circulation,* 116, 706–13.

Pochampally, R. 2008. Colony forming unit assays for MSCs. *Methods Mol Biol,* 449, 83–91.

Popov, B. V., Serikov, V. B., Petrov, N. S., Izusova, T. V., Gupta, N., and Matthay, M. A. 2007. Lung epithelial cells induce endodermal differentiation in mouse mesenchymal bone marrow stem cells by paracrine mechanism. *Tissue Eng,* 13, 2441–50.

Prockop, D. J. 1997. Marrow stromal cells as stem cells for nonhematopoietic tissues. *Science,* 276, 71–4.

Prockop, D. J. 2007. "Stemness" does not explain the repair of many tissues by mesenchymal stem/multi-potent stromal cells (MSCs). *Clin Pharmacol Ther,* Sep; 82(3), 241–3.

Psaltis, P. J., Zannettino, A. C., Worthley, S. G., and Gronthos, S. 2008. Concise review: Mesenchymal stromal cells: Potential for cardiovascular repair. *Stem Cells,* 26, 2201–10.

Rafii, S. and Lyden, D. 2003. Therapeutic stem and progenitor cell transplantation for organ vascularization and regeneration. *Nat Med,* 9, 702–12.

Ramasamy, R., Fazekasova, H., Lam, E. W., Soeiro, I., Lombardi, G., and Dazzi, F. 2007. Mesenchymal stem cells inhibit dendritic cell differentiation and function by preventing entry into the cell cycle. *Transplantation,* 83, 71–6.

Ren, C., Kumar, S., Chanda, D., Kallman, L., Chen, J., Mountz, J. D., and Ponnazhagan, S. 2008. Cancer gene therapy using mesenchymal stem cells expressing interferon-beta in a mouse prostate cancer lung metastasis model. *Gene Ther,* 15, 1446–53.

Rubio, D., Garcia-Castro, J., Martin, M. C., De La Fuente, R., Cigudosa, J. C., Lloyd, A. C., and Bernad, A. 2005. Spontaneous human adult stem cell transformation. *Cancer Res,* 65, 3035–9.

Sekiguchi, H., Li, M., and Losordo, D. W. 2009. The relative potency and safety of endothelial progenitor cells and unselected mononuclear cells for recovery from myocardial infarction and ischemia. *J Cell Physiol,* 219, 235–42.

Sekiya, I., Larson, B. L., Smith, J. R., Pochampally, R., Cui, J. G., and Prockop, D. J. 2002. Expansion of human adult stem cells from bone marrow stroma: Conditions that maximize the yields of early progenitors and evaluate their quality. *Stem Cells,* 20, 530–41.

Shi, M., Li, J., Liao, L., Chen, B., Li, B., Chen, L., Jia, H., and Zhao, R. C. 2007. Regulation of CXCR4 expression in human mesenchymal stem cells by cytokine treatment: Role in homing efficiency in NOD/SCID mice. *Haematologica,* 92, 897–904.

Shi, S. and Gronthos, S. 2003. Perivascular niche of postnatal mesenchymal stem cells in human bone marrow and dental pulp. *J Bone Miner Res,* 18, 696–704.

Smith, J. R., Pochampally, R., Perry, A., Hsu, S. C., and Prockop, D. J. 2004. Isolation of a highly clonogenic and multipotential subfraction of adult stem cells from bone marrow stroma. *Stem Cells,* 22, 823–31.

Song, L. and Tuan, R. S. 2004. Transdifferentiation potential of human mesenchymal stem cells derived from bone marrow. *FASEB J,* 18, 980–2.

Song, L., Webb, N. E., Song, Y., and Tuan, R. S. 2006. Identification and functional analysis of candidate genes regulating mesenchymal stem cell self-renewal and multipotency. *Stem Cells,* 24, 1707–18.

Spaggiari, G. M., Capobianco, A., Becchetti, S., Mingari, M. C., and Moretta, L. 2006. Mesenchymal stem cell-natural killer cell interactions: Evidence that activated NK cells are capable of killing MSCs, whereas MSCs can inhibit IL-2-induced NK-cell proliferation. *Blood,* 107, 1484–90.

Studeny, M., Marini, F. C., Champlin, R. E., Zompetta, C., Fidler, I. J., and Andreeff, M. 2002. Bone marrow-derived mesenchymal stem cells as vehicles for interferon-beta delivery into tumors. *Cancer Res,* 62, 3603–8.

Takahashi, K., Okita, K., Nakagawa, M., and Yamanaka, S. 2007. Induction of pluripotent stem cells from fibroblast cultures. *Nat Protoc,* 2, 3081–9.

Takahashi, K. and Yamanaka, S. 2006. Induction of pluripotent stem cells from mouse embryonic and adult fibroblast cultures by defined factors. *Cell,* 126, 663–76.

Thomson, J. A., Itskovitz-Eldor, J., Shapiro, S. S., Waknitz, M. A., Swiergiel, J. J., Marshall, V. S., and Jones, J. M. 1998. Embryonic stem cell lines derived from human blastocysts. *Science,* 282, 1145–7.

Tian, H., Bharadwaj, S., Liu, Y., Ma, P. X., Atala, A., and Zhang, Y. 2010. Differentiation of human bone marrow mesenchymal stem cells into bladder cells: Potential for urological tissue engineering. *Tissue Eng Part A,* 16, 1769–79.

Uccelli, A., Pistoia, V., and Moretta, L. 2007. Mesenchymal stem cells: A new strategy for immunosuppression? *Trends Immunol,* 28, 219–26.

Valarmathi, M. T., Goodwin, R. L., Fuseler, J. W., Davis, J. M., Yost, M. J., and Potts, J. D. 2010. A 3-D cardiac muscle construct for exploring adult marrow stem cell based myocardial regeneration. *Biomaterials,* 31, 3185–200.

Van Damme, A. et al. 2006. Efficient lentiviral transduction and improved engraftment of human bone marrow mesenchymal cells. *Stem Cells,* 24, 896–907.

Wakitani, S., Saito, T., and Caplan, A. I. 1995. Myogenic cells derived from rat bone marrow mesenchymal stem cells exposed to 5-azacytidine. *Muscle Nerve,* 18, 1417–26.

Wakitani, S., Takaoka, K., Hattori, T., Miyazawa, N., Iwanaga, T., Takeda, S., Watanabe, T. K., and Tanigami, A. 2003. Embryonic stem cells injected into the mouse knee joint form teratomas and subsequently destroy the joint. *Rheumatology (Oxford),* 42, 162–5.

Weiss, D. J., Kolls, J. K., Ortiz, L. A., Panoskaltsis-Mortari, A., and Prockop, D. J. 2008. Stem cells and cell therapies in lung biology and lung diseases. *Proc Am Thorac Soc,* 5, 637–67.

Ying, Q. L., Nichols, J., Chambers, I., and Smith, A. 2003. BMP induction of Id proteins suppresses differentiation and sustains embryonic stem cell self-renewal in collaboration with STAT3. *Cell,* 115, 281–92.

Yu, J. et al. 2007. Induced pluripotent stem cell lines derived from human somatic cells. *Science,* 318, 1917–20.

Zhao, Z. G., Li, W. M., Chen, Z. C., You, Y., and Zou, P. 2008. Hematopoiesis capacity, immunomodulatory effect and ex vivo expansion potential of mesenchymal stem cells are not impaired by cryopreservation. *Cancer Invest,* 26, 391–400.

Zipori, D. 2005. The stem state: Plasticity is essential, whereas self-renewal and hierarchy are optional. *Stem Cells,* 23, 719–26.

Zuk, P. A., Zhu, M., Mizuno, H., Huang, J., Futrell, J. W., Katz, A. J., Benhaim, P., Lorenz, H. P., and Hedrick, M. H. 2001. Multilineage cells from human adipose tissue: Implications for cell-based therapies. *Tissue Eng,* 7, 211–28.

# II

# Enabling Technologies

**11 Nanobiomaterials for Tissue Engineering** *Pramod K. Avti, Sunny C. Patel, Pushpinder Uppal, Grace O'Malley, Joseph Garlow, and Balaji Sitharaman* ................... 11-1
Introduction • Nanobiomaterials to Improve Bulk and Surface Properties of Tissue Engineering Scaffolds • Nanobiomaterials for Therapeutic Delivery • Nanobiomaterials to Image the Process of Tissue Formation • Continuing and Future Developments • Abbreviations • References

**12 Biomimetic Approaches in Tissue Engineering** *Indong Jun, Min Sup Kim, Ji-Hye Lee, Young Min Shin, and Heungsoo Shin* .............................................. 12-1
Introduction • Biomimetic Surface Modifications • Growth Factor-Presenting Materials • Biomimetic Hydrogels and Controlled Cell Interactions • Composite Scaffolds Used to Mimic Specific Cellular Environments • Scaffolds Mimicking the Structure of ECM • Conclusions • References

**13 Molecular Biology Techniques** *X.G. Chen, Y.L. Fang, and W.T. Godbey* ..................... 13-1
Histochemistry • Gel Electrophoresis • Restriction Enzymes • Other DNA Modification Enzymes • The Polymerase Chain Reaction • Blotting • References

**14 Biomaterial Mechanics** *Kimberly M. Stroka, Leann L. Norman, and Helim Aranda-Espinoza* ......................................................................... 14-1
Introduction • Cellular Mechanotransduction • Mechanics of Biomaterials • Potential Target and Applications • Summary • References

**15 Mechanical Conditioning** *Elaine L. Lee and Horst A. von Recum* .............................. 15-1
Why Do We Need Mechanical Conditioning? • Cellular Response to Mechanical Stimuli versus the Living Cell as a Mechanical Structure • Mechanotransduction and Mechanical Conditioning Terminology • Current Technologies—Advantages and Disadvantages • Upcoming Technologies • Conclusion • References

**16 Micropatterned Biomaterials for Cell and Tissue Engineering** *Murugan Ramalingam and Ali Khademhosseini* ............................................................. 16-1
Introduction • Surface Modification and Patterning Approaches • Techniques for Chemical Patterning and Applications to Cell Studies • Techniques for Topographical Patterning and Applications to Cell Studies • Techniques for Three-Dimensional Patterning and Applications to Tissue Engineering • Concluding Remarks • References

**17 Drug Delivery** *Prinda Wanakule and Krishnendu Roy* .................................... 17-1
Introduction • Mechanisms of Drug Delivery • Drugs of Interest in Tissue Engineering • Drug Delivery in Tissue Engineering • Outlook • References

**18 Gene Therapy** *C. Holladay, M. Kulkarni, W. Minor, and Abhay Pandit*...................... **18**-1
Introduction • Delivery Technique (Vector) • Systemic and Local Gene Delivery •
Therapeutic Preclinical or Clinical Trials • Summary • Acknowledgments • References

**19 Nanotechnology-Based Cell Engineering Strategies for Tissue Engineering and
Regenerative Medicine Applications** *Joaquim Miguel Oliveira, João Filipe Mano,
and Rui Luís Reis*..................................................................................................... **19**-1
Introduction • Cell Engineering Strategies • Concluding Remarks • References

**20 Cell Encapsulation** *Stephanie J. Bryant*.......................................................... **20**-1
Introduction • Gelation Mechanisms Employed in Cell Encapsulation • Hydrogel
Structure and Degradation • Concluding Remarks • References

**21 Coculture Systems for Mesenchymal Stem Cells** *Song P. Seto and Johnna S. Temenoff* .. **21**-1
Introduction • Cells of Interest • Overview of Coculture Methods • Cocultures
with Chondrocytes • Osteoblast Coculture with MSCs • Myoblast Coculture with
MSCs • Communication between Mesenchymal and Endothelial Lineages • Future
Outlook • Acknowledgments • References

**22 Tissue Engineering Bioreactors** *Sarindr Bhumiratana, Elisa Cimetta,
Nina Tandon, Warren Grayson, Milica Radisic, and Gordana Vunjak-Novakovic* ....... **22**-1
Introduction • Overview of the Field • Principles of Bioreactor Design • Microscale
Technologies • Cardiac Tissue Engineering Bioreactors • Vascular
Bioreactors • Bone Tissue Engineering Bioreactor • Cartilage Tissue Engineering
Bioreactors • Tendon/Ligament Tissue Engineering Bioreactors • Summary and
Challenges • Acknowledgment • References

**23 Shear Forces** *Jose F. Alvarez-Barreto, Samuel B. VanGordon,
Brandon W. Engebretson, and Vasillios I. Sikavitsas*........................................... **23**-1
Introduction: Cells and Shear Forces • Effect of Shear Forces on Tissue-Specific
Cells • References

**24 Vascularization of Engineered Tissues** *Monica L. Moya and Eric M. Brey*............... **24**-1
Introduction • Neovascularization • Strategies for Vascularizing Engineered
Tissues • Conclusions • References

**25 Biomedical Imaging of Engineered Tissue** *Nicholas E. Simpson and
Athanassios Sambanis*.............................................................................................. **25**-1
Introduction • Optical Imaging • Radiation-Based Imaging • Ultrasound • Infrared
Imaging • Nuclear Magnetic Resonance • Conclusion • Acknowledgments • References

**26 Multiscale Modeling of *In Vitro* Tissue Cultivation** *Kyriacos Zygourakis*................. **26**-1
Introduction • Model Detail and Abstraction • Cell Proliferation and
Migration • Cell Population Dynamics and Mass Transport • Continuous, Discrete,
and Hybrid Models for Tissue Growth • A Modeling Framework for *In Vitro*
Tissue Cultivation • Components of the Hybrid Multiscale Model • Results and
Discussion • References

# 11

# Nanobiomaterials for Tissue Engineering

Pramod K. Avti
*Stony Brook University*

Sunny C. Patel
*Stony Brook University*

Pushpinder Uppal
*Stony Brook University*

Grace O'Malley
*Stony Brook University*

Joseph Garlow
*Stony Brook University*

Balaji Sitharaman
*Stony Brook University*

11.1 Introduction ........................................................................... 11-1
11.2 Nanobiomaterials to Improve Bulk and Surface Properties of Tissue Engineering Scaffolds...................................................... 11-2
  Nanofibrous Scaffolds • Nanobiomaterial-Incorporated Polymer Scaffolds
11.3 Nanobiomaterials for Therapeutic Delivery ............................. 11-5
11.4 Nanobiomaterials to Image the Process of Tissue Formation .... 11-9
11.5 Continuing and Future Developments....................................... 11-13
Abbreviations ...................................................................................... 11-13
References............................................................................................ 11-15

## 11.1 Introduction

Tissue engineering (TE) is an emerging interdisciplinary field that seeks to restore, improve and maintain normal tissue or organ functions. To these ends, one or more of the following three components: progenitor cells, signaling molecules, and engineered biomaterials or scaffolds are applied (Langer and Vacanti, 1993). The advancement of TE requires new biomaterials to deliver important biochemical moieties (e.g., growth factors) to the engineered tissues, to direct tissue growth, and to improve monitoring and evaluating of the regenerating tissue.

Nanotechnology-based approaches are currently being pursued for a variety of biomedical applications. Nanotechnology is a relatively new field of science broadly defined as research and technology development at length scales between 1 and 100 nm to create materials, gain fundamental insights into their properties, and to use the nanoscale materials as components or building blocks to create novel structures, or devices (Rodgers et al., 2006). At these length scales, materials show unique properties and functions. However, in certain cases, the length scales for these novel properties maybe under 1 nm (down to 0.1 nm for atomic and molecular manipulation) or over 100 nm (up to 300 nm in case of nanopolymers and nanocomposites). Nanotechnology is a convergent technology in which, the boundaries separating discrete disciplines become blurred. Biochemists, materials scientists, electrical engineers, and molecular biologists may all be considered experts in the field if they are involved in the development of nanosized structures.

Specifically for TE, nanotechnology-based approaches allow the synthesis of unique nanobiomaterials having nanoscale features that can mimic the natural extracellular matrix to affect the cellular functions (e.g., adhesion, mobility, and differentiation) (Harrison and Atala, 2007; Kim and Fisher, 2007). Further, these nanobiomaterials could be developed with multifunctional capabilities as delivery agents of signaling molecules and genes as well as efficient imaging probes to noninvasively monitor implanted cells, and the process of tissue regeneration in tissue-engineered constructs. This chapter provides the reader a perspective of nanobiomaterials for TE. It discusses the various nanobiomaterials been developed to (a) improve bulk and surface properties of TE scaffolds; (b) deliver biochemical moieties (e.g., genes, growth factors); and (c) image the process of tissue formation.

## 11.2 Nanobiomaterials to Improve Bulk and Surface Properties of Tissue Engineering Scaffolds

Nanobiomaterial-based approaches have been used in the developments of two types of TE structures: (1) Nanofibrous scaffolds and (2) Nanobiomaterial-incorporated polymer composite scaffolds.

### 11.2.1 Nanofibrous Scaffolds

Scaffolds are porous biomaterials and play a pivotal role in the TE paradigm by providing temporary structural support, guiding cells to grow, assisting the transport of essential nutrients and waste products, and facilitating the formation of functional tissues and organs. Nanofiber scaffolds are TE scaffolds with nanoscopic structure and morphologies fabricated using natural and synthetic materials. These materials are biodegradable or nonbiodegradable polymers and generally biocompatible. Some examples of the natural materials used as starting materials for the development of nanofiber scaffolds are self-assembling polypeptides, DNA, RNA, carbohydrates, peptides, collagen, fibrin, glycosaminoglycans, fibrinogen, gelatin, elastin, silk, hyaluronan, and chitosan (Matthews et al., 2002; Min et al., 2004; Silva et al., 2004; Bhattarai et al., 2005; Li et al., 2005; Hamdi et al., 2009; Carneiro et al., 2010). Examples of synthetic materials include poly(ethylene glycol) (PEG), poly(vinyl alcohol) (PVA), poly(hydroxyethyl methacrylate), poly(lactic acid) (PLA), poly(glycolic acid), poly(lactic-*co*-glycolic acid) (PLGA), poly(ε-caprolactone) (PCL), poly(methyl methacrylate) (PMMA), poly(propylene fumarate) (PPF) (Ding et al., 2002; Kenawy et al., 2003; Gupta et al., 2005; Kim et al., 2005; Chen et al., 2008; Choi et al., 2008; Corey et al., 2008; Powell and Boyce, 2008). Nanofiber scaffolds have special characteristics such as high surface area to volume ratio, functional groups for high density functionalization, and high porosities. The nanofibers can also mimic natural extracellular matrix (ECM). The fabrication techniques used in synthesizing these scaffolds are phase separation (Smith and Ma, 2004), melt-blowing, template synthesis, electrospinning (Li et al., 2002), and self-assembly (Whitesides and Boncheva, 2002). Among these methods, nanofibers obtained from electrospinning and self-assembly have widespread applications in bone, skin, neural, cartilage, vascular heart, and lung TE (Pham et al., 2006; Rubenstein et al., 2007; Chew et al., 2008; Venugopal et al., 2008).

The electrospinning method allows the fabrication of solid, hollow, or core–shell nanofiber scaffolds, where the nanofibers can be randomly arranged or aligned along a particular direction (Bini et al., 2004; Corey et al., 2007). The hollow fiber scaffolds (Figure 11.1) are suitable for loading drugs, and enzymes to improve tissue regeneration (Bini et al., 2004).

The core–shell fibers are also well suited for drug-delivery applications as the core helps in loading the drug and the shell controls release kinetics. Synthetic and overexpressed peptide and protein precursors have been widely used as starting materials for the development of self-assembled nanofiber scaffolds (Koide et al., 2005; Kotch and Raines, 2006; Paramonov et al., 2006; Woolfson and Ryadnov, 2006; Gauba and Hartgerink, 2007). For instance, elastin is a self-assembling polymeric protein with good mechanical strength properties with potential applications for vascular TE (Bellingham et al., 2003; Miao et al., 2005; Daamen et al., 2007). Recently, recombinant (synthetic) polypeptides of elastin were self-assembled to form novel macromolecular nanostructures (Bellingham et al., 2003; Vieth et al., 2007). Self-assembled nanofiber scaffolds are well-suited to incorporate cell signaling molecules that can affect progenitor cell behavior such as their attachment, differentiation, and proliferation (Hofmann et al., 2006; Meinel et al., 2006, 2009). The complexity of the self-assembly techniques leads to low yields and relatively high cost; its main limitations compared to the electrospinning method. Table 11.1 lists some of the recent advances in the development of nanofibrous scaffolds for TE.

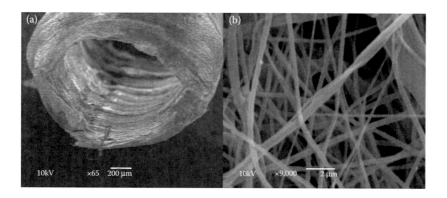

**FIGURE 11.1** SEM imaging of micro- and nanofiber electrospun poly(1-caprolactone)/poly(D,L-lactic-*co*-glycolic acid) tubular scaffolds designed for regenerating sciatic nerve transections. (a) Tube lumen and (b) zoomed details of the tube wall. Both nano- and microfibers are visible. Fiber links are obtained via partial solvent evaporation and polymer annealing subsequent to electrospinning in order to increase the overall prosthesis mechanical properties. (Reprinted from *Biomaterials* 26(31), Bhattarai N. et al. Electrospun chitosan based nanofibers and their cellular compatibility, 6176–84. Copyright 2005, with permission from Elsevier.)

**TABLE 11.1** Nanofibrous Scaffolds

| Nanofiber Material | Intended Application | Functions and Biological Response/Improvements | Reference |
|---|---|---|---|
| PLGA | Neural TE | Neurite formation and elongation | Lee et al. (2009) |
| | Bladder tissue engineering | Increased bladder cell adhesion and growth, increased production of elastin, and collagen proteins enhance in urinary bladder wall replacement | Pattison et al. (2005) |
| PGS | Retinal transplantation | Improved the growth of graft-host cells without signs of inflammation | Pritchard et al. (2010) |
| | Vascular regeneration | Decreased thrombogenecity (platelet adhesion and aggregation) and inflammatory response when used as blood contacting surface | Motlagh et al. (2006) |
| | Cardiac tissue engineering | Bioinert, biocompatible, wide degradation properties, good mechanical properties matching the physical characteristics of heart tissue | Chen et al. (2008) |
| PEG | Cartilage regeneration | Improved cellularity, collagen and glycosaminoglycan content | Mahmood et al. (2006) |
| | Wound healing | Fibronectin-coupled PEG are cytocompatible, improves proliferation and migration of fibroblasts both *in vitro* and *in vivo* | Ghosh et al. (2006) |
| PLLA | Neural tissue engineering | Improves neurite growth, elongation, and differentiation | Corey et al. (2007); Yang et al. (2004, 2005) |
| | Cardiac tissue engineering | Increased contractile machinery (sarcomeres) in cardiomyocytes | Zong et al. (2005) |
| | Bone tissue engineering | Increased osteoblast adhesion, proliferation, mineralization, and protein marker expression | Woo et al. (2003, 2006) |
| CNFs | Neural tissue engineering | Increased elastic modulus, neuronal cell adhesion, neurite extension, and decreased astrocyte adhesion | McKenzie et al. (2004) |
| | Vascular tissue engineering | Supports the aggregation and enhances the migration ability of endothelial cells | Han et al. (2009) |

*continued*

**TABLE 11.1**    (continued) Nanofibrous Scaffold

| Nanofiber Material | Intended Application | Functions and Biological Response/Improvements | Reference |
|---|---|---|---|
| Peptide nanofibers | Bone tissue engineering | Increased osteoblast adhesion, enhanced mineral deposition, decreased fibroblast adhesion | Khang et al. (2006); Price et al. (2003) |
| | Bladder tissue regeneration | Promotes bladder smooth muscle cells attachment, matrix production and spindled morphology | Harrington et al. (2006) |
| | Neural regeneration | IKVAV-Peptide nanofibers increased the neural progenitor cells attachment, migration, neurite outgrowth and undergo selective and rapid differentiation. | Silva et al. (2004) |
| | Vascular tissue regeneration | Heparin binding-peptide nanofibers influenced the tube formation in endothelial cells | Rajangam et al. (2006, 2008) |
| | Cardiac tissue engineering | Heparin binding-peptide nanofibers restored the hemodynamic functions in acute myocardial infarction | Rajangam et al. (2006, 2008) |
| PCL | Skin grafting | Improved growth, longevity of keratinocytes and fibroblasts during wound healing | Reed et al. (2009) |
| | Vascular tissue engineering | Modulated smooth muscle cells behavior to express contractile phenotype, attained spindle shape, oriented and directional migration | Xu et al. (2004) |
| | Cardiac tissue engineering | Enhanced cardiomyocytes attachment, growth and proliferation. Increased synchronized contraction and contractile machinery (actin, tropomyosin, cardiac troponin) | Ishii et al. (2005); Shin et al. (2004) |
| | Bone tissue engineering | Improved cellular adhesion, penetration into the scaffold thereby releasing ECM and helps in differentiation | Yoshimoto et al. (2003); Shin et al. (2004); Li et al. (2005a,b) |
| Polyurethane | Skin grafting | Increased rate of epithelialization, well organized dermis formation | Khil et al. (2003) |
| Chitin nanofiber | Skin tissue engineering | Promoted keratinocyte and fibroblast cellular attachment and proliferation | Noh et al. (2006) |
| SF | Skin tissue engineering | Highly porous, high surface area and improved mechanical properties of SFs responsible for use in wound dressing material and skin regeneration application | Kim et al. (2003) |
| PET | Vascular tissue engineering | Increased hydrophobicity of scaffold enables endothelial cells to attain polygonal morphology and express cell adhesion markers PECAM, ICAM, VCAM responsible for vascularization | Ma et al. (2005) |

## 11.2.2 Nanobiomaterial-Incorporated Polymer Scaffolds

Nanoparticles have also been incorporated into porous scaffolds to improve their bulk and surface properties. A large number of porous scaffolds do not possess mechanical properties (a bulk property) necessary for *in vivo* applications (Mistry and Mikos, 2005). Thus, nanobiomaterials are incorporated into these scaffolds to improve their mechanical properties. For instance, carbon nanotubes have high Young's modulus (~1 TPa), and therefore, have been incorporated as reinforcing agents into porous polymer scaffolds to improve their mechanical properties (Lukic et al., 2005; Shi et al., 2005) (Figure 11.2).

Further, organic or inorganic nanomaterials have also been incorporated to induce bioactive properties (a surface property) into the scaffolds. The rationale here is that the physical interface between biological systems (e.g., proteins, DNA) and nanobiomaterials share a number of common (e.g., similar size scales) as well as complementary (e.g., inorganic/organic versus biological composition) attributes. Since, the

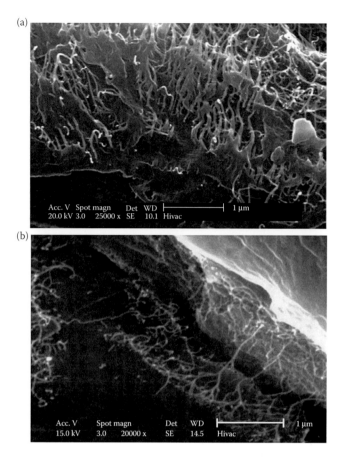

**FIGURE 11.2** SEM images of single-walled carbon nanotubes (SWCNTs) incorporated polymer scaffolds. (a) SWCNT bundles pulled out of the fracture surface from SWCNT polymer scaffold (0.05% by weight of SWCNT was dispersed in the scaffold). (b) Crack region propagation is prevented by spanning the SWCNT bundles. (Shi, X. et al. Rheological behaviour and mechanical characterization of injectable poly(propylene fumarate)/single-walled carbon nanotube composites for bone tissue engineering. *Nanotechnology.* 16: S531–8. Copyright 2005 IOP Science.)

nanoscale interactions in tissues (e.g., protein–protein interaction) are crucial for controlling many cellular functions such as cell–cell interactions, migration, proliferation, and ECM production (Benoit and Anseth, 2005), the nanomaterials could affect these interactions to achieve the desired result. For instance, incorporating ceramic nanoparticles into polymer scaffolds has been shown to induce bioactive properties into the scaffolds (Liu et al., 2006). The bioactive properties are induced by the ceramic nanoparticles by improving the adsorption characteristics of proteins such as fibronectin, vitronectin, laminin, and collagen involved in osteoblast functions (Webster et al., 1999, 2000, 2001). Some of the common fabrication techniques to incorporate nanoparticles into scaffolds include solvent casting, salt leaching, and freeze drying. Using all these methods, the individual nanoparticles are randomly distributed into the scaffolds. More examples of the nanoparticle-incorporated scaffolds examples and their applications are listed in Table 11.2.

## 11.3 Nanobiomaterials for Therapeutic Delivery

Controlled production and/or delivery of tissue-inducing macromolecules such as cytokines and growth factors are widely applied strategies in regenerative medicine. The physical and chemical properties of a large number of nanobiomaterials make them suitable for a variety of therapeutic and drug-delivery applications in TE (Figure 11.3). The external surfaces of the nanobiomaterials can be covalently or noncovalently functionalized with biological moieties that target specific cell or tissues types and/or pharmaceutical agents. Here, the nanobiomaterials target a specific cell or tissue type, and act as biological cargo vehicles to transport, and deliver therapeutic agents via a biochemical or biophysical stimulus (Langer and Tirrell, 2004).

Furthermore, the nanobiomaterial themselves can be used as a therapeutic agent by exploiting their unique physical properties (Shi et al., 2010). For example, the strong optical absorption properties of SWCNTs and gold nanoparticles render them capable of generating acoustic waves upon irradiation. These waves have shown to affect the process of osteoinduction (Green et al., 2009). Other advantages of using nanobiomaterials for therapeutic purposes, and as delivery vehicles include their nanoscale dimensions, which enhance their retention and permeability in the regenerating tissues (Gannon et al.,

**TABLE 11.2**   Nanobiomaterial-Based Polymer/Composite Scaffolds

| Nanoparticle Material | Intended Applications | Function and Biological Improvements | Reference |
|---|---|---|---|
| *n*-HA/PA, *n*-HA/PA/ MSC | Bone Tissue engineering | Enhanced osteogenesis than pure *n*-HA/PA scaffolds | Wang et al. (2007) |
| Bioactive-glass ceramic nanoparticles | Bone tissue engineering | Higher amount of mineral deposited on the composite scaffold, which increased with increasing time of incubation | Peter et al. (2010) |
| Bioglass-based glass-ceramic pellets | General applications | Bioactive and resorbable nanofibrous coatings can be used to tailor the surface topography of bioactive glass-ceramics | Bretcanu et al. (2009) |
| Mesoporous bioactive glasses | Bone tissue engineering | *In vitro* bioactivity of these MBGs scaffolds was dependent on the chemical composition | Zhu et al. (2008), Yan et al. (2006) |
| Forsterite | Bone tissue engineering | Significantly promoted cell proliferations, cell adhesion, spread, and growth on the surface of the nanostructured forsterite ceramic | Kharaziha and Fathi (2010) |
| Chitosan–nanohydroxyapatite | Bone tissue engineering | Well-developed structure morphology, physicochemical properties and superior cytocompatibility seen in chitosan–*n*HA porous scaffolds | Thein-Han and Misra (2009) |
| HA and PEG/PBT | Bone tissue engineering | Increased Young's modulus, tensile strength, and elongation at break of composite scaffold | Liu et al. (1998) |
| HA/PLLA | Bone tissue engineering | Increased compressive modulus and protein adsorption | Wei and Ma (2004) |
| HA/PLGA | Bone tissue engineering | Stimulated cell proliferation and osteogenic differentiation | Kim et al. (2006) |
| HA/PLGA | Bone tissue engineering | *In vivo* bone formation after 8 weeks of implantation to critical size defects in rat skulls | Kim et al. (2007) |
| POC | Cardiac tissue engineering | Decreased porosity caused a rise in the elastic modulus, ECM proteins promoted cell adhesion in a protein-type- and concentration-dependent manner | Hidalgo-Bastida et al. (2007) |
| Cellulose acetate, regenerated cellulose | Cardiac tissue engineering | Cellulose acetate and regenerated cellulose surfaces promoted cardiac cell growth, enhanced cell connectivity (gap junctions) and electrical functionality | Entcheva et al. (2004) |
| Fibrin | Cardiac tissue engineering | Dense fibrin scaffolds had mechanical properties closer to native myocardium than fibrin gels | Robinson et al. (2008), Thomson et al. (2010) |
| PF | Cardiac tissue engineering | PF hydrogel biomaterial can be used as an *in situ* polymerizable biomaterial for stem cells and their cardiomyocyte derivatives | Shapira-Schweitzer et al. (2009) |

**TABLE 11.2**  (continued) Nanobiomaterial-Based Polymer/Composite Scaffolds

| Nanoparticle Material | Intended Applications | Function and Biological Improvements | Reference |
|---|---|---|---|
| Fibrin, Collagen | Neural tissue engineering | Cells showed high viability after printing, which was equivalent to that of manually plated cells, cells printed within 1 mm from the border of VEGF releasing fibrin gel showed GF-induced changes in their morphology | Lee et al. (2010) |
| SWCNT/PPF | Bone tissue engineering | Significantly improved flexural and compressive modulus, compressive offset yield strength, flexural strength | Shi et al. (2006) |
| HA/collagen dip-coated in aqueous ferrofluids containing iron oxide nanoparticles | Bone tissue engineering | Magnetic scaffolds supported adhesion and proliferation of human bone marrow stem cells *in vitro* | Bock et al. (2010) |
| Gold colloid/chitosan film | Skin tissue engineering | Significantly increased the attachment of keratinocytes and promote their growth; a good candidate for wound dressing in skin tissue engineering | Zhang et al. (2009) |
| Silver and collagen type 1 | Neural tissue engineering | Superior functionality of the nano-silver–collagen scaffold in the adsorption to laminin and subsequent regeneration of damaged peripheral nerves | Ding et al. (2010) |
| Titanium, CoCrMo | Vascular stent applications | Vascular stents composed of nanometer compared with micron-sized metal particles invoked cellular responses important for improved vascular stent applications | Choudhary et al. (2006) |
| Titanium | Vascular stent applications | Enhanced endothelial and vascular smooth muscle cell functions compared with those of conventional-sized particles | Choudhary et al. (2007) |
| Titanium | Bone tissue engineering | Superior compressive strength, and osteoconductivity of PMMA composite | Goto et al. (2005) |
| Titanium | Bone tissue engineering | Enhanced cellular adhesion | Webster et al. (1999), Kay et al. (2002) |
| Titanium | Bone tissue engineering | Increased osteogenic functions in PLGA composite scaffolds | Webster and Smith (2005), Liu et al. (2005, 2006) |
| Surface-modified alumoxane, PPF/ PF-DA | Bone tissue engineering | Demonstrated feasibility of fabricating degradable nanocomposite scaffolds for bone tissue engineering by photo-crosslinking fumarate-based polymers, alumoxane nanoparticles | Mistry et al. (2009) |
| Aluminum | Bone tissue engineering | Increased flexural, and compressive strength of PPF composite scaffold | Horch et al. (2004) |
| Polyurethane | Cardiac tissue engineering | Cells cultured on laminin and collagen IV exhibited preferential attachment | Alperin et al. (2005) |
| PGS | Cardiac tissue engineering | Showed a wide range of degradability | Chen et al. (2008) |
| PGS | Cardiac tissue engineering | Strain amplifications were lower in ALH versus rectangular honeycomb scaffolds, appearing to be inversely correlated with previously measured strains-to-failure | Jean and Engelmayr (2010) |
| Alginate | Cardiac tissue engineering | Immobilized RGD peptide promoted cell adherence to the matrix, prevented cell apoptosis and accelerated cardiac tissue regeneration | Shachar et al. (2011) |

*continued*

**TABLE 11.2**    (continued) Nanobiomaterial-Based Polymer/Composite Scaffolds

| Nanoparticle Material | Intended Applications | Function and Biological Improvements | Reference |
|---|---|---|---|
| PEG | Neural tissue engineering | Initial presence of fibrin did not influence the cell-fate decisions of the encapsulated precursor cells (fibrin degraded enzymatically) | Namba et al. (2009) |
| PVA/PAA IPN films, PDMS | Neural tissue engineering | Glial fibrillary acidic protein immunoreactivity in animals receiving coated implants was significantly lower compared to that of uncoated implants, neurite extension of rat pheochromocytoma cells was clearly greater on PVA/PAA IPN films than on PDMS substrates | Lu et al. (2009) |
| Melanin | Neural tissue engineering | Enhanced Schwann cell growth and neurite extension compared to collagen films *in vitro*; induced an inflammation response that was comparable to silicone implants; implants were significantly resorbed after 8 weeks | Bettinger et al. (2009) |
| Silica/PCL | Bone tissue engineering | Similar mechanical properties of natural bone | Yoo and Rhee (2004) |
| PCL, PCL/Matrigel | Neural tissue engineering | Covalently functionalized PCL/Matrigel nanofibrous scaffolds promoted the proliferation and neurite outgrowth of NPCs compared to PCL | Ghasemi-Mobarakeh et al. (2010) |
| PCL | Neural tissue engineering | Cells on nanowire surfaces expressed key neuronal markers and demonstrated neuronal phenotypic behavior as compared to the cells on control surfaces, significantly higher cell adhesion, proliferation and viability of cells cultured on nanowire surfaces | Bechara et al. (2010) |
| PCL/gelatin | Neural tissue engineering | Increased hydrophilicity of nanofibrous scaffolds and yielded better mechanical properties compared to PCL alone | Gupta et al. (2009) |
| PCL | Cardiac tissue engineering | Low stiffness in the range of 300–400 kPa for soft-tissue engineering achieved; high density of cells was recorded after 4 days of culture. Fusion and differentiation observed as early as 6 days *in vitro* and was confirmed after 11 days | Yeong et al. (2010) |
| PCL | Cardiac tissue engineering | Honeycomb structures and the pore sizes influenced the morphology, cytoskeletal organization and focal adhesion of the cardiac myocytes | Arai et al. (2008) |
| PLGA | Bone tissue engineering | Collagen mineralization process induced the formation of nanosize carbonated hydroxyapatite, while nanosize hydroxyapatite is formed during PLGA mineralization | Liao et al. (2008) |
| PLLA | Bladder tissue engineering | Provided an optimal microenvironment for facilitating cell-matrix penetration and retention of myogenic-differentiated BMSCs | Tian et al. (2010) |
| | Cardiac tissue engineering | Better cell adhesion and mature cytoskeleton structure with well-defined periodic units in the contractile machinery (sarcomeres) in PLLA, superior response in PLLA, CM cell density was lower on hydrophilic and faster degrading electrospun scaffolds | Zong et al. (2005) |
| | Neural tissue engineering | Directed neuronal stem cell elongation and its neurite outgrowth is parallel to the direction of PLLA fibers | Yang et al. (2005) |
| | Bone tissue engineering | Dual-scale scaffold structures provided a better choice for tissue engineering and 3-D cell culture applications with | Cheng and Kisaalita (2010) |

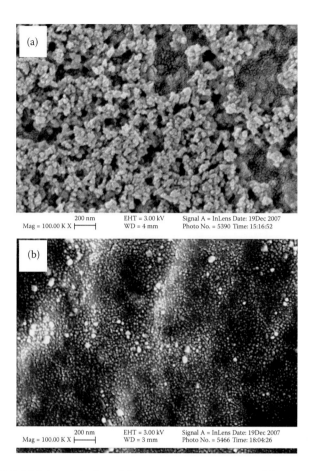

**FIGURE 11.3** Nano-HA-PLGA-peptide drug delivery system. SEM images of the (a) HA-PLGA nanoparticles with peptides physically adsorbed on the nanoparticles and (b) HA/PLGA nanoparticles with peptides covalently immobilized on the nanoparticles. (Liu, H. and T. J. Webster. Ceramic/polymer nanocomposites with tunable drug delivery capability at specific disease sites. *J Biomed Mater Res A*. 93(3): 1180–92. Copyright 2010 Wiley Interscience. Reproduced with permission.)

2007). Additionally, in case of certain types of nanomaterials (e.g., nanorods or nanotubes), their large aspect ratio allows attachment of multiple functional groups for the targeted delivery of multiple therapeutic entities. Table 11.3 represents some of the developed nanobiomaterial systems for delivery and therapeutic applications.

## 11.4 Nanobiomaterials to Image the Process of Tissue Formation

The limitations of standard diagnostic tools and techniques for detecting, and monitoring the process of tissue regeneration in small animals are well known (Greco, 2008). The most robust technique for the evaluation of *de novo* tissue formation, neo-vascularization or monitoring the fate of transplanted cells is histological analysis. Because histology is an endpoint evaluation, and large variation is observed, it is difficult to assess temporal results in a statistically significant manner. In search of alternatives, much progress has been made on new approaches for noninvasive *in vivo* imaging using positron emission tomography (PET), magnetic resonance imaging (MRI), and x-ray computed tomography (CT).

These imaging modalities offer scientists the spatial and temporal information in a faster and more convenient manner. For each imaging modality, substantial attention has been devoted to the development of contrast agents. Novel nanobiomaterial-based contrast agents may enhance molecular imaging by improving detection sensitivity and selectivity. The strategies developed for design of these nanobiomaterial-based contrast agents for imaging tissue regeneration include encapsulation or coating of medically relevant metal ions within hollow nanomaterials (Figure 11.4), the functionalization of the exterior surface of the nanobiomaterials with a variety of imaging agents (e.g., organic

**TABLE 11.3** Nanobiomaterial-Based Drug Delivery System in Tissue Engineering

| Nanoparticle System | Intended Application | Delivery | Function and Biological Improvements | Reference |
|---|---|---|---|---|
| Dendrimer | Bone tissue engineering | Gene delivery | LacZ gene transduction in human chondrocyte-like cell without cytotoxic effect and morphological changes | Ohashi et al. (2001) |
| | Bone tissue engineering | Gene delivery | Increased nucleus penetration and enhanced gene transfection using dexamethasone conjugated PAMAM | Choi et al. (2006) |
| | Bone tissue engineering | Gene delivery | Targeted delivery of antiarthritic drug with folate–PAMAM dendrimer | Chandrasekar et al. (2007) |
| | Bone tissue engineering | Gene delivery | Improved bone formation in a rat bone-defect model using magnetic rhBMP-2 liposomes | Matsuo et al. (2003) |
| | Bone tissue engineering | Gene delivery | Enhanced bone formation in cranial defect on rabbit model using cationic liposome loading BMP-2 cDNA plasmids | Ono et al. (2004) |
| Liposome | Bone tissue engineering | Gene delivery | Critical size defect healing in rat model | Park et al. (2003) |
| Micelle | Bone tissue engineering | Gene delivery | Improved efficiency, and less toxic transfection toward primary osteoblast cells using polyplex micelles | Kanayama et al. (2006) |
| | Bone tissue engineering | Gene delivery | Allowed adherence of aldehyde-terminated PEG–PLA block polymer to a tissue surface *in vivo* | Murakami et al. (2007) |
| PEGylation | Bone tissue engineering | Gene delivery | Extended half-life of BSA with PEG–PLGA nanoparticle | Li et al. (2001) |
| | Neurons tissue engineering | Drug delivery | TTC was conjugated to nanoparticles using neutravidin, and the resulting nanoparticles were shown to selectively target neuroblastoma cells *in vitro* | Townsend et al. (2007) |
| | | Drug delivery | The amount of lipid coverage affected its drug release kinetics | Chan et al. (2009) |
| | | Gene delivery | Variable transfection activity can be achieved over extended periods of time upon release of pDNA and nonviral gene delivery vectors from electrospun coaxial fiber mesh scaffolds | Saraf et al. (2010) |
| | Bone tissue engineering | Gene delivery | Showed effective gene release with AMPEG/PCL nanoparticle with low density of primary amine groups | Jang et al. (2006) |
| | Bone tissue engineering | Gene delivery | Demonstrated higher DNA protection to enzymatic degradation and higher reporter gene expression with PEG-cationized gelatin | Kushibiki and Tabata (2005) |
| Polymeric | Intra ocular | Device delivery | Photo-crosslinked PPF-based matrices showed promise as long-term delivery devices for intraocular drug delivery. | Haesslein et al. (2006) |

**TABLE 11.3**    (continued) Nanobiomaterial-Based Drug Delivery System in Tissue Engineering

| Nanoparticle System | Intended Application | Delivery | Function and Biological Improvements | Reference |
|---|---|---|---|---|
| | Ophthalmic | Drug delivery | Combination of the nanoparticles with bioadhesive polymers increased the ocular drug bioavailability | Langer et al. (1997) |
| | Cancer treatment | Drug delivery | Surface functionalization of NPs with the A10 PSMA Apt significantly enhanced delivery of NPs to tumors versus equivalent NPs lacking the A10 PSMA Apt | Cheng et al. (2007) |
| | Tumor treatment | Drug delivery | PEO-modified poly-1 nanoparticles could provide increased therapeutic benefit by delivering the encapsulated drug to solid tumors | Potineni et al. (2003) |
| | | Drug delivery | NPs with methoxyl surface groups might be an ideal candidate for drug delivery applications | Salvador-Morales et al. (2009) |
| | Horomone therapy | Hormone delivery | Blood glucose levels of diabetic rats can be effectively controlled by oral SS-ILP administration | Morishita et al. (2006) |
| | Hormone therapy | Hormone delivery | Particle size and delivery site are very important factors for ILP with respect to increasing the bioavailability of insulin following oral administration. | Morishita et al. (2004), Huang and Wang (2006) |
| | Bone tissue engineering | Gene delivery | Increased DNA penetration into the cells and luciferase activity with DNA–PEG–gelatin nanoparticle | Hosseinkhani and Tabata (2006) |
| Polymeric nanoparticle + DNA | Bone tissue engineering | Gene delivery | Up to 70% high DNA encapsulation efficiency with sustained release both *in vitro* and *in vivo* | Cohen et al. (2000) |
| | Bone tissue engineering | Gene delivery | PLGA nanoparticle with tetracycline with affinity for HA | Choi et al. (2005) |
| | Tissue specific | Gene delivery | Variations in nanoparticle peptide coating density can alter the tissue-specificity of gene delivery *in vivo* | Harris et al. (2010) |
| | Bone tissue engineering | Gene delivery | Polymerized nanogel with stability in aqueous media, low toxicity, and enhanced DNA uptake in HeLa cell | McAllister et al. (2002) |
| | Bone tissue engineering | Gene delivery | Penetration of PLGA–VEGF nanoparticle carrier in myocardial cells and successful *in vivo* angiogenesis | Yi et al. (2006) |
| | Bone tissue engineering | Gene delivery | Higher gene expression level with smaller size of PLGA | Prabha et al. (2002) |
| Nanosized inorganic material | Bone tissue engineering | Gene delivery | Enhanced DNA internalization of DNA mediated byfolate receptor binding, improved gene transfection rate subsequently | Mansouri et al. (2006) |
| | Bone tissue engineering | Gene delivery | *In vitro* DNA transfection using DNA—chitosan nanoparticle | Erbacher et al. (1998) |
| | Bone tissue engineering | Gene delivery | Co-precipitated DNA with calcium phosphate nanocomposites onto the cell-culture surface enhanced b-gal expression level in MG-63 and Saos-2 cells | Shen et al. (2004) |
| Nanosized metallic material | Renal regeneration | Gene delivery | Synthesized shRNA that is specific to the p53 gene was efficiently delivered into HEK293 and HeLa human cell lines | Ryou et al. (2010) |

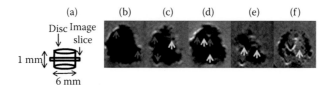

**FIGURE 11.4** MRI of Gadonanotube-reinforced biodegradable polymer nanocomposites. (a) Schematic of the sample arrangement within the MRI. Representation two-dimensional images through a nanocomposite disc after (b) 2 h, (c) 24 h, (d) 3 days, (e) 5 days, and (f) 7 days. The higher (white) pixel intensities within the dark disc represent regions of higher water concentration. The MRI showed enhanced water penetration, which increased with time. Beyond day 1, the discs swelled considerably, the dark parts on the MRI slowly disappeared, and by day 5, there was an increase in image brightness throughout the disc indicating that the water was homogenously distributed throughout the sample. (Sitharaman, B. et al. Magnetic resonance imaging studies on gadonanotube-reinforced biodegradable polymer nanocomposites. *J Biomed Mater Res A*. 93(4): 1454–62. Copyright 2010 Wiley Interscience. Reproduced with permission.)

dyes, radiopharmaceuticals), and exploiting the intrinsic physical properties of the nanobiomaterials (e.g., intrinsic fluorescence of quantum dots). The charge and the nature of coating material determine the stability, biodistribution, metabolism, pharmacokinetics, and pharmacodynamics of these imaging agents (Corot et al., 2006). Table 11.4 lists some of the recent advances in the development of nanobio-material-based imaging systems for TE.

**TABLE 11.4** Nanobiomaterials Based Imaging in Tissue Engineering

| Imaging System | Nanoparticle/Polymer Materials | Functions and Biological Response/ Improvements | Reference |
|---|---|---|---|
| MRI | Perfluorocarbons-conjugated RGD-peptide nanoparticles | Vascular disease specific targeting, easy cellular internalization, molecular imaging, cellular tracking and *in vivo* imaging | Kok et al. (2011) |
| | SPION nanoparticles in agar based stem cell implants | Cellular tracking of labeled stem cells and noninvasive *in vivo* MRI during cartilage regeneration | Nedopil et al. (2010) |
| | SPION (Ferridex) nanoparticles in chondrocyte-hydrogel constructs | Approach towards understanding the fate of chondrocyte labeled iron oxide nanoparticles in tissue-engineering constructs for cartilage tissue regeneration | Ramaswamy et al. (2009) |
| | SPION (Ferrumoxide) | SPION labeled BMSCs do not undergo differentiation *in vivo* and provides nontoxic MRI contrast agents | Balakumaran et al. (2010) |
| | SPION | Direct injection of SPION-ESCs into infarct myocardium improves cardiac functions | Au et al. (2009) |
| | Gadolinium-SWCNTs nanoparticles | Gadolinium catalyzed SWCNTs reinforced PLGA nanocomposites is used for noninvasive MRI and to study the fate of the nanoparticles upon degradation from polymer scaffolds | Sitharaman et al. (2010); Van der Zande et al. (2011) |
| microPET | [18F]FB-PEG-RGD | These particles have fast blood clearance rates, rapid and high uptake by tumors, lower organ accumulation, and image the process of angiogenesis | Chen et al. (2004) |

**TABLE 11.4**    (continued) Nanobiomaterials Based Imaging in Tissue Engineering

| Imaging System | Nanoparticle/Polymer Materials | Functions and Biological Response/ Improvements | Reference |
|---|---|---|---|
| Optical imaging | Rare earth doped nanoparticles conjugated with human serum albumin and RGD peptide | Biocompatible, and biologically targetable nanoshell complexes useful for disease targeting and NIR imaging | Naczynski et al. (2010) |
| | Gold nanoparticles-conjugated to dye labeled targeting peptides and PEG | Noninvasive NIR imaging to study the protease activity mediated disease progression. | Mu et al. (2010) |
| | Silicon nanocrystals coated with amphiphilic polymers | Stable and bright photoluminescence in the pH range of 7–10 for biological tissue imaging | Hessel et al. (2010) |
| CT | Gold nanoparticles functionalized with glutamic acid | Targeting damaged bone tissue | Zhang et al. (2010) |

# 11.5  Continuing and Future Developments

Nanobiomaterials show promise and potential towards the development of tools and techniques for TE. A number of nanobiomaterials have been investigated for applications in cellular and molecular imaging/sensing such as *in vivo* monitoring and tracking of transplanted cells and engineered tissues; therapeutic drug-delivery to deliver genes, signaling proteins, and growth factors; improving the bulk and surface properties of TE scaffolds. In a number of these applications, nanobiomaterials have been used in combination with other biomaterials and have demonstrated suitability in enabling components of various electronic, biochemical, and mechanical structures, devices or implants for TE.

Advancements in synthesis of high-quality nanobiomaterials and the availability in bulk quantities for a number of these nanobiomaterials have facilitated research and the development of a number of nanobiomaterial-driven biomedical technologies. For some TE applications, products that utilize nanobiomaterials *in vitro* are already commercially available. For example, Invitrogen Inc. (Carlsbad, California), has developed miniaturized sensor systems that utilizes quantum dots to detect a wide variety of proteins and antibodies *in vitro*. Nanoprobes Inc. (Yaphank, New York) has developed proprietary technology utilizes the stability and unique structure of gold nanoparticles for immunoassays in a variety of tissues. However, progress has been slow in developing nanobiomaterial-based products for *in vivo* TE applications. The *in vivo* toxicity and biodistribution of a large number of nanobiomaterials still needs to be thoroughly understood before their translation into clinic. Additionally, high costs and time constraints associated with nanobiomaterial production and processing (purification and sorting) are barriers for some applications. However, these costs are highly dependent on the specific application of a particular nanobiomaterial. Nevertheless, the development of nanobiomaterial-based TE technologies represents a challenging, but potentially rewarding opportunity to develop the next generation biomedical products.

# Abbreviations

| | |
|---|---|
| ALH | Accordion-like honeycomb |
| ALP | Alkaline phosphatase |
| AMPEG | Amine-terminated methoxy poly(ethylene glycol) |
| Apt | A10 RNA aptamer |
| BMP | Bone morphogenetic protein |
| BMSC | Bone marrow mesenchymal stem cells |
| BSA | Bovine serum albumin |
| CG | Chitosan–gelatin |

| | |
|---|---|
| CH | Pure chitosan scaffolds |
| CH1 | nHA-chitosan scaffold |
| CM | Chitosan scaffolds of varying% nHA weight |
| CNFs | Carbon nanofibers |
| CPC | Calcium phosphate cement |
| CT | Computed tomography |
| DOTA | 1,4,7,10-tetraazacyclododecane-N,N′,N″,N‴-tetraacetic acid |
| ECM | Extracellular matrix |
| ESCs | Embryonic stem cells |
| FB | Fluorobenzoyl |
| GF | Growth factor |
| HA | Hydroxyapatite |
| HA-coll | Hyaluronic acid–collagen |
| HBDC | Human bone-derived cells |
| HCA | Hydroxylcarbonate apatite |
| hMSC | Human mesenchymal stem cell |
| ICAM | Inter-cellular adhesion molecule |
| IPNs | Interpenetrating polymer networks |
| IKVAV | Isolucinelysine-valine-alanine-valine |
| MBGs | Mesoporous bioactive glass |
| microPET | micro Positron emission tomography |
| MMA | Methylmethacrylate |
| MPEG | Methoxy poly(ethylene glycol) |
| MSCs | Marrow stem cells or mesenchymal stem cells |
| n-HA/PA | Nano-hydroxyapatite/polyamide |
| nHA | Chitosan–nanohydroxyapatite |
| nBGC | Bioactive glass ceramic nanoparticles |
| NIR | Near infrared |
| NP | Nanoparticles |
| NSC | Neural stem cells |
| NT-3 | Neurotrophin-3 |
| P3HB | Poly(3-hydroxybutyrate) |
| PAMAM | Polyamidoamine |
| PBT | Poly(butylene terephthalate) |
| PCL | Poly(1-caprolactone) |
| PDMS | Poly-(dimethylsiloxane) |
| pDNA | Plasmid DNA |
| PECAM | Platelet endothelial cell adhesion molecule |
| PEG | Poly(ethylene glycol) |
| PEI-HA | Poly(ethylenimine)-hyaluronic acid |
| PEO | Poly(ethylene oxide) |
| PET | Polyethylene terephthalate |
| PF | PEGylated fibrinogen |
| PHBV | Poly(3-hydroxybutyrate-*co*-hydroxyvalerate) |
| PGS | Poly(glycerol-co-sebacic acid) |
| PLA | Poly(lactic acid) |
| PLGA | Poly(D,L-lactic-*co*-glycolic acid) |
| PLLA | Poly(L-lactic acid) |
| PMMA | Poly(methyl methacrylate) |
| POC | Poly(1,8-octanediol-*co*-citric acid) |

| PPF | Poly(propylene fumarate) |
| PPF/PF-DA | Poly(propylene fumarate)/propylene fumarate-diacrylate |
| Ppy | Polypyrrole |
| PSMA | Prostate specific membrane antigen |
| PVA/PAA | Poly(vinyl alcohol)/poly(acrylic acid) |
| RGD | L-arginine, glycine, and L-aspartic acid peptide |
| rh | Recombinant human |
| SBF | Simulated body fluid |
| SEM | Scanning electron microscope |
| SF | Silk fibroin |
| SPION | Super paramagnetic iron oxide nanoparticles |
| SPM | Sulfopropylmethacrylate |
| SS-ILP | Super small–insulin-loaded polymer microparticle |
| SWCNT | Single-walled carbon nanotubes |
| TTC | Tetanus toxin C |
| VCAM | Vascular cell adhesion molecule |
| VEGF | Vascular endothelial growth factor |

# References

Alperin, C., P. W. Zandstra, and K. A. Woodhouse. 2005. Polyurethane films seeded with embryonic stem cell-derived cardiomyocytes for use in cardiac tissue engineering applications. *Biomaterials* 26(35): 7377–86.

Arai, K., M. Tanaka, S. Yamamoto, and M. Shimomura. 2008. Effect of pore size of honeycomb films on the morphology, adhesion and cytoskeletal organization of cardiac myocytes. *Colloids and Surfaces A: Physicochem Eng Aspects* 313–314: 530–35.

Au, K. W., S. Y. Liao, Y. K. Lee, W. H. Lai, K. M. Ng, Y. C. Chan, M. C. Yip et al. 2009. Effects of iron oxide nanoparticles on cardiac differentiation of embryonic stem cells. *Biochem Biophys Res Commun* 379(4): 898–903.

Balakumaran, A., E. Pawelczyk, J. Ren , B. Sworder, A. Chaudhry, M. Sabatino, D. Stroncek, J. A. Frank, and P. G. Robey. 2010. Superparamagnetic iron oxide nanoparticles labeling of bone marrow stromal (mesenchymal) cells does not affect their "stemness". *PLoS One* 5(7): e11462.

Bechara, S. L., A. Judson, and K. C. Popat. 2010. Template synthesized poly(3-caprolactone) nanowire surfaces for neural tissue engineering. *Biomaterials* 31: 3492–501.

Bellingham, C. M., M. A. Lillie, J. M. Gosline, G. M. Wright, B. C. Starcher, A. J. Bailey, K. A. Woodhouse, and F. W. Keeley. 2003. Recombinant human elastin polypeptides self-assemble into biomaterials with elastin-like properties. *Biopolymers* 70(4): 445–55.

Benoit, D. S., and K. S. Anseth. 2005. Heparin functionalized PEG gels that modulate protein. *Biochem Eng Biotechnol* 94: 1–22.

Bettinger, C. J., J. P. Bruggeman, A. Misra, J. T. Borenstein, and R. Langer. 2009. Biocompatibility of biodegradable semiconducting melanin films for nerve tissue engineering. *Biomaterials* 30(17): 3050–57.

Bhattarai, N., D. Edmondson, O. Veiseh, F. A. Matsen, and M. Zhang. 2005. Electrospun chitosan based nanofibers and their cellular compatibility. *Biomaterials* 26(31): 6176–84.

Bini, T. B., S. Gao, X. Xu, S. Wang, S. Ramakrishna, and K. W. Leong. 2004. Peripheral nerve regeneration by microbraided poly(L-lactide-*co*-glycolide) biodegradable polymer fibers. *J Biomed Mater Res A* 68(2): 286–95.

Bock, N., A. Riminucci, C. Dionigi et al. 2010. A novel route in bone tissue engineering: Magnetic biomimetic scaffolds. *Acta Biomater* 6: 786–96.

Bretcanu, O., S. K. Misra, D. M. Yunos, A. R. Boccaccini, I. Roy, T. Kowalczyk, S. Blonski, and T. A. Kowalewski. 2009. Electrospun nanofibrous biodegradable polyester coatings on Bioglass®-based glass-ceramics for tissue engineering. *Mater Chem Phys* 118: 420–26.

Carneiro, K. M., F. A. Aldaye, and H. F. Sleiman. 2010. Long-range assembly of DNA into nanofibers and highly ordered networks using a block copolymer approach. *J Am Chem Soc* 132(2): 679–85.

Chan, J. M., L. Zhang, K. P. Yuet, G. Liao, J. W. Rhee, R. Langer, and O. C. Farokhzad. 2009. PLGA–lecithin–PEG core–shell nanoparticles for controlled drug delivery. *Biomaterials* 30(8): 1627–34.

Chandrasekar, D., R. Sistla, F. J. Ahmad, R. K. Khar, and P. V. Diwan. 2007. The development of folate-PAMAM dendrimer conjugates for targeted delivery of anti-arthritic drugs and their pharmacokinetics and biodistribution in arthritic rats. *Biomaterials* 28(3): 504–12.

Chen, F., X. Li, X. Mo, C. He, H. Wang, and Y. Ikada. 2008. Electrospun chitosan-P(LLA-CL) nanofibers for biomimetic extracellular matrix. *J Biomater Sci Polym Ed* 19: 677–91.

Chen, Q. Z., A. Bismarck, U. Hansen, S. Junaid, M. Q. Tran, S. E. Harding, N. N. Ali, and A. R. Boccaccini. 2008. Characterisation of a soft elastomer poly(glycerol sebacate) designed to match the mechanical properties of myocardial tissue. *Biomaterials* 29(1): 47–57.

Chen, V. J. and P. X. Ma. 2004. Nano-fibrous poly(L-lactic acid) scaffolds with interconnected spherical macropores. *Biomaterials* 25: 2065–73.

Chen, X., R. Park, Y. Hou, V. Khankaldyyan, I. Gonzales-Gomez, M. Tohme, J. R. Bading, W. E. Laug, and P. S. Conti. 2004. MicroPET imaging of brain tumor angiogenesis with 18F-labeled PEGylated RGD peptide. *Eur J Nucl Med Mol Imaging* 31(8): 1081–9.

Chen, X., Y. Hou, M. Tohme, R. Park, V. Khankaldyyan, I. Gonzales-Gomez, J. R. Bading, W. E. Laug, and P. S. Conti. 2004. Pegylated Arg-Gly-Asp peptide: 64Cu labeling and PET imaging of brain tumor alphavbeta3-integrin expression. *J Nucl Med* 45(10): 1776–83.

Cheng, J., B. A. Teply, I. Sherifi, J. Sung, G. Luther, F. X. Gu, E. Levy-Nissenbaum, A. F. Radovic-Moreno, R. Langer, and O. C. Farokhzad. 2007. Formulation of functionalized PLGA–PEG nanoparticles for *in vivo* targeted drug delivery. *Biomaterials* 28(5): 869–76.

Cheng, K. and W. S. Kisaalita. 2010. Exploring cellular adhesion and differentiation in a micro-/nano-hybrid polymer scaffold. *Biotechnol Prog* 26(3): 838–46.

Chew, S. Y., R. Mi, A. Hoke A, and K. W. Leong. 2008. The effect of the alignment of electrospun fi brous scaffolds on Schwann cell maturation. *Biomaterials* 29: 653–61.

Choi, J. S., K. S. Ko, J. S. Park, Y. H. Kim, S. W. Kim, and M. Lee. 2006. Dexamethasone conjugated poly(amidoamine) dendrimer as a gene carrier for efficient nuclear translocation. *Int J Pharm* 320(1/2): 171–8.

Choi, J. S., S. J. Lee, G. J. Christ, A. Atala, and J. J. Yoo. 2008. The influence of electrospun aligned poly(varepsilon-caprolactone)/collagen nanofiber meshes on the formation of self-aligned skeletal muscle myotubes. *Biomaterials* 29: 2899–906.

Choi, S. W., W. S. Kim, and J. H. Kim. 2005. Surface-functionalized nanoparticles for controlled drug delivery. *Methods Mol Biol* 303: 121–31.

Choudhary, S., M. Berhe, K. M. Haberstroh, and T. J. Webster. 2006. Increased endothelial and vascular smooth muscle cell adhesion on nanostructured titanium and CoCrMo. *Int J Nanomed* 1(1): 41–9.

Choudhary, S., K. M. Haberstroh, and T. J. Webster. 2007. Enhanced functions of vascular cells on nano-structured Ti for improved stent applications. *Tissue Eng* 13(7): 1421–30.

Cohen, H., R. J. Levy, J. Gao, I. Fishbein, V. Kousaev, S. Sosnowski, S. Slomkowski, and G. Golomb. 2000. Sustained delivery and expression of DNA encapsulated in polymeric nanoparticles. *Gene Ther* 7(22): 1896–905.

Corey, J. M., C. C. Gertz, B. S. Wang, L. K. Birrell, S. L. Johnson, D. C. Martin, and E. L. Feldman. 2008. The design of electrospun PLLA nanofi ber scaffolds compatible with serum-free growth of primary motor and sensory neurons. *Acta Biomater* 4(4): 863–75.

Corey, J. M., D. Y. Lin, K. B. Mycek, Q. Chen, S. Samuel, E. L. Feldman, and D. C. Martin. 2007. Aligned electrospun nanofibers specify the direction of dorsal root ganglia neurite growth. *J Biomed Mater Res A* 83(3): 636–45.

Corot, C., P. Robert, J. M. Idée, and M. Port. 2006. Recent advances in iron oxide nanocrystal technology for medical imaging. *Adv Drug Deliv Rev* 58(14): 1471–504.

Daamen, W. F., J. H. Veerkamp, J. C. van Hest, and T. H. van Kuppevelt. 2007. Elastin as a biomaterial for tissue engineering. *Biomaterials* 28(30): 4378–98.

Ding, B., H. Y. Kim, S. C. Lee, C.-L. Shao, D.-R. Lee, S.-J. Park, G.-B. Kwag, and K.-J. Choi. 2002. Preparation and characterization of a nanoscale poly(vinyl alcohol) fiber aggregate produced by an electrospinning method. *J Polym Sci B-Polym Phys* 40: 1261–8.

Ding, T., Z. J. Luo, Y. Zheng, X. Y. Hu, and Z. X. Ye. 2010. Rapid repair and regeneration of damaged rabbit sciatic nerves by tissue-engineered scaffold made from nano-silver and collagen type I. *Injury* 41: 522–7.

Entcheva, E., H. Bien, L. Yin, C. Y. Chung, M. Farrell, and Y. Kostov. 2004. Functional cardiac cell constructs on cellulose-based scaffolding. *Biomaterials* 25: 5753–62.

Erbacher, P., S. Zou, T. Bettinger, A. M. Steffan, and J. S. Remy. 1998. Chitosan-based vector/DNA complexes for gene delivery: Biophysical characteristics and transfection ability. *Pharm Res* 15(9): 1332–9.

Gannon, C. J., P. Cherukuri, B. I. Yakobson, L. Cognet, J. S. Kanzius, C. Kittrell, R. B. Weisman et al. 2007. Carbon nanotube-enhanced thermal destruction of cancer cells in a noninvasive radiofrequency field. *Cancer* 110(12): 2654–65.

Gauba, V. and J. D. Hartgerink. 2007. Self-assembled heterotrimeric collagen triple helices directed through electrostatic interactions. *J Am Chem Soc* 129: 2683–90.

Ghasemi-Mobarakeh, L., M. P. Prabhakaran, M. Morshed, M. H. Nasr-Esfahani, and S. Ramakrishna. 2010. Bio-functionalized PCL nanofibrous scaffolds for nerve tissue engineering. *Mater Sci Eng C* 30: 1129–36.

Ghosh, K., X. D. Ren, X. Z. Shu, G. D. Prestwich, and R. A. Clark. 2006. Fibronectin functional domains coupled to hyaluronan stimulate adult human dermal fibroblast responses critical for wound healing. *Tissue Eng* 12(3): 601–13.

Goto, K., J. Tamura, S. Shinzato, S. Fujibayashi, M. Hashimoto, M. Kawashita, T. Kokubo, and T. Nakamura. 2005. Bioactive bone cements containing nano-sized titania particles for use as bone substitutes. *Biomaterials* 26(33): 6496–505.

Greco, G. N. (ed.). 2008. *Tissue Engineering Research Trends*. Nova Science Publishers, New York.

Green, D. E., J. P. Longtin, and B. Sitharaman. 2009. The effect of nanoparticle-enhanced photoacoustic stimulation on multipotent marrow stromal cells. *ACS Nano* 3(8): 2065–72.

Gupta, D., J. Venugopal, M. P. Prabhakaran, V. R. Dev, S. Low, A. T. Choon, and S. Ramakrishna. 2009. Aligned and random nanofibrous substrate for the *in vitro* culture of Schwann cells for neural tissue engineering. *Acta Biomater* 5(7): 2560–9.

Gupta, P., C. Elkins, T. E. Long, and G. L. Wilkes. 2005. Electrospinning of linear homopolymers of poly(methyl methacrylate): Exploring relationships between fiber formation, viscosity, molecular weight and concentration in a good solvent. *Polymer* 46: 4799.

Haesslein, A., H. Ueda, M. C. Hacker, S. Jo, D. M. Ammon, R. N. Borazjani, J. F. Kunzler, J. C. Salamone, and A. G. Mikos. 2006. Long-term release of fluocinolone acetonide using biodegradable fumarate-based polymers. *J Control Release* 114(2): 251–60.

Hamdi, H., A. Furuta, V. Bellamy, A. Bel, E. Puymirat, S. Peyrard, O. Agbulut, and P. Menasché. 2009. Cell delivery: Intramyocardial injections or epicardial deposition? Ahead-to-head comparison. *Ann Thorac Surg.* 87(4): 1196–203.

Han, Z., H. Kong, J. Meng, C. Wang, S. Xie, and H. Xu. 2009. Electrospun aligned nanofibrous scaffold of carbon nanotubes-polyurethane composite for endothelial cells. *J Nanosci Nanotechnol* 9(2): 1400–2.

Harrington, D. A., E. Y. Cheng, M. O. Guler, L. K. Lee, J. L. Donovan, R. C. Claussen, and S. I. Stupp. 2006. Branched peptide-amphiphiles as self-assembling coatings for tissue engineering scaffolds. *J Biomed Mater Res A* 78(1): 157–67.

Harris, T. J., J. J. Green, P. W. Fung, R. Langer, D. G. Anderson, and S. N. Bhatia. 2010. Tissue-specific gene delivery via nanoparticle coating. *Biomaterials* 31(5): 998–1006.

Harrison, B. S. and A. Atala. 2007. Carbon nanotube applications for tissue engineering. *Biomaterials* 28(2): 344–53.

Hessel, C. M., M. R. Rasch, J. L. Hueso, B. W. Goodfellow, V. A. Akhavan, P. Puvanakrishnan, J. W. Tunnel, and B. A. Korgel. 2010. Alkyl passivation and amphiphilic polymer coating of silicon nanocrystals for diagnostic imaging. *Small* 6(18): 2026–34.

Hidalgo-Bastida, L. A., J. J. A. Barry, N. M. Everitt, F. R. Rose, L. D. Buttery, I. P. Hall, W. C. Claycomb, and K. M. Shakesheff. 2007. Cell adhesion and mechanical properties of a flexible scaffold for cardiac tissue engineering. *Acta Biomater* 3(4): 457–62.

Hofmann, S., S. Knecht, R. Langer, D. L. Kaplan, G. Vunjak-Novakovic, H. P. Merkle, and L. Meinel. 2006. Cartilage-like tissue engineering using silk scaffolds and mesenchymal stem cells. *Tissue Eng* 12(10): 2729–38.

Horch, R. A., N. Shahid, A. S. Mistrry, M. D. Timmer, A. G. Mikos, and A. R. Rarron. 2004. Nanoreinforcement of poly(propylene fumarate)- based networks with surface modified alumoxane nanoparticles for bone tissue engineering. *Biomacromolecules* 5: 1990–8.

Hosseinkhani, H. and Y. Tabata. 2006. Self assembly of DNA nanoparticles with polycations for the delivery of genetic materials into cells. *J Nanosci Nanotechnol* 6(8): 2320–8.

Huang, Y. Y. and C. H. Wang. 2006. Pulmonary delivery of insulin by liposomal carriers. *J Control Release* 113(1): 9–14.

Ishii, O., M. Shin, T. Sueda, and J. P. Vacanti. 2005. *In vitro* tissue engineering of a cardiac graft using a degradable scaffold with an extracellular matrix-like topography. *J Thorac Cardiovasc Surg* 130: 1358–63.

Jang, J. S., S. Y. Kim, S. B. Lee, K. O. Kim, J. S. Han, and Y. M. Lee. 2006. Poly(ethylene glycol)/poly(1-caprolactone) diblock copolymeric nanoparticles for non-viral gene delivery: The role of charge group and molecular weight in particle formation, cytotoxicity and transfection. *J Control Release* 113(2): 173–82.

Jean, A. and G. C. Engelmayr Jr. 2010. Finite element analysis of an accordion-like honey comb scaffold for cardiac tissue engineering. *J Biomech* 31 July 2010. Ahead of print.

Kanayama, N., S. Fukushima, N. Nishiyama, K. Itaka, W. D. Jang, K. Miyata, Y. Yamasaki, U. I. Chung, and K. Kataoka. 2006. A PEG based biocompatible block catiomer with high 17 buffering capacity for the construction of polyplex micelles showing efficient gene transfer toward primary cells. *Chem Med Chem* 1(4): 439–44.

Kay, S., A. Thapa, K. M. Haberstroh, and T. J. Webster. 2002. Nanostructured polymer/nanophase ceramic composites enhance osteoblast and chondrocyte adhesion. *Tissue Eng* 8(5): 753–61.

Kenawy, E. R., J. M. Layman, J. R. Watkins, G. L. Bowlin, J. A. Matthews, D. G. Simpson, and G. E. Wnek. 2003. Electrospinning of poly(ethyleneco-vinyl alcohol) fibers. *Biomaterials* 24(6): 907–13.

Khang, D., M. Sato, R. L. Price, A. E. Ribbe, and T. J. Webster. 2006. Selective adhesion and mineral deposition by osteoblasts on carbon nanofiber patterns. *Int J Nanomed* 1(1): 65–72.

Kharaziha, M. and M. H. Fathi. 2010. Improvement of mechanical properties and biocompatibility of forsterite bioceramic addressed to bone tissue engineering materials. *J Mech Behav Biomed Mater* 3(7): 530–7.

Khil, M. S., D. I. Cha, H. Y. Kim, I. S. Kim, and N. Bhattarai. 2003. Electrospun nanofibrous polyurethane membrane as wound dressing. *J Biomed Mater Res B Appl Biomater* 67: 675–9.

Kim, S. S., K. M. Ahn, M. S. Park, J. H. Lee, C. Y. Choi, and B. S. Kim. 2007. A poly(lactide-co-glycolide)/hydroxyapatite composite scaffold with enhanced osteoconductivity. *J Biomed Mater Res A* 80(1): 206–15.

Kim, H. S., K. Kim, H. J. Jin, and I. J. Chin. 2005. Morphological characterization of electrospun nano-fibrous membranes of biodegradable poly(L-lactide) and poly(lactide-*co*-glycolide). *Macromol Symp* 224: 145.

Kim, K. and J. P. Fisher. 2007. Nanoparticle technology in bone tissue engineering. *J Drug Target* 15(4): 241–52.

Kim, S. H., Y. S. Nam, T. S. Lee, and W. H. Park. 2003. Silk fibroin nanofiber Electrospinning, properties, and structure. *Polym J* 35: 185–90.

Kim, S. S., P. M. Sun, O. Jeon, Yong Choi C, and B. S. Kim. 2006. Poly(lactide-co-glycolide)/hydroxyapatite composite scaffolds for bone tissue engineering. *Biomaterials* 27(8): 1399–409.

Koide, T., D. L. Homma, S. Asada, and K. Kitagawa. 2005. Self-complementary peptides for the formation of collagen-like triple helical supramolecules. *Bioorg Med Chem Lett* 15: 5230–3.

Kok, M. B., A. de Vries, D. Abdurrachim, J. J. Prompers, H. Grüll, K. Nicolay, and G. J. Strijkers. 2011. Quantitative (1)H MRI, (19)F MRI, and (19)F MRS of cell-internalized perfluorocarbon paramagnetic nanoparticles. *Contrast Media Mol Imaging* 6(1): 19–27.

Kotch, F. W. and R. T. Raines. 2006. Self-assembly of synthetic collagen triple helices. *Proc Natl Acad Sci USA* 103: 3028–33.

Kushibiki, T. and Y. Tabata. 2005. Preparation of poly(ethylene glycol)-introduced cationized gelatin as a non-viral gene carrier. *J Biomater Sci Polym Ed* 16(11): 1447–61.

Langer, K., E. Mutschler, G. Lambrecht, D. Mayer, G. Troschau, F. Stieneker, and J. Kreuter. 1997. Methyl methacrylate sulfopropyl methacrylate copolymer nano particles for drug delivery: Part III: Evaluationas drug delivery system for ophthalmic applications. *Int J Pharm.* 158(2): 219–31.

Langer, R. and D. A. Tirrell. 2004. Designing materials for biology and medicine. *Nature* 428 (6982): 487–92.

Langer, R. and Vacanti, J. P. 1993. Tissue engineering. *Science* 260(5110): 920–6.

Lee, J. Y., C. A. Bashur, A. S. Goldstein, and C. E. Schmidt. 2009. Polypyrrole-coated electrospun PLGA nanofibers for neural tissue applications. *Biomaterials* 30(26): 4325–35.

Lee, Y. B., S. Polio, W. Lee, G. Dai, L. Menon, R. S. Carroll, and S. S. Yoo. 2010. Bio-printing of collagen and VEGF-releasing fibrin gel scaffolds for neural stem cell culture. *Exp Neurol* 223(2): 645–52.

Li, M. Y., M. J. Mondrinos, M. R. Gandhi, F. K. Ko, A. S. Weiss, and P. I. Lelkes. 2005. Electrospun protein fibers as matrices for tissue engineering. *Biomaterials* 26(30): 5999–6008.

Li, W. J., C. T. Laurencin, E. J. Caterson, R. S. Tuan, and F. K. Ko. 2002. Electrospun nanofibrous structure: A novel scaffold for tissue engineering. *J Biomed Mater Res* 60(4): 613–21.

Li, W. J., R. Tuli, X. Huang, P. Laquerriere, and R. S. Tuan. 2005a. Multilineage differentiation of human mesenchymal stem cells in a three-dimensional nanofibrous scaffold. *Biomaterials* 26(5): 5158–66.

Li, W. J., R. Tuli, C. Okafor, A. Derfoul, K. G. Danielson, D. J. Hall, and R. S. Tuan. 2005b. A three-dimensional nanofibrous scaffold for cartilage tissue engineering using human mesenchymal stem cells. *Biomaterials* 26(6): 599–609.

Li, Y.-P., Y.-Y. Pei, X.-Y. Zhang, Z.-H. Gu, Z. H. Zhou, W.-F. Yuan, J.-J. Zhao, J.-H. Zhu, and X.-J. Gao. 2001. PEGylated PLGA nanoparticles as protein carriers: synthesis, preparation and biodistribution in rats. *J Control Release* 71: 203–11.

Liao, S., R. Murugan, C. K. Chan, and S. Ramakrishna. 2008. Processing nanoengineered scaffolds through electrospinning and mineralization suitable for biomimetic bone tissue engineering. *J Mech Behav Biomed Mater* 1(3): 252–60.

Liu, H., E. B. Slamovich, and T. J. Webster. 2005. Increased osteoblast functions on nanophase titania dispersed in poly-lactic-coglycolicacid composites. *Nanotechnology* 16(7): S601–S608.

Liu, H., E. B. Slamovich, and T. J. Webster. 2006. Increased osteoblast functions among nanophase titania/poly(lactide-co-glycolide) composites of the highest nanometer surface roughness. *J Biomed Mater Res A* 78A(4): 798–807.

Liu, H. and T. J. Webster. 2010. Ceramic/polymer nanocomposites with tunable drug delivery capability at specific disease sites. *J Biomed Mater Res A* 93(3): 1180–92.

Liu, Q., J. R. de Wijn, and C. A. van Blitterswijk. 1998. Composite biomaterials with chemical bonding between hydroxyapatite filler particles and PEG/PBT copolymer matrix. *J Biomed Mater Res A* 40(3): 490–7.

Lu, Y., D. Wang, T. Li, X. Zhao, Y. Cao, H. Yang, and Y. Y. Duan. 2009. Poly(vinyl alcohol)/poly(acrylic acid) hydrogel coatings for improving electrode–neuralt issue interface. *Biomaterials* 30(25): 4143–51.

Lukic, B., J. W. Seo, R. R. Bacsa, S. Delpeux, F. Béguin, G. Bister, A. Fonseca et al. 2005. Catalytically grown carbon nanotubes of small diameter have a high Young's modulus. *Nano Lett* 5(10): 2074–7.

Ma, Z., M. Kotaki, T. Yong, W. He, and S. Ramakrishna. 2005. Surface engineering of electrospun polyethylene terephthalate (PET) nanofibers towards development of a new material for blood vessel engineering. *Biomaterials* 26: 2527–36.

Mahmood, T. A., V. P. Shastri, C. A. van Blitterswijk, R. Langer, and J. Riesle. 2006. Evaluation of chondrogenesis within PEGT: PBT scaffolds with high PEG content. *J Biomed Mater Res A* 79(1): 216–22.

Mansouri, S., Y. Cuie, F. Winnik, Q. Shi, P. Lavigne, M. Benderdour, E. Beaumont, and J. C. Fernandes. 2006. Characterization of folate–chitosan–DNA nanoparticles for gene therapy. *Biomaterials* 27(9): 2060–5.

Matsuo, T., T. Sugita, T. Kubo, Y. Yasunaga, M. Ochi, and T. Murakami. 2003. Injectable magnetic liposomes as a novel carrier of recombinant human BMP-2 for bone formation in a rat bone defect model. *J Biomed Mater Res A* 66(4): 747–54.

Matthews, J. A., G. E. Wnek, D. G. Simpson, and G. L. Bowlin. 2002. Electrospinning of collagen nanofibers. *Biomacromolecules* 3(2): 232–8.

McAllister, K., P. Sazani, M. Adam, M. J. Cho, M. Rubinstein, R. J. Samulski, and J. M. DeSimone. 2002. Polymeric nanogels produced via inverse microemulsion polymerization as potential gene and antisense delivery agents. *J Am Chem Soc* 124(51): 15198–207.

McKenzie, J. L., M. C. Waid, R. Shi, and T. J. Webster. 2004. Decreased functions of astrocytes on carbon nanofiber materials. *Biomaterials* 25(7–8): 1309–17.

Meinel, L., O. Betz, R. Fajardo, S. Hofmann, A. Nazarian, E. Cory, M. Hilbe et al. 2006. Silk based biomaterial to heal critical sized femur defects. *Bone* 39: 922–31.

Meinel, A. J., K. E. Kubow, E. Klotzsch, M. Garcia-Fuentes, M. L. Smith, V. Vogel, H. P. Merkle, and L. Meinel. 2009. Optimization strategies for electrospun silk fibroin tissue engineering scaffolds. *Biomaterials* 30(17): 3058–67.

Miao, M., J. T. Cirulis, S. Lee, and F. W. Keeley. 2005. Structural determinants of cross-linking and hydrophobic domains for self-assembly of elastin-like polypeptides. *Biochemistry* 44(43): 14367–75.

Min, B. M., G. Lee, S. H. Kim, Y. S. Nam, T. S. Lee, and W. H. Park. 2004. Electrospinning of silk fibroin nanofibers and its effect on the adhesion and spreading of normal human keratinocytes and fibroblasts *in vitro*. *Biomaterials* 25(7–8):1289–97.

Mistry, A. S., S. H. Cheng, T. Yeh, E. Christenson, J. A. Jansen, and A. G. Mikos. 2009. Fabrication and *in vitro* degradation of porous fumarate-based polymer/alumoxane nanocomposite scaffolds for bone tissue engineering. *J Biomed Mater Res A* 89(1): 68–79.

Mistry, A. S. and A. G. Mikos. 2005. Tissue engineering strategies for bone regeneration. *Adv Biochem Eng Biotechnol* 94:1–22.

Morishita, M., T. Goto, K. Nakamura, A. M. Lowman, K. Takayama, N. A. Peppas. 2006. Novel oral insulin delivery systems based on complexation polymer hydrogels: Single and multiple administration studiesintype1 and 2 diabeticrats. *J Control Release* 110(3): 587–94.

Morishita, M., T. Goto, N. A. Peppas, J. I. Joseph, M. C. Torjman, C. Munsick, K. Nakamura, T. Yamagata, K. Takayama, and A. M. Lowman. 2004. Mucosal insulin delivery systems based on complexation polymer hydrogels: Effect of particle size on insulin enteral absorption. *J Control Release* 97(1): 115–24.

Motlagh, D., Y. Yang, K. Y. Lui, A. R. Webb, and G. A. Ameer. 2006. Hemocompatibility evaluation of poly(glycerol-sebacate) *in vitro* for vascular tissue engineering. *Biomaterials* 27(24): 4315–24.

Mu, C. J., D. A. LaVan, R. S. Langer, and B. R. Zetter. 2010. Self-assembled gold nanoparticles molecular probes for detecting proteolytic activity *in vivo*. *ACS Nano* 4(3): 1511–20.

Murakami, Y., M. Yokoyama, T. Okano, H. Nishida, Y. Tomizawa, M. Endo, and H. Kurosawa. 2007. A novel synthetic tissue-adhesive hydrogel using a crosslinkable polymeric micelle. *J Biomed Mater Res A* 80(2): 421–7.

Naczynski, D. J., T. Andelman, D. Pal, S. Chen, R. E. Riman, C. M. Roth, and P. V. Moghe. 2010. Albumin nanoshell encapsulation of near-infrared-excitable rare-Earth nanoparticles enhances biocompatibility and enables targeted cell imaging. *Small* 6(15): 1631–40.

Namba, R. M., A. A. Cole, K. B. Bjugstad, and M. J. Mahoney. 2009. Development of porous PEG hydrogels that enable efficient, uniform cell-seeding and permit early neural process extension. *Acta Biomater* 5(6): 1884–97.

Nedopil, A. J., L. G. Mandrussow, and H. E. Daldrup-Link. 2010. Implantation of ferumoxides labeled human mesenchymal stem cells in cartilage defects. *J Vis Exp* 38: 1793.

Noh, H. K., S. W. Lee, J. M. Kim, J. E. Oh, K. H. Kim, C. P. Chung, S. C. Choi, W. H. Park, and B. M. Min. 2006. Electrospinning of chitin nanofibers: Degradation behavior and cellular response to normal human keratinocytes and fibroblasts. *Biomaterials* 27(21): 3934–44.

Ohashi, S., T. Kubo, T. Ikeda, Y. Arai, K. Takahashi, Y. Hirasawa, M. Takigawa, E. Satoh, J. Imanishi, and O. Mazda. 2001. Cationic polymer-mediated genetic transduction into cultured human chondrosarcoma-derived HCS-2/8 cells. *J Orthop Sci* 6(1): 75–81.

Ono, I., T. Yamashita, H. Y. Jin, Y. Ito, H. Hamada, Y. Akasaka, M. Nakasu, T. Ogawa, and K. Jimbow. 2004. Combination of porous hydroxyapatite and cationic liposomes as a vector for BMP-2 gene therapy. *Biomaterials* 25(19): 4709–18.

Paramonov, S. E., H. W. Jun, and J. D. Hartgerink. 2006. Self-assembly of peptide-amphiphile nanofibers: The roles of hydrogen bonding and amphiphilic packing. *J Am Chem Soc* 128(22): 7291–98.

Park, J., J. Ries, K. Gelse, F. Kloss, K. von der Mark, J. Wiltfang, F. W. Neukam, and H. Schneider. 2003. Bone regeneration in critical size defects by cell-mediated BMP-2 gene transfer: A comparison of adenoviral vectors and liposomes. *Gene Ther* 10(13): 1089–98.

Pattison, M. A., S. Wurster, T. J. Webster, and K. M. Haberstroh. 2005. Three-dimensional, nano-structured PLGA scaffolds for bladder tissue replacement applications. *Biomaterials* 26(15): 2491–500.

Peter, M., N. S. Binulala, S. V. Naira, N. Selvamurugana, H. Tamura, and R. Jayakumara. 2010. Novel biodegradable chitosan–gelatin/nano-bioactive glass ceramic composite scaffolds for alveolar bone tissue engineering. *Chem Eng J* 158: 353–61.

Pham, Q. P., U. Sharma, and A. G. Mikos. 2006. Electrospinning of polymeric nanofibers for tissue engineering applications: A review. *Tissue Eng* 12: 1197–211.

Potineni, A., D. M. Lynn, R. Langer, and M. M. Amiji. 2003. Poly(ethyleneoxide)-modified poly(β-aminoester) nanoparticles asapH-sensitive biodegradable system for paclitaxel delivery. *J Control Release* 86(2–3): 223–34.

Powell, H. M. and S. T. Boyce. 2008. Fiber density of electrospun gelatin scaffolds regulates morphogenesis of dermal-epidermal skin substitutes. *J Biomed Mater Res A* 84: 1078–86.

Prabha, S., W. Z. Zhou, J. Panyam, and V. Labhasetwar. 2002. Sizedependency of nanoparticle-mediated gene transfection: Studies with fractionated nanoparticles. *Int J Pharm* 244(1/2): 105–15.

Price, R. L., M. C. Waid, K. M. Haberstroh, and T. J. Webster. 2003. Selective bone cell adhesion on formulations containing carbon nanofibers. *Biomaterials* 24(11): 1877–87.

Pritchard, C. D., K. M. Arnér, R. A. Neal, W. L. Neeley, P. Bojo, E. Bachelder, J. Holz et al. 2010. The use of surface modified poly(glycerol-co-sebacic acid) in retinal transplantation. *Biomaterials* 31(8): 2153–62.

Rajangam, K., M. S. Arnold, M. A. Rocco, and S. I. Stupp. 2008. Peptide amphiphile nanostructure-heparin interactions and their relationship to bioactivity. *Biomaterials* 29(23): 3298–305.

Rajangam, K., H. A. Behanna, M. J. Hui, X. Han, J. F. Hulvat, J. W. Lomasney, and S. I. Stupp. 2006. Heparin binding nanostructures to promote growth of blood vessels. *Nano Lett* 6(9): 2086–90.

Ramaswamy, S., J. B. Greco, M. C. Uluer, Z. Zhang, Z. Zhang, K. W. Fishbein, and R. G. Spencer. 2009. Magnetic resonance imaging of chondrocytes labeled with superparamagnetic iron oxide nanoparticles in tissue-engineered cartilage. *Tissue Eng Part A* 15(12): 3899–910.

Reed, C. R., L. Han, A. Andrady, M. Caballero, M. C. Jack, J. B. Collins, S. C. Saba, E. G. Loboa, B. A. Cairns, and J. A. van Aalst. 2009. Composite tissue engineering on polycaprolactone nanofiber scaffolds. *Ann Plast Surg* 62(5): 505–12.

Robinson, P. S., S. L. Johnson, M. C. Evans, V. H. Barocas, and R. T. Tranquillo. 2008. Functional tissue-engineered valves from cell-remodeled fibrin with commissural alignment of cell-produced collagen. *Tissue Eng Part A*. 14(1): 83–95.

Rodgers, P., A. L. Chun, S. Cantrill, and J. Thomas. 2006. Small is different. *Nature Nanotechnol* 1(1): 1–9.

Rubenstein, D., D. Han, S. Goldgraben, H. El-Gendi, P. I. Gouma, and M. D. Frame. 2007. Bioassay chamber for angiogenesis with perfused explanted arteries and electrospun scaffolding. *Microcirculation* 14(7): 723–37.

Ryou, S. M., S. Kim, H. H. Jang, J. H. Kim, J. H. Yeom, M. S. Eom, J. Bae, M. S. Han, and K. Lee. 2010. Delivery of shRNA using gold nanoparticle–DNA oligonucleotide conjugates as a universal carrier. *Biochem Biophys Res Commun* 398(3): 542–6.

Salvador-Morales, C., L. Zhang, R. Langer, and O. C. Farokhzad. 2009. Immuno compatibility properties of lipid–polymer hybrid nanoparticles with heterogeneous surface functional groups. *Biomaterials* 30(12): 2231–40.

Saraf, A., L. S. Baggett, R. M. Raphael, F. K. Kasper, and A. G. Mikos. 2010. Regulatednon-viral genedelivery from coaxial electrospun fiber mesh scaffolds. *J Control Release* 143(1): 95–103.

Shachar, M., O. Tsur-Gang, T. Dvir, J. Leor, and S. Cohen. 2011. The effect of immobilized RGD peptide in alginate scaffolds on cardiac tissue engineering. *Acta Biomater* 7(1): 152–62.

Shapira-Schweitzer, K., M. Habib, L. Gepstein, and D. Seliktar. 2009. A photopolymerizable hydrogel for 3-D culture of human embryonic stemcell-derived cardio myocytes and rat neonatal cardiac cells. *J Mol Cell Cardiol* 46(2): 213–24.

Shen, H., J. Tan, and W. M. Saltzman. 2004. Surface-mediated gene transfer from nanocomposites of controlled texture. *Nat Mater* 3(8): 569–74.

Shi, J., A. R. Votruba, O. C. Farokhzad, and R. Langer. 2010. Nanotechnology in drug delivery and tissue engineering: from discovery to applications. *Nano Lett* 10(9): 3223–30.

Shi, X., J. L. Hudson, P. P. Spicer, J. M. Tour, R. Krishnamoorti, and A. G. Mikos. 2005. Rheological behaviour and mechanical characterization of injectable poly(propylene fumarate)/single-walled carbon nanotube composites for bone tissue engineering. *Nanotechnology* 16: S531–8.

Shi, X., J. L. Hudson, P. P Spicer, J. M. Tour, R. Krishnamoorti, and A. G. Mikos. 2006. Injectable nanocomposites of single-walled carbon nanotubes and biodegradable polymers for bone tissue engineering. *Biomacromolecules* 7(7): 2237–42.

Shin, M., O. Ishii, T. Sueda, and J. P. Vacanti. 2004. Contractile cardiac grafts using a novel nanofibrous mesh. *Biomaterials* 25: 3717–23.

Shin, M., H. Yoshimoto, and J. P. Vacanti. 2004. *In vivo* bone tissue engineering using mesenchymal stem cells on a novel electrospun nanofibrous scaffold. *Tissue Eng* 10(1/2): 33–41.

Silva, G. A., C. Czeisler, K. L. Niece, E. Beniash, D. A. Harrington, J. A. Kessler, and S. I. Stupp. 2004. Selective differentiation of neural progenitor cells by high-epitope density nanofibers. *Science* 303(5662): 1352–5.

Sitharaman, B., M. Van Der Zande, J. S. Ananta, X. Shi, A. Veltien, X. F. Walboomers, L. J. Wilson, A. G. Mikos, A. Heerschap, and J. A. Jansen. 2010. Magnetic resonance imaging studies on gadonanotube-reinforced biodegradable polymer nanocomposites. *J Biomed Mater Res A* 93(4): 1454–62.

Smith, L. A. and P. X. Ma. 2004. Nano-fibrous scaffolds for tissue engineering. *Coll Surf B Biointerf* 39: 125–31.

Thein-Han, W. W. and R. D. K. Misra. 2009. Biomimetic chitosan- nanohydroxyapatite composite scaffolds for bone tissue engineering. *Acta Biomaterialia* 5: 1182–97.

Thomson, K. S., G. Robinson, F. S. Korte et al. 2010. Cell-seeded fibrin scaffolds for cardiac tissue engineering. *Biophys J* 98(3): 718a.

Tian, H., S. Bharadwaj, Y. Liu, H. Ma, P. X. Ma, Z. Atala, and Y. Zhang. 2010. Myogenic differentiation of human bone marrow mesenchymal stem cells on a 3D nano fibrous scaffold for bladder tissue engineering. *Biomaterials* 31(5): 870–7.

Townsend, S. A., G. D. Evrony, F. X. Gu, M. P. Schulz, R. H. Brown Jr, and R. Langer. 2007. Tetanus toxin C fragment-conjugated nanoparticles for targeted drug delivery to neurons. *Biomaterials* 28(34): 5176–84.

van der Zande, M., B. Sitharaman, X. F. Walboomers, L. Tran, J. S. Ananta, A. Veltien, L. J. Wilson et al. 2011. *In vivo* Magnetic resonance imaging of the distribution pattern of gadonanotubes released from a degrading poly(Lactic-Co-Glycolic Acid) scaffold. *Tissue Eng Part C Methods* 17(1): 19–26.

Venugopal, J. R., S. Low, A. T. Choon, A. B. Kumar, and S. Ramakrishna. 2008. Nanobioengineered electrospun composite nanofibers and osteoblasts for bone regeneration. *Artif Organs* 32: 388–97.

Venugopal, J., S. Low, A. T. Choon, A. B. Kumar, and S. Ramakrishna. 2008. Electrospun-modified nanofibrous scaffolds for the mineralization of osteoblast cells. *J Biomed Mater Res A* 85(2): 408–17.

Vieth, S., C. M. Bellingham, F. W. Keeley, S. M. Hodge, and D. Rousseau. 2007. Microstructural and tensile properties of elastinbased polypeptides crosslinked with genipin and pyrroloquinoline quinone. *Biopolymers* 85(3): 199–206.

Wang, H., Y. Li, Y. Zuo, J. Li, S. Ma, and L. Cheng. 2007. Biocompatibility and osteogenesis of biomimetic nanohydroxyapatite/polyamide composite scaffolds for bone tissue engineering. *Biomaterials* 28: 3338–48.

Webster, T. J., C. Ergun, R. H. Doremus, R. W. Siegel, and R. Bizios. 2000. Specific proteins mediate enhanced osteoblast adhesion on nanophase ceramics. *J Biomed Mater Res* 51(3): 475–83.

Webster, T. J., L. S. Schadler, and R. W. Siegel, and R. Bizios. 2001. Mechanisms of enhanced osteoblast adhesion on nanophase alumina involve vitronectin. *Tissue Eng* 7(3): 291–301.

Webster, T. J., R. W. Siegel, R. Bizios. 1999. Osteoblast adhesion on nanophase ceramics. *Biomaterials* 10(13): 1221–27.

Webster, T. J. and T. A. Smith. 2005. Increased osteoblast function on PLGA composites containing nanophase titania. *J Biomed Mater Res A* 74(4): 677–86.

Wei, G. and P. X. Ma. 2004. Structure and properties of nanohydroxyapatite/polymer composite scaffolds for bone tissue engineering. *Biomaterials* 25(19): 4749–57.

Whitesides, G. M. and M. Boncheva. 2002. Beyond molecules: Self-assembly of mesoscopic and macroscopic components. *Proc Natl Acad Sci USA* 99: 4769–74.

Woo, K. M., V. J. Chen, and P. X. Ma. 2003. Nano-fibrous scaffolding architecture selectively enhances protein adsorption contributing to cell attachment. *J Biomed Mater Res A* 67(2): 531–7.

Woo, K. M., J. H. Jun, V. J. Chen, J. Seo, J. H. Baek, H. M. Ryoo, G. S. Kim, M. J. Somerman, and P. X. Ma. 2007. Nano-fibrous scaffolding promotes osteoblast differentiation and biomineralization. *Biomaterials* 28(2): 335–43.

Woolfson, D. N. and M. G. Ryadnov. 2006. Peptide-based fibrous biomaterials: Some things old, new and borrowed. *Curr Opin Chem Biol* 10: 559–67.

Xu, C. Y., R. Inai, M. Kotaki, and S. Ramakrishna. 2004. Aligned biodegradable nanofibrous structure: A potential scaffold for blood vessel engineering. *Biomaterials* 25: 877–86.

Yan, X., X. Huang, C. Yu, H. Deng, Y. Wang, Z. Zhang, S. Qiao, G. Lu, and D. Zhao. 2006. The in-vitro bioactivity of mesoporous bioactive glasses. *Biomaterials* 27(18): 3396–403.

Yang, F., C. Y. Xu, M. Kotaki, S. Wang, S. Ramakrishna S. 2004. Characterization of neural stem cells on electrospun poly(L-lactic acid) nanofibrous scaffold. *J Biomater Sci Polym Ed.* 15(12): 1483–97.

Yang, F., R. Murugan, S. Wang, and S. Ramakrishna. 2005. Electrospinning of nano/micro scale poly(L-lactic acid) aligned fibers and their potential in neural tissue engineering. *Biomaterials* 26: 2603–10.

Yeong, W. Y., N. Sudarmadji, H. Y. Yu, C. K. Chua, K. F. Leong, S. S. Venkatraman, Y. C. Boey, and L. P. Tan. 2010. Porous polycaprolactone scaffold for cardiac tissue engineering fabricated by selective laser sintering. *Acta Biomater* 6: 2028–34.

Yi, F., H. Wu, and G. L. Jia. 2006. Formulation and characterization of poly(D, L-lactide-co-glycolide) nanoparticle containing vascular endothelial growth factor for gene delivery. *J Clin Pharm Ther* 31(1): 43–8.

Yoo, J. J., and S. H. Rhee. 2004. Evaluations of bioactivity and mechanical properties of poly (e-caprolactone)/silica nanocomposite following heat treatment. *J Biomed Mater Res A* 68(3): 401–10.

Yoshimoto, H., Y. M. Shin, H. Terai, and J. P. Vacanti. 2003. A biodegradable nanofiber scaffold by electrospinning and its potential for bone tissue engineering. *Biomaterials* 24(12): 2077–82.

Zhang, Y., H. He, W. J. Gao, S. Y. Lu, Y. Liu, and H. Y. Gu. 2009. Rapid adhesion and proliferation of keratinocytes on the gold colloid/chitosan film scaffolds. *Mater Sci Eng C* 29(3): 908–12.

Zhang, Z., R. D. Ross, and R. K. Roeder. 2010. Preparation of functionalized gold nanoparticles as a targeted X-ray contrast agent for damaged bone tissue. *Nanoscale* 2(4): 582–6.

Zhu, Y., C. Wu, Y. Ramaswamy et al. 2008. Preparation, characterization and *in vitro* bioactivity of mesoporous bioactive glasses (MBGs) scaffolds for bone tissue engineering. *Microporous and Mesoporous Materials* 112: 494–503.

Zong, X., H. Bien, C. Y. Chung, L. Yin, D. Fang, B. S. Hsiao, B. Chu, and E. Entcheva. 2005. Electrospun fine-textured scaffolds for heart tissue constructs. *Biomaterials* 26(26): 5330–8.

# 12

# Biomimetic Approaches in Tissue Engineering

Indong Jun
*Hanyang University*

Min Sup Kim
*Hanyang University*

Ji-Hye Lee
*Hanyang University*

Young Min Shin
*Hanyang University*

Heungsoo Shin
*Hanyang University*

12.1 Introduction ................................................................................ **12**-1
12.2 Biomimetic Surface Modifications ............................................ **12**-3
12.3 Growth Factor-Presenting Materials......................................... **12**-5
12.4 Biomimetic Hydrogels and Controlled Cell Interactions ........ **12**-6
12.5 Composite Scaffolds Used to Mimic Specific Cellular
     Environments....................................................................... **12**-8
12.6 Scaffolds Mimicking the Structure of ECM ............................ **12**-10
12.7 Conclusions.............................................................................. **12**-11
References.......................................................................................... **12**-12

## 12.1 Introduction

Tissue engineering aims to direct regeneration or repair of damaged tissue through the use of cells, biomaterials, and bioactive signals. During the last several decades, many tissue engineering products have been in clinical use for treating patients suffering from tissue loss or dysfunction in skin, bone, or cartilage, and increasing numbers of clinical trials are currently waiting for approval and commercialization to treat more challenging diseases in nerves and pancreatic tissue (Place et al., 2009). Previously developed tissue engineering products include biomaterial derived from natural as well as synthetic origins, growth factors stimulating tissue morphogenesis, differentiated or progenitor cells, or combinations of these. In particular, for full recovery of biological function of engineered tissues, the strategy of implanting a combination of biomaterials, cells, and growth factors together has been considered the most feasible compared to separate applications of the individual components (Huebsch and Mooney, 2009). However, this strategy has often failed due to lack or absence of an ideal biomaterial that is able to actively control the many functions of native cellular microenvironments.

The roles of biomaterials in tissue engineering are diverse as shown in Figure 12.1; they primarily provide structural support (scaffolds) for cell adhesion and expansion during *ex vivo* cultivation of biopsied cells prior to transplantation (Shin et al., 2003). Cells isolated from patients or donors could be directly injected into patients, and, in some circumstances, biomaterials, including fibrin or collagen, have been coinjected to prevent initial cell loss and to improve graft survival rate (Wang and Guan, 2010a). In some cases, application of cells can be excluded and the scaffold alone can be implanted in order to recruit endogenous progenitors and to prompt them to undergo repair and regeneration processes (Shin et al., 2003). In either approach, appropriate porosity and pore distribution within scaffolds are imperative for the free exchange of gases and cellular by-products, and the scaffolds themselves should be degraded by coordination of tissue in-growth and remodeling with minimal adverse effects. Additionally, scaffolds have been utilized as carriers of tissue-specific chemokines and morphogens (Lee and Shin, 2007). Many of these growth factors are proteins that have a low circulation

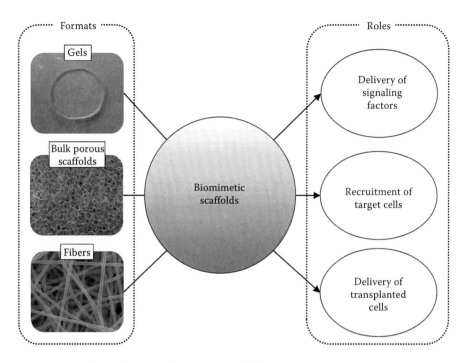

**FIGURE 12.1**    Major roles and formats of biomimetic scaffolds in tissue engineering.

half-life in blood, resulting in abrupt denaturation and loss of biological activities upon systemic injection. Dosage optimization is also important for the retention of therapeutic concentration during specific regeneration or the occurrence of repair events (it could be days or months depending on target tissues). Scaffolds have been designed to incorporate several growth factors and to control their temporal and spatial presentations in order to maximize tissue regeneration. In addition to these relatively simple roles, regeneration of complex tissues requires more defined chemical, mechanical, and physiological characteristics of scaffolds; this has become more evident with improved knowledge of the regulatory mechanisms of the cellular microenvironment in normal tissues that actively govern cell homeostasis and survival (Marklein and Burdick, 2010). In particular, utilization of embryonic and adult stem cells as cell sources has been a major paradigm in tissue engineering, and being able to design scaffolds to precisely control key functions of stem cells may have enormous impact on the full exploitation of their therapeutic potential.

Under normal conditions, cells have intimate contact with neighboring cells via mechanical binding of membrane-bound proteins, allowing for the operation of metabolic machinery via interactions with soluble factors. The main components in cellular microenvironment and how they are interacting with cells are illustrated in Figure 12.2. In addition, cells are surrounded by the extracellular matrix (ECM), conglomerates of biomacromolecules, including polysaccharides and proteins, which provide structural support and trigger biochemical signaling. Many biomacromolecules in the ECM are crosslinked and assembled as fibrous bundles, which are also involved in multiple bindings with residing cells to control diverse cellular activities. The key cellular components involved in adhesion are proteins that exist on the cell surface. Several classes of cell adhesion proteins have been identified, including cadherins, selectins, immunoglobulin-like adhesion molecules, and integrins. Among them, integrins are one of the major glycoproteins able to sense external signals through specific binding with numerous ligands (Hynes, 2002). Some domains, such as the arginine–glycine–aspartic acid (RGD) domain, can specifically bind to integrins, which are widely used to modulate cell adhesion and proliferation on scaffolds (Shin et al., 2003; Marklein and Burdick, 2010). Extracellular domains of transmembrane receptors

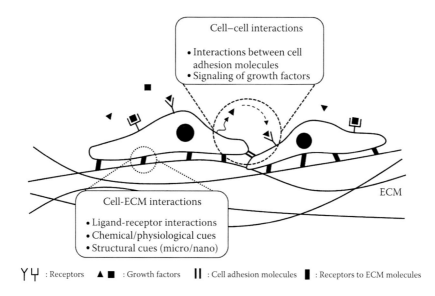

**FIGURE 12.2** Main components in cellular microenvironment.

have specific ligands for receptor-mediated binding, presumably regulating a myriad of cell functions; these have attracted significant attention in scaffold design. Recent reports have demonstrated that not only chemical composition and conformation of proteins and polysaccharides within the context of the cellular microenvironment, but also the overall organization and mechanical properties of the ECM are involved in the regulation of intrinsic cell properties (Engler et al., 2006; Huebsch et al., 2010). For example, subtle changes in the presentation of spatially distributed ligands on a nanometer scale can modulate the clustering of transmembrane receptors and subsequently affect intercellular signaling. Intrinsic elasticity within the cellular environment directs the specificity of the stem cell lineage from soft to hard tissue.

In this chapter, biomimetic approaches in tissue engineering are defined as combined efforts to design scaffolds with defined features that mimic structure and function of the native cellular microenvironment (compared to conventional scaffolds). Particularly, this chapter will focus on the most widely reported themes in biomimetic scaffold design, how they have been exploited in several tissue engineering applications, and the remaining challenges for their use. The main strategies covered in the chapter are summarized in Figure 12.3.

## 12.2 Biomimetic Surface Modifications

The appropriate cellular environment properly regulates cell survival, including adhesion, spreading, proliferation, and differentiation activities. During the development of a tissue engineering strategy, as a structural platform to support tissue homeostasis, biodegradable poly($\alpha$-hydroxy)esters such as poly(lactic-*co*-glycolic acid) (PLGA), poly(L-lactide) (PLLA), and polycaprolactone (PCL) have been widely used as scaffolds due to their biocompatibilities and good mechanical properties (Jeong et al., 2005, 2008; Hutmacher, 2000; Jin et al., 2009). Even though these materials have been useful in the fabrication of controlled porous and/or nanofibrous structures, active control of cellular behaviors has been limited due to the absence of cellular interactivity (Shin et al., 2003; Cheung et al., 2007). In fact, these materials are hydrophobic and lack surface functional groups to modulate cell–material interactions. Therefore, surface modification techniques to immobilize hydrophilic groups and to further incorporate bioactive molecules have attracted significant attention (Furth et al., 2007).

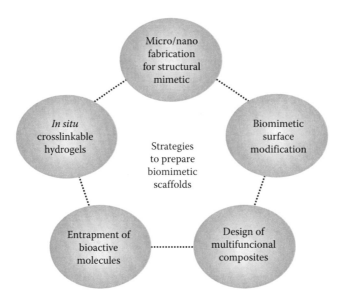

**FIGURE 12.3**    Strategies to prepare biomimetic scaffolds.

The most simple surface modification technique is physical protein adsorption. In these processes, proteins are physically absorbed onto the scaffold surface via ionic bonding and electrostatic interactions, and the substrates with absorbed proteins are simply and easily obtained through dipping into a protein solution (Wilson et al., 2005). For example, PLLA film and nanofibrous mesh were immersed in a 20 g/mL fibronectin and laminin solution for 12 h; the protein-coated substrates exhibited four times greater adhesion of mouse skeletal muscle cells (c2c12) than did the nonmodified substrates (Cui et al., 2003). However, the interactions between the materials and the physically adsorbed proteins are relatively weak and are insufficient to organize long-term cellular behaviors because the proteins can be easily detached from the material surface. To address the problem of physical protein adsorption, covalent immobilization of proteins has also been attempted. To accomplish covalent immobilization, the surfaces of synthetic polymers were pretreated via several processes to enhance the surface functional groups so that covalent immobilization is more favorable, since most synthetic polymers used as scaffolding materials are relatively inert. One previous approach involved surface etching (aminolysis), in which carboxyl (–COOH) groups were simply exposed on the surface by immersing scaffolds in an alkaline solution such as 0.1 or 1 M NaOH, and amide bonds were formed with primary amine groups in most proteins (Zhu et al., 2002). Previously, PLLA films were immersed in 1 M NaOH, and then gelatin was covalently conjugated with EDC/NHS chemistry. The gelatin-conjugated PLLA films accelerated the proliferation of chondrocytes as well as the expressions of collagen type II and GAG (Cui et al., 2003).

Introduction of surface functional groups can be achieved using plasma treatment by altering exposure power, time, and types of gases. High-energy plasma generates free radicals on the surfaces of scaffolds in the presence of argon gas, and hyperoxide is generated on the surfaces. The activated surfaces sequentially react with acrylic acid (AAc), and AAc-grafted surfaces exhibiting COOH group are finally obtained. Klee et al. (2003) previously obtained PVDF–PAAc films by exposing cells to argon plasma (900 W, 30 s) and 20% AAc, and a twofold increase in human osteoblasts over an 8-day period of cultivation was observed after fibronectin conjugation. In addition, AAc was grafted onto PCL films after argon plasma exposure, and collagen was subsequently conjugated on the AAc–PCL films, directing significant enhancement of human dermal fibroblast and myoblast proliferation on the substrates (Cheng and Teoh, 2004). AAc–PLCL films have also been prepared using gamma-ray irradiation (5–15 kGy), and gelatin (2 mg/mL) was further immobilized on the films, which modulated human mesenchymal stem cells (hMSCs) behaviors, including adhesion, spreading, proliferation, and differentiation (Shin et al., 2008). Recently, electron beams, as a source for precise control of high resolution and power, have also been used to induce graft polymerization of AAc (Sun et al., 2004).

As previously mentioned, a potential strategy to enhance cell interactivity using tissue engineering scaffolds is secondary immobilization of adhesion-related proteins. Since major proteins involved in the construction of ECM environments, such as fibronectin, collagen, laminin, and vitronectin, play roles in modulating cell behaviors, they are popular targets of immobilization. For instance, fibronectin was conjugated on PLLA, PCL, and silicone rubber scaffolds and exhibited significantly enhanced survivals for osteoblasts, chondrocytes, and myoblasts (Volcker et al., 2001; Bhati et al., 2001; Lan et al., 2005; Cronin et al., 2004; Klee et al., 2003). Similarly, specific domains present in these proteins have been widely used to enhance cell interactivity using scaffolds (Kim and Park, 2006). The RGD derived from fibronectin peptide has been widely conjugated on prefunctionalized scaffolds; the scaffolds can successfully organize adhesion and proliferation of osteoblasts, myoblasts, fibroblasts, hMSCs, as well as osteogenic differentiation of osteoblasts (Smith and Ma, 2004; Hill et al., 2006; Shin et al., 2010). In addition, nonintegrin-mediated sequences, including Tyr–Ile–Gly–Ser–Arg (YIGSR) peptide, derived from laminin, also control adhesion and proliferation of cells similar to that of the RGD peptide; YIGSR peptide-immobilized polyurethane–polyethylene glycol (PEG) reduced platelet deposition and facilitated endothelialization (Jun and West, 2005). Similarly, when the Arg–Glu–Asp–Val (REDV) peptide was conjugated on a lactide–polyethylene glycol base scaffold, adhesion of human umbilical vein endothelial cells (HUVEC) was enhanced (Park et al., 2010a). Tissue engineering scaffolds functionalized with bioactive molecules have been used in many tissues, including defective bone, cartilage, muscle, and nerve. RGD peptide-conjugated nanofibers modulated differentiation of osteoblasts and showed significant potential to trigger faster bone growth (Shin et al., 2010). Moreover, collagen-modified PLLA scaffolds were shown to facilitate proliferation of chondrocytes for 20 days, suggesting that it would potentially be a more favorable cartilage regeneration system (Ma et al., 2005). In addition, biomimicked nanofibers with collagen demonstrated greater nerve regeneration, with a two times higher survival of neural stem cells (Li et al., 2008). Therefore, incorporation of a variety of ECM proteins and peptides could be the simplest method for modulating a wide range of cellular activities and tissue responses.

## 12.3 Growth Factor-Presenting Materials

Growth factors play a crucial role in information transfer between cells and their ECM in tissue regeneration. Growth factors can also stimulate or inhibit cellular proliferation, differentiation, migration, adhesion, and gene expression. Therefore, many researchers have been interested in the delivery of growth factors to regulate cellular metabolism in order to regenerate the desired tissue from the cells (Babensee et al., 2000). However, many growth factors are rapidly degraded and deactivated by enzymes or other chemical and physical degrading reactions occurring at body temperature and hence have short biological half-lives (Lee et al., 2000). To address these problems, polymeric materials have been frequently used to allow for controlled, sustained, and localized delivery of growth factors, providing the necessary spatial and temporal gradients to regulate cellular metabolism. Polymeric delivery vehicles (as scaffolds) allow for controlled kinetics and dosing of growth factor release, while also protecting the protein from degradation (Tayalia and Mooney, 2009). Growth factors could be incorporated within the scaffolds by simple mixing during the preparation of the scaffolds or could be reversibly introduced by exploiting physiological interactions. Heparin is commonly used as a natural polymer to capture many growth factors in their heparin-binding domains. Another strategy to introduce growth factors in an engineered cellular environment is direct immobilization of growth factors onto scaffolds. However, some growth factors are sensitive to conformational changes, and forced presentation of an active domain during the immobilization process may be a major concern.

Nonetheless, the simplest method for encapsulating growth factors into a polymer matrix is by mixing the factors with the polymer prior to the gelation or crosslinking process. In hydrogels, growth factors are typically encapsulated, and their encapsulation and release profiles from gels are controlled by crosslinking density or shape and by the density of pores in the polymer network. Also, the biological activity and distribution of growth factors after gelation are critical factors. Murphy et al. (2000) fabricated three-dimensional (3D), porous scaffolds of the copolymer 85:15 poly(lactide-*co*-glycolide), including vascular endothelial growth factor (VEGF), into a gas foaming/particulate leaching process, from which VEGF was released slowly and maintained its biological activity over a 15 day period. In another study, epidermal growth factor (EGF) delivery vehicles were made of chitosan, and, during *in vivo* testing, EGF released from the chitosan hydrogels accelerated the decrease of skin defects compared to those of groups without EGF (Alemdaroglu et al., 2006). There have been other studies performed with growth factors encapsulated or imbedded within scaffolds for effective neoepithelialization and bone formation using bFGF and bone morphogenetic protein-2 (BMP-2), respectively (Miyoshi et al., 2005; Pitukmanorom et al., 2008).

Although physical entrapment of growth factors within scaffolds may be simple and easy, control over release kinetic can sometimes be difficult to achieve. In ECM, heparin is a highly sulfated glycosaminoglycan, with lysine-rich heparin-binding domains that are capable of high-affinity binding to several growth factors, including fibroblast growth factors (FGF), VEGF, BMP-2, and others. The interactions between heparin and heparin-binding growth factors are reversible depending on the physiological properties of the surrounding environment. Thus, various growth factor delivery systems have exploited heparin to actively capture and liberate heparin-binding growth factors. Patel et al. (2007) fabricated heparin conjugated PLLA nanofibers, and these nanofibers stored and released bFGF in a controlled manner. Using these nanofibers, they determined that released bFGF enhanced neurite outgrowth from DRG tissues and migration of fibroblasts compared to groups without bFGF. Similar studies have demonstrated that heparin immobilization onto scaffolds is effective for the controlled release of bFGF and other heparin-binding growth factors (Jeon et al., 2006; Freeman et al., 2008).

As described above, growth factors regulate cellular behaviors, and many researchers have focused on regenerating the desired tissue from cells in *in vivo* experiments targeted for wound healing, angiogenesis, and regeneration of bone and nerve. Although the majority of studies using growth factors were based on a system in which growth factors are released in a soluble form, Choi et al. (2008) fabricated EGF immobilized on PCL–PEG copolymer nanofibers for the purpose of treating diabetic ulcers. The EGF-nanofibers showed enhanced *in vivo* wound healing activities compared to those of control groups (without EGF) or those of EGF solutions alone, indicating that this particular growth factor can be activated from an immobilized state. Hosseinkhani et al. (2007) fabricated a self-assembled peptide-amphiphile (PA) to induce enhanced ectopic bone formation through the controlled release of BMP-2. During *in vivo* testing, the injection of PA together with BMP-2 into the back subcutis of rats resulted in significant bone formation around the injection site compared to those of BMP-2 injection alone or PA injection alone. Heparin-conjugated fibrin gel was also effective for the controlled delivery of nerve growth factor (NGF); after *in vivo* testing of rats, groups receiving heparin and NGF demonstrated that controlled release of NGF factors enhanced significant peripheral nerve regeneration (Lee et al., 2003). Another study combined heparin and PA to deliver VEGF and bFGF, demonstrating that the released dual-growth factors induced greater blood vessel formation compared to those of groups with mono-growth factor (Rajangam et al., 2006).

## 12.4 Biomimetic Hydrogels and Controlled Cell Interactions

Hydrogels are 3D networks of polymeric chains which are formed via covalent or noncovalent crosslinking reactions. They provide a favorable environment for cell growth due to high biocompatibility and could be used as an injectable format to fill tissue defects. Moreover, many hydrogels are resistant to nonspecific protein adsorption and therefore have been widely studied as potential platforms for the incorporation of proteins and peptides in ECM to control cell–scaffolds interactions. The capability to absorb large amounts of water allows for the entrapment and sustainability of the release of growth factors or chemokines for suitable tissue growth via diffusion-mediated mechanisms (Lutolf, 2009; Slaughter et al., 2009).

Early work with PEG hydrogels focused on immobilization of cell-adhesive and nonadhesive peptide sequences derived from ECM proteins to modulate cell adhesion, spreading, and proliferation. The peptide sequences Arg–Gly–Asp (RGD, fibronectin), Tyr–Ile–Gly–Ser–Arg (YIGSR, laminin), Ile–Lys–Val–Ala–Val (IKVAV, fibrinogen), Ile–Lys–Leu–Leu–Ile (IKLLI), and Pro–Asp–Ser–Gly– Arg (PDSGR) were widely studied for specific cell–matrix interactions (Meiners and Mercado, 2003). The pioneering work with these themes was reported by Hubbell and his colleagues, suggesting that incorporation of the cell-adhesive peptide domain is critical for *in vitro* neurite extension and *in vivo* bone formation (Hubbell, 1999). Other types of hydrogels have also been synthesized. Recent work by Benton et al. (2009) reported that valvular interstitial cells cultured within hydrogels composed of PEG-norbornene as a photo-polymerizable polymer along with various concentrations of RGD peptide (0 ~ 2000 μM) increased the projected area and spreading of the cells with increasing peptide concentration. Hydrogels can serve as a reservoir to entrap growth factors and regulate cellular behavior. For example, precursor solutions consisting of primary hepatocytes, thermosensitive PEG–DA, thiolated heparin, and hepatocyte growth factor (HGF) (capable of binding with heparin via electrostatic interactions) were used to prepare hydrogels to control the release of HGF. As a result, the encapsulated primary hepatocytes produced statistically increased levels of albumin and urea as an important factor of liver metabolism (Kim et al., 2010b). These results indicate that hydrogels coupled with appropriate signals can provide an optimal cellular growth environment. In addition, in an ischemia model, a microbead-like hydrogel system incorporating HGF was injected into the hind limb, revealing relatively higher levels of ischemic leg limb perfusion, alpha SMA expression, and blood vessel formation (Ruvinov et al., 2010).

One of the most interesting features of hydrogels is their versatility of mechanical properties with minimal alteration of other environmental factors. Analysis with alginate hydrogels using diverse stiffness suggests that the mechanics of adhesive substrates may regulate the cell proliferation and transfection efficiency of nonviral vectors (Kong et al., 2005). Acrylamide gels with immobilized collagen possess a broad range of elasticity, which has been used to demonstrate that stem cells can be differentiated into myogenic, neurogenic, and osteogenic lineages upon elasticity sensing. Recently, modified gelatin with 3-(4-hydroxyphenyl) propionic acid (HPA) was synthesized and prepared as a hydrogel via enzyme polymerization using $H_2O_2$ and horseradish peroxidase (HRP). hMSCs were cultured with gelatin-modified hydrogels prepared as soft (281 Pa) and hard (841 Pa) types; it was reported that the neurogenic differentiation within 3D gelatin hydrogels showed different levels of several neurogenic differentiation markers such as β3-tubulin, NFH, NFL, and MAP2 (Wang et al., 2010b). These results suggest that biomimetic hydrogels with tunable mechanical properties can serve as useful tools to address fundamental questions regarding the mechanobiological regulation of cellular microenvironments of various cell types and as regulators of specific cell functions for tissue regeneration. Cellular behaviors, including cell adhesion, spreading, differentiation, and ECM deposition, are known to be dictated by micro- or nanoscale arrangements and by geographical patterns of the underlying matrices. Under physiological conditions, muscle tissue has anisotropic alignment, and many studies have shown that differentiation of myoblasts is affected by these anisotropically patterned hydrogels. For example, myocytes cultured on nanoscale-patterned anisotropic PEG hydrogels showed greater expression of connexin 43 protein and increased conduction velocity of connexin gap junctions, an important parameter in the characterization of biologically functional cardiac tissue formation (Kim et al., 2010a). In addition, cultured myoblasts revealed higher differentiation characteristics on PDMS hydrogels using a master mold and fabricated using electron-beam lithography (EBL) to form an array of 120 nm diameter pits of 100 nm depth and 300 nm pitch in hexagonal and square arrangements than they did on nonpatterned hydrogels with respect to the expression of α-actinin, a characteristic gene of myogenic differentiation (Shimizu et al., 2009). In addition to muscle cells, Matthew et al. reported that hMSCs cultured on nanoscale symmetry hydrogels or with disorder patterning showed higher bone mineralization on a substrate with disordered patterns (Dalby et al., 2007). These results indicate that providing geometrical signals to hydrogels may synergistically guide tissue formation.

Cells cultured on the surfaces of hydrogels may be useful as an *in vitro* defined culture system to investigate the physiology and pathophysiology of both cells and tissues. The two-dimensional culture system, however, does not provide a microenvironment close to that *in vivo* and therefore may not represent an accurate model. The main drawbacks of the two-dimensional culture hydrogel system are the insufficient regulation of 3D architecture and the variations in biochemical cues from those of the *in vivo* environment, which may alter metabolism and reduce the functionalities of cells (Lutolf et al., 2009; Tibbitt and Anseth, 2009).

The movements and polarizations of cells are dynamically controlled by degradation of crosslinked ECM biomolecules in the vicinity of cells in response to specific enzymes secreted by the cells themselves. Specifically, matrix metalloproteinases (MMP) cause a disruption in the physical barrier inside the ECM, which may allow for cellular invasion, intravasation, extravastion, and migration. Although encapsulation of cells in natural hydrogels such as collagen and fibrin can be successful, these natural hydrogels can be degraded by secreted enzymes, including collagenase, stromelysin, and gelatinase, to enhance 3D migration; thus they are intrinsically lacking in mechanical properties. To address this problem, synthetic hydrogels that mimic proteolytic degradation properties have been developed. Using a Michael-type addition reaction, 4-arm-PEG-tetravinyl sulfone, mono-cysteine adhesion peptide, and bis-cysteine MMP substrate peptide (GPQGIWGQK) were combined to prepare hydrogels with encapsulated human foreskin fibroblasts (HFF). The hydrogels were degraded in response to proteases secreted from HFF residing within the hydrogels, resulting in free cell migration into the partially degraded hydrogel network (Lutolf et al., 2003). Similarly, using hydrogels consisting of PEG–DA, cell-adhesive peptide (CGRGDS), primary chick aortas cells, and MMP-sensitive peptide, researchers demonstrated that the angiogenic sprout of an aorta was regulated by the MMP-susceptibility of the hydrogel backbone (Miller et al., 2010). Recently, more advanced approaches have been reported, in which the angiogenic growth factor VEGF was genetically modified to have a terminal thiol group that was covalently incorporated into the hydrogel through photopolymerization, with a proteolytic sequence as a spacer. When subcutaneously implanted into male Lewis rats *in vivo*, the hydrogels were degraded by the activity of the proteases secreted by the cells, and the VEGF was released in response to the proteolytic enzymes that controlled the release rate (Phelps et al., 2010).

## 12.5 Composite Scaffolds Used to Mimic Specific Cellular Environments

In the development of scaffolds for tissue regeneration, the use of composite materials with diverse chemical and physical properties may be plausible to mimic the complex cellular microenvironment. In general, composite scaffolds can be prepared using a simple combination of both natural and synthetic polymers and both organic and inorganic materials, which are desired for their unique properties. Here, we will briefly discuss composite scaffolds used in bone, muscle, and neural tissue regeneration.

As discussed in the previous section, one major drawback of using synthetic polymers as a scaffold material is the limited cellular interaction capability due to the absence of a bioactive domain. Immobilization of proteins and peptides present in the ECM may partially alleviate these problems. The preparation of composite materials by physically mixing synthetic biodegradable polymers with natural polymers such as chitosan or collagen has been sought as an alternative strategy. In a study of composite materials by Ghasemi-Mobarakeh et al. (2008), poly(ε-carprolactone) and gelatin were mixed in a 70:30 ratio and electrospun to fabricate random and aligned fibers. The results showed increased neural cell proliferation in gelatin-containing fibers in both random and aligned structures. It was also reported that the introduction of gelatin into synthetic polymers affected differentiation of hMSCs (Rim et al., 2009). The incorporation of gelatin into a poly[(L-lactide)-*co*-(e-caprolactone)] (PLCL) matrix increased the cellularity and controlled morphology of cultured hMSCs as a function of the concentration of gelatin in the matrix compared to those of PLCL-only nanofibers. Moreover, under osteogenic differentiation conditions, the expression of osteogenic differentiation-associated genes, alkaline phosphatase activity, and calcium deposition were enhanced in the gelatin-containing PLCL nanofibers compared to those of the PLCL group, indicating that physical mixing of natural and synthetic polymers can regulate many cell functions, including adhesion and osteogenic differentiation of stem cells. A similar approach was applied to the development of scaffolds for cardiac tissue engineering, in which three different materials were combined to mimic the chemical and mechanical properties of myocardium; PLCL was used as a basic matrix to provide stable mechanical properties and elasticity, PLGA was incorporated to retard the overall degradation rate of the matrix, and collagen was added to improve the bioactivities of the scaffolds (Park et al., 2005). Other groups developed composites of synthetic and natural polymers for articular cartilage regeneration in which thin knitted PLGA meshes were used as a skeleton for mechanical support and collagen was incorporated as a thick layer on both sides of the PLGA skeleton to increase the overall thickness. The results showed improved syntheses of aggrecan and type-2 collagen on the composite forms when the chondrocytes were cultured for 8 weeks (Dai et al., 2010). These results suggest that composites of natural and synthetic polymers can easily recapitulate appropriate cellular events for successful tissue regeneration.

It is well known that proliferation or differentiation of nerve or muscle tissue can be enhanced by electrical stimulation, which is in part attributed to the propagation of action potentials upon stimulation. To exploit these physiological events, composites of biodegradable polymers with electroconductive materials have been investigated for effective transmission of electrical signals to the cells cultured on them. PLCL and polyaniline, one of the widely used electrically conductive materials, were mixed to fabricate the nanofiber meshes, illustrating that myotube formation was accelerated when the myoblasts were cultured on polyaniline-containing nanofibers compared to that of PLCL-only nanofibers, even without electrical stimulation (Jun et al., 2009). Another electroconductive polymer, polypyrrole, was also used as a composite with other synthetic polymers. For example, polypyrrole was incorporated as particles into polylactide scaffolds, and the fibroblasts cultured on them with various intensities of DC current showed controlled proliferation in a current-dependent manner (Shi et al., 2004).

Unlike other tissues, bone is composed of over 70% inorganic constituents rich in calcium and phosphate ions. This unique chemical composition has been known to influence bone development and repair. Therefore, composites of synthetic polymer matrices with bone-like inorganic chemicals have been widely used to facilitate bone formation. For example, when hydroxyapatites were incorporated into PLGA nanofibers, the osteogenic differentiation of hMSCs was better than that in cells cultured on pure PLGA nanofibers, as shown by their osteoconductive effect (Lee et al., 2010). The composite nanofibers of tricalcium phosphates and PLLA were also reported as a scaffold for the culture of adipose-derived stem cells (ADSC), demonstrating enhanced cellular proliferation and ALP activity, suggesting that chemicals with structures similar to bone can modulate the osteogenic differentiation of ADSC (McCullen et al., 2009). Instead of using composites, carbonated hydroxyapatite crystals can be formed in simulated body fluid (SBF); PCL nanofibers were incubated in SBF solution to produce a bone-like mineral film, which can also control cell adhesion and proliferation (Araujo et al., 2008). The composites of calcium phosphates can be formulated as a gel as well as a solid type of scaffold. When hydroxyapatite and tricalcium phosphate or biphasic calcium phosphate (BCP) were mixed with fibrin gel and subsequently injected into sheep muscle, formation of mineralized bone was observed 6 months after implantation (Le Nihouannen et al., 2008). Similarly, biphasic calcium phosphate/PLGA composite scaffolds improved the regeneration of alveolar bone 24 weeks after implantation (Ajdukovic et al., 2007).

Although tissue engineering approaches have led to regeneration or repair of damaged tissue, the success is often only partial; the original biological function is often not regained due to limited integration with native tissue or incomplete recovery of chemical and biological compositions of the tissue interface. Geometrically, the tissue interface, that is, cartilage–bone, tendon/ligament–bone, or muscle–tendon, is placed between two dissimilar tissues; however, the chemical composition, orientation, and structure of the ECMs exhibit profound differences. In order to engineer such a complicated tissue structure, biphasic scaffolds are also required for effective regeneration of two types of tissues and their interfaces. For example, polycaprolactone(PCL)-poly(glycolic acid)(PGA) hybrid scaffolds were fabricated for reconstruction of the tooth and gingival interface. The scaffolds were fabricated using a 3D printing technique; PGA was targeted for the periodontal ligament region, and PCL was targeted for bone regeneration. The human gingival fibroblasts and human periodontal ligament cells were separately seeded onto each side of the scaffold, and the *in vivo* results showed that the formed structure appeared to be similar to those of tooth cementum-like tissue, ligament, and bone (Park et al., 2010b). To mimic the epi/endothelium (collagen-rich connective tissue/muscle layer that exists in hollow organs), collagen matrices were stitched onto PGA scaffolds using threaded collagen fibers. Urothelial and bladder smooth muscle cells were seeded onto composite scaffolds, and the construct formed a bladder tissue-like structure, showing histological evidence of the presence of both layers 4 weeks after *in vivo* implantation into mice (Eberli et al., 2009). Osteochondral composite scaffolds were also developed for the treatment of defects in both bone and cartilage; the upper layer of the scaffolds was made of a mixture of hyaluronic acid and collagen, and the bottom layer was of collagen with a high composition of hydroxyapatite. In addition, the intermediate layer was composed of collagen with a relatively lower content of hydroxyapatite. When bone marrow stem cells were seeded onto the scaffolds, the cells differentiated into different types of cells in response to the local chemical composition of the matrix. Chondrocytes were seen on the upper layer, with osteoblasts on the bottom (Tampieri et al., 2008). Composite scaffolds of multiple components may also be useful for other applications. For example, tripolyphosphate was mixed with PLGA to neutralize the acidic degradation product of PLGA after *in vivo* implantation (Xie et al., 2010). Incorporation of PEO into a nanofibrous system was effective for control and porosity of fibers after coelectrospinning using 50% EtOH (Ionescu et al., 2010). Thus, the method to prepare composite combined scaffolds is useful for mimicking the complex microenvironment of the body through full exploitation of mechanical, chemical, and physiological properties of the constituent materials.

## 12.6 Scaffolds Mimicking the Structure of ECM

In tissue engineering, the regeneration of tissue can be obtained through the cultivation of cells on the appropriate scaffolds. These scaffolds play the role of the native ECM and mimic its fibrous and porous structures (size: from micro- to nanometer), which are composed of various biomolecules. Thus, scaffolds with various structural alterations have been developed to modulate cellular behaviors via property control, including morphology, porosity, pore density, surface, and mechanical properties.

Generally, control over pore structure and distribution and micro/nanoscale structures have been achieved using several scaffold-preparation methods, including salt leaching, phase separation, peptide assembly, knitting fibers, and electrospinning. Kang et al. (2006) fabricated gelatin scaffolds with dual pores using a modified overrun process for closed pores and a particle-leaching technique (NaCl and sucrose) for open pores. These gelatin scaffolds could also easily modulate the distribution and shapes of dual pores. A report by Liu et al. (2000) showed that the pore shape of macroporous poly(2-hydroxyethyl methacrylate) (p(HEMA)) hydrogels with NaCl was dependent on the concentration of NaCl. They found that the swelling ratio increased with increasing equilibrium water content and hydrogel porosity. Cooper et al. (2005) developed a PLGA graft with microfibrous scaffolds for the anterior cruciate ligament (ACL). These PLGA grafts had easily controllable architecture, porosity, degradability, and mechanical properties for regeneration of the ligament. Moreover, their microfibrous scaffolds exhibited optimal pore diameters (175–233 micron) for ligament tissue ingrowth, and initial mechanical properties of the construct approximated those of the native ligament. The arrangement of fibers regulates the overall mechanical properties and matrix deposition patterns of cultured cells. A 3D weaving technique was used to generate anisotropic 3D woven structures for cartilage tissue constructs, and these scaffolds showed mechanical properties on the same order of magnitude as values for native articular cartilage, as measured by compressive, tensile, and shear testing. Moreover, they observed that the developed scaffolds had the potential for direct implantation *in vivo* with biological support without requiring cultivation *in vitro* (Moutos et al., 2007).

Biomolecules with distinct hydrophobic and hydrophilic domains such as peptides can form self-assembled nanostructures via weak interactions, such as hydrogen bonding, hydrophobic interactions, and Van der Waals interactions. For application as a cell culture substrate and drug delivery vehicle, self-assembled nanostructures could easily be functionalized by incorporating peptide sequences that direct cell behavior into the buildup molecule. Gelain et al. (2007) developed self-assembling peptide nanofibers that were able to be utilized as a cell culture substrate and drug delivery vehicles for the regeneration of peripheral nerve and cardiomyocytes. Electrospinning is an additional method of producing nano/microscale fibers, and it provides a simple and versatile method to fabricate nanofibrous scaffolds with various biocompatible polymers. This method has been widely modified for nonwoven and oriented fiber development for cell culture substrates and for tubular fibers used as vehicles in the delivery of therapeutic proteins. Using nonwoven and oriented fibers, researchers investigated the control of cellular responses according to polymer composition, porosity, physical properties, and fiber morphology. Also, using tubular fibers, they investigated the delivery efficiencies of drug or protein target cells and tissues. Kim et al. (2010c) fabricated a polycaprolactone-gelatin (PG) composite of nonwoven fibers and evaluated its physical properties based on the content of gelatin in the fibers. They observed enhanced myogenesis on the PG composite nonwoven fibers with increasing contents of gelatin. The electrospinning process is advantageous for controlling porosity and fiber diameter, major parameters in the regulation of cell function. For example, a study using nonwoven fibers that were able to control porosity using PCL and water-soluble PEO particles in which the porosity of nonwoven fibers was effectively modulated by leaching PEO particles demonstrated that nonwoven fibers with high porosity induced higher differentiation of osteoblasts (Ekaputra et al., 2008). Polyethersulfone nonwoven fibers with various fiber diameters used to investigate the behaviors of neural stem cells on fibers were effective in modulating differentiation and migration of neural stem cells as a function of fiber diameter (Christopherson et al., 2009).

There is an increasing body of evidence that suggesting that surface geometry and topography affect the regulatory mechanisms of certain type of cells. Charest et al. (2007) developed topographic patterns on scaffolds consisting of embossed ridges and grooves or arrays of holes to investigate the differentiation of myoblasts. They observed higher alignment of myoblasts on grooves and the highest degree of differentiation at 5 ~ 25 µm patterns. Also, they found that microscale topography modulates myoblast alignment but did not have an effect on cell density. To mimic the mechanical properties of the ventricular myocardium recognized as anisotropic tissue, microfabrication techniques were used to create an accordion-like honeycomb microstructure in poly(glycerol sebacate). These scaffolds show similar mechanical properties and microstructures to the native myocardium, which may be dictated by the fiber orientation (Engelmayr et al., 2008). Using an electrospinning technique, oriented fibers can be produced easily by modulating the velocity of the collecting drum. These oriented fibers allowed for the induction of fibroblast migration (Kurpinski et al., 2010), differentiation of human coronary artery smooth muscle cells (Xu et al., 2004) and cardiomyocytes (Zong et al., 2005) and have been further utilized as vascular graft materials (Hashi et al., 2007).

## 12.7 Conclusions

The detailed understanding of regulatory mechanisms of cellular interaction with the microenvironment and how these mutual communications translate to the development, repair, and regeneration of certain types of tissues has long been a goal of many biologists and medical scientists. Although the goal has not been completely achieved and many challenges still remain, the gradual understanding in the field has spurred scientists in material engineering to create novel biomaterials that can be recognized by cells and that are responsive to cellular secretions and production in ways similar to those occurring in the native cellular microenvironment. These materials can be used in many biological applications, particularly holding great potential as scaffolds for tissue engineering. With conventional properties such as biocompatibility and degradability, the scaffold should be designed to manipulate the fates of implanted and endogenous cells and to actively modulate tissue regeneration. Biomimetic approaches discussed in this chapter and other creative methods to be developed would definitely open a new era for redefining new roles for biological scaffold.

# References

Ajdukovic, Z., Ignjatovic, N., Petrovic, D. et al. 2007. Substitution of osteoporotic alveolar bone by biphasic calcium phosphate/poly-DL-lactide-*co*-glycolide biomaterials. *J Biomater Appl* 21: 317–28.

Alemdaroglu, C., Degim, Z., Celebi, N. et al. 2006. An investigation on burn wound healing in rats with chitosan gel formulation containing epidermal growth factor. *Burns* 32: 319–27.

Araujo, J. V., Martins, A., Leonor, I. B. et al. 2008. Surface controlled biomimetic coating of polycaprolactone nanofiber meshes to be used as bone extracellular matrix analogues. *J Biomater Sci Polym Ed* 19: 1261–78.

Babensee, J. E., Mcintire, L. V., and Mikos, A. G. 2000. Growth factor delivery for tissue engineering. *Pharmaceut Res* 17: 497–504.

Benton, J. A., Fairbanks, B. D., and Anseth, K. S. 2009. Characterization of valvular interstitial cell function in three dimensional matrix metalloproteinase degradable PEG hydrogels. *Biomaterials* 30: 6593–603.

Bhati, R. S., Mukherjee, D. P., Mccarthy, K. J. et al. 2001. The growth of chondrocytes into a fibronectin-coated biodegradable scaffold. *J Biomed Mater Res* 56: 74–82.

Charest, J. L., Garcia, A. J., and King, W. P. 2007. Myoblast alignment and differentiation on cell culture substrates with microscale topography and model chemistries. *Biomaterials* 28: 2202–10.

Cheng, Z. and Teoh, S. H. 2004. Surface modification of ultra thin poly (epsilon-caprolactone) films using acrylic acid and collagen. *Biomaterials* 25: 1991–2001.

Cheung, H. Y., Lau, K. T., Lu, T. P. et al. 2007. A critical review on polymer-based bio-engineered materials for scaffold development. *Composites Part B-Eng* 38: 291–300.

Choi, J. S., Leong, K. W., and Yoo, H. S. 2008. *in vivo* wound healing of diabetic ulcers using electrospun nanofibers immobilized with human epidermal growth factor (EGF). *Biomaterials* 29: 587–96.

Christopherson, G. T., Song, H., and Mao, H. Q. 2009. The influence of fiber diameter of electrospun substrates on neural stem cell differentiation and proliferation. *Biomaterials* 30: 556–64.

Cooper, J. A., Lu, H. H., Ko, F. K. et al. 2005. Fiber-based tissue-engineered scaffold for ligament replacement: Design considerations and *in vitro* evaluation. *Biomaterials* 26: 1523–32.

Cronin, E. M., Thurmond, F. A., Bassel-Duby, R. et al. 2004. Protein-coated poly(L-lactic acid) fibers provide a substrate for differentiation of human skeletal muscle cells. *J Biomed Mater Res Part A* 69A: 373–81.

Cui, Y. L., Hou, X., Qi, A. D. et al. 2003. Biomimetic surface modification of poly(L-lactic acid) with gelatin and its effects on articular chondrocytes in vitro. *J Biomed Mater Res A* 66: 770–8.

Dai, W., Kawazoe, N., Lin, X. et al. 2010. The influence of structural design of PLGA/collagen hybrid scaffolds in cartilage tissue engineering. *Biomaterials* 31: 2141–52.

Dalby, M. J., Gadegaard, N., Tare, R. et al. 2007. The control of human mesenchymal cell differentiation using nanoscale symmetry and disorder. *Nat Mater* 6: 997–1003.

Eberli, D., Freitas Filho, L., Atala, A. et al. 2009. Composite scaffolds for the engineering of hollow organs and tissues. *Methods* 47: 109–15.

Ekaputra, A. K., Prestwich, G. D., Cool, S. M. et al. 2008. Combining electrospun scaffolds with electrosprayed hydrogels leads to three-dimensional cellularization of hybrid constructs. *Biomacromolecules* 9: 2097–103.

Engelmayr, G. C., JR., Cheng, M., Bettinger, C. J. et al. 2008. Accordion-like honeycombs for tissue engineering of cardiac anisotropy. *Nat Mater* 7: 1003–10.

Engler, A. J., Sen, S., Sweeney, H. L. et al. 2006. Matrix elasticity directs stem cell lineage specification. *Cell* 126: 677–89.

Freeman, I., Kedem, A., and Cohen, S. 2008. The effect of sulfation of alginate hydrogels on the specific binding and controlled release of heparin-binding proteins. *Biomaterials* 29: 3260–8.

Furth, M. E., Atala, A., and Van Dyke, M. E. 2007. Smart biomaterials design for tissue engineering and regenerative medicine. *Biomaterials* 28: 5068–73.

Gelain, F., Horii, A., and Zhang, S. G. 2007. Designer self-assembling peptide scaffolds for 3-D tissue cell cultures and regenerative medicine. *Macromol Biosci* 7: 544–51.

Ghasemi-Mobarakeh, L., Prabhakaran, M. P., Morshed, M. et al. 2008. Electrospun poly(epsilon-caprolactone)/gelatin nanofibrous scaffolds for nerve tissue engineering. *Biomaterials* 29: 4532–9.

Hashi, C. K., Zhu, Y., Yang, G. Y. et al. 2007. Antithrombogenic property of bone marrow mesenchymal stem cells in nanofibrous vascular grafts. *Proc Natl Acad Sci USA* 104: 11915–20.

Hill, E., Boontheekul, T., and Mooney, D. J. 2006. Regulating activation of transplanted cells controls tissue regeneration. *Proc Natl Acad Sci USA* 103: 2494–9.

Hosseinkhani, H., Hosseinkhani, M., Khademhosseini, A. et al. 2007. Bone regeneration through controlled release of bone morphogenetic protein-2 from 3-D tissue engineered nano-scaffold. *J Contr Rel* 117: 380–6.

Hubbell, J. A. 1999. Bioactive biomaterials. *Curr Opin Biotechnol* 10: 123–9.

Huebsch, N., Arany, P. R., Mao, A. S. et al. 2010. Harnessing traction-mediated manipulation of the cell/matrix interface to control stem-cell fate. *Nat Mater* 9: 518–26.

Huebsch, N. and Mooney, D. J. 2009. Inspiration and application in the evolution of biomaterials. *Nature* 462: 426–32.

Hutmacher, D. W. 2000. Scaffolds in tissue engineering bone and cartilage. *Biomaterials* 21: 2529–43.

Hynes, R. O. 2002. Integrins: Bidirectional, allosteric signaling machines. *Cell* 110: 673–87.

Ionescu, L. C., Lee, G. C., Sennett, B. J. et al. 2010. An anisotropic nanofiber/microsphere composite with controlled release of biomolecules for fibrous tissue engineering. *Biomaterials* 31: 4113–20.

Jeon, O., Kang, S. W., Lim, H. W. et al. 2006. Long-term and zero-order release of basic fibroblast growth factor from heparin-conjugated poly(L-lactide-*co*-glycolide) nanospheres and fibrin gel. *Biomaterials* 27: 1598–607.

Jeong, S. I., Kwon, J. H., Lim, J. I. et al. 2005. Mechano-active tissue engineering of vascular smooth muscle using pulsatile perfusion bioreactors and elastic Plcl scaffolds. *Biomaterials* 26: 1405–11.

Jeong, S. I., Lee, A. Y., Lee, Y. M. et al. 2008. Electrospun gelatin/poly(L-lactide-*co*-epsilon-caprolactone) nanofibers for mechanically functional tissue-engineering scaffolds. *J Biomater Sci Polym Ed* 19: 339–57.

Jin, J., Jeong, S. I., Shin, Y. M. et al. 2009. Transplantation of mesenchymal stem cells within a poly(lactide-*co*-epsilon-caprolactone) scaffold improves cardiac function in a rat myocardial infarction model. *Eur J Heart Fail* 11: 147–53.

Jun, H. W. and West, J. L. 2005. Modification of polyurethaneurea with Peg and Yigsr peptide to enhance endothelialization without platelet adhesion. *J Biomed Mater Res B Appl Biomater* 72: 131–9.

Jun, I., Jeong, S., and Shin, H. 2009. The stimulation of myoblast differentiation by electrically conductive sub-micron fibers. *Biomaterials* 30: 2038–47.

Kang, H. G., Kim, S. Y., and Lee, Y. M. 2006. Novel porous gelatin scaffolds by overrun/particle leaching process for tissue engineering applications. *J Biomed Mater Res B Appl Biomater* 79B: 388–97.

Kim, D. H., Lipke, E. A., Kim, P. et al. 2010a. Nanoscale cues regulate the structure and function of macroscopic cardiac tissue constructs. *Proc Natl Acad Sci USA* 107: 565–70.

Kim, M., Lee, J. Y., Jones, C. N. et al. 2010b. Heparin-based hydrogel as a matrix for encapsulation and cultivation of primary hepatocytes. *Biomaterials* 31: 3596–603.

Kim, M. S., Jun, I., Shin, Y. M. et al. 2010c. The development of genipin-crosslinked poly(caprolactone) (PCL)/gelatin nanofibers for tissue engineering applications. *Macromol Biosci* 10: 91–100.

Kim, T. G. and Park, T. G. 2006. Biomimicking extracellular matrix: Cell adhesive Rgd peptide modified electrospun poly(D,L-lactic-*co*-glycolic acid) nanofiber mesh. *Tissue Eng* 12: 221–33.

Klee, D., Ademovic, Z., Bosserhoff, A. et al. 2003. Surface modification of poly(vinylidenefluoride) to improve the osteoblast adhesion. *Biomaterials* 24: 3663–70.

Kong, H. J., Liu, J. D., Riddle, K. et al. 2005. Non-viral gene delivery regulated by stiffness of cell adhesion substrates. *Nat Mater* 4: 460–4.

Kurpinski, K. T., Stephenson, J. T., Janairo, R. R. et al. 2010. The effect of fiber alignment and heparin coating on cell infiltration into nanofibrous Plla scaffolds. *Biomaterials* 31: 3536–42.

Lan, M. A., Gersbach, C. A., Michael, K. E. et al. 2005. Myoblast proliferation and differentiation on fibronectin-coated self assembled monolayers presenting different surface chemistries. *Biomaterials* 26: 4523–31.

Le Nihouannen, D., Saffarzadeh, A., Gauthier, O. et al. 2008. Bone tissue formation in sheep muscles induced by a biphasic calcium phosphate ceramic and fibrin glue composite. *J Mater Sci Mater Med* 19: 667–75.

Lee, A. C., Yu, V. M., Lowe, J. B. et al. 2003. Controlled release of nerve growth factor enhances sciatic nerve regeneration. *Exp Neurol* 184: 295–303.

Lee, J. H., Rim, N. G., Jung, H. S. et al. 2010. Control of osteogenic differentiation and mineralization of human mesenchymal stem cells on composite nanofibers containing poly[lactic-*co*-(glycolic acid)] and hydroxyapatite. *Macromol Biosci* 10: 173–82.

Lee, K. Y., Peters, M. C., Anderson, K. W. et al. 2000. Controlled growth factor release from synthetic extracellular matrices. *Nature* 408: 998–1000.

Lee, S. H. and Shin, H. 2007. Matrices and scaffolds for delivery of bioactive molecules in bone and cartilage tissue engineering. *Adv Drug Deliv Rev* 59: 339–59.

Li, W., Guo, Y., Wang, H. et al. 2008. Electrospun nanofibers immobilized with collagen for neural stem cells culture. *J Mater Sci Mater Med* 19: 847–54.

Liu, Q., Hedberg, E. L., Liu, Z. W. et al. 2000. Preparation of macroporous poly(2-hydroxyethyl methacrylate) hydrogels by enhanced phase separation. *Biomaterials* 21: 2163–9.

Lutolf, M. P. 2009. Spotlight on hydrogels. *Nat Mater* 8: 451–3.

Lutolf, M. P., Gilbert, P. M., and Blau, H. M. 2009. Designing materials to direct stem-cell fate. *Nature* 462: 433–41.

Lutolf, M. P., Lauer-Fields, J. L., Schmoekel, H. G. et al. 2003. Synthetic matrix metalloproteinase-sensitive hydrogels for the conduction of tissue regeneration: Engineering cell-invasion characteristics. *Proc Natl Acad Sci USA* 100: 5413–8.

Ma, Z., Gao, C., Gong, Y. et al. 2005. Cartilage tissue engineering Plla scaffold with surface immobilized collagen and basic fibroblast growth factor. *Biomaterials* 26: 1253–9.

Marklein, R. A. and Burdick, J. A. 2010. Controlling stem cell fate with material design. *Adv Mater* 22: 175–89.

McCullen, S. D., Zhu, Y., Bernacki, S. H. et al. 2009. Electrospun composite poly(L-lactic acid)/tricalcium phosphate scaffolds induce proliferation and osteogenic differentiation of human adipose-derived stem cells. *Biomed Mater* 4: 035002.

Meiners, S. and Mercado, M. L. T. 2003. Functional peptide sequences derived from extracellular matrix glycoproteins and their receptors—Strategies to improve neuronal regeneration. *Mol Neurobiol* 27: 177–95.

Miller, J. S., Shen, C. J., Legant, W. R. et al. 2010. Bioactive hydrogels made from step-growth derived Peg-peptide macromers. *Biomaterials* 31: 3736–43.

Miyoshi, M., Kawazoe, T., Igawa, H. H. et al. 2005. Effects of bfgf incorporated into a gelatin sheet on wound healing. *J Biomater Sci Polym Ed* 16: 893–907.

Moutos, F. T., Freed, L. E., and Guilak, F. 2007. A biomimetic three-dimensional woven composite scaffold for functional tissue engineering of cartilage. *Nat Mater* 6: 162–7.

Murphy, W. L., Peters, M. C., Kohn, D. H. et al. 2000. Sustained release of vascular endothelial growth factor from mineralized poly(lactide-*co*-glycolide) scaffolds for tissue engineering. *Biomaterials* 21: 2521–7.

Park, C. H., Hong, Y. J., Park, K. et al. 2010a. Peptide-grafted lactide-based poly(ethylene glycol) porous scaffolds for specific cell adhesion. *Macromol Res* 18: 526–32.

Park, C. H., Rios, H. F., Jin, Q. et al. 2010b. Biomimetic hybrid scaffolds for engineering human tooth-ligament interfaces. *Biomaterials* 31: 5945–52.

Park, H., Radisic, M., Lim, J. O. et al. 2005. A novel composite scaffold for cardiac tissue engineering. *In Vitro Cell Dev Biol Anim* 41: 188–96.

Patel, S., Kurpinski, K., Quigley, R. et al. 2007. Bioactive nanofibers: Synergistic effects of nanotopography and chemical signaling on cell guidance. *Nano Lett* 7: 2122–8.

Phelps, E. A., Landazuri, N., Thule, P. M. et al. 2010. Bioartificial matrices for therapeutic vascularization. *Proc Natl Acad Sci USA* 107: 3323–8.

Pitukmanorom, P., Yong, T. H., and Ying, J. Y. 2008. Tunable release of proteins with polymer-inorganic nanocomposite microspheres. *Adv Mater* 20: 3504–9.

Place, E. S., Evans, N. D., and Stevens, M. M. 2009. Complexity in biomaterials for tissue engineering. *Nat Mater* 8: 457–70.

Rajangam, K., Behanna, H. A., Hui, M. J. et al. 2006. Heparin binding nanostructures to promote growth of blood vessels. *Nano Lett* 6: 2086–90.

Rim, N. G., Lee, J. H., Jeong, S. I. et al. 2009. Modulation of osteogenic differentiation of human mesenchymal stem cells by poly[(L-lactide)-*co*-(epsilon-caprolactone)]/gelatin nanofibers. *Macromol Biosci* 9: 795–804.

Ruvinov, E., Leor, J., and Cohen, S. 2010. The effects of controlled Hgf delivery from an affinity-binding alginate biomaterial on angiogenesis and blood perfusion in a hindlimb ischemia model. *Biomaterials* 31: 4573–82.

Shi, G., Rouabhia, M., Wang, Z. et al. 2004. A novel electrically conductive and biodegradable composite made of polypyrrole nanoparticles and polylactide. *Biomaterials* 25: 2477–88.

Shimizu, K., Fujita, H., and Nagamori, E. 2009. Alignment of skeletal muscle myoblasts and myotubes using linear micropatterned surfaces ground with abrasives. *Biotechnol Bioeng* 103: 631–8.

Shin, H., Jo, S., and Mikos, A. G. 2003. Biomimetic materials for tissue engineering. *Biomaterials* 24: 4353–64.

Shin, Y. M., Kim, K. S., Lim, Y. M. et al. 2008. Modulation of spreading, proliferation, and differentiation of human mesenchymal stem cells on gelatin-immobilized poly(L-lactide-*co*-caprolactone) substrates. *Biomacromolecules* 9: 1772–81.

Shin, Y. M., Shin, H., and Lim, Y. M. 2010. Surface modification of electrospun poly(L-lactide-*co*-ε-caprolactone) fibrous meshes with a rgd peptide for the control of adhesion, proliferation and differentiation of the preosteoblastic cells. *Macromol Res* 18: 472–81.

Slaughter, B. V., Khurshid, S. S., Fisher, O. Z. et al. 2009. Hydrogels in regenerative medicine. *Adv Mater* 21: 3307–29.

Smith, L. A. and Ma, P. X. 2004. Nano-fibrous scaffolds for tissue engineering. *Coll Surf B-Biointerfaces* 39: 125–31.

Sun, H., Wirsen, A. and Albertsson, A. C. 2004. Electron beam-induced graft polymerization of acrylic acid and immobilization of arginine-glycine-aspartic acid-containing peptide onto nanopatterned polycaprolactone. *Biomacromolecules* 5: 2275–80.

Tampieri, A., Sandri, M., Landi, E. et al. 2008. Design of graded biomimetic osteochondral composite scaffolds. *Biomaterials* 29: 3539–46.

Tayalia, P. and Mooney, D. J. 2009. Controlled growth factor delivery for tissue engineering. *Adv Mater* 21: 3269–85.

Tibbitt, M. W. and Anseth, K. S. 2009. Hydrogels as extracellular matrix mimics for 3D cell culture. *Biotechnol Bioeng* 103: 655–63.

Volcker, N., Klee, D., Hocker, H. et al. 2001. Functionalization of silicone rubber for the covalent immobilization of fibronectin. *J Mater Sci Mater Med* 12: 111–9.

Wang, F. and Guan, J. 2010a. Cellular cardiomyoplasty and cardiac tissue engineering for myocardial therapy. *Adv Drug Deliv Rev* 62: 784–97.

Wang, L. S., Chung, J. E., Chan, P. P. Y. et al. 2010b. Injectable biodegradable hydrogels with tunable mechanical properties for the stimulation of neurogenesic differentiation of human mesenchymal stem cells in 3D culture. *Biomaterials* 31: 1148–57.

Wilson, C. J., Clegg, R. E., Leavesley, D. I. et al. 2005. Mediation of biomaterial-cell interactions by adsorbed proteins: A review. *Tissue Eng* 11: 1–18.

Xie, S., Zhu, Q., Wang, B. et al. 2010. Incorporation of tripolyphosphate nanoparticles into fibrous poly(lactide-*co*-glycolide) scaffolds for tissue engineering. *Biomaterials* 31: 5100–9.

Xu, C. Y., Inai, R., Kotaki, M. et al. 2004. Aligned biodegradable nanotibrous structure: A potential scaffold for blood vessel engineering. *Biomaterials* 25: 877–86.

Zhu, Y., Gao, C., Liu, X. et al. 2002. Surface modification of polycaprolactone membrane via aminolysis and biomacromolecule immobilization for promoting cytocompatibility of human endothelial cells. *Biomacromolecules* 3: 1312–9.

Zong, X. H., Bien, H., Chung, C. Y. et al. 2005. Electrospun fine-textured scaffolds for heart tissue constructs. *Biomaterials* 26: 5330–8.

# 13

# Molecular Biology Techniques

13.1 Histochemistry.................................................................13-1
Hematoxylin and Eosin • Toluidine Blue • Crystal
Violet • Alkaline Phosphatase Assay • Oil Red O
13.2 Gel Electrophoresis..........................................................13-4
Agarose Gel Electrophoresis • Polyacrylamide Gel
Electrophoresis • SDS-PAGE
13.3 Restriction Enzymes .......................................................13-9
Introduction to the Technique • Technical Considerations
13.4 Other DNA Modification Enzymes.........................13-10
DNA Ligase • Blunting Enzymes • Calf Intestinal Phosphatase
13.5 The Polymerase Chain Reaction................................13-14
The Traditional Polymerase Chain Reaction • Real-Time
Quantitative PCR
13.6 Blotting............................................................................13-20
The Southern Blot • The Northern Blot • The Western
Blot • The Eastern Blot
References..........................................................................13-24

X.G. Chen
*Tulane University*

Y.L. Fang
*Tulane University*

W.T. Godbey
*Tulane University*

Biomedical engineering covers many facets, from chemistry for the development of biodegradable tissue scaffolds, to physics to describe the mechanical properties of an implanted material, to biology for the manipulation of cells for implantation as well as the understanding of the host organism that will receive the implant, to mathematics for analysis and modeling applications. This chapter will focus on molecular biology techniques that are commonly employed in biomedical engineering. It will cover different ways of analyzing proteins, RNA, and DNA, as well as an introduction to DNA manipulation techniques that are used in genetic engineering.

The chapter is by no means a comprehensive presentation of techniques; only a small subset of the most common techniques is presented. In doing so, a technique will be introduced and broadly described, followed by some technical considerations one might want to keep in mind when performing the laboratory procedures. For more detailed protocols, the reader might be interested in consulting one of several laboratory manuals that have done an excellent job of compiling and explaining a broad range of molecular biology techniques. These manuals include *Molecular Cloning: A Laboratory Manual* by Sambrook and Russell, *Conn's Biological Stains: A Handbook of Dyes, Stains and Fluorochromes for Use in Biology and Medicine* by Horobin, Kiernan, and Kiernan, and *Gene Cloning* by Lodge, Lund, and Minchin.

## 13.1 Histochemistry

Cells and tissues are relatively colorless under microscopy. To aid with visualization and analysis, a variety of stains have been developed to enhance the details of structures of particular interest. Stains can also be used to detect and determine the location of specific substances in a sample. In this section, five stains used in common practice are introduced and outlined.

### 13.1.1  Hematoxylin and Eosin

#### 13.1.1.1  Introduction to the Technology

The dyes hematoxylin and eosin (H&E) are typically used together because the cellular structures that they label are complimentary. Hematoxylin is obtained via extraction from logwood. Eosin is an artificial stain.

The extracted form of hematoxylin is not endowed with staining ability until it has been oxidized into hematein. There are two common methods used for the oxidation. "Ripening" is one strategy that leaves hematoxylin in the air and under light, thus allowing oxidation to take place naturally. Although the process is slow, the oxidized product can maintain an enduring property of staining. The second common strategy shortens the time of reaction via the use of oxidizing agents such as sodium iodate. This method makes hematein available whenever it is needed, but the resulting solution may suffer from over-oxidization or later degradation by natural oxidation (Bancroft and Gamble, 2008). The addition of a mordant to a sample stained with hematein will yield a positively charged complex that will bind to negatively charged structures in the prepared sample, including nuclear chromatin. A mordant in this case is a substance that has an affinity with a particular dye that will help to form an insoluble material upon interaction with the dye (Bourne and Danielli, 1970). Mordants often used in hematein staining are metal salts including aluminum, iron, copper, and chromium salts. Although oxidation and the use of a mordent are required to convert hematoxylin into a positively charged hematein complex, hematoxylin itself is said to be a nuclear stain.

There are several forms of eosin that are commercially available. One of the most popular types, eosin Y, is soluble in both water and alcohol. As opposed to hematoxylin, eosin is an anionic stain that forms a complex with acidophilic sites such as the cytoplasm, connective tissue fibers, and collagen fibers, which will be stained red or pink (Cormack, 2001). Usually acetic acid is added to eosin solutions to act as an accelerant to enhance staining.

#### 13.1.1.2  Technical Considerations

The following is a simple procedure for staining using H&E (Nagy, 2008, Dhein et al., 2005, Bronner-Fraser, 1996):

1. *Dewaxing and rehydration:* For samples that have been embedded in paraffin, sectioned, and mounted on slides, the mounted sections are soaked in xylene to dissolve the wax. Several immersions in a series of ethanol/water solutions with descending percentages of ethanol (100%, 95%, 80% then 70%) are sequentially performed to rehydrate the section for staining. Finally, the sections are washed with tap water and soaked in distilled water.
2. *Hematoxylin staining:* The section is next stained for 5 min using alum hematoxylin (50 g aluminum potassium sulfate, 11 g hematoxylin, 0.1 g sodium iodate, 1.0 g citric acid and 50 g chloral hydrate) and washed by tap water. It is recommended that the slide is next dipped in a solution of acid alcohol (ethanol containing 1% hydrochloric acid) to sharpen the contrast of the stain. After rinsing with tap water, the section may change from light red to gray-blue if the tap water is alkaline. This process is commonly known as "bluing."
3. *Eosin counterstaining:* The treated section is immersed in an eosin solution (2.5 g eosin, 0.5 mL glacial acetic acid and 495 mL water) for 3 min and rinsed with tap water.
4. *Dehydration and mounting:* The stained section is immersed in a series of ethanol/water solutions with increasing percentages of ethanol (70%, 80%, 95%, and 100%) to remove water because the presence of water can refract light and prevent clear observation of fine structures under microscopy. Xylene is an effective clearing agent and is suggested to be employed to allow the refraction coefficient of the tissue to increase. The resulting slide can then be mounted for preservation using a medium such as Permount.

## 13.1.2 Toluidine Blue

### 13.1.2.1 Introduction to the Technology

Toluidine blue is a synthetic dye that is frequently used as a nuclear stain. It is a typical alkaline dye and the cation in it has affinity for acidic substances contained in cell and tissue samples. For example, toluidine blue can be used to detect cell nuclei by staining the nucleic acids therein. The dye is also used for staining mucin and mast cells (Humason, 1972).

In histology, stains can be categorized into two groups: orthochromatic and metachromatic. Orthochromatic stains pass on the color themselves to specific components in cells or tissues. Fast green and Orange G are two orthochromatic dyes. Metachromatic stains take on a different color after binding to their targets. Methylene blue is an example of a metachromatic dye (Krishnamurthy, 1999, Humason, 1972). Toluidine blue can be either orthochromatic or metachromatic, depending on the chemical reaction that takes place during the staining process. When toluidine blue reacts with lignin, a molecule common used by some plants to make their cell walls stronger, the dye will take on the orthochromatic blue color. However, when the dye reacts with sulfated proteoglycans such as those found in mast cells and basophilic granules, the dye will metachromatically stain the structures purple/red at acid pH.

### 13.1.2.2 Technical Considerations

A brief protocol for the use of toluidine blue for the detection of mast cells follows (Humason, 1972):

1. Slides are deparaffinized and immersed in alcohol in the same fashion as that described for H&E staining.
2. Slides are immersed for 1–2 min in the staining solution, comprised of 0.2 g toluidine blue O in 100 mL or 60% ethanol in water.
3. Tap water is used for rinsing.
4. The samples are dehydrated in acetone.
5. Xylene is added for the purpose of clearing tissues followed by slide mounting.

Toluidine blue can also be used to locate cells in a biodegradable three-dimensional matrix when hydrolysis is a concern (Godbey et al., 2004):

1. Incubate the scaffold containing cells in 10% neutral-buffered formalin overnight
2. Rinse 3 × 15 min with phosphate-buffered saline.
3. Dehydrate the scaffolds by passing them 2 × 10 min through each of a series of dilutions of 70%, 80%, 90%, 95%, and 100% ethanol.
4. The scaffolds are now ready for embedding and sectioning. (JB-4 polymethacrylate embedding is recommended.)
5. Sections can then be stained using 1% toluidine blue in sodium acetate followed by rinsing with water.

## 13.1.3 Crystal Violet

### 13.1.3.1 Introduction to the Technology

Crystal violet is an excellent stain that is widely used in cytology, histology, and bacteriology. It is a typical basic dye that can be dissolved in both water and alcohol, allowing the staining of cell nuclei. Crystal violet staining is often used in the evaluation of cytotoxicity and growth inhibition assays.

### 13.1.3.2 Technical Considerations (Saotome et al., 1989)

1. Wash cells with PBS. The cells should not be fixed—this is an assay to be performed on intact cells.
2. Add 50 μL of 0.5% crystal violet in methanol to the cell culture.
3. Incubate for 10 min at room temperature.

4. Discard the staining solution and wash the culture gently with tap water.
5. Add 1% sodium dodecyl sulfate solution to the sample to solubilize the stain and agitate lightly.
6. Quantify via absorbance readings at 570 nm versus control cultures.

### 13.1.4 Alkaline Phosphatase Assay

#### 13.1.4.1 Introduction to the Technology

Alkaline phosphatase is a specific enzyme that can remove the phosphate groups from nucleotides or proteins. The total level of serum alkaline phosphatase is a good indicator for the activity of a series of isoenzymes in liver and bone, and the placenta during pregnancy (Campbell et al., 1993). For the tissue engineer, the alkaline phosphatase assay is used as a marker of bone tissue production, including the osteogenic differentiation of stem or progenitor cells into bone cells.

#### 13.1.4.2 Technical Considerations

A procedure for measuring alkaline phosphatase activity via a colorimetric assay follows (Holtorf et al., 2005):

1. Mix 80 μL of cell lysate with 20 μL of alkaline buffer solution (1.5 M 2-amino-2- methyl-1-propanol at pH 10.3).
2. Add 100 μL of p-nitrophenyl phosphate 100× stock substrate solution (100× stock is made by adding 40 mg of 4-nitrophenyl phosphate disodium salt hexahydrate into 10 mL of $ddH_2O$).
3. Incubate at 37°C for 1 h.
4. Stop the reaction with 100 μL of 0.3 M NaOH.
5. Measure absorbance at 405 nm.

### 13.1.5 Oil Red O

#### 13.1.5.1 Introduction to the Technology

Oil red O is used to stain lipids, fatty acids, triglycerides, and cholesterol to make them visible under light microscopy. Like other lysochromes (fat stains), oil red O is more soluble in lipids than in its alcohol solvent which causes it to preferentially stay in lipid droplets (Kiernan, 1981). This stain is often used to demonstrate adipogenic differentiation of stem or progenitor cells.

#### 13.1.5.2 Technical Considerations

Oil red O is has an intense color and the staining procedure is convenient to perform on sectioned preparations (Humason, 1972):

1. Rinse the frozen section in 60% isopropanol for 30 s.
2. Stain the section by immersion in oil red O solution (0.7 g oil red O in 200 mL pure isopropanol) for 10 min.
3. Rinse the section in 60% isopropanol for few seconds and then wash in tap water for 2–3 min.
4. A hematoxylin counterstain can be performed at this point.

## 13.2 Gel Electrophoresis

Gel electrophoresis is widely used in molecular biology to separate macromolecules, such as polynucleotides or proteins, via physical characteristics such as size, shape, or isoelectric point. The technique has been an essential tool in the biosciences for analyzing protein molecular weights, determining the number of bases in a DNA fragment, preparing samples for blotting, visualizing results of the polymerase chain reaction, and more.

Both proteins and polynucleotides have electrostatic charges. When in the presence of an electric field, they will move toward the anode or cathode according to the net charge of the molecule. The gel matrix serves as a barrier to slow the movement of the macromolecules. Molecules with different sizes, shapes, or net charges will migrate at different rates through the matrix, thereby being sorted into different bands. Dyes, radiolabeling, or immunoblotting can be used to visualize the separated bands of macromolecules. The bands can be compared to a reference marker of the same material (nucleotide or protein) to ascertain fundamental information such as molecular weight.

## 13.2.1 Agarose Gel Electrophoresis

### 13.2.1.1 Introduction to the Technique

Agarose gel electrophoresis is often used to separate polynucleotides. Agarose is a polysaccharide isolated from seaweed, which is remarkably suitable for serving as gel matrix because of its neutral charge and relatively low degree of chemical complexity. Agarose melts and dissolves at a relatively high temperature and forms a gel matrix upon cooling. The gel is made in a buffer solution such as Tris-acetate-EDTA (TAE) to match the buffer that will be used for the electrophoresis procedure. Upon application of an electric field, polynucleotides of different sizes can pass through the porous agarose matrix at different rates according to their size because of the uniform negative charge distribution of the molecules. The resulting bands are visualized via the use of fluorescent molecules.

### 13.2.1.2 Technical Considerations

#### 13.2.1.2.1 Concentration of Agarose

When used to separate polynucleotides, agarose is used at concentrations in the range of 0.3–2% (w/v). Agarose concentration determines pore size within the gel matrix, which in turn determines the optimal range of polynucleotide sizes that can be efficiently separated. The following table is a convenient way to determine the concentration of agarose to use for various DNA separations (Mitra, 2003):

| Concentration of Agarose | Fragment Sizes (bp) |
| --- | --- |
| 0.3% | 5000–60,000 |
| 0.6% | 1000–20,000 |
| 0.7% | 800–10,000 |
| 0.9% | 500–7000 |
| 1.2% | 400–6000 |
| 1.5% | 200–3000 |
| 2.0% | 100–2000 |

#### 13.2.1.2.2 Applied Voltage

The rate of polynucleotide movement is dependent upon applied voltage (Rapley and Walker, 1998). The higher the voltage, the faster the DNA moves. However, higher voltages are associated with higher currents within the gel, which translates into higher temperatures. High temperatures accelerate the migration rates of fragments in the sample, which would increase band widths and thereby reduce resolution. An inhomogeneous temperature distribution would produce convection and possibly mix fragments that are to be separated. If the temperatures are high enough, double-stranded fragments can denature and produce unexpected results. Therefore, an appropriate voltage should be used, or cooling methods should be employed when the high voltage is required.

Recommended voltage settings are as follows (Brown, 2000):

| Recommended Voltage (V/cm)[a] | Fragment Sizes (bp) |
| --- | --- |
| 5 | ≤1000 |
| 4–10 | 1000–12,000 |
| 1–2 | ≥12,000 |

[a] cm refers to the distance from cathode to anode, in centimeters.

While it may be counterintuitive to use a lower voltage for larger fragment sizes, this is the usual practice to prevent streaking of the bands.

#### 13.2.1.2.3 *Visualization of Bands*

Ethidium bromide (EB) is a DNA intercalating dye that fluoresces orange upon exposure to ultraviolet light. EB can be added to the hot agarose solution (~4 µL/100 mL of solution) before it is cooled to form the gel. Alternatively, EB can be added to the buffer reservoir closest to the anode just prior to turning on the electrical current for running the gel. Being positively charged, EB will migrate toward the cathode as the DNA migrates toward the anode. When the two molecules meet, the EB will bind to the DNA. One could also immerse the gel into a solution of buffer containing EB after the sample has been run. While soaking the gel after separation allows for less use of the neurotoxic and carcinogenic EB over time since the soaking solution can be reused, DNA can diffuse during the soak which will decrease the sharpness of the observed bands.

PicoGreen is another fluorophore that is used to bind to double-stranded DNA (dsDNA) for visualization of separated DNA bands after electrophoresis. This technique is sensitive enough to detect 1ng of DNA even when RNA and protein contaminants are present (Kieleczawa, 2006). Because of its sensitivity, the dye can be used to quantify dsDNA concentrations. One must avoid contamination with divalent metal ions such as $Mg^{2+}$, $Ca^{2+}$, and $Zn^{2+}$ because they can quench the fluorescence of the dye (Singer et al., 1997, Saunders et al., 1999).

#### 13.2.1.2.4 *DNA Loading Buffer*

There are two or three main reasons for mixing a DNA sample with loading buffer before loading it into a gel for electrophoresis. First, loading buffer will contain an agent such as glycerol or ficoll to increase the density of the sample so that the sample will settle to the bottom of the well upon loading. Second, the loading buffer will contain one or more dyes to aid the user with monitoring the progress of migration without having to halt the electrophoretic process. A common dye pair is bromophenol blue/xylene cyanol, which will migrate at rates similar to 300 and 4000 base-pair DNA, respectively (Kumar and Garg, 2005). Third, some loading buffers will incorporate 6 mM EDTA, which serves as a chelating agent for divalent cations and therefore indirectly inhibits the action of many enzymes.

A recipe for a common 6× loading buffer (which will be used at 2 µL of loading buffer per 10 µL of DNA sample) follows (Sambrook and Russell, 2001):

0.25% (w/v) bromophenol blue
0.25% (w/v) xylene cyanol FF
30% (v/v) glycerol in water (15% Ficoll (w/v) can be used, instead)

## 13.2.2 Polyacrylamide Gel Electrophoresis

### 13.2.2.1 Introduction to the Technique

Polyacrylamide gel electrophoresis (PAGE) is an electrophoresis technique that can be used for separating small macromolecules such as proteins or small oligonucleotides. To form the cross-linked gel, acrylamide monomers are polymerized with ethylene bisacrylamide, using tetramethylethylenediamine as the catalyst and ammonium persulfate as the initiator. Polyacrylamide gels can be classified into two categories: continuous and discontinuous systems. The continuous system has a single gel separating tanks containing the same buffer as that used in the gel. The separation of macro molecules occurs by the sieve effect. The discontinuous system contains two gels—a stacking gel and a separating gel—each made with a different buffer. The stacking gel operates by the concentration effect, where leading ions (generally Cl⁻) move more quickly through the gel than does the protein sample. In contrast, trailing ions (commonly glycine in the electrophoresis buffer) migrate more slowly than the protein. Between the two ion layers the protein molecules are concentrated into a sharp band. The separating gel consists of smaller pores in which the sieve effect is the determining factor. After the protein moves from the stacking gel into the separating gel, the smaller pores separate the protein based on size (and shape, when the proteins are not denatured).

### 13.2.2.2 Technical Considerations

#### 13.2.2.2.1 Pore Size

The pore size of gel can be controlled by monomer concentration ($T$) and cross-linker concentration ($C$). $T$ and $C$ could be calculated by the following equations (Hjerten, 1962):

$$T = \frac{a + b}{m} \times 100\%; \quad \text{and} \quad C = \frac{b}{a + b} \times 100\%,$$

where

$a$ = the mass of acrylamide
$b$ = the mass of ethylene bisacrylamide
$m$ = the buffer volume

The following table can serve as a guide for preparing the appropriate polyacrylamide gels for protein separation (Hames, 1998):

| $M_r$ range of Proteins in the Sample | Acrylamide Concentration | |
|---|---|---|
| | %T | %C |
| 25,000–300,000 | 5 | 2.6 |
| 15,000–100,000 | 10 | 2.6 |
| 12,000–50,000 | 15 | 2.6 |
| 13,000–1,000,000 | 3–30 | 8.4 |
| 14,000–210,000 | 5–20 | 2.6 |
| 14,000–330,000 | 8–15 | 1.0 |

#### 13.2.2.2.2 Visualization of Bands

The separated polypeptide bands can be visualized through staining with Coomassie Brilliant Blue or silver salts (Roe, 2001). Coomassie blue staining follows three straightforward steps: fixation, staining, and destaining. Fixation locks the proteins inside the gel to prevent their diffusion during staining and destaining. Staining entails the submersion of the entire gel into a solution of a solvent mixture (45 mL water + 45 mL methanol + 10 mL glacial acetic acid) plus Coomassie Brilliant Blue (0.25 g), causing the entire gel to turn blue. Because of the methanol and acetic acid in the solution, the fixation and staining steps are performed simultaneously. Destaining entails the submersion of the gel into solvent solution without dye, which will remove dye molecules that are not bound to protein.

## 13.2.3 SDS-PAGE

Sodium dodecyl sulfate polyacrylamide gel electrophoresis (SDS-PAGE) is a technique used for analyzing proteins. SDS is a detergent with a hydrophobic, saturated 12-carbon tail and a sulfate head group (and sodium as a counterion) (Clark, 2005). When proteins are treated with SDS, the hydrocarbon tail binds to the polypeptides via the polypeptide backbones, leaving the sulfate head groups to interact with water. This interaction disrupts the secondary and tertiary structure of the proteins and they will denature. Approximately one SDS molecule will bind for every two amino acid residues, so the negatively charged dodecyl sulfate molecules can completely shield the charge of protein. While the overall charge will be roughly proportional to protein size, the charge to mass ratio will be the same for large versus small proteins (Figure 13.1). As a result of roughly equivalent charge concentrations, electrophoresis can be used to separate mixed samples of proteins based on size. Comparing the resulting bands to a set of standards will yield the approximate molecular weights of the proteins in a sample.

It is relatively easy to treat proteins with SDS. First, a 2× sample buffer—composed of 0.92 g SDS, 2 mL β-mercaptoethanol, 4.0 g glycerol, 0.3 g Tris, and 2 mL bromophenol blue (0.1% w/v in water)

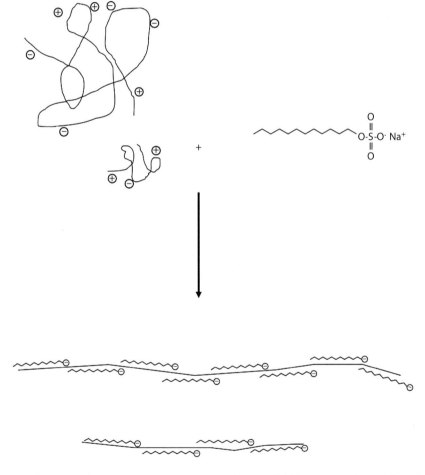

**FIGURE 13.1** The action of SDS on proteins. Proteins in solution will fold and carry charges dependently upon their primary amino acid sequences. In the presence of SDS, they will denature and carry a uniform coating of negative charges. The charges of the amino acid side chains will be masked by the SDS. This example shows SDS molecules interacting with two proteins of different net charge and differing in mass by approximately twofold. The end result is two polypeptides with equal charge-to-mass ratios that can be separated by PAGE according to size.

in water to 20 mL total volume, with pH adjusted to 6.8 with HCl—is mixed with the protein sample at 1:1 buffer to sample (Walker, 1994). The β-mercaptoethanol is a reducing agent used to break any disulfide bonds within the proteins. Glycerol is used to increase the sample density, and bromophenol blue is used to aid with the visualization process during electrophoresis. Tris is used to buffer the pH of the mixture. The solution is then boiled for two minutes to completely denature the proteins. After the sample is cooled, it can then be placed into the wells of a polyacrylamide gel for electrophoresis.

# 13.3 Restriction Enzymes

## 13.3.1 Introduction to the Technique

Restriction enzymes are bacterial endonucleases that get their name from the early finding that they restrict the propagation of bacteriophages on culture plates. Their native function is to cut dsDNA, such as what may be transduced into a bacterium by a bacteriophage, via the recognition of specific DNA sequences. Since the first restriction enzyme was isolated at 1968 (Menninger et al., 1968) this class of enzymes has been one of the most significant tools in molecular biology and has allowed the development of recombinant DNA technology. Custom stretches of DNA, such as engineered plasmids with bioactive promoter or exon sequences, can be formed though the cutting of target fragments from genomic or plasmid DNA followed by fragment transfer into a gene vector (a process that utilizes additional enzymes such as the Klenow fragment or DNA ligase). Another application of restriction enzymes is in verifying plasmid identities through affirmation of specific base sequences within the plasmids, and the distance between such sequences via the lengths of fragments that are generated by the cuts. In brief, restriction enzymes are indispensable tools for modern gene engineering.

There is a systematic way in which restriction enzymes are named (Smith and Nathans, 1973). The first three letters are in italics, and represent the genus and species names of the host bacterium. A nonitalicized letter may appear next, representing the particular strain from which the isolate was purified. The name will end with a roman numeral to indicate the order of discovery for multiple restriction enzymes arising from the same bacterium. For example, *Eco*RI was isolated from *Escherichia coli* **R**Y13, while *Hin*dIII was isolated from *Haemophilus influenzae* strain **d**, and was the third enzyme isolated from this strain. (Note that the strain for *Hin*dIII can be found in older publications listed as Rd. The "R" is part of an R–M system, which denotes **R**estriction endonuclease versus **M**odification enzymes. The R and M strain designations are routinely dropped.)

Restriction enzymes can be classified into three types, type I, II, or III, based on their enzymology and cofactor requirements (Wilson, 1988). Because types I and III cut DNA variably or with low efficiency, they are not typically used for genetic engineering. Type II enzymes can reproducibly and efficiently cleave specific nucleotide sequences ("restriction sites"), making them the most reliable set of restriction enzymes for DNA manipulation.

Type II restriction enzymes typically have two similar subunits that can recognize and cleave DNA in the presence of the cofactor $Mg^{2+}$ (Pingoud and Jeltsch, 2001). The enzyme initially binds to the DNA recognition site directly or will bind randomly to the DNA and then linearly diffuse to the recognition site. Once at the recognition site, the conformation of the enzyme would change to allow for catalysis of the digestion reaction. After strand cleavage, the enzyme detaches from the DNA molecule or moves on to another recognition site on the same dsDNA (Pingoud and Jeltsch, 2001).

A restriction enzyme can produce one of two types of cuts: sticky or blunt. A sticky cut produces sticky ends, or two DNA overhangs that are complimentary to one another. *Eco*RI produces sticky ends as follows (triangles indicate cleavage points):

5′ ... XXX**G**▾**AATTC**XXX ⋯ 3′         ⋯ XXX**G**         **and**         **AATTC**XXX ⋯

3′ ... XXX**CTTAA**▴**G**XXX ⋯ 5′         ⋯ XXX**CTTAA**         **G**XXX ⋯

Blunt ends result when the DNA cuts are at the same position on both sides of the double strand. For example, an AluI cut would produce two blunt ends as follows:

5′ ⋯ XXXAG▾CTXXX ⋯ 3′                    ⋯ XXXAG        **and**        CTXXX ⋯

$$\longrightarrow$$

3′ ⋯ XXXTC▴GAXXX ⋯ 5′                    ⋯ XXXTC                GAXXX ⋯

Regardless of whether a blunt or sticky cut has been made, there will be a phosphate group on the 5′ end and a hydroxyl group on the 3′ end of each strands. This is important for ligation purposes. In general, sticky ends are easier to insert and ligate than are blunt ends.

## 13.3.2 Technical Considerations

It is a relatively simple matter to use restriction enzymes to cut DNA. All that is required is a suitable buffer (supplied by the company that provides the enzyme), any required cofactors for the enzyme being used (such as bovine serum albumin), some DNA, and the appropriate temperature for incubation of the reaction. In determining the correct amount of enzyme to use for a particular reaction, one should be aware of enzyme activity, which is reported as "units" of enzyme. One unit of commercial restriction enzyme is typically defined as the amount of enzyme needed to digest 1 μg of λ DNA in 1 h at optimal temperature (usually 37°C) in a total reaction volume of 50 μL (New England Biolabs, 2009a). As an example, if the restriction enzyme is supplied in glycerol at a concentration of 20,000 U/mL and one wishes to digest 1 μg of DNA, 0.05 μL of restriction enzyme would work for the particular reaction. However, measuring 0.05 μL of solution is impractical, so 0.5 μL is often used instead. While one could dilute the enzyme stock solution, this practice generally yields poor results and is not recommended.

A typical endonuclease digestion reaction takes place in 10 μL total volume. Volumes for the reaction are given below, in the order in which the reaction solution is mixed:

$10.0 - \Sigma$ (all other reagents) μL     water
1.0 μL         $10 \times$ buffer
$x$ μL          $10 \times$ additives (such as bovine serum albumin). $x = 0.0$ or $1.0$
$y$ μL          DNA, 1 μg (although 0.1 μg may be enough to faintly visualize large fragments)
0.5 μL        enzyme 1
(0.5 μL      enzyme 2, if used)

10.0 μL total volume

# 13.4 Other DNA Modification Enzymes

Restriction enzymes are often used for the construction of engineered plasmids. At this point in the chapter it might be useful to mention other enzymes that are commonly used for DNA manipulation, namely DNA ligase, blunting enzymes, and calf intestinal phosphatase.

## 13.4.1 DNA Ligase

### 13.4.1.1 Introduction to the Technique

For plasmid construction, simply putting two fragments with sticky ends together is not enough. There will still be a gap in the phosphodeoxyribose backbone unless steps are taken to conjugate the free 3′ hydroxyl of one fragment with the 5′ phosphate group of the next (Figure 13.2). This can be accomplished using a DNA ligase. T4 DNA ligase, isolated from bacteriophage T4-infected *Escherichia coli*, is a convenient choice for this purpose. It can catalyze the conjugation of the two end groups into a single

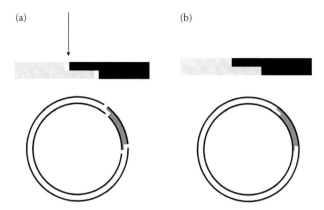

**FIGURE 13.2** An overview of DNA ligase. (a) Although DNA fragments with sticky ends can fit like a puzzle piece into a vector with complimentary sticky ends, the plasmids cannot be replicated because of the molecular gaps between the two pieces. (b) DNA ligase seals the molecular gaps by creation of new phosphodiester bonds. Top—two DNA fragments with complimentary 5′ overhangs. The arrow indicates a discontinuous gap in the DNA backbone. Bottom—a larger view, showing the interaction of an insert with a plasmid vector.

phosphodiester bond (Figure 13.3). Blunt ends can also be recombined by T4 DNA ligase, but the efficiency of ligation is much lower than for sticky end ligation.

### 13.4.1.2 Technical Considerations

The ligation reaction takes place by mixing reaction buffer, the DNA to be ligated, and an appropriate amount of enzyme, and incubating at 16°C for 4–16 h (Sambrook and Russell, 2001). A 10× reaction buffer is supplied with commercial T4 DNA ligases. To determine the appropriate amount of enzyme, use the definition of one unit: the amount of DNA ligase needed to ligate 50% of HindIII fragments of λ DNA with a 5′ DNA termini concentration of 0.12 μM (300 μg/mL) in a 20 μL reaction volume in 30 min at 16°C using 1× T4 DNA ligase reaction buffer (New England Biolabs, 2009b). Thus the required amount of enzyme depends on the DNA content in the sample.

Following is a typical ligation reaction setup (Sambrook and Russell, 2001, New England Biolabs, 2009b):

10.0 – Σ (all other reagents) μL      water
1.0 μL      10 × T4 DNA ligase reaction buffer
*x* μL      vector DNA
*y* μL      insert DNA
1 μL      T4 DNA ligase (400,000 cohesive end units/ml)

10.0 μL total volume

Note that the total concentration of vector plus insert should be 1–10 μg/mL.

### 13.4.2 Blunting Enzymes

#### 13.4.2.1 Introduction to the Technique

Sometimes it is necessary to ligate fragments that do not have complementary base pair overhangs (the sticky ends do not match up). In this case T4 DNA ligase cannot be used for ligation because the fragments will not be held in close proximity to one another by hydrogen bonds. However, the fragments can be made to have blunt ends via the DNA polymerase activity or the exonuclease activity of either the Klenow fragment or T4 DNA polymerase.

The Klenow fragment is the large proteolytic fragment of *E. coli* DNA polymerase. This enzyme has 5′ to 3′ polymerization and 3′ to 5′ exonuclease activities, which are important to note with respect to the

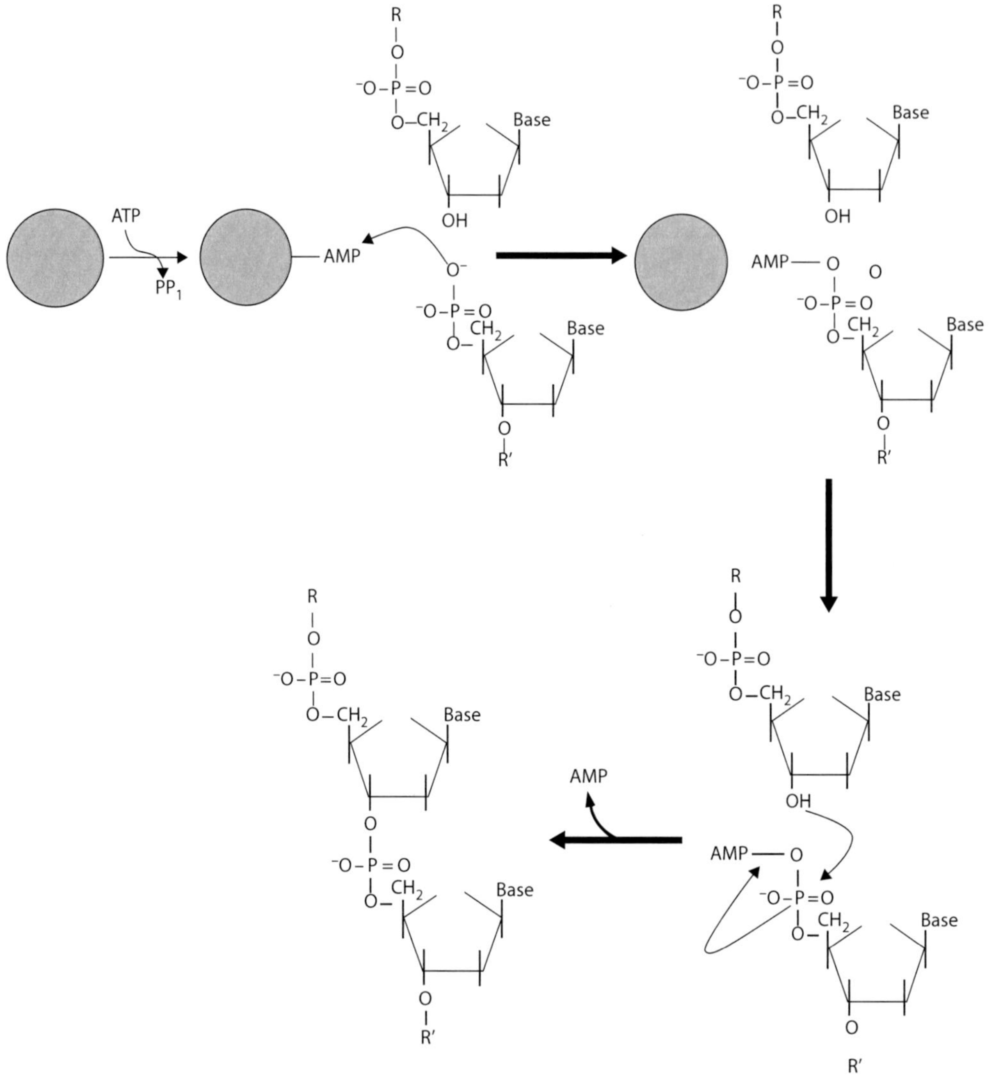

**FIGURE 13.3** The mechanism of DNA ligase. After being activated by the addition of an AMP molecule by cleavage of an ATP, DNA ligase catalyzes attachment of a phosphate on a 5′ DNA terminus to the phosphate of AMP, followed by the transfer of the terminal phosphate to the hydroxyl of a 3′ DNA terminus and the release of the AMP molecule.

type of overhang the DNA fragment of interest has (Steitz, 1993). The Klenow fragment can utilize dNTPs to complementarily fill in the gap of a 5′ overhang to form a blunt end (Sambrook and Russell, 2001). Although the Klenow fragment also has 3′ to 5′ exonuclease activity, it is not recommended for blunting 3′ overhangs because of lower reaction efficiency (Sambrook and Russell, 2001). Versions of the enzyme are available that have lost their 3′ to 5′ exonuclease activity altogether (Derbyshire et al., 1988).

To make blunt ends out of DNA fragments having 3′ overhangs, T4 DNA polymerase is recommended. T4 DNA polymerase is an enzyme isolated from bacteriophage T4-infected *E. coli*. Like the Klenow fragment, it also has 5′ to 3′polymerization and 3′ to 5′ exonuclease activities (Sambrook and Russell, 2001). However, the activity of 3′ to 5′ exonuclease is 200-fold greater than that of the Klenow fragment.

After treatment with the Klenow fragment or T4 DNA polymerase, the resulting blunt-ended fragments can be cloned into an open blunt-ended vector using T4 DNA ligase.

### 13.4.2.2 Technical Considerations

| Klenow Fragment (Sambrook and Russell, 2001) | | T4 DNA Polymerase (Brown, 2000) | |
| --- | --- | --- | --- |
| Water | $\times$ μL | Water | $\times$ μL |
| 10× buffer | 2.5 μL | 10 × buffer | 2.5 μL |
| DNA | 1 μg | DNA | 1 μg |
| | | BSA | 1.25 μL 10× restriction enz. |
| dNTP | 133 μM final conc.[a] | dNTP | 100 μM final conc.[b] |
| Enzyme | 1.0 μL | Enzyme | 1.0 μL |
| Total | 25 μL | Total | 25 μL |
| Incubate 15 min at room temperature | | Incubate 15–30 min at 15°C | |

[a] 133 μM final concentration = 1.66 μL of 2 mM dNTP
[b] 100 μM final concentration = 1.25 μL of 2 mM dNTP

## 13.4.3 Calf Intestinal Phosphatase

### 13.4.3.1 Introduction to the Technique

Calf intestinal alkaline phosphatase (CIP) is a dimeric metalloenzyme whose function in genetic engineering is to dephosphorylate the 5′ end of a plasmid vector after a restriction cut to prevent the plasmid from being ligated without a DNA insert (Eun, 1996). The DNA fragment to be inserted into the plasmid will not be exposed to CIP to preserve its 5′ phosphate groups. The result of combining the unmodified insert with the dephosphorylated vector is that ligation will produce only vector–insert combinations, thus easing the burden of screening for plasmids containing the inserted DNA in subsequent steps.

### 13.4.3.2 Technical Considerations

CIP is a powerful enzyme, and many molecular biologists will avoid using it because it is hard to deactivate or remove completely from reaction mixtures, which would have a deleterious effect on subsequent ligation efforts. Others might suggest that the amount of enzyme needed is so small that simply dipping a pipette tip into stock enzyme solution will usually transfer enough enzyme for the reaction to take place. Incubation of a heat-killed restriction cut or blunting reaction mixture for 60 min at 37°C could suffice, with purification via gel electrophoresis, phenol extraction, or spin column taking place immediately after the incubation.

A more formal method of using CIP has the reaction mixture incubated in a two-step manner. The amount of enzyme and reaction time will depend on the amount and type of fragment end that is produced by restriction cutting. Details are given in the following table (Sambrook and Russell, 2001):

| Termius Type | Amount of CIP per Mole DNA Ends | Reaction Times and Temperatures |
| --- | --- | --- |
| 5′-overhang | 0.01 unit | 37°C for 30 min, then |
| | | 37°C for 30 min[a] |
| 3′-overhang | 0.1–0.5 unit | 37°C 15 min, then |
| | | 55°C 45 min |
| Blunt end | 0.1–0.5 unit | 37°C 15 min, then |
| | | 55°C 45 min |

[a] The procedure is to add the given amount of enzyme and incubate at the first time and temperature shown, then to add an additional aliquot of the same amount of enzyme and incubate at the second time and temperature.

After the final incubation, the enzyme should be inactivated or removed (or both). Inactivation can occur by heating the solution to 65°C for 30 min, or to 75°C for 10 min (Sambrook and Russell, 2001). Commercially available purification kits can be used to remove the enzyme and salts from the DNA solution.

# 13.5  The Polymerase Chain Reaction

## 13.5.1  The Traditional Polymerase Chain Reaction

### 13.5.1.1  Introduction to the Technique

The polymerase chain reaction (PCR) is a means to amplify a given stretch of nucleotides to determine their relative concentration in different cell samples, or to produce usable quantities of a sequence of nucleotides for DNA cloning. The technique allows for the amplification of a few copies (in theory, only one copy is needed) of a specific piece of DNA into perhaps billions of copies in a relatively short time. The procedure is relatively inexpensive, requiring only a thermocycler and the appropriate enzymes and reagents for processing. The first description of PCR was published in 1985 (Saiki et al., 1985), and has proven to be such an important technique that the Nobel Prize in 1993 was awarded to Kary Banks Mullis for its discovery.

PCR is an enzymatic process that is repeated over multiple cycles. The enzyme can be one of many commercially available versions of DNA polymerase, and it is used to catalyze the synthesis of a DNA sequence complimentary to a single-stranded template to yield a double-stranded DNA fragment composed of the original DNA template plus the newly synthesized strand. Double-stranded DNA is required for DNA polymerase to bind to and commence synthesis of the complimentary strand. This double-stranded region is provided by the binding of short (~20 base) primers to the single-stranded DNA template. The primers also give specificity to PCR because they are designed to bind only in regions flanking the particular DNA sequence of interest.

### 13.5.1.2  Technical Considerations

#### 13.5.1.2.1  Cycle Parameters

One cycle of this traditional form of PCR contains three steps: denaturation, annealing, and elongation. Each of the three PCR steps takes place under a different temperature for specific reasons, as outlined below.

*Denature*: This step is performed at 90–98°C to separate dsDNA into single-stranded chains (ssDNA) (Saiki et al., 1988). Heating allows the DNA duplexes to melt through the dissociation of the hydrogen bond between the complementary bases in each strand. It is important to keep the temperature high in this step to prevent re-association of the strands, but it must be kept below 100°C to prevent the removal of water molecules from the DNA.

*Anneal*: The goal of this step is to permit association of the primers with the ssDNA fragments. The temperature used for this step is critical to the PCR process, and varies with the base composition of the dsDNA sequence being amplified. If the temperature is too low, the ssDNA fragments will reassociate and not be amplified. If the temperature is too high, then there will be too much energy in the system to allow for hydrogen bonding to hold primer and template strands together. There is a relatively small temperature range whereby the ssDNA fragments will associate with the primers preferentially over their complimentary (and longer) ssDNA counterparts, typically 50–65°C. However, even this range is not exact enough because temperatures slightly too low will allow association of primers to sequences of DNA in a less-specific fashion (termed "nonspecific binding"), which will result in the amplification of unwanted DNA sequences. The optimal temperature for annealing can be determined by the following formula (Rychlik et al., 1990):

$$T_a = 0.3 \cdot T_m(\text{primer}) + 0.7 \cdot T_m(\text{product}) - 14.9,$$

where

$T_a$ = annealing temperature, and

$T_m$ = melting temperature of the primers or product, defined as the temperature at which 50% of the oligonucleotides and the associated complimentary strand are in duplex. $T_m$ can be calculated by:

For short sequences (≤20 bases), such as primers,

$$T_m = 2(A + T) + 4(G + C),$$

where $A$, $T$, $G$, and $C$ are the number of adenine, thymine, guanine, and cytosine bases in the sequence, respectively (Marmur and Doty, 1962).

For longer sequences, such as amplicons,

$$T_m = 81.5 + 16.6(\log M) + 0.41(\%G + \%C) - 0.63(\%\text{formamide}) - \left(\frac{600}{n}\right),$$

where $M$ = the concentration of monovalent cations (such as $Na^+$ and $K^+$), %G and %C are the mole fractions of guanine and cytosine, respectively, % formamide = the percentage of formamide in the solution, and $n$ = the number of nucleotides in the sequence (Newton and Graham, 1997).

*Extend*: This step allows the DNA polymerase to create a complimentary fragment to the template strand, yielding a dsDNA fragment with "new" DNA bases. Since the original dsDNA was separated into two ssDNA chains using the double-stranded primer/template pair as a primer, the net result will be twice as many dsDNA fragments of interest, with each fragment containing a newly synthesized DNA polymer. The extension step is carried out at the optimal temperature for the DNA polymerase being used. For instance, 72°C would be used for Taq DNA polymerase (Sambrook and Russell, 2001), because this is the temperature at which the parent organism, *Thermus aquaticus*, lives.

Theoretically, the number of fragments of the target DNA is doubled after each cycle, which implies an exponential relation between the number of cycles and the amount of PCR product. For instance, after 30 PCR cycles one could theoretically obtain up to $2^{30}$ copies of the target DNA sequence. This does not mean that one could easily perform 100 cycles of PCR to obtain $2^{100}$ copies of the original fragment. DNA polymerase uses deoxyribonucleotide triphosphates (dNTPs) as high-energy monomers for building the polymeric DNA copies, and the amount of starting materials required are infeasible due, in part, to the osmolarity of the solution that would contain them (or the cost of the system that would require greater volumes or reagents and enzyme).

### 13.5.1.2.2 Primer Design

Primers are the main determinant of PCR specificity, so great care must be taken for their proper design. There exist many computer programs, both free and for purchase, that were written to assist with the task of primers design. Outputs generally list many possibilities for primer sets so the investigator must be prepared to analyze the results for proper selection. Following are some guidelines to aid with selecting successful and unique primer sets (McPherson and Hames, 1995, Pelt-Verkuil et al., 2008, Newton and Graham, 1997):

1. Primers lengths should be in the range of 18 and 30 nucleotides. Shorter primers could decrease the specificity of the PCR and therefore cause amplification of sequences that are not of interest. Primers that are too long will require higher annealing temperatures, which could affect DNA polymerase activity during elongation.
2. The sequences of primer sets should not be complementary, which would lead to the self-annealing of primers into structures known as primer-dimers. Primer-dimers cannot bind to template DNA strands and are therefore useless for PCR.

3. One should avoid having complementary regions in any individual primer, otherwise hairpin structures could form within the primer itself.
4. Regions of repeated bases should be avoided, such as CCCCC or TTTTT. Such sequences are prone to mismatching.
5. The annealing temperatures of the two primers in a set should be roughly the same (within 5°C of each other).

## 13.5.2 Real-Time Quantitative PCR

As a cornerstone of modern molecular biology techniques, the polymerase chain reaction has undergone persistent development during the past 20 years. The advent of real-time quantitative PCR has brought the potential of the PCR into full play, allowing a shift from qualitative to quantitative analyses. It can measure the starting concentration of DNA, cDNA, or RNA templates. As opposed to traditional PCR, the process of real-time PCR is monitored via fluorescence readings once per replication cycle to allow for direct measurements of PCR amplifications without the need for postprocessing.

### 13.5.2.1 Introduction to the Technique

The introduction of fluorescent chemistries into reaction systems has made it possible to detect PCR product concentration through its relation to fluorescence intensity. The fluorescent chemistries that are used in real-time quantitative PCR will be introduced in detail later. First, a discussion of the DNA amplification process is needed to acquire a basic understanding of the principles underlying PCR.

The curve of DNA concentration versus cycle number typically has four distinct regions, termed the linear, early exponential, exponential, and plateau phases (Wong and Medrano, 2005). In the beginning of the process (generally the first 5 or 10 cycles), the amount of PCR product is insufficient to yield fluorescence emission above the background level. Baseline fluorescence is calculated at this stage. Upon entering the early exponential phase, the accumulated fluorescence intensity has increased to a level that exceeds background levels—ordinarily 10 times the standard deviation of the background levels observed. At this point the target (amplicon) can be reliably detected. The PCR cycle number at which the observed fluorescence first exceeds this value is referred to as the cycle threshold ($C_t$). The $C_t$ value is what is used for subsequent calculations of relative and quantitative DNA or RNA concentrations.

In the exponential phase, the number of DNA copies increases exponentially under ideal reaction conditions. As the reaction cycles continue to increase, reagents are used and the efficiency of template amplification decreases. Amplification fails to occur in an exponential way, and the PCR enters into the plateau stage. Since it is the $C_t$ value that will be used for analyses, log-linear and plateau data serve as little more than confirmation that the amplification process proceeded in a standard way.

In traditional PCR, the amplified target is detected by postprocessing that includes gel electrophoresis. Real-time PCR produces more reliable results than the traditional method because the error-generating steps of postprocessing are not performed. In addition, obtaining $C_t$ data from the early exponential phase is associated with less variance than data obtained at the end of the exponential phase. Another advantage of real-time PCR is that it is not plagued by the problem of determining whether data from different samples were gathered from different phases of the amplification curve (where plateau values for all samples may be equal if the number of cycles used is high enough). Studies have supported the theoretical statement that the $C_t$ value has a linear relation to the logarithm of the original DNA template concentration (Hilario and Mackay, 2007).

If one were to start with a greater amount of target DNA, a significant increase in fluorescence signal will appear more quickly, which would be reflected by a lower $C_t$ value. The curve of fluorescence intensity versus cycle number for standard samples of known concentrations can be used to generate data that can be used to determine the starting concentrations of unknown samples. This technique is termed real-time quantitative PCR, or qPCR.

### 13.5.2.2 Fluorescence Chemistries

In the early stage of real-time qPCR development, sequence-unspecific detection based on DNA binding dyes like SYBR green was widely applied. SYBR green is a DNA-intercalating dye that dramatically increases in fluorescence when associated with dsDNA. During the PCR reaction set, as cycle number increases so does the accumulation of dsDNA, so there is more dsDNA around to bind the dye to make it fluorescent. Fluorescence intensity correlates with dsDNA concentration and will therefore increase proportionally with DNA amplification. This technique is useful for detecting the amplification of any dsDNA without designing probes (discussed below) so it is convenient and economical. However, dyes can also bind nonspecifically to any dsDNA such as primer dimers to possibly yield false-positive signals. To resolve this problem, dissociation curve analysis must be performed to address the possible presence of multiple PCR products via the number of first-derivative melting peaks (Osborn and Smith, 2005).

The technique that uses hydrolysis probes is an indirect means to detect PCR products. A pair of primers (the same primers as can be designed and used for the Traditional PCR method described earlier) is added to the system along with a sequence-specific probe—designed to bind between the two primers—that is labeled with a reporter dye on the 5′ end and a quencher dye on the 3′ end. Before the probe unfolds and binds to its DNA target sequence, the light energy emitted by the reporter can be absorbed by the quencher group, thus reducing observable reporter fluorescence intensity. However, after the probe has bound to its complimentary sequence on the target DNA strand, the extension step of PCR will utilize the 5′ to 3′ nuclease activity of the DNA polymerase and the probe will be degraded, thus releasing the nucleotides holding the reporter and quencher groups and separating the fluorophore from its quencher. Unshielded by the quencher dye, more of the emitted fluorescence signal can be observed. Every time a DNA strand is amplified a fluorescent molecule is released, so PCR product formation can be inferred through fluorescence. An advantage of this technique is that multiple probes, with different fluorophore/quencher pairs, can be used in the same tube to detect multiple DNA sequences in the same sample.

The molecular beacon technique also utilizes probes for hybridization. The beacons are comprised of a sequence-specific region flanked by two inverted repeats that will hybridize with each other to form a hairpin structure. They contain a fluorophore and a quencher that act as a fluorescence resonance energy transfer (FRET) pair. When the molecular beacon is in a hairpin structure the fluorophore and quencher that are bound to each end of the molecule will result in a reduction of fluorescence intensity via FRET. When the complementary sequence becomes exposed on the ssDNA molecule to be amplified after the melting step of PCR, the beacon will hybridize with the target DNA and transform into an open structure that includes the separation of the reporter and quencher. Reporter emission will then occur without energy transfer to the quencher. The molecular beacon probes have greater specificity than the hydrolysis probes mentioned above because of the presence of the complimentary flanking sequences that are used to form hairpins. This yields a situation where, thermodynamically, the probe bound to the ssDNA target complex must be more stable than probe bound to itself to form the hairpin for the hybridization to occur (Wong and Medrano, 2005).

Evolving from molecular beacons, fluorescence-labeled primers link both the PCR primer and detection mechanism together in the same molecule, thus allowing the fluorophore to directly appear in PCR products. Scorpion primers are one type of such primers. They are composed of a reporter dye on the 5′ end, internal complementary sequences for forming a hairpin loop, a quencher dye, a DNA-polymerase-blocker, and a primer complimentary to the DNA target sequence on the 3′ end (Figure 13.4a). Initially, the primer portion of the Scorpion probe binds to the target template and chain extension takes place. Then the probe transforms from a hairpin loop structure to an open structure after exposure to a second heat denaturing step, and the newly exposed bases on the probe are able to hybridize with the newly synthesized DNA after the extension step (Figure 13.4b through c) (Thelwell et al., 2000). The fluorophore, being on the 5′ end of the probe, is relocated to the far end of the probe–new DNA hybrid as the hairpin denatures and the 5′ end of the probe binds with the 3′ end of the new DNA (Figure 13.4d). With the reporter molecule being far removed from the quencher molecule, fluorescence will be readily detectable. This unimolecular fluorescent chemistry has the advantage of rapid detection with fewer molecules versus methods utilizing primer-probe sets.

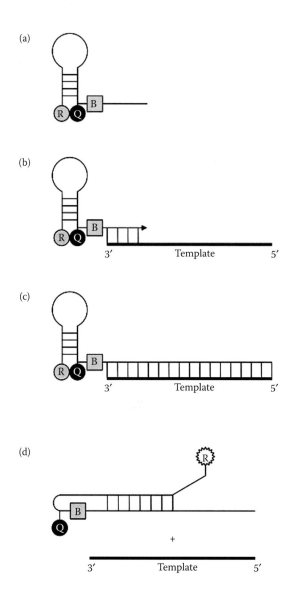

**FIGURE 13.4** Scorpion primers. (a) Scorpion primers contain a reporter dye (R) on the 5′ end, internal complementary sequences for forming a hairpin loop, a quencher dye (Q), a DNA-polymerase-blocker (B), and a primer complimentary to the DNA target sequence on the 3′ end of the primer. (b) The primer binds to the target DNA sequence via the 3′ primer sequence. (c) DNA polymerase extends the primer to make a new sequence complimentary to the DNA template. (d) After heating and denaturation, the scorpion primer is released from the DNA template and denatures to lose its hairpin structure. The internal sequence is free to bond with the new DNA bases, thus separating the reporter and the quencher and yielding an increase in detectable reporter fluorescence.

### 13.5.2.3 Technical Considerations

As with the traditional PCR method, real-time PCR also utilizes the repeated three steps of denature, anneal, and extend. The technical considerations presented earlier are also valid for this PCR method. However, there are differences between the two methods, which are noted below.

Fluorescent probes or DNA intercalating dyes are used in real-time PCR because an assessment of DNA concentration is made during each cycle via fluorescence intensity. As a result, primer design is slightly more complicated than that for traditional PCR. In particular, more attention must be paid to the possible secondary structures that the primers and probes can form, such as hairpins or primer-dimers. These structures are of especial concern when SYBR Green-based qPCR is being used, since short dsDNA fragments will result which will be detected by the intercalating dye.

The optimal amplicon size for real-time PCR is in the range of 50–150 base pairs. A larger target, in particular greater than 300 base pairs, will result in a delayed emergence of the $C_t$. Concerning probe design, the melting temperature of the probe is recommended to be 10°C higher than that of the primer set to obtain a priority for probe binding to the target. The probe should bind on the same strand and somewhat close to one of the primers to allow for detectible changes to the fluorescent signal soon after extension begins (Pestana et al., 2009).

Real-time PCR also requires a more complex thermocycler than does traditional PCR because a light source and a fluorescence detection system are required. Adding to the expense of real-time PCR are the costs of SYBR green or labeled primer/probe sets, a computer, and an analytical software package.

### 13.5.2.4 Quantification

There are two strategies for template quantification in real-time qPCR: absolute and relative. In the absolute quantification method, the amplification signal is associated with DNA copy number by employing a calibration curve (Pestana et al., 2009). A series of diluted standards of known concentrations, determined by light absorption at 260 nm using a spectrophotometer, are prepared and used to obtain the calibration curve (Walker and Rapley, 2009). The standards should be the same material as the samples of unknown concentration. Samples concentrations can be determined via matching their $C_t$ values against the calibration curve. In absolute quantification it is assumed that all standards and samples have equal amplification efficiencies. Taking into account the difficulty related to preparing reliable standards for quantification, the absolute quantification strategy requires considerable effort. It is highly recommended that a fresh calibration curve is generated for each experiment, especially in cases where data are collected and compared on different days or in different laboratories.

In the relative quantification method, a calibrator is utilized to measure the relative change of samples in gene expression. The calibrator can be an endogenous control, an exogenous control, or a reference gene (Dorak, 2006).

When a standard curve is used for relative quantification, the sample quantities are calculated based on the standard curve and then reported as *n*-fold differences relative to the calibrator (which is defined as 1-fold). This method can be employed even though the amplification efficiencies of the calibrator and target genes may not be equal (Wong and Medrano, 2005). An endogenous control—typically a house-keeping gene such as β-actin, GAPDH, or 18s rRNA—is routinely introduced and amplified along with the gene of interest.

The comparative $C_t$ method, another popular method of relative quantification, makes use of mathematical equations to calculate the relative differences between samples and the reference gene (Schmittgen and Livak, 2008). The values of $C_t$ obtained in the early-exponential phase of PCR can reflect the amounts of the initial templates. Various models may take nonideal PCR efficiencies into account, but assume equal amplification kinetics for both the gene of interest and the reference gene. A standard curve is not required in this method, so it is a convenient way of testing a great number of samples. A variety of relative quantification methods have been proposed in recent years for the purpose of improving the accuracy of PCR product quantification, including those put forth by Pfaffl (2001),

Godbey et al. (2008), and Liu and Saint (2002), plus other models termed Amplification plot (Peirson et al., 2003), and Q-gene (Muller et al., 2002).

Real-time PCR has multiple advantages, including high sensitivity, great specificity, good reproducibility, and a wide dynamic quantification range (Dorak, 2006). In consideration of these advantages, the method is viewed as one of the most popular molecular biological techniques for analytical and quantitative study.

# 13.6 Blotting

## 13.6.1 The Southern Blot

### 13.6.1.1 Introduction to the Technique

The Southern blot is a useful technique for determining the presence of a specific sequence in DNA samples. While it is not used much for tissue engineering, the fundamental principal of separating a sample and then hybridizing a probe to a specific sequence is common to other blots that are useful to the tissue engineer. This technique is presented before the other blots for historical perspective.

The Southern blot is a basic molecular biological technique that was invented by the British biologist Edwin Mellor Southern in 1975 (Southern, 1975). It has been applied extensively for the detection of major gene arrangements, thus playing an important role in DNA chromatographic analysis, diagnosis of genetic diseases, and the analysis of PCR products.

### 13.6.1.2 Technical Considerations (Southern, 1975, Hoy, 2003)

1. *Preparation of sample: DNA* Genomic DNA is extracted directly from animal cells or tissues. The DNA obtained will be too long to be used in hybridization analyses, so the sample should be digested by restriction endonucleases into a series of smaller fragments.

2. *Gel electrophoresis:* Agarose gel electrophoresis is used to separate DNA fragments from step 1 by size. Fragments that have the same size will occupy the same band within the gel. The molecular weights of different fragments can be determined based on DNA molecular weight standards that are introduced into the gel adjacent to the sample.

3. *Pretreatment:* Before the DNA is transferred from the gel onto the blotting membrane, it is important to process the separated DNA beforehand because of the amount of time required to completely transfer DNA fragments. It takes much longer for fragments in excess of 10 kilobase pairs (kbp) to be transferred than small fragments (<1 kbp). When there are DNA fragments larger than 10 kbp, the gel should be treated with dilute HCl to depurinate the large fragments and break them into small pieces (Slater, 1986).

   During steps 1 and 2, the DNA in the sample maintains a double-stranded configuration. However, single-stranded DNA is required for hybridization. To denature dsDNA into ssDNA, the gel is incubated with an alkaline solution (commonly sodium hydroxide), followed by neutralization via a buffer. After denaturing, binding between the negatively charged DNA and the positively charged membrane in step 4 will be enhanced. In addition, any residual RNA that may exist in the DNA sample will be hydrolyzed.

4. *Transfer:* The material used for the transfer membrane is an important factor for retaining DNA following transfer. Nitrocellulose was the first material to be used for nucleic acid blots. Buffers with high ionic strength are indispensable for the binding of nucleic acids to these membranes because nitrocellulose interacts with nucleic acids via hydrophobic interactions. As such, nitrocellulose does not have a strong affinity for nucleic acids, so DNA can easily dissolve into solution (particularly the small fragments). Nitrocellulose membranes are also quite brittle when dry, which complicates the procedure further. An alternative to the nitrocellulose membrane is the nylon membrane, which has stronger DNA binding capability than nitrocellulose because it

interacts with DNA via charge–charge interactions (Avison, 2007). Furthermore, it can be reused for detection of different nucleic acids sequences without preparing a new sample. The probe previously used is rinsed at high temperature and a different probe is later introduced to detect another sequence.

A large filter paper is soaked in saline–sodium citrate buffer (0.15 M NaCl, 0.015 M sodium citrate) and placed on a glass or plastic support. The gel strip is laid on top of the wet paper and covered by a sheet of nitrocellulose or nylon membrane. Many layers of dry filter paper (or paper towels) are placed on top of the membrane. Capillary action causes the movement of buffer through the membrane to the dry paper. The DNA fragments are carried along with the buffer, but the fragments are deposited on the membrane through the interactions just mentioned.

Electrophoretic transfer is also an effective strategy for performing the blotting procedure, and is especially suited for transferring large DNA fragments. One must keep in mind that the ionic strength of buffer is related to its conductance, so the buffer composition has an influence on electrophoretic transfer efficiency and the binding ability with membrane (Butler, 1991). A vacuum pump can also be used to facilitate the blot transfer. No matter which method is applied, the separation pattern of the DNA fragments is preserved as they travel from the gel to the membrane.

The membrane is next baked in an oven, placed in a vacuum or exposed to ultraviolet light to strengthen the attachment of the DNA that has been transferred.

5. *Pre-hybridization:* The membrane used to trap the restriction fragments can also bind the probe, which is also made from DNA. The membrane is therefore soaked in pre-hybridization solution containing salmon or herring sperm DNA to nonspecifically block all remaining DNA-binding sites on the membrane. The blocking DNAs are heterogenic with mammalian DNA, so they will not bind with the hybridization probe.

6. *Southern hybridization:* The labeled DNA probe should be denatured via heating to transform it into a ssDNA structure, then used to wash the filter membrane. If the sample DNA contains a sequence complementary to that of the probe, the probe will bind to the sample DNA. Hybridization is carried out in a salt buffer with comparatively high ionic strength. The stringency of the hybridization can be increased by increasing the hybridization temperature or decreasing the salt concentration (Gearhart, 2003, Walker and Rapley, 2000).

7. *Wash:* Excessive probe should be washed from the membrane with saline–sodium citrate buffer. During the wash process, if radiolabeled probes were used, the radioactive intensity of the membrane is monitored. Rinsing is halted when the radiation intensity of the membrane is within one- to two-fold that of background. If the membrane is not rinsed sufficiently there will be reduced contrast upon detection.

8. *Detection:* If a radioactive probe is used, hybridization can be detected via exposure of x-ray film to the membrane. Note that fluorescent and chromogenic probes are also available.

## 13.6.2 The Northern Blot

### 13.6.2.1 Introduction to the Technique

Inspired by the Southern blot, James Alwine, David Kemp, and George Stark at Stanford University developed the northern blot technique in 1977 (Alwine et al., 1977). The northern blot is used to analyze gene expression via RNA detection. It can be used to monitor transcriptional activity of an endogenous or exogenous gene in cells or tissues.

There are three significant advantages to use the northern blotting technique for measuring the level of RNA. First, one gene can sometimes generate different RNA species. Northern blotting can provide a comparison between multiple RNAs derived from a single gene, yielding detailed information including size and relative copy number. Second, after an RNA sample has been bound to a membrane, multiple hybridizations with different probes can be performed to analyze the expression of several genes on the same RNA sample (Murray, 1991). Third, the technique is relatively simple to perform and all required equipments are inexpensive.

Northern blot analysis can also be associated with several drawbacks. Measures should be taken to prevent samples from being contaminated by RNase, a prevalent enzyme that is responsible for RNA degradation. The presence of RNases would affect data quality and render the quantification of gene expression unreliable. In addition, northern blotting is not as sensitive as other techniques such as nuclease protection assays or PCR. Although simple to perform, the technique is time consuming, especially when a great number of samples are to be analyzed, even though more than one gene can be detected per blot (Perdew et al., 2006).

### 13.6.2.2 Technical Considerations

The main procedure of northern blotting is very similar to that of Southern blotting in that both contain steps of sample preparation, gel electrophoresis, transfer from gel to membrane, probe hybridization, and detection. Northern blotting differs from the Southern procedure in the following ways:

1. *Preparation of sample:* Detergents are used to lyse cells and then solvents are required to extract RNA. RNA is separated from proteins and DNA by means of liquid-phase separation or oligo (dT) chromatography. Considering that RNase is ubiquitous, RNase inhibition must be performed to prevent RNA degradation. Guanidine isothiocyanate can be used lyse cells and simultaneously inactivate RNases (Bird and Smith, 2002). Because RNA molecules are comparatively small, there is no need to use restriction endonucleases to break the RNA into smaller fragments.

2. *Gel electrophoresis:* Denaturing agents are incorporated into the agarose gels to limit RNA secondary structures (as opposed to performing the gel electrophoresis first and denaturing in a subsequent step). Formaldehyde and glyoxal are two commonly used denaturants. Sodium hydroxide should be avoided because it tends to hydrolyze the 2′-hydroxyl groups of RNA. In addition, it has been reported that the use of ethidium bromide in gels can hinder the subsequent transfer of RNA from gel to membrane, thus and alternative such as alcidine orange should be used for RNA visualization (Coleman and Tsongalis, 2006).

## 13.6.3 The Western Blot

### 13.6.3.1 Introduction to the Technique

The western blot, also known as the immunoblot, is used to identify and relatively quantify the amount of a specific protein within a sample containing multiple proteins, such as what is obtained following cell lysis. An immunochemical assay is used for protein identification. The technique is often used to detect the downstream product of specific gene expression. Due to high sensitivity, efficiency, and convenience, the western blot has been widely used by researchers through the world.

There are three basic steps to the western blot procedure: separation of proteins by gel electrophoresis, transfer of the separated samples from the gel to a membrane, and probing the membrane with antibodies. Proteins carry highly variable charges which are not easy to separate by simple gel electrophoresis. Therefore, sodium dodecyl sulfate (SDS) is often applied to denature the proteins and apply a uniform negative charge concentration to all of the polypeptides. The polypeptides can then be separated via polyacrylamide gel electrophoresis according to size.

After gel electrophoresis, the polypeptides are transferred electrophoretically from the gel to a membrane which serves as a support for the immunoreactions to follow. The fractionated polypeptides are adsorbed onto the membrane by noncovalent bonds and then exposed to a primary antibody which will bind specifically to the protein in question. The primary antibody will be detected through the binding of a labeled secondary antibody. The label is visualized via staining or radioactive assay.

### 13.6.3.2 Technical Considerations

The main procedures of western blotting are similar to those of Southern and northern blotting, including gel electrophoresis, transfer to a membrane, and probe hybridization. However, there are differences of particular note:

1. *Gel electrophoresis:* The gel electrophoresis used for the western blot is SDS-PAGE. The proteins in the sample are denatured by mixing them with SDS and then boiling. Details for SDS-PAGE are given in Section 13.2.3.

2. *Transfer:* Typically, electrophoretic transfer is the more preferable method for western blotting due to its high efficiency. Electro-transfer of the separated polypeptides onto the membrane can be accomplished by either semi-dry blotting or tank transferring systems (Walker, 2002). Tank transferring is more convenient and efficient than semi-dry blotting, but semi-dry blotting is more suitable for large gels because fewer buffers are required. For semi-dry blotting, two stacks of filter paper pre-wet with buffer are placed into contact with the gel and membrane to form a sandwich. The membrane is on the side of the anode, while the gel is by the cathode. Applying an electric current will cause the polypeptides to be transferred from the gel to the membrane because of the SDS that was used to denature them while providing a uniform negative charge. The tank transfer system is similar, utilizing a blotting sandwich with filter paper, membrane and gel submerged in a tank. The polypeptides will be similarly transferred by applied electrical current.

   Nitrocellulose or polyvinylidene difluoride membranes are often utilized for western blotting. Because of their moderate levels of protein retention and comparably low price, nitrocellulose membranes have been well accepted for basic detection. However, polyvinylidene difluoride membranes possess better protein retention, physical strength, and chemical resistance. Thus they are often used when reprobing or protein sequencing will be performed because they will not be affected by repeated washing with organic solvents.

3. *Blocking:* Before applying the probes, the membrane must be blocked with proteins that will not be recognized by the probes. Blocking buffer or even dry instant milk can be used. This step is necessary because the portions of the membrane that did not receive the electrically transferred sample would still be charged, which could lead to nonspecific binding of the primary antibody probe.

4. *Probe hybridization:* Unlike in Southern and northern blots, the probes of the western blot are antibodies. Primary antibodies specific for the target polypeptides are required, and can be produced from animal species that are different from the origin of the protein sample. For example, if we are investigating the expression of mouse protein XYZ, we might use a primary immunoglobulin G (IgG) antibody raised in rabbits termed rabbit anti-mouse XYZ. Secondary antibodies could be tagged as antibody–enzyme conjugates or [125]I-labeled antibodies. The secondary antibodies will detect the primary antibodies, and be raised in a species different from what produced the primary antibodies. In our example, we might use labeled goat anti-rabbit IgG.

There are many commercially available labeled secondary antibody products. The most common conjugated enzymes are alkaline phosphatase and horseradish peroxidase. Alkaline phosphatase, discussed earlier in the section on histochemistry, dephosphorylates the substrate 5-bromo-4-chloro-3-indolyl phosphate which can be oxidized by nitroblue tetrazolium. The resulting signal would appear as a blue/purple dye. Horseradish peroxidase can catalyze the oxidation of 4-(chloro-1-naphthol), in the presence of hydrogen peroxide, into an insoluble blue dye. Apart from using antibody–enzyme conjugates, secondary antibodies can be labeled with [125]I to permit detection by autoradiography.

## 13.6.4 The Eastern Blot

After the development of the Southern and northern blots, and after the western blotting technique was developed by Towbin in 1979 (Towbin et al., 1979), many scholars have attempted to use "Eastern" in the name of their own blotting techniques. As examples, Wreschner et al. (Wreschner and Herzberg, 1984), and Ishikawa et al. (Taki et al., 1994, Ishikawa and Taki, 2000) have put forth techniques termed Middle Eastern blotting, Eastern–Western blotting, and Far-Eastern blotting, respectively. In 2001, Shan et al. (2001) proposed their own "Eastern blotting" technique for the visualization of small molecules by means of thin layer chromatography (TLC). In the technique, the TLC plate is dried, followed by blotting of small molecules to a poly(vinylidene fluoride) (PVDF) membrane (Crocker and Murray, 2003). In general, eastern blotting is used to analyze proteins, lipoproteins, or glycoproteins, to detect posttranslational protein modifications. Samples are separated via SDS-PAGE and transferred to PVDF or nitrocellulose membranes for detection and analysis. So far, however, the scientific community has not reached a consensus for the definition of eastern blotting. Some researchers insist that eastern blotting does not exist at all.

# References

Alwine, J. C., Kemp, D. J., and Stark, G. R. 1977. Method for detection of specific RNAs in agarose gels by transfer to diazobenzyloxymethyl-paper and hybridization with DNA probes. *Proc Natl Acad Sci USA,* 74: 5350–4.

Avison, M. B. 2007. *Measuring Gene Expression,* New York; Abingdon [England], Taylor & Francis.

Bancroft, J. D. and Gamble, M. 2008. *Theory and Practice of Histological Techniques,* Edinburgh; New York, Churchill Livingstone.

Bird, R. C. and Smith, B. F. 2002. *Genetic Library Construction and Screening : Advanced Techniques and Applications,* Berlin; New York, Springer.

Bourne, G. H. and Danielli, J. F. (ed.) 1970. *International Review of Cytology,* New York: Academic Press, Inc..

Bronner-Fraser, M. (ed.) 1996. *Methods in Cell Biology,* San Diego: Academic Press, Inc.

Brown, T. A. 2000. *Essential Molecular Biology: A Practical Approach,* Oxford; New York, Oxford University Press.

Butler, J. E. 1991. *Immunochemistry of Solid-Phase Immunoassay,* Boca Raton, CRC Press.

Campbell, G., Compston, J., and Crisp, A. 1993. *The Management of Common Metabolic Bone Disorders,* Cambridge [England]; New York, Cambridge University Press.

Clark, D. P. 2005. *Molecular Biology,* Amsterdam; Boston, Elsevier Academic Press.

Coleman, W. B. and Tsongalis, G. J. 2006. *Molecular Diagnostics: For the Clinical Laboratorian,* Totowa, NJ, Humana Press.

Cormack, D. H. 2001. *Essential Histology,* Philadelphia, Lippincott Williams & Wilkins.

Crocker, J. and Murray, P. 2003. *Molecular Biology in Cellular Pathology,* Chichester, West Sussex, England; Hoboken, NJ, John Wiley & Sons.

Derbyshire, V. et al. 1988. Genetic and crystallographic studies of the $3',5'$-exonucleolytic site of DNA polymerase I. *Science,* 240: 199–201.

Dhein, S., Mohr, F. W., and Delmar, M. 2005. *Practical Methods in Cardiovascular Research,* Berlin; New York, Springer.

Dorak, M. T. 2006. *Real-Time PCR,* New York, Taylor & Francis.

Eun, H.-M. 1996. *Enzymology Primer for Recombinant DNA Technology,* San Diego, Academic Press.

Gearhart, J. P. (ed.) 2003. *Pediatric Urology,* Totowa, Humana Press Inc.

Godbey, W. T., Hindy, S. B., Sherman, M. E., and Atala, A. 2004. A novel use of centrifugal force for cell seeding into porous scaffolds. *Biomaterials,* 25: 2799–805.

Godbey, W. T., Zhang, X., and CHANG, F. 2008. The importance of and a method for including transfection efficiency into real-time PCR data analyses. *Biotechnol Bioeng,* 100: 765–72.

Hames, B. D. 1998. *Gel Electrophoresis of Proteins: A Practical Approach,* Oxford; New York, Oxford University Press.

Hilario, E. and Mackay, J. 2007. *Protocols for Nucleic Acid Analysis by Nonradioactive Probes,* Totowa, NJ, Humana Press.

Hjerten, S. 1962. "Molecular sieve" chromatography on polyacrylamide gels, prepared according to a simplified method. *Arch Biochem Biophys,* Suppl 1: 147–51.

Holtorf, H. L., Jansen, J. A., and Mikos, A. G. 2005. Flow perfusion culture induces the osteoblastic differentiation of marrow stroma cell-scaffold constructs in the absence of dexamethasone. *J Biomed Mater Res A,* 72: 326–34.

Hoy, M. A. 2003. *Insect Molecular Genetics: An Introduction to Principles and Applications,* Amsterdam; Boston, Academic Press.

Humason, G. L. 1972. *Animal Tissue Techniques,* San Francisco, W. H. Freeman.

Ishikawa, D. and Taki, T. 2000. Thin-layer chromatography blotting using polyvinylidene difluoride membrane (Far-Eastern blotting) and its applications. *Sphingolipid Metabolism and Cell Signaling, Pt B,* 312: 145–57.

Kieleczawa, J. 2006. *DNA Sequencing II: Optimizing Preparation and Cleanup,* Sudbury, MA, Jones and Bartlett Publishers.

Kiernan, J. A. 1981. *Histological and Histochemical Methods: Theory and Practice,* Oxford, England; New York, Pergamon Press.

Krishnamurthy, K. V. 1999. *Methods in Cell Wall Cytochemistry,* Boca Raton, FL, CRC Press.

Kumar, A. and Garg, N. 2005. *Genetic Engineering,* New York, Nova Biomedical Books.

Liu, W. and Saint, D. A. 2002. A new quantitative method of real time reverse transcription polymerase chain reaction assay based on simulation of polymerase chain reaction kinetics. *Anal Biochem,* 302: 52–9.

Marmur, J. and Doty, P. 1962. Determination of the base composition of deoxyribonucleic acid from its thermal denaturation temperature. *J Mol Biol,* 5: 109–18.

McPherson, M. J. and Hames, B. D. 1995. *PCR 2 : A Practical Approach,* Oxford; New York, IRL Press at Oxford University Press.

Menninger, J. R., Wright, M., Menninger, L., and Meselson, M. 1968. Attachment and detachment of bacteriophage lambda DNA in lysogenization and induction. *J Mol Biol,* 32: 631–7.

Mitra, S. 2003. *Sample Preparation Techniques in Analytical Chemistry,* Hoboken, NJ, J. Wiley.

Muller, P. Y., Janovjak, H., Miserez, A. R., and Dobbie, Z. 2002. Processing of gene expression data generated by quantitative real-time RT-PCR. *Biotechniques,* 32: 1372–4, 1376, 1378–9.

Murray, E. J. 1991. *Gene Transfer and Expression Protocols,* Clifton, NJ, Humana Press.

Nagy, L. E. 2008. *Alcohol: Methods and Protocols,* Totowa, NJ, Humana Press.

New England Biolabs. 2009a. *Optimizing Restriction Endonuclease Reactions* [Online]. Available at http://www.neb.com/nebecomm/tech_reference/restriction_enzymes/setting_up_reaction.asp

New England Biolabs. 2009b. *T4 DNA Ligase FAQ* [Online]. Available at http://www.neb.com/nebecomm/products/faqproductM0202.asp

Newton, C. R. and Graham, A. 1997. *PCR,* Oxford, OX, UK New York, BIOS Scientific Publishers; Springer.

Osborn, A. M. and Smith, C. J. 2005. *Molecular Microbial Ecology,* New York; Abingdon [England], Taylor & Francis.

Peirson, S. N., Butler, J. N., and Foster, R. G. 2003. Experimental validation of novel and conventional approaches to quantitative real-time PCR data analysis. *Nucleic Acids Res,* 31: e73.

Pelt-Verkuil, E. V., Belkum, A. V., and Hays, J. P. 2008. *Principles and Technical Aspects of PCR Amplification,* Dordrecht, Springer.

Perdew, G. H., Vanden Heuvel, J. P., and Peters, J. M. 2006. *Regulation of Gene Expression: Molecular Mechanisms,* Totowa, NJ, Humana Press.

Pestana, E. A., Adama Diallo, S. B., Crowther, J. R., and Viljoen, G. J. 2009. *Early, Rapid and Sensitive Veterinary Molecular Diagnostics—Real Time pcr Applications,* New York, Springer.

Pfaffl, M. W. 2001. A new mathematical model for relative quantification in real-time RT-PCR. *Nucleic Acids Res,* 29: e45.

Pingoud, A. and Jeltsch, A. 2001. Structure and function of type II restriction endonucleases. *Nucleic Acids Res,* 29: 3705–27.

Rapley, R. and Walker, J. M. 1998. *Molecular Biomethods Handbook,* Totowa, NJ, Humana Press.

Roe, S. 2001. *Protein Purification Techniques : A Practical Approach,* Oxford; New York, Oxford University Press.

Rychlik, W., Spencer, W. J., and Rhoads, R. E. 1990. Optimization of the annealing temperature for DNA amplification in vitro. *Nucleic Acids Res,* 18: 6409–12.

Saiki, R. K., Gelfand, D. H., Stoffel, S. et al. 1988. Primer-directed enzymatic amplification of DNA with a thermostable DNA polymerase. *Science,* 239: 487–91.

Saiki, R. K., Scharf, S., Faloona, F. et al. 1985. Enzymatic amplification of beta-globin genomic sequences and restriction site analysis for diagnosis of sickle cell anemia. *Science,* 230: 1350–4.

Sambrook, J. and Russell, D. W. 2001. *Molecular Cloning : A Laboratory Manual,* Cold Spring Harbor, NY, Cold Spring Harbor Laboratory Press.

Saotome, K., Morita, H., and Umeda, M. 1989. Cytotoxicity test with simplified crystal violet staining method using microtitre plates and its application to injection-drugs. *Toxicology in Vitro,* 3: 317–21.

Saunders, G. C., Parkes, H. C., and Laboratory of the Government Chemist (Great Britain) 1999. *Analytical Molecular Biology: Quality and Validation,* Cambridge, Published for Laboratory of the Government Chemist by the Royal Society of Chemistry.

Schmittgen, T. D. and Livak, K. J. 2008. Analyzing real-time PCR data by the comparative C(T) method. *Nat Protoc,* 3: 1101–8.

Shan, S. J., Tanaka, H., and Shoyama, Y. 2001. Enzyme-linked immunosorbent assay for glycyrrhizin using anti-glycyrrhizin monoclonal antibody and an eastern blotting technique for glucuronides of glyc-yrrhetic acid. *Anal Chem,* 73: 5784–90.

Singer, V. L., Jones, L. J., Yue, S. T., and Haugland, R. P. 1997. Characterization of PicoGreen reagent and development of a fluorescence-based solution assay for double-stranded DNA quantitation. *Anal Biochem,* 249: 228–38.

Slater, R. J. 1986. *Experiments in Molecular Biology,* Clinton, NJ, Humana Press.

Smith, H. O. and Nathans, D. 1973. Letter: A suggested nomenclature for bacterial host modification and restriction systems and their enzymes. *J Mol Biol,* 81: 419–23.

Southern, E. M. 1975. Detection of specific sequences among DNA fragments separated by gel electropho-resis. *J Mol Biol,* 98: 503–17.

Steitz, T. A. 1993. *Structural Studies of Protein-Nucleic Acid Interaction : The Sources of Sequence-Specific Binding,* New York, NY, USA, Cambridge University Press.

Taki, T., Handa, S., and Ishikawa, D. 1994. Blotting of glycolipids and phospholipids from a high-perfor-mance thin-layer chromatogram to a polyvinylidene difluoride membrane. *Analytical Biochemistry,* 221: 312–16.

Thelwell, N., Millington, S., Solinas, A., Booth, J., and Brown, T. 2000. Mode of action and application of Scorpion primers to mutation detection. *Nucleic Acids Res,* 28: 3752–61.

Towbin, H., Staehelin, T., and Gordon, J. 1979. Electrophoretic transfer of proteins from polyacrylamide gels to nitrocellulose sheets—Procedure and some applications. *Proc Natl Acad Sci USA,* 76: 4350–4.

Walker, J. M. 1994. *Basic Protein and Peptide Protocols,* Totowa, NJ, Humana Press.

Walker, J. M. 2002. *The Protein Protocols Handbook,* Totowa, NJ, Humana Press.

Walker, J. M. and Rapley, R. 2000. *Molecular Biology and Biotechnology,* Cambridge, Royal Society of Chemistry.

Walker, J. M. and Rapley, R. 2009. *Molecular Biology and Biotechnology,* Cambridge, Royal Society of Chemistry.

Wilson, G. G. 1988. Type II restriction- modification systems. *Trends Genet,* 4: 314–8.

Wong, M. L. and Medrano, J. F. 2005. Real-time PCR for mRNA quantitation. *Biotechniques,* 39: 75–85.

Wreschner, D. H. and Herzberg, M. 1984. A new blotting medium for the simple isolation and identifica-tion of highly resolved messenger-RNA. *Nucl Acids Res,* 12: 1349–59.

# 14

# Biomaterial Mechanics

Kimberly M. Stroka
*University of Maryland*

Leann L. Norman
*University of Maryland*

Helim
Aranda-Espinoza
*University of Maryland*

14.1 Introduction ................................................................. 14-1
14.2 Cellular Mechanotransduction ....................................... 14-1
   Overview • Mechanobiology • Mechanical Changes Influence
   Cellular Behavior • Mechanotransduction in Disease
14.3 Mechanics of Biomaterials ........................................... 14-6
   Cell–Substrate Interactions • Parameters That Affect Cell–Substrate
   Interactions • Approaches for Regulating Cellular Behavior
14.4 Potential Target and Applications .................................. 14-10
   Neural Engineering • Cardiovascular Engineering • Suppression
   of Cancerous Tumors • Engineering with Stem Cells
14.5 Summary .................................................................... 14-12
References .......................................................................... 14-12

## 14.1 Introduction

The interaction of cells with surfaces is a complicated phenomenon that has been widely studied from many different angles, including those relevant to biology, chemistry, physics, and engineering. An understanding of how cells interact with surfaces of varying physical and chemical properties is important for applications in human health, biomaterial development, and tissue engineering. An aspect of biomaterial fabrication that just recently has been addressed is the importance of the mechanical properties of the biomaterial in relation to cell–surface interactions. Here, we present a short review of the state of the art in biomaterial mechanics. We start by reviewing cellular mechanotransduction (how cells convert mechanical forces to biochemical signaling pathways) and then overview the mechanics of biomaterials. This review is far from extensive given the tremendous amount of work in this area and we regret that many interesting aspects have been left out.

## 14.2 Cellular Mechanotransduction

### 14.2.1 Overview

From bacteria to mammals, all living organisms are subjected to physical forces. Mechanotransduction is referred to as the process of translating these mechanical forces into useful biochemical signals and cellular responses. The translation of physical forces into cellular responses is fundamental to development and physiology (Davidson et al. 2002; Farge 2003; Keller et al. 2003), cell migration (Pelham and Wang 1997; Stroka and Aranda-Espinoza 2009), and differentiation (Engler et al. 2007, 2008b; Oh et al. 2009), as well as certain diseases (Hahn and Schwartz 2008; Ingber 2003; Lammerding et al. 2004; Spence et al. 2002). In the case of development and physiology, the continuous translation of physical forces into meaningful biochemical responses ensures not only structural stability among cells and organisms, but also a way to generate specific three-dimensional structures, such as the formation of tissues and organs (Orr et al. 2006). Mechanotransduction also plays a role in the migration of numerous cell types, including neutrophils (Stroka and Aranda-Espinoza 2009), neurons (Balgude et al. 2001; Flanagan et al. 2002; Leach et al. 2007; Norman and Aranda-Espinoza 2010), and endothelial cells (ECs) (Yeung et al. 2005). In the case of neutrophils, the migratory behavior of these immune response cells can be directly affected by the mechanical properties of the extracellular matrix (ECM), which in turn can inhibit the speed of migration (Stroka and Aranda-Espinoza 2009) as well as the ability to target infection through transmigration (Rabodzey et al. 2008; Stroka and Aranda-Espinoza 2010). The differentiation of stem cells has also been recently related to the mechanical properties of the ECM (Engler et al. 2006; Saha et al. 2008; Shi et al. 2009). Remarkably, the stiffness of the ECM can direct stem cell lineage, with softer substrates inducing the differentiation of "neuron-like" cells, intermediate substrates inducing "muscle-like" cells, and stiff substrates directing the differentiation of "bone-like" cells (Engler et al. 2006). This behavior emphasizes the importance of matrix compliance and mechanotransduction in the development of stem cell therapeutics, since the mechanical environment alone is enough to direct their lineage. Although the above mentioned behaviors highlight some of the beneficial aspects of cellular mechanotransduction, multiple diseases and disorders can also be attributed to defects and abnormalities associated with mechanotransduction components and pathways. These diseases and disorders are further addressed below.

## 14.2.2 Mechanobiology

Numerous cellular components have been identified as mediators of mechanotransduction. Some of these elements include the cell membrane, cytoskeleton, nuclei, and surface processes (i.e., cilia), as well as cell–cell and cell–ECM adhesions. The ECM plays a particularly critical role in mechanoregulation of tissues and cells by serving as a scaffold through which the stresses applied to the tissue can be distributed (Balaban et al. 2001; Wang et al. 1993). These stresses are typically focused on cell–ECM adhesions, which occur through integrin binding. Integrins serve as a site for the transfer of an extracellular mechanical signal across the plasma membrane and to the cytoskeleton, triggering a specific molecular pathway and cellular response (Balaban et al. 2001; Choquet et al. 1997; Wang et al. 1993). In addition to integrin signaling, general mechanisms by which physical force can regulate cellular responses can occur through changes in protein conformation and the regulation of stretch-sensitive channels (Byfield et al. 2006; Martinac 2004; Orr et al. 2006). External forces can induce the unfolding of specific ECM proteins, which in turn can stimulate mechanotransduction signaling pathways. Alternatively, in the plasma membrane of cells, stretch-activated channels can respond to strain by opening and closing, allowing the regulation of calcium and ions and initiation of specific signaling cascades (Munevar et al. 2004). For example, the regulation of stretch-activated channels contributes to the mechanical response of cardiomyocytes as well as sensory cells (Jaalouk and Lammerding 2009). In general, the regulation of mechanosensors (including stretch-activate channels, as well as integrins, integrin-associated proteins, and cell–surface receptors) can activate multiple signaling pathways, which in turn, contribute to specific gene expression or cellular behavior changes.

## 14.2.3 Mechanical Changes Influence Cellular Behavior

As briefly mentioned above, modification of the ECM and cell–ECM adhesions both *in vivo* and *in vitro* can significantly influence the morphology, growth, differentiation, and/or migration of numerous cell types (Chicurel et al. 1998), including neurons (Balgude et al. 2001; Flanagan et al. 2002; Leach et al. 2007; Leann L. Norman and Aranda-Espinoza 2010), endothelial (Yeung et al. 2005), fibroblasts (Pelham and Wang 1997; Yeung et al. 2005), neutrophils (Stroka and Aranda-Espinoza 2009), and stem cells (Engler et al. 2006; Saha et al. 2008; Shi et al. 2009). For example, the endothelium can directly respond to fluid shear stress by altering the expression of specific immune response binding proteins (i.e., ICAM) (Davies 1995), while kidney epithelial cells modify their calcium influx in response to the fluid shear stress of urine (Nauli et al. 2003; Park et al. 1999). Mechanical load and strain can also trigger changes in cellular behavior, as seen with the increase in the production of proteoglycans by chondrocytes after compressive loading (Grodzinsky et al. 2000), and the increase in growth and/or size of bone and muscle cells (Hatton et al. 2003; Hove et al. 2003; Miller et al. 2000a).

Interestingly, both micro- and macromechanical properties of substrates and cellular environments can influence mechanotransduction. For example, forces applied at the macroscale can propagate microscale modifications of the ECM and cytoskeletal mechanics. This is seen in the case of blood vessel mechanics, which become more rigid when distended under high blood pressure conditions, and also in the case of increased osmotic forces following injury, which can trigger the stiffening of interstitial matrix (Ingber 2003). The microscale changes that occur due to macroscale forces are not applied uniformly across clusters of cells; instead, the forces are felt on the ECM through focal adhesions (Balaban et al. 2001). Cells that experience mechanical stress through integrin adhesions can respond to these stresses by recruiting focal adhesion proteins, therefore strengthening it against future stresses (Schmidt et al. 1993; Wang et al. 1993). One of the most referenced models of mechanotransduction is hearing and balance within the auditory system (Chalfie 2009). In this system, mechanical stimulus within the inner ear causes small displacements of the stereocilia of hair cells, which initiates tension in adjacent stereocilia tips, and triggers the opening of mechanically gated ion channels (Holt and Corey 2000). The opening of these channels can initiate a calcium influx, which triggers further downstream signaling (Holt and Corey 2000). Resting tension can be restored through the relaxation of motor proteins also located on the stereocilia tips (Vollrath et al. 2007). Mechanotransduction pathways involved with proprioception and sensation have been identified to follow similar mechanisms to that of the auditory system as well (Eberl et al. 2000; Jaalouk and Lammerding 2009). Since mechanotransduction signaling is crucial for the normal functioning of almost all cell types, impaired mechanosensing can significantly affect many tissues and organs.

## 14.2.4 Mechanotransduction in Disease

Defects in cellular mechanotransduction have been associated with a vast and seemingly dissimilar variety of diseases and disorders. Modifications in the extracellular environment, as well as changes in cellular structure, organization, sensing, and/or signaling can trigger aberrant mechanotransduction signaling, which in turn, can lead to disease (Ingber 2003; Jaalouk and Lammerding 2009). Changes in the extracellular environment may include variations in stiffness or porosity, or alterations in fluid shear stress or applied forces. Alterations in cell structure may include changes in integrin, ion channels, or other transmembrane proteins, as well as changes in cytoskeletal, and nuclear proteins. Lastly, changes in cellular sensing and signaling, such as modifications of stretch-activated channels or other mechanosensors, and alterations in the Rho or mitogen-activated protein kinase (MAPK) pathways may alter mechanotransduction signaling (Martineau and Gardiner 2001). Diseases including, but not limited to, developmental disorders (Hove et al. 2003; Patwari and Lee 2008), arteriosclerosis (Cheng et al. 2006; Matsumoto et al. 2002), asthma and lung dysfunctions (Ichimura et al. 2003; Uhlig 2002), deafness (Vollrath et al. 2007), liver fibrosis (Georges et al. 2007), osteoporosis (Klein-Nulend et al. 2003), premature aging (Capell et al. 2007; Verstraeten et al. 2008), and cancer (Liang et al. 2008; Paszek et al. 2005a; Suresh 2007; Wolf et al. 2007) have all been associated with some type of mechanotransduction deficiency.

Defects in mechanotransduction components may arise due to genetic mutations, such as muscular dystrophy, which results from a laminin α2 mutation that eventually leads to the degeneration of muscle and potential hearing loss (Pillers et al. 2002). Additional conditions such as pulmonary fibrosis, vascular hypertension, diabetic nephropathy, and scleroderma all involve abnormal tissue function and mechanics due to the accumulation of atypical ECM (Ingber 2003). Genetic mutations in myosin (Lynch et al. 1997; Redowicz 2002), β-actin (Boulassel et al. 2001), and integrin α8β1 (Evans and Muller 2000) contribute to some of the genetic causes of deafness, primarily due to alterations of hair cell composition and mechanics. Various forms of heart disease as well as vascular smooth muscle and cardiac muscle contractility abnormalities have been identified to arise due to the genetic mutation of integrins and/or ECM molecules (Balogh et al. 2002; Keller et al. 2001). Some of the major diseases and disorders that are associated with mechanotransduction abnormalities include cardiac diseases, muscular dystrophies, and cancer.

### 14.2.4.1 Cardiac Myopathy

The mechanosensitive capabilities of the heart allow this organ to respond to the necessary increases in growth required through life. Unfortunately, the same machinery that allows the body to adapt to physiological changes can also contribute to serious cardiac diseases and potential heart failure. Cardiac myocytes are responsive to axial stretch and are remarkably able to react to stretching by changing their function and increasing in size, referred to as hypertrophy (Weckstrom and Tavi 2007). The key mechanosensors believed to be responsible for this behavior include integrins (and their associated proteins), stretch-sensitive ion channels, sarcomeric proteins (i.e., titin and myosin), and cell–surface receptors (Jaalouk and Lammerding 2009). The increase in cardiac myocyte size is generally classified as physiological or pathological hypertrophy, and in both cases, cells sense enhanced stresses placed on the ventricular wall and respond by increasing in size (Zhong et al. 2006). Physiological hypertrophy refers to normal and healthy increases in cardiac wall thickness and architecture due to regular events such as pregnancy or aerobic exercise, while pathological hypertrophy occurs due to a deviation in cardiac activity (Iemitsu et al. 2001; McMullen and Jennings 2007). It has recently been identified that regulating the signaling pathways involved in hypertrophic response may prevent pathological hypertrophy (Heineke and Molkentin 2006), suggesting a target for cardiac therapeutics.

### 14.2.4.2 Atherosclerosis

Atherosclerosis is a disease associated with the stiffening of arteries and is another example of disease associated with changes in cell/tissue mechanics. Initiation of atherosclerosis occurs due to increased low-density lipoproteins (LDLs), which promote plaque formation and damage to the endothelium. Typically, the formation of these plaques occurs in regions of disturbed blood flow, such as near branching locations (Davies 1995). After damage to the endothelium, the immune system sends leukocytes to this area; however, they are typically unable to process the oxidized LDLs, leading to a cascade of more oxidized LDL deposits and the development of disease. The increasing size of these developed plaques slowly narrow the artery, causing a reduction in blood flow as well as potential functional deficiencies, pain, heart failure, and/or peripheral vascular disease (Hahn and Schwartz 2009). Most severely, these plaques are capable of rupturing, which can lead to blockage of the vessel or thrombus formation, and cause heart attack or stroke. The regulation of mechanical forces, the response of the surrounding endothelium, and the changes in blood flow are all critical components of this disease and require consideration in both treatment and prevention options. It has been observed that in athero-resistant arteries, ECs are aligned with the direction of blood flow, have low proliferation and death rates, and do not strongly attract leukocytes due to low adhesion receptor and cytokine levels (Cunningham and Gotlieb 2005; Hahn and Schwartz 2009). On the other hand, in more atherosclerosis-susceptible locations, blood flow is abnormal, the alignment of ECs is poor, and high expression of leukocyte adhesion receptors (i.e., E-selectin, VCAM-1, and ICAM-1) is presented, causing the adhesion of increased leukocyte binding described above (Cunningham and Gotlieb 2005; Hahn and Schwartz 2009). A more thorough understanding of mechanical forces involved in endothelial cell alignment, signaling cascades, and change in cell stiffness may aid in the prevention of several cardiac malfunctions triggered by the development of atherosclerosis.

### 14.2.4.3 Muscular Dystrophies

Disruption of intracellular structure and the proper transmission and signaling of forces can contribute to multiple muscular diseases. In the case of Duchenne muscular dystrophy, progressive muscle degeneration occurs due to a mutation in the gene that encodes dystrophin, a component that contributes to the coupling of the cytoskeleton to the ECM (Spence et al. 2002). Dystrophin also plays a role in the fluid-shear-stress-mediated dilation of arteries (Loufrani et al. 2001). In the case of a dystrophin deficiency, the mechanotransduction signaling of ECs caused by fluid shear stress is impaired, and results in the loss of artery dilation and vascular density, which can add to muscle loss (Loufrani et al. 2004). Other muscular abnormalities have been associated with mutations in cytoskeletal proteins desmin, titin, and myosin. Abnormalities in these critical cytoskeletal components results in disorganized sarcomeres, which cause the disruption of cellular mechanics, including changes in cytoskeletal stiffness and force generation (Jaalouk and Lammerding 2009). Mutations in other components critical to the load-bearing components of muscle include nuclear envelope proteins (lamins A and C, as well as emerin and nesprins) (Brodsky et al. 2000; Zhang et al. 2005), as well as other ECM and adhesion complex proteins and integrins (Burkin et al. 2001; Pillers et al. 2002; Spence et al. 2002). These abnormalities emphasize the vital importance of proper signaling pathways necessary in regulating force transmission within the muscular system.

### 14.2.4.4 Cancer

Normal tissue function and structure requires a tensional homeostasis, maintained by cells through the forces exerted on the ECM (Petroll et al. 2004; Polte et al. 2004). Disturbing the balance of these forces has been suggested to contribute to cancer formation (Ingber et al. 1981; Paszek et al. 2005a). This is seen through the dramatic remodeling of the ECM and its mechanical properties, and the resulting changes in mechanotransduction signaling, which contribute to malignant transformation, tumorigenesis, and cancer metastasis (Huang and Ingber 2005; Suresh 2007; Wolf et al. 2007). Numerous studies have illustrated that the ECM stiffness affects the cytoskeletal tension in tumors (Huang and Ingber 2005; Paszek et al. 2005a; Suresh 2007). Interestingly, the stiffness of tumors is typically much higher than the nearby tissue; for example, the mammary gland has a typical stiffness of ~150 Pa, while tumors are more than 4000 Pa in stiffness (Levental et al. 2007). This change in stiffness has led many to question whether increased stiffness in tissues could promote malignant phenotypes through the regulation of integrins, since these are the critical components in linking the cytoskeleton of cells to the ECM. Paszek and colleagues (Paszek et al. 2005a) discovered that both the matrix stiffness and the cytoskeletal tension function together through the regulation of Rho and ERK signaling pathways. In the case of stiff substrates, increased forces encourage integrin clustering, promoting focal adhesion formation and stabilization due to increased cytoskeletal tension resulting from Rho–ROCK signaling (Paszek et al. 2005a). The increase in focal adhesion assembly triggers specific events that can contribute to cancer development. This includes the initiation of focal adhesion kinase signaling, disruption of adherens junctions, disturbance of basal polarity, and in turn, remodeling of the tissue architecture (Paszek et al. 2005a). Most interestingly, interfering with ERK and Rho signaling leads to reduced tumor cell proliferation due to a decrease in the cytoskeletal tension (Paszek et al. 2005a). This work emphasizes that even small increases in matrix stiffness can trigger Rho-generated cytoskeletal tension, which in turn modifies tissue architecture and enhances tumor cell growth. The ability to control these signaling pathways and therefore regulate the cytoskeletal tension may appear to be critical targets in cancer therapeutics; however, much more work remains to be done to fully understand the complete model of tensional homeostasis and force-dependent tumorigenesis.

### 14.2.4.5 Mechanical Therapies

This broad span of diseases suggests that a more thorough understanding of the relationship between tissue structure and function may lead to a vast array of potential therapeutic interventions. Presently, there are numerous therapies in use or in development that focus on targeting cellular mechanotransduction and/or cell and tissue mechanics. These "mechanical therapies" include treatments such as tissue expansion methods, muscle relaxants, cardiac perfusion, botox, lung ventilation, and tissue engineering and manufacturing (Ingber 2003). These treatments illustrate the critical importance of mechanobiology in relation to disease, and the appreciation of this field in the clinical world. Further identification of key molecules involved in mediating mechanotransduction may prove to be potential therapeutic targets. Because it is now known that mechanotransduction plays such a significant role in development of disease, it is necessary to have a more complete understanding of how the mechanical properties of engineered biomaterials regulate cell and tissue behavior.

## 14.3 Mechanics of Biomaterials

### 14.3.1 Cell–Substrate Interactions

A major issue in tissue engineering is biocompatibility. Whether cells are being implanted along with the tissue-engineered construct, or whether the construct is simply interacting with the native cells in the region where it is placed, it must be designed to optimize the desired cellular response. Because cells have the ability to sense and respond to both chemical and mechanical stimuli (as discussed above), the mechanical properties of engineered constructs have significant effects on cellular spreading, migration, proliferation, signaling, and other behaviors. Many of these changes in behavior have been recognized using both *in vitro* and *in vivo* techniques which manipulate biomaterial stiffness, porosity, and topography.

### 14.3.2 Parameters That Affect Cell–Substrate Interactions

#### 14.3.2.1 Stiffness

The mechanical properties of a tissue-engineered construct significantly affect the outcome of the repair. For example, the construct or scaffold must be stiff enough at the macroscale to hold up through daily activities, but it must employ the optimum stiffness for the desired cellular behavior at the microscale. This is a key parameter in influencing cell behavior, as a range of cell types sense and respond to environmental stiffness in many different ways.

A significant amount of past *in vitro* work has studied cellular behavior using glass as a substrate. However, glass is not physiologically relevant, as the body is composed of a diverse array of different stiffnesses, from soft brain tissue to stiff bone tissue (Figure 14.1) (Levental et al. 2007). To address this concern, in recent years, much attention has been placed on the effects of substrate stiffness on cellular behavior. Commonly, polyacrylamide gels are used because their stiffness can easily be changed by modifying the amount of cross-linker in the gel composition, and the gel stiffness can be studied independent of the ECM chemical composition. However, other materials, such as collagen gels and polydimethylsiloxane (PDMS) have also been used. Of course, in terms of tissue engineering, biocompatibility, biodegradability, and toxicity are all relevant concerns and must be addressed prior to *in vivo* use.

The effects of substrate stiffness can be seen in the morphology of cells, from cells as simple as neutrophils (Figure 14.2; Stroka and Aranda-Espinoza 2009), to many other cell types (Califano and Reinhart-King 2008; Engler et al. 2004a; Isenberg et al. 2009; Pelham and Wang 1997; Ulrich et al. 2009; Yeung et al. 2005). Substrate stiffness also influences cell motility (de Rooij et al. 2005; Oakes et al. 2009; Pelham and Wang 1997; Peyton and Putnam 2005; Stroka and Aranda-Espinoza 2009), cell–substrate adhesion (Pelham and Wang 1997), cell–cell adhesion (Califano and Reinhart-King 2008; de Rooij et al. 2005), cell mechanical properties (Byfield et al. 2009a; Ghosh et al. 2007; Solon et al. 2007), proliferation (Ulrich et al. 2009), differentiation (Engler et al. 2006), cytoskeletal organization (Pelham and Wang 1997; Yeung et al. 2005), traction forces (Califano and Reinhart-King 2010; Lo et al. 2000; Wang et al. 2002), and biochemical signaling (Pelham and Wang 1997). Each of these behaviors is a crucial component of tissue-engineered scaffolds. For example, many cell types display increased spreading area on stiffer surfaces (Califano and Reinhart-King 2008; Engler et al. 2004b; Isenberg et al. 2009; Stroka

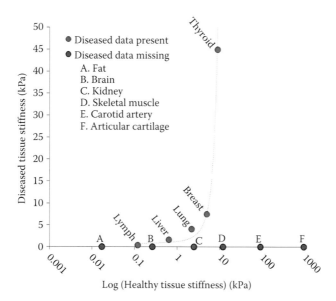

**FIGURE 14.1** (**See color insert.**) Stiffness (Young's modulus) of diseased tissue versus the log10 of healthy tissue. Blue data points indicate tissues for which the stiffnesses of both the healthy and diseased conditions are known. These points seem to follow an exponential trend, with equation $E_{dis} = 755e^{-0.0005}E_{healthy}$. This trend suggests that there exists an underlying mechanism which regulates tissue biomechanics during disease development. Diseases of the tissues shown include lymph containing metastases, fibrotic liver, lung fibrosis, breast tumor, and thyroid cancer. Red data points indicate tissues for which the stiffness of only the healthy condition is known. Further work is necessary to fill in the stiffnesses of diseased conditions for these tissues. (This data was pooled from the following sources: Dolhnikoff, M., T. Mauad, and M.S. Ludwig. 1999. *American Journal of Respiratory and Critical Care Medicine* 160(5): 1750–7; Engler, A.J. et al. 2004b. *Journal of Cell Biology* 166(6): 877–87; Freed, L.E. et al. 1997. *Proceedings of the National Academy of Sciences of the United States of America* 94(25): 13885–90; Guo, X.M. et al. 2006b. *American Journal of Physiology-Heart and Circulatory Physiology* 290(5): H1788–97; Lyshchik, A. et al. 2005. *Ultrasonic Imaging* 27(2): 101–10; Miller, K. et al. 2000b. *Journal of Biomechanics* 33(11): 1369–76; Miyaji, K. et al. 1997. *Cancer* 80(10): 1920–5; Nasseri, S., L.E. Bilston, and N. Phan-Thien. 2002. *Rheologica Acta* 41(1–2): 180–92; Norman, L.L. and H. Aranda-Espinoza. 2010. *Cellular and Molecular Bioengineering* (accepted); Paszek, M.J. et al. 2005b. *Cancer Cell* 8(3): 241–54; Wellman, P. et al. 1999. Harvard Biorobotics Laboratory Technical Report; Yeh, W.C. et al. 2002. *Ultrasound in Medicine and Biology* 28(4): 467–74; Yuan, H.C. et al. 2000. *Journal of Applied Physiology* 89(1): 3–14.)

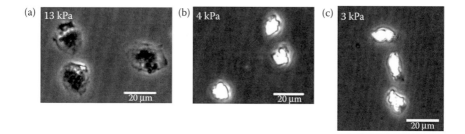

**FIGURE 14.2** Human neutrophil morphology varies with substrate stiffness. Neutrophils were plated on fibronectin-coated polyacrylamide gels of stiffness, ranging from (a) stiff (13 kPa), to (b) intermediate (5 kPa), to (c) soft (3 kPa), as indicated on each image. After activation with a peptide chemoattractant, neutrophils spread well onto a stiff surface (a), while most neutrophils do not spread on softer surfaces (b and c). (These images were taken with permission from Stroka, K.M. and H. Aranda-Espinoza. 2009. *Cell Motility and the Cytoskeleton* 66(6): 328–41.)

and Aranda-Espinoza 2009; Ulrich et al. 2009; Yeung et al. 2005), as shown in Figure 14.2, which is an indication of stronger adhesion. Obviously, if cells are being incorporated into an engineered construct, it is desirable for them to stick to it, and thus adhesion strength is important. However, stiffness could also be used to deter certain harmful cell types from adhering to the construct, possibly by minimizing the immune response or preventing fibroblast proliferation in the defected area.

Cell migration is also affected by substrate stiffness, as neutrophils (Stroka and Aranda-Espinoza 2009), smooth muscle cells (Peyton and Putnam 2005), and epithelial cells (de Rooij et al. 2005) display a biphasic migration speed with substrate stiffness; that is, there exists an intermediate stiffness where migration is at a maximum. Thus, if a tissue engineering strategy relies on effective cell migration, the construct could be mechanically manipulated for the given cell type to produce maximal migration. Also, substrate stiffness can be used to influence the stiffness of the cells themselves. For example, both ECs (Byfield et al. 2009a) and fibroblasts (Ghosh et al. 2007; Solon et al. 2007) increase in stiffness as their substrate stiffness increases. In terms of tissue engineering, this suggests that cell stiffness can be modulated by tuning the stiffness of the biomaterial, an effect which may be important in diseases where tissue stiffness changes, such as in cancer or atherosclerosis. Interestingly, there seems to be an exponential relationship between the stiffness of healthy tissue and the stiffness of diseased tissue (Figure 14.1), which may suggest an underlying mechanism for tissue biomechanics during development of disease. Further work is necessary to complete this plot for tissues in which only the healthy stiffness is known. Finally, cells can actually communicate with each other through the substrate; they are able to deform the matrix through traction force generation, which creates a local increase in matrix stiffness. Nearby cells can feel this change in stiffness and respond accordingly (Reinhart-King et al. 2008). Thus, cell–cell communication through biomaterial mechanical properties could be used to direct the behavior of cells at the site of an implant.

Many different types of cells, including fibroblasts (Ghosh et al. 2007; Pelham and Wang 1997; Solon et al. 2007), ECs (Byfield et al. 2009a; Califano and Reinhart-King 2008, 2010; Deroanne et al. 2001; Kumar et al. 2006; Reinhart-King et al. 2008; Sieminski et al. 2004; Stroka and Aranda-Espinoza 2010; Yamamura et al. 2007; Yeung et al. 2005), epithelial cells (de Rooij et al. 2005; Pelham and Wang 1997), cardiomyocytes (Bhana et al. 2010; Engler et al. 2008a; Jacot et al. 2008), dorsal root ganglia neurons (Balgude et al. 2001; Willits and Skornia 2004), neutrophils (Oakes et al. 2009; Stroka and Aranda-Espinoza 2009), cancer cells (Ulrich et al. 2009), and stem cells (Engler et al. 2006), are sensitive to substrate stiffness, while cells such as cortical neurons are not able to detect differences in substrate stiffness (Norman and Aranda-Espinoza 2010). Later in this chapter, we focus on the effects of substrate stiffness on neurons, cardiovascular and immune cells, cancer cells, and stem cells. We relate these behaviors to potential targets and applications for diseases related to each different cell type.

### 14.3.2.2 Porosity

Porosity is another physical parameter which can be varied in engineered biomaterials for various medical applications. There seems to be a shift away from synthetic implants and grafts, toward porous biodegradable scaffolds, with pores in the range of 10–1000 microns (Hollister 2005). One advantage of these porous scaffolds is that cells and molecules can be easily incorporated, and then as the tissue regenerates with the help of the added cells and molecules, the scaffold degrades over time. The pores allow for bulk transport of material into and out of the scaffold, and they also facilitate cell migration, proliferation, and signaling (Yoon and Fisher 2006). Current research focuses on establishing the optimum size, geometry, and density of pores, along with the appropriate base scaffold material, cell density, and bound or soluble molecules integrated in the scaffold. For example, porous scaffolds for bone repairs need a small enough pore density to maintain sound mechanical properties in multiple directions, but large enough pore density to allow for bulk transport of soluble materials and cell migration through the scaffold (Karageorgiou and Kaplan 2005).

The microstructure of these scaffolds includes hydrogels, open pore structures, and fibrous matrices. Methods for creating the scaffolds include freeze drying, gas-foaming, stereolithography, porogen-leaching, and the simple, conventional method of combining a water-soluble porogen with a hydrophobic polymer scaffold (Chen et al. 2010). Of course, once the scaffolds are created, it is also necessary to characterize their architecture in terms of pore size, porosity, and pore interconnectivity. Methods for porous scaffold characterization include mercury intrusion porosimetry (Karageorgiou and Kaplan 2005), the liquid displacement method (Nazarov et al. 2004), scanning electron microscopy (Park et al. 2002), microcomputed tomography (Moore et al. 2004), and, more recently, optical coherence tomography (Chen et al. 2010).

### 14.3.2.3 Topography

Topographic cues can significantly affect cell behavior, both in the native environment and also in a tissue-engineered scaffold. As cells migrate, they must navigate a complex three-dimensional environment. They are able to sense and respond to grooves, platforms, plateaus, roughness, and other three-dimensional structures within a scaffold, and thus it could be advantageous to incorporate topographic cues into engineered biomaterials. The ability to investigate this behavior has recently been accomplished with the aid of newly developed devices to pattern materials, including electron beam lithography (Diehl et al. 2003), colloidal lithography (Dalby et al. 2004), dip pen lithography (Piner et al. 1999), and nano- or microcontact printing (Kulangara and Leong 2009; Sniadecki et al. 2006). Often, the size, shape, and density of these nano- or micron-sized structures are varied in order to explore the range of cell behavior and to achieve a particular behavior, depending on the cell type and application. For example, these structures can be used to control cell spreading, migration velocity, and alignment.

Topography can be used to control cell behavior in a large array of medical applications. In cardiovascular engineering, x-ray lithography can be used to etch nanoscale grooves in polyurethane substrates, in order to produce patterns which resemble the native basement membrane below the endothelium in blood vessels (Karuri et al. 2004; Liliensiek et al. 2010). Interestingly, ECs from large and small blood vessels respond differently to topographic cues (Liliensiek et al. 2010). Nanogrooves direct the alignment of calcium phosphate mineralization driven by osteoblasts, an effect which could control bone cell growth at the interface between an implant and bone (Lamers et al. 2010). Skeletal muscle orientation and myotube development can be guided through topographic features on grafts (Altomare et al. 2010). Further, human mesenchymal stem cells respond to nanograted substrates by decreasing expression of integrin subunits, aligning and decreasing density of the F-actin cytoskeleton, and changing mechanical properties (Yim et al. 2010).

Topographic control of scaffolds for neural engineering applications also seems promising. Neonatal dorsal root ganglion neurons, if presented with optimum groove dimensions, can span across the grooves to the next plateau (Goldner et al. 2006). Human neuroblastoma cells can sense changes in roughness on the length scale of a few nanometers and respond to roughness by displaying a loss of polarity, fragmentation of Golgi apparatus, nuclear condensation, and loss of actin cytoskeleton organization (Brunetti et al. 2010). In these applications, neuronal polarization and contact guidance depend on focal adhesion geometry and are influenced by ROCK-mediated signaling to control cell contractility (Ferrari et al. 2010).

## 14.3.3 Approaches for Regulating Cellular Behavior

For the reason that cellular behavior depends so much on a wide variety of chemical and mechanical cues, regulating cellular behavior in tissue engineering applications can be quite difficult. Much *in vitro* work has focused on isolating one cue at a time, such as substrate stiffness, chemical soluble factors (e.g., cytokines and growth factors), substrate ligand density, or topography. However, because each of these variables contributes to the complex behavior of cells *in vivo*, integrated approaches which combine multiple cues at once are becoming more effective and appropriate tissue engineering strategies for regulating cellular behavior.

### 14.3.3.1 Heterogeneous Materials/Gradients

In the body, the cellular environment is very heterogeneous, and cells are capable of migrating preferentially toward surface-attached and soluble stimuli. Thus, when designing a tissue scaffold to support cell growth and native function, one approach is to engineer a heterogeneous material. Examples of heterogeneous materials include those containing gradients in stiffness, which cells sense through mechanotaxis, and also gradients in adhesion protein density, which cells sense through haptotaxis. Many cell types display decreased speed on and increased adhesion to stiff surfaces coated with a large density of ECM protein; therefore, using gradients in stiffness or protein could be an effective strategy for trapping cells in a particular location on an engineered graft.

One of the first studies to analyze mechanotaxis utilized a polyacrylamide gel with a gradient in stiffness generated through a discontinuity in the bis-acrylamide cross-linker (Lo et al. 2000). When migrating from the soft side, fibroblasts easily crossed the mechanical gradient to the stiff side; however, when migrating from the stiff side, fibroblasts turned around or retracted upon encountering the gradient. Gradients in gel stiffness have also been created using microfluidic devices (Byfield et al. 2009b; Cheung et al. 2009; Zaari et al. 2004) and photolithographic microelastic patterning methods using styrenated gelatin (Kidoaki and Matsuda 2008). In most cases, the stiffness of these elastic gradients was quantified locally using atomic force microscopy, where an indenter was used to measure the response of the gel to an applied force.

In addition to gradients in stiffness, cells can also detect sharp changes in environmental stiffness. Microfabrication of PDMS substrates (Chou et al. 2009) or PDMS molds with polyacrylamide patterns (Gray et al. 2003) of varying stiffness have been used to show that certain cell types accumulate on the stiffer regions. This response is mostly due to preferential migration of cells to stiffer areas and is not due to increased proliferation of cells on stiffer surfaces (Gray et al. 2003). Thus, both sharp and gentle gradients in stiffness are capable of spatially controlling cell adhesion.

### 14.3.3.2 Combinatorial Designs

In addition to constructs with heterogeneous properties of one parameter such as stiffness, it could also be beneficial to utilize combinatorial designs. Examples of this strategy include merging optimum substrate stiffness and ECM protein parameters (Charest et al. 2006), combining mechanical and soluble cues, and selecting optimum topography, stiffness, and porosity parameters in a single construct. Also, each of these combinatorial designs could also integrate specific cell types, possibly through initial seeding of the cells into the construct prior to placing the construct into the body. In general, the combinatorial design strategy takes the results of several independent optimum parameters and merges them to create the most favorable environment for the desired cellular response. This approach will likely be the most effective in creating engineered tissues for medication of defects *in vivo*. Of course, another source of heterogeneity comes from the cells themselves, since, for example, their response to biomaterial stiffness is cell type-dependent.

## 14.4 Potential Target and Applications

### 14.4.1 Neural Engineering

One of the greatest challenges in the field of neural engineering is gaining the ability to repair injuries to the central nervous system. While the peripheral nervous system is capable of repairing itself after injury, the central nervous system (brain and spinal cord) has not been shown to be capable of repairing axonal damage. One approach to overcome this difficulty is to engineer a biomaterial as an implant to encourage axon outgrowth and also functionality. For example, biomaterial stiffness could be chosen to maximize axon length, outgrowth rate, persistence, and to minimize axon branching and turning (for summary, see Table 1 in Norman et al. 2009). This would encourage axons to cross the injured area. At the same time, however, the biomaterial must address functionality, since the regenerated axons must create a functional synapse with another neuron at the far side of the gap. It is believed that this strategy will necessitate a heterogeneous, combinatorial biomaterial which incorporates both attractive and repulsive signaling mechanisms (Norman et al. 2009). However, design strategy must also take into account the cell-dependent response, since cortical neurons do not sense substrate stiffness, while others have demonstrated that hypocampal and dorsal root ganglia neurons do sense stiffness.

## 14.4.2 Cardiovascular Engineering

ECs, which form a single layer at the luminal surface of blood vessels, are capable of sensing the mechanical properties of their environment. For example, in two dimensions, EC morphology changes from a tube-like network to a monolayer with increasing substrate stiffness (Deroanne et al. 2001); however, this transition also depends on a balance between substrate compliance and amount of bound ligand on the surface of the substrate (Califano and Reinhart-King 2008). As discussed above, EC size (Yeung et al. 2005), stiffness (Byfield et al. 2009a), cytoskeleton, and focal adhesion size (Deroanne et al. 2001) can also be controlled through manipulation of substrate compliance. In three dimensions, increased matrix stiffness leads to larger lumens, thicker and deeper EC networks, and high vinculin expression at the tips of branching networks.

The ability of ECs to respond to environmental stiffness in both two- and three-dimensional *in vitro* systems has significant ramifications for cardiovascular engineering applications. For example, these results, along with optimum topography, could be incorporated into the design of vascular grafts to bypass blocked or damaged blood vessels. In addition, the mechanical properties of stents, devices used to prop open occluded arteries during angioplasty, could be tailored to promote re-endothelialization of the artery. Further, a major hurdle in the field of tissue engineering is how to induce vasculogenesis (formation of new blood vessels) and also angiogenesis (formation of vascular trees) in engineered tissues. Manipulation of construct stiffness, topography, and porosity, along with proper molecular cues, could help to overcome this hurdle.

## 14.4.3 Suppression of Cancerous Tumors

The mechanics of biomaterials may also have applications in suppression of malignant tumors, as many types of cancer cells are also sensitive to substrate stiffness (Kostic et al. 2009; Krndija et al. 2010; Ulrich et al. 2009). Thus, one approach to control tumor size could be to encapsulate the tumor with a nonpermissive material for cancer cell migration. Thus, the cells would not be able to break away from the primary tumor site and metastasize to other parts of the body. Another approach could be to prevent the formation of a vascular system within the tumor, possibly by applying a material with mechanical properties which are nonpermissive for endothelial cell migration. These strategies could be effective in controlling tumor development and size.

One of the major problems in cancer is cell metastasis, where the cancer cells migrate away from the tumor, enter the bloodstream, exit the bloodstream at another part of the body, and infect the surrounding tissue. In order for cancer cells to metastasize, they must first break away from the primary tumor site. This process involves tight regulation of cell–cell adhesions. While there are many different proteins which line the junctions between cancer cells, a promising strategy for controlling cell–cell adhesion could rely on biomaterial mechanics. Evidence for this is that both fibroblasts and epithelial cells scatter (i.e., *cell–cell adhesions break*) more on stiffer surfaces (de Rooij et al. 2005; Guo et al. 2006a). Thus, a very soft biomaterial implanted at the tumor site could prevent cell scattering and be effective in stopping or slowing cancer cell metastasis.

### 14.4.4 Engineering with Stem Cells

The incorporation of stem cells into engineered constructs is another promising strategy for tissue engineering applications to repair nonfunctioning or damaged parts of the body. An advantage of integrating stem cells is that they are self-renewing, and thus they can promote self-healing and tissue replacement. In recent years, it was discovered that stem cell differentiation can be directed through manipulation of cell–substrate interactions, as discussed above. Specifically, stem cells on very soft gels (~1 kPa; approximate stiffness of brain) differentiate into neurons, stem cells on intermediate stiff gels (~10 kPa; approximate stiffness of muscle) differentiate into muscle cells, and stem cells on stiff gels (~100 kPa; approximate stiffness of collagenous bone) differentiate into bone cells (Engler et al. 2006). In each case, the cells expressed distinguishing molecular markers for the specific differentiated cell type. Thus, manipulation of biomaterial stiffness, along with incorporation of soluble, diffusible molecules, could effectively direct the spatiotemporal differentiation of stem cells. Of course, it is critical to know the stiffness of the target tissue *in vivo* so that the stiffness of the biomaterial can be tailored appropriately.

## 14.5 Summary

The mechanical properties (stiffness, porosity, topography) of biomaterials can significantly affect the behavior (spreading, migration, differentiation, cell–cell communication) and phenotype (morphology, cytoskeletal arrangement, stiffness) of many different cell types (endothelial cells, immune cells, cancer cells, stem cells, neurons). Cells sense the mechanical properties of their surroundings through mechanotransduction, the process by which they convert physical forces to biochemical signaling pathways. Thus, tissue engineers can take advantage of the mechanosensitive nature of many different cell types, and along with signaling through chemical cues, create biomaterials of varying mechanical and chemical properties which optimize the desired cellular response. This combinatorial approach will likely be the key in developing more effective treatments for cardiovascular disease, central nervous system repair, and cancer.

## References

Altomare, L., N. Gadegaard, L. Visai, M.C. Tanzi, and S. Fare. 2010. Biodegradable microgrooved polymeric surfaces obtained by photolithography for skeletal muscle cell orientation and myotube development. *Acta Biomaterialia* 6(6): 1948–57.

Balaban, N.Q., U.S. Schwarz, D. Riveline, P. Goichberg, G. Tzur, I. Sabanay, D. Mahalu, S. Safran, A. Bershadsky, L. Addadi, and B. Geiger. 2001. Force and focal adhesion assembly: A close relationship studied using elastic micropatterned substrates. *Nature Cell Biology* 3(5): 466–72.

Balgude, A.P., X. Yu, A. Szymanski, and R.V. Bellamkonda. 2001. Agarose gel stiffness determines rate of DRG neurite extension in 3d cultures. *Biomaterials* 22(10): 1077–84.

Balogh, J., M. Merisckay, Z. Li, D. Paulin, and A. Arner. 2002. Hearts from mice lacking desmin have a myopathy with impaired active force generation and unaltered wall compliance. *Cardiovascular Research* 53(2): 439–50.

Bhana, B., R.K. Iyer, W.L.K. Chen, R.G. Zhao, K.L. Sider, M. Likhitpanichkul, C.A. Simmons, and M. Radisic. 2010. Influence of substrate stiffness on the phenotype of heart cells. *Biotechnology and Bioengineering* 105(6): 1148–60.

Boulassel, M.R., N. Deggouj, J.P. Tomasi, and M. Gersdorff. 2001. Inner ear autoantibodies and their targets in patients with autoimmune inner ear diseases. *Acta Oto-Laryngologica* 121(1): 28–34.

Brodsky, G.L., F. Muntoni, S. Miocic, G. Sinagra, C. Sewry, and L. Mestroni. 2000. Lamin a/c gene mutation associated with dilated cardiomyopathy with variable skeletal muscle involvement. *Circulation* 101(5): 473–6.

Brunetti, V., G. Maiorano, L. Rizzello, B. Sorce, S. Sabella, R. Cingolani, and P.P. Pompa. 2010. Neurons sense nanoscale roughness with nanometer sensitivity. *Proceedings of the National Academy of Sciences of the United States of America* 107(14): 6264–9.

Burkin, D.J., G.Q. Wallace, K.J. Nicol, D.J. Kaufman, and S.J. Kaufman. 2001. Enhanced expression of the alpha 7 beta 1 integrin reduces muscular dystrophy and restores viability in dystrophic mice. *Journal of Cell Biology* 152(6): 1207–18.

Byfield, F.J., R.K. Reen, T.P. Shentu, I. Levitan, and K.J. Gooch. 2009a. Endothelial actin and cell stiffness is modulated by substrate stiffness in 2d and 3d. *Journal of Biomechanics* 42(8): 1114–9.

Byfield, F.J., S. Tikku, G.H. Rothblat, K.J. Gooch, and I. Levitan. 2006. Oxldl increases endothelial stiffness, force generation, and network formation. *Journal of Lipid Research* 47(4): 715–23.

Byfield, F.J., Q. Wen, I. Levental, K. Nordstrom, P.E. Arratia, R.T. Miller, and P.A. Janmey. 2009b. Absence of filamin a prevents cells from responding to stiffness gradients on gels coated with collagen but not fibronectin. *Biophysics Journal* 96(12): 5095–102.

Califano, J.P. and C.A. Reinhart-King. 2008. A balance of substrate mechanics and matrix chemistry regulates endothelial cell network assembly. *Cellular and Molecular Bioengineering* 1(2–3): 122–32.

Califano, J.P. and C.A. Reinhart-King. 2010. Substrate stiffness and cell area predict cellular traction stresses in single cells and cells in contact. *Cellular and Molecular Bioengineering* 3(1): 68–75.

Capell, B.C., F.S. Collins, and E.G. Nabel. 2007. Mechanisms of cardiovascular disease in accelerated aging syndromes. *Circulation Research* 101(1): 13–26.

Chalfie, M. 2009. Neurosensory mechanotransduction. *Nature Reviews Molecular Cell Biology* 10(1): 44–52.

Charest, J.L., M.T. Eliason, A.J. Garcia, and W.P. King. 2006. Combined microscale mechanical topography and chemical patterns on polymer cell culture substrates. *Biomaterials* 27(11): 2487–94.

Chen, C.-W., M.W. Betz, J.P. Fisher, A. Paek, and Y. Chen. 2010. Macroporous hydrogel scaffolds and their characterization by optical coherence tomography. *Tissue Engineering Part C: Methods* 17(1): 101–12.

Cheng, C., D. Tempel, R. Van Haperen, A. Van Der Baan, F. Grosveld, M.J. Daemen, R. Krams, and R. De Crom. 2006. Atherosclerotic lesion size and vulnerability are determined by patterns of fluid shear stress. *Circulation* 113(23): 2744–53.

Cheung, Y.K., E.U. Azeloglu, D.A. Shiovitz, K.D. Costa, D. Seliktar, and S.K. Sia. 2009. Microscale control of stiffness in a cell-adhesive substrate using microfluidics-based lithography. *Angewandte Chemie-International Edition* 48(39): 7188–92.

Chicurel, M.E., C.S. Chen, and D.E. Ingber. 1998. Cellular control lies in the balance of forces. *Current Opinion in Cell Biology* 10(2): 232–9.

Choquet, D., D.P. Felsenfeld, and M.P. Sheetz. 1997. Extracellular matrix rigidity causes strengthening of integrin-cytoskeleton linkages. *Cell* 88(1): 39–48.

Chou, S.Y., C.M. Cheng, and P.R. Leduc. 2009. Composite polymer systems with control of local substrate elasticity and their effect on cytoskeletal and morphological characteristics of adherent cells. *Biomaterials* 30(18): 3136–42.

Cunningham, K.S. and A.I. Gotlieb. 2005. The role of shear stress in the pathogenesis of atherosclerosis. *Laboratory Investigation* 85(1): 9–23.

Dalby, M.J., C.C. Berry, M.O. Riehle, D.S. Sutherland, H. Agheli, and A.S.G. Curtis. 2004. Attempted endocytosis of nano-environment produced by colloidal lithography by human fibroblasts. *Experimental Cell Research* 295(2): 387–94.

Davidson, L.A., A.M. Ezin, and R. Keller. 2002. Embryonic wound healing by apical contraction and ingression in xenopus laevis. *Cell Motility and the Cytoskeleton* 53(3): 163–76.

Davies, P.F. 1995. Flow-mediated endothelial mechanotransduction. *Physiological Reviews* 75(3): 519–60.

De Rooij, J., A. Kerstens, G. Danuser, M.A. Schwartz, and C.M. Waterman-Storer. 2005. Integrin-dependent actomyosin contraction regulates epithelial cell scattering. *Journal of Cell Biology* 171(1): 153–64.

Deroanne, C.F., C.M. Lapiere, and B.V. Nusgens. 2001. *In vitro* tubulogenesis of endothelial cells by relaxation of the coupling extracellular matrix-cytoskeleton. *Cardiovascular Research* 49(3): 647–58.

Diehl, K.A., J.D. Foley, G. Zhang, P. Podsiadlo, P.F. Nealy, and C.J. Murphy. 2003. Nanoscale topography modulates corneal epithelial cell migration. *Investigative Ophthalmology and Visual Science* 44: U216–U16.

Dolhnikoff, M., T. Mauad, and M.S. Ludwig. 1999. Extracellular matrix and oscillatory mechanics of rat lung parenchyma in bleomycin-induced fibrosis. *American Journal of Respiratory and Critical Care Medicine* 160(5): 1750–7.

Eberl, D.F., R.W. Hardy, and M.J. Kernan. 2000. Genetically similar transduction mechanisms for touch and hearing in drosophila. *Journal of Neuroscience* 20(16): 5981–8.

Engler, A., L. Bacakova, C. Newman, A. Hategan, M. Griffin, and D. Discher. 2004a. Substrate compliance versus ligand density in cell on gel responses. *Biophysics Journal* 86(1 Pt 1): 617–28.

Engler, A.J., C. Carag-Krieger, C.P. Johnson, M. Raab, H.Y. Tang, D.W. Speicher, J.W. Sanger, J.M. Sanger, and D.E. Discher. 2008a. Embryonic cardiomyocytes beat best on a matrix with heart-like elasticity: Scar-like rigidity inhibits beating. *Journal of Cell Science* 121(22): 3794–802.

Engler, A.J., C. Carag-Krieger, C.P. Johnson, M. Raab, H.Y. Tang, D.W. Speicher, J.W. Sanger, J.M. Sanger, and D.E. Discher. 2008b. Embryonic cardiomyocytes beat best on a matrix with heart-like elasticity: Scar-like rigidity inhibits beating. *Journal of Cell Science* 121(Pt 22): 3794–802.

Engler, A.J., M.A. Griffin, S. Sen, C.G. Bonnetnann, H.L. Sweeney, and D.E. Discher. 2004b. Myotubes differentiate optimally on substrates with tissue-like stiffness: Pathological implications for soft or stiff microenvironments. *Journal of Cell Biology* 166(6): 877–87.

Engler, A.J., S. Sen, H.L. Sweeney, and D.E. Discher. 2006. Matrix elasticity directs stem cell lineage specification. *Cell* 126(4): 677–89.

Engler, A.J., H.L. Sweeney, D.E. Discher, and J.E. Schwarzbauer. 2007. Extracellular matrix elasticity directs stem cell differentiation. *Journal of Musculoskeletal and Neuronal Interactions* 7(4): 335.

Evans, A.L. and U. Muller. 2000. Stereocilia defects in the sensory hair cells of the inner ear in mice deficient in integrin alpha 8 beta 1. *Nature Genetics* 24(4): 424–8.

Farge, E. 2003. Mechanical induction of twist in the drosophila foregut/stomodeal primordium. *Current Biology* 13(16): 1365–77.

Ferrari, A., M. Cecchini, M. Serresi, P. Faraci, D. Pisignano, and F. Beltram. 2010. Neuronal polarity selection by topography-induced focal adhesion control. *Biomaterials* 31(17): 4682–94.

Flanagan, L.A., Y.E. Ju, B. Marg, M. Osterfield, and P.A. Janmey. 2002. Neurite branching on deformable substrates. *Neuroreport* 13(18): 2411–5.

Freed, L.E., R. Langer, I. Martin, N.R. Pellis, and G. Vunjaknovakovic. 1997. Tissue engineering of cartilage in space. *Proceedings of the National Academy of Sciences of the United States of America* 94(25): 13885–90.

Georges, P.C., J.J. Hui, Z. Gombos, M.E. Mccormick, A.Y. Wang, M. Uemura, R. Mick, P.A. Janmey, E.E. Furth, and R.G. Wells. 2007. Increased stiffness of the rat liver precedes matrix deposition: Implications for fibrosis. *American Journal of Physiology. Gastrointestinal and Liver Physiology* 293(6): G1147–54.

Ghosh, K., Z. Pan, E. Guan, S. Ge, Y. Liu, T. Nakamura, X.D. Ren, M. Rafailovich, and R.A. Clark. 2007. Cell adaptation to a physiologically relevant ECM mimic with different viscoelastic properties. *Biomaterials* 28(4): 671–9.

Goldner, J.S., J.M. Bruder, G. Li, D. Gazzola, and D. Hoffman-Kim. 2006. Neurite bridging across micropatterned grooves. *Biomaterials* 27(3): 460–72.

Gray, D.S., J. Tien, and C.S. Chen. 2003. Repositioning of cells by mechanotaxis on surfaces with micropatterned young's modulus. *Journal of Biomedical Materials Research Part A* 66A(3): 605–14.

Grodzinsky, A.J., M.E. Levenston, M. Jin, and E.H. Frank. 2000. Cartilage tissue remodeling in response to mechanical forces. *Annual Review of Biomedical Engineering* 2: 691–713.

Guo, W.H., M.T. Frey, N.A. Burnham, and Y.L. Wang. 2006a. Substrate rigidity regulates the formation and maintenance of tissues. *Biophysical Journal* 90(6): 2213–20.

Guo, X.M., X. Lu, H.M. Ren, E.R. Levin, and G.S. Kassab. 2006b. Estrogen modulates the mechanical homeostasis of mouse arterial vessels through nitric oxide. *American Journal of Physiology-Heart and Circulatory Physiology* 290(5): H1788–97.

Hahn, C. and M.A. Schwartz. 2008. The role of cellular adaptation to mechanical forces in atherosclerosis. *Arteriosclerosis, Thrombosis and Vascular Biology* 28(12): 2101–7.

Hahn, C. and M.A. Schwartz. 2009. Mechanotransduction in vascular physiology and atherogenesis. *Nature Reviews Molecular Cell Biology* 10(1): 53–62.

Hatton, J.P., M. Pooran, C.F. Li, C. Luzzio, and M. Hughes-Fulford. 2003. A short pulse of mechanical force induces gene expression and growth in mc3t3-e1 osteoblasts via an ERK 1/2 pathway. *Journal of Bone and Mineral Research* 18(1): 58–66.

Heineke, J. and J.D. Molkentin. 2006. Regulation of cardiac hypertrophy by intracellular signalling pathways. *Nature Reviews Molecular Cell Biology* 7(8): 589–600.

Hollister, S.J. 2005. Porous scaffold design for tissue engineering. *Nature Materials* 4(7): 518–24.

Holt, J.R. and D.P. Corey. 2000. Two mechanisms for transducer adaptation in vertebrate hair cells. *Proceedings of the National Academy of Sciences of the United States of America* 97(22): 11730–5.

Hove, J.R., R.W. Koster, A.S. Forouhar, G. Acevedo-Bolton, S.E. Fraser, and M. Gharib. 2003. Intracardiac fluid forces are an essential epigenetic factor for embryonic cardiogenesis. *Nature* 421(6919): 172–7.

Huang, S. and D.E. Ingber. 2005. Cell tension, matrix mechanics, and cancer development. *Cancer Cell* 8(3): 175–6.

Ichimura, H., K. Parthasarathi, S. Quadri, A.C. Issekutz, and J. Bhattacharya. 2003. Mechano-oxidative coupling by mitochondria induces proinflammatory responses in lung venular capillaries. *Journal of Clinical Investigation* 111(5): 691–9.

Iemitsu, M., T. Miyauchi, S. Maeda, S. Sakai, T. Kobayashi, N. Fujii, H. Miyazaki, M. Matsuda, and I. Yamaguchi. 2001. Physiological and pathological cardiac hypertrophy induce different molecular phenotypes in the rat. *American Journal of Physiology-Regulatory Integrative and Comparative Physiology* 281(6): R2029–36.

Ingber, D.E. 2003. Mechanobiology and diseases of mechanotransduction. *Annals of Medicine* 35(8): 564–77.

Ingber, D.E., J.A. Madri, and J.D. Jamieson. 1981. Role of basal lamina in neoplastic disorganization of tissue architecture. *Proceedings of the National Academy of Sciences of the United States of America-Biological Sciences* 78(6): 3901–5.

Isenberg, B.C., P.A. Dimilla, M. Walker, S. Kim, and J.Y. Wong. 2009. Vascular smooth muscle cell durotaxis depends on substrate stiffness gradient strength. *Biophysical Journal* 97(5): 1313–22.

Jaalouk, D.E. and J. Lammerding. 2009. Mechanotransduction gone awry. *Nature Reviews Molecular Cell Biology* 10(1): 63–73.

Jacot, J.G., A.D. Mcculloch, and J.H. Omens. 2008. Substrate stiffness affects the functional maturation of neonatal rat ventricular myocytes. *Biophysical Journal* 95(7): 3479–87.

Karageorgiou, V. and D. Kaplan. 2005. Porosity of 3d biomaterial scaffolds and osteogenesis. *Biomaterials* 26(27): 5474–91.

Karuri, N.W., S. Liliensiek, A.I. Teixeira, G. Abrams, S. Campbell, P.F. Nealey, and C.J. Murphy. 2004. Biological length scale topography enhances cell-substratum adhesion of human corneal epithelial cells. *Journal of Cell Science* 117(15): 3153–64.

Keller, R., L.A. Davidson, and D.R. Shook. 2003. How we are shaped: The biomechanics of gastrulation. *Differentiation* 71(3): 171–205.

Keller, R.S., S.Y. Shai, C.J. Babbitt, C.G. Pham, R.J. Solaro, M.L. Valencik, J.C. Loftus, and R.S. Ross. 2001. Disruption of integrin function in the murine myocardium leads to perinatal lethality, fibrosis, and abnormal cardiac performance. *American Journal of Pathology* 158(3): 1079–90.

Kidoaki, A. and T. Matsuda. 2008. Microelastic gradient gelatinous gels to induce cellular mechanotaxis. *Journal of Biotechnology* 133(2): 225–30.

Klein-Nulend, J., R.G. Bacabac, J.P. Veldhuijzen, and J.J. Van Loon. 2003. Microgravity and bone cell mechanosensitivity. *Advances in Space Research* 32(8): 1551–9.

Kostic, A., C.D. Lynch, and M.P. Sheetz. 2009. Differential matrix rigidity response in breast cancer cell lines correlates with the tissue tropism. *PloS One* 4(7): e6361.

Krndija, D., H. Schmid, J.L. Eismann, U. Lother, G. Adler, F. Oswald, T. Seufferlein, and G. Von Wichert. 2010. Substrate stiffness and the receptor-type tyrosine-protein phosphatase alpha regulate spreading of colon cancer cells through cytoskeletal contractility. *Oncogene* 29(18): 2724–38.

Kulangara, K. and K.W. Leong. 2009. Substrate topography shapes cell function. *Soft Matter* 5(21): 4072–6.

Kumar, S., I.Z. Maxwell, A. Heisterkamp, T.R. Polte, T.P. Lele, M. Salanga, E. Mazur, and D.E. Ingber. 2006. Viscoelastic retraction of single living stress fibers and its impact on cell shape, cytoskeletal organization, and extracellular matrix mechanics. *Biophysics Journal* 90(10): 3762–73.

Lamers, E., X.F. Walboomers, M. Domanski, J. Te Riet, F.C.M.J.M. Van Delft, R. Luttge, L.A.J.A. Winnubst, H.J.G.E. Gardeniers, and J.A. Jansen. 2010. The influence of nanoscale grooved substrates on osteoblast behavior and extracellular matrix deposition. *Biomaterials* 31(12): 3307–16.

Lammerding, J., P.C. Schulze, T. Takahashi, S. Kozlov, T. Sullivan, R.D. Kamm, C.L. Stewart, and R.T. Lee. 2004. Lamin a/c deficiency causes defective nuclear mechanics and mechanotransduction. *Journal of Clinical Investigation* 113(3): 370–8.

Leach, J.B., X.Q. Brown, J.G. Jacot, P.A. Dimilla, and J.Y. Wong. 2007. Neurite outgrowth and branching of pc12 cells on very soft substrates sharply decreases below a threshold of substrate rigidity. *Journal of Neural Engineering* 4(2): 26–34.

Levental, I., P.C. Georges, and P.A. Janmey. 2007. Soft biological materials and their impact on cell function. *Soft Matter* 3(3): 299–306.

Liang, S., M.J. Slattery, D. Wagner, S.I. Simon, and C. Dong. 2008. Hydrodynamic shear rate regulates melanoma-leukocyte aggregation, melanoma adhesion to the endothelium, and subsequent extravasation. *Annals of Biomedical Engineering* 36(4): 661–71.

Liliensiek, S.J., J.A. Wood, J.A. Yong, R. Auerbach, P.F. Nealey, and C.J. Murphy. 2010. Modulation of human vascular endothelial cell behaviors by nanotopographic cues. *Biomaterials* 31(20): 5418–26.

Lo, C.-M., H.-B. Wang, M. Dembo and Y.-L. Wang. 2000. Cell movement is guided by the rigidity of the substrate. *Biophysical Journal* 79: 144–52.

Loufrani, L., C. Dubroca, D. You, Z. Li, B. Levy, D. Paulin, and D. Henrion. 2004. Absence of dystrophin in mice reduces no-dependent vascular function and vascular density: Total recovery after a treatment with the aminoglycoside gentamicin. *Arteriosclerosis Thrombosis and Vascular Biology* 24(4): 671–6.

Loufrani, L., K. Matrougui, D. Gorny, M. Duriez, I. Blanc, B.I. Levy, and D. Henrion. 2001. Flow (shear stress)-induced endothelium-dependent dilation is altered in mice lacking the gene encoding for dystrophin. *Circulation* 103(6): 864–70.

Lynch, E.D., M.K. Lee, J.E. Morrow, P.L. Welcsh, P.E. Leon, and M.C. King. 1997. Nonsyndromic deafness dfna1 associated with mutation of a human homolog of the drosophila gene diaphanous. *Science* 278(5341): 1315–8.

Lyshchik, A., T. Higashi, R. Asato, S. Tanaka, J. Ito, M. Hiraoka, A.B. Brill, T. Saga, and K. Togashi. 2005. Elastic moduli of thyroid tissues under compression. *Ultrasonic Imaging* 27(2): 101–10.

Martinac, B. 2004. Mechanosensitive ion channels: Molecules of mechanotransduction. *Journal of Cell Science* 117(Pt 12): 2449–60.

Martineau, L.C. and P.F. Gardiner. 2001. Insight into skeletal muscle mechanotransduction: Mapk activation is quantitatively related to tension. *Journal of Applied Physiology* 91(2): 693–702.

Matsumoto, T., H. Abe, T. Ohashi, Y. Kato, and M. Sato. 2002. Local elastic modulus of atherosclerotic lesions of rabbit thoracic aortas measured by pipette aspiration method. *Physiological Measurement* 23(4): 635–48.

McMullen, J.R. and G.L. Jennings. 2007. Differences between pathological and physiological cardiac hypertrophy: Novel therapeutic strategies to treat heart failure. *Clinical and Experimental Pharmacology and Physiology* 34(4): 255–62.

Miller, C.E., K.J. Donlon, L. Toia, C.L. Wong, and P.R. Chess. 2000a. Cyclic strain induces proliferation of cultured embryonic heart cells. *In Vitro Cellular and Developmental Biology-Animal* 36(10): 633–9.

Miller, K., K. Chinzei, G. Orssengo, and P. Bednarz. 2000b. Mechanical properties of brain tissue in-vivo: Experiment and computer simulation. *Journal of Biomechanics* 33(11): 1369–76.

Miyaji, K., A. Furuse, J. Nakajima, T. Kohno, T. Ohtsuka, K. Yagyu, T. Oka, and S. Omata. 1997. The stiffness of lymph nodes containing lung carcinoma metastases—A new diagnostic parameter measured by a tactile sensor. *Cancer* 80(10): 1920–5.

Moore, M.J., E. Jabbari, E.L. Ritman, L.C. Lu, B.L. Currier, A.J. Windebank, and M.J. Yaszemski. 2004. Quantitative analysis of interconnectivity of porous biodegradable scaffolds with micro-computed tomography. *Journal of Biomedical Materials Research Part A* 71A(2): 258–67.

Munevar, S., Y.L. Wang, and M. Dembo. 2004. Regulation of mechanical interactions between fibroblasts and the substratum by stretch-activated ca2+ entry. *Journal of Cell Science* 117(1): 85–92.

Nasseri, S., L.E. Bilston, and N. Phan-Thien. 2002. Viscoelastic properties of pig kidney in shear, experimental results and modelling. *Rheologica Acta* 41(1–2): 180–92.

Nauli, S.M., F.J. Alenghat, Y. Luo, E. Williams, P. Vassilev, X. Li, A.E. Elia, W. Lu, E.M. Brown, S.J. Quinn, D.E. Ingber, and J. Zhou. 2003. Polycystins 1 and 2 mediate mechanosensation in the primary cilium of kidney cells. *Nature Genetics* 33(2): 129–37.

Nazarov, R., H.J. Jin, and D.L. Kaplan. 2004. Porous 3-d scaffolds from regenerated silk fibroin. *Biomacromolecules* 5(3): 718–26.

Norman, L.L. and H. Aranda-Espinoza. 2010. Cortical neuron outgrowth is insensitive to substrate stiffness. *Cellular and Molecular Bioengineering* 3: 398–414.

Norman, L.L., K. Stroka, and H. Aranda-Espinoza. 2009. Guiding axons in the central nervous system: A tissue engineering approach. *Tissue Engineering Part B-Reviews* 15(3): 291–305.

Oakes, P.W., D.C. Patel, N.A. Morin, D.P. Zitterbart, B. Fabry, J.S. Reichner, and J.X. Tang. 2009. Neutrophil morphology and migration are affected by substrate elasticity. *Blood* 114(7): 1387–95.

Oh, S., K.S. Brammer, Y.S. Li, D. Teng, A.J. Engler, S. Chien, and S. Jin. 2009. Stem cell fate dictated solely by altered nanotube dimension. *Proceedings of the National Academy of Sciences of the United States of America* 106(7): 2130–5.

Orr, A.W., B.P. Helmke, B.R. Blackman, and M.A. Schwartz. 2006. Mechanisms of mechanotransduction. *Developmental Cell* 10(1): 11–20.

Park, J.M., T. Yang, L.J. Arend, J.B. Schnermann, C.A. Peters, M.R. Freeman, and J.P. Briggs. 1999. Obstruction stimulates cox-2 expression in bladder smooth muscle cells via increased mechanical stretch. *American Journal of Physiology* 276(1 Pt 2): F129–36.

Park, S.N., J.C. Park, H.O. Kim, M.J. Song, and H. Suh. 2002. Characterization of porous collagen/hyaluronic acid scaffold modified by 1-ethyl-3-(3-dimethylaminopropyl)carbodiimide cross-linking. *Biomaterials* 23(4): 1205–12.

Paszek, M.J., N. Zahir, K.R. Johnson, J.N. Lakins, G.I. Rozenberg, A. Gefen, C.A. Reinhart-King, S.S. Margulies, M. Dembo, D. Boettiger, D.A. Hammer, and V.M. Weaver. 2005a. Tensional homeostasis and the malignant phenotype. *Cancer Cell* 8(3): 241–54.

Paszek, M.J., N. Zahir, K.R. Johnson, J.N. Lakins, G.I. Rozenberg, A. Gefen, C.A. Reinhart-King, S.S. Margulies, M. Dembo, D. Boettiger, D.A. Hammer, and V.M. Weaver. 2005b. Tensional homeostasis and the malignant phenotype. *Cancer Cell* 8(3): 241–54.

Patwari, P. and R.T. Lee. 2008. Mechanical control of tissue morphogenesis. *Circulation Research* 103(3): 234–43.

Pelham, R.J., Jr. and Y. Wang. 1997. Cell locomotion and focal adhesions are regulated by substrate flexibility. *Proceedings of the National Academy of Sciences of the United States of America* 94(25): 13661–5.

Petroll, W.M., M. Vishwanath, and L.S. Ma. 2004. Corneal fibroblasts respond rapidly to changes in local mechanical stress. *Investigative Ophthalmology and Visual Science* 45(10): 3466–74.

Peyton, S.R. and A.J. Putnam. 2005. Extracellular matrix rigidity governs smooth muscle cell motility in a biphasic fashion. *Journal of Cellular Physiology* 204: 198–209.

Pillers, D.M., J.B. Kempton, N.M. Duncan, J.Q. Pang, S.J. Dwinnell, and D.R. Trune. 2002. Hearing loss in the laminin-deficient dy mouse model of congenital muscular dystrophy. *Molecular Genetics and Metabolism* 76(3): 217–24.

Piner, R.D., J. Zhu, F. Xu, S.H. Hong, and C.A. Mirkin. 1999. "Dip-pen" nanolithography. *Science* 283(5402): 661–3.

Polte, T.R., G.S. Eichler, N. Wang, and D.E. Ingber. 2004. Extracellular matrix controls myosin light chain phosphorylation and cell contractility through modulation of cell shape and cytoskeletal prestress. *American Journal of Physiology-Cell Physiology* 286(3): C518–28.

Rabodzey, A., P. Alcaide, F.W. Luscinskas, and B. Ladoux. 2008. Mechanical forces induced by the transendothelial migration of human neutrophils. *Biophysics Journal* 95(3): 1428–38.

Redowicz, M.J. 2002. Myosins and pathology: Genetics and biology. *Acta Biochimica Polonica* 49(4): 789–804.

Reinhart-King, C.A., M. Dembo, and D.A. Hammer. 2008. Cell-cell mechanical communication through compliant substrates. *Biophysics Journal* 95(12): 6044–51.

Saha, K., A.J. Keung, E.F. Irwin, Y. Li, L. Little, D.V. Schaffer, and K.E. Healy. 2008. Substrate modulus directs neural stem cell behavior. *Biophysics Journal* 95(9): 4426–38.

Schmidt, C.E., A.F. Horwitz, D.A. Lauffenburger, and M.P. Sheetz. 1993. Integrin cytoskeletal interactions in migrating fibroblasts are dynamic, asymmetric, and regulated. *Journal of Cell Biology* 123(4): 977–91.

Shi, P., K. Shen, S. Ghassemi, J. Hone, and L.C. Kam. 2009. Dynamic force generation by neural stem cells. *Cell and Molecular Bioengineering* 2(4): 464–74.

Sieminski, A.L., R.P. Hebbel, and K.J. Gooch. 2004. The relative magnitudes of endothelial force generation and matrix stiffness modulate capillary morphogenesis *in vitro*. *Experimental Cell Research* 297(2): 574–84.

Sniadecki, N., R.A. Desai, S.A. Ruiz, and C.S. Chen. 2006. Nanotechnology for cell-substrate interactions. *Annals of Biomedical Engineering* 34(1): 59–74.

Solon, J., I. Levental, K. Sengupta, P.C. Georges, and P.A. Janmey. 2007. Fibroblast adaptation and stiffness matching to soft elastic substrates. *Biophysics Journal* 93(12): 4453–61.

Spence, H.J., Y.J. Chen, and S.J. Winder. 2002. Muscular dystrophies, the cytoskeleton and cell adhesion. *Bioessays* 24(6): 542–52.

Stroka, K.M. and H. Aranda-Espinoza. 2009. Neutrophils display biphasic relationship between migration and substrate stiffness. *Cell Motility and the Cytoskeleton* 66(6): 328–41.

Stroka, K.M. and H. Aranda-Espinoza. 2010. A biophysical view of the interplay between mechanical forces and signaling pathways during transendothelial cell migration. *FEBS Journal* 277(5): 1145–58.

Suresh, S. 2007. Biomechanics and biophysics of cancer cells. *Acta Biomaterials* 3(4): 413–38.

Uhlig, S. 2002. Ventilation-induced lung injury and mechanotransduction: Stretching it too far? *American Journal of Physiology-Lung Cellular and Molecular Physiology* 282(5): L892–6.

Ulrich, T.A., E.M.D. Pardo, and S. Kumar. 2009. The mechanical rigidity of the extracellular matrix regulates the structure, motility, and proliferation of glioma cells. *Cancer Research* 69(10): 4167–74.

Verstraeten, V.L., J.Y. Ji, K.S. Cummings, R.T. Lee, and J. Lammerding. 2008. Increased mechanosensitivity and nuclear stiffness in hutchinson-gilford progeria cells: Effects of farnesyltransferase inhibitors. *Aging Cell* 7(3): 383–93.

Vollrath, M.A., K.Y. Kwan, and D.P. Corey. 2007. The micromachinery of mechanotransduction in hair cells. *Annual Reviews of Neuroscience* 30: 339–65.

Wang, N., J.P. Butler, and D.E. Ingber. 1993. Mechanotransduction across the cell-surface and through the cytoskeleton. *Science* 260(5111): 1124–7.

Wang, N., I.M. Tolic-Norrelykke, J. Chen, S.M. Mijailovich, J.P. Butler, J.J. Fredberg, and D. Stamenovic. 2002. Cell prestress. I. Stiffness and prestress are closely associated in adherent contractile cells. *American Journal of Physiology-Cell Physiology* 282(3): C606–16.

Weckstrom, M. and P. Tavi. 2007. *Cardiac Mechanotransduction*. Austin, Texas: Springer.

Wellman, P., R. Howe, E. Dalton, and K. Kern. 1999. Harvard Biorobotics Laboratory Technical Report.

Willits, R.K. and S.L. Skornia. 2004. Effect of collagen gel stiffness on neurite extension. *Journal of Biomaterials Science-Polymer Edition* 15(12): 1521–31.

Wolf, K., Y.I. Wu, Y. Liu, J. Geiger, E. Tam, C. Overall, M.S. Stack, and P. Friedl. 2007. Multi-step pericellular proteolysis controls the transition from individual to collective cancer cell invasion. *Nature Cell Biology* 9(8): 893–904.

Yamamura, N., R. Sudo, M. Ikeda, and K. Tanishita. 2007. Effects of the mechanical properties of collagen gel on the *in vitro* formation of microvessel networks by endothelial cells. *Tissue Engineering* 13(7): 1443–53.

Yeh, W.C., P.C. Li, Y.M. Jeng, H.C. Hsu, P.L. Kuo, M.L. Li, P.M. Yang, and P.H. Lee. 2002. Elastic modulus measurements of human liver and correlation with pathology. *Ultrasound in Medicine and Biology* 28(4): 467–74.

Yeung, T., P.C. Georges, L.A. Flanagan, B. Marg, M. Ortiz, M. Funaki, N. Zahir, W. Ming, V. Weaver, and P.A. Janmey. 2005. Effects of substrate stiffness on cell morphology, cytoskeletal structure, and adhesion. *Cell Motility and the Cytoskeleton* 60(1): 24–34.

Yim, E.K.F., E.M. Darling, K. Kulangara, F. Guilak, and K.W. Leong. 2010. Nanotopography-induced changes in focal adhesions, cytoskeletal organization, and mechanical properties of human mesenchymal stem cells. *Biomaterials* 31(6): 1299–306.

Yoon, D.M. and J.P. Fisher. 2006. Chondrocyte signaling and artificial matrices for articular cartilage engineering. *Tissue Engineering* 585: 67–86.

Yuan, H.C., S. Kononov, F.S.A. Cavalcante, K.R. Lutchen, E.P. Ingenito, and B. Suki. 2000. Effects of collagenase and elastase on the mechanical properties of lung tissue strips. *Journal of Applied Physiology* 89(1): 3–14.

Zaari, N., P. Rajagopalan, S.K. Kim, A.J. Engler, and J.Y. Wong. 2004. Photopolymerization in microfluidic gradient generators: Microscale control of substrate compliance to manipulate cell response. *Advanced Materials* 16(23–24): 2133–7.

Zhang, Q.P., C.D. Ragnauth, J.N. Skepper, N.F. Worth, D.T. Warren, R.G. Roberts, P.L. Weissberg, J.A. Ellis, and C.M. Shanahan. 2005. Nesprin-2 is a multi-isomeric protein that binds lamin and emerin at the nuclear envelope and forms a subcellular network in skeletal muscle. *Journal of Cell Science* 118(4): 673–87.

Zhong, W.G., S.Y. Mao, S. Tobis, E. Angelis, M.C. Jordan, K.P. Roos, M.C. Fishbein, I.M. De Alboran, and W.R. Maclellan. 2006. Hypertrophic growth in cardiac myocytes is mediated by myc through a cyclin d2-dependent pathway. *EMBO Journal* 25(16): 3869–79.

# 15

# Mechanical Conditioning

Elaine L. Lee
*Case Western Reserve University*

Horst A. von Recum
*Case Western Reserve University*

15.1 Why Do We Need Mechanical Conditioning? .......................... **15**-1
15.2 Cellular Response to Mechanical Stimuli versus the Living Cell as a Mechanical Structure ................................................... **15**-1
15.3 Mechanotransduction and Mechanical Conditioning Terminology ...................................................................................**15**-4
15.4 Current Technologies—Advantages and Disadvantages .........**15**-6
Fluid Shear Systems • Tensile Loading Systems • Compressive Loading Systems
15.5 Upcoming Technologies ...............................................................**15**-18
15.6 Conclusion ....................................................................................**15**-18
References....................................................................................**15**-18

## 15.1 Why Do We Need Mechanical Conditioning?

The body's tissues and organs are subjected to multiple types of forces: gravitational, static, dynamic, and cyclical. The whole body is affected by the pull of Earth's gravity (or lack thereof in space), which in turn applies hydrostatic pressure to all organs and tissues. Under a static force of constant magnitude, organs such as the liver are able to maintain tone. Conversely, other parts of the body are made to withstand gradual or sudden changes in force, like the bones when different stresses are applied in the act of walking compared to running. Still yet, the function of other organs is to repeatedly resist against stress, such as the beating of the heart.

Just as a new paper clip and one bent to the point before fracture will have different stiffnesses to hold sheets of paper together, the rupture of the extracellular matrix (ECM) and the cells when a tissue or organ is injured causes a change in the mechanical force at the site of injury (Ingber 2008a, Sims et al. 1992). The body must remodel to compensate for the unbalanced mechanical function and to eventually restore the normal function to an unstressed state. However, in some cases, the organ may never fully remodel or may even propagate improper stresses and cause greater injury, such as hypertrophy of the heart from hypertension. Consequently, the inquisitive scientist can use a mechanical cell stimulator to manipulate stresses that deviate from normal conditions in a controlled environment to determine the subsequent trajectory of a tissue from a healthy to a diseased state. Similarly, to the innovative biomedical engineer, the goal is to engineer functionally viable replacement or regenerative tissues using stress parameters that mimic the native environment to induce the desired ECM remodeling and to reduce the recovery time.

## 15.2 Cellular Response to Mechanical Stimuli versus the Living Cell as a Mechanical Structure

The living cell is an adaptive mechanical structure that both receives and responds to biochemical, biomechanical, and bioelectrical signals; and its responsiveness on the cellular level influences the mechanical function on the tissue and organ level (Chiquet et al. 2007, Sarasa-Renedo and Chiquet 2005, Chiquet et al. 1996). By the same token, physical forces acting at the level of the organ can influence the function on the cellular level. In other words, form follows function: the cell increases transcription and assembly of proteins into architecture such that the function of the tissue or organ is optimal (Russell et al. 2000). For example, when the work load exceeds the preexisting capacity of the muscle fiber, such as during a workout exercise, the stretched muscle cell will undergo hypertrophy (i.e., an increase in mass and cross-sectional area) by the increasing production of contractile proteins such as actin and myosin (van Wamel et al. 2000, Russell et al. 2000). As a result, the muscle cell has an increased potential for force production that is directly proportional to the amount of hypertrophy. In the absence of such a stimulus, the muscle will atrophy.

The mechanical stimulation of cells results in cell-generated responses for a variety of cell processes (Figure 15.1) (Trepat et al. 2007):

1. Directing cell lineage, such as directing bone marrow-derived stromal cells to regenerate bone, cartilage, or ligaments (Potier et al. 2010, Guilak et al. 2009).
2. Increasing cell proliferation, such as the proliferation of fibroblasts in forming scar tissue following an injury (Palatinus et al. 2010).
3. Increasing ECM production, such as the longitudinal growth of long bones where chondrocytes synthesize cartilage (composed of Type II collagen, proteoglycans, and elastin) before ossification (Villemure and Stokes 2009).
4. Inducing cellular alignment, such as cyclic stretching of cardiomyocytes to induce alignment perpendicular to the direction of strain (Shimko and Claycomb 2008, Ingber 2010).
5. Cell migration, such as the inhibition of vascular smooth muscle cell migration under laminar shear stress (Wang et al. 2006a).
6. Cell adhesion, such as the upregulation of α-actin for cell-cell and cell-matrix adhesion (Wang et al. 2010).
7. Cell signaling, such as the mechanical deformation of a sensory neuron's plasma membrane that can cause stretch-activated ion channels to be opened to ion flow (Martinac 2004, Fan and Walsh 1999, Nishimura et al. 2008).
8. Cell morphology, such as when the membrane is perturbed, causing actin filaments in the cytoskeleton to reorganize and reinforce the area of perturbation (Nishimura et al. 2008).

In relation to Newton's third law (i.e., every action has an equal and opposite reaction), the cell shape is controlled by the cytoskeleton, which counterbalances the forces exerted by the neighboring cells and

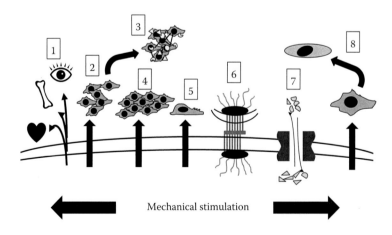

**FIGURE 15.1**  Mechanical stimulation can affect a variety of cell responses: (1) differentiation, (2) proliferation, (3) extracellular matrix production, (4) alignment, (5) migration, (6) adhesion, (7) signaling, and (8) morphology.

the environment, such as the rigidity of the adhesion substrate (Sims et al. 1992, Fletcher and Mullins 2010). Ingber modeled the cell as an architecture that is constantly under tension to stabilize its shape, known as the "tensegrity" model (Figure 15.2a) (Ingber 2008b, 2010). The actin cytoskeleton within the cell acts as rods attached to the cell membrane that are under constant tension. When these internal struts are unanchored to a culture substrate or another cell structure, the cell has a rounded shape

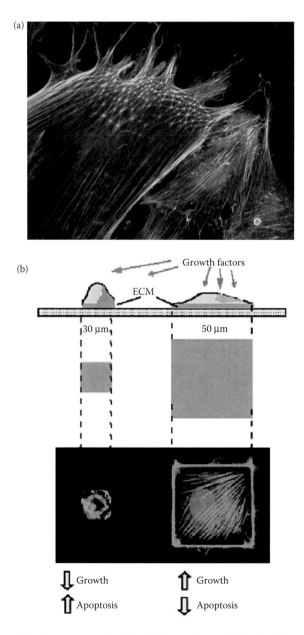

**FIGURE 15.2** (a) Internal structs composed of cytoskeletal actin filaments in Ingber's tensegrity model are extended under constant tension when the cell is adhered to a substrate. (b) The cell's growth and function are dictated by its interactions with the extracellular matrix. The cell's cycle can be modulated by the membrane's tension. The adhered cells spread over a large area will experience high tension, signaling cell growth; conversely, cells that are prevented from spreading will experience low tension and become apoptotic. (Reprinted with permission from Ingber, D. E. 2008. *Prog Biophys Mol Biol* 97: 163–79.)

maintained only by the resistance of the struts against the membrane, such as when the cells are trypsinized. When these struts are anchored to a rigid substrate, the cell model flattens and spreads, much like the adherence of a cell to a substrate. Indeed, the disruption of actin polymerization by pharmacological treatment with cytochalasin D will lead to disruption of the membrane's potential response to stretching via stretch-activated channels, thus preventing changes in cell morphology (Nishimura et al. 2008). Conversely, microtubules have been shown to bear compression, and resist the forces generated by the contracting actin cytoskeleton. Brangwynne et al. (2006) demonstrated this phenomenon using cardiomyocytes transfected with GFP-tubulin, where the microtubules buckle in unison with each contraction and straighten when the cells relax. Similarly, several groups have shown that excessive microtubule proliferation in hypertrophied hearts leads to passive stiffening and contractile dysfunction, which can be restored using colchicine to disrupt the microtubules (Tagawa et al. 1998, Nishimura et al. 2006, Zile et al. 1999, Ishibashi et al. 1996, Tsutsui et al. 1993).

The tensegrity model and the micromechanical cell response to physical distortion have been elegantly demonstrated using several different cell types by Ingber's group (Huang et al. 1998, Parker et al. 2002, Chen et al. 1997, Singhvi et al. 1994, Ingber 2008a,b, Huang and Ingber 2000). An elastomeric stamp was used to micropattern a gold substrate with defined shapes of different sizes to allow uniform absorption of ECM and resist absorption of proteins elsewhere (Figure 15.2b). Cells that typically demonstrate spread lamellipodia under standard culture substrates (e.g., hepatocytes, capillary endothelial cells, fibroblasts, and smooth muscle cells) attached preferentially to the adhesive domains and conformed to the specific shapes. The cells spread over larger surface areas exhibited the highest rates of cell growth, while cells on intermediate-sized domains became quiescent and differentiated, and cells prevented from spreading underwent apoptosis under the same conditions (Chen et al. 1997). Thus, the degree of mechanical distention can control the cell growth and death. In addition, cells spread over angular polygon domains reoriented the cytoskeletons and focal adhesions to concentrate tractional forces at the corners (Parker et al. 2002). When cell tension was released, the lamellipodia extended first from the corners, whereas cells on circular domains had no preferential direction of spreading, indicating that the direction of cell movement is influenced directly by the interaction between the cell and ECM, which is critical in embryonic and tissue development. Similar studies also demonstrated that contractility (e.g., heart cells) can also be altered as a result of changes to the matrix (Polte et al. 2004).

How does the cell "sense" these changes in physical force? The transmembrane cell surface receptors (i.e., integrins) physically link the load-responsive cytoskeleton to the ECM and are theorized to be capable of mediating mechanosensing (Gov 2009, Yeung et al. 2005, Ingber 2010, Fletcher and Mullins 2010, Guilak et al. 2009). Through the integrins, the cell transfers mechanical signals from the macroscale to the nanoscale. The conversion of external mechanical signals to changes in intracellular biochemical signals and gene expression is known as mechanotransduction. Thus, if the external mechanical signal transmitted to the cell can be controlled *in vitro*, we can steer cell development to express proteins and matrix desirable to functional tissues.

## 15.3 Mechanotransduction and Mechanical Conditioning Terminology

Cells can be mechanically stimulated by tensile, compressive, or shear forces. *Force* (*F*) is a vector with magnitude (mass times acceleration or $F = ma$) and direction. *Tension* is an applied force (or stress) external to the cell that pulls and causes it to elongate, and can also cause an increase in volume. Conversely, *compression* decreases the length of the cell. To apply compression, pressure is usually applied. *Pressure* (*P*) is a three-dimensional, isotropic, compressive stress that describes the force per unit area:

$$P = \frac{F_n}{A}$$

(15.1)

*Isotropy* describes a material property in which the values are the same when measured along the axes in all directions; *anisotropy* describes a material property in which the values along the axes are different. An example of anisotropy is the induced alignment of cells with repeated applications of stress in one direction.

*Stress* ($\sigma$) is the measure of average normal force per unit area, assumed to be uniformly distributed within a deformable body:

$$\sigma_{avg} = \frac{F_n}{A} \tag{15.2}$$

Thus, pressure is a type of stress. The SI unit for stress is *pascal* (Pa), which is equivalent to one Newton-force per square meter (1 N/m²). A normal force or stress is considered to be *tensile* if it is stretched perpendicularly out of the plane or *compressive* if it is acting inward. Tensile stresses are usually denoted by a positive sign convention, and compressive stresses are negative. For example, the vertical cables supporting a suspension bridge are under tension, being pulled downward by the weight of the bridge. The concrete pillars supporting a bridge from underneath experience compressive stress.

Forces acting on the transverse plane are *shear forces*, which can be normalized over the unit area to obtain the *shear stress* ($\tau$):

$$\tau_{avg} = \frac{F_s}{A} \tag{15.3}$$

Shear stress is usually described by a "sliding" motion, such as when blocks from the game Jenga® are pulled from the tower or a log is pulled longitudinally out of a stack of firewood.

*Strain* is a dimensionless quantity defined as elongation per unit length:

$$\varepsilon = \frac{\delta}{L}$$

or

$$e = \frac{\Delta L}{L} = \frac{\ell - L}{L} \tag{15.4}$$

where $\varepsilon$ is the true strain and $e$ is the engineering strain. $\delta$ is defined as the total elongation and $L$ is the total length. Similarly, imagine a fiber being pulled. To measure $e$, the original length of the fiber $L$ and the final length $\ell$ need to be measured. As with tensile and compressive stresses, strains can also be tensile or compressive and follow the same sign convention. A *linearly elastic* material will assume that for infinitesimally small strains or deformations, the relationship between stress and strain is linear.

*Stiffness* ($k$) describes how much a material can resist deformation:

$$k = \frac{AE}{L} \tag{15.5}$$

where $A$ is the cross-sectional area, $E$ is the elastic or Young's modulus, and $L$ is the length. *Young's modulus* ($E$) describes the ratio of uniaxial stress to uniaxial strain for an isotropic material:

$$E = \frac{\text{tensile stress}}{\text{tensile strain}} = \frac{\sigma}{\varepsilon} = \frac{F/A_0}{\Delta L/L_0} \tag{15.6}$$

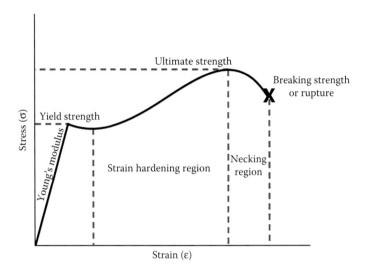

**FIGURE 15.3**  A material's relationship between stress and strain can be represented graphically.

where $A_0$ and $L_0$ are the original cross-sectional area and length, respectively, to which the force is applied. Conversely, *compliance* is the inverse of stiffness.

The relationship between stress and strain of a material can be graphically represented on a *stress-strain curve* (Figure 15.3). Along the first portion of the curve, the relationship is linear, indicating the linearly elastic region or the Young's modulus. Imagine eating ice cream with a stainless steel spoon: the spoon may deform slightly as it scoops more ice cream from the bowl, but ultimately it returns to its original configuration. When the material reaches its *yield strength*, the material will no longer return to its original shape when the applied force is removed and thus permanently deforms. *Strength* refers to the stress at which the material permanently deforms or fractures. Imagine that more ice cream is desired, but scooping the ice cream directly from the carton fresh out of the freezer causes the spoon to reach its *yield strength* and bend permanently. The material *strain hardens* (i.e., material strengthens as it plastically deforms) until it reaches its *ultimate strength*, which is the maximum amount of stress the material can withstand. Beyond this point, a *neck* forms, where the cross-sectional area quickly decreases before reaching the *breaking strength*, where the material ruptures. Continuing to scoop the frozen ice cream will cause the shaft of the spoon to become harder until the stainless steel ultimately breaks.

*Uniaxial* or *axial force* is a load directed along one principal axis of an object, and *biaxial force* is a load directed perpendicularly to two principal axes in the same plane. *Equibiaxial* refers to equal loads directed along all axes in all directions (i.e., isotropy). *Static* refers to loads in equilibrium, whereas *dynamic* refers to loads in motion. For example, a gymnast in perfect balance on a beam will have a static load on her bones, compared to when her bones will be dynamically loading when she tumbles to dismount off the beam.

## 15.4 Current Technologies—Advantages and Disadvantages

Brown (2000) presents an excellent review of the types of mechanical stimulation systems. More detail can also be found in Gooch and Tennant (1997). A summary of the devices and methods used to study the effects of physical forces on cells in culture can be found in Table 15.1.

**TABLE 15.1** Summary of Devices Used to Study Effects of Physical Forces on Cells in Culture

| Name of Device/Method of Developing Force | Primary Force | Stress Profile | Comments |
|---|---|---|---|
| Parallel-plate flow chamber | Shear | • Parabolic velocity profile[a] <br> • Greatest at plate surfaces <br><br> • Wall stress:[b] $\tau_w = \dfrac{6\mu Q}{bh^2}$ <br><br> • Homogeneous <br> • Not a function of position <br> • Linear decrease of pressure as a function of position, usually negligible | • Possible presence of not fully developed laminar flow where the fluid enters the device[c] <br> • Requires a significant number of cells at the start of the experiment[d] <br> • Simple hardware <br> • Easy to visualize |
| Radial flow chamber | Shear | • Linearly decreasing velocity profile <br> • Greatest near center, minimum at outer edge <br><br> • Wall stress:[e] $\tau_w = \dfrac{3\mu Q}{\pi r h^2}$ <br><br> • Varies as a function of position | • Possible presence of not fully developed laminar flow where the fluid enters the device[c] <br> • Requires a significant number of cells at the start of the experiment <br> • Simple hardware <br> • Easy to visualize |
| Cone-and-plate viscometer[f] | Shear | • Flow determined by Reynolds' number:[f] <br><br> $Re = \dfrac{r^2 \omega \alpha^2}{12\nu} = \dfrac{r^2 \omega \alpha^2 \rho}{12\mu}$ <br><br> • For $Re \ll 1$: <br>    • Laminar flow <br>    • Linearly proportional gradient velocity to $\alpha$ <br>    • Spatially homogeneous flow <br><br> • Wall stress: [f] $\tau_w = \mu \left.\dfrac{\partial U}{\partial y}\right|_{y=0} = \dfrac{\mu \omega}{\alpha}$ <br><br> • Ideal stress not a function of position | • Possible presence of secondary flows <br> • Simple hardware <br> • Difficult to visualize |
| Rotary orbital shaker[g,h] | Shear | • Average stress dependent on rotary speed:[h] <br>    • 25 rpm: $0.67 \pm 0.23$ dyn/cm$^2$ <br>    • 40 rpm: $1.68 \pm 0.14$ dyn/cm$^2$ <br>    • 55 rpm: $2.54 \pm 0.31$ dyn/cm$^2$ <br> • Laminar flow <br> • Uniform hydrodynamic environment | • Spatial embryoid body distribution dependent on rotary speed <br> • EB size dependent on rotary speed (decreases as the rotary speed increases) <br> • Simple hardware <br> • Easy to visualize |
| Longitudinal stretch[a] | Tension | • Dynamic or static load <br> • Anisotropic <br> • Peak strain typically ranges from 1–10% <br> • Greatest at the center of the device <br> • Four-point bending systems deliver low and homogeneous strains | • Creates corresponding compressive stress in perpendicular direction <br> • Boundary condition created at grips <br> • May also generate shear stress due to the motion of cells relative to the fluid <br> • Complicated hardware <br> • Difficult to visualize |
| Out-of-plane circular substrate stretch[a] | Tension | • Usually a dynamic load <br> • Heterogeneous radial strain unless the membrane is very thin[i,j] <br> • Greatest at the center of the device | • May be subjected to other stresses depending on signal input, media movement, or preexisting system tension <br> • Simple hardware <br> • Difficult to visualize |

*continued*

**TABLE 15.1** (continued) Summary of Devices Used to Study Effects of Physical Forces on Cells in Culture

| Name of Device/Method of Developing Force | Primary Force | Stress Profile | Comments |
|---|---|---|---|
| In-plane substrate stretch[a] | Tension | • Isotropic<br>• Homogeneous equibiaxial strain | • Plate approach<br>  • Simple hardware<br>  • Easy visualization<br>• Biaxial grip approach[k]<br>  • Complicated hardware<br>  • Difficult to visualize |
| Matrix-contracting gel system[a] | Tension | • Dependent on the cell's contractile response[l–n] | • Can embed a strain gauge |
| Compression of gas/liquid phase | Compression | • Static or dynamic load<br>• Spatially homogeneous[a,o] | • Cells do not need to be adhered<br>• Change in concentration of dissolved gas due to increase in oxygen and carbon dioxide partial pressures or osmotic balance[p]<br>• May require different media composition to accommodate pressure changes[q]<br>• Proper humidification required[r]<br>• Simple hardware |
| Direct compression of the specimen phase | Compression | • Static or dynamic load<br>• Spatially homogeneous | • Accommodates explanted tissue specimens[s–v] or polymeric carriers[a]<br>• May cause anisotropic strain deformation from flat-plate abutment<br>• Simple hardware |

*Source:* With kind permission from Springer Science+Business Media: *Mechanical Forces: Their Effects on Cells and Tissues,* 1997, Gooch, K. J. and C. J. Tennant. New York: Springer.

[a] Brown TD. *J Biomech* 2000;33:3–14.
[b] Bacabac RG et al. *J Biomech* 2005;38:159–67.
[c] Gooch KJ, Tennant CJ. *Mechanical Forces: Their Effects on Cells and Tissues.* New York: Springer; 1997.
[d] Brown D, Larson R. *BMC Immunol* 2001;2:9.
[e] Kandlikar SG et al. *Heat Transfer and Fluid Flow in Minichannels and Microchannels.* Kidlington, Oxford: Elsevier; 2005.
[f] Einav S et al. *Experiments in Fluids* 1994;16:196–202.
[g] Carpenedo RL et al. *Stem Cells* 2007;25:2224–34.
[h] Sargent CY et al. *Biotechnol Bioeng* 2010;105:611–26.
[i] Brown TD et al. *Am J Med Sci* 1998;316:162–8.
[j] Brown TD et al. *Comput Methods Biomech Biomed Engin* 2000;3:65–78.
[k] Eastwood M et al. *Biochim Biophys Acta* 1994;1201(2):186–92.
[l] Dahlmann-Noor AH et al. *Exp Cell Res* 2007;313:4158–69.
[m] Lambert CA et al. *Lab Invest* 1992;66:444–51.
[n] Chamson A et al. *Arch Dermatol Res* 1997;289:596–9.
[o] Myers KA et al. *Biochem Cell Biol* 2007;85:543–51.
[p] Ozawa H et al. *J Cell Physiol* 1990;142:177–85.
[q] Tanck E et al. *J Biomech* 1999;32:153–61.
[r] Maul TM et al. *J Biomech Eng* 2007;129:110–6.
[s] Aufderheide AC, Athanasiou KA. *Ann Biomed Eng* 2006;34:1463–74.
[t] Guilak F et al. *Osteoarthritis Cartilage* 1994;2:91–101.
[u] Burton-Wurster N et al. *J Orthop Res* 1993;11:717–29.
[v] Torzilli PA et al. *J Biomech* 1997;30:1–9.

## 15.4.1 Fluid Shear Systems

Fluid shear influences a number of cellular phenomena, including but not limited to vasoconstriction via vascular smooth muscle cells, mechanoreception via plasma membrane receptors or ion channels, and nitric oxide release via endothelial cells. Two main types of systems dominate the application of fluid shear stress: parallel plate and cone-and-plate systems. These systems are most useful for studying cell adhesion and engineering vasculature under physiological flow conditions; however, the main challenge of these systems is keeping a homogeneous fluid flow to produce uniform shear stress.

The parallel plate system is a flow chamber that applies laminar shear flow with an incompressible fluid (i.e., homogeneous and has constant density throughout) by a pressure differential (Figure 15.4a), where the wall shear stress ($\tau_w$) is given by (Bacabac et al. 2005):

$$\tau_w = \frac{6\mu Q}{bh^2} \tag{15.7}$$

where $\mu$ is the fluid viscosity, $Q$ is the volumetric flow rate, $b$ is the width of the chamber, and $h$ is the distance between the plates for rectangular flow chambers. The parabolic velocity profile will generate a shear stress profile that has the maximum magnitude at the plate surfaces, with >85% exposed to homogeneous shear wall stress for $b/h > 20$. For radial parallel plate systems, $\tau_w$ is given as a function of radial position $r$ by (Figure 15.4b) (Kandlikar et al. 2006):

$$\tau_w = \frac{3\mu Q}{\pi r h^2} \tag{15.8}$$

Radial parallel plate systems have a flow inlet from the center of the plate that flows radially outward, covering a larger surface area and having a linearly decreasing velocity profile as it flows from the inner

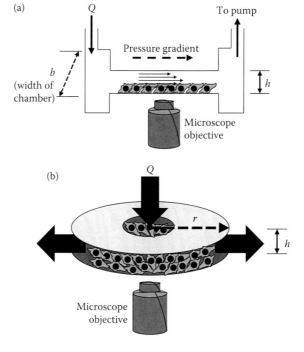

**FIGURE 15.4** (a) Parallel plate flow chamber systems apply homogeneous laminar shear stress. (b) Radial parallel plate flow chamber systems apply the highest shear stress near the center and minimum shear stress at the outer edge.

to the outer region. Thus, the highest shear stress is near the center, and the minimum shear stress is at the outer edge. This shear stress profile is most useful for examining a range of stress values with a single experiment, as opposed to several different experiments at different flow rates.

Two slits are formed at opposite ends of a rectangular or radial chamber, between which the pressure difference is created where the lowest speed will occur where the pressure is highest (i.e., the chamber is most narrow) (Brown 2000). Fluid flow can be created by a gravity pressure head (i.e., steady shear stress) or an active pump (i.e., transient shear stress). The parallel plate system requires minimal equipment (fluid flow chamber, tubing, pump if required) and requires a minimal amount of media, which can easily be accessed for changing media. If desired, the media can also be recirculated. The chamber construction is made to allow easy visualization under a microscope. The system should produce homogeneous fluid flow in the absence of bubbles in the tubing, which can cause cells to be stripped from the substrate. Also, depending on the substrate, the initial adhesion of cells may be low and thus require a significant number of cells (approximately $10^6$–$10^7$ cells), which can be problematic when studying rare cell populations (Brown and Larson 2001). In addition, for inhibition studies, chambers that do not recirculate media may require large quantities of expensive inhibitors.

The second most common system to study shear stress is the cone-and-plate fluid shear system, which places a cone's axis perpendicular to a flat plate to rotate the cone (Figure 15.5) (Brown 2000, Einav et al. 1994). By controlling the angular velocity of the cone rotation, a spatially homogeneous fluid shear stress can be achieved over the plate on which the cone rotates. To determine laminar flow, the Reynolds number ($Re$) can be obtained by:

$$Re = \frac{r^2 \omega \alpha^2}{12\nu} = \frac{r^2 \omega \alpha^2 \rho}{12\mu} \tag{15.9}$$

where $r$ is the radial distance from the cone's surface, $\omega$ is the angular velocity of the cone, $\alpha$ is the angle between the cone and the plate in radians, $\nu$ is the kinematic viscosity, $\mu$ is the dynamic viscosity, and $\rho$ is density. For values of $Re \ll 1$, the centrifugal force is small, the fluid velocity is a linearly proportional gradient to $\alpha$, and the fluid shear stress is constant over the entire plate. As $Re$ increases, centrifugal force increases, creating flow in the radial direction near the rotating cone, but the corresponding centripetal flow close to the stationary plate negates it. The shear stress thus changes in magnitude and direction; for $Re > 4$, flow becomes turbulent, which can be achieved via the conic taper and the imposed angular velocity. For $Re \ll 1$, the fluid wall stress ($\tau_w$) is constant over the flat plate and is given by:

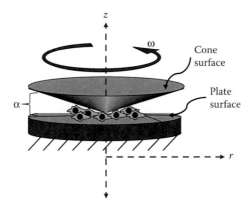

**FIGURE 15.5** Cone-and-plate systems apply homogenous laminar shear stress.

$$\tau_w = \mu \left.\frac{\partial U}{\partial y}\right|_{y=0} = \frac{\mu\omega}{\alpha} \tag{15.10}$$

where $U$ is the fluid velocity parallel to the wall and $y$ is the distance to the wall. Although the hardware for the system is simple, it also makes modulating a constant shear stress for sustained periods of time difficult since the flow field will often develop transient peaks in shear stresses. In addition, microscopic visualization can be challenging.

More recently, several groups have used fluid shear via rotary suspension culture bioreactors to induce embryonic stem cell aggregation into embryoid bodies (EBs) and differentiation on a large scale (Kim and von Recum 2009, 2010, Cormier et al. 2006, Sargent et al. 2010, Carpenedo et al. 2007). EBs recapitulate the path of cellular morphogenic events of embryos as in the native development environment, from embryo to the formation of the three germ layers (ectoderm, endoderm, and mesoderm) (Coucouvanis and Martin 1995, Keller 1995). Other methods of EB formation are problematic: (a) Hanging drop formation is tedious, has low yield, and is not easily scalable (Maltsev et al. 1994); (b) centrifugation into 96-well plates also has the same issue as hanging drop formation (Ng et al. 2005); and (c) static suspension cultures produce heterogeneous-sized EBs, which lead to heterogeneous differentiation and thus lower yield (Dang et al. 2002). Many groups have turned to large rotary suspension culture bioreactors and spinner flask methods to increase EB production with excellent results (Chen et al. 2006, Dang et al. 2002, Gerecht-Nir et al. 2004, Wang et al. 2006b, Zandstra et al. 2003). However, as a consequence of space constraints, a few groups have reduced the scale to simply that of a 10-cm Petri dish, achieving suspension through a rotary orbital shaker (Kim and von Recum 2009, 2010, Carpenedo et al. 2007, Sargent et al. 2010). Carpenedo et al. (2007) reported the first successful large-scale, size-controllable production of EBs using this method, and Kim and von Recum (2009, 2010) demonstrated successful differentiation of early, middle, and late progenitors for endothelial cells, illustrating the effects of shear mechanical stimulation on endothelial differentiation. Sargent et al. (2010) later characterized the hydrodynamic conditions necessary for EB formation with optimal and uniform distribution for rotary orbital shaker suspension cultures. EBs decrease in size but increased in yield as the speed increases (20–25 rpm gives 500 µm diameter EBs; 40–50 rpm, 225 µm; 55–60 rpm, 140 µm). More importantly, the rotary orbital conditions did not hinder the normal progression of differentiation, and differentiation markers for all three germ layers increased. Thus, compared to the static culture conditions, hydrodynamic forces significantly influence gene expression and impact the internal organization of cells within EBs.

## 15.4.2 Tensile Loading Systems

The most common biologic stressor studied is tensile stress (see terminology section for definitions and equations), and examples of biologic phenomena are numerous. Microscopic tears in tendon fibrils may disrupt homeostatic tension, and the subsequent stress absence may induce apoptosis to tendon cells (Egerbacher et al. 2008). Ventricular myocytes undergoing tensile deformations can stimulate mechanosensitive currents that lead to spontaneous contraction (Bett and Sachs 2000). When the skin is stretched, mRNA for collagen synthesis and other ECM proteins increases, indicating upregulation at a pretranslational level (Lambert et al. 1992).

Tensile loading systems can be categorized into four different groups: longitudinal stretch, out-of-plane circular substrate distention, in-plane substrate distention, and contracting systems (Brown 2000). Longitudinal stretch systems apply uniaxial or anisotropic deformations, while out-of-plane circular substrate systems apply radial distention. In-plane substrate systems allow for biaxial or equibiaxial stretching. The last system involves matrix contraction to study cell responsive behavior.

Longitudinal stretch systems generally employ gripped substrates that are run by a stimulating driver (Figure 15.6a) (see Table 15.2 for descriptions) (Brown 2000). Most mechanical conditioning systems are designed to deliver peak strains in the range of 1–10% (Brown 2000). Tensile loading

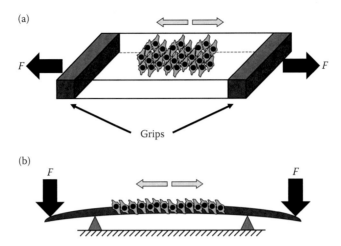

**FIGURE 15.6** Longitudinal tensile loading systems apply uniaxial stress by (a) gripping and pulling on a substrate or (b) bending a substrate.

**TABLE 15.2** Methods to Apply Tension

| Method | Description | Select References |
|---|---|---|
| | Longitudinal Strain (Uniaxial Strain) | |
| Immobilized specimens | • Frame supports the stretched specimen<br>• Static stretch applied | • Weiser et al. (1995)<br>• Somjen et al. (1980)<br>• Meikle et al. (1979) |
| Thumbscrew-driven stretch frame | • Frame with thumbscrews supports substrate<br>• Strain increases with each turn of the screw<br>• Quasi-static stretch applied | • Komuro et al. (1990) |
| Cam systems | • Eccentric disks rotated axially by a motor<br>• Translates rotary motion into oscillatory linear motion<br>• Dynamic stretch applied | • Gupta et al. (2008)<br>• Eastwood et al. (1994)<br>• Ives et al. (1986)<br>• De Witt et al. (1984)<br>• Leung et al. (1977) |
| Linear actuators | • Applies cyclic force in a controlled and linear manner<br>• Based on the principle of an inclined plane turned into a screw thread<br>• Dynamic stretch applied | • Alexander et al. (1999)<br>• Ozerdem and Tözeren (1995) |
| Solenoid-driven and electromagnetically driven metal bars | • Coil of wire through which current passes to generate energy via a magnetic field<br>• The magnetic field attracts metal bars embedded within the substrate<br>• Dynamic stretch applied | • Forth and Layne (2008)<br>• Smalt et al. (1997)<br>• Xu et al. (1996)<br>• Alexander (1976) |
| Pneumatic pistons | • Converts the potential energy of compressed air into kinetic energy<br>• Transfers the energy to piston to impart force<br>• Dynamic stretch applied | • Chokalingam et al. (2009)<br>• Gustafson et al. (2006)<br>• Sotoudeh et al. (1998) |
| Mounted substrate-substrate bending | • Cells seeded on a rectangular substrate<br>• Substrates mounted to a base substrate attached to an outrigger arm<br>• Powered by stepper motor, which allows waveforms to be varied easily<br>• Dynamic stretch applied | • Neidlinger-Wilke et al. (2009)<br>• Neidlinger-Wilke et al. (1994)<br>• Murray and Rushton (1990)<br>• Vandenburgh and Karlisch (1989) |

**TABLE 15.2** (continued) Methods to Apply Tension

| Method | Description | Select References |
|---|---|---|
| Four-point bending systems | • Does not need grips for the substrate (no boundary condition)<br>• Deliver low and homogeneous strains<br>• Maneuvers the substrate using shielded electromagnetic actuators or can seed plastic strips as substrates<br>• Can also embed strain gauges | • Li et al. (2010)<br>• Carpenter et al. (2006)<br>• Jessop et al. (2002)<br>• Robling et al. (2001)<br>• Bottlang et al. (1997)<br>• Pitsillides et al. (1995)<br>• Jones et al. (1991) |
| | Out-of-Plane Circular Substrate (Radial Strain) | |
| Template displacement | • The convex template prong is pressed vertically against the underside of the substrate for displacement<br>• Static or dynamic load | • Rana et al. (2008)<br>• Felix et al. (1996)<br>• Matsuo et al. (1996)<br>• Williams et al. (1992)<br>• Vandenburgh and Karlisch (1989)<br>• Hasegawa et al. (1985) |
| Flexible bottom substrate using vacuum | • Vacuum is applied underneath the membrane<br>• Distends below the original position<br>• Imparts strain to cells seeded on top of the membrane<br>• Controllable parameters include percent strain (vacuum magnitude), waveform, frequency, and duty cycle<br>• Uniform strain only for thin membranes | • Banes et al. (1985) |
| Positive pressure displacement (fluid) on a flexible substrate | • Flexible sheets clamped down into a circular shape<br>• Pressure from the fluid causes an upward displacement from the origin position<br>• Can be driven by pneumatic cylinders or solenoid-based devices | • Ellis et al. (1995)<br>• Brighton et al. (1991)<br>• Winston et al. (1989) |
| | In-Plane Distention (Equibiaxial Strain) | |
| Flat plate upward displacement | • Flat plate is frictionless (e.g., lubricated)<br>• The plate is driven upward (e.g., piston) | • Hung and Williams (1994)<br>• Schaffer et al. (1994) |
| Flat plate with applied vacuum | • Modification of out-of-plane, flexible bottom system using vacuum<br>• Insert a frictionless flat plate and apply vacuum for periphery downward displacement | • Gilbert et al. (1994) |
| Multiaxial tension loading system | • Applies stretch on two axes perpendicular to each other<br>• Cells seeded in intersection of two membranes | • Gupta et al. (2008)<br>• Norton et al. (1995)<br>• Eastwood et al. (1994) |
| | Matrix-Contracting Systems | |
| Acid-soluble gel matrices | • Metabolite secretion causes gel dissolution<br>• Cell tension will cause contractile response<br>• Gel contracts as a result of cellular contraction | • Dahlmann-Noor et al. (2007)<br>• Chamson et al. (1997)<br>• Lambert et al. (1992)<br>• Tomasek et al. (1992) |

systems have advanced from simple static stretch to complex systems that can allow control of parameters such as duty cycle, stress magnitude, frequency, and waveform. However, these loading systems still have limitations. The tensile stress of the substrate causes a corresponding compressive stress in the perpendicular direction. Additionally, because the substrates must be gripped, a boundary condition is created.

Alternatively, to circumvent the boundary problem, some groups have designed four-point bending systems (Figure 15.6b) that typically deliver low, homogeneous strains (Robling et al. 2001, Jessop et al. 2002, Li et al. 2010), which may not load in the physiological range (such as with osteoclasts entombed in mineralized matrices). Groups have driven the substrate stretch using a number of options, such as shielded electromagnetic actuators (Bottlang et al. 1997) and cell-seeded plastic strips (Pitsillides et al. 1995). The substrates in four-point bending systems often engage strain gauges to quantify the amount of strain (Jones et al. 1991).

Out-of-plane circular substrate systems typically create deformations proportionate with respect to the radius, with the maximum strain occurring at the center and zero strain at the periphery. The substrate is flexible and displaced from its originating position via template displacement (Figure 15.7a), vacuum of substrate (Figure 15.7b), or positive fluid displacement of substrate (Figure 15.7c) (see Table 15.2 for descriptions) (Brown 2000).

The first to report using a template to displace a substrate, Hasegawa et al. (1985) claimed that the curvature of convex templates governed distention in the membrane, and therefore the input strain. However, although the group claimed that their template produced uniform strain, they did not provide

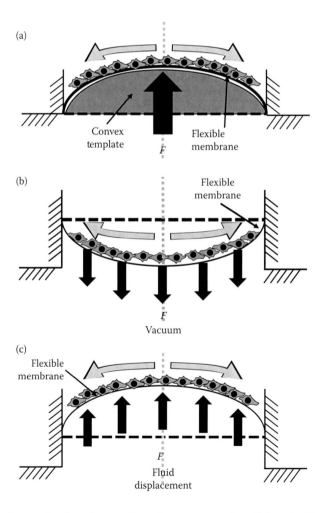

**FIGURE 15.7** Out-of-plane circular substrate distention systems apply radial strain (linearly decreasing with respect to the center) by (a) physical displacement with a solid template, (b) downward displacement with applied vacuum, or (c) upward displacement with a positive pressure fluid flow.

any means (calculated or measured) to verify the specific template used, and Williams et al. (1992) disputed Hasegawa et al.'s claim through analytical solutions that demonstrate surface strains due to bending are not negligible. Nevertheless, the design inspired several subsequent modifications, such as changing the substrate area (Felix et al. 1996), applying static stretch via thumbscrew-driven stretch frame (Rana et al. 2008), or using pulsating rounded prongs (Vandenburgh and Karlisch 1989) or flat-ended circular pistons (Matsuo et al. 1996).

Banes et al. (1985) first introduced the concept of applying a vacuum to a flexible bottom substrate. The device became one of the most requested mechanostimulus devices and is now marketed as the Flexcell Tension System (Flexcell International Corporation, Hillsborough, NC). Its popularity with the scientific community outpaced a thorough analysis by the engineering community, who later determined that the substrate had inhomogeneous radial strain (Gilbert et al. 1990, 1994, Brown et al. 2000). Redesigned in 1995, the current iteration is a very thin substrate that closely resembles an ideal membrane behavior and has radial strain homogeneity (Brown et al. 1998, 2000). Converse to vacuum application, a positive-pressure displacement can be done using a flowing fluid (Winston et al. 1989, Brighton et al. 1991).

Several factors may influence the cells in these systems to be subjected to stresses other than tension. For example, cells on diaphragmatic substrates subjected to pressure differentials may also be exposed to shear stresses due to media movement relative to the cells. Other factors may include the input signal magnitude, frequency, and waveform; the depth and viscosity of the nutrient media; and any preexisting tension in the system (Brown 2000). The constant movement in these systems also makes cellular observation under microscopy difficult.

Alternative solutions to work around strain heterogeneity in out-of-plane circular deformation systems feature in-plane distention to achieve homogeneous biaxial or equibiaxial strain. A few groups physically limit cell adhesion to a specific spot by spot-plating or masking to achieve uniform deformation; however, the most common method is to change the area impacted by deformation while keeping the culture plane level. One approach axially and upwardly punctuates a large area of the substrate from underneath using a frictionless plate (e.g., lubricated) (Figure 15.8a) (Hung and Williams 1994, Schaffer et al. 1994); the other approach modifies the Flexcell, using a large area frictionless plate and applying vacuum from underneath along the periphery (Figure 15.8b). Cells centered over the plate are stretched in an outwardly radial direction when the deforming component causes the overlying substrate to slide over plate edges with negligible friction, and both methods allow easy access for visualization. In an entirely different approach, some groups grip a membrane or substrate (e.g., collagen) and pull in two perpendicular directions, where the cells seeded in the intersection of both membranes are exposed to an isotropic stretch (Figure 15.8c,d) (Eastwood et al. 1994, Gupta et al. 2007, 2008, Norton et al. 1995). Although friction is negligible, the hardware necessary to implement this approach is challenging and does not allow easy access for microscopy.

Finally, matrix-contracting systems use acid-soluble gel matrices seeded with cells as a way to study cellular response to tension. The secretion of metabolites will cause gel dissolution (Lambert et al. 1992, Dahlmann-Noor et al. 2007, Tomasek et al. 1992, Chamson et al. 1997, Brown 2000), and the subsequent residual stress from the adherent cell results in spontaneous cellular contraction and thus gel contraction. The gel may also be embedded with a strain gauge as a way to quantify the contractile response.

## 15.4.3 Compressive Loading Systems

Chondrocytes that decrease aggrecan expression in articular cartilage (Lammi et al. 1994), osteocytes that signal a decrease in bone resorption by inhibiting osteoclast formation (Lau et al. 2010), and irritant receptors lining the inside of the epithelium of the airways that are activated by sustained inflation of the lungs (Kappagoda and Ravi 2006) are all examples of biologic phenomena response to compressive stresses (see terminology section for definitions and equations). To study

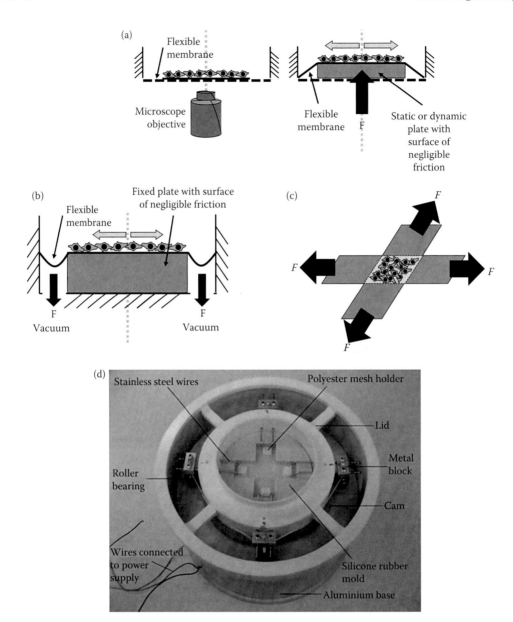

**FIGURE 15.8** In-plane displacement systems apply homogeneous equibiaxial strain to flexible membranes by (a) upward plate displacement or (b) downward vacuum displacement. Alternatively, (c) isotropic strain may be applied with two axes of stretch, situated perpendicular to each other. (d) Gives an example of such a system. (Reprinted with permission from Gupta V. et al. 2008 *Ann Biomed Eng* 36: 1092–103.)

cell behavior to compression in a variety of tissues (e.g., cartilage, bone, airways, and vasculature), scientists frequently use positive or negative hydrostatic pressure, the pressure exerted by a fluid at equilibrium due to the force of gravity, to apply mechanical stress to the tissue or cell culture (Myers et al. 2007, Brown 2000).

Hydrostatic pressure systems have relatively simple equipment setup in comparison to tensile loading systems: a flat plate is used to press down on the contained culture (Figure 15.9a). The system may or may not also have an incubator gas phase pressurized on top of the media. The simplicity in the

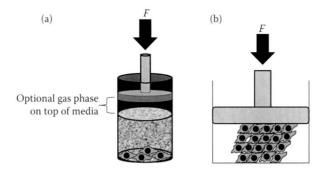

**FIGURE 15.9**  Compressive loading systems using a plate to apply pressure (a) directly to the liquid phase or on top of a buffering gaseous phase. (b) Specimens can also be loaded by directly abutting the plate to the sample.

equipment allows replicate experiments to be run simultaneously using a manifold design (Brown 2000). The load application may be static or transient and is spatially homogeneous. Unlike fluid shear and tensile loading systems, cells in compressive loading systems do not need to be adhered to a substrate to be subjected to hydrostatic pressure. In addition, hydrostatic pressure systems generally do not require a direct contact with the flat plate, which guarantees that the specimen is not impacted by the plate and that metabolite transfer between cells and media is not impeded physically. On the other hand, incubator partial pressures of oxygen and carbon dioxide must increase to reach physiologic stress levels under normal culture conditions (Ozawa et al. 1990). Consequential to the increase in gas pressures, different media composition or alterations to the physical chemistry may be required unless the load is low in magnitude or high in frequency (Tanck et al. 1999). In cyclic pressure systems, the constant movement of air can cause a change in osmotic balance as water from culture media evaporates, leading to disruption in cell processes and even cell death (Maul et al. 2007). In conjunction with this problem, proper humidification of the chamber is difficult to preserve for long-term experiments (>2 days). Finally, compressive loading systems are limited in use for engineering tissues since very few tissues experience purely hydrostatic pressures.

Alternatively, some approaches have placed the specimens directly against a hydraulically operated flat plate, such as with cartilage, which mimics direct contact *in vivo* loading (Figure 15.9b) (Brown 2000, Aufderheide and Athanasiou 2006, Guilak et al. 1994, Burton-Wurster et al. 1993, Torzilli et al. 1997). This method accommodates a variety of three-dimensional specimens, such as tissue explants or cells seeded within a matrix or polymeric carrier, a distinct advantage over noncontact pressure application since interactions between cells and a carrier can be studied (Brown 2000). Again, the hardware required is simple, although the plate's direct abutment to the specimen may cause strain deformations as a result of friction, not uniaxial compression. The specimens may be unconfined or confined during compression; the latter conditions more closely mimic physiologic conditions but may impede diffusion of nutrients and metabolites. In addition, because the uniaxial loading application induces an anisotropic strain field (as opposed to isotropic in noncontact compression), competing cellular or molecular response mechanisms may be activated.

Only a few novel systems have been custom-designed (Hasel et al. 2002, Nagatomi et al. 2002, Pugin et al. 1998, Sumpio et al. 1994, Parkkinen et al. 1995, Maul et al. 2007, Shaikh et al. 2010), since pressure application is conceptually different from tensile systems. Hydrostatic pressure is generally nondirectional in its application (except for gravity), and the actual compressibility of fluid-filled cellular structures is orders of magnitude smaller than tensile deformations (Myers et al. 2007). For example, an erythrocyte experiencing a 10 MPa load (the upper limit of loads experienced *in vivo*) will only result in a roughly 0.4% volume change due to compression. Despite its small-magnitude stress contribution in comparison to shear and tensile stresses, cyclic hydrostatic pressure is thought to be an important stimulus in determining cell phenotype (Myers et al. 2007).

## 15.5 Upcoming Technologies

The mechanical stimulation systems described previously have been used to distinguish the effects of the applied stress independent from other stress parameters. The next level of complexity in mechanical stimulation systems combines these technologies with independent control to understand interactions between simultaneous stresses and to provide tools to the tissue engineer. Novel systems for application of both fluid shear and longitudinal distention have been used to study stretch-activated membrane ion channels in chondrocytes (Wright et al. 1996), to understand the response of tendon cells to cyclic loading (Lavagnino et al. 2008), and to engineer heart valve tissue (Engelmayr Jr. et al. 2008). Other groups have grown cells inside distensible tubular constructions and applied fluid shear to study the vasculature responses to wall strain (Ayajiki et al. 1996, Moore et al. 1994, Benbrahim et al. 1994). With the constant, dynamic loading undertaken, bone and cartilage have been studied for the interaction between compressive and shear forces (Heiner and Martin 2004, Orr and Burg 2008). In addition, these groups designed their devices with the forethought to become culture systems for tissue engineering.

Translation is limited until we can recover the mechanically conditioned cells without damage. For example, by modifying the surface of the silicone substrate with an *N*-isopropylacrylamide (NIPAAm)-based polymer, Lee and von Recum (2010) introduced a nondamaging cellular detachment component to the existing baseplate substrate for a commercially available mechanical culture tension system. NIPAAm-based polymers have advantageous properties to tissue engineers. Above 32°C (e.g., body temperature), cells preferentially and viably attach and grow on these materials. Below 32°C, the polymer resumes hydrophilic behavior, and swells to allow spontaneous cellular detachment, thus avoiding enzymatic (e.g., trypsinization) or mechanical (e.g., scraping) damage to the cells and ECM. Thus, cells may be mechanically stimulated on NIPAAm-modified substrates at parameters specific to the engineered regenerative or replacement tissue to induce synthesis of ECM that can withstand native stresses. The resulting cellular sheet with the synthesized matrix can then be detached intact with cells and subsequently layered with other sheets to create a three-dimensional tissue. The current engineered tissues will reach diffusion limits for oxygen and nutrient delivery without a blood supply nearby. The cell-sheet-layering method is promising since it can circumvent the diffusion limiting problem (Okano et al. 1993, Shimizu et al. 2006): layers of vasculature or layers of cells with high angiogenic potential can be placed between sheets of the target tissue.

## 15.6 Conclusion

The human body has an amazing capacity to regenerate after an injury. But sometimes, the remodeling environment presents an unnatural mechanical stimuli that may promote maladaptation instead of healing. By understanding how cells respond to the mechanical stimuli is a critical step in learning how to direct cells *in vitro* to produce regenerative tissues. Additionally, the current and future mechanical-conditioning technologies that reconstruct the fluid shear, tensile, and compressive forces of the *in vivo* environment can enable tissue engineers in improving patient recovery.

## References

Alexander, D. E., K. L. Ratzlaff, R. J. Roggero, and J. S. Hsieh. 1999. Inexpensive, semi-automated system for measuring mechanical properties of soft tissues. *J Exp Zoo* 284: 374–78.

Alexander, R. S. 1976. Series elasticity of urinary bladder smooth muscle. *Am J Physiol* 231: 1337–42.

Aufderheide, A. C. and K. A. Athanasiou. 2006. A direct compression stimulator for articular cartilage and meniscal explants. *Ann Biomed Eng* 34: 1463–74.

Ayajiki, K., M. Kindermann, M. Hecker, I. Fleming, and R. Busse. 1996. Intracellular pH and tyrosine phosphorylation but not calcium determine shear stress-induced nitric oxide production in native endothelial cells. *Circ Res* 78: 750–58.

Bacabac, R. G., T. H. Smit, S. C. Cowin et al. 2005. Dynamic shear stress in parallel-plate flow chambers. *J Biomech* 38: 159–67.

Banes, A., J. Gilbert, D. Taylor, and O. Monbureau. 1985. A new vacuum-operated stress-providing instrument that applies static or variable duration cyclic tension or compression to cells in vitro. *J Cell Sci* 42: 35–42.

Benbrahim, A., G. J. L'Italien, B. B. Milinazzo et al. 1994. A compliant tubular device to study the influences of wall strain and fluid shear stress on cells of the vascular wall. *J Vasc Surg* 20: 184–94.

Bett, G. and F. Sachs. 2000. Whole-cell mechanosensitive currents in rat ventricular myocytes activated by direct stimulation. *J Membr Biol* 173: 255–263.

Bottlang, M., M. Simnacher, H. Schmitt, R. A. Brand, and L. Claes. 1997. A cell strain system for small homogeneous strain applications. *Biomed Tech (Berl)* 42: 305–9.

Brangwynne, C. P., F. C. MacKintash, S. Kumar et al. 2006. Microtubes can bear enhanced compressive loading in living cells because of lateral reinforcement. *J Cell Biol* 173: 733–41.

Brighton, C. T., B. Strafford, S. B. Gross, D. F. Leatherwood, J. L. Williams, and S. R. Pollack. 1991. The proliferative and synthetic response of isolated calvarial bone cells of rats to cyclic biaxial mechanical strain. *J Bone Joint Surg* 73: 320–31.

Brown, T. D. 2000. Techniques for mechanical stimulation of cells in vitro: A review. *J Biomech* 33: 3–14.

Brown, T. D., M. Bottlang, D. R. Pedersen, and A. J. Banes. 1998. Loading paradigms— intentional and unintentional— for cell culture mechanostimulus. *Am J Med Sci* 316: 162–68.

Brown, T. D., M. Bottlang, D. R. Pedersen, and A. J. Banes. 2000. Development and experimental validation of a fluid/structure-interaction finite element model of a vacuum-driven cell culture mechanostimulus system. *Comput Methods Biomech Biomed Engin* 3: 65–78.

Brown, D. and R. Larson. 2001. Improvements to parallel plate flow chambers to reduce reagent and cellular requirements. *BMC Immunol* 2: 9.

Burton-Wurster, N., M. Vernier-Singer, T. Farquhar, and G. Lust. 1993. Effect of compressive loading and unloading on the synthesis of total protein, proteoglycan, and fibronectin by canine cartilage explants. *J Orthop Res* 11: 717–29.

Carpenedo, R. L., C. Y. Sargent, and T. C. McDevitt. 2007. Rotary suspension culture enhances the efficiency, yield, and homogeneity of embryoid body differentiation. *Stem Cells* 25: 2224–34.

Carpenter, A. E., T. R. Jones, M. R. Lamprecht et al. 2006. CellProfiler: Image analysis software for identifying and quantifying cell phenotypes. *Genome Biol* 7: R100.

Chamson, A., F. C. Sudre, . J. Le Guen, Le, A. Rattner, and J. Frey. 1997. Morphological alteration of fibroblasts mechanically stressed in a collagen lattice. *Arch Dermatol Res* 289: 596–99.

Chen, C. S., M. Mrksich, S. Huang, G. M. Whitesides, and D. E. Ingber. 1997. Geometric control of cell life and death. *Science* 276: 1425–28.

Chen, X., H. Xu, C. Wan, M. McCaigue, and G. Li. 2006. Bioreactor expansion of human adult bone marrow-derived mesenchymal stem cells. *Stem Cells* 24: 2052–59.

Chiquet, M., M. Matthisson, M. Koch, M. Tannheimer, and R. Chiquet-Ehrismann. 1996. Regulation of extracellular matrix synthesis by mechanical stress. *Biochem Cell Biol* 74: 737–44.

Chiquet, M., V. Tunc-Civelek, and A. Sarasa-Renedo. 2007. Gene regulation by mechanotransduction in fibroblasts. *Appl Physiol Nutr Metab* 32: 967–73.

Chokalingam, K., N. Juncosa-Melvin, S. A. Hunter et al. 2009. Tensile stimulation of murine stem cell-collagen sponge constructs increases collagen type I gene expression and linear stiffness. *Tissue Eng Part A* 15: 2561–70.

Cormier, J. T., N. I. Zur Nieden, D. E. Rancourt, and M. S. Kallos. 2006. Expansion of undifferentiated murine embryonic stem cells as aggregates in suspension culture bioreactors. *Tissue Eng* 12: 3233–45.

Coucouvanis, E. and G. R. Martin. 1995. Signals for death and survival: A two-step mechanism for cavitation in the vertebrate embryo. *Cell* 83: 279–87.

Dahlmann-Noor, A. H., B. Martin-Martin, M. Eastwood, P. T. Khaw, and M. Bailly. 2007. Dynamic protrusive cell behaviour generates force and drives early matrix contraction by fibroblasts. *Exp Cell Res* 313: 4158–69.

Dang, S. M., M. Kyba, R. Perlingeiro, G. Q. Daley, and P. W. Zandstra. 2002. Efficiency of embryoid body formation and hematopoietic development from embryonic stem cells in different culture systems. *Biotechnol Bioeng* 78: 442–53.

De Witt, M. T., C. J. Handley, B. W. Oakes, and D. A. Lowther. 1984. *In vitro* response of chondrocytes to mechanical loading. The effect of short term mechanical tension. *Connect Tissue Res* 12: 97–109.

Eastwood, M., D. A. McGrouther, and R. A. Brown. 1994. A culture force monitor for measurement of contraction forces generated in human dermal fibroblast cultures: Evidence for cell-matrix mechanical signalling. *Biochim Biophys Acta* 1201: 186–92.

Egerbacher, M., S. P. Arnoczky, O. Caballero, M. Lavagnino, and K. L. Gardner. 2008. Loss of homeostatic tension induces apoptosis in tendon cells: An *in vitro* study. *Clin Orthop Relat Res* 466: 1562–68.

Einav, S., C. Dewey, and H. Hartenbaum. 1994. Cone-and-plate apparatus: A compact system for studying well-characterized turbulent flow fields. *Exp Fluids* 16: 196–202.

Ellis, E. F., J. S. McKinney, K. A. Willoughby, S. Liang, and J. T. Povlishock. 1995. A new model for rapid stretch-induced injury of cells in culture: Characterization of the model using astrocytes. *J Neurotrauma* 12: 325–39.

Engelmayr Jr., G. C., L. Soletti, S. C. Vigmostad et al. 2008. A novel flex-stretch-flow bioreactor for the study of engineered heart valve tissue mechanobiology. *Ann Biomed Eng* 36: 700–12.

Fan, J. and K. B. Walsh. 1999. Mechanical stimulation regulates voltage-gated potassium currents in cardiac microvascular endothelial cells. *Circ Res* 84: 451–17.

Felix, J. A., M. L. Woodruff, and E. R. Dirksen. 1996. Stretch increases inositol 1,4,5-trisphosphate concentration in airway epithelial cells. *Am J Respir Cell Mol Biol* 14: 296–301.

Fletcher, D. A. and R. D. Mullins. 2010. Cell mechanics and the cytoskeleton. *Nature* 463: 485–92.

Forth, K. E. and C. S. Layne. 2008. Neuromuscular responses to mechanical foot stimulation: The influence of loading and postural context. *Aviat Space Environ Med* 79: 844–51.

Gerecht-Nir, S., S. Cohen, and J. Itskovitz-Eldor. 2004. Bioreactor cultivation enhances the efficiency of human embryoid body (hEB) formation and differentiation. *Biotechnol Bioeng* 86: 493–502.

Gilbert, J. A., A. J. Banes, G. W. Link, and G. L. Jones. 1990. Video analysis of membrane strain: An application in cell stretching. *Exp Tech* 14: 43–5.

Gilbert, J. A., P. S. Weinhold, A. J. Banes, G. W. Link, and G. L. Jones. 1994. Strain profiles for circular cell culture plates containing flexible surfaces employed to mechanically deform cells in vitro. *J Biomech* 27: 1169–77.

Gooch, K. J. and C. J. Tennant. 1997. *Mechanical Forces: Their Effects on Cells and Tissues*. New York: Springer.

Gov, N. 2009. Traction forces during collective cell motion. *HFSP J* 3: 223–27.

Grande-Allen, K. J., A. Calabro, V. Gupta, T. N. Wight, V. C. Hascall, and I. Vesely. 2004. Glycosaminoglycans and proteoglycans in normal mitral valve leaflets and chordae: Association with regions of tensile and compressive loading. *Glycobiology* 14: 621–33.

Guilak, F., D. M. Cohen, B. T. Estes, J. M. Gimble, W. Liedtke, and C. S. Chen. 2009. Control of stem cell fate by physical interactions with the extracellular matrix. *Cell stem cell* 5: 17–26.

Guilak, F., B. C. Meyer, A. Ratcliffe, and V. C. Mow. 1994. The effects of matrix compression on proteoglycan metabolism in articular cartilage explants. *Osteoarthritis Cartilage* 2: 91–101.

Gupta, V., J. A. Werdenberg, T. L. Blevins, and K. J. Grande-Allen. 2007. Synthesis of glycosaminoglycans in differently loaded regions of collagen gels seeded with valvular interstitial cells. *Tissue Eng* 13: 41–9.

Gupta, V., J. A. Werdenberg, B. D. Lawrence, J. S. Mendez, E. H. Stephens, and K. J. Grande-Allen. 2008. Reversible secretion of glycosaminoglycans and proteoglycans by cyclically stretched valvular cells in 3D culture. *Ann Biomed Eng* 36: 1092–103.

Gustafson, K. J., J. D. Sweeney, J. Gibney, and L. A. Fiebig-Mathine. 2006. Performance of dynamic and isovolumetric trained skeletal muscle ventricles. *J Surg Res* 134: 198–204.

Hasegawa, S., S. Sato, S. Saito, Y. Suzuki, and D. Brunette. 1985. Mechanical stretching increases the number of cultured bone cells synthesizing DNA and alters their pattern of protein synthesis. *Calcif Tissue Int* 37: 431–6.

Hasel, C., S. Dürr, S. Brüderlein, I. Melzner, and P. Möller. 2002. A cell-culture system for long-term maintenance of elevated hydrostatic pressure with the option of additional tension. *J Biomech* 35: 579–84.

Heiner, A. and J. Martin. 2004. Cartilage responses to a novel triaxial mechanostimulatory culture system. *J Biomech* 37: 689–95.

Huang, S., C. S. Chen, and D. E. Ingber. 1998. Control of cyclin D1, p27(Kip1), and cell cycle progression in human capillary endothelial cells by cell shape and cytoskeletal tension. *Mol Biol Cell* 9: 3179–93.

Huang, S. and D. E. Ingber. 2000. Shape-dependent control of cell growth, differentiation, and apoptosis: Switching between attractors in cell regulatory networks. *Exp Cell Res* 261: 91–103.

Hung, C. T. and J. L. Williams. 1994. A method for inducing equi-biaxial and uniform strains in elastomeric membranes used as cell substrates. *J Biomech* 27: 227–32.

Ingber, D. E. 2008a. Tensegrity-based mechanosensing from macro to micro. *Prog Biophys Mol Biol* 97: 163–79.

Ingber, D. E. 2008b. Tensegrity and mechanotransduction. *J Bodyw Mov Ther* 12: 198–200.

Ingber, D. E. 2010. From cellular mechanotransduction to biologically inspired engineering. *Ann Biomed Eng* 38: 1148–61.

Ishibashi, Y., H. Tsutsui, S. Yamamoto et al. 1996. Role of microtubules in myocyte contractile dysfunction during cardiac hypertrophy in the rat. *Am J Physiol* 271: H1978–87.

Ives, C. L., S. G. Eskin, and L. V. McIntire. 1986. Mechanical effects on endothelial cell morphology: *In vitro* assessment. *In Vitro Cell Dev Biol* 22: 500–7.

Jessop, H. L., S. C. F. Rawlinson, A. A. Pitsillides, and L. E. Lanyon. 2002. Mechanical strain and fluid movement both activate extracellular regulated kinase (ERK) in osteoblast-like cells but via different signaling pathways. *Bone* 31: 186–94.

Jones, D. B., H. Nolte, J. G. Schölübbers, E. Turner, and D. Veltel. 1991. Biochemical signal transduction of mechanical strain in osteoblast-like cells. *Biomaterials* 12: 101–10.

Kandlikar, S. G., S. Garimella, D. Li, S. Colin, and M. R. King. 2006. *Heat Transfer and Fluid Flow in Minichannels and Microchannels*. Kidlington, Oxford: Elsevier.

Kappagoda, C. T. and K. Ravi. 2006. The rapidly adapting receptors in mammalian airways and their responses to changes in extravascular fluid volume. *Experiment Physiol* 91: 647–54.

Keller, G. M. 1995. *In vitro* differentiation of embryonic stem cells. *Curr Opin Cell Biol* 7: 862–69.

Kim, S. and H. A. Von Recum. 2009. Endothelial progenitor populations in differentiating embryonic stem cells I: Identification and differentiation kinetics. *Tissue Eng Part A* 15: 3709–18.

Kim, S. and H. A. Von Recum. 2010. Endothelial progenitor populations in differentiating embryonic stem cells. II. Drug selection and functional characterization. *Tissue Eng Part A* 16: 1065–74.

Komuro, I., T. Kaida, Y. Shibazaki et al. 1990. Stretching cardiac myocytes stimulates protooncogene expression. *J Biol Chem* 265: 3595–98.

Lambert, C. A., E. P. Soudant, B. V. Nusgens, and C. M. Lapière. 1992. Pretranslational regulation of extracellular matrix macromolecules and collagenase expression in fibroblasts by mechanical forces. *Lab Invest* 66: 444–51.

Lammi, M. J., R. Inkinen, J. J. Parkkinen et al. 1994. Expression of reduced amounts of structurally altered aggrecan in articular cartilage chondrocytes exposed to high hydrostatic pressure. *Biochem J* 304: 723–30.

Lau, E., S. Al-Dujaili, A. Guenther, D. Liu, L. Wang, and L. You. 2010. Effect of low-magnitude, high-frequency vibration on osteocytes in the regulation of osteoclasts. *Bone* 46: 1508–15.

Lavagnino, M., S. P. Arnoczky, E. Kepich, O. Caballero, and R. C. Haut. 2008. A finite element model predicts the mechanotransduction response of tendon cells to cyclic tensile loading. *Biomech Model Mechanobiol* 7: 405–16.

Lee, E. L. and H. A. Von Recum. 2010. Cell culture platform with mechanical conditioning and non-damaging cellular detachment. *J Biomed Mater Res A* 93: 411–8.

Leung, D. Y., S. Glagov, and M. B. Mathews. 1977. A new *in vitro* system for studying cell response to mechanical stimulation. Different effects of cyclic stretching and agitation on smooth muscle cell biosynthesis. *Experiment Cell Res* 109: 285–98.

Li, H., H.S. Yang, T.J. Wu et al. 2010. Proteomic analysis of early-response to mechanical stress in neonatal rat mandibular condylar chondrocytes. *J Cell Physiol* 223: 610–22.

Maltsev, V. A., A. M. Wobus, J. Rohwedel, M. Bader, and J. Hescheler. 1994. Cardiomyocytes differentiated *in vitro* from embryonic stem cells developmentally express cardiac-specific genes and ionic currents. *Circ Res* 75: 233–44.

Martinac, B. 2004. Mechanosensitive ion channels: Molecules of mechanotransduction. *J Cell Sci* 117: 2449–60.

Matsuo, T., H. Uchida, and N. Matsuo. 1996. Bovine and porcine trabecular cells produce prostaglandin F2 alpha in response to cyclic mechanical stretching. *Jpn J Ophthalmol* 40: 289–96.

Maul, T. M., D. W. Hamilton, A. Nieponice, L. Soletti, and D. A. Vorp. 2007. A new experimental system for the extended application of cyclic hydrostatic pressure to cell culture. *J Biomech Eng* 129: 110–16.

Meikle, M. C., J. J. Reynolds, A. Sellers, and J. T. Dingle. 1979. Rabbit cranial sutures in vitro: A new experimental model for studying the response of fibrous joints to mechanical stress. *Calcif Tissue Int* 28: 137–44.

Moore, J. E., E. Bürki, A. Suciu et al. 1994. A device for subjecting vascular endothelial cells to both fluid shear stress and circumferential cyclic stretch. *Ann Biomed Eng* 22: 416–22.

Murray, D. and N. Rushton. 1990. The effect of strain on bone cell prostaglandin E 2 release: A new experimental method. *Calcif Tissue Int* 47: 35–9.

Myers, K. A., J. B. Rattner, N. G. Shrive, and D. A. Hart. 2007. Hydrostatic pressure sensation in cells: Integration into the tensegrity model. *Biochem Cell Biol* 85: 543–51.

Nagatomi, J., B. P. Arulanandam, D. W. Metzger, A. Meunier, and R. Bizios. 2002. Effects of cyclic pressure on bone marrow cell cultures. *J Biomech Eng* 124: 308–14.

Neidlinger-Wilke, C., A. Liedert, K. Wuertz et al. 2009. Mechanical stimulation alters pleiotrophin and aggrecan expression by human intervertebral disc cells and influences their capacity to stimulate endothelial migration. *Spine* 34: 663–9.

Neidlinger-Wilke, C., H. J. Wilke, and L. Claes. 1994. Cyclic stretching of human osteoblasts affects proliferation and metabolism: A new experimental method and its application. *J Orthop Res* 12: 70–8.

Ng, E., R. Davis, L. Azzola, E. Stanley, and A. Elefanty. 2005. Forced aggregation of defined numbers of human embryonic stem cells into embryoid bodies fosters robust, reproducible hematopoietic differentiation. *Blood* 106: 1601–3.

Nishimura, S., S. Nagai, M. Katoh et al. 2006. Microtubules modulate the stiffness of cardiomyocytes against shear stress. *Circ Res* 98: 81–7.

Nishimura, S., K. Seo, M. Nagasaki et al. 2008. Responses of single-ventricular myocytes to dynamic axial stretching. *Prog Biophys Mol Biol* 97: 282–97.

Norton, L. A., K. L. Andersen, D. Arenholt-Bindslev, L. Andersen, and B. Melsen. 1995. A methodical study of shape changes in human oral cells perturbed by a simulated orthodontic strain in vitro. *Arch Oral Biol* 40: 863–72.

Okano, T., N. Yamada, H. Sakai, and Y. Sakurai. 1993. A novel recovery system for cultured cells using plasma-treated polystyrene dishes grafted with poly(N-isopropylacrylamide). *J Biomed Mater Res* 27: 1243–51.

Orr, D. E. and K. J. L. Burg. 2008. Design of a modular bioreactor to incorporate both perfusion flow and hydrostatic compression for tissue engineering applications. *Ann Biomed Eng* 36: 1228–41.

Ozawa, H., K. Imamura, E. Abe et al. 1990. Effect of a continuously applied compressive pressure on mouse osteoblast-like cells (MC3T3-E1) in vitro. *J Cell Physiol* 142: 177–85.

Ozerdem, B. and A. Tözeren. 1995. Physical response of collagen gels to tensile strain. *J Biomech Eng* 117: 397–401.

Palatinus, J. A., J. M. Rhett, and R. G. Gourdie. 2010. Translational lessons from scarless healing of cutaneous wounds and regenerative repair of the myocardium. *J Mol Cell Cardiol* 48: 550–7.

Parker, K. K., A. L. Brock, C. Brangwynne et al. 2002. Directional control of lamellipodia extension by constraining cell shape and orienting cell tractional forces. *FASEB J* 16: 1195–204.

Parkkinen, J. J., M. J. Lammi, R. Inkinen et al. 1995. Influence of short-term hydrostatic pressure on organization of stress fibers in cultured chondrocytes. *J Orthop Res* 13: 495–502.

Pitsillides, A., S. Rawlinson, R. Suswillo, and S. Bourrin. 1995. Mechanical strain-induced NO production by bone cells: A possible role in adaptive bone (re) modeling? *FASEB J* 9: 1614–22.

Polte, T. R., G. S. Eichler, N. Wang, and D. E. Ingber. 2004. Extracellular matrix controls myosin light chain phosphorylation and cell contractility through modulation of cell shape and cytoskeletal prestress. *Am J Physiol Cell Physiol* 286: C518–28.

Potier, E., J. Noailly, and K. Ito. 2010. Directing bone marrow-derived stromal cell function with mechanics. *J Biomech* 43: 807–17.

Pugin, J., I. Dunn, P. Jolliet et al. 1998. Activation of human macrophages by mechanical ventilation in vitro. *Am J Physiol* 275: L1040–50.

Rana, O. R., C. Zobel, E. Saygili et al. 2008. A simple device to apply equibiaxial strain to cells cultured on flexible membranes. *Am J Physiol Heart Circ Physiol* 294: H532–40.

Robling, A. G., D. B. Burr, and C. H. Turner. 2001. Recovery periods restore mechanosensitivity to dynamically loaded bone. *J Experiment Biol* 204: 3389–99.

Russell, B., D. Motlagh, and W. W. Ashley. 2000. Form follows function: How muscle shape is regulated by work. *J App Physiol* 88: 1127–32.

Sarasa-Renedo, A. and M. Chiquet. 2005. Mechanical signals regulating extracellular matrix gene expression in fibroblasts. *Scand J Med Sci Sports* 15: 223–30.

Sargent, C. Y., G. Y. Berguig, M. A. Kinney et al. 2010. Hydrodynamic modulation of embryonic stem cell differentiation by rotary orbital suspension culture. *Biotechnol Bioeng* 105: 611–26.

Schaffer, J. L., M. Rizen, G. J. L'Italien et al. 1994. Device for the application of a dynamic biaxially uniform and isotropic strain to a flexible cell culture membrane. *J Orthop Res* 12: 709–19.

Shaikh, F. M., T. P. O'Brien, A. Callanan et al. 2010. New pulsatile hydrostatic pressure bioreactor for vascular tissue-engineered constructs. *Artif Organs* 34: 153–8.

Shimizu, T., H. Sekine, Y. Isoi, M. Yamato, A. Kikuchi, and T. Okano. 2006. Long-term survival and growth of pulsatile myocardial tissue grafts engineered by the layering of cardiomyocyte sheets. *Tissue Eng* 12: 499–507.

Shimko, V. F. and W. C. Claycomb. 2008. Effect of mechanical loading on three-dimensional cultures of embryonic stem cell-derived cardiomyocytes. *Tissue Eng Part A* 14: 49–58.

Sims, J. R., S. Karp, and D. E. Ingber. 1992. Altering the cellular mechanical force balance results in integrated changes in cell, cytoskeletal and nuclear shape. *J Cell Sci* 103: 1215–22.

Singhvi, R., A. Kumar, G. P. Lopez et al. 1994. Engineering cell shape and function. *Science* 264: 696–8.

Sumpio, B. E., M. D. Widmann, J. Ricotta, M. A. Awolesi, and M. Watase. 1994. Increased ambient pressure stimulates proliferation and morphologic changes in cultured endothelial cells. *J Cell Physiol* 158: 133–9.

Tagawa, H., M. Koide, H. Sato, M. R. Zile, B. A. Carabello, and G. Cooper IV. 1998. Cytoskeletal role in the transition from compensated to decompensated hypertrophy during adult canine left ventricular pressure overloading. *Circ Res* 82: 751–61.

Tanck, E., W. D. Van Driel, J. W. Hagen, E. H. Burger, L. Blankevoort, and R. Huiskes. 1999. Why does intermittent hydrostatic pressure enhance the mineralization process in fetal cartilage? *J Biomech* 32: 153–61.

Tomasek, J. J., C. J. Haaksma, R. J. Eddy, and M. B. Vaughan. 1992. Fibroblast contraction occurs on release of tension in attached collagen lattices: Dependency on an organized actin cytoskeleton and serum. *Anat Rec* 232: 359–68.

Torzilli, P. A., R. Grigiene, C. Huang et al. 1997. Characterization of cartilage metabolic response to static and dynamic stress using a mechanical explant test system. *J Biomech* 30: 1–9.

Trepat, X., L. Deng, S. S. An et al. 2007. Universal physical responses to stretch in the living cell. *Nature* 447: 592–95.

Tsutsui, H., K. Ishihara, and G. Cooper IV. 1993. Cytoskeletal role in the contractile dysfunction of hypertrophied myocardium. *Science* 260: 682–7.

Van Wamel, J. E., C. Ruwhof, E. J. Van der Valk-Kokshoorn, P. I. Schrier, and A. Van der Laarse. 2000. Rapid gene transcription induced by stretch in cardiac myocytes and fibroblasts and their paracrine influence on stationary myocytes and fibroblasts. *Pflugers Arch* 439: 781–8.

Vandenburgh, H. H. and P. Karlisch. 1989. Longitudinal growth of skeletal myotubes *in vitro* in a new horizontal mechanical cell stimulator. *In Vitro Cell Dev Biol* 25: 607–16.

Villemure, I. and I. A. Stokes. 2009. Growth plate mechanics and mechanobiology. A survey of present understanding. *J Biomech* 42: 1793–803.

Wang, H., L. Huang, M. Qu et al. 2006a. Shear stress protects against endothelial regulation of vascular smooth muscle cell migration in a coculture system. *Endothelium* 2: 171–80.

Wang, X., G. Wei, W. Yu, Y. Zhao, X. Yu, and X. Ma. 2006b. Scalable producing embryoid bodies by rotary cell culture system and constructing engineered cardiac tissue with ES-derived cardiomyocytes in vitro. *Biotechnol Prog* 22: 811–8.

Wang, Y., Z. Zhao, Y. Li et al. 2010. Up-regulated alpha-actin expression is associated with cell adhesion ability in 3-D cultured myocytes subjected to mechanical stimulation. *Mol Cell Biochem* 338: 175–81.

Williams, J. L., J. H. Chen, and D. M. Belloli. 1992. Strain fields on cell stressing devices employing clamped circular elastic diaphragms as substrates. *J Biomech Eng* 114: 377–84.

Winston, F. K., E. J. Macarak, S. F. Gorfien, and L. E. Thibault. 1989. A system to reproduce and quantify the biomechanical environment of the cell. *J App Physiol* 67: 397–405.

Wright, M., P. Jobanputra, C. Bavington, D. M. Salter, and G. Nuki. 1996. Effects of intermittent pressure-induced strain on the electrophysiology of cultured human chondrocytes: Evidence for the presence of stretch-activated membrane ion channels. *Clin Sci (London)* 90: 61–71.

Yeung, T., P. C. Georges, L. A. Flanagan et al. 2005. Effects of substrate stiffness on cell morphology, cytoskeletal structure, and adhesion. *Cell Motil Cytoskeleton* 60: 24–34.

Zandstra, P. W., C. Bauwens, T. Yin et al. 2003. Scalable production of embryonic stem cell-derived cardiomyocytes. *Tissue Eng* 9: 767–78.

Zile, M. R., M. Koide, H. Sato et al. 1999. Role of microtubules in the contractile dysfunction of hypertrophied myocardium. *J Am Coll Cardiol* 33: 250–60.

# 16

# Micropatterned Biomaterials for Cell and Tissue Engineering

Murugan
Ramalingam
*Tohoku University*

Ali Khademhosseini
*Tohoku University*

*Harvard University*

*Massachusetts Institute of Technology*

16.1 Introduction ................................................................ 16-1
16.2 Surface Modification and Patterning Approaches .................. 16-2
16.3 Techniques for Chemical Patterning and Applications
to Cell Studies.......................................................... 16-2
  Photolithography • Microcontact Printing • Micromolding
16.4 Techniques for Topographical Patterning and Applications
to Cell Studies.......................................................... 16-6
  Imprint Lithography • Colloidal Lithography
16.5 Techniques for Three-Dimensional Patterning
and Applications to Tissue Engineering ................................ 16-10
  Microfluidics • Stamping/Printing • Self-Assembly
16.6 Concluding Remarks.................................................. 16-14
References.................................................................... 16-14

## 16.1 Introduction

Control of the cellular microenvironment is a key requirement for understanding cell biology as well as to develop new substrates for using cell and tissue engineering (Khademhosseini et al. 2006, 2009). The cues derived from the surrounding microenvironment regulate cellular behaviors such as attachment, spreading, proliferation, migration, and differentiation. The cells in our body are arranged in distinct patterns during their development that are subsequently regulated by spatial and temporal environmental cues over many length scales. The cellular microenvironment is comprised of a complex mixture of extracellular matrix (ECM) molecules, soluble factors, nonsoluble factors, and other cell types. It is known that the microenvironment of cells is critical for maintaining their normal function. Regulating cell behavior by modulating the cellular microenvironment such as the cell–substrate interaction is therefore of great importance to enable such a defined biological activity.

Engineering cell–substrate interactions requires strict control over a material's surface properties, such as chemical, physical, and architectural features. This is because the cultured cells' initial response to the material mainly depends upon its surface properties. The modification of the surface of a material by patterning (chemical or topographical) can thus be used to mimic the native cellular environment. It should also be noted that most cellular components and biological structures possess length scales that range from a few tens of nanometers to a few centimeters. Therefore, patterning material surfaces with features on similar length scales can be used to regulate cell behavior and study the interactions of cells with a substrate. Microfabrication technology offers the capability to design a well-defined chemical composition and topology of the material substrate, suitable to control cell–substrate, cell–cell, and cell–soluble factor interactions. In this chapter, we discuss some aspects of surface patterning of biomaterials, both chemical and topographical, suitable for cell studies. In particular, the design strategies and methodologies involved in surface patterning process are discussed with specific examples on how the patterned surfaces influence cell behavior in two-dimensional (2D) and three-dimensional (3D) systems.

## 16.2 Surface Modification and Patterning Approaches

Surface modification is a process that considerably changes the surface of a material in terms of chemical composition and/or physical structure. Surface modification can be performed either by chemically or physically altering the atoms or molecules on the surface, or alternatively by coating the surface with chemicals or biological agents. There are numerous methods to modify the surface of the biomaterials by using various chemical and topographical modifications (Craighead 2001; Stevens and George 2005). Surface chemistry and topography of a material have a great influence on regulating cell behavior, such as adhesion, migration, orientation, guidance, proliferation, and differentiation (Jenney and Anderson 1999; Saneinejad and Shoichet 2000; Craighead et al. 2001; Andersson et al. 2003). Therefore, surface patterning of biomaterials, suitable to regulate the organization and assembly of cells, is of great importance for a variety of biological applications.

Surface patterning is an approach for controlling a substrate's surface chemistry and/or topography in a spatially controlled manner. Surface patterning allows a direct control over cell placement to the desired regions of a substrate material, and inhibits their attachment to the undesired regions of the same substrate (Kumar et al. 2003; Tourovskaia et al. 2003; Veiseh et al. 2004; Welle et al. 2005; Falconnet et al. 2006; Khademhosseini et al. 2006). By patterning cells on a substrate, not only will cell location and shape be controlled but also its survival, proliferation, differentiation, and subsequent function (Mrksich et al. 1996; Chen et al. 1997; Oliva et al. 2003; Kaehr et al. 2004; Romanova et al. 2004; Sanjana and Fuller 2004; Li and Folch 2005). Thus, patterned surfaces can serve as a model system to study the fundamental aspects of cell–substrate and cell–cell interaction, which is necessary for engineering physiologically functional cellular systems. A wide range of microfabrication techniques have been developed to fabricate biologically relevant devices or substrates with micro- and nanometer scale resolution (Mrksich and Whitesides 1995; Grayson et al. 2004; Chung 2007; Nakanishi et al. 2008; Murugan et al. 2009). Although most of these techniques were initially developed for the semiconductor industry to fabricate integrated circuits and other components, they have been adopted and modified to fabricate a large variety of devices and substrates suitable for biological applications. In the following sections, we will discuss the most commonly used techniques in the preparation of chemical, topographical, and 3D patterns suitable for cell studies.

## 16.3 Techniques for Chemical Patterning and Applications to Cell Studies

Chemical patterning refers to modifying a substrate with patterns of different chemistries. An example of a commonly used patterning material is self-assembled monolayers (SAMs) (Mrksich and Whitesides 1995; Mrksich et al. 1996; Smith et al. 2004; Yan et al. 2004; Senaratne et al. 2005). SAMs are versatile molecular assemblies that are formed spontaneously by the adsorption of a surfactant with a specific affinity of its one end of a molecule (called "head group") to a substrate. SAMs also consist of a tail with a specific functional group at the other end of the same molecule (called "tail group"). SAMs are known to influence cell attachment and other functions (Georger et al. 1992; Stenger et al. 1993; Spargo et al. 1994; Mrksich and Whitesides 1996; Ostuni et al. 1999). The use of SAMs facilitates the assembly of unidirectional, ultra-thin layers on a solid surface using the appropriate chemicals by the spontaneous organization of their constituents via covalent bonding (called chemisorption) or noncovalent bonding (called physisorption) (Ulman 1991, 1991, 1996). There are a variety of organic SAMs developed with different functional groups for various biological applications. Among them, silane- and thiol-based SAMs are well- characterized systems for cell and tissue engineering applications. SAMs are generally prepared on a metal (e.g., gold) or hydroxyl-terminated substrates (e.g., silica glass). In this approach, the solid substrate is first cleaned with acids (e.g., HCl or $H_2SO_4$) and then gently dipped into a solution containing the SAMs precursors under ambient conditions to facilitate the self-assembly process. This method has provided a straightforward way to obtain well-ordered monolayers and the SAMs formed by this method are chemically stable (Schlenoff et al. 1995). In the following sections, the most widely used techniques for patterning of SAMs, such as photolithography and microcontact printing (μCP), are discussed with experimental examples in the context of cell engineering. In addition, the patterning of cellular cocultures by using micromolding techniques is also highlighted.

## 16.3.1 Photolithography

Photolithography is a well-established technique that utilizes light to generate patterns with the desired geometry. This method involves three key components, namely a light source, a photosensitive material (also called photoresist), and a photomask. The light source provides the energy required for the exposure of photoresist or ablation of SAMs over the selected regions of the substrate. Ultraviolet (UV) light has been the source often used for patterning. Photoresists are often made from organic compounds, whose molecular chains are capable of reorganizing or crosslinking upon exposure to energy. A photomask is a solid substrate (planar) usually made of quartz and coated with a thin layer (~1 μm) of chrome with the desired pattern geometry. Some of the early studies in the use of microfabricated structures and cells were done by using this approach. For example, in the late 1980s, Kleinfield et al., demonstrated that neurons can be spatially cultured onto the photolithographically patterned substrates (Kleinfeld et al. 1988). The processing steps involved in the chemical patterning of a silica glass substrate by conventional photolithography (i.e., photoresist-based) is schematically shown in Figure 16.1a (Kleinfeld et al. 1988). The spin coating with the photoresist was carried out after cleaning the surface of the substrate (Figure 16.1a, Step 1). The photoresist-coated substrate was exposed to UV light through the photomask (Figure 16.1a, Step 2). Note that the light rays were transmitted only through the quartz background, but not through the chrome pattern on the mask. This chemically altered the solubility of the photoresist in certain developer solutions due to the molecular chain rearrangement. The light-exposed part of the photoresist was then solubilized in a developer solution, which yielded a photoresist pattern that corresponds to the image of the pattern designed on the mask (Figure 16.1a, Step 3). Consequently, the material of interest (e.g., alkylchlorosilane, a cell nonadhesive agent) to be patterned was applied on the photoresist pattern (Figure 16.1a, Step 4) and then the photoresist was carefully removed (Figure 16.1a, Step 5), and the open areas (the area other than the cell's nonadhesive region) were backfilled with another material of interest (e.g., alkylaminosilane, a cell-adhesive agent) (Figure 16.1a, Step 6). This lithographic process led to a chemically defined substrate with patterns of cell-adhesive and nonadhesive regions. By using this photolithographic technique, the authors constructed simplified neuronal patterns with synoptically active neurons *in vitro*. The study revealed that dissociated neurons can be directed to adhere and grow in high-resolution patterns and the cells underwent normal morphological and physiological development during their culture period of 12 days.

In the early 1990s, a direct ablation of SAMs, without the use of a photoresist, was introduced for patterning biomaterials. This is because the use of a photoresist in patterning led to many practical complications. For example, a small dust particle, or other forms of ultra-fine debris, greatly destroys the uniformity of a thin layer of a photoresist during spin-coating; thus, this step must be carried out in a clean room facility. Some biological solutions are banned from use in a clean room facility, which further limits its usage in many biological applications. In addition, some of the chemicals that are used as a photoresist are toxic to cells. In a notable study, Dulcey et al., introduced the use of direct ablation by a deep UV light (193 nm) for pattering silane-based SAMs, without a photoresist (Dulcey

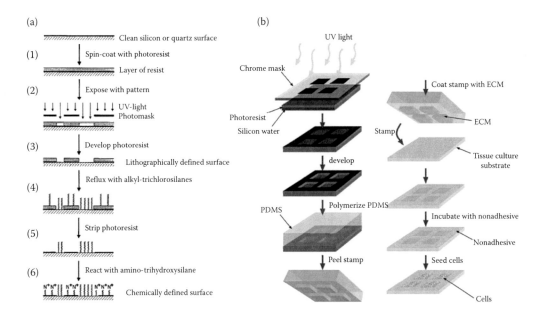

**FIGURE 16.1** (a) Schematic representation of the processing steps involved in chemically patterning silicon or silicon dioxide (quartz) substrates by photolithography and (b) schematic representation of the soft lithographic approach for micropatterning a substrate using microcontact printing. PDMS stamps were generated by photolithography (left column) and were used to print ECM proteins onto tissue-culture substrates to generate cell patterns (right column). (Figure 16.1a is adapted with permission from Kleinfeld D. et al. 1988. *Journal of Neuroscience* **8**(11): 4098–4120.)

et al. 1991). In their study, monolayers of *N*-(2-aminoethyl-3-aminopropyl) trimethoxysilane (EDA) were exposed to deep UV radiation, which induced photochemical changes in the cell-adhesive EDA monolayers. The exposed substrates were then reacted with perfluorinated alkylsilane (tridecafluoro-1,1,2,2-tetrabydrooctyl)-1-dimethylchlorosilane (13F) to form the cell's nonadhesive regions. The patterned surfaces were used to spatially control the cell's adhesion as well as direct the outgrowth of human neuroblastoma cells. This study revealed that a large change occurred in the shape and growth of the cells cultured on the patterned surfaces. For instance, the cells maintained a relatively spherical shape with visible contact points on a 40 μm wide EDA region, while a low width (12 μm) EDA region cells were elongated and confined to the line width. This is because the line width of the EDA is smaller than the cell diameter and this greatly affects the shape and size of the cell. Therefore, the use of UV photolithography is a good choice for patterning cells to control their behavior.

## 16.3.2 Microcontact Printing

μCP is a technique in which patterns with high spatial resolution are transferred to a substrate by direct contact (Kane et al. 1999; Lahiri et al. 1999; James et al. 2000; Hyun et al. 2001). This technique is well-suited for biological applications because it can be used to place cells or proteins into specified locations on the substrate material to control their shape, growth, and function. μCP is a widely used microfabrication technique because of its simplicity, flexibility, and ability to pattern many biomaterials with feature sizes down to 1 μm without using any expensive equipment. In addition, this technique can be extended to pattern nonplanar surfaces (i.e., 3D assembly), unlike the conventional photolithography method where it is not feasible, and the material to be patterned need not be photosensitive. This technique was initially popularized by Whitesides and colleagues as it was introduced to pattern SAMs of alkanethiols onto gold surfaces to control cell behavior and for engineering cell shape and function (Singhvi et al. 1994).

The major processing steps involved in the pattern formation by using μCP is schematically shown in Figure 16.1b (Liu and Chen 2005). This method uses an elastomeric stamp to print a pattern of the material of interest (cell-adhesive compounds, for example) on a solid substrate. There are three major components associated with this technique, namely master, stamp, and ink. The "master" is a solid substrate (silicon, for example), often created by standard photolithography with a desired geometry with high-resolution features that are specific to a particular application. The "stamp" is a soft elastomeric material, frequently created by casting an elastomeric material (e.g., polydimethylsiloxane [PDMS]) over a predesigned master). The "ink" is a functional material chosen to be patterned onto a substrate material. In the patterning process, the stamp is first inked with a solution made from the materials of interest (cell-adhesive compounds, for example) and the stamp is then brought into contact with the surface of the substrate material. For a period of time, the stamp and the substrate remain undisturbed, which ultimately yields a geometrical pattern of the stamp on the substrate material. The result of the stamping process is the formation of patterns on the surface of the substrate material, in those regions where the stamp has come into contact with the substrate. The unstamped regions are then backfilled with another material of interest (noncell-adhesive compounds, for example) to ensure that the resultant patterned surfaces have both cell-adhesive and nonadhesive regions, which directs the cells to grow only on the cell-adhesive regions. The resultant patterned surface can be used to study the fundamental aspects of cell behavior that can be eventually applied to engineering the physiologically functional tissues. In a notable study, Chen et al., revealed that micropatterned surfaces can be used to control cellular viability and apoptosis decisions (Chen et al. 1997). The authors used a μCP technique to fabricate planar adhesive regions of a defined size and shape, separated by nonadhesive regions. When the cells were plated on circular fibronectin (FN)-coated regions, 10 or 20 μm in diameter, they tend to align themselves to the shape of the underlying adhesive region. They also noticed that more cells entered apoptosis when held in a round form on 20 μm circles than when spread on identically fabricated unpatterned substrates. The shape change induces changes in the cytoskeletal features and has been shown to influence apoptosis and proliferation. Because of their original studies, a number of other publications have used similar techniques to decipher important features of the underlying cell biology (McBeath et al. 2004). It is anticipated that a further use of the patterned substrates will have a tremendous potential in controlling as well as understanding the effects of the microenvironment on cell shape, growth, and the subsequent function.

## 16.3.3 Micromolding

Engineering complex tissue structures often requires the culture of multiple cell types in physiologically relevant geometrical patterns to restore and maintain their normal cellular functions. Patterning cellular cocultures is therefore an exciting and emerging area in cell and tissue engineering. Microscale technologies have been used to pattern heterotypic cells to study their cell–cell and cell–substrate interactions on different substrates (Bhatia et al. 1998, 1999; Fukuda et al. 2006). Micromolding techniques (and variations such as capillary force lithography) are soft lithographic-based methods, in which different layers of cell-responsive and cell-repellent components, suitable for patterning multiple cells, can be fabricated. For example, Fukuda et al., reported micropatterned cell cocultures using various ECM components such as hyaluronic acid (HA), FN, and collagen (Fukuda et al. 2006). The authors introduced a capillary force lithographic method in combination with layer-by-layer deposition. A schematic illustration of the steps involved in the patterning of cellular cocultures is shown in Figure 16.2a (Fukuda et al. 2006). As shown, HA was first patterned on a glass substrate and the regions of the exposed glass substrate were then coated with FN (more cell-adhesive relative to HA) to generate cell-adhesive and nonadhesive regions to regulate the cell growth. The primary cell type (embryonic stem [ES] cells, for example) was immobilized on the adhesive regions, the subsequent electrostatic adsorption of collagen to HA patterns switched the cell-repellent HA surfaces to cell-adherent, thereby facilitating the adhesion of a secondary cell type (NIH-3T3 fibroblasts, for example). Figure 16.2b shows optical images of

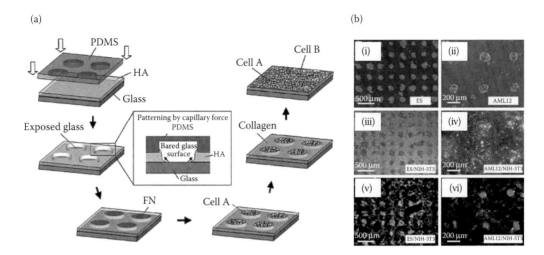

**FIGURE 16.2** (**See color insert.**) (a) The scheme for patterning of cellular cocultures by using capillary force lithography and layer-by-layer deposition. A few drops of HA solution were spun coated onto a glass slide, and a PDMS mold was immediately placed on the thin layer of HA. HA under the void space of the PDMS mold receded until the glass surface became exposed. The exposed region of a glass substrate was coated with FN, where primary cells could be selectively adhered. Subsequently, the HA surface was complexed with collagen, allowing for the subsequent adhesion of secondary cells. (b) Images of patterned cells and patterned cell cocultures on HA/collagen surfaces. (i) Murine ES cells and (ii) AML12 murine hepatocytes selectively adhered to the FN-coated region on HA-patterned surface after an 8 h incubation. The HA surface including the primary cells was treated with collagen and seeded with NIH-3T3 fibroblasts. After 3 days of culture, ES cells formed dense spherical aggregates and were clearly distinct from the surrounding fibroblasts monolayer. (iii) The coculture of AML12 hepatocytes and NIH-3T3 fibroblasts was difficult to distinguish under a light microscope. (iv) Fluorescently stained primary cells (green) and secondary cells (red) were visualized for ES/NIH-3T3 (v) and AML12/NIH-3T3. (vi) Cocultures at 3 days of culture. (Adapted with permission from Fukuda, J. et al. 2006. *Biomaterials* **27**(8): 1479–1486.)

patterned cocultures. Figures 16.2b (a and b) show that both cell types deposited preferentially to the FN-coated cell-adhesive regions. ES cells formed multilayer aggregates potentially as a result of strong cell–cell interactions. Although ES cells formed multilayer dense spherical aggregates and were clearly distinct from the surrounding fibroblast monolayer (see Figure 16.2b(iii)), hepatocyte/fibroblast cocultures were difficult to distinguish under a light microscope (Figure 16.2b(iv)). Therefore, fluorescence staining with a cytoplasmic tracer (CFSE-green) and a membrane labeling dye (PHK26-red) was carried out to visualize and to validate the cocultures (see Figure 16.2b (v and vi). As seen from the figure, after 3 days of culture, the spherically aggregated dense ES cells were clearly distinguishable from the surrounding fibroblasts. Thus, patterned cocultures could be achieved which is independent of the cell types. This patterned coculturing method can be useful for controlling cellular microenvironments for studying the effects of heterotypic and homotypic cell–cell interactions on cell-fate decisions.

## 16.4 Techniques for Topographical Patterning and Applications to Cell Studies

Topographical patterning refers to the physical modification of a substrate with a predefined texture by modulating their shape and size. The topographical features of the substrate have long been known to play a critical role in dictating cell behavior. Cells, in general, have the ability to sense and respond to the surface structural features of the substrates where they are cultured (Curtis and Wilkinson 1997; Dalby et al. 2002a,b, 2004a,b). For example, fibroblasts sense the substrate's topography by a sensory element called filopodia and accordingly respond to them (Dalby et al. 2002). When a suitable site for adhesion is sensed, other cellular activities such as focal adhesions, stress fibers, and microtubules are developed, which stabilize the contact between the cells and surfaces. In the early 1960s, Curtis and Varde proposed that cells responded to the microscale topographical environments and their behavior can be controlled by modulating the surface topography (Curtis and Varde 1964). This study revealed that cells are sensitive to the degree of curvature of the underlying substrate and are capable of aligning on a cylindrical glass with diameters of less than 100 μm. These data indicate that surface topography at the microscale has a significant influence on cell behavior. Recent investigations have shown that nanoscale topography also greatly affects cellular behavior. For example, Yang et al., reported that nanofibers of poly(L-lactic acid) promotes neural cell adhesion, neurite outgrowth, and other cellular processes compared to other surfaces (Yang et al. 2005). These findings suggested that topographical features can be used as cues to modulate cell orientation, growth, and its subsequent function.

The shape of the underlying topography also affects cell orientation and growth. As anchorage-dependent cells adhere to a substrate, they tend to align themselves to the shape of the substrate's topography, such as grooves and ridges. For example, Johansson et al. (2006) reported that patterns consisting of grooves and ridges can be used for axonal guidance. This is because axons preferred to grow on ridge edges and elevations on the patterned surfaces rather than in the grooves. They also found that the nerve cell processes, particularly axons of the peripheral neurons, might be guided by patterns of poly(methyl methacrylate) (PMMA) when the lateral features are 100 nm or larger. In another study, Gadegaard et al., reported the effect of grooves on the shape of the cells. They found that the orientation of fibroblasts greatly differed with respect to the grooves' dimensions (depth and width, for example) (Gadegaard et al. 2006) as cells that were on the grooved surfaces had an elongated spindle shape, but not on the flat surface. The cells were also found to preferentially migrate as guided by the grooves (Gadegaard et al. 2006). In a cell grown on a flat surface (control sample), microfilaments extended in all directions, while the microfilament bundles are predominately aligned along the groove ridge transitions on the grooved surface. This confirmed that the topography of the substrate significantly influenced the cytoskeletal organization. The experimental examples highlighted here, and others, clearly demonstrate the impact of the topography of the substrate on controlling cell behavior.

There are a variety of other techniques also employed for patterning of cells on various topographically modified substrates to investigate cell–substrate interactions *in vitro* (Hoffman-Kim et al.; Dalby et al. 2004; Yim et al. 2005; Gadegaard et al. 2006; Healy 2009; Zamanian et al. 2010). These include electron beam lithography (Gadegaard et al. 2006), imprint lithography (IL) (Yim et al. 2005), colloidal lithography (CL) (Dalby et al. 2004), and phase separation (Healy 2009). The ability to implement these technologies in a manner that is cost-effective, high-throughput, and scalable to commercial production of cellular substrates is still a challenge and requires continued efforts. Although electron beam lithography can be used to produce pattered surfaces with micro- and nanoscale features, this method has been somewhat expensive and time consuming as well as too slow for the patterning of large areas. Phase separation is a simple method that could be employed to pattern large areas, but the control of feature size and surface geometry is poor. Lithographic techniques, particularly CL and IL, have recently been developed and shown a great promise in patterning surfaces with the desired topography, with features less than 100 nm in resolution, in a convenient, rapid, and inexpensive manner. In the following sections, the methodology of IL and CL and their efficacy in studying cellular responses, utilizing patterned surfaces, are briefly discussed.

## 16.4.1 Imprint Lithography

IL is a versatile technique for patterning surfaces with topographical features that are less than 100 nm in size. IL is simple and cost-effective since it does not require any expensive equipment or sophisticated clean room facilities. This technique can be applied to pattern 2D or 3D topography of different geometrical patterns on a wide range of biomaterial substrates suitable for cell and tissue engineering. This patterning technique, in principle, replicates topographical patterns by the means of applied pressure and temperature, in which a rigid master (silicon, for example) with topographical features is imprinted onto a polymer resist (PMMA, for example), that results in a relief replica of the master on the substrate's surface. There are two basic steps involved in this lithographic technique. First is the imprint step, in which a master (also called a "mold") with a custom-designed geometrical pattern is pressed onto a polymer resist (usually in the form of a thin film), layered on a substrate material, and followed by the removal of the master. This step duplicates the topography of the master on the polymer resist. During the process, the polymer resist is heated to a temperature above its glass transition ($T_g$), because the resist becomes a viscous liquid at the temperature that facilitates the polymer to flow and easily mold into the shape of the master. For example, to transfer the pattern from a rigid master onto a PMMA resist requires a temperature of around 110°C. PMMA has proven to be an excellent material as a resist for IL, because it has a low thermal expansion and pressure shrinkage coefficient. The second step is the pattern transfer, where an anisotropic etching process is used to remove the residual resist in the compressed region. This step transfers the thickness of the contrast pattern onto the entire resist, leaving polymer patterns on the substrate material. It should be noted that the process of IL is fundamentally different from stamping μCP which uses a monolayer of self-assembled molecules because it is more like a physical than a chemical process.

Numerous studies demonstrated the efficiency of imprint technique in controlling cell behavior. For example, Yim et al., developed a patterned silicon substrate using a polymeric thin film of PMMA (comprised of gratings with a 350 nm line width, 700 nm pitch, and 350 nm depth) by IL to study the efficacy of the patterned substrates in regulating cell behavior (Yim et al. 2005). Smooth muscle cells (SMC) were cultured on these patterned substrates and their morphology and a concomitant orientation was studied, with respect to their elongation and alignment. This study revealed that a patterned substrate with nanoscale topographical features can effectively direct cell orientation and function (see Figure 16.3a) (Yim et al. 2005). The cells cultured on the patterned surfaces showed an elongated morphology and were mostly parallel to one another (Figure 16.3a(i through iv)). In contrast, the SMC cultured on unpatterned surfaces showed neither elongation nor orientation at both low and high cell densities (see Figures 16.3a(v and vi), respectively). The orientation of the cells along the axis of the gratings could be seen more clearly in Figure 16.3a(vii), in comparison to unpatterned surfaces where they were randomly spread as shown in Figure 16.3a(viii). In addition, the cytoskeleton and nuclei of the cells were also found to elongate and align to the long axis of the cell (see Figures 16.3a(i and ii)). The cells were significantly elongated on the patterned substrates compared to the nonpatterned substrates. This study, in addition to others, suggest that IL-patterned substrates can be used as a model substrate to study cell–substrate interactions with respect to topographical changes.

## 16.4.2 Colloidal Lithography

CL is a simple and an efficient technique to produce topographical patterns on biomaterial substrates, which utilizes the ability of colloidal particles to self-organize on surfaces via electrostatic forces. This makes them suitable as a mask for pattern transfer onto the substrate materials and well-ordered micro- and nanoscale topographical features with a large surface area can eventually be obtained. Dalby et al., utilized the colloidal lithographic technique to modify the surface of the PMMA with cylindrical columnar topographical features (160 nm height and 100 nm diameter) (Dalby et al. 2004). The efficacy of the patterned substrates in promoting cell adhesion and cytoskeleton development was evaluated using fibroblasts. The changes in the fibroblasts' morphology and their cellular functions in response to a geometrical pattern were studied. The results of this study showed that the cells grown on the geometrical patterns exhibited many peripheral protrusions, whereas they were absent in cells on planar

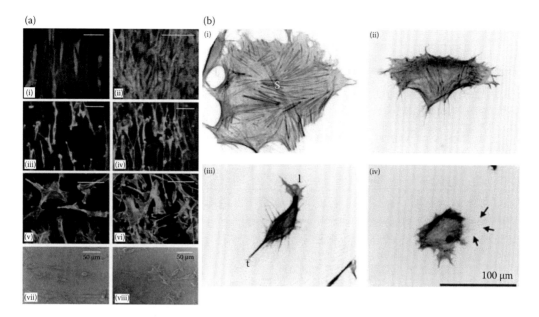

**FIGURE 16.3** (**See color insert**.) (a) Confocal micrographs of F-actin stained SMCs on (i) nano-imprinted PMMA at a low cell density, (ii) nano-imprinted PMMA at a high cell density, (iii) nanopatterned PDMS at a low cell density, (iv) nanopatterned PDMS at a high cell density, (v) nonpatterned PMMA, and (vi) glass cover slip. SEM micrographs of SMC cultured on (vii) nano-imprinted gratings on PMMA coated on $SiO_2$ wafer and (viii) nonpatterned PMMA coated on $SiO_2$ wafer. Bar = 50 μm for all except (ii) Bar = 100 μm. (b) Fluorescent actin staining (images inverted to show filopodia more clearly). (i and ii) Fibroblasts on control, (iii and iv) fibroblasts on nano-columns. (i) A well-spread cell with many stress fibers (s); (ii) cells becoming well-spread, but still with a polarized morphology; (iii) a rounded cell that is clearly polarized with lamellipodia at the leading edge (l) and a trailing tail (t); (iv) spreading cell, which is still notably smaller, and has fewer stress fibers than the cells seen in (i and ii) (arrows point to faint filopodia). (Figure 16.3a is adapted with permission from Yim E. K. F. et al. 2005. *Biomaterials* **26**(26): 5405–5413; Figure 16.3b is adapted with permission from Dalby, M. J. et al. 2004b. *Biomaterials* **25**(23): 5415–5422.)

surfaces. For example, fibroblasts produced a higher number of filopodia per micron of cell perimeter than in planar surfaces and an interaction between the filopodia and the nano-columns could often be seen. The results also showed that the number of filopodia significantly increased in fibroblasts cultured on the nanoscale's columnar structures compared to the planar surfaces, which indicated a stronger cellular response and interaction toward patterned substrates. During the initial stage, the fibroblasts that were in contact with the nano-columnar substrates stimulated the formation of cytoskeleton faster than the fibroblasts on the planar-controlled surfaces. However, over a longer period of time, the organization of cytoskeleton became more diffuse and the morphology of fibroblasts appeared more rounded, thicker, and smaller in size. On the other hand, fibroblasts on the planar surfaces had a clearly defined intermediate filament-like structure. Thus, it appears that, rather than adhering and spreading as that of the cells on the planar surfaces, fibroblasts on the columnar structures were more polarized with rounded cell bodies having a higher density of filopodia, with the filopodia probing the nano-structured environment surrounding the cell.

The behavior of a cell, particularly morphology, cytoskeletal organization, and focal contacts, in relation to topography and planar surfaces were also assessed by determining the protein distribution using immunochemistry and confocal microscopy. The observation of filamentous actin clearly showed different cell morphologies between the cells on the nano-columnar surfaces compared to planar surfaces (see Figure 16.3b) (Dalby et al. 2004). The cells on the planar surfaces appear to spread with signs of many stress fibers formed at the lamellae region (Figures 16.3b(i and ii)). The cellular growth behavior on the nano-columnar surfaces appeared to spread less (Figures 16.3b(iii and iv)) and many of them were highly polarized with areas of dense filopodia extensions that could be observed interacting with the nano-columns (see Figure 16.3b(iii)), compared to planar surfaces (see Figure 16.3b(iv)). This is of particular interest when considering cell responses to topographical features. This study demonstrated that control of the cellular environment might lead to increased levels of endocytosis and the topographical patterns may be able to alter the cell morphology, growth, and subsequent functions. On the basis of this experimental example, and others, CL can be utilized to fabricate topographical patterns to study the fundamental aspects of cell behaviors.

## 16.5 Techniques for Three-Dimensional Patterning and Applications to Tissue Engineering

While 2D patterning of biomaterials continues to be widely used for the fundamental studies of cell and tissue engineering, the most promising and versatile methods for constructing mimics of native tissues are those techniques that enable the creation of 3D substrates. Most tissue engineering approaches at present use random seeding of cells within porous polymer structures. While this has yielded major advances in the field, the generation of complex tissue structures may require control over the localization of the behavior of multiple cell types in 3D. Moreover, often, the cells cultured in 3D behave more physiologically compared to the cells cultured onto 2D surfaces (Sun et al. 2006; Yang et al. 2008; May 2010), which eventually leads to the concept of 3D cell patterning. Indeed, tissues in our body are composed of a complex mixture of multiple cells arranged in geometrically organized patterns. Researchers have long sought to mimic these patterns to engineer the tissues in the laboratory conditions. In the following sections, the most frequently used techniques for fabricating 3D patterning are briefly discussed.

### 16.5.1 Microfluidics

Microfluidic techniques can be used to pattern cells in 3D structures. Microfluidic patterning is a process in which microchannels are used to deliver fluids to selected areas of a substrate, resulting in patterning of the material. This method is frequently used to pattern multiple components on a single substrate and allows a directed delivery of cells and soluble factors onto the substrate; thereby it has significant implications for the fields of cell biology and cell-based assay. Unlike the conventional *in vitro* cell-culture methods, microfluidics can provide miniature and complex structures mimicking the *in vivo* cellular environment. Among the numerous types of biomaterials, hydrogels are particularly attractive for generating the cell containing 3D patterns as they are biocompatible, degradable in a controlled manner, possesses adequate mechanical properties, flexibility in designing, feasible to surface modification, and functionalization. The use of hydrogels in a microfluidic system plays a critical role as well in controlling cell behavior. Previously, contractile cardiac organoids have been engineered by using microfluidic patterning of HA (Khademhosseini et al. 2007). HA micropatterns served as inductive templates for organoid assembly. A schematic representation for fabricating cardiomyocyte organoids using a microfluidic patterning is shown in Figure 16.4a (Khademhosseini et al. 2007). In this approach, a PDMS microfluidic mold was placed on a glass substrate, and the HA solution was injected into the microchannels (having 100 μm in width and 60 μm in height). When HA regions were formed, the PDMS mold was removed, and the resulting substrate was treated with FN to generate cell-adhesive regions. The resultant patterns had both cell-adhesive and nonadhesive regions, which could be used for controlling cell behavior *invitro*. The efficacy of the microfluidic pattern was tested by culturing primary cardiomyocytes onto the predesigned microlanes. It was found that cardiomyocytes elongated and aligned along the pattern direction attaching preferentially to the glass substrate and the interface between HA patterns and the glass substrate. After 3 days in culture, the linearly aligned myocytes

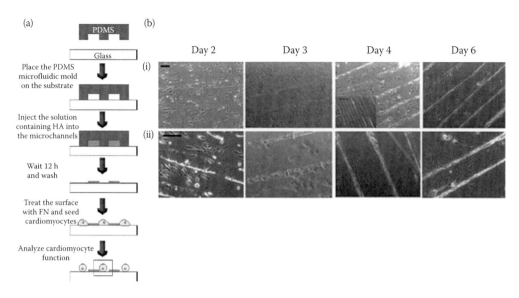

**FIGURE 16.4** (a) Schematic diagram of the approach used to fabricate cardiomyocyte organoids and (b) progression of cardiac–organoid formation on HA-patterned surfaces. (i) Images taken at 100×. Day 4 inset image taken at 40× illustrates several millimeter-long cardiac organoids. (ii) Images taken at 200×. Scale bars (i and ii) 100 μm. Inset scale bar 1 mm. (Adapted with permission from Khademhosseini, A. et al. 2007. *Biomedical Microdevices* **9**(2): 149–157.)

detached from the substrate and formed contractile cardiac organoids (see Figure 16.4b). This study demonstrated that microfludic patterning can be used to generate patterns that can be used to construct cardiac tissue models *in vitro*.

For 3D tissue engineering, the *in vivo*-like properties of 3D patterned structure with multiple cell types are necessary to generate a biomimetic cellular structure. Microfluidic patterning also allows for the formation of 3D structures consisting of multiple cell types Tan and Desai 2003, 2004). In this approach, a desired cell type resuspended in an appropriate ECM component was applied into a microfluidic network. Next, following the contraction of the biopolymer matrix by cells, another layer with a different cell type was applied into the microfluidic network, which is able to create a tissue assembly with multiple cell types arranged in 3D (z-direction). The 3D topology of the microfluidic network in the stamp makes this technique versatile with which multiple cell types can be patterned even in the complex structures. To demonstrate the capability of a microfluidic system to generate complex 3D patterns, Chiu et al., developed a two-layer stamp for the deposition of two cell types in a concentric square pattern (see Figure 16.5a) (Chiu et al. 2000). Bovine adrenal capillary endothelial cells (BCEs) and human bladder cancer cells (ECVs) were used for patterning. Coating of the channels with a noncell-adhesive agent as bovine serum albumin, (BSA) prevented the cell's attachment to the undesired regions. The cell-culture data demonstrated the cell viability and spreading of patterned cells only on the channels. The authors suggested that the ability to pattern multiple cell types will pave the way to study the functional significance of tissue architecture at the resolution of individual cells, and the molecular interactions between different cell types. On the basis of the experimental examples discussed here, and others, the microfluidic-based 3D cell patterning is a useful tool for cellular analysis.

## 16.5.2 Stamping/Printing

In tissue engineering, the goal of a hierarchical organization of cells to promote the *in vitro* development of a functional tissue may benefit from the spatially controlled placement of cells in specific locations

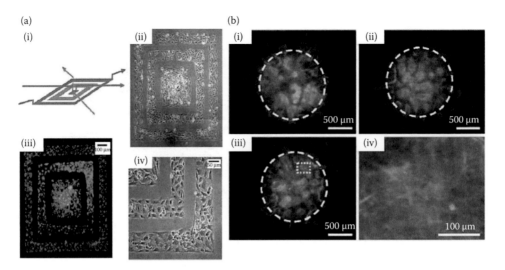

**FIGURE 16.5** (**See color insert**.) (i) Fluorescence (ii) and phase-contrast (iii and iv) pictures of two cell types deposited on a tissue culture dish in a concentric square pattern by using the 3D stamp depicted in (a). The cells that appear green are (ECVs) labeled with 5-chloromethylfluorescein diacetate (CMFDA); the cells that appear red are BCEs labeled with DiI-conjugated acetylated low density lipoprotein. Suspensions of cells were introduced into the three sets of channels and were allowed to sediment and attach to the surface of the tissue-culture dish. These cells were cultured with the stamp in place for ≈24 h to grow and spread into a confluent layer. An expanded view of the lower right corner of (iii) is shown in (iv). (b) Different regions of a hydroxyapatite scaffold patterned with osteoblasts using a single agarose stamp with 1000 µm diameter circular features. Images (i through iii) show an area on the top surface of the same scaffold that was patterned during the same stamping event. The dashed white lines indicate the areas patterned with cells. (iv) Higher magnification of the area within the white box in (iii). Actin was stained bright green with phalloidin and DNA stained bright blue with Hoescht 33342. The dark blue/grey features in the unpatterned background of the images in (i through iii) are artifacts of fluorescence microscopy, resulting from the light reflected from the white hydroxyapatite scaffolds. The images were acquired 24 h after patterning. (Figure 16.5a is adapted with permission from Chiu D. T. et al. 2000. *Proceedings of the National Academy of Sciences of the United States of America* **97**(6): 2408–2413; Figure 16.5b is adapted with permission from Stevens, M. M. et al. 2005. *Biomaterials* **26**(36): 7636–7641.)

on a cellular substrate. In a notable study, Stevens et al., demonstrated a new methodology for generating patterns of osteoblasts with circular shapes (diameters of 200, 700, or 1000 mm) on hydroxyapatite substrates and glass slides, using replica stamping/printing (Stevens et al. 2005). The cells (human osteoblasts) were transferred directly from a topographically patterned agarose (hydrogel) stamp onto the surface of hydroxyapatite (a compound rich in bone mineral). The use of a hydrogel for the stamp provided a "wet" surface that kept cells hydrated and maintained cell viability throughout the stamping process. Figure 16.5b shows spots of osteoblasts patterned on the surface of hydroxyapatite substrates. These patterns were printed with an agarose stamp having 1 mm diameter posts and a pitch of 2.5 mm. The technique transferred the material to the surface of the substrate in parallel, making it possible to pattern multiple spots of cells simultaneously. Figures 16.5b(i through iii) show three spots of cells patterned at the same time on the same scaffold, which demonstrates the reproducibility of the pattern transfer on 3D substrates. The viability of the patterned cells was also confirmed by imaging the adhesion of cells and spreading the actin cytoskeleton on the surface (see Figure 16.5b(iv)). This study suggested that stamping of mammalian cells directly onto tissue engineering scaffolds may find their use in controlling the spatial invasion of scaffolds, promoting the hierarchical organization of cells, and in controlling cell–cell interactions. Furthermore, the field of bioprinting has gained a significant momentum over the past few years to demonstrate the potential of printing cells, gels, or a combination of both in a controlled manner on a substrate (Boland et al. 2003; Mironov et al. 2003; Jakab et al. 2004). On the basis of these findings, and others, direct patterning of cells on a 3D substrate has a unique advantage for engineering functional tissues.

## 16.5.3 Self-Assembly

Self-assembly is a process that can be utilized to enable assembly of 3D tissues with building blocks of hydrogels encapsulated with desired cell types (also called cell-laden hydrogels) with desired microstructural features. Basically self-assembly is a bottom-up approach, which plays a critical role in the development of a complex cellular microenvironment that mimics *in vivo*-like microarchitectural features to spatially control the cells and direct their growth into a specific tissue. Self-assembly process is scalable and controllable, and thus it can be used to engineer functional tissues under laboratory conditions (Whitesides and Grzybowski 2002). Recently, Du et al., demonstrated a self-assembly process which assembles engineered tissues through the control of hydrophilic/hydrophobic interactions of cell-laden hydrogels with control over the microarchitectural features (Du et al. 2008). A schematic diagram of the hydrogel assembly process is shown in Figure 16.6a. In this method, NIH-3T3 mouse fibroblast cells were encapsulated in polyethylene glycol methacrylate (PEG-MA) hydrogels and these hydrophilic building blocks were randomly placed on the surface of a high-density hydrophobic solution (mineral oil, for instance) where they migrated toward each other by surface tension. This process caused the hydrophilic hydrogels to aggregate to form tissue-like features of varying dimensions, which could then be gelled together through a secondary UV polymerization. Varying the aspect ratio of the modules demonstrated the ability to control the ultimate size and shape of the resulting aggregate tissues as the number of hydrogels per tissue increased proportionally with the module aspect ratio (see Figure 16.6b). The culture

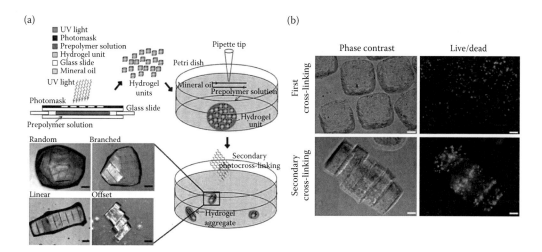

**FIGURE 16.6** **(See color insert.)** (a) Schematic diagram of microgel (micron-sized hydrogel) self-assembly process. Microgel units were synthesized by photolithography, transferred into a dish containing mineral oil, and subjected to mechanical agitation applied by manually manipulating a pipette-tip in a back-and-forth manner. Four structural types of microgel assemblies were observed: linear, branched, random, and offset. Secondary cross-linking was achieved by exposing the microgel assemblies to UV light. (Scale bars, 200 μm.) (b) Phase-contrast and fluorescence images of cell-laden (NIH 3T3) microgel assemblies. (Adapted with permission from Du, Y. A. et al. 2008. *Proceedings of the National Academy of Sciences of the United States of America* **105**(28): 9522–9527.)

data confirmed that the high fraction of cells remained viable immediately after cell encapsulation. The self-assembly process can also be used to induce a directed assembly of cell-laden hydrogels while maintaining high cell viability. The subsequent work in this area are simple and versatile since most of the biocompatible materials with these characteristics (hydrophilic–hydrophobic interfaces) can be utilized to construct cell-laden complex tissue-like system (Fernandez and Khademhosseini 2010; Zamanian et al. 2010). In overall, self-assembly process could be a powerful and highly scalable approach for the directed assembly of cell-laden hydrogels to construct 3D tissues *in vitro*.

## 16.6 Concluding Remarks

Micro- and nanopatterning of biomaterials that are suitable to study cell behavior and engineer tissue-mimetic systems are discussed in this chapter. The data summarized in this chapter represent some of the developments of cell patterning from a variety of approaches, conventional to nonconventional. The results of all these experimental examples, in addition to others, clearly demonstrate the efficacy of patterned biomaterials to regulate cell organization and development. Cell patterning is an emerging area of applied research and an enabling technology for manipulating cellular assemblies in a controlled fashion and to understand the cell behavior toward new surfaces/substrates. Therefore, patterning cells on biomaterials will continue to be of importance in various biological applications, in particular to engineer the transplantable tissue constructs or as a tool for understanding the mechanism of how cells respond to synthetic materials.

## References

Andersson, A. S., P. Olsson et al. 2003. The effects of continuous and discontinuous groove edges on cell shape and alignment. *Experimental Cell Research* **288**(1): 177–188.

Bhatia, S. N., U. J. Balis et al. 1998. Microfabrication of hepatocyte/fibroblast co-cultures: Role of homotypic cell interactions. *Biotechnology Progress* **14**(3): 378–387.

Bhatia, S. N., U. J. Balis et al. 1999. Effect of cell–cell interactions in preservation of cellular phenotype: Cocultivation of hepatocytes and nonparenchymal cells. *The FASEB Journal* **13**: 1883–1900.

Boland, T., V. Mironov et al. 2003. Cell and organ printing 2: Fusion of cell aggregates in three-dimensional gels. *The Anatomical Record. Part A, Discoveries in Molecular, Cellular, and Evolutionary Biology* **272**(2): 497–502.

Chen, C. S., M. Mrksich et al. 1997. Geometric control of cell life and death. *Science* **276**(5317): 1425–1428.

Chiu, D. T., N. L. Jeon et al. 2000. Patterned deposition of cells and proteins onto surfaces by using three-dimensional microfluidic systems. *Proceedings of the National Academy of Sciences of the United States of America* **97**(6): 2408–2413.

Chung, B. G., L. F. Kang et al. 2007. Micro- and nanoscale technologies for tissue engineering and drug discovery applications. *Expert Opinion on Drug Discovery* **2**(12): 1653–1668.

Craighead, H. G., C. D. James et al. 2001. Chemical and topographical patterning for directed cell attachment. *Current Opinion in Solid State & Materials Science* **5**(2–3): 177–184.

Curtis, A. S. G. and M. Varde 1964. Control of cell behavior: Topographical factors. *Journal of National Cancer Research Institute* **33**: 15.

Curtis, A. and C. Wilkinson 1997. Topographical control of cells. *Biomaterials* **18**(24): 1573–1583.

Dalby, M. J., D. Giannaras et al. 2004a. Rapid fibroblast adhesion to 27 nm high polymer demixed nanotopography. *Biomaterials* **25**(1): 77–83.

Dalby, M. J., M. O. Riehle et al. 2004b. Changes in fibroblast morphology in response to nano-columns produced by colloidal lithography. *Biomaterials* **25**(23): 5415–5422.

Dalby, M. J., M. O. Riehle et al. 2002a. In vitro reaction of endothelial cells to polymer demixed nanotopography. *Biomaterials* **23**(14): 2945–2954.

Dalby, M. J., M. O. Riehle et al. 2002b. Polymer-demixed nanotopography: Control of fibroblast spreading and proliferation. *Tissue Engineering* **8**(6): 1099–1108.

Du, Y. A., E. Lo et al. 2008. Directed assembly of cell-laden microgels for fabrication of 3D tissue constructs. *Proceedings of the National Academy of Sciences of the United States of America* **105**(28): 9522–9527.

Dulcey, C. S., J. H. Georger, Jr. et al. 1991. Deep UV photochemistry of chemisorbed monolayers: Patterned coplanar molecular assemblies. *Science* **252**(5005): 551–554.

Falconnet, D., G. Csucs et al. 2006. Surface engineering approaches to micropattern surfaces for cell-based assays. *Biomaterials* **27**(16): 3044–3063.

Fernandez, J. G. and A. Khademhosseini 2010. Micro-masonry: Construction of 3D structures by microscale self-assembly. *Advanced Materials* **22**(23): 2538–2541.

Fukuda, J., A. Khademhosseini et al. 2006. Micropatterned cell co-cultures using layer-by-layer deposition of extracellular matrix components. *Biomaterials* **27**(8): 1479–1486.

Gadegaard, N., E. Martines et al. 2006. Applications of nano-patterning to tissue engineering. *Microelectronic Engineering* **83**(4–9): 1577–1581.

Georger, J. H., D. A. Stenger et al. 1992. Coplanar patterns of self-assembled monolayers for selective cell-adhesion and outgrowth. *Thin Solid Films* **210**(1–2): 716–719.

Grayson, A. C. R., R. S. Shawgo et al. 2004. A BioMEMS review: MEMS technology for physiologically integrated devices. *Proceedings of the IEEE* **92**(1): 6–21.

Healy, K. E. 2009. Patterning: Cells nourished by nanodrops. *Nature Materials* **8**(9): 700–702.

Hoffman-Kim, D., J. A. Mitchel et al. Topography, cell response, and nerve regeneration. *Annual Review of Biomedical Engineering* **12**: 203–231.

Hyun, J., Y. J. Zhu et al. 2001. Microstamping on an activated polymer surface: Patterning biotin and streptavidin onto common polymeric biomaterials. *Langmuir* **17**(20): 6358–6367.

Jakab, K., A. Neagu et al. 2004. Organ printing: Fiction or science. *Biorheology* **41**(3–4): 371–375.

James, C. D., R. Davis et al. 2000. Aligned microcontact printing of micrometer-scale poly-L-lysine structures for controlled growth of cultured neurons on planar microelectrode arrays. *IEEE Transactions on Biomedical Engineering* **47**(1): 17–21.

Jenney, C. R. and J. M. Anderson 1999. Alkylsilane-modified surfaces: Inhibition of human macrophage adhesion and foreign body giant cell formation. *Journal of Biomedical Materials Research* **46**(1): 11–21.

Johansson, F., P. Carlberg et al. 2006. Axonal outgrowth on nano-imprinted patterns. *Biomaterials* **27**(8): 1251–1258.

Kaehr, B., R. Allen et al. 2004. Guiding neuronal development with *in situ* microfabrication. *Proceedings of the National Academy of Sciences of the United States of America* **101**(46): 16104–16108.

Kane, R. S., S. Takayama et al. 1999. Patterning proteins and cells using soft lithography. *Biomaterials* **20**(23–24): 2363–2376.

Khademhosseini, A., G. Eng et al. 2007. Microfluidic patterning for fabrication of contractile cardiac organoids. *Biomedical Microdevices* **9**(2): 149–157.

Khademhosseini, A., R. Langer et al. 2006. Microscale technologies for tissue engineering and biology. *Proceedings of the National Academy of Sciences of the United States of America* **103**(8): 2480–2487.

Khademhosseini, A., J. Vacanti et al. 2009. Tissue engineering: Next generation tissue constructs and challenges to clinical practice. *Scientific American* **300**: 64–71.

Kleinfeld, D., K. H. Kahler et al. 1988. Controlled outgrowth of dissociated neurons on patterned substrates. *Journal of Neuroscience* **8**(11): 4098–4120.

Kumar, G., Y. C. Wang et al. 2003. Spatially controlled cell engineering on biomaterials using polyelectrolytes. *Langmuir* **19**(25): 10550–10556.

Lahiri, J., E. Ostuni et al. 1999. Patterning ligands on reactive SAMs by microcontact printing. *Langmuir* **15**(6): 2055–2060.

Li, N. and A. Folch 2005. Integration of topographical and biochemical cues by axons during growth on microfabricated 3-D substrates. *Experimental Cell Research* **311**: 307–316.

Liu, W. F. and C. S. Chen 2005. Engineering biomaterials to control cell function. *Materials Today* **8**(12): 28–35.

May, M. 2010. Taking control of 3D cell culture. *Drug Discovery and Development* **13**: 10–10.

McBeath, R., D. M. Pirone et al. 2004. Cell shape, cytoskeletal tension, and RhoA regulate stem cell lineage commitment. *Developmental Cell* **6**(4): 483–495.

Mironov, V., T. Boland et al. 2003. Organ printing: Computer-aided jet-based 3D tissue engineering. *Trends in Biotechnology* **21**(4): 157–161.

Mrksich, M., C. S. Chen et al. 1996. Controlling cell attachment on contoured surfaces with self-assembled monolayers of alkanethiolates on gold. *Proceedings of the National Academy of Science USA* **93**(20): 10775–10778.

Mrksich, M. and G. M. Whitesides 1995. Patterning self-assembled monolayers using microcontact printing—A new technology for biosensors. *Trends in Biotechnology* **13**(6): 228–235.

Mrksich, M. and G. M. Whitesides 1996. Using self-assembled monolayers to understand the interactions of man-made surfaces with proteins and cells. *Annual Review of Biophysics and Biomolecular Structure* **25**: 55–78.

Murugan, R., P. Molnar et al. 2009. Biomaterial surface patterning of self assembled monolayers for controlling neuronal cell behavior. *International Journal of Biomedical Enginnering Technology* **2**(2): 104–134.

Nakanishi, J., T. Takarada et al. 2008. Recent advances in cell micropatterning techniques for bioanalytical and biomedical sciences. *Analytical Sciences* **24**(1): 67–72.

Oliva, A. A., C. D. James et al. 2003. Patterning axonal guidance molecules using a novel strategy for micro-contact printing. *Neurochemical Research* **28**(11): 1639–1648.

Ostuni, E., L. Yan et al. 1999. The interaction of proteins and cells with self-assembled monolayers of alka-nethiolates on gold and silver. *Colloids and Surfaces B-Biointerfaces* **15**(1): 3–30.

Romanova, E. V., K. A. Fosser et al. 2004. Engineering the morphology and electrophysiological parameters of cultured neurons by microfluidic surface patterning. *FASEB J*: 03–1368fje.

Saneinejad, S. and M. S. Shoichet 2000. Patterned poly(chlorotrifluoroethylene) guides primary nerve cell adhesion and neurite outgrowth. *Journal of Biomedical Materials Research* **50**(4): 465–474.

Sanjana, N. E. and S. B. Fuller 2004. A fast flexible ink-jet printing method for patterning dissociated neurons in culture. *Journal of Neuroscience Methods* **136**(2): 151–163.

Schlenoff, J. B., M. Li et al. 1995. Stability and self-exchange in alkanethiol monolayers. *Journal of the American Chemical Society* **117**(50): 12528–12536.

Senaratne, W., L. Andruzzi et al. 2005. Self-assembled monolayers and polymer brushes in biotechnology: Current applications and future perspectives. *Biomacromolecules* **6**(5): 2427–2448.

Singhvi, R., A. Kumar et al. 1994. Engineering cell shape and function. *Science* **264**(5159): 696–698.

Smith, R. K., P. A. Lewis et al. 2004. Patterning self-assembled monolayers. *Progress In Surface Science* **75**(1–2): 1–68.

Spargo, B. J., M. A. Testoff et al. 1994. Spatially controlled adhesion, spreading, and differentiation of endothelial cells on self-assembled molecular monolayers. *Proceedings of the National Academy of Sciences* **91**: 11070–11074.

Stenger, D. A., C. J. Pike et al. 1993. Surface determinants of neuronal survival and growth on self- assembled monolayers in culture. *Brain Research* **630**(1–2): 136–147.

Stevens, M. M. and J. H. George 2005. Exploring and engineering the cell surface interface. *Science* **310**(5751): 1135–1138.

Stevens, M. M., M. Mayer et al. 2005. Direct patterning of mammalian cells onto porous tissue engineering substrates using agarose stamps. *Biomaterials* **26**(36): 7636–7641.

Sun, T., S. Jackson et al. 2006. Culture of skin cells in 3D rather than 2D improves their ability to survive exposure to cytotoxic agents. *Journal of Biotechnology* **122**(3): 372–381.

Tan, W. and T. A. Desai 2003. Microfluidic patterning of cells in extracellular matrix biopolymers: Effects of channel size, cell type, and matrix composition on pattern integrity. *Tissue Engineering* **9**(2): 255–267.

Tan, W. and T. A. Desai 2004. Layer-by-layer microfluidics for biomimetic three-dimensional structures. *Biomaterials* **25**(7–8): 1355–1364.

Tourovskaia, A., T. Barber et al. 2003. Micropatterns of chemisorbed cell adhesion-repellent films using oxygen plasma etching and elastomeric masks. *Langmuir* **19**(11): 4754–4764.

Ulman, A. 1991. *Introduction to Ultrathin Organic Films*, San Diego, Academic Press.

Ulman, A. 1991. *Ultrathin Organic Films: From Langmuir-Blodgett to Self-Assembly*, Boston Academic Press..

Ulman, A. 1996. Formation and structure of self-assembled monolayers. *Chemical Review* **96**(4): 1533–1554.

Veiseh, M., B. T. Wickes et al. 2004. Guided cell patterning on gold-silicon dioxide substrates by surface molecular engineering. *Biomaterials* **25**(16): 3315–3324.

Welle, A., S. Horn et al. 2005. Photo-chemically patterned polymer surfaces for controlled PC-12 adhesion and neurite guidance. *Journal of Neuroscience Methods* **142**(2): 243–250.

Whitesides, G. M. and B. Grzybowski 2002. Self-assembly at all scales. *Science* **295**(5564): 2418–2421.

Yan, L., W. T. S. Huck et al. 2004. Self-assembled monolayers (SAMS) and synthesis of planar micro- and nanostructures. *Journal of Macromolecular Science-Polymer Reviews* **C44**(2): 175–206.

Yang, F., R. Murugan et al. 2005. Electrospinning of nano/micro scale poly(L-lactic acid) aligned fibers and their potential in neural tissue engineering. *Biomaterials* **26**(15): 2603–2610.

Yang, Y., D. Bolikal et al. 2008. Combinatorial polymer scaffold libraries for screening cell-biomaterial interactions in 3D. *Advanced Materials* **20**(11): 2037.

Yim, E. K. F., R. M. Reano et al. 2005. Nanopattern-induced changes in morphology and motility of smooth muscle cells. *Biomaterials* **26**(26): 5405–5413.

Zamanian, B., M. Masaeli et al. 2010. Interface-directed self-assembly of cell-laden microgels. *Small* **6**(8): 937–944.

# 17

# Drug Delivery

17.1 Introduction ........................................................ 17-1
17.2 Mechanisms of Drug Delivery.................................. 17-2
    Diffusion from Nondegradable Systems • Bioerosion •
    Stimuli-Responsive Systems • Overall Release Profiles
17.3 Drugs of Interest in Tissue Engineering ..................... 17-6
    Drug Properties and Design Considerations
17.4 Drug Delivery in Tissue Engineering......................... 17-8
    Classical Drug Delivery Systems • Drug Delivery from Tissue
    Engineering Scaffolds and Matrices
17.5 Outlook............................................................ 17-13
References................................................................17-14

**Prinda Wanakule**
*University of Texas, Austin*

**Krishnendu Roy**
*University of Texas, Austin*

## 17.1 Introduction

The study and practice of tissue engineering requires a multidisciplinary approach in order to create new cells and tissues for the treatment of diseases (Langer and Vacanti 1993, Becker and Göpferich 2007). Drug delivery has proven to be an integral part in directing the development and differentiation of progenitor cells into functional tissues, specifically, the controlled delivery of pharmacologically active or bioactive agents, such as cytokines, growth factors, morphogens, and nucleic acids. By controlling the delivery of these drugs at different time points and concentrations, a direct effect is exerted on the cell proliferation, differentiation, or migration, with the potential for controlling the phenotype and functionality of developing tissues (Biondi et al. 2008, Boontheekul and Mooney 2003, Fisher et al. 2010, Langer and Vacanti 1993, Nomi et al. 2002, Saltzman and Olbricht 2002, Tabata 2003, Uebersax et al. 2009).

The goals of drug delivery, in general, are manifold, and include the targeting of drug to specific cells or sites in the body, overcoming tissue barriers associated with delivery routes, overcoming cellular barriers which control cellular uptake, and controlled release. Controlled release concepts encompass the ability to control release of bioactive molecules at target sites, the effective concentration of drug in the body, as well as its duration of activity.

In tissue engineering, controlled delivery encompasses "the provision of a bioactive molecule over time in a manner such that its biological activity can be productively harnessed" (Hubbell 2008). The use of controlled drug delivery, more so than the other goals of drug delivery, has come into greater use in tissue engineering in recent years (Biondi et al. 2008, Fisher et al. 2010, Uebersax et al. 2009). In this context, there are three major applications of drug delivery concepts that are being widely used to engineer tissue constructs: (a) spatially and temporally controlled delivery of proteins, peptides, lipids, and small molecules (e.g., growth factors, enzymes, and morphogens), (b) spatially patterned presentation of cell-signaling ligands, and (c) delivery of nucleic acids to direct progenitor cells to specific pathways (e.g., through either ectopic gene expression or targeted gene silencing).

While it is possible to directly infuse these bioactive molecules into culture flasks and plates (*in vitro*) or by injection (*in vivo*), this may be undesirable for several reasons. For example, many proteins and

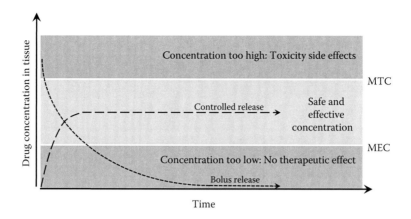

**FIGURE 17.1**   In classical drug delivery, controlled release systems aim to achieve a constant concentration of bioactive drug that is both safe and effective. MEC = minimum effective concentration; MTC = minimum toxic concentration.

peptides have short half-lives in serum or media due to inactivation by proteases and enzymes, and thus, need continual replenishment to maintain a certain minimum effective concentration (see Figure 17.1). Additionally, unconstrained repeated doses may result in toxic effects. Delivery of nucleic acids also poses the additional challenge of intracellular targeting. The controlled temporal and spatial release of these drugs could reduce the amount of expensive drug and chemical signals required, as well as the potential toxic effects (Hubbell 2008, Biondi et al. 2008, Boontheekul and Mooney 2003, Caldorera-Moore and Peppas 2009, Fisher et al. 2010, Saltzman and Olbricht 2002, Uebersax et al. 2009) and at the same time increase their bioavailability. This temporal and spatial control has also given rise to new possibilities and advances in tissue engineering, for example, the use of three-dimensional scaffolds to spatially differentiate cells into various "zones" consisting of different cell types (Mapili et al. 2005, Klein et al. 2009).

The objective of this chapter is to provide the reader with a basic understanding of drug delivery, an overview of controlled drug delivery technologies, as well as their applicability to and significance in the field of tissue engineering. We first begin by providing a brief review on the modes of drug delivery, or drug release, from drug delivery systems. Next, we move on to discuss some drugs of interest in tissue engineering applications, as well as their properties that affect the design of the delivery system. We then explore the methods used to control the release of drugs in tissue engineering, with special emphasis on the release of drugs from tissue engineering scaffolds and matrices. Finally, we provide an outlook on the future of drug delivery in tissue engineering, and follow with references.

## 17.2  Mechanisms of Drug Delivery

There are myriad mechanisms to direct the release of drugs in a controlled manner. We can classify the drug delivery mechanisms of special interest in tissue engineering into three main categories: diffusion from nondegradable systems, bioerodible systems, and stimuli-responsive systems. Several other strategies have been employed to create desirable release profiles; however, an exhaustive description is certainly beyond the scope of this chapter, and may be found in excellent reviews in the literature (Caldorera-Moore and Peppas 2009, Langer and Peppas 2003, Lavan et al. 2003, Saltzman and Olbricht 2002).

### 17.2.1  Diffusion from Nondegradable Systems

Diffusion is one of the most kinetically well-defined concepts of transport phenomena, and is especially applicable in the diffusion of drug molecules from nondegradable drug delivery systems (Truskey et al.

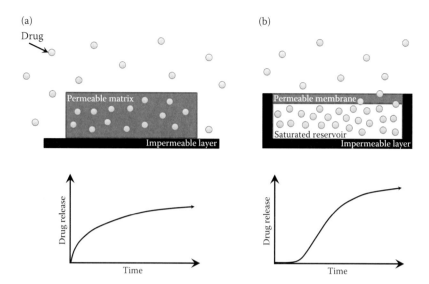

**FIGURE 17.2** (a) Diffusion-driven release of drug from a matrix. (b) Diffusion-driven release of drug from a saturated reservoir through a membrane.

2004, Becker and Göpferich 2007). Thermodynamically driven, it is the result of the random walk of submicron particles, called Brownian motion. Although movement may seem random at the microscopic level, at the macroscopic level, movement of particles along a concentration gradient is observed. Fick's second law of diffusion describes the temporal and spatial net movement of particles by diffusion:

$$\frac{\partial C(x,y,z,t)}{\partial t} = \frac{\partial^2 C}{\partial x^2} + \frac{\partial^2 C}{\partial y^2} + \frac{\partial^2 C}{\partial z^2}$$

Numerous solutions for this equation have been derived in order to describe the diffusion of drug molecules from several types of drug delivery devices under several conditions; for details, we refer the reader to an excellent text by Truskey et al. (2004). However, the two main diffusive conditions of special interest in drug delivery for tissue engineering are the diffusion of drug from a polymer matrix and the diffusion of drug from a reservoir through a membrane (see Figure 17.2), both of which are predictably well defined. The solutions to the problem are highly dependent on the initial drug concentration and the geometry of the device, and as such, the diffusion of drug out of the system may be changed by altering the device geometry, and prolonged by increasing the initial concentration (Truskey et al. 2004, Becker and Göpferich 2007).

Along the same lines, however, the disadvantage of this system lies in its dependence on drug concentration to define the flux of drug out of the system. As the drug concentration decreases over time and there is less of a concentration gradient, the release rate also decreases over time. This is especially pronounced in the diffusion of drug from a polymer matrix. However, by using a highly saturated drug reservoir with diffusion of drug driven through a membrane, a constant release of drug may be achieved over an extended period of time—longer than may be typically achieved through use of a matrix alone (Truskey et al. 2004, Becker and Göpferich 2007, Hubbell 2008).

### 17.2.1.1 Diffusion from Swellable Polymers

Diffusion of drugs may also be controlled by the use of swellable polymers, including swellable cross-linked hydrogels. In this case, there is an increase in polymer chain mobility due to the uptake of a solvent, such as water, that decreases the glass transition of the polymer ($T_g$). Drugs that are entrapped

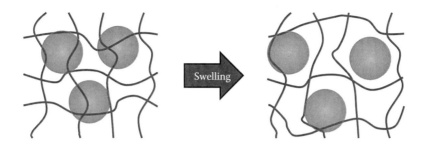

**FIGURE 17.3** Diffusion of drug from a swellable polymer matrix. In the preswollen state, drug molecules are entrapped within the network structure. Swelling of the polymer network results in increased polymer chain mobility and pore size, increasing the rate of diffusion of drugs out of the network.

and immobilized by the nonswollen polymer matrix may then begin to diffuse out due to the increased flexibility, resulting in a heightened release rate. In order to achieve this, the pore size of the polymer matrix must be sufficiently small so as to restrict a drug of known hydrodynamic radius. Upon swelling, the pore size increases, thus allowing movement and diffusion of the drug out from the matrix (see Figure 17.3) (Becker and Göpferich 2007, Hubbell 2008, Lustig and Peppas 1988). The diffusion of drugs from swellable polymer matrices has been well studied for macroporous (pore size between 0.1 and 1.0 μm), microporous (100–1000Å), and nonporous (10–100Å) hydrogels by several groups, and tunable drug release profiles from swellable polymers have been achieved (Hubbell 2008, Annabi et al. 2010).

## 17.2.2 Bioerosion

By definition, bioerosion refers to the erosion of a polymer into water-soluble products under physiological conditions, including both physical and chemical processes (according to the European Society for Biomaterials Consensus Conference in 1986) (Williams 1986). As a side note, biodegradation refers to the degradation by biological molecules, such as enzymes, which will be covered in the following section on stimuli-responsive systems. The most common mechanism of bioerosion is by hydrolysis of a polymer backbone by neutral water; however, accelerated hydrolysis may occur in the presence of ion catalysts and acidic pH. Erosion may proceed by either surface erosion or bulk erosion (see Figure 17.4). In surface erosion, the rate at which water is able to penetrate the device is slower than the erosion rate.

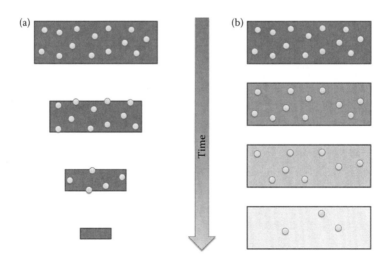

**FIGURE 17.4** Surface erosion (a) and bulk erosion (b) of polymeric devices.

On the other hand, bulk erosion occurs when the rate of water penetration into the device is greater than the rate of erosion (Gombotz and Pettit 1995, Göpferich 1996, Steinbüchel and Matsumura 2003).

Bioerodible drug delivery systems have been designed to both provide a mechanism of controlled drug release and to eliminate the need for device extraction after the lifetime of the system. As the device erodes, drug that has been solubilized or suspended within the device is slowly released. In general, surface eroding systems (heterogeneous) have a release rate proportional to the surface erosion rate, are driven primarily by erosion rather than diffusion, and can be varied according to device geometry. Bulk eroding systems (homogeneous) are driven by a combination of erosion and diffusion kinetics, with first-order kinetics for the rate of erosion, as well as the permeability of the device. Several parameters affect the rate of hydrolysis, and thus, release rate, including lability of the polymer backbone, hydrophobicity or hydrophilicity of the polymer, morphology, and molecular weight (Gombotz and Pettit 1995, Göpferich 1996, Heller 1985, Jain et al. 2005, Steinbüchel and Matsumura 2003).

## 17.2.3 Stimuli-Responsive Systems

In recent decades, a greater interest in the stimuli-responsive subfield in controlled drug delivery has been developing as a means to deliver drug only when or where it is needed. These stimuli-responsive types of systems often rely on physicochemical changes due to disease pathology or the cell microenvironment. Common stimuli include pH, temperature, ions, enzymes, light, and biomolecules, all of which have been designed to illicit a response in drug carriers to trigger drug release (Caldorera-Moore et al. 2010, Caldorera-Moore and Peppas 2009, Fisher et al. 2010, Jia and Kiick 2009, Löwik et al. 2010, Wanakule and Roy 2012).

### 17.2.3.1 pH-Responsive Systems

Several hydrogel-based drug delivery systems with the ability to swell or shrink in response to pH changes have been developed as triggered-release delivery systems. The pH-triggered swelling and shrinking mechanisms are primarily due to the properties of the side chain pendant group, which are cationic or anionic (Caldorera-Moore and Peppas 2009, Khare and Peppas 1993, 1995). Anionic hydrogels are ionized at pHs above their $pK_a$, and thus exhibit high swelling at these higher pHs due to repulsion of the ionized groups (Khare and Peppas 1995). In contrast, cationic hydrogels are ionized at pHs below their $pK_a$, exhibiting high swelling below their $pK_a$ (Khare and Peppas 1993).

Changes in pH exist throughout the body at the organ, tissue, and cellular level, and even due to various disease states. For example, pH-triggered drug delivery systems have been developed that are capable of triggering drug release when moving from the acidic gastric cavity to the more neutral small intestine (Gallardo et al. 2008, Liu and Basit 2010), where much drug absorption occurs, as well as from the neutral extracellular environment to the slightly more acidic early endosome (intracellular) (Boussif et al. 1995, Putnam et al. 2001). Thus, pH-responsive systems offer a versatile way in which to trigger drug release in response to environmental cues.

### 17.2.3.2 Enzyme-Responsive Systems

A relatively new strategy in drug delivery is to incorporate enzyme-sensitive components into the drug carriers, which are primarily hydrogel-based. Enzyme-degradable hydrogels have been shown to exhibit minimal release without the presence of enzyme, and triggered release in the presence of enzyme (Caldorera-Moore and Peppas 2009, Gobin and West 2002, Miyata et al. 2002, Peppas et al. 2000, Vartak and Gemeinhart 2007). This strategy has been used extensively in tissue engineering applications (Gobin and West 2002, Zisch et al. 2003a); however, it also provides an effective means of physiologically controlled release of drugs (Aimetti et al. 2009, Vartak and Gemeinhart 2007). Enzyme-responsive systems are suitable for site-specific delivery because enzymatic cleavage is highly specific, and many enzymes are upregulated in several diseases, such as various cancers and inflammatory diseases (Aimetti et al. 2009, Caldorera-Moore et al. 2010, Caldorera-Moore and Peppas 2009, Glangchai et al. 2008, Vartak and

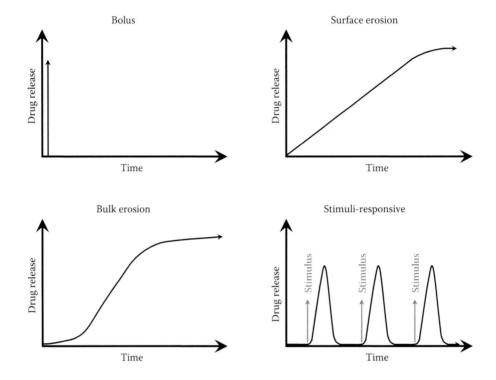

**FIGURE 17.5**   Release profiles of various delivery mechanisms. See Figure 17.2 for diffusion-driven release profiles.

Gemeinhart 2007). In most cases, enzyme-cleavable proteins, peptides, or extracellular matrix (ECM) components are incorporated into the hydrogel cross-links (Gobin and West 2002, Miyata et al. 2002, Zisch et al. 2003a). In another set-up, enzyme-degradable components are used as covalent linkers to conjugate drugs as pendant groups off the polymer backbone (Caldorera-Moore and Peppas 2009, Tauro et al. 2008). Upon encountering the enzyme, the cross-links are broken, releasing any encapsulated drug.

### 17.2.4  Overall Release Profiles

Oftentimes, the overall drug release mechanism may be due to a combination of the aforementioned modes. For example, diffusion plays a role in each of these mechanisms in that the drug must diffuse out of eroding scaffolds, or swollen matrices. Stimuli-responsive carriers may also release drug by stimuli-induced erosion or swelling. In choosing a release mechanism, the temporal requirements of drug in the system, as well as drug pharmacokinetics, must be considered.

There are several release profiles that may be achieved by the delivery systems described here (Figure 17.5). Several classical drug delivery systems were designed with the aim of achieving a zero order, or linear, release rate, which results in a constant level of drug in the tissues. However, newer drug delivery systems are designed to release drug when and where it is needed, thereby reducing side effects (Truskey et al. 2004, Hubbell 2008, Biondi et al. 2008, Becker and Göpferich 2007). Since spatial and temporal control over drug release is often required to guide the differentiation of cells into their appropriate niches, highly ordered systems with a combination of mechanisms may be required.

## 17.3  Drugs of Interest in Tissue Engineering

The primary drugs of interest for tissue engineering applications may be roughly divided into three groups: growth factors, adhesion factors, and nucleic acids. Growth factors are cell signaling proteins or

**TABLE 17.1**  Common Drugs or Bioactive Agents Used in Tissue Engineering

| Abbreviation | Bioactive Agent | Application |
|---|---|---|
| BMP | Bone morphogenetic protein | Osteogenesis |
| PTH | Human parathyroid hormone | Osteogeneisis |
| TGF-β | Transforming growth factor beta | Differentiation, anti-proliferation |
| HGF | Hepatocyte growth factor | Proliferation |
| G-CSF | Granulocyte colony-stimulating factor | Proliferation |
| GM-CSF | Granulocyte-macrophage colony-stimulating factor | Proliferation |
| VEGF | Vascular endothelial growth factor | Angiogenesis |
| FGF | Fibroblast growth factor | Angiogenesis |
| EPO | Erythropoietin | Angiogenesis |
| OPG | Osteoprotegerin | Angiogenesis |
| Ang1 | Angiopoietin-1 | Angiogenesis, vessel maturation |
| PDGF | Platelet-derived growth factor | Angiogenesis, vessel maturation |
| NGF | Nerve growth factor | Nerve regeneration |
| GDNF | Glial-derived neurotrophic factor | Nerve regeneration |
| | Fibronectin | Adhesion, cell substrate |
| | Vitronectin | Adhesion, cell substrate |
| | Fibrinogen | Adhesion, cell substrate |
| | Laminin | Adhesion, cell substrate |
| RGD | Arginine–Glycine–Asparagine | Adhesion |
| S1P | Sphingosine 1-phosphate | Chemoattractant |
| MIP3α | Macrophage inflammatory protein 3 alpha | Chemoattractant |

hormones that have an effect on cell differentiation, proliferation, and maturation through a process of ligand–receptor binding. Some examples of growth factors include bone morphogenetic proteins, vascular endothelial growth factors, and some cytokines. Adhesion factors are proteins and peptides that are typically bound to the ECM and relay mechanical stress feedback to the cell. Adhesion factors include vitronectin and fibronectin, as well as the fibronectin-derived peptide sequence, RGD. Some common proteins used in tissue engineering, as well as the intended function or purpose, are summarized in Table 17.1 (Hubbell 2008, Biondi et al. 2008, Chen and Mooney 2003, Haller and Saltzman 1998, Becker and Göpferich 2007, Robinson and Talmadge 2002, Tabata 2003, Zisch et al. 2003b). Nucleic acids (plasmid DNA, oligonucleotides, and siRNA) are used in tissue engineering primarily to direct progenitor cells into a specific phenotype or to express growth factors and morphogens *in situ* (Amiji 2005, Reynolds et al. 2004). A detailed discussion of this modality is beyond the scope of this chapter and can be found in the Gene Therapy (Chapter 18) and Cell Engineering (Chapter 19) chapters of this text. This chapter will predominantly focus on protein, peptide, and small-molecule drugs used directly as growth factors or adhesion factors.

## 17.3.1 Drug Properties and Design Considerations

Given that the majority of growth factors and adhesion factors are composed of bioactive proteins, or derivatives thereof, there are many considerations that must be made in order to design suitable systems for the delivery of these proteins in active forms. The most prominent consideration is the need to deliver the proteins in their native forms, that is, with their tertiary structure intact. Several methods of drug incorporation into delivery systems may cause protein denaturation from processing and encapsulation conditions, such as the application of heat, high shear forces, pH changes, UV, and exposure to organic solvents. Also considering that the majority of these proteins are hydrophilic, the choice of delivery materials is important in that exposure to hydrophobic materials may cause protein denaturation (Manning et al. 1989, 2010, Wang 1999). Lastly, the conditions that lead to drug release must also be evaluated to verify that they do not damage the protein. For example, in the case of hydrolytically degradable polyester drug carriers, a slightly acidic microenvironment is often created, which could affect protein activity (Fu et al. 2000). The final conformation of the protein must be such that its bioactivity is not affected, and there are no forms present that may elicit ill effects or immunogenicity (Hubbell 2008).

Along the same lines, the biological environment that the protein drugs are exposed to, whether *in vitro* or *in vivo*, may affect the protein conformation and activity. Several components in serum, including enzymes and peptidases, cause protein degradation often within minutes, decreasing the half-life dramatically. Glomerular, or renal, filtration also plays a key role in decreasing the half-life of proteins. For example, *in vivo*, the half-lives of PDGF, bFGF, and VEGF are approximately 2, 3, and 50 min respectively. A common strategy to improve the circulating half-lives of these proteins is to encapsulate them within polymers, however, care must be taken to ensure that the encapsulating material does not cause protein agglomeration or activate clotting factors (Manning et al. 1989, 2010, Wang 1999). Another common strategy is the conjugation of poly(ethylene glycol), or PEG, referred to as PEGylation (Eliason 2001, Molineux 2002, Roberts et al. 2002, Sato 2002). PEGylation of proteins has been shown to increase circulation time *in vivo* and decrease the rate of protein degradation by enzymes (Molineux 2003, Yang et al. 2004).

Aside from classical cell culture flasks and dishes, there has recently been an increased usage of ECM-mimicking gel matrices to serve both as a cell scaffold and as a controlled drug delivery device (Gobin and West 2002, Lutolf et al. 2003). These bioinspired matrices may be either hybrid synthetic and biomaterial or biomaterial alone, offer improved compatibility and stability with proteins, and have been designed to mimic the ways in which growth factors are released in the body (Wee and Gombotz 1998, Sano et al. 1998, Ikada and Tabata 1998, Lutolf et al. 2003). In the body, growth factors are either stored within the ECM or secreted by cells for short-term signaling. The ECM serves as a responsive delivery system for these growth factors, which may be controlled dynamically by cell movement and secretion of enzymes that degrade the matrix (Gobin and West 2002, Hubbell 2008). Adhesion factors in the ECM also relay mechanical feedback to the cells, and help the cells migrate as controlled by cellular signals (Wacker et al. 2008, Jia and Kiick 2009, Saltzman and Baldwin 1998). These ECM-mimicking systems offer several advantages over classical systems, as we will discuss in the following section.

## 17.4 Drug Delivery in Tissue Engineering

Given the complex temporal and spatial control of drug delivery required in tissue engineering, several strategies have been developed to meet the needs of this growing field. The strategies may be roughly classified into four major categories:

1. Classical drug delivery systems for use in cell culture or *in vivo* at local sites
2. Drug delivery from tissue engineering scaffolds and matrices
3. Cells (genetically altered or otherwise) to produce drugs in the system
4. Biomimetic systems with conjugated drugs

The primary focus of this chapter will be to discuss in greater detail the first two strategies, the use of classical drug delivery systems, and especially the delivery of drugs from the cell scaffolds and matrices. The latter two strategies are discussed in great lengths within the Gene Therapy (Chapter 18), and Cell Engineering (Chapter 19), and Biomimetics (Chapter 12) chapters.

### 17.4.1 Classical Drug Delivery Systems

Several classical drug delivery systems for tissue engineering are still in use for a wide variety of applications. The majority of these systems are employed to provide a means of long-term, controlled release of drugs into the local environment, whether *in vitro* or *in vivo*, for example, the use of poly(lactic-*co*-glycolic) acid (PLGA), microparticles for the controlled delivery of encapsulated growth factor. The required release profile may be chosen based on several factors including the rate of drug clearance from the system, pharmacokinetics, and stability. Thereafter, a system will be designed or chosen based on these requirements, considering parameters such as material properties, degradation rate, and device geometry. Generally, the major types of classical systems used include monolithic or slab-type systems, particulate systems, and gel-like systems.

### 17.4.1.1 Monolithic Systems

Monolithic polymer systems have a long history in drug delivery in that they were the first types of systems to be used for the controlled release of bioactive proteins and peptides. Among the first systems reported for controlled release was the polymeric membrane system composed of poly(ethylene-*co*-vinyl acetate) or EVAc, as described by Folkman and Langer in 1976 (Cao and Langer 2008). Although these systems were not biodegradable, the excellent controlled release profiles set the stage for an entirely new strategy of controlled release. In the following decade, several new biodegradable or bioerodible materials were developed with the aim of achieving sustained release *in vivo* without the need for removal after transplantation. Some of the materials included polyanhydrides (Jain et al. 2005), poly(ortho esters) (Heller 1985), and poly($\alpha$-hydroxyesters) (Lucke et al. 2002), with several more described in the literature. However, with the advent of these erodible systems came new unforeseen challenges due to the new intricacies of the system, including pH changes and side reactions with encapsulated drug due to the degraded products (Brunner et al. 1999, Fu et al. 2000, Van De Weert et al. 2000).

These early delivery systems were made in the form of monolithic devices because of their ease of manufacture by solvent casting, extrusion, and injection molding. These bulk devices were also able to carry a large payload of drug, and could be tailored for different release rates by changing material composition, drug loading, or including dispersants. As discussed in the previous section on the mechanisms of drug release, release from nondegradable systems is controlled primarily by diffusion. Erosion-controlled release provided more control over the release rate, which could be changed by the degradation rate, or by choosing between surface or bulk erosion. Monolithic devices based on the poly(lactic-*co*-glycolic acid) copolymer, PLGA, were and still are commonly used in the erodible systems because erosion may be well controlled by changing crystallinity, copolymer composition, and molecular weight (Athanasiou et al. 1998, Fu et al. 2000, Mohamed and Van Der Walle 2008, Sánchez et al. 2003, Thissen et al. 2006, Van De Weert et al. 2000). Other monolithic devices have been based on cross-linked hydrogels, and will be discussed in more detail in the following sections.

### 17.4.1.2 Particulate Systems

Following the progress made in monolithic and erodible devices, microparticulate systems began to surface in the field. Whereas monolithic systems required surgical implantation *in vivo* and are associated with a strong drug gradient, particulate systems offered the possibility of an injectable system and more even distribution in the tissue *in vivo*, or in cell culture. Microparticles also provided the flexibility for cell microencapsulation, or combinatorial delivery from microparticle distribution within monolithic systems or gels (Truskey et al. 2004, Becker and Göpferich 2007, Singh et al. 2009). Aside from microparticles, nanoparticles, liposomes, and other similar particulate technologies have also been explored; however, microparticles have been most widely applied to tissue engineering, and some of these other technologies will be discussed in other chapters.

Microparticulate systems have been widely used for the delivery of growth factors for directing cell differentiation and proliferation. One application that has been extensively studied is the use of both EVAc and PLGA microparticles to deliver nerve growth factor (NGF) for supporting cellular therapy in neurodegenerative diseases (Haller and Saltzman 1998). PLGA microparticles are also still in use for delivery of several other proteins, including BMP-2 (Kempen et al. 2008) and interferon-$\alpha$ (Sánchez et al. 2003). Poly(phosphoester) microspheres with encapsulated NGF loaded within silicone nerve conduits showed greater peripheral nerve regeneration as compared to conduits with free NGF loaded (Xu et al. 2003). Pfister et al. (2007) has reviewed other similar systems of NGF loaded microspheres for nerve regeneration. Excellent reviews may be found in the contemporary literature on the important considerations with protein encapsulation within polymer systems (Mohamed and Van Der Walle 2008, Van De Weert et al. 2000).

Hydrogel microparticles have also been used extensively to encapsulate proteins for drug delivery in tissue engineering. Some of the earliest hydrogel microparticle, or microgel, systems were the alginate beads, easily formed by dropping or spraying into cationic solutions, such as calcium (Wee and Gombotz 1998, Tønnesen and Karlsen 2002). Alginate microbeads are still widely used for delivery of FGF and osteogenic proteins (Lee et al. 2009, Moya et al. 2010a,b), as well as for microencapsulation of chondrocytes for coculture with bone marrow stem cells for osteogenic differentiation (Thompson et al. 2009). Along with alginate, microgels based on collagen (Nagai et al. 2010), gelatin (Li et al. 2010), and hyaluronan and its derivatives (Gaffney et al. 2010) are all used to deliver a variety of proteins.

Aside from encapsulation of proteins, much work has been done on the surface functionalization of microparticles for cellular interaction and proliferative effects. Surface modification of PLGA microspheres with an amine-terminated dendrimer improved long-term proliferation of chondrocytes without observed changes in the cell phenotype, as compared to monolayer culture systems (Thissen et al. 2006). Additionally, surface functionalization of polystyrene magnetic microbeads with the DLL4 notch ligand used in coculture has been shown to efficiently generate T cells from mouse bone marrow hematopoietic stem cells (Taqvi et al. 2006).

### 17.4.1.3 Gel-Based and Gel-Like Systems

Several gel-based and gel-like systems also offer the advantage of being injectable *in vivo*, taking on the shape of the tissue cavity. Additionally, the hydrophilic matrix structures of gels offer the advantage of high compatibility with the majority of proteins and peptides of interest in tissue engineering. Gelation occurs by several methods, including thermally- or pH-induced cross-linking (Zisch et al. 2003a,b), sol–gel transitions, and physical gelation. Early injectable gel-like systems include those composed of alginate, gelatin, and collagen (Wee and Gombotz 1998, Sano et al. 1998, Ikada and Tabata 1998). Although gel systems for protein delivery are a classical form of drug delivery, they have in recent decades gained much significance as a combinatorial tissue engineering substrate and drug delivery medium. As such, much attention will be directed toward these systems in the following section.

## 17.4.2 Drug Delivery from Tissue Engineering Scaffolds and Matrices

As the previous systems focused on controlled delivery strategies separate from a tissue engineering substrate, herein referred to as the substrate, much work has been done in using the substrate itself as a controlled release medium. Both scaffolds and matrices have been used to achieve desirable release strategies, where scaffolds refer to macro- or microporous substrates to provide structural support, and matrices refer to more or less continuous nanoporous substrates, such as gels. Several strategies may be used to achieve the desired effect, including the admixing of drugs within matrices, entrapment of drugs within matrices, covalent binding of drugs to the matrix, affinity binding of drugs to the matrix, and microparticles embedded in matrices for delivery of drug.

### 17.4.2.1 Drugs Admixed with Cell Substrate

A common form of drug delivery from the tissue engineering substrate is by simply admixing the drug with the cell substrate. As previously discussed, various mechanisms may be used to control the release, with the desired effect usually being prolongation of the release. In the case of prolongation, even a small degree of affinity between the substrate materials may serve to slow the release rate. Additionally, poorly soluble drugs may dissolve over time and provide a sustained release profile. The cell substrate may also serve as a diffusion-limiting factor, providing drug release in a localized area of the scaffold, also known as zonal release.

Several examples of drugs admixed within a cell substrate have already resulted in commercial products, especially the release of bone morphogenetic proteins from collagen sponges and matrices (Seeherman and Wozney 2005). Aside from the collagen sponge, other substrates for BMP delivery have included calcium phosphate cement, both of which have shown excellent orthopedic tissue regeneration *in vivo* (Seeherman and Wozney 2005, Seeherman et al. 2006, 2008, 2010). Gelatin, a form of denatured collagen, has also been used both in its native self-assembled gel form and as a cross-linked gel to deliver growth factors. During fabrication, gelatin may be modified into either negatively or positively charged gels at physiological pH in order to create low-affinity electrostatic interactions with a protein drug (Thyagarajapuram et al. 2007, Young et al. 2005, Ikada and Tabata 1998). These low-affinity electrostatic interactions of proteins with gelatin have been shown to prolong release rates as compared to nonelectrostatic gelatin (Thyagarajapuram et al. 2007, Yamamoto et al. 2006, Ozeki and Tabata 2006, Guo et al. 2010).

Growth factors have also been admixed with hydrophobic polymers, such as PLGA, to provide a sustained release profile. For example, early work by Richardson et al., used combinatorial PLGA scaffold and particulate systems to achieve dual growth factor delivery. In this case, one growth factor (VEGF) is admixed with particulate polymer along with microsphere-encapsulated growth factor (PDGF), which is then processed into a porous cell scaffold. By successfully achieving sustained release of both growth factors, improved angiogenesis was observed as compared to either growth factor alone (Richardson et al. 2001).

### 17.4.2.2 Drugs Entrapped within Cell Substrate

It is also possible to engineer hydrogel cell carriers with structures capable of physically trapping drug molecules within the cell carrier's molecular structure, most commonly, with hydrogels. Hydrogels form somewhat of a three-dimensional network structure, where the molecular weight and structure of the cross-linking molecule determines the pore size. If the pore size of the hydrogel is sufficiently close to the size of the drug of interest, then the release of the drug from the matrix could then be inhibited by the network structure (Lustig and Peppas 1988). In this case, drug release would be driven either by polymer swelling or degradation of cross-links. Commonly, the drug is loaded with the polymer precursor solutions, and the hydrogel network is then reacted to form around the drug (Lin and Anseth 2009, Jia and Kiick 2009, Metters and Hubbell 2005).

Common materials used for these systems include PEG, fibrin, collagen, and hyaluronic acid (Suri and Schmidt 2009, Lin and Anseth 2009, Jia and Kiick 2009, Metters and Hubbell 2005, Lutolf et al. 2003, Sakiyama-Elbert and Hubbell 2000). A study by van de Wettering et al. illustrated the ability to tune the release of human growth hormone (hGH) from various PEG-based hydrogels using different cross-linked network architectures. Tighter cross-linked networks were able to significantly prolong the release of hGH over loosely formed networks (Van De Wetering et al. 2005). In addition to single-component hydrogel networks, hybrid hydrogels of interpenetrated networks or semi-interpenetrated networks are similarly able to form diverse network structures of varying pore sizes and cross-linking densities (Suri and Schmidt 2009).

Due to the tight nanoporous properties of these hydrogels, which may prevent cell intergrowth, these systems are often employed as particulate systems within a scaffold. Scott et al. created PEG-based scaffolds using a modular assembly system of hydrogel microspheres with encapsulated sphingosine 1-phosphate (S1P), microspheres for structural support, and porogen particles. The resulting macroporous scaffolds with incorporated S1P-loaded microspheres showed an approximate twofold increase in rate of cell migration into the scaffold as compared to scaffolds without S1P-loaded microspheres (Scott et al. 2010). Alternatively, cell ingrowth into such nanoporous hydrogels may be achieved by incorporating enzyme-cleavable moieties into the network structure, thus allowing a cell to easily infiltrate the hydrogel by secreting ECM-degrading enzymes. Examples of these ingrowth matrices with entrapped drug include fibrin-based matrices for controlled release of NGF (Sakiyama-Elbert and Hubbell 2000) and

PEG-based matrices with matrix metalloproteinase substrates as cross-linkers with entrapped rhBMP (Lutolf et al. 2003).

### 17.4.2.3 Covalent Binding of Drugs to Cell Substrate

It is oftentimes advantageous, if not required, to covalently bind drugs to the cell substrate itself. For example, adhesion peptides must be bound to the substrate in order to elicit the correct response in the cell for migration. Although adhesion sites are already present in naturally derived materials, such as collagen and fibrin, cell substrates composed of synthetic components (such as PEG) must include adhesion peptides to effectively promote cell adhesion and signaling. Scaffolds of naturally derived materials may also benefit from adhesion peptide or growth factor incorporation to provide a higher degree of control over cell migration and differentiation.

In a study by Hern and Hubbell, the cell adhesion peptide RGD (Arg–Gly–Asp) was covalently bound to PEG-based hydrogels either directly or using a PEG spacer arm, and compared to a nonadhesive control peptide (Hern and Hubbell 1998). Due to the greater steric availability of the adhesion peptide bound to the PEG spacer arm, specific mediation of cell spreading was observed in contrast to nonspecific cell spreading observed in direct conjugation of the peptide to the scaffold. Wacker et al. compared S1P-induced endothelial cell migration in PEG hydrogels with either linear or cyclic RGD peptide sequences for implications in implant endothelialization speed following implantation (Wacker et al. 2008). Although linear RGD produced greater adhesion strength and long-term adhesion on exposure to shear stress from fluid flow, cyclic RGD produced a faster rate of endothelial cell migration. These studies illustrate the complexity in the incorporation of adhesion peptides into scaffolds, from determining the optimal conformation for steric availability, and finding the balance between high adhesion strength and higher migration rates for tissue regeneration.

In addition to covalent binding of adhesion peptides into cell substrates, drugs may also be covalently bound to the substrates in order to achieve directed differentiation, interaction, or promote migration of a specific cell phenotype. For example, vascularization of regenerated tissues is necessary for nutrient delivery *in vivo*, and requires high-order cell and tissue arrangement controlled by growth factors. Leslie-Barbick et al. were able to achieve endothelial cell tubulogenesis in 2D and 3D PEG-based scaffolds by covalently attaching VEGF and an RGD adhesion peptide, in comparison to RGD-immobilized scaffolds alone (Leslie-Barbick et al. 2009). Similarly, a study by Chiu and Radisic showed enhanced vascularization of endothelial cells in collagen scaffolds with immobilized VEGF and angiopoietin-1 over collagen scaffolds alone and soluble factor in collagen scaffolds alone (Chiu and Radisic 2010).

Furthermore, some drugs require binding to the substrate such that they are released only in response to cell ingrowth, for example, by enzymatic cleavage, providing on-demand delivery of the drug. In the case of bone regeneration, high concentrations of drug may result in overactivation of cells locally, and thus, abnormal tissue regeneration. By incorporating an enzyme-cleavable prodrug of a parathyroid hormone fragment into a cell ingrowth matrix, Arrighi et al. (2009) were able to circumvent osteoclast overactivation and show dose-dependent bone healing *in vivo*.

### 17.4.2.4 Affinity Binding of Drugs to Cell Substrate

Another strategy for binding drugs to a cell substrate involves the use of affinity binding molecules that have strong interactions with several growth factors and other proteins. A comprehensive review of the myriad molecules is outside the scope of this chapter, and we refer the reader to excellent reviews in the literature (Uebersax et al. 2009, Maxwell et al. 2005). Instead, we will focus on two groups of common affinity binding molecules: heparin/heparan sulfate and fibrin/fibrinogen. Other molecules of interest include laminins, collagens, glycosaminoglycans (GAGs), DNA, poly(amino acids), avidin-biotin (Baeza et al. 2010, Clapper et al. 2008, Segura et al. 2005), and other polysaccharides.

Heparan sulfate and heparin are GAGs that are present in a variety of tissues throughout the body, regulate many processes, and bind a variety of proteins or growth factors. There are several growth factors that bind to both heparan sulfate and heparin, and are known as heparin binding growth factors (HBGFs). Commonly noted HBGFs include members of the families of FGF, HGF, and VEGFs. Heparan sulfate has been used in micropatterned PEG-based scaffolds for spatiotemporal release of growth factors and multilineage differentiation (Mapili et al. 2005), and widely in other applications (Woodruff et al. 2007, Pieper et al. 2002, Chintala et al. 1995). However, due to lower costs, heparin is more widely used in cell substrates for HBGFs, and has been incorporated into gels for osteogenic differentiation (Benoit et al. 2007, Benoit and Anseth 2005), endothelialization (Mcgonigle et al. 2008, Tae et al. 2006), nerve regeneration (Wood et al. 2009, 2010), and a variety of other applications (Uebersax et al. 2009, Kiick 2008, Nie et al. 2007, Zhang et al. 2006).

Fibrin and fibrinogen are proteins found in the blood that are critical in the clotting and wound sealing process; cleavage of fibrinogen by thrombin yields fibrin (Spicer and Mikos 2010, Uebersax et al. 2009, Sierra 1993). Fibrinogen is used primarily in fibrin glue systems, where a mixture of fibrinogen solution and calcium-rich thrombin solution are codelivered for surgical use as a sealant or hemostatic agent (Sierra 1993, Spicer and Mikos 2010), but has recently gained more interest as a cell substrate with protein immobilization capabilities (Spicer and Mikos 2010). Fibrin is widely used for its affinity binding characteristics with other proteins to slowly release growth factors, particularly VEGF and FGF, to loaded cells within the gel (Ehrbar et al. 2008, Losi et al. 2010). Work by the Swartz group used VEGF bound to fibrin-based matrices along with interstitial fluid flow in order to direct blood and lymphatic capillary morphogenesis, resulting in organized tubular structures (Helm et al. 2005, 2007). Hybrid PEG and fibrin matrices have also been used to create cell substrates with the ability to entrap, covalently conjugate, and affinity bind growth factors, and have tunable mechanical properties for directed differentiation (Drinnan et al. 2010, Zhang et al. 2010). PEG-based materials that mimic the fibrin clotting cascade, known as fibrin analogs, have also been created for tissue engineering applications (Ehrbar et al. 2007).

### 17.4.2.5 Particulate Systems within Cell Substrate

Microparticles, and to a lesser extent, nanoparticles, may often be incorporated into cell substrates to provide another mechanism of controlled drug release to the cells. The complexities in these systems are vast when considering the combinations of material properties, release profiles, release mechanisms, or substrate construct. In some cases, the particles may be hydrophobic and rely on hydrolysis to control the release of growth factors, as in the release of BMPs from PLGA microspheres in scaffolds and matrices (Ji et al. 2010, Gavenis et al. 2010, Li et al. 2009a, Wang et al. 2009). In other cases, the particles provide a facile means in which to provide controlled delivery of growth factors *in vivo*, for example, by injection (Li et al. 2009b, Sasaki et al. 2008, Inoue et al. 2006) or intratracheally (Hirose et al. 2008). Particles may also serve as cell carriers themselves, or assemble into a cell substrate at a later stage (Scott et al. 2010).

## 17.5 Outlook

The concepts of controlled release and controlled ligand presentation in tissue engineering are gaining increasing interest and are now considered to be integral to the success of tissue regeneration and cell engineering. The merging of the two complementary fields, tissue engineering and drug delivery, is providing exciting new directions in regenerative medicine. Although significant progress has been made in incorporating temporally controlled growth factor release from scaffolds, as well as in efficient presentation of adhesive ligands, there remain considerable challenges in mimicking the complex, spatially and temporally patterned microenvironments of tissues *in vivo*. The complicated milieu of growth factors, morphogens, extracellular matrix components, and cell signaling must be accurately reproduced if complex, functionally relevant tissue structures are to be regenerated and engineered. Future directions in tissue engineering therefore must incorporate and develop new drug delivery concepts where multiple bioactive agents can be available to progenitor cells in a highly spatially controlled manner and at levels and sequences relevant to the differentiation kinetics of specific tissues.

# References

Aimetti, A. A., A. J. Machen, and K. S. Anseth. 2009. Poly(ethylene glycol) hydrogels formed by thiol-ene photopolymerization for enzyme-responsive protein delivery. *Biomaterials* 30: 6048–54.

Amiji, M. M. 2005. *Polymeric Gene Delivery: Principles and Applications.* Boca Raton, FL: CRC Press.

Annabi, N., J. W. Nichol, X. Zhong et al. 2010. Controlling the porosity and microarchitecture of hydrogels for tissue engineering. *Tissue Eng Pt B Rev* 16: 371–83.

Arrighi, I., S. Mark, M. Alvisi et al. 2009. Bone healing induced by local delivery of an engineered parathyroid hormone prodrug. *Biomaterials* 30: 1763–71.

Athanasiou, K. A., C. M. Agrawal, F. A. Barber, and S. S. Burkhart. 1998. Orthopaedic applications for pla-pga biodegradable polymers. *Arthroscopy* 14: 726–37.

Baeza, A., I. Izquierdo-Barba, and M. Vallet-Regí. 2010. Biotinylation of silicon-doped hydroxyapatite: A new approach to protein fixation for bone tissue regeneration. *Acta Biomater* 6: 743–49.

Becker, C. and A. Göpferich. 2007. Drug delivery. In *Tissue Engineering,* ed. Fisher, J. P., A. G. Mikos and J. D. Bronzino (Eds.) 600. Boca Raton: CRC Press.

Benoit, D. S. W. and K. S. Anseth. 2005. Heparin functionalized PEG gels that modulate protein adsorption for hmsc adhesion and differentiation. *Acta Biomater* 1: 461–70.

Benoit, D. S. W., A. R. Durney, and K. S. Anseth. 2007. The effect of heparin-functionalized PEG hydrogels on three-dimensional human mesenchymal stem cell osteogenic differentiation. *Biomaterials* 28: 66–77.

Biondi, M., F. Ungaro, F. Quaglia, and P. A. Netti. 2008. Controlled drug delivery in tissue engineering. *Adv Drug Deliv Rev* 60: 229–42.

Boontheekul, T. and D. J. Mooney. 2003. Protein-based signaling systems in tissue engineering. *Curr Opin Biotechnol* 14: 559–65.

Boussif, O., F. Lezoualc'h, M. A. Zanta et al. 1995. A versatile vector for gene and oligonucleotide transfer into cells in culture and *in vivo*: Polyethylenimine. *PNAS* 92: 7297–301.

Brunner, A., K. Mäder, and A. Göpferich. 1999. Ph and osmotic pressure inside biodegradable microspheres during erosion. *Pharm Res* 16: 847–53.

Caldorera-Moore, M., N. Guimard, L. Shi, and K. Roy. 2010. Designer nanoparticles: Incorporating size, shape and triggered release into nanoscale drug carriers. *Expert Opin Drug Deliv* 7: 479–95.

Caldorera-Moore, M. and N. A. Peppas. 2009. Micro- and nanotechnologies for intelligent and responsive biomaterial-based medical systems. *Adv Drug Deliv Rev* 61: 1391–401.

Cao, Y. and R. Langer. 2008. A review of Judah Folkman's remarkable achievements in biomedicine. *PNAS* 105: 13203.

Chen, R. R. and D. J. Mooney. 2003. Polymeric growth factor delivery strategies for tissue engineering. *Pharm Res* 20: 1103–12.

Chintala, S. K., R. R. Miller, and C. A. Mcdevitt. 1995. Role of heparan sulfate in the terminal differentiation of growth plate chondrocytes. *Arch Biochem Biophys* 316: 227–34.

Chiu, L. L. Y. and M. Radisic. 2010. Scaffolds with covalently immobilized VEGF and angiopoietin-1 for vascularization of engineered tissues. *Biomaterials* 31: 226–41.

Clapper, J. D., M. E. Pearce, C. A. Guymon, and A. K. Salem. 2008. Biotinylated biodegradable nanotemplated hydrogel networks for cell interactive applications. *Biomacromolecules* 9: 1188–94.

Drinnan, C. T., G. Zhang, M. A. Alexander, A. S. Pulido, and L. J. Suggs. 2010. Multimodal release of transforming growth factor-beta1 and the bb isoform of platelet derived growth factor from pegylated fibrin gels. *J Control Release* 147: 180–86.

Ehrbar, M., S. C. Rizzi, R. Hlushchuk et al. 2007. Enzymatic formation of modular cell-instructive fibrin analogs for tissue engineering. *Biomaterials* 28: 3856–66.

Ehrbar, M., S. M. Zeisberger, G. P. Raeber et al. 2008. The role of actively released fibrin-conjugated VEGF for VEGF receptor 2 gene activation and the enhancement of angiogenesis. *Biomaterials* 29: 1720–29.

Eliason, J. F. 2001. Pegylated cytokines: Potential application in immunotherapy of cancer. *BioDrugs* 15: 705–11.

Fisher, O. Z., A. Khademhosseini, R. Langer, and N. A. Peppas. 2010. Bioinspired materials for controlling stem cell fate. *Acc Chem Res* 43: 419–28.

Fu, K., D. W. Pack, A. M. Klibanov, and R. Langer. 2000. Visual evidence of acidic environment within degrading poly(lactic-*co*-glycolic acid) (PLGA) microspheres. *Pharm Res* 17: 100–16.

Gaffney, J., S. Matou-Nasri, M. Grau-Olivares and M. Slevin. 2010. Therapeutic applications of hyaluronan. *Mol Biosyst* 6: 437–43.

Gallardo, D., B. Skalsky, and P. Kleinebudde. 2008. Controlled release solid dosage forms using combinations of (meth)acrylate copolymers. *Pharm Dev Technol* 13: 413–23.

Gavenis, K., U. Schneider, J. Groll, and B. Schmidt-Rohlfing. 2010. BMP-7-loaded PGLA microspheres as a new delivery system for the cultivation of human chondrocytes in a collagen type I gel: The common nude mouse model. *Int J Artif Organs* 33: 45–53.

Glangchai, L. C., M. Caldorera-Moore, L. Shi, and K. Roy. 2008. Nanoimprint lithography based fabrication of shape-specific, enzymatically-triggered smart nanoparticles. *J Control Release* 125: 263–72.

Gobin, A. S. and J. L. West. 2002. Cell migration through defined, synthetic ecm analogs. *FASEB J* 16: 751–53.

Gombotz, W. R. and D. K. Pettit. 1995. Biodegradable polymers for protein and peptide drug delivery. *Bioconjug Chem* 6: 332–51.

Göpferich, A. 1996. Mechanisms of polymer degradation and erosion. *Biomaterials* 17: 103–14.

Guo, X., H. Park, S. Young et al. 2010. Repair of osteochondral defects with biodegradable hydrogel composites encapsulating marrow mesenchymal stem cells in a rabbit model. *Acta Biomater* 6: 39–47.

Haller, M. F. and W. M. Saltzman. 1998. Nerve growth factor delivery systems. *J Control Release* 53: 1–6.

Heller, J. 1985. Controlled drug release from poly(ortho esters). *Ann N Y Acad Sci* 446: 51–66.

Helm, C.-L. E., M. E. Fleury, A. H. Zisch, F. Boschetti, and M. A. Swartz. 2005. Synergy between interstitial flow and VEGF directs capillary morphogenesis *in vitro* through a gradient amplification mechanism. *PNAS* 102: 15779–84.

Helm, C.-L. E., A. Zisch, and M. A. Swartz. 2007. Engineered blood and lymphatic capillaries in 3-d VEGF-fibrin-collagen matrices with interstitial flow. *Biotechnol Bioeng* 96: 167–76.

Hern, D. and J. Hubbell. 1998. Incorporation of adhesion peptides into nonadhesive hydrogels useful for tissue resurfacing. *J Biomed Mater Res* 39: 266–76.

Hirose, K., A. Marui, Y. Arai et al. 2008. Novel approach with intratracheal administration of microgelatin hydrogel microspheres incorporating basic fibroblast growth factor for rescue of rats with monocrotaline-induced pulmonary hypertension. *J Thorac Cardiovasc Surg* 136: 1250–56.

Hubbell, J. 2008. Controlled release strategies in tissue engineering. In *Tissue Engineering*, ed. Blitterswijk, C. A. V. and P. Thomsen (Eds.) 740. Boston: Elsevier/Academic Press.

Ikada, Y. and Y. Tabata. 1998. Protein release from gelatin matrices. *Adv Drug Deliv Rev* 31: 287–301.

Inoue, A., K. A. Takahashi, Y. Arai et al. 2006. The therapeutic effects of basic fibroblast growth factor contained in gelatin hydrogel microspheres on experimental osteoarthritis in the rabbit knee. *Arthritis Rheum* 54: 264–70.

Jain, J. P., S. Modi, A. J. Domb, and N. Kumar. 2005. Role of polyanhydrides as localized drug carriers. *J Control Release* 103: 541–63.

Ji, Y., G. P. Xu, Z. P. Zhang et al. 2010. BMP-2/PLGA delayed-release microspheres composite graft, selection of bone particulate diameters, and prevention of aseptic inflammation for bone tissue engineering. *Ann Biomed Eng* 38: 632–39.

Jia, X. and K. L. Kiick. 2009. Hybrid multicomponent hydrogels for tissue engineering. *Macromol Biosci* 9: 140–56.

Kempen, D. H. R., L. Lu, T. E. Hefferan et al. 2008. Retention of *in vitro* and *in vivo* BMP-2 bioactivities in sustained delivery vehicles for bone tissue engineering. *Biomaterials* 29: 3245–52.

Khare, A. R. and N. A. Peppas. 1993. Release behavior of bioactive agents from pH-sensitive hydrogels. *J Biomater Sci Polym Ed* 4: 275–89.

Khare, A. R. and N. A. Peppas. 1995. Swelling/deswelling of anionic copolymer gels. *Biomaterials* 16: 559–67.

Kiick, K. L. 2008. Peptide- and protein-mediated assembly of heparinized hydrogels. *Soft Matter* 4: 29–37.

Klein, T. J., J. Malda, R. L. Sah, and D. W. Hutmacher. 2009. Tissue engineering of articular cartilage with biomimetic zones. *Tissue Eng Part B Rev* 15: 143–57.

Langer, R. and N. Peppas. 2003. Advances in biomaterials, drug delivery, and bionanotechnology. *AIChE J* 49: 2990–3006.

Langer, R. and J. P. Vacanti. 1993. Tissue engineering. *Science* 260: 920–26.

Lavan, D. A., T. Mcguire, and R. Langer. 2003. Small-scale systems for *in vivo* drug delivery. *Nat Biotechnol* 21: 1184–91.

Lee, M., W. Li, R. K. Siu et al. 2009. Biomimetic apatite-coated alginate/chitosan microparticles as osteogenic protein carriers. *Biomaterials* 30: 6094–101.

Leslie-Barbick, J. E., J. J. Moon, and J. L. West. 2009. Covalently-immobilized vascular endothelial growth factor promotes endothelial cell tubulogenesis in poly(ethylene glycol) diacrylate hydrogels. *J Biomater Sci Polym Ed* 20: 1763–79.

Li, B., T. Yoshii, A. E. Hafeman et al. 2009a. The effects of rhbmp-2 released from biodegradable polyurethane/microsphere composite scaffolds on new bone formation in rat femora. *Biomaterials* 30: 6768–79.

Li, L., H. Okada, G. Takemura et al. 2009b. Sustained release of erythropoietin using biodegradable gelatin hydrogel microspheres persistently improves lower leg ischemia. *J Am Coll Cardiol* 53: 2378–88.

Li, M., X. Liu, X. Liu, and B. Ge. 2010. Calcium phosphate cement with BMP-2-loaded gelatin microspheres enhances bone healing in osteoporosis: A pilot study. *Clin Orthop Relat Res* 468: 1978–85.

Lin, C.-C. and K. S. Anseth. 2009. PEG hydrogels for the controlled release of biomolecules in regenerative medicine. *Pharm Res* 26: 631–43.

Liu, F. and A. W. Basit. 2010. A paradigm shift in enteric coating: Achieving rapid release in the proximal small intestine of man. *J Control Release* 147: 242–45.

Losi, P., E. Briganti, A. Magera et al. 2010. Tissue response to poly(ether)urethane-polydimethylsiloxane-fibrin composite scaffolds for controlled delivery of pro-angiogenic growth factors. *Biomaterials* 31: 5336–44.

Löwik, D. W. P. M., E. H. P. Leunissen, M. Van Den Heuvel, M. B. Hansen, and J. C. M. Van Hest. 2010. Stimulus responsive peptide based materials. *Chem Soc Rev* 39: 3394–412.

Lucke, A., J. Kiermaier, and A. Göpferich. 2002. Peptide acylation by poly(alpha-hydroxy esters). *Pharm Res* 19: 175–81.

Lustig, S. and N. Peppas. 1988. Solute diffusion in swollen membranes. Ix. Scaling laws for solute diffusion in gels. *J Appl Polym Sci* 36: 735–47.

Lutolf, M. P., F. E. Weber, H. G. Schmoekel et al. 2003. Repair of bone defects using synthetic mimetics of collagenous extracellular matrices. *Nat Biotechnol* 21: 513–18.

Manning, M. C., D. K. Chou, B. M. Murphy, R. W. Payne, and D. S. Katayama. 2010. Stability of protein pharmaceuticals: An update. *Pharm Res* 27: 544–75.

Manning, M. C., K. Patel, and R. T. Borchardt. 1989. Stability of protein pharmaceuticals. *Pharm Res* 6: 903–18.

Mapili, G., Y. Lu, S. Chen, and K. Roy. 2005. Laser-layered microfabrication of spatially patterned functionalized tissue-engineering scaffolds. *J Biomed Mater Res B* 75: 414–24.

Maxwell, D. J., B. C. Hicks, S. Parsons, and S. E. Sakiyama-Elbert. 2005. Development of rationally designed affinity-based drug delivery systems. *Acta Biomater* 1: 101–13.

McGonigle, J. S., G. Tae, P. S. Stayton, A. S. Hoffman, and M. Scatena. 2008. Heparin-regulated delivery of osteoprotegerin promotes vascularization of implanted hydrogels. *J Biomater Sci Polym Ed* 19: 1021–34.

Metters, A. and J. A. Hubbell. 2005. Network formation and degradation behavior of hydrogels formed by michael-type addition reactions. *Biomacromolecules* 6: 290–301.

Miyata, T., T. Uragami, and K. Nakamae. 2002. Biomolecule-sensitive hydrogels. *Adv Drug Deliv Rev* 54: 79–98.

Mohamed, F. and C. F. Van Der Walle. 2008. Engineering biodegradable polyester particles with specific drug targeting and drug release properties. *J Pharm Sci* 97: 71–87.

Molineux, G. 2002. Pegylation: Engineering improved pharmaceuticals for enhanced therapy. *Cancer Treat Rev* 28 Suppl A: 13–16.

Molineux, G. 2003. Pegylation: Engineering improved biopharmaceuticals for oncology. *Pharmacotherapy* 23: 3S-8S.

Moya, M. L., M.-H. Cheng, J.-J. Huang et al. 2010a. The effect of fgf-1 loaded alginate microbeads on neovascularization and adipogenesis in a vascular pedicle model of adipose tissue engineering. *Biomaterials* 31: 2816–26.

Moya, M. L., M. R. Garfinkel, X. Liu et al. 2010b. Fibroblast growth factor-1 (fgf-1) loaded microbeads enhance local capillary neovascularization. *J Surg Res* 160: 208–12.

Nagai, N., N. Kumasaka, T. Kawashima et al. 2010. Preparation and characterization of collagen microspheres for sustained release of VEGF. *J Mater Sci Mater Med* 21: 1891–98.

Nie, T., A. Baldwin, N. Yamaguchi, and K. L. Kiick. 2007. Production of heparin-functionalized hydrogels for the development of responsive and controlled growth factor delivery systems. *J Control Release* 122: 287–96.

Nomi, M., A. Atala, P. D. Coppi, and S. Soker. 2002. Principals of neovascularization for tissue engineering. *Mol Aspects Med* 23: 463–83.

Ozeki, M. and Y. Tabata. 2006. Interaction of hepatocyte growth factor with gelatin as the carrier material. *J Biomater Sci Polym Ed* 17: 163–75.

Peppas, N. A., P. Bures, W. Leobandung, and H. Ichikawa. 2000. Hydrogels in pharmaceutical formulations. *Eur J Pharm Biopharm* 50: 27–46.

Pfister, L. A., M. Papaloïzos, H. P. Merkle, and B. Gander. 2007. Nerve conduits and growth factor delivery in peripheral nerve repair. *J Peripher Nerv Syst* 12: 65–82.

Pieper, J. S., T. Hafmans, P. B. Van Wachem et al. 2002. Loading of collagen-heparan sulfate matrices with bFGF promotes angiogenesis and tissue generation in rats. *J Biomed Mater Res* 62: 185–94.

Putnam, D., C. A. Gentry, D. W. Pack, and R. Langer. 2001. Polymer-based gene delivery with low cytotoxicity by a unique balance of side-chain termini. *PNAS* 98: 1200–5.

Reynolds, A., D. Leake, Q. Boese et al. 2004. Rational siRNA design for RNA interference. *Nat Biotechnol* 22: 326–30.

Richardson, T. P., M. C. Peters, A. B. Ennett, and D. J. Mooney. 2001. Polymeric system for dual growth factor delivery. *Nat Biotechnol* 19: 1029–34.

Roberts, M. J., M. D. Bentley, and J. M. Harris. 2002. Chemistry for peptide and protein pegylation. *Adv Drug Deliv Rev* 54: 459–76.

Robinson, S. N. and J. E. Talmadge. 2002. Sustained release of growth factors. *In Vivo* 16: 535–40.

Sakiyama-Elbert, S. E., and J. A. Hubbell. 2000. Controlled release of nerve growth factor from a heparin-containing fibrin-based cell ingrowth matrix. *J Control Release* 69: 149–58.

Saltzman, W. M. and S. Baldwin. 1998. Materials for protein delivery in tissue engineering. *Adv Drug Deliv Rev* 33: 71–86.

Saltzman, W. M. and W. L. Olbricht. 2002. Building drug delivery into tissue engineering. *Nat Rev Drug Discov* 1: 177–86.

Sánchez, A., M. Tobío, L. González, A. Fabra, and M. J. Alonso. 2003. Biodegradable micro- and nanoparticles as long-term delivery vehicles for interferon-alpha. *Eur J Pharm Sci* 18: 221–29.

Sano, A., T. Hojo, M. Maeda, and K. Fujioka. 1998. Protein release from collagen matrices. *Adv Drug Deliv Rev* 31: 247–66.

Sasaki, N., T. Minami, K. Yamada et al. 2008. *In vivo* effects of intra-articular injection of gelatin hydrogen microspheres containing basic fibroblast growth factor on experimentally induced defects in third metacarpal bones of horses. *Am J Vet Res* 69: 1555–59.

Sato, H. 2002. Enzymatic procedure for site-specific pegylation of proteins. *Adv Drug Deliv Rev* 54: 487–504.

Scott, E. A., M. D. Nichols, R. Kuntz-Willits, and D. L. Elbert. 2010. Modular scaffolds assembled around living cells using poly(ethylene glycol) microspheres with macroporation via a non-cytotoxic porogen. *Acta Biomater* 6: 29–38.

Seeherman, H. J., J. M. Archambault, S. A. Rodeo et al. 2008. Rhbmp-12 accelerates healing of rotator cuff repairs in a sheep model. *J Bone Joint Surg Am* 90: 2206–19.

Seeherman, H., R. Li, M. Bouxsein et al. 2006. Rhbmp-2/calcium phosphate matrix accelerates osteotomy-site healing in a nonhuman primate model at multiple treatment times and concentrations. *J Bone Joint Surg Am* 88: 144–60.

Seeherman, H. J., X. J. Li, M. L. Bouxsein, and J. M. Wozney. 2010. Rhbmp-2 induces transient bone resorption followed by bone formation in a nonhuman primate core-defect model. *J Bone Joint Surg Am* 92: 411–26.

Seeherman, H. and J. M. Wozney. 2005. Delivery of bone morphogenetic proteins for orthopedic tissue regeneration. *Cytokine Growth Factor Rev* 16: 329–45.

Segura, T., B. C. Anderson, P. H. Chung et al. 2005. Crosslinked hyaluronic acid hydrogels: A strategy to functionalize and pattern. *Biomaterials* 26: 359–71.

Sierra, D. H. 1993. Fibrin sealant adhesive systems: A review of their chemistry, material properties and clinical applications. *J Biomater Appl* 7: 309–52.

Singh, A., S. Suri, and K. Roy. 2009. In-situ crosslinking hydrogels for combinatorial delivery of chemokines and sirna-DNA carrying microparticles to dendritic cells. *Biomaterials* 30: 5187–200.

Spicer, P. P. and A. G. Mikos. 2010. Fibrin glue as a drug delivery system. *J Control Release* 148: 49–55.

Steinbüchel, A. and S. Matsumura. 2003. *Biopolymers: Miscellaneous Biopolymers and Biodegradation of Synthetic Polymers*. Weinheim: Wiley-VCH.

Suri, S. and C. E. Schmidt. 2009. Photopatterned collagen-hyaluronic acid interpenetrating polymer network hydrogels. *Acta Biomater* 5: 2385–97.

Tabata, Y. 2003. Tissue regeneration based on growth factor release. *Tissue Eng* 9 Suppl 1: S5–15.

Tae, G., M. Scatena, P. S. Stayton, and A. S. Hoffman. 2006. PEG-cross-linked heparin is an affinity hydrogel for sustained release of vascular endothelial growth factor. *J Biomater Sci Polym Ed* 17: 187–97.

Taqvi, S., L. Dixit, and K. Roy. 2006. Biomaterial-based notch signaling for the differentiation of hematopoietic stem cells into t cells. *J Biomed Mater Res A* 79: 689–97.

Tauro, J. R., B.-S. Lee, S. S. Lateef, and R. A. Gemeinhart. 2008. Matrix metalloprotease selective peptide substrates cleavage within hydrogel matrices for cancer chemotherapy activation. *Peptides* 29: 1965–73.

Thissen, H., K.-Y. Chang, T. A. Tebb et al. 2006. Synthetic biodegradable microparticles for articular cartilage tissue engineering. *J Biomed Mater Res A* 77: 590–98.

Thompson, A. D., M. W. Betz, D. M. Yoon, and J. P. Fisher. 2009. Osteogenic differentiation of bone marrow stromal cells induced by coculture with chondrocytes encapsulated in three-dimensional matrices. *Tissue Eng Pt A* 15: 1181–90.

Thyagarajapuram, N., D. Olsen, and C. R. Middaugh. 2007. The structure, stability, and complex behavior of recombinant human gelatins. *J Pharm Sci* 96: 3363–78.

Tønnesen, H. H. and J. Karlsen. 2002. Alginate in drug delivery systems. *Drug Dev Ind Pharm* 28: 621–30.

Truskey, G. A., F. Yuan, and D. F. Katz. 2004. *Transport Phenomena in Biological Systems*. Upper Saddle River: Pearson/Prentice Hall.

Uebersax, L., H. P. Merkle, and L. Meinel. 2009. Biopolymer-based growth factor delivery for tissue repair: From natural concepts to engineered systems. *Tissue Eng Pt B Rev* 15: 263–89.

Van De Weert, M., W. E. Hennink, and W. Jiskoot. 2000. Protein instability in poly(lactic-*co*-glycolic acid) microparticles. *Pharm Res* 17: 1159–67.

Van De Wetering, P., A. T. Metters, R. G. Schoenmakers, and J. A. Hubbell. 2005. Poly(ethylene glycol) hydrogels formed by conjugate addition with controllable swelling, degradation, and release of pharmaceutically active proteins. *J Control Release* 102: 619–27.

Vartak, D. G. and R. A. Gemeinhart. 2007. Matrix metalloproteases: Underutilized targets for drug delivery. *J Drug Target* 15: 1–20.

Wacker, B. K., S. K. Alford, E. A. Scott et al. 2008. Endothelial cell migration on RGD-peptide-containing PEG hydrogels in the presence of sphingosine 1-phosphate. *Biophys J* 94: 273–85.

Wanakule, P. and K. Roy. 2012. Disease-responsive drug delivery: The next generation of smart delivery devices. *Curr Drug Metab* 13: 42–9.

Wang, C.-K., M.-L. Ho, G.-J. Wang et al. 2009. Controlled-release of rhbmp-2 carriers in the regeneration of osteonecrotic bone. *Biomaterials* 30: 4178–86.

Wang, W. 1999. Instability, stabilization, and formulation of liquid protein pharmaceuticals. *Int J Pharm* 185: 129–88.

Wee, S. and W. Gombotz. 1998. Protein release from alginate matrices. *Adv Drug Deliv Rev* 31: 267–85.

Williams, D. F. 1986. Definitions in biomaterials. Proceedings of The European Society for Biomaterials Consensus Conference in Chester, England.

Wood, M. D., M. R. Macewan, A. R. French et al. 2010. Fibrin matrices with affinity-based delivery systems and neurotrophic factors promote functional nerve regeneration. *Biotechnol Bioeng* 106: 970–79.

Wood, M. D., A. M. Moore, D. A. Hunter et al. 2009. Affinity-based release of glial-derived neurotrophic factor from fibrin matrices enhances sciatic nerve regeneration. *Acta Biomater* 5: 959–68.

Woodruff, M. A., S. N. Rath, E. Susanto et al. 2007. Sustained release and osteogenic potential of heparan sulfate-doped fibrin glue scaffolds within a rat cranial model. *J Mol Histol* 38: 425–33.

Xu, X., W.-C. Yee, P. Y. K. Hwang et al. 2003. Peripheral nerve regeneration with sustained release of poly(phosphoester) microencapsulated nerve growth factor within nerve guide conduits. *Biomaterials* 24: 2405–12.

Yamamoto, M., Y. Takahashi, and Y. Tabata. 2006. Enhanced bone regeneration at a segmental bone defect by controlled release of bone morphogenetic protein-2 from a biodegradable hydrogel. *Tissue Eng.* 12: 1305–11.

Yang, B.-B., P. K. Lum, M. M. Hayashi, and L. K. Roskos. 2004. Polyethylene glycol modification of filgrastim results in decreased renal clearance of the protein in rats. *J Pharm Sci* 93: 1367–73.

Young, S., M. Wong, Y. Tabata, and A. G. Mikos. 2005. Gelatin as a delivery vehicle for the controlled release of bioactive molecules. *J Control Release* 109: 256–74.

Zhang, G., C. T. Drinnan, L. R. Geuss, and L. J. Suggs. 2010. Vascular differentiation of bone marrow stem cells is directed by a tunable three-dimensional matrix. *Acta Biomater* 6: 3395–403.

Zhang, L., E. M. Furst, and K. L. Kiick. 2006. Manipulation of hydrogel assembly and growth factor delivery via the use of peptide-polysaccharide interactions. *J Control Release* 114: 130–42.

Zisch, A. H., M. P. Lutolf, M. Ehrbar et al. 2003a. Cell-demanded release of VEGF from synthetic, biointeractive cell ingrowth matrices for vascularized tissue growth. *FASEB J* 17: 2260–62.

Zisch, A. H., M. P. Lutolf, and J. A. Hubbell. 2003b. Biopolymeric delivery matrices for angiogenic growth factors. *Cardiovasc Pathol* 12: 295–310.

# 18

# Gene Therapy

C. Holladay
*National University of Ireland, Galway*

M. Kulkarni
*National University of Ireland, Galway*

W. Minor
*National University of Ireland, Galway*

Abhay Pandit
*National University of Ireland, Galway*

18.1 Introduction .................................................................. 18-1
18.2 Delivery Technique (Vector) ..................................... 18-2
 Viral • Nonviral • Scaffolds • Cell-Mediated Gene Therapy
18.3 Systemic and Local Gene Delivery .......................... 18-6
 Dose
18.4 Therapeutic Preclinical or Clinical Trials ............... 18-8
 Bone • Diabetic Wound Healing • Lower-Limb
 Ischemia • Myocardial Infarction • Cancer
18.5 Summary .................................................................... 18-18
Acknowledgments ................................................................ 18-19
References .............................................................................. 18-19

## 18.1 Introduction

The area of gene therapy is considered to have its roots in the early 1960s with the birth of genetic transformation of eukaryotic cells *in vitro* (Friedmann, 1992), although it could be argued that it was the transformation of pneumococcal cells in the 1940s that really inspired the concept (Avery et al., 1944). Another critical leap was made in the early 1980s with the work of Spradling and Rubin in Drosophilia, where exogeneous DNA sequences were introduced into germ line cells in order to correct a genetic defect (Rubin and Spradling, 1982, Spradling and Rubin, 1982). In the subsequent years, gene therapy has been proposed for a variety of genetic diseases (Friedmann, 1989) as well as other, more organ-specific pathologies.

> Gene therapy broadly encompasses any technique used to regulate eukaryotic protein expression by manipulation of the genetic machinery. This includes everything from delivery of DNA sequences to miRNA interference of mRNA translation to delivery of cells with altered genomes.

This can take the form of permanently inserting a gene into a nonspecific location on a chromosome in order to replace a nonfunctional gene, regulating a specific gene, temporarily placing a gene in the nucleus to be expressed for a short period, replacing an original, impaired gene or gene promoter with a functioning sequence using homologous recombination, or repairing an impaired gene using selective reverse mutation to return a gene to normal function.

Unlike drug delivery, a cell transfected by gene delivery to produce a specific protein can continuously release the bioactive chemical. Epigenetic promoters can even be used so that expression will only occur under certain conditions. Gene vectors can be tailored to preferentially transfect specific cells. In contrast, local drug injections expose the drug to the surrounding area, possibly causing unnecessary side effects.

The aim of this work is to provide a general overview of the field as well as the recent advances and techniques. To that end, the vectors used in gene therapy, the advantages and disadvantages of systemic vs. local delivery, and a variety of examples of clinical and preclinical studies using gene therapy for the treatment of disease will be discussed.

# 18.2 Delivery Technique (Vector)

The genes must enter the nuclease of a cell to be effective. Gene therapy vectors are not required, but greatly increase transfection efficiency. Genes can be delivered to a host through modified viruses, lipid or polymer complexes, cells modified *ex vivo,* or released from a scaffold. These methods are described in detail below (see Figure 18.1).

## 18.2.1 Viral

Viral gene delivery exploits the highly evolved ability of viruses to infect cells and thereby deliver exogenous nucleic acids.

While there may be other drawbacks associated with their use, viruses represent the most effective method for introducing exogenous DNA into eukaryotic cells. As early as the 1960s, evidence existed that viruses could be used to genetically modify cells (Friedmann, 1992). By the mid-1980s, evidence existed that nearly 100% efficiency could be obtained with available viral systems. Over the last few decades, a variety of different viruses have become common tools cited in gene therapy literature. Both retroviruses (such as Maloney murine leukemia virus, lentivirus and semliki forest virus) and DNA viruses (which include adenovirus and adeno-associated virus [AAV]) have been applied in both *in vitro* and *in vivo* gene-therapy studies.

### 18.2.1.1 Adenovirus

Adenoviruses are DNA viruses commonly used in gene therapy which do not incorporate their DNA into the host's genome.

As a result, it will not be duplicated with the host DNA and cell division will produce daughter cells without the transfected genetic material. This makes the effects of the adenovirus temporary, but removes the risk of damage to the host's genome. Gendicine, a cancer treatment using adenovirus delivered

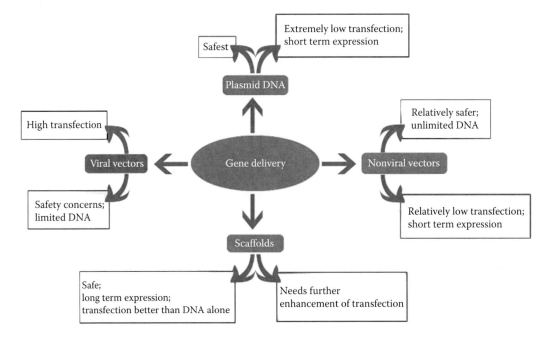

**FIGURE 18.1**   Vectors of gene delivery.

gene therapy has been licensed in China, but not approved in the European Union or the United States (Pearson et al., 2004). Adenovirus vectors were used in the 1999 gene therapy that resulted in the death of a patient, Jesse Gelsinger. This was the first, and as of yet, only death as the result of gene therapy in the United States. After the death of Mr. Gelsinger, an altered, genetically crippled version of the adenovirus has been used in gene therapy trials (Pollner, 2000).

The major advantages of adenoviral vectors compared to other viral vectors include ease of manipulation, relatively large transgene cloning capacity, and the ability to produce high titers (Vinge et al., 2008). These vectors are relatively efficient, *in vitro* and *in vivo*, and capable of transfecting nondividing cells (Davis et al., 2008). An additional advantage of adenoviruses is that they can be made replication deficient to improve safety and can be "gutted" to increase the cloning capacity. The major disadvantage of these vectors is the inflammatory and immune response seen upon *in vivo* delivery, as this limits the gene expression time and can induce further complications (Vinge et al., 2008). Gutted adenoviruses have lower immunogenicity, but they still trigger a reasonably significant cellular immune response (Davis et al., 2008). Coating adenoviruses with polyethylene glycol (PEG) has been suggested as a strategy to reduce the immune response to the proteins in the viral capsid. This method could also allow control of targeting by masking certain receptor-binding domains and presenting others (Gray and Samulski, 2008).

### 18.2.1.2 Adeno-Associated Virus

The AAV is a very small virus incapable of replication in a host cell without the assistance of a helper-virus.

AAVs are the most difficult of all the viral delivery vectors to produce, but new production techniques are increasing the ease of mass producing these small vectors. AAVs have been shown to be able to transfect quiescent cells.

AAVs are single-stranded DNA viruses (unlike adenoviruses which are double-stranded DNA viruses) (Gray and Samulski, 2008). They are somewhat analogous to gutted adenovirus in that they are usually incapable of replication in a host cell without the assistance of a helper virus (Davis et al., 2008). The recombinant AAVs used in gene therapy lack the ability to integrate into host genomes, persisting instead as episomal DNA in target cells (Lyon et al., 2008).Thus, there is theoretically a negligible risk of mutagenesis although long-term clinical trials would be required to confirm this. Importantly, no AAV serotype has been found to cause human disease (Davis et al., 2008). However, AAV vectors do elicit immune responses *in vivo* and some argue that they can cause insertional mutagenesis (Hacein-Bey-Abina et al., 2003) and their cloning capacity is also somewhat limited (4–5 kb) (Davis et al., 2008, Vinge et al., 2008).

Another feature, which could be advantageous or disadvantageous depending on the application, is that the expression kinetics of AAVs are relatively slow. Transgene expression generally peaks between 2 and 4 weeks after transfection (Lyon et al., 2008). Self-complementary AAVs have higher transfection levels—sometimes reported as more than 100 times over normal AAVs—but the packaging capacity of the virus is necessarily halved (~2.3 kb), which limits the applicability of such vectors (Gray and Samulski, 2008). A final concern is that 20–40% of the human population has antibodies to AAV2 serotype and thus can neutralize the vectors, drastically reducing transfection. It is also possible that, with repeated treatment, patients could develop antibodies to the vectors and thus the treatment would lose effectiveness over time (Lyon et al., 2008).

### 18.2.1.3 Retrovirus

Retroviruses are RNA carrying viruses that use reverse transcriptase to create DNA for incorporation into the host's genome.

A complication arising from the use of retroviruses in genetic engineering is that they add DNA to a random section of the altered chromosome. There is a small chance that the new genetic material will be inserted within gene or gene promoter, disrupting gene production.

Lentivirus has shown reasonable promise for cardiac applications because it can transduce nondividing cells like cardiomyocytes (Davis et al., 2008). The sequence delivered by the lentivirus integrates into host genome, which means that transfection is "stable" but also introduces the risk of mutagenesis, carcinogenesis, and immune response induction (Haider et al., 2008). Another disadvantage of lentivirus is that only low titres can be prepared (Davis et al., 2008). Furthermore, lentiviruses are less stable than other vectors and thus are more difficult to work with (Davis et al., 2008). A final drawback is that these vectors have very high efficiency *in vitro* (80–100%) but only up to about 30% efficiency *in vivo* (Davis et al., 2008).

## 18.2.2 Nonviral

While viral systems are among the most effective agents available for gene transfer, they have associated health risks, high production costs, and a variety of other drawbacks. Thus, the gene therapy field has focused on the development of nonviral gene delivery systems. A variety of agents have been investigated.

While viral systems are among the most effective agents available for gene transfer, they have associated health risks, high production costs, and a variety of other drawbacks. Thus, the gene therapy field has focused on the development of nonviral gene delivery systems. A variety of agents have been investigated (see Figure 18.2).

### 18.2.2.1 Naked DNA

DNA can transfect a cell without a delivery vector when simply injected intramuscularly or intravenously. However, this technique has a much lower efficiency than other methods. To improve transfection efficiency, physical methods can be used to improve gene delivery. Electroporation using an electric current or calcium ions temporarily increases the permeability of the plasma membrane and allows DNA to pass into the cell (Neumann et al., 1982). Sonoporation uses ultrasonic sound to

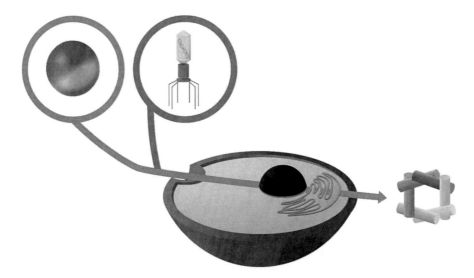

**FIGURE 18.2** Hypothesized route of polymeric or liposomal complex internalization in a eukaryotic cell. Initially, particles bind to the surface of the cell. This can occur via charge interaction or ligand binding. A pit forms and becomes an endosome. This endosome then combines with an acidic lysosome. This swelling may be responsible for the bursting of the endosomal membrane and release of the complexes. These complexes then may enter the nucleus via nuclear pores. Once in the nucleus, normal transcription and translation are hypothesized to occur. It should be noted that at each step the vast majority of complexes are likely degraded or excreted, leaving only a very small fraction that actually reaches the nucleus. (From Dennig, J. and Duncan, E. 2002. *Journal of Biotechnology*, 90, 339–347; Dufes, C., Uchegbu, I. F., and Schatzlein, A. G. 2005. *Advanced Drug Delivery Reviews*, 57, 2177–2202.)

induce a similar increase in permeability of the plasma membrane and allowing large molecules to pass into the cell (Song et al., 2007).

### 18.2.2.2 Lipids

> Lipoplexes are complexes arising from the combination of nucleic acids and lipids which form condensed structures capable of passing through cell membranes.

Under normal conditions, DNA is too negatively charged from the phosphates within its chemical structure to pass through a cell membrane. Naked DNA either requires a membrane to be chemically or electrically disrupted or enters the cell during cytokinesis. Lipoplexes and polyplexes form a positively charged sheath around a plasmid and allow the DNA to pass through the plasma membrane. Anion and neutral lipids can be used to form lipoplexes, but cationic lipids have increased lipoplex stability and cellular uptake and are more popular. Unfortunately, lipoplexes formed with cationic lipids exhibit cell toxicity at high levels. This dose-dependent toxicity limits the genetic load that can be delivered and, until it can be solved, limits the therapeutic uses of lipoplexes.

Lipoplexes are commonly used in gene therapy to transfer genetic material into a cancer cell, either by suppressing oncogenes or activating tumor suppression control genes. Lipoplexes have also been used to successfully transfect respiratory endothelial cells leading to studies to treat respiratory diseases such as cystic fibrosis.

### 18.2.2.3 Polymers

> Polyplexes are complexes arising from the interaction between nucleic acids and polymers, where the polymers condense the nucleic acids and mediate their passage through the cell membrane.

Polyplexes are similar to lipoplexes in that most of the interactions between the polymer and the genetic sequence are ionic chemical interactions. Most polymers used for DNA complexation are cationic and interact with the anionic phosphates in nucleic acid.

In most cases, the DNA used in polyplexes and lipoplexes is not inserted into the host genome, but is delivered in plasmid form which, when inserted into the nucleus, is transcribed along with the genome. In addition to minimizing the risk of mutating a healthy gene with random insertion, using a noninserting plasmid means that the gene therapy will only cause a temporary alteration of gene expression. While this is a limitation when the desired effect in gene therapy is the replacement of a defective gene, it does allow gene therapy to be used when a permanent alteration to gene expression is not desired. For example, transient gene therapy can be used to increase the growth of nerve axons or increase the healing of a diabetic patient without resulting in a permanent increase in the natural growth rate of cells.

## 18.2.3 Scaffolds

Scaffolds can also be used as a delivery device for genetic information. As gene therapy has applications for tissue engineering and regenerative medicine, combining gene therapy with tissue-engineered scaffolds (a biocompatible framework for growing tissue on and within it) is a natural approach. Scaffolds can be used to control the dose and duration of exposure. They can be used with cell-mediated gene therapy to localize the delivery of the altered cells. As previously mentioned, many vectors for gene delivery have dose-dependent cytotoxicity or immune response. Using scaffolds as a secondary release mechanism causes a gradual release while keeping the high transfection efficiency of the other vectors (Jawad et al., 2007) (Simpson et al., 2007). Scaffold-mediated gene therapy is used in the treatment of cancer as well as regenerative medicine. In this case, the goal is either to increase the expression of antioncogenes or by using gene therapy to modify immune cells to more readily attack tumor cells. Gene delivery scaffolds can be inserted near cancer cells or into the dead space remaining after a tumor is removed (Kusumoto et al., 2001).

### 18.2.4 Cell-Mediated Gene Therapy

> Cell-mediated gene therapy relies upon the delivery of cells genetically modified *ex vivo* to modulate the protein expression for therapeutic purposes.

Cell-mediated gene therapy differs from other vector-mediated techniques in a variety of ways. First, the genetic manipulation occurs *ex vivo*, before the cells are implanted. Second, the transgene production depends entirely on the viability of the implanted cells, so the delivery technique of the cell suspension must be carefully considered. Finally, the source, preparation, and characterization of the cells represent an additional level of complication. There are several important implications of these differences, as compared to vector-mediated gene delivery. For example, the cell type that produces the transgene depends on the experimental or therapeutic strategy rather than on the vector or administration technique used. The isolation and expansion of these cells may determine the overall efficacy of the treatment as the viability of the cells is critical. Intelligent choice of cell type may also augment the efficacy of the therapy; for example, using stem cells to deliver factors to infarcted myocardium means that the paracrine benefits of stem cells in such a situation are included in addition to the benefits associated with the gene therapy (Baraniak and McDevitt, 2010).

A significant advantage of *ex vivo* gene delivery is that selection protocols can be used to select the transfected cells over the unmodified cells, essentially eliminating the importance of transfection efficiency. Furthermore, the immunogenicity of the vector is less problematic as it does not have to be introduced *in vivo*. While it is possible that *ex vivo* manipulation could alter the expression of molecules such as MHC class I or II on the cell surface, these effects tend to be less problematic than, for example, the immune response to systemically administered virus (Shayakhmetov et al., 2010). However, the potential danger of tumorigenicity is not eliminated. As the vector is not introduced into the host, it is unlikely to induce tumor formation in the host tissue; however, the transplanted cells are genetically modified to permanently express the transgene which implies a modification in their genetic structure. Insertional mutagenesis is thus quite likely, which can lead to the uncontrolled proliferation of these cells (Themis et al., 2003, Shi et al., 2001, Haviernik and Bunting, 2004, Ali et al., 1994).

As the delivery technique is so critical to the success of cell-mediated therapy, significant research has gone into development of an "optimal" cell delivery technique. The simplest method, injection of cell suspension, offers minimal opportunity to augment the survival rate of the cells or to direct their engraftment. Indeed, very low retention rates of injected cells have been observed in certain settings (Pons et al., 2009). The use of biomaterial scaffolds presents a solution to both of these concerns, as the cells can be physically protected and their migration limited by using a cell-seeded scaffold to deliver the modified cells (Sales et al., 2007, Jawad et al., 2007, Simpson et al., 2007). Modification and functionalization of the scaffold can further enhance the viability and control the differentiation of the implanted cells (Hosseinkhani et al., 2006a,b, 2005, 2008, Hosseinkhani and Tabata, 2006, Hosseinkhani, 2006, Zhang et al., 2006, Simpson et al., 2007). Considering the benefits associated with the incorporation of the scaffold, as well as the potential for added functionality, the future of effective cell-mediated gene therapy will likely include scaffold-based delivery.

## 18.3  Systemic and Local Gene Delivery

While the administration technique and the actual gene therapy vector may seem less important than the gene being delivered, they can have a significant impact. Certain administration techniques are more effective than others and the choice of local or systemic delivery may determine the efficacy of the therapy.

The successful treatment of certain diseases requires systemic gene delivery. However, the viral and nonviral vectors administered systemically, mostly by intravenous injection, meet with a number of barriers that hinder their ability to reach the target tissues, including interactions with proteins and cells in blood, serum stability, first pass metabolism in liver, nonspecific delivery to unintended tissues and/or attacked by macrophages, digestive enzymes such as proteases and nucleases, suffer destruction by immune responses. A number of studies have investigated the methods to determine and modulate the viral tropism (Ylosmaki et al., 2008, Michelfelder and Trepel, 2009, Tan et al., 2007, Yang et al., 2009, Li et al., 2008a, Bakker et al., 2001). In case of nonviral vectors, a number of approaches have shown promising results. Generally, when naked DNA is used for systemic delivery, large doses are employed. However, a study has shown successful delivery to kidney when comparatively much lower dose is administered via inferior vena cava (Wu et al., 2005). For liposomal systems, PEGylation is a commonly used method which increases the circulation time by protecting them from attack by macrophages. Various such stealth technologies have been described (Immordino et al., 2006). PEGylated nanoparticles have shown promising results for systemic nonviral delivery (Kaul and Amiji, 2004, 2005). A wide range of targeting strategies such peptide (Li and Huang, 2006, Zhang et al., 2008a), antibody (Zhang et al., 2008b, Peer et al., 2008) or antibody fragment (Kim et al., 2008) linkage or substrates for specific receptors (Hattori et al., 2004), have been employed for targeted delivery to tissue/cells of interest.

Some diseased conditions only need local gene therapy and the use of tissue engineered scaffolds becomes more evident in these cases. Tissue-engineered scaffolds can act as reservoir or depot systems to keep the gene vectors from having systemic effect while, at the same time, release the genes in a controlled manner for extended periods of protein expression (Kulkarni et al., 2010) or suppression. A number of studies have shown localized sustained release of DNA (Guo et al., 2006, Chun et al., 2005, Chen et al., 2007a). Tissue-engineered scaffolds also provide protection to the DNA which partially explains the enhancement of the transfection observed by delivery via gene activated matrices (GAM) (Bonadio et al., 1999a, Bonadio, 2000). The enhanced efficacy and therapeutic benefits has been observed in various studies employing tissue engineered scaffolds with either plasmid DNA alone (Andree et al., 2001) or complexed with liposomes/polymers (Winn et al., 2005b, Peng et al., 2009, Wang et al., 2009) or with virus (Breen et al., 2008).

## 18.3.1 Dose

When considering a treatment regimen, the dose of the therapeutic agent is an extremely important issue. It can, in fact, represent the difference between massive therapeutic benefit and complete ineffectiveness. A further consideration is that in gene delivery, a higher dose is not necessarily associated with a higher level of transgene expression. As with many biological systems, there appears to be both an upper and lower limit or a "window" of efficacy (Bonadio et al., 1999b).

Comparing the dose of viral and nonviral therapies is not trivial. As the transfection efficiency of viruses is far higher than that observed with nonviral vectors, far less virus is required to stimulate comparable levels of transgene expression. In general, the transfection efficiency of a vector is inversely related to the required dose (Holladay et al., 2009). The cytotoxicity of the vector is another important consideration. Naked plasmid DNA elicits very little immune or inflammatory response, while many polymers and viruses are significantly antigenic (Breunig et al., 2007). Thus, the maximum dose of a virus might be determined by the host response to the vector rather than the optimal transgene expression. Indeed, viral therapies are now regarded with caution after isolated incidences of fatalities and other "serious adverse events" (SAEs) were associated with viral clinical trials (Lyon et al., 2008, Lehrman, 1999, Marshall, 2000, Check, 2003, Porteus et al., 2006). The earliest fatality reported to be associated with a viral clinical trial used one of the highest doses cited in the literature, $3.8 \times 10^{13}$ virus particles of an adenovirus variant (Lehrman, 1999). Naked plasmids, conversely, can be administered in very high doses but are unlikely to induce significant transgene expression. For example, 4 mg of plasmid induced no adverse reactions in an early angiogenic clinical trial (Kalka et al., 2000) as was a total of 8 mg delivered over the course of a more recent angiogenic clinical trial (Shigematsu et al., 2010). The doses of nonviral vectors are generally lower than naked plasmid, as most vectors have some antigenicity. The most popular nonviral vector used in clinical trials are cationic lipid/plasmid complexes (Edelstein et al., 2007).

Comparing animal studies to human clinical trials is also problematic, as differences in size and weight logically translate to differences in optimal dose. The doses used in clinical trials do not always reflect this, however. For example, in the cardiac area, approximately the same average dose of naked plasmid (~0.75 mg) is used in rats, pigs, and humans, despite orders of magnitude differences in overall mass.

## 18.4 Therapeutic Preclinical or Clinical Trials

A wide range of disease states have been investigated as potential candidates for gene therapy. Some of the areas with more significant recent advances are discussed, including gene therapy for bone regeneration, diabetic wound healing, lower-limb ischemia, myocardial infarction, and cancer.

### 18.4.1 Bone

The regeneration of bone tissue presents an interesting problem for the tissue-engineering and biomaterials field. Bone defects are relatively common, whether due to injury, disease, or as a by-product of surgery. While many types of fractures and small defects can be fully regenerated without intervention, others require replacement or other therapy in order to heal. The natural healing process involves primarily osteoinduction—the stimulation of bone tissue formation by undifferentiated or progenitor cell types. The other major method of bone tissue formation depends on osteoconduction, where bone tissue forms over a surface. This is more commonly observed in response to implants than in natural bone regeneration (Albrektsson and Johansson, 2001). The current gold standard in bone tissue engineering is the use of autografts (Ahlmann et al., 2002). Essentially, bone from a less critical area (i.e., pelvis) is harvested and used to replace the missing bone elsewhere. This has obvious drawbacks, as two injury sites result, and the harvest site must then regenerate. Allografts—bone harvested from donors—are an alternative, but in order to minimize the chance of immune rejection, fresh allografts are freeze-dried, frozen, gamma irradiated or treated with ethylene oxide. This significantly decreases the osteoinductive and osteoconductive properties of the allografts (Keating and McQueen, 2001). However, allografts are a commercially available alternative to autografts. Xenografts, bone harvested from animals, represents a third option. There are a number of bovine-derived bone substitutes available on the market, such as Cerabone®, Endobon®, and Osteograf® (Gisep, 2002, Tadic and Epple, 2004). As these xenografts are composed of the natural hydroxyapatite structure which is common to all vertebrates, they are osteoconductive. However, they do not possess the osteoinductive properties of autografts, which may be largely due to the presence of natural signaling molecules on unmodified bone. Tissue engineering products for bone regeneration are available commercially, OP-1® and INFUSE®, which use recombinant human bone morphogenic protein-7 (rhBMP-7) and recombinant human bone morphogenic protein-2 (rhBMP-2), respectively.

Gene therapy approaches for the regeneration of bone predominantly focus on the upregulation of growth factors such as bone morphogenic protein 2 (BMP-2). Naked plasmid DNA delivery has been shown to improve bone formation, epithelialization and the formation of blood vessels, as discussed in Table 18.1. Viral gene delivery has been shown to induce bone formation when adenovirus encoding BMP-2 was injected into mouse skeletal muscle (Musgrave et al., 1999).

Scaffold-based approaches have found a significant benefit to be associated with loading the plasmid (naked or complexed) or virus into a biomaterial. Higher transfection efficiencies have been observed as compared to direct delivery of the vector (Winn et al., 2005a). In fact, the delivery and transgene expression profiles were found to depend on the complexation reagent, implying a potential mechanism for control of transfection and gene expression (Winn et al., 2005a, Xie et al., 2001). The term "Gene Activated Matrix," often abbreviated as GAM, has emerged as a descriptor for some of the collagen-scaffold-based systems used for the delivery of plasmid DNA (Fang et al., 1996, Bonadio et al., 1999b). These matrices were found to significantly increase bone regeneration when used to deliver a secreted peptide

**TABLE 18.1** Summary of Therapeutic Trials Using Gene Therapy for Bone Tissue Engineering

| Mode of Delivery | Gene | Reference |
|---|---|---|
| Adenovirus | BMP-2 | Egermann et al., 2006a,b, Baltzer et al., 2000 |
| Adenovirus | BMP-2 | Musgrave et al., 1999 |
| Polylactic coglycolic acid/ polypropylene fumarate scaffold | BMP-7 | Rivard et al., 1995 |
| Retrovirus | BMP-4, BMP-6 | Jane et al., 2002 |
| Retrovirus | MDS1-EVI1, PRDM16, SETBP1 | Schwarzwaelder et al., 2006, Ott et al., 2006 |
| Naked DNA/ Electroporation | BMP-4 | Kishimoto et al., 2002 |
| Lipoplex | LIM Mineralization Protein (LMP-1) | Yoon and Boden, 2004, Sangadala et al., 2003, Minamide et al., 2003, Kim et al., 2003, Viggeswarapu et al., 2002, 2005, 2001, Minamide et al., 2001, Boden et al., 1998, Liu et al., 2010 |
| Collagen calcium-phosphate scaffold | VEGF | Keeney et al., 2010 |
| Collagen scaffold | BMP-2 or secreted peptide fragment of human parathyroid hormone (hPTH 1-34) | Fang et al., 1996 |
| Collagen scaffold | Secreted peptide fragment of human parathyroid hormone (hPTH 1-34) | Bonadio et al., 1999b |
| Cell-mediated | BMP-7 | Nussenbaum et al., 2005 |
| Cell-mediated | BMP-2 | Blum et al., 2003 |
| Cell-mediated | BMP-2 | Wang et al., 2003 |
| Cell-mediated | BMP-2 | Laurencin et al., 2001 |
| Cell mediated | BMP-2 | Jiang et al., 2009 |

fragment of human parathyroid hormone (hPTH) in the treatment of critical gap defects. Collagen calcium-phosphate scaffolds, which naturally have osteoconductive properties, were found to act as both a reservoir system and a transfection reagent when used to deliver VEGF plasmid (Keeney et al., 2010). Filling of the femoral cavity was increased in the groups treated with the plasmid, implying a beneficial effect of VEGF upregulation in the regenerating bone and suggesting a potential gene of interest for future studies. Functionalized decellularized, or demineralized bone has also been studied as a carrier for cell-mediated gene therapy (Wang et al., 2003).

While efficacy has been established in a variety of preclinical studies, gene therapy for bone regeneration is still in development. Scaffold-mediated delivery of genes or cells may represent a major future direction in the field, whether the scaffold is used simplistically as a delivery vehicle or is functionalized with osteoinductive or osteoconductive factors such as calcium phosphate or recombinant growth factors.

## 18.4.2 Diabetic Wound Healing

Wound healing is a classic example of a complex and highly intricate response in the repair and regeneration of damaged tissue. Under physiological conditions, normal adult skin has a considerable capacity for structural and functional repair via a highly orchestrated process tightly regulated by growth factors and cytokines (Werner and Grose, 2003) and characterized by distinct but overlapping phases of wound healing, namely hemostasis, inflammation, proliferation, and remodeling (Diegelmann and Evans, 2004). When the wounds fail to progress through the normal phases of healing and enter to a state of chronic pathologic inflammation, they are termed as "chronic," "impaired," or "compromised" (Menke et al., 2007). Diabetes is one of most common causes of chronic wounds, others being venous and pressure ulcers (Mustoe et al., 2006, Nwomeh et al., 1998). Diabetes is a major health problem and disease prevalence is growing at a phenomenal rate. Management of diabetic foot disease is very expensive and the cost of managing the diabetic foot complications is estimated to be in billions of US dollars (Giurini and Lyons, 2005, Dorresteijn et al., 2010, Wukich, 2010). In Europe, the average cost per episode is €6,650 for leg ulcers and €10,000 for foot ulcers, which accounts for 2–4% of health-care budgets (Gottrup et al., 2010). The altered molecular mechanisms leading to chronic healing are being extensively studied (Blakytny and Jude, 2006, 2009, Brem and Tomic-Canic, 2007, Galkowska et al., 2006), unraveling the pathogenesis of diabetic wound healing and opening new avenues, complementary to the standard treatment protocol, for successful management of diabetic ulcers. To date, a number of studies have investigated the role of growth factors and cytokines, such as VEGF, FGF, PDGF, TGF-α, IGF-1, NGF, GM-CSF, in the management of diabetic wounds either as individual factors (Fernandez-Montequin et al., 2007, 2009, Saba et al., 2002, Pandit et al., 2000, Mustoe et al., 1991, Judith et al., 2010, Li et al., 2008b, Matsuda et al., 1998, Fang et al., 2010) or as combination of factors (Kiritsy et al., 1995, Greenhalgh et al., 1993, Brown et al., 1994, Davidson et al., 1997, Jazwa et al., 2010b, Cao et al., 2010). In recent years, gene therapy is being investigated extensively in recent years, majorly due to failure to achieve the clinical promise of growth factors/cytokines delivery despite of intensive research (Eming et al., 2004). The limited success of growth factors/cytokines delivery can be attributed to a number of factors which include their short half-lives, degradation by proteases, toxicity at high doses and lack of effective delivery (Steed, 1998, Grinnell et al., 1992, Barrick et al., 1999, Lauer et al., 2000, Bowler, 2002). A number of studies have shown promising results in normalizing various pathological aspects of diabetic wound healing. Some recent salient examples have been details in Table 18.2.

Recently, tissue-engineered biological dressings have gained significant attention, not only because they fill the wound gap by extracellular matrix and induce expression of cytokines and growth factors which accelerate wound healing (Veves et al., 2001), but also due to the fact that they provide opportunity to combine other wound therapeutics such as antimicrobial agents, growth factors and/or cytokines as recombinant proteins, genes, or live cells (Andreadis and Geer, 2006, Horch et al., 2005, Supp and Boyce, 2005). One such tissue-engineered scaffold which employs human platelet-derived growth factor (PDGF)-B with replication-defective adenovirus in bovine collagen gel (GAM501) is being investigated in human patients. The clinical phase I/II results of this study showed that 93% of patients had a positive-biologic response to GAM501, as assessed by a decrease in ulcer size and GAM501 did not appear to have any toxicity at doses that showed biologic activity (Mulder et al., 2009).

### 18.4.3 Lower-Limb Ischemia

Peripheral arterial disease (PAD) is an increasingly common disease, affecting approximately 4.3% of people over the age of 40 in the United States (Selvin and Erlinger, 2004), and 12–20% of people over the age of 65 (Bakal et al., 2000). The most severe form of this disease is critical limb ischemia (CLI) which affects 0.05–0.1% of people worldwide (Shigematsu et al., 2010). Current treatment strategies include surgical and endovascular revascularization, but more than one in four patients will require major amputation within a year of treatment and current mortality rates exceed 20% per annum (Shigematsu et al., 2010). Thus, this is an excellent candidate for gene therapy trials as the current gold standard of treatment has extremely limited success.

Delivery of angiogenic genes is the most popular gene therapy treatment for CLI. VEGF, HGF, eNOS and FGF have all been investigated as potential angiogenic genes in preclinical and clinical trials (see Table 18.3).

Randomized, multi-center meta-analyses have indicated significant improvements in odds ratios associated with angiogenic gene therapy (Haro et al., 2009). In a recent trial involving diabetic patients, an apparent improvement was observed, but due to the small numbers the primary end point of

**TABLE 18.2** Summary of Therapeutic Trials Using Gene Therapy for Diabetic Wound Healing

| Vector | Gene | Animal Model | Wound Type | Significant Finding | Reference |
|---|---|---|---|---|---|
| Viral vectors | | | | | |
| AAV vector | Simultaneous transfer of VEGF-A and fibroblast growth factor 4 | C57BLKS mice homozygous for a mutation in the leptin receptor (Lepr[db]) | Full-thickness excisional circular wounds (4 mm in diameter) | Simultaneous delivery VEGF-A and FGF-4 gene therapy leads to significantly faster wound closure, increased granulation tissue formation, vascularity and dermal matrix deposition | Jazwa et al., 2010a |
| rAAV | Ang-1 (angiopoietin-1) | C57BL/KsJ *Lep*[db] mice | full-thickness longitudinal incisions (4 cm) on dorsum | Ang-1 gene transfer improves the delayed wound repair in diabetes by stimulating angiogenesis, apparently without VEGF involvement | Bitto et al., 2008 |
| Adenovirus | c-Met gene | Organ cultured human diabetic corneas | 5-mm epithelial wounds | Recombinant AV-driven c-met transduction into diabetic corneas appears to restore HGF signaling, normalize diabetic marker patterns, and accelerate wound healing | Saghizadeh et al., 2010 |
| Adenovirus in fibrin scaffold | Endothelial nitric oxide synthase (eNOS) | Alloxan-induced diabetic New Zealand white rabbits | 6-mm punch biopsy wounds on the ears | Fibrin delivery of AdeNOS resulted in enhanced eNOS expression, inflammatory response, and a faster rate of re-epithelialization | Breen AM, 2008 |
| Adenovirus vector (ADV/VEGF165) | VEGF 165 | BKS.Cg-m +/+ Lepr[db] type 2 diabetic mice | Full-thickness excisional wounds, 1.4 cm in diameter on the dorsum | ADV/VEGF165 improves healing enhancing tensile stiffness and/or increasing epithelialization and collagen deposition, as well as by decreasing time to wound closure | Brem et al., 2009 |
| Adenovirus | Placenta growth factor (PlGF) | Streptozotocin induced diabetic C57Bl/6 male mice | 6 mm-diameter full-thickness punch biopsy wound | PlGF gene transfer improved granulation tissue formation, maturation, and vascularization, as well as monocytes/macrophages local recruitment | Cianfarani et al., 2006 |
| Adenovirus | Platelet-derived growth factor (PDGF)-B | C57BLKS/J-m +/+ Lepr(db) and streptozotocin induced | 8 mm full-thickness flank wounds | Adenoviral-mediated gene therapy with PDGF-B significantly enhanced wound healing and neovascularization in diabetic wounds with augmentation of EPC recruitment | Keswani et al., 2004 |

*continued*

**TABLE 18.2** (continued) Summary of Therapeutic Trials Using Gene Therapy for Diabetic Wound Healing

| Vector | Gene | Animal Model | Wound Type | Significant Finding | Reference |
|---|---|---|---|---|---|
| Lentivirus | Stromal-derived growth factor-1α (SDF-1α). | BKS.Cg-m$^{+/+}$ Lepr$^{db}$/J mice | 8-mm full-thickness wound | SDF-1α treatment exhibited a decrease in wound surface area with more cellular wounds and increased granulation tissue volume and resulted in complete epithelialization at 2 weeks | Badillo et al., 2007 |
| Lentivirus | Platelet-derived growth factor (PDGF)-B | *db/db* mice | 2 × 2-cm full-thickness dermal wound | Statistically significant increase in angiogenesis and substantially thicker, more coherently aligned collagen fibers | Lee et al., 2005, Man et al., 2005 |
| | | | **Non-Viral Vectors** | | |
| Naked plasmid injection | HSP47 | Alloxan-induced diabetic rat | Excisional skin wounds | Increased collagen I production around the wound during repair process | Wang and Li, 2009 |
| Plasmid vector with electroporation | Hypoxia-inducible factor 1α (HIF-1α) | BKS.Cg-m$^{+/+}$ Lepr$^{db}$/J mice | 5-mm full-thickness circular excisional wounds on the dorsum | Electroporation with HIF-1α increased levels of HIF-1α mRNA on day 3 and increased levels of VEGF, PLGF, PDGF-B, and ANGPT2 mRNA on day 7 and ten folds increase in circulating angiogenic cells after HIF-1α treatment | Liu et al., 2008 |
| Plasmid vector with electroporation | Keratinocyte growth factor-1 (KGF-1) | BKS.Cg-m. Lepr$^{db}$-db mice | Excisional wounds | Results showed improvement in healing rate, quality of epithelialization and density of new blood vessels | Marti et al., 2004, 2008 |
| Sonoporation of minicircle DNA | VEGF$_{165}$ | Streptozotocin-Induced diabetic C57BL/6J mice | 6 mm punch biopsy wounds on the dorsum | Sonoporation of minicircle-VEGF$_{165}$ resulted in Accelerated wound closure with markedly increased skin blood perfusion and CD31 expression and full restoration of normal architecture | Yoon et al., 2009 |
| Plasmid pellet (1% methyl cellulose) | HOXA3 | db/db mice | 8-mm full thickness excisional wound on the dorsum | HOXA3 accelerates wound repair by mobilizing endothelial progenitor cells and attenuating the excessive inflammatory response of chronic wounds | Mace et al., 2009 |

| DNA/Methylcellulose Pellets | Sonic hedgehog (Shh) | C57BLKS/J-m$^{+/+}$Lepr$^{db}$ mice | 8 mm full-thickness excisional skin wounds | Topical gene therapy resulted in acceleration of wound recovery with increased wound vascularity | Asai et al., 2006 |
|---|---|---|---|---|---|
| Gold particles and gene gun | Rat opioid growth factor receptor (OGFr) complementary DNA | Adult male rats | 3-mm corneal abrasions | Excess OGFr delays reepithelialization, whereas attenuation of OGFr accelerates repair of the corneal surface | Zagon et al., 2006 |
| RGDK-lipopeptide | rhPDGF-B | Streptozotocin-Induced Diabetic Sprague-Dawley Rats | 2.1 cm (radii) circular dorsal skin incision to the level of the loose subcutaneous tissues | A single subcutaneous administration of the electrostatic complex of RGDK-lipopeptide and rhPDGF-B plasmid is capable of healing incisional wounds in streptozotocin-induced diabetic rats with significantly higher degree of epithelization, keratization, fibrocollagenation and blood vessel formation | Bhattacharyya et al., 2009 |
| Lipofectin and Lipofectamine 2000 | Human insulin-like growth factor (hIGF)-1 (with keratinocytes) | Streptozotocin-Induced Diabetic Yorkshire pigs | Full-thickness excisional wounds (15 × 1.5 × 0.8 cm) on the dorsum | Nonviral gene transfer increased IGF-1 expression in diabetic wounds by up to 900-fold and 83% wound closure achieved with combined gene and cell therapy | Hirsch et al., 2008 |
| Plasmid/liposome | aFGF | Db/db mouse | Excisional and incisional | Accelerated closure of excisional wounds and increased wound breaking strength in incisional wounds | Sun et al., 1997 |
| Plasmid in PEG-PLGAPEG tri-block co-polymer | TGFβ1 | Db/db mouse | 7 x 7 mm excisional | Enhanced closure, re-epithelialization and cell proliferation | Lee et al., 2003 |

**TABLE 18.3**   Summary of Selected Trials Using Angiogenic Gene Therapy to Treat CLI

| Gene | Delivery Method | Dose | Reference |
|------|-----------------|------|-----------|
| VEGF-121 | Adenovirus | $4 \times 10^{9.5}$–$4 \times 10^{10}$ particles | Rajagopalan et al., 2001 |
| HGF | Hemagglutinating virus of Japan (HVJ)-liposome | 20–40 μg | Taniyama et al., 2001 |
| FGF-1 | Naked plasmid (clinical trial) | 0.5–32 mg in total (16 mg per injection maximum, 2 injections in some cases) | Comerota et al., 2002 |
| eNOS | Naked plasmid | 500 μg | Namba et al., 2003 |
| VEGF-165 | Naked plasmid (clinical trial) | 0.4–2 mg | Shyu et al., 2003 |
| FGF-1 | Naked plasmid (clinical trial) | 0.5,2, 4 mg | Baumgartner et al., 2009 |
| VEGF-165 | Naked plasmid (case study) | 2 mg | Isner et al., 1996 |
| VEGF-165 | Naked plasmid (clinical trial) | 2 mg | Isner et al., 1998 |
| VEGF-165 | Naked plasmid (clinical trial) | 4 mg | Baumgartner et al., 1998 |
| VEGF-165 | Adenovirus and naked plasmid | $2 \times 10^{10}$ pfu or 2 mg plasmid | Makinen et al., 2002 |
| VEGF-165 | Naked plasmid (clinical trial) | 2 mg | Kusumanto et al., 2006 |

reduction in the number of amputations was not observed (Kusumanto et al., 2006). Overall, while there does appear to be a small but significant improvement, the therapeutic potential originally envisioned by Baumgartner et al. has not yet been achieved (Baumgartner et al., 1998). Improvements such as polymeric transfection reagents or biomaterial-based systems which improve the specificity of the gene delivery could represent future directions for this area.

## 18.4.4  Myocardial Infarction

There are two predominant forms of ischemic heart disease, namely acute damage due to myocardial infarction (MI) and chronic damage due to restricted perfusion of tissue due to atherosclerosis. These two forms of heart disease accounts for 35% of deaths reported in the United States every year (Guyton and Hall, 2000) and approximately a third of deaths worldwide, making it the most common cause of death in developed countries (Gray and Samulski, 2008).

Cardiac gene therapy has been under investigation for more than two decades. In the 1990s, trials established that cardiac tissue could be genetically modified with viruses, naked plasmids and liposomes (Acsadi et al., 1991, Barnes et al., 1993, Guzman et al., 1993, French et al., 1994, Baru et al., 1995, Nabel, 1995). Since then, gene therapy has been proposed as a treatment for conditions ranging myocarditis to advanced congestive heart failure. The goals of cardiac gene therapy are essentially to minimize damage, to promote regeneration, or some combination thereof. The late Dr. Jeffrey Isner and his colleagues were responsible for much of the ground-breaking work in the area, conducting a number of clinical trials starting in 1995, focusing on delivery of vascular endothelial growth factor (VEGF-A) plasmid (Isner, 1998, Losordo et al., 1998, 2002, Ashare et al., 1999, Lathi et al., 1999, Symes et al., 1999, Schwarz et al., 2000, Henry et al., 2001, Vale et al., 2001, Fortuin et al., 2003, Yoon et al., 2005). A variety of other genes have been investigated since, although no major breakthroughs in clinical studies have yet been reported. A variety of viral vectors have been employed as well as naked plasmids and lipid or polymer-mediated delivery (see Table 18.4).

A variety of cardiac disorders have been treated with adenoviral systems, including cardiomyopathy (Bathgate et al., 2008), ventricular arrhythmia (Prunier et al., 2008), and, most significantly, damage after myocardial infarction (Shah et al., 2001, White et al., 2000) (Gupta et al., 2008a, Pleger et al., 2007). Adenovirus vectors have been used to study calcium handling in the myocardium by modulating expression of sarcoplasmic reticulum Ca2+ ATPase pump (SERCA2a) (del Monte et al., 2001, Miyamoto et al., 2000, Schmidt et al., 2000, Gupta et al., 2008b). Myocardial delivery of a variety of growth factors with adenovirus has also been investigated, including human hepatocyte growth factor (hHGF) (Chen et al., 2007b), placental growth factor (PlGF) (Roncal et al., 2008), human vascular endothelial growth

**TABLE 18.4** Summary of Reported Gene Therapy Clinical Trials

| Mode of Delivery | Gene | Lead Author | Reference |
|---|---|---|---|
| Naked plasmid | VEGF-A165 | Ripa | Ripa et al., 2006 |
| Naked plasmid | VEGF-A165 | Gyongyosi | Gyongyosi et al., 2005 |
| Naked plasmid | VEGF-A165 | Kastrup | Kastrup et al., 2005 |
| Naked plasmid | VEGF-A165 | Losordo | Losordo et al., 1998 |
| Naked plasmid | VEGF-A165 and GSF (granulocyte stimulating factor) | Wang | Wang et al., 2007 |
| Naked plasmid | VEGF-C | Vale | Vale et al., 2001 |
| Lipid-mediated | VEGF-A165 | Hedman | Hedman et al., 2003, 2008 |
| AAV | SERCA2a | Hajjar | Hajjar et al., 2008 |
| Adenovirus | HGF | Yuan | Yuan et al., 2008b |
| Adenovirus | FGF | Lyon, Flynn, Rosengart, Grines, Kapur | Lyon et al., 2008, Flynn and O'Brien, 2008, Rosengart et al., 1999, Kapur and Rade, 2008, Grines et al., 2002 |

**TABLE 18.5** Summary of *In Vivo* Preclinical Cardiac Studies Using Viral Gene Therapy

| Mode of Delivery | Gene | Reference |
|---|---|---|
| Adenovirus | SERCA2a | Prunier et al., 2008, Gupta et al., 2008b, Sabbah et al., 2003, del Monte et al., 2001, Schmidt et al., 2000, Miyamoto et al., 2000 |
| Adenovirus | Human HGF | Miyagawa et al., 2006, Chen et al., 2007b |
| Adenovirus | PlGF | Roncal et al., 2008 |
| Adenovirus | VEGF | Guerrero et al., 2008 |
| Adenovirus | HGF | Yuan et al., 2008a |
| AAV | IL-10 | Nonaka-Sarukawa et al., 2008 |
| AAV | Antisense phospholamban (asPLB) | Zhao et al., 2008 |
| Lentivirus | Angiotensin converting enzyme 2 (ACE2) | Sarkissian et al., 2008 |

factor (VEGF) (Guerrero et al., 2008). A summary of selected preclinical studies using viruses to transfect the myocardium is described in Table 18.5.

Approximately half of the ongoing and completed clinical trials in cardiac gene therapy have used adenoviral vectors. The adenovirus-based clinical trials with the acronym AGENT were the largest and first myocardial gene therapy trials conducted on humans (Kapur and Rade, 2008, Grines et al., 2002). VEGF delivery via adenoviral vectors was demonstrated by Rosengart et al. to be safe, with clinically significant therapeutic effects (Rosengart et al., 1999). However, Phase II and III clinical trials in humans were largely inconclusive (Lyon et al., 2008).

Naked plasmid delivery accounts for about 41% of the reported clinical trials (Holladay et al., 2009), while lipid and cell-mediated gene delivery account for approximately 3% and 2%, respectively. The success rate has been relatively high considering that the transfection efficiency of non-viral gene delivery techniques is much lower than that of viruses. Neither treatment technique has significantly improved cardiac function in large-scale clinical trials, but both have shown promise. A wide variety of genes have been investigated in non-viral preclinical trials, as shown in Table 18.6, but clinical trials have focused solely on VEGF (Holladay et al., 2009) (Figure 18.3).

**TABLE 18.6**　Summary of *In Vivo* Cardiac Studies Using Lipid- or Polymer-Mediated Delivery of Plasmid DNA

| Gene | Lead Author | Reference |
|---|---|---|
| Anti-angiotensin converting enzyme (ACE) siRNA | Kim | Kim et al., 2007 |
| IL-4 | Furukawa | Furukawa et al., 2005, 2008 |
| IL-10 | Sen, Hong, Oshima, Furukawa | Sen et al., 2001, Hong et al., 2002, Oshima et al., 2002, 2007, Furukawa et al., 2005, 2008 |
| Antisense cyclin-dependent kinase cdk2, E2F decoy | Kawauchi | Kawauchi et al., 2000 |
| Cis element decoy against NFkB | Sawa | Sawa et al., 1997 |
| Heat-shock protein (HSP70) | Suzuki | Suzuki et al., 1997 |
| Heat-shock protein (HSP70) | Jayakumar | Jayakumar et al., 2000 |
| Heat-shock protein (HSP70) | Jayakumar | Jayakumar et al., 2001 |
| eNOS | Iwata | Iwata et al., 2001 |
| VEGF-A165 | Pelisek | Pelisek et al., 2003 |
| VEGF-A121 | Wang | Wang et al., 2004 |

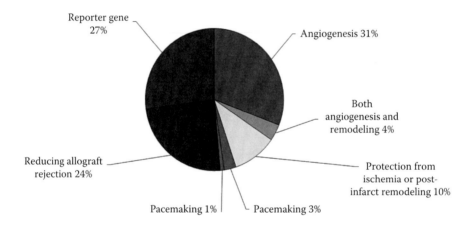

**FIGURE 18.3**　Summary of genes studied in preclinical cardiac trials.

Another growing area of interest in myocardial gene therapy is cell-mediated delivery of therapeutics, as summarized in Table 18.7. *Ex vivo* transfection of cells such as mesenchymal stem cells or skeletal myoblasts has been shown to improve cardiac function in a variety of preclinical models. Overexpression of elastin fragments (Mizuno et al., 2005b,a), VEGF (Ye et al., 2007, Suzuki et al., 2001, Yang et al., 2007), HGF (Miyagawa et al., 2006), adrenomedullin (Jo et al., 2007, Nagaya et al., 2003), MHC class I (Geissler et al., 2000), hyperpolarization-activated cyclic nucleotide-gated (HCN) channels (Potapova et al., 2004), and β2-adrenergic receptor (Edelberg et al., 1998) have all been investigated using cell-mediated gene therapy.

One of the disadvantages of cell injection is that great precision is required for the effective administration of the cells. Furthermore, very low retention rates are generally observed using these techniques. While the reason for this is not completely understood, it is likely that inflammation, nutrient limitations, and damage due to the injection procedure could be responsible. Scaffold-based cell therapy approaches for the treatment of the myocardium could present a possible solution to this problem. A number of recent studies have described using cell-seeded scaffolds instead of cell injections for cell-based therapy of the myocardium cells. Delivery of cardiomyocytes (Zimmermann et al., 2004), mesenchymal stem

**TABLE 18.7**    Summary of Studies Using Cell-Mediated Delivery of Therapeutics

| Gene | Lead Author | Reference |
|------|-------------|-----------|
| Elastin | Mizuno | Mizuno et al., 2005b |
| Elastin | Mizuno | Mizuno et al., 2005a |
| VEGF-A165 and Ang-1 | Ye | Ye et al., 2007 |
| VEGF-A165 | Suzuki | Suzuki et al., 2001 |
| HGF | Miyagawa | Miyagawa et al., 2006 |
| VEGF-A165 | Yang | Yang et al., 2007 |
| Adrenomedullin (AM) | Jo Ji | Jo et al., 2007 |
| Adrenomedullin (AM) | Nagaya | Nagaya et al., 2003 |
| MHC class I | Geissler | Geissler et al., 2000 |
| Hyperpolarization-activated cyclic nucleotide-gated (HCN) channels | Potapova | Potapova et al., 2004 |
| β2-Adrenergic receptor | Edelberg | Edelberg et al., 1998 |
| VEGF, PDGF | Das | Das et al., 2009 |
| VEGF | Goncalves | Goncalves et al., 2010 |
| VEGF, HGF, SDF-1, Akt1 | Blumenthal | Blumenthal et al., 2010 |

cells (Xiang et al., 2006, Potapova et al., 2008, Wei et al., 2008), fibroblasts (Kellar et al., 2005) and bone marrow cells (Chachques et al., 2007) has been achieved. The observed benefits included significant improvements in ejection fraction (Chachques et al., 2007, Kellar et al., 2005), increases in infarcted wall thickness (Chachques et al., 2007), higher levels of angiogenic and cardioprotective factors (Wei et al., 2008) and improved electrical properties (Potapova et al., 2008). The use of biomaterial scaffolds to deliver genetically modified cells has also been demonstrated using a fibrin gel to deliver VEGF-expressing cardiac fibroblasts (Goncalves et al., 2010) and polyurethane to deliver skeletal myoblasts expressing a variety of different factors (Blumenthal et al., 2010). The use of scaffold-based gene therapy without a cellular component represents a potential new direction for cardiac gene therapy. A proof-of-concept study used fibrin glue as a delivery vehicle for plasmid DNA encoding pleiotrophin. Enhanced neovasculature was found to be associated with the therapy, but overall functional effects were not reported (Christman et al., 2005).

While the progress of gene therapy approaches for myocardial regeneration may be closer to clinical realization than some other areas, significant advances remain to be made. The role of nonviral approaches, especially cell and scaffold-mediated, are likely to be key to clinical translation of many therapies.

## 18.4.5 Cancer

Gene therapy can treat cancer by directly reducing the amount of tumor cells by lysing them with oncolytic viruses (Norman and Lee, 2005), regulating the expression of bioactive molecules that affect cell growth and development (Duval et al., 2006), or by inciting the immune system to react against antigens found in tumor cells (Clarke et al., 2010). These therapies can be combined, but the limiting size of the capsid and the dose-dependent responses to gene therapy make this difficult. It is more likely to combine a single technique with standard therapies. Gene therapy treatments are still in the early clinical trial phase, and while some trials show partial patient improvement, they have not resulted in full regression. Such trials are shown in Table 18.8.

The systemic administration of cytokines show a clinical response in treating cancer (Lotze et al., 1986, Shau et al., 1990, Motzer et al., 1998, Ozer et al., 1998), but natural toxicity makes administering cytokines as a treatment unfeasible. Cytokine gene therapy is one of the methods being developed

**TABLE 18.8**    Clinical Trials of Gene Therapy Treating Cancer

| Type of Cancer | Gene | Mode of Delivery | Reference |
|---|---|---|---|
| Melanoma | IL-2 | Cell-mediated | Duval et al., 2006 |
| | GM-CSF | Cell-mediated | Kusumoto et al., 2001 |
| Renal cancer | GM-CSF | Cell-mediated | Tani et al., 2004 |
| | IL-2 | Cell-mediated | Uemura et al., 2006 |
| Small-cell lung cancer | IL-2 | Adenovirus | Griscelli et al., 2003 |
| | P-53 | Adenovirus | Chiappori et al., 2010 |
| Prostate | IL-2 | Adenovirus | Trudel et al., 2003 |
| | — — — — - | Wild-type reovirus | Norman and Lee, 2005 |
| Breast | IL-2 | Adenovirus | Stewart et al., 1999 |
| Solid tumors | TNF | Adenovirus | Gregorc et al., 2009 |
| Sarcoma | TNF | Adenovirus | Mundt et al., 2004 |

for a more efficient, less toxic use of cytokines. Not only does this result in a more gradual, continuous exposure to cytokines, but the use of promoters give more control over the rate or duration of cytokine production (Lopez et al., 2004).

Tumor-associated antigens (TAAs) are chemical markers to identify tumor cells and can be used to specifically target tumor cells. Antitumor immunotherapy involves inciting the immune system, usually cytotoxic T cells (CTC), to attack cells with TAAs. Viruses are encoded with transgenes for TAAs and are administered to infect host cells. The immune response to the viral load will lead to specific immune responses against the transgene product, causing the virus to act as a vaccine (Woo et al., 2006).

Oncolytic virus therapy exploits tumor cells' susceptibility to viruses to target them and transfect only the tumor cells. By using viruses very unlikely to transfect healthy human cells, the viruses specificity makes it a useful anticancer agent. Some wild-type viruses, such as the reovirus, can be used as an oncolytic virus (Comins et al., 2008).

## 18.5  Summary

To conclude, gene therapy can be administered using effective but immunogenic viruses or less antigenic nonviral techniques with associated lower levels of transfection. Gradual, continuous release can be mediated by the use of scaffolds as reservoirs. Another alternative is cells already altered *ex vivo*. Gene therapy is currently limited to clinical trials and more basic research, but multiple treatments are showing marked improvement with acceptable side effects.

The future of gene therapy requires a significant decrease in side effects while providing effective treatment. This is necessary both to compete against other therapies and to obtain regulatory approval. As new methods of avoiding dangerous doses, such as the gradual release of vectors with scaffolds, become more widespread, gene therapy will become a more viable form of treatment. Further research into nonviral vectors will develop new materials with limited cytotoxicity and high transfection efficiency. As viruses become less necessary for gene therapy the stigma against them will no longer hurt gene therapy when it comes to patient approval and regulation.

The use of scaffolds will likely become more pronounced in gene therapy as it integrates with other therapies. Scaffolds can support increased loads of DNA or cells transfected *in vitro*, leading to increased expression, or the scaffold can be designed for a slow degradation, resulting in long-term modified gene expression. They are improving to where a high DNA complex load, highly controlled and adjustable degradation rate, biocompatibility, angiogenic properties, and differentiation induction can be achieved in the same structure without sacrificing any of the desired qualities.

# Acknowledgments

This material is based upon works supported by the Science Foundation Ireland under grant no. 07/SRC/B1163.

Health Research Board (HRB/2008/188) for financial support of this work.

# References

2008. First gene therapy clinical trial for heart failure. *Molecular Therapy,* 16, 1353–1353.

Acsadi, G., Jiao, S., Jani, A., Duke, D., Williams, P., Chong, W., and Wolff, J. A. 1991. Direct gene-transfer and expression into rat-heart in vivo. *New Biologist,* 3, 71–81.

Ahlmann, E., Patzakis, M., Roidis, N., Shepherd, L., and Holtom, P. 2002. Comparison of anterior and posterior iliac crest bone grafts in terms of harvest-site morbidity and functional outcomes. *Journal of Bone and Joint Surgery-American Volume,* 84A, 716–720.

Albrektsson and Johansson 2001. Osteoinduction, osteoconduction and osseointegration. *European Spine Journal,* 10, S96-S101-S101.

Ali, M., Lemoine, N. R., and Ring, C. J. A. 1994. The use of Dna viruses as vectors for gene-therapy. *Gene Therapy,* 1, 367–384.

Andreadis, S. T. and Geer, D. J. 2006. Biomimetic approaches to protein and gene delivery for tissue regeneration. *Trends in Biotechnology,* 24, 331–337.

Andree, C., Voigt, M., Wenger, A., Erichsen, T., Bittner, K., Schaefer, D., Walgenbach, K. J., Borges, J., Horch, R. E., Eriksson, E., and Stark, G. B. 2001. Plasmid gene delivery to human keratinocytes through a fibrin-mediated transfection system. *Tissue Eng,* 7, 757–766.

Asai, J., Takenaka, H., Kusano, K. F., II, M., Luedemann, C., Curry, C., Eaton, E., Iwakura, A., Tsutsumi, Y., Hamada, H., Kishimoto, S., Thorne, T., Kishore, R., and Losordo, D. W. 2006. Topical sonic hedgehog gene therapy accelerates wound healing in diabetes by enhancing endothelial progenitor cell-mediated microvascular remodeling. *Circulation,* 113, 2413–2424.

Ashare, A. B., Maysky, M., Vale, P. R., Losordo, D. W., Symes, J. F., and Isner, J. M. 1999. Quantitative evaluation of gene therapy for myocardial angiogenesis. *Journal of Nuclear Medicine,* 40, 760.

Avery, O. T., Mcleod, C. M., and Mccarty, M. 1944. Studies on the chemical nature of the substance inducing transformation of pneumococcal types. *Journal of Experimental Medicine,* 79, 137–158.

Badillo, A. T., Chung, S., Zhang, L., Zoltick, P., and Liechty, K. W. 2007. Lentiviral gene transfer of Sdf-1alpha to wounds improves diabetic wound healing. *Journal of Surgery and Research,* 143, 35–42.

Bakal, C., Becker, G., Clement, D. L., Cronenwett, J., Durand-Zaleski, I., Diehm, C., Harris, K., Hiatt, W. R., Hunink, M., Isner, J., Lammer, J., Norgren, L., Novo, S., Ricco, J. B., Verstraete, M., and White, J. 2000. Management of peripheral arterial disease (Pad). *European Journal of Vascular and Endovascular Surgery,* 19 Suppl A, S115–S143.

Bakker, A. C., Van DE Loo, F. A., Joosten, L. A., Bennink, M. B., Arntz, O. J., Dmitriev, I. P., Kashentsera, E. A., Curiel, D. T., and Van DEN Berg, W. B. 2001. A tropism-modified adenoviral vector increased the effectiveness of gene therapy for arthritis. *Gene Therapy,* 8, 1785–1793.

Baltzer, A. W. A., Lattermann, C., Whalen, J. D., Wooley, P., Weiss, K., Grimm, M., Ghivizzani, S. C., Robbins, P. D., and Evans, C. H. 2000. Genetic enhancement of fracture repair: healing of an experimental segmental defect by adenoviral transfer of the Bmp-2 gene. *Gene Therapy,* 7, 734–739.

Baraniak, P. R. and Mcdevitt, T. C. 2010. Stem cell paracrine actions and tissue regeneration. *Regenerative Medicine,* 5, 121–143.

Barnes, P. F., Abrams, J. S., LU, S. Z., Sieling, P. A., Rea, T. H., and Modlin, R. L. 1993. Patterns of cytokine production by Mycobacterium-reactive human T-cell clones. *Infection and Immunity,* 61, 197–203.

Barrick, B., Campbell, E. J., and Owen, C. A. 1999. Leukocyte proteinases in wound healing: Roles in physiologic and pathologic processes. *Wound Repair Regen,* 7, 410–422.

Baru, M., Axelrod, J. H., and Nur, I. 1995. Liposome-encapsulated DNA-mediated gene-transfer and synthesis of human factor-IX in mice. *Gene*, 161, 143–150.

Bathgate, R. A. D., Lekgabe, E. D., Mcguane, J. T., SU, Y., Pham, T., Ferraro, T., Layfield, S., Hannan, R. D., Thomas, W. G., Samuel, C. S., and DU, X. J. 2008. Adenovirus-mediated delivery of relaxin reverses cardiac fibrosis. *Molecular and Cellular Endocrinology*, 280, 30–38.

Baumgartner, I., Chronos, N., Comerota, A., Henry, T., Pasquet, J. P., Finiels, F., Caron, A., Dedieu, J. F., Pilsudski, R., and Delaä¨RE, P. 2009. Local gene transfer and expression following intramuscular administration of Fgf-1 plasmid DNA in patients with critical limb ischemia. *Molecular Therapy*, 17, 914–921.

Baumgartner, I., Pieczek, A., Manor, O., Blair, R., Kearney, M., Walsh, K., and Isner, J. M. 1998. Constitutive expression of phvegf165 after intramuscular gene transfer promotes collateral vessel development in patients with critical limb ischemia. *Circulation*, 97, 1114–1123.

Bhattacharyya, J., Mondal, G., Madhusudana, K., Agawane, S. B., Ramakrishna, S., Gangireddy, S. R., Madhavi, R. D., Reddy, P. K., Konda, V. R., Rao, S. R., Udaykumar, P., and Chaudhuri, A. 2009. Single subcutaneous administration of Rgdk-lipopeptide:rhpdgf-B gene complex heals wounds in streptozotocin-induced diabetic rats. *Molecular Pharmacology*, 6, 918–927.

Bitto, A., Minutoli, L., Galeano, M. R., Altavilla, D., Polito, F., Fiumara, T., Calo, M., LO Cascio, P., Zentilin, L., Giacca, M., and Squadrito, F. 2008. Angiopoietin-1 gene transfer improves impaired wound healing in genetically diabetic mice without increasing Vegf expression. *Clinical Science (Lond)*, 114, 707–718.

Blakytny, R. and Jude, E. 2006. The molecular biology of chronic wounds and delayed healing in diabetes. *Diabetes Medicine*, 23, 594–608.

Blakytny, R. and Jude, E. B. 2009. Altered molecular mechanisms of diabetic foot ulcers. *International Journal of Low Extreme Wounds*, 8, 95–104.

Blum, J. S., Barry, M. A., Mikos, A. G., and Jansen, J. A. 2003. *In vivo* evaluation of gene therapy vectors in ex vivo-derived marrow stromal cells for bone regeneration in a rat critical-size calvarial defect model. *Human Gene Therapy*, 14, 1689–1701.

Blumenthal, B., Golsong, P., Poppe, A., Heilmann, C., Schlensak, C., Beyersdorf, F., and Siepe, M. 2010. Polyurethane scaffolds seeded with genetically engineered skeletal myoblasts: A promising tool to regenerate myocardial function. *Artificial Organs*, 34(2), E46–E54.

Boden, S. D., Liu, Y. S., Hair, G. A., Helms, J. A., HU, D., Racine, M., Nanes, M. S., and Titus, L. 1998. Lmp-1, a Lim-domain protein, mediates Bmp-6 effects on bone formation. *Endocrinology*, 139, 5125–5134.

Bonadio, J. 2000. Tissue engineering via local gene delivery: Update and future prospects for enhancing the technology. *Advances in Drug Delivery Reviews*, 44, 185–194.

Bonadio, J., Smiley, E., Patil, P., and Goldstein, S. 1999a. Localized, direct plasmid gene delivery in vivo: prolonged therapy results in reproducible tissue regeneration. *Nature Medicine*, 5, 753–759.

Bonadio, J., Smiley, E., Patil, P., and Goldstein, S. 1999b. Localized, direct plasmid gene delivery in vivo: prolonged therapy results in reproducible tissue regeneration. *Nature Medicine*, 5, 753–759.

Bowler, P. G. 2002. Wound pathophysiology, infection and therapeutic options. *Annals in Medicine*, 34, 419–427.

Breen, A., Dockery, P., O'brien, T., and Pandit, A. 2008. The use of therapeutic gene enos delivered via a fibrin scaffold enhances wound healing in a compromised wound model. *Biomaterials*, 29, 3143–3151.

Breen AM, D. P., O'Brien T, Pandit AS 2008. The use of therapeutic gene enos delivered via a fibrin scaffold enhances wound healing in a compromised wound model. *Biomaterials*, 29, 3143–3151.

Brem, H., Kodra, A., Golinko, M. S., Entero, H., Stojadinovic, O., Wang, V. M., Sheahan, C. M., Weinberg, A. D., Woo, S. L., Ehrlich, H. P., and Tomic-Canic, M. 2009. Mechanism of sustained release of vascular endothelial growth factor in accelerating experimental diabetic healing. *Journal of Investigative Dermatology*, 129, 2275–2287.

Brem, H. and Tomic-Canic, M. 2007. Cellular and molecular basis of wound healing in diabetes. *Journal of Clinical Investigation*, 117, 1219–1222.

Breunig, M., Lungwitz, U., Liebl, R., and Goepferich, A. 2007. Breaking up the correlation between efficacy and toxicity for nonviral gene delivery. *Proceedings of the National Academy of Sciences of the United States of America*, 104, 14454–14459.

Brown, R. L., Breeden, M. P., and Greenhalgh, D. G. 1994. Pdgf and Tgf-alpha act synergistically to improve wound healing in the genetically diabetic mouse. *Journal of Surgical Research,* 56, 562–70.

Cao, L., Arany, P. R., Kim, J., Rivera-Feliciano, J., Wang, Y. S., He, Z., Rask-Madsen, C., King, G. L., and Mooney, D. J. 2010. Modulating Notch signaling to enhance neovascularization and reperfusion in diabetic mice. *Biomaterials,* 34, 9048–9056.

Chachques, J. C., Trainini, J. C., Lago, N., Masoli, O. H., Barisani, J. L., Cortes-Morichetti, M., Schussler, O., and Carpentier, A. Year. Myocardial assistance by grafting a new bioartificial upgraded myocardium (Magnum clinical trial): One year follow-up. In: *3rd International Conference on Cell Therapy for Cardiovascular Diseases,* 2007 New York, NY, pp. 927–934.

Check, E. 2003. Cancer risk prompts US to curb gene therapy. *Nature,* 422, 7–7.

Chen, J., Huang, S. W., Lin, W. H., and Zhuo, R. X. 2007a. Tunable film degradation and sustained release of plasmid DNA from cleavable polycation/plasmid DNa multilayers under reductive conditions. *Small,* 3, 636–643.

Chen, X. H., Minatoguchi, S., Kosai, K., Yuge, K., Takahashi, T., Arai, M., Wang, N. Y., Misao, Y., Lu, C. J., Onogi, H., Kobayashi, H., Yasuda, S., Ezaki, M., Ushikoshi, H., Takemura, G., Fujiwara, T., and Fujiwara, H. 2007b. *In vivo* hepatocyte growth factor gene transfer reduces myocardial ischemia – reperfusion injury through its multiple actions. *Journal of Cardiac Failure,* 13, 874–883.

Chiappori, A. A., Soliman, H., Janssen, W. E., Antonia, S. J., and Gabrilovich, D. I. 2010. Ingn-225: A dendritic cell-based p53 vaccine (Ad.p53-DC) in small cell lung cancer: Observed association between immune response and enhanced chemotherapy effect. *Expert Opin Biol Ther,* 10, 983–991.

Christman, K. L., Fang, Q. Z., Yee, M. S., Johnson, K. R., Sievers, R. E., and Lee, R. J. 2005. Enhanced neovasculature formation in ischemic myocardium following delivery of pleiotrophin plasmid in a biopolymer. *Biomaterials,* 26, 1139–1144.

Chun, K. W., Lee, J. B., Kim, S. H., and Park, T. G. 2005. Controlled release of plasmid DNA from photo-cross-linked pluronic hydrogels. *Biomaterials,* 26, 3319–3326.

Cianfarani, F., Zambruno, G., Brogelli, L., Sera, F., Lacal, P. M., Pesce, M., Capogrossi, M. C., Failla, C. M., Napolitano, M., and Odorisio, T. 2006. Placenta growth factor in diabetic wound healing: Altered expression and therapeutic potential. *American Journal of Pathology,* 169, 1167–1182.

Clarke, J. M., Morse, M. A., Lyerly, H. K., Clay, T., and Osada, T. 2010. Adenovirus vaccine immunotherapy targeting Wt1-expressing tumors. *Expert Opinion in Biological Therapy,* 10, 875–883.

Comerota, A. J., Throm, R. C., Miller, K. A., Henry, T., Chronos, N., Laird, J., Sequeira, R., Kent, C. K., Bacchetta, M., Goldman, C., Salenius, J. P., Schmieder, F. A., and Pilsudski, R. 2002. Naked plasmid Dna encoding fibroblast growth factor type 1 for the treatment of end-stage unreconstructible lower extremity ischemia: Preliminary results of a phase I trial. *Journal of Vascular Surgery,* 35, 930–936.

Comins, C., Heinemann, L., Harrington, K., Melcher, A., DE Bono, J., and Pandha, H. 2008. Reovirus: Viral therapy for cancer 'as nature intended'. *Clinical Oncology (R Coll Radiol),* 20, 548–554.

Das, H., George, J. C., Joseph, M., Das, M., Abdulhameed, N., Blitz, A., Khan, M., Sakthivel, R., Mao, H. Q., Hoit, B. D., Kuppusamy, P., and Pompili, V. J. 2009. Stem cell therapy with overexpressed Vegf and Pdgf genes improves cardiac function in a rat infarct model. *Plos One,* 4(10), e7325.

Davidson, J. M., Broadley, K. N., and Quaglino, D. 1997. Reversal of the wound healing deficit in diabetic rats by combined basic fibroblast growth and transforming factor-beta1 therapy. *Wound Repair Regeneration,* 5, 77–88.

Davis, J., Westfall, M. V., Townsend, D., Blankinship, M., Herron, T. J., Guerrero-Serna, G., Wang, W., Devaney, E., and Metzger, J. M. 2008. Designing heart performance by gene transfer. *Physiological Reviews,* 88, 1567–1651.

Del Monte, F., Williams, E., Lebeche, D., Schmidt, U., Rosenzweig, A., Gwathmey, J. K., Lewandowski, E. D., and Hajjar, R. J. 2001. Improvement in survival and cardiac metabolism after gene transfer of sarcoplasmic reticulum Ca2 + -ATPase in a rat model of heart failure. *Circulation,* 104, 1424–1429.

Dennig, J. and Duncan, E. 2002. Gene transfer into eukaryotic cells using activated polyamidoamine dendrimers. *Journal of Biotechnology*, 90, 339–347.

Diegelmann, R. F. and Evans, M. C. 2004. Wound healing: An overview of acute, fibrotic and delayed healing. *Frontiers in Bioscience*, 9, 283–289.

Dorresteijn, J. A., Kriegsman, D. M., and Valk, G. D. 2010. Complex interventions for preventing diabetic foot ulceration. *Cochrane Database Systems Reviews*, 1, Cd007610.

Dufes, C., Uchegbu, I. F., and Schatzlein, A. G. 2005. Dendrimers in gene delivery. *Advanced Drug Delivery Reviews*, 57, 2177–2202.

Duval, L., Schmidt, H., Kaltoft, K., Fode, K., Jensen, J. J., Sorensen, S. M., Nishimura, M. I., and Von DER Maase, H. 2006. Adoptive transfer of allogeneic cytotoxic T lymphocytes equipped with a Hla-A2 restricted Mart-1 T-cell receptor: A phase I trial in metastatic melanoma. *Clinical Cancer Research*, 12, 1229–1236.

Edelberg, J. M., Aird, W. C., and Rosenberg, R. D. 1998. Enhancement of murine cardiac chronotropy by the molecular transfer of the human beta(2) adrenergic receptor cdna. *Journal of Clinical Investigation*, 101, 337–343.

Edelstein, M. L., Abedi, M. R., and Wixon, J. 2007. Gene therapy clinical trials worldwide to 2007—An update. *The Journal of Gene Medicine*, 9, 833–842.

Egermann, M., Baltzer, A. W., Adamaszek, S., Evans, C., Robbins, P., Schneider, E., and Lill, C. A. 2006a. Direct adenoviral transfer of bone morphogenetic protein-2 cdna enhances fracture healing in osteoporotic sheep. *Human Gene Therapy*, 17, 507–517.

Egermann, M., Lill, C. A., Griesbeck, K., Evans, C. H., Robbins, P. D., Schneider, E., and Baltzer, A. W. 2006b. Effect of Bmp-2 gene transfer on bone healing in sheep. *Gene Therapy*, 13, 1290–1299.

Eming, S. A., Krieg, T., and Davidson, J. M. 2004. Gene transfer in tissue repair: status, challenges and future directions. *Expert Opinion in Biological Therapy*, 4, 1373–1386.

Fang, J. M., Zhu, Y. Y., Smiley, E., Bonadio, J., Rouleau, J. P., Goldstein, S. A., Mccauley, L. K., Davidson, B. L., and Roessler, B. J. 1996. Stimulation of new bone formation by direct transfer of osteogenic plasmid genes. *Proceedings of the National Academy of Sciences of the United States of America*, 93, 5753–5758.

Fang, Y., Shen, J., Yao, M., Beagley, K. W., Hambly, B. D., and Bao, S. 2010. Granulocyte–macrophage colony-stimulating factor enhances wound healing in diabetes via upregulation of proinflammatory cytokines. *British Journal of Dermatology*, 162, 478–486.

Fernandez-Montequin, J. I., Infante-Cristia, E., Valenzuela-Silva, C., Franco-Perez, N., Savigne-Gutierrez, W., Artaza-Sanz, H., Morejon-Vega, L., Gonzalez-Benavides, C., Eliseo-Musenden, O., Garcia-Iglesias, E., Berlanga-Acosta, J., Silva-Rodriguez, R., Betancourt, B. Y., and Lopez-Saura, P. A. 2007. Intralesional injections of Citoprot-P (recombinant human epidermal growth factor) in advanced diabetic foot ulcers with risk of amputation. *International Wound Journal*, 4, 333–343.

Fernandez-Montequin, J. I., Valenzuela-Silva, C. M., Diaz, O. G., Savigne, W., Sancho-Soutelo, N., Rivero-Fernandez, F., Sanchez-Penton, P., Morejon-Vega, L., Artaza-Sanz, H., Garcia-Herrera, A., Gonzalez-Benavides, C., Hernandez-Canete, C. M., Vazquez-Proenza, A., Berlanga-Acosta, J., and Lopez-Saura, P. A. 2009. Intra-lesional injections of recombinant human epidermal growth factor promote granulation and healing in advanced diabetic foot ulcers: multicenter, randomised, placebo-controlled, double-blind study. *International Wound Journal*, 6, 432–443.

Flynn, A. and O'brien, T. 2008. Alferminogene tadenovec, an angiogenic Fgf4 gene therapy for coronary artery disease. *Idrugs*, 11, 283–293.

Fortuin, F. D., Vale, P., Losordo, D. W., Symes, J., Delaria, G. A., Tyner, J. J., Schaer, G. L., March, R., Snell, R. J., Henry, T. D., Van Camp, J., Lopez, J. J., Richenbacher, W., Isner, J. M., and Schatz, R. A. 2003. One-year follow-up of direct myocardial gene transfer of vascular endothelial growth factor-2 using naked plasmid deoxyribonucleic acid by way of thoracotomy in no-option patients. *American Journal of Cardiology*, 92, 436–439.

French, B. A., Mazur, W., Geske, R. S., and Bolli, R. 1994. Direct *in vivo* gene-transfer into porcine myocardium using replication-deficient adenoviral vectors. *Circulation*, 90, 2414–2424.

Friedmann, T. 1989. Progress toward human gene therapy. *Science,* 244, 1275–1281.

Friedmann, T. 1992. A brief history of gene therapy. *Nature Genetics,* 2, 93–98.

Furukawa, H., Oshima, K., Tung, T., Cui, G. G., Laks, H., and Sen, L. 2005. Liposome-mediated combinatorial cytokine gene therapy induces localized synergistic immunosuppression and promotes long-term survival of cardiac allografts. *Journal of Immunology,* 174, 6983–6992.

Furukawa, H., Oshima, K., Tung, T., Cui, G. G., Laks, H., and Sen, L. Y. 2008. Overexpressed exogenous IL-4 and IL-10 paradoxically regulate allogenic T-Cell and cardiac myocytes apoptosis through Fas/Fasl pathway. *Transplantation,* 85, 437–446.

Galkowska, H., Wojewodzka, U., and Olszewski, W. L. 2006. Chemokines, cytokines, and growth factors in keratinocytes and dermal endothelial cells in the margin of chronic diabetic foot ulcers. *Wound Repair and Regeneration,* 14, 558–565.

Geissler, E. K., Graeb, C., Tange, S., Guba, M., Jauch, K. W., and Scherer, M. N. 2000. Effective use of donor Mhc class I gene therapy in organ transplantation: Prevention of antibody-mediated hyperacute heart allograft rejection in highly sensitized rat recipients. *Human Gene Therapy,* 11, 459–469.

Gisep, A. 2002. Research on ceramic bone substitutes: Current status. *Injury-International Journal of the Care of the Injured,* 33, 88–92.

Giurini, J. M. and Lyons, T. E. 2005. Diabetic foot complications: Diagnosis and management. *Int J Low Extreme Wounds,* 4, 171–182.

Goncalves, G. A., Vassallo, P. F., Dos Santos, L., Schettert, I. T., Nakamuta, J. S., Becker, C., Tucci, P. J. F., and Krieger, J. E. 2010. Intramyocardial transplantation of fibroblasts expressing vascular endothelial growth factor attenuates cardiac dysfunction. *Gene Therapy,* 17, 305–314.

Gottrup, F., Apelqvist, J., and Price, P. 2010. Outcomes in controlled and comparative studies on non-healing wounds: Recommendations to improve the quality of evidence in wound management. *J Wound Care,* 19, 237–268.

Gray, S. J. and Samulski, R. J. 2008. Optimizing gene delivery vectors for the treatment of heart disease. *Expert Opinion on Biological Therapy,* 8, 911–922.

Greenhalgh, D. G., Hummel, R. P., Albertson, S., and Breeden, M. P. 1993. Synergistic actions of platelet-derived growth factor and the insulin-like growth factors in vivo. *Wound Repair Regen,* 1, 69–81.

Gregorc, V., Santoro, A., Bennicelli, E., Punt, C. J., Citterio, G., Timmer-Bonte, J. N., Caligaris Cappio, F., Lambiase, A., Bordignon, C., and Van Herpen, C. M. 2009. Phase Ib study of Ngr-htnf, a selective vascular targeting agent, administered at low doses in combination with doxorubicin to patients with advanced solid tumours. *British Journal of Cancer,* 101, 219–224.

Grines, C., Rubanyi, G. M., Kleiman, N. S., Marrott, P., and Watkins, M. W. Year. Angiogenic gene therapy with adenovirus 5 fibroblast growth factor-4 (Ad5fgf = 4): A new option for the treatment of coronary artery disease. In: *Workshop on Angiogenic Gene Therapy,* Dec 13–15, 2002 New York, New York. 24N–31N.

Grinnell, F., Ho, C. H., and Wysocki, A. 1992. Degradation of fibronectin and vitronectin in chronic wound fluid: analysis by cell blotting, immunoblotting, and cell adhesion assays. *Journal of Investigative Dermatology,* 98, 410–416.

Griscelli, F., Opolon, P., Saulnier, P., Mami-Chouaib, F., Gautier, E., Echchakir, H., Angevin, E., LE Chevalier, T., Bataille, V., Squiban, P., Tursz, T., and Escudier, B. 2003. Recombinant adenovirus shedding after intratumoral gene transfer in lung cancer patients. *Gene Therapy,* 10, 386–395.

Guerrero, M., Athota, K., Moy, J., Mehta, L. S., Laguens, R., Crottogini, A., Borrelli, M., Corry, P., Schoenherr, D., Gentry, R., Boura, J., Grines, C. L., Raff, G. L., Shanley, C. J., and O'neill, W. W. 2008. Vascular endothelial growth factor-165 gene therapy promotes cardiomyogenesis in reperfused myocardial infarction. *Journal of Interventional Cardiology,* 21, 242–251.

Guo, T., Zhao, J., Chang, J., Ding, Z., Hong, H., Chen, J., and Zhang, J. 2006. Porous chitosan-gelatin scaffold containing plasmid Dna encoding transforming growth factor-beta1 for chondrocytes proliferation. *Biomaterials,* 27, 1095–1103.

Gupta, D., Molina, E. J., Palma, J., Gaughan, J. P., Long, W., and Macha, M. 2008a. Adenoviral beta-adrenergic receptor kinase inhibitor gene transfer improves exercise capacity, cardiac contractility, and systemic inflammation in a model of pressure overload hypertrophy. *Cardiovascular Drugs and Therapy,* 22, 373–381.

Gupta, D., Palma, J., Molina, E., Gaughan, J. P., Long, W., Houser, S., and Macha, M. 2008b. Improved exercise capacity and reduced systemic inflammation after adenoviral-mediated Serca-2a gene transfer. *Journal of Surgical Research,* 145, 257–265.

Guyton, A. C. and Hall, J. E. 2000. Unit IV: The circulation. *Textbook of Medical Physiology.* 10th ed. Philadelphia, Pennsylvania: W.B. Saunders Company.

Guzman, R. J., Lemarchand, P., Crystal, R. G., Epstein, S. E., and Finkel, T. 1993. Efficient gene transfer into myocardium by direct-injection of adenovirus vectors. *Circulation Research,* 73, 1202–1207.

Gyongyosi, M., Khorsand, A., Zamini, S., Sperker, W., Strehblow, C., Kastrup, J., Jorgensen, E., Hesse, B., Tagil, K., Botker, H. E., Ruzyllo, W., Teresinska, A., Dudek, D., Hubalewska, A., Ruck, A., Nielsen, S. S., Graf, S., Mundigler, G., Novak, J., Sochor, H., Maurer, G., Glogar, D., and Sylven, C. 2005. Noga-guided analysis of regional myocardial perfusion abnormalities treated with intramyocardial injections of plasmid encoding vascular endothelial growth factor A-165 in patients with chronic myocardial ischemia—Subanalysis of the Euroinject-One multicenter double-blind randomized study. *Circulation,* 112, I157–I165.

Hacein-Bey-Abina, S., Von Kalle, C., Schmidt, M., LE Deist, F., Wulffraat, N., Mcintyre, E., Radford, I., Villeval, J.-L., Fraser, C. C., Cavazzana-Calvo, M., and Fischer, A. 2003. A serious adverse event after successful gene therapy for X-linked severe combined immunodeficiency. *The New England Journal of Medicine,* 348, 255–256.

Haider, H. K., Elmadbouh, I., Jean-Baptiste, M., and Ashraf, M. 2008. Nonviral vector gene modification of stem cells for myocardial repair. *Molecular Medicine,* 14, 79–86.

Hajjar, R. J., Zsebo, K., Deckelbaum, L., Thompson, C., Rudy, J., Yaroshinsky, A., Ly, H., Kawase, Y., Wagner, K., Borow, K., Jaski, B., London, B., Greenberg, B., Pauly, D. F., Patten, R., Starling, R., Mancini, D., and Jessup, M. 2008. Design of a phase 1/2 trial of intracoronary administration of Aav1/SERCA2a in patients with heart failure. *Journal of Cardiac Failure,* 14, 355–367.

Haro, J., Acin, F., Lopez-Quintana, A., Florez, A., Martinez-Aguilar, E., and Varela, C. 2009. Meta-analysis of randomized, controlled clinical trials in angiogenesis: Gene and cell therapy in peripheral arterial disease. *Heart and Vessels,* 24, 321–328.

Hattori, Y., Kawakami, S., Suzuki, S., Yamashita, F., and Hashida, M. 2004. Enhancement of immune responses by Dna vaccination through targeted gene delivery using mannosylated cationic liposome formulations following intravenous administration in mice. *Biochemistry and Biophysics Research Communication,* 317, 992–999.

Haviernik, P. and Bunting, K. D. 2004. Safety concerns related to hematopoietic stem cell gene transfer using retroviral vectors. *Current Gene Therapy,* 4, 263–276.

Hedman, M., Hartikainen, J., Syvanne, M., Stjernvall, J., Hedman, A., Kivela, A., Vanninen, E., Mussalo, H., Kauppila, E., Simula, S., Narvanen, O., Rantala, A., Peuhkurinen, K., Nieminen, M. S., Laakso, M., and Yla-Herttuala, S. 2003. Safety and feasibility of catheter-based local intracoronary vascular endothelial growth factor gene transfer in the prevention of postangioplasty and in-stent restenosis and in the treatment of chronic myocardial ischemia—Phase II results of the Kuopio Angiogenesis Trial (Kat). *Circulation,* 107, 2677–2683.

Henry, T. D., Rocha-Singh, K., Isner, J. M., Kereiakes, D. J., Giordano, F. J., Simons, M., Losordo, D. W., Hendel, R. C., Bonow, R. O., Eppler, S. M., Zioncheck, T. F., Holmgren, E. B., and Mccluskey, E. R. 2001. Intracoronary administration of recombinant human vascular endothelial growth factor to patients with coronary artery disease. *American Heart Journal,* 142, 872–880.

Hirsch, T., Spielmann, M., Velander, P., Zuhaili, B., Bleiziffer, O., Fossum, M., Steinstraesser, L., Yao, F., and Eriksson, E. 2008. Insulin-like growth factor-1 gene therapy and cell transplantation in diabetic wounds. *Journal of Gene Medicine,* 10, 1247–1252.

Holladay, C. A., O'brien, T., and Pandit, A. 2009. Non-viral gene therapy for myocardial engineering. *Wiley Interdisciplinary Reviews: Nanomedicine and Nanobiotechnology,* 2, 232–248.

Hong, Y. S., Laks, H., Cui, G. G., Chong, T., and Sen, L. Y. 2002. Localized immunosuppression in the cardiac allograft induced by a new liposome-mediated IL-10 gene therapy. *Journal of Heart and Lung Transplantation,* 21, 1188–1200.

Horch, R. E., Kopp, J., Kneser, U., Beier, J., and Bach, A. D. 2005. Tissue engineering of cultured skin substitutes. *Journal of Cellular and Molecular Medicine,* 9, 592–608.

Hosseinkhani, H. 2006. Dna nanoparticles for gene delivery to cells and tissue. *International Journal of Nanotechnology,* 3, 416–461.

Hosseinkhani, H., Azzam, T., Kobayashi, H., Hiraoka, Y., Shimokawa, H., Domb, A. J., and Tabata, Y. 2006a. Combination of 3D tissue engineered scaffold and non-viral gene carrier enhance *in vitro* Dna expression of mesenchymal stem cells. *Biomaterials,* 27, 4269–4278.

Hosseinkhani, H., Hosseinkhani, M., Gabrielson, N. P., Pack, D. W., Khademhosseini, A., and Kobayashi, H. 2008. Dna nanoparticles encapsulated in 3D tissue-engineered scaffolds enhance osteogenic differentiation of mesenchymal stem cells. *Journal of Biomedical Materials Research Part A,* 85A, 47–60.

Hosseinkhani, H., Inatsugu, Y., Hiraoka, Y., Inoue, S., Shimokawa, H., and Tabata, Y. 2005. Impregnation of plasmid Dna into three-dimensional scaffolds and medium perfusion enhance *in vitro* Dna expression of mesenchymal stem cells. *Tissue Engineering,* 11, 1459–1475.

Hosseinkhani, H. and Tabata, Y. 2006. Self assembly of Dna nanoparticles with polycations for the delivery of genetic materials into cells. *Journal of Nanoscience and Nanotechnology,* 6, 2320–2328.

Hosseinkhani, H., Yamamoto, M., Inatsugu, Y., Hiraoka, Y., Inoue, S., Shimokawa, H., and Tabata, Y. 2006b. Enhanced ectopic bone formation using a combination of plasmid Dna impregnation into 3-D scaffold and bioreactor perfusion culture. *Biomaterials,* 27, 1387–1398.

Immordino, M. L., Dosio, F., and Cattel, L. 2006. Stealth liposomes: Review of the basic science, rationale, and clinical applications, existing and potential. *International Journal of Nanomedicine,* 1, 297–315.

Isner, J. M. 1998. Arterial gene transfer of naked Dna for therapeutic angiogenesis: Early clinical results. *Advanced Drug Delivery Reviews,* 30, 185–197.

Isner, J. M., Baumgartner, I., Rauh, G., Schainfeld, R., Blair, R., Manor, O., Razvi, S., and Symes, J. F. 1998. Treatment of thromboangiitis obliterans (Buerger's disease) by intramuscular gene transfer of vascular endothelial growth factor: Preliminary clinical results. *Journal of Vascular Surgery,* 28, 964–975.

Isner, J. M., Pieczek, A., Schainfeld, R., Blair, R., Haley, L., Asahara, T., Rosenfield, K., Razvi, S., Walsh, K., and Symes, J. F. 1996. Clinical evidence of angiogenesis after arterial gene transfer of phvegf165 in patient with ischaemic limb. *Lancet,* 348, 370–374.

Iwata, A., Sai, S., Nitta, Y., Chen, M., DE Fries-Hallstrand, R., Dalesandro, J., Thomas, R., and Allen, M. D. 2001. Liposome-mediated gene transfection of endothelial nitric oxide synthase reduces endothelial activation and leukocyte infiltration in transplanted hearts. *Circulation,* 103, 2753–2759.

Jane, J. A., Dunford, B. A., Kron, A., Pittman, D. D., Sasaki, T., Li, J. Z., Li, H. W., Alden, T. D., Dayoub, H., Hankins, G. R., Kallmes, D. F., and Helm, G. A. 2002. Ectopic osteogenesis using adenoviral bone morphogenetic protein (Bmp)-4 and Bmp-6 gene transfer. *Molecular Therapy,* 6, 464–470.

Jawad, H., Ali, N. N., Lyon, A. R., Chen, Q. Z., Harding, S. E., and Boccaccini, A. R. 2007. Myocardial tissue engineering: A review. *Journal of Tissue Engineering and Regenerative Medicine,* 1, 327–342.

Jayakumar, J., Suzuki, K., Khan, M., Smolenski, R. T., Farrell, A., Latif, N., Raisky, O., Abunasra, H., Sammut, I. A., Murtuza, B., Amrani, M., and Yacoub, M. H. 2000. Gene therapy for myocardial protection—Transfection of donor hearts with heat shock protein 70 gene protects cardiac function against ischemia – reperfusion injury. *Circulation,* 102, 302–306.

Jayakumar, J., Suzuki, K., Sammut, I. A., Smolenski, R. T., Khan, M., Latif, N., Abunasra, H., Murtuza, B., Amrani, M., and Yacoub, M. H. 2001. Heat shock protein 70 gene transfection protects mitochondrial and ventricular function against ischemia – reperfusion injury. *Circulation,* 104, I303–I307.

Jazwa, A., Kucharzewska, P., Leja, J., Zagorska, A., Sierpniowska, A., Stepniewski, J., Kozakowska, M., Taha, H., Ochiya, T., Derlacz, R., Vahakangas, E., Yla-Herttuala, S., Jozkowicz, A., and Dulak, J. 2010a. Combined vascular endothelial growth factor-A and fibroblast growth factor 4 gene transfer improves wound healing in diabetic mice. *Genetic Vaccines Therapy,* 8, 6.

Jazwa, A., Kucharzewska, P., Leja, J., Zagorska, A., Sierpniowska, A., Stepniewski, J., Kozakowska, M., Taha, H., Ochiya, T., Derlacz, R., Vahakangas, E., Yla-Herttuala, S., Jozkowicz, A., and Dulak, J. 2010b. Combined vascular endothelial growth factor-A and fibroblast growth factor 4 gene transfer improves wound healing in diabetic mice. *Genetic Vaccines Therapy*, 8, 6.

Jiang, X. Q., Zhao, J., Wang, S. Y., Sun, X. J., Zhang, X. L., Chen, J., Kaplan, D. L., and Zhang, Z. Y. 2009. Mandibular repair in rats with premineralized silk scaffolds and Bmp-2-modified bMSCs. *Biomaterials*, 30, 4522–4532.

Jo, J. I., Nagaya, N., Miyahara, Y., Kataoka, M., Harada-Shiba, M., Kangawa, K., and Tabata, Y. 2007. Transplantation of genetically engineered mesenchymal stem cells improves cardiac function in rats with myocardial infarction: Benefit of a novel nonviral vector, cationized dextran. *Tissue Engineering*, 13, 313–322.

Judith, R., Nithya, M., Rose, C., and Mandal, A. B. 2010. Application of a Pdgf-containing novel gel for cutaneous wound healing. *Life Science*, 87, 1–8.

Kalka, C., Masuda, H., Takahashi, T., Gordon, R., Tepper, O., Gravereaux, E., Pieczek, A., Iwaguro, H., Hayashi, S.-I., Isner, J. M., and Asahara, T. 2000. Vascular endothelial growth factor165 gene transfer augments circulating endothelial progenitor cells in human subjects. *Circulation Research*, 86, 1198–1202.

Kapur, N. K. and Rade, J. J. 2008. Fibroblast growth factor 4 gene therapy for chronic ischemic heart disease. *Trends in Cardiovascular Medicine*, 18, 133–141.

Kastrup, J., Jorgensen, E., Ruck, A., Tagil, K., Glogar, D., Ruzyllo, W., Botker, H. E., Dudek, D., Drvota, V., Hesse, B., Thuesen, L., Blomberg, P., Gyongyosi, M., and Sylven, C. 2005. Direct intramyocardial plasmid vascular endothelial growth factor-A(165)-gene therapy in patients with stable severe angina pectoris–A randomized double-blind placebo-controlled study: The Euroinject One trial. *Journal of the American College of Cardiology*, 45, 982–988.

Kaul, G. and Amiji, M. 2004. Biodistribution and targeting potential of poly(ethylene glycol)-modified gelatin nanoparticles in subcutaneous murine tumor model. *Journal of Drug Target*, 12, 585–591.

Kaul, G. and Amiji, M. 2005. Tumor-targeted gene delivery using poly(ethylene glycol)-modified gelatin nanoparticles: *In vitro* and *in vivo* studies. *Pharmaceutical Research*, 22, 951–961.

Kawauchi, M., Suzuki, J., Morishita, R., Wada, Y., Izawa, A., Tomita, N., Amano, J., Kaneda, Y., Ogihara, T., Takamoto, S., and Isobe, M. 2000. Gene therapy for attenuating cardiac allograft arteriopathy using ex vivo E2F decoy transfection by Hvj-Ave-liposome method in mice and nonhuman primates. *Circulation Research*, 87, 1063–1068.

Keating, J. F. and Mcqueen, M. M. 2001. Substitutes for autologous bone graft in orthopaedic trauma. *Journal of Bone and Joint Surgery-British Volume*, 83B, 3–8.

Keeney, M., Van DEN Beucken, J., Van DER Kraan, P. M., Jansen, J. A., and Pandit, A. 2010. The ability of a collagen/calcium phosphate scaffold to act as its own vector for gene delivery and to promote bone formation via transfection with Vegf(165). *Biomaterials*, 31, 2893–2902.

Kellar, R. S., Shepherd, B. R., Larson, D. F., Naughton, G. K., and Williams, S. K. 2005. Cardiac patch constructed from human fibroblasts attenuates reduction in cardiac function after acute infarct. *Tissue Engineering*, 11, 1678–1687.

Keswani, S. G., Katz, A. B., Lim, F. Y., Zoltick, P., Radu, A., Alaee, D., Herlyn, M., and Crombleholme, T. M. 2004. Adenoviral mediated gene transfer of Pdgf-B enhances wound healing in type I and type II diabetic wounds. *Wound Repair and Regeneration*, 12, 497–504.

Kim, H. S., Viggeswarapu, M., Boden, S. D., Liu, Y. S., Hair, G. A., Louis-Ugbo, J., Murakami, H., Minamide, A., Suh, D. Y., and Titus, L. 2003. Overcoming the immune response to permit ex vivo gene therapy for spine fusion with human type 5 adenoviral delivery of the Lim mineralization protein-1 cdna. *Spine*, 28, 219–226.

Kim, K. S., Lee, Y. K., Kim, J. S., Koo, K. H., Hong, H. J., and Park, Y. S. 2008. Targeted gene therapy of Ls174 T human colon carcinoma by anti-Tag-72 immunoliposomes. *Cancer Gene Therapy*, 15, 331–340.

Kim, W. J., Chang, C. W., Lee, M., and Kim, S. W. 2007. Efficient sirna delivery using water soluble lipopolymer for anti-angiogenic gene therapy. *Journal of Controlled Release*, 118, 357–363.

Kiritsy, C. P., Antoniades, H. N., Carlson, M. R., Beaulieu, M. T., and D'andrea, M. 1995. Combination of platelet-derived growth factor-BB and insulin-like growth factor-I is more effective than platelet-derived growth factor-BB alone in stimulating complete healing of full-thickness wounds in "older" diabetic mice. *Wound Repair Regeneration,* 3, 340–350.

Kishimoto, K. N., Watanabe, Y., Nakamura, H., and Kokubun, S. 2002. Ectopic bone formation by electroporatic transfer of bone morphogenetic protein-4 gene. *Bone,* 31, 340–347.

Kulkarni, M., Greiser, U., O'brien, T., and Pandit, A. 2010. Liposomal gene delivery mediated by tissue-engineered scaffolds. *Trends in Biotechnology,* 28, 28–36.

Kusumanto, Y. H., Van Weel, V., Mulder, N. H., Smit, A. J., Van DEN Dungen, J. J. A. M., Hooymans, J. M. M., Sluiter, W. J., Tio, R. A., Quax, P. H. A., Gans, R. O. B., Dullaart, R. P. F., and Hospers, G. A. P. 2006. Treatment with intramuscular vascular endothelial growth factor gene compared with placebo for patients with diabetes mellitus and critical limb ischemia: A double-blind randomized trial. *Human Gene Therapy,* 17, 683–691.

Kusumoto, M., Umeda, S., Ikubo, A., Aoki, Y., Tawfik, O., Oben, R., Williamson, S., Jewell, W., and Suzuki, T. 2001. Phase 1 clinical trial of irradiated autologous melanoma cells adenovirally transduced with human GM-Csf gene. *Cancer Immunology and Immunotherapy,* 50, 373–381.

Lathi, K. G., Cespedes, R. M., Losordo, D. W., Vale, P. R., Symes, J. F., and Isner, J. M. 1999. Direct intra-myocardial gene therapy with Vegf for inoperable coronary artery disease: Preliminary clinical results. *Anesthesia and Analgesia,* 88, U78–U78.

Lauer, G., Sollberg, S., Cole, M., Flamme, I., Sturzebecher, J., Mann, K., Krieg, T., and Eming, S. A. 2000. Expression and proteolysis of vascular endothelial growth factor is increased in chronic wounds. *Journal of Investigative Dermatology,* 115, 12–18.

Laurencin, C. T., Attawia, M. A., Lu, L. Q., Borden, M. D., Lu, H. H., Gorum, W. J., and Lieberman, J. R. 2001. Poly(lactide-*co*-glycolide)/hydroxyapatite delivery of Bmp-2-producing cells: A regional gene therapy approach to bone regeneration. *Biomaterials,* 22, 1271–1277.

Lee, J. A., Conejero, J. A., Mason, J. M., Parrett, B. M., Wear-Maggitti, K. D., Grant, R. T., and Breitbart, A. S. 2005. Lentiviral transfection with the Pdgf-B gene improves diabetic wound healing. *Plastic Reconstruction Surgery,* 116, 532–538.

Lee, P. Y., Li, Z., and Huang, L. 2003. Thermosensitive hydrogel as a Tgf-beta1 gene delivery vehicle enhances diabetic wound healing. *Pharmaceutical Research,* 20, 1995–2000.

Lehrman, S. 1999. Virus treatment questioned after gene therapy death. *Nature,* 401, 517–518.

Li, D., Guang, W., Abuzeid, W. M., Roy, S., Gao, G. P., Sauk, J. J., and O'Malley, B. W., JR. 2008a. Novel adenoviral gene delivery system targeted against head and neck cancer. *Laryngoscope,* 118, 650–658.

Li, H., Fu, X., Zhang, L., Huang, Q., Wu, Z., and Sun, T. 2008b. Research of Pdgf-BB gel on the wound healing of diabetic rats and its pharmacodynamics. *Journal of Surgery and Research,* 145, 41–48.

Li, S. D. and Huang, L. 2006. Surface-modified Lpd nanoparticles for tumor targeting. *Annals of New York Academy of Sciences,* 1082, 1–8.

Liu, H., Bargouti, M., Zughaier, S., Zheng, Z. M., Liu, Y. S., Sangadala, S., Boden, S. D., and Titus, L. 2010. Osteoinductive Lim mineralization protein-1 suppresses activation of NF-kappa B and selectively regulates Mapk pathways in pre-osteoclasts. *Bone,* 46, 1328–1335.

Liu, L., Marti, G. P., Wei, X., Zhang, X., Zhang, H., Liu, Y. V., Nastai, M., Semenza, G. L., and Harmon, J. W. 2008. Age-dependent impairment of Hif-1alpha expression in diabetic mice: Correction with electroporation-facilitated gene therapy increases wound healing, angiogenesis, and circulating angiogenic cells. *Journal of Cell Physiology,* 217, 319–327.

Lopez, C. A., Kimchi, E. T., Mauceri, H. J., Park, J. O., Mehta, N., Murphy, K. T., Beckett, M. A., Hellman, S., Posner, M. C., Kufe, D. W., and Weichselbaum, R. R. 2004. Chemoinducible gene therapy: A strategy to enhance doxorubicin antitumor activity. *Molecular Cancer Therapy,* 3, 1167–1175.

Losordo, D. W., Vale, P. R., Hendel, R. C., Milliken, C. E., Fortuin, F. D., Cummings, N., Schatz, R. A., Asahara, T., Isner, J. M., and Kuntz, R. E. 2002. Phase 1/2 placebo-controlled, double-blind, dose-escalating trial of myocardial vascular endothelial growth factor 2 gene transfer by catheter delivery in patients with chronic myocardial ischemia. *Circulation,* 105, 2012–2018.

Losordo, D. W., Vale, P. R., Symes, J. F., Dunnington, C. H., Esakof, D. D., Maysky, M., Ashare, A. B., Lathi, K., and Isner, J. M. 1998. Gene therapy for myocardial angiogenesis—Initial clinical results with direct myocardial injection of phvegf(165) as sole therapy for myocardial ischemia. *Circulation,* 98, 2800–2804.

Lotze, M. T., Chang, A. E., Seipp, C. A., Simpson, C., Vetto, J. T., and Rosenberg, S. A. 1986. High-dose recombinant interleukin 2 in the treatment of patients with disseminated cancer. Responses, treatment-related morbidity, and histologic findings. *JAMA,* 256, 3117–3124.

Lyon, A. R., Sato, M., Hajjar, R. J., Samulski, R. J., and Harding, S. E. 2008. Gene therapy: Targeting the myocardium. *Heart,* 94, 89–99.

Mace, K. A., Restivo, T. E., Rinn, J. L., Paquet, A. C., Chang, H. Y., Young, D. M., and Boudreau, N. J. 2009. Hoxa3 modulates injury-induced mobilization and recruitment of bone marrow-derived cells. *Stem Cells,* 27, 1654–65.

Makinen, K., Manninen, H., Hedman, M., Matsi, P., Mussalo, H., Alhava, E., and Yla-Herttuala, S. 2002. Increased vascularity detected by digital subtraction angiography after Vegf gene transfer to human lower limb artery: a randomized, placebo-controlled, double-blinded phase II study. *Molecular Therapy,* 6, 127–133.

Man, L. X., Park, J. C., Terry, M. J., Mason, J. M., Burrell, W. A., Liu, F., Kimball, B. Y., Moorji, S. M., Lee, J. A., and Breitbart, A. S. 2005. Lentiviral gene therapy with platelet-derived growth factor B sustains accelerated healing of diabetic wounds over time. *Annals in Plastic Surgery,* 55, 81–86; discussion 86.

Marshall, E. 2000. Biomedicine: Gene therapy on trial. *Science,* 288, 951–957.

Marti, G., Ferguson, M., Wang, J., Byrnes, C., Dieb, R., Qaiser, R., Bonde, P., Duncan, M. D., and Harmon, J. W. 2004. Electroporative transfection with Kgf-1 Dna improves wound healing in a diabetic mouse model. *Gene Therapy,* 11, 1780–1785.

Marti, G. P., Mohebi, P., Liu, L., Wang, J., Miyashita, T., and Harmon, J. W. 2008. Kgf-1 for wound healing in animal models. *Methods in Molecular Biology,* 423, 383–391.

Matsuda, H., Koyama, H., Sato, H., Sawada, J., Itakura, A., Tanaka, A., Matsumoto, M., Konno, K., Ushio, H., and Matsuda, K. 1998. Role of nerve growth factor in cutaneous wound healing: Accelerating effects in normal and healing-impaired diabetic mice. *Journal of Experimental Medicine,* 187, 297–306.

Menke, N. B., Ward, K. R., Witten, T. M., Bonchev, D. G., and Diegelmann, R. F. 2007. Impaired wound healing. *Clinical Dermatology,* 25, 19–25.

Michelfelder, S. and Trepel, M. 2009. Adeno-associated viral vectors and their redirection to cell-type specific receptors. *Advances in Genetics,* 67, 29–60.

Minamide, A., Boden, S. D., Viggeswarapu, M., Hair, G. A., Oliver, C., and Titus, L. 2003. Mechanism of bone formation with gene transfer of the cdna encoding for the intracellular protein Lmp-1. *Journal of Bone and Joint Surgery-American Volume,* 85A, 1030–1039.

Minamide, A., Titus, L., Viggeswarapu, M., Oliver, C., Hair, G., and Boden, S. D. 2001. Bone formation induced by Ad5-Lmp-1: Histological and immunohistochemical analysis. *Journal of Bone and Mineral Research,* 16, S477–S477.

Miyagawa, S., Sawa, Y., Fukuda, K., Hisaka, Y., Taketani, S., Memon, I. A., and Matsuda, H. 2006. Angiogenic gene cell therapy using suicide gene system regulates the effect of angiogenesis in infarcted rat heart. *Transplantation,* 81, 902–907.

Miyamoto, M. I., Del Monte, F., Schmidt, U., Disalvo, T. S., Kang, Z. B., Matsui, T., Guerrero, J. L., Gwathmey, J. K., Rosenzweig, A., and Hajjar, R. J. 2000. Adenoviral gene transfer of SERCA2a improves left-ventricular function in aortic-banded rats in transition to heart failure. *Proceedings of the National Academy of Sciences of the United States of America,* 97, 793–798.

Mizuno, T., Mickle, D. A. G., Kiani, C. G., and LI, R. K. 2005a. Overexpression of elastin fragments in infarcted myocardium attenuates scar expansion and heart dysfunction. *American Journal of Physiology-Heart and Circulatory Physiology,* 288, H2819–H2827.

Mizuno, T., Yau, T. M., Weisel, R. D., Kiani, C. G., and LI, R. K. 2005b. Elastin stabilizes an infarct and preserves ventricular function. *Circulation,* 112, I81–I88.

Motzer, R. J., Rakhit, A., Schwartz, L. H., Olencki, T., Malone, T. M., Sandstrom, K., Nadeau, R., Parmar, H., and Bukowski, R. 1998. Phase I trial of subcutaneous recombinant human interleukin-12 in patients with advanced renal cell carcinoma. *Clinical Cancer Research,* 4, 1183–1191.

Mulder, G., Tallis, A. J., Marshall, V. T., Mozingo, D., Phillips, L., Pierce, G. F., Chandler, L. A., and Sosnowski, B. K. 2009. Treatment of nonhealing diabetic foot ulcers with a platelet-derived growth factor gene-activated matrix (Gam501): Results of a phase 1/2 trial. *Wound Repair and Regeneration,* 17, 772–779.

Mundt, A. J., Vijayakumar, S., Nemunaitis, J., Sandler, A., Schwartz, H., Hanna, N., Peabody, T., Senzer, N., Chu, K., Rasmussen, C. S., Kessler, P. D., Rasmussen, H. S., Warso, M., Kufe, D. W., Gupta, T. D., and Weichselbaum, R. R. 2004. A Phase I trial of TNFerade biologic in patients with soft tissue sarcoma in the extremities. *Clinical Cancer Research,* 10, 5747–5753.

Musgrave, D. S., Bosch, P., Ghivizzani, S., Robbins, P. D., Evans, C. H., and Huard, J. 1999. Adenovirus-mediated direct gene therapy with bone morphogenetic protein-2 produces bone. *Bone,* 24, 541–547.

Mustoe, T. A., O'Shaughnessy, K., and Kloeters, O. 2006. Chronic wound pathogenesis and current treatment strategies: A unifying hypothesis. *Plastic Reconstruction Surgery,* 117, 35S–41S.

Mustoe, T. A., Pierce, G. F., Morishima, C., and Deuel, T. F. 1991. Growth factor-induced acceleration of tissue repair through direct and inductive activities in a rabbit dermal ulcer model. *Journal of Clinical Investigation,* 87, 694–703.

Nabel, E. G. 1995. Gene therapy for cardiovascular disease. *Circulation,* 91, 541–548.

Nagaya, N., Kangawa, K., Kanda, M., Uematsu, M., Horio, T., Fukuyama, N., Hino, J., Harada-Shiba, M., Okumura, H., Tabata, Y., Mochizuki, N., Chiba, Y., Nishioka, K., Miyatake, K., Asahara, T., Hara, H., and Mori, H. 2003. Hybrid cell − gene therapy for pulmonary hypertension based on phagocytosing action of endothelial progenitor cells. *Circulation,* 108, 889–895.

Namba, T., Koike, H., Murakami, K., Aoki, M., Makino, H., Hashiya, N., Ogihara, T., Kaneda, Y., Kohno, M., and Morishita, R. 2003. Angiogenesis induced by endothelial nitric oxide synthase gene through vascular endothelial growth factor expression in a rat hindlimb ischemia model. *Circulation,* 108, 2250–2257.

Neumann, E., Schaefer-Ridder, M., Wang, Y., and Hofschneider, P. H. 1982. Gene transfer into mouse lyoma cells by electroporation in high electric fields. *EMBO Journal,* 1, 841–845.

Nonaka-Sarukawa, M., Okada, T., Ito, T., Yamamoto, K., Yoshioka, T., Nomoto, T., Hojo, Y., Shimpo, M., Urabe, M., Mizukami, H., Kume, A., Keda, U., Shimada, K., and Ozawa, K. 2008. Adeno-associated virus vector-mediated systemic interleukin-10 expression ameliorates hypertensive organ damage in Dahl salt-sensitive rats. *Journal of Gene Medicine,* 10, 368–374.

Norman, K. L., and Lee, P. W. 2005. Not all viruses are bad guys: The case for reovirus in cancer therapy. *Drug Discov Today,* 10, 847–855.

Nussenbaum, B., Rutherford, R. B., and Krebsbach, P. H. 2005. Bone regeneration in cranial defects previously treated with radiation. *Laryngoscope,* 115, 1170–1177.

Nwomeh, B. C., Yager, D. R., and Cohen, I. K. 1998. Physiology of the chronic wound. *Clinical and Plastic Surgery,* 25, 341–356.

Oshima, K., Cui, G. G., Tung, T., Okotie, O., Laks, H., and Sen, L. Y. 2007. Exogenous IL-10 overexpression reduces perforin production by activated allogenic Cd8+ cells and prolongs cardiac allograft survival. *American Journal of Physiology-Heart and Circulatory Physiology,* 292, H277–H284.

Oshima, K., Sen, L., Cui, G. G., Tung, T., Sacks, B. M., Arellano-Kruse, A., and Laks, H. 2002. Localized interleukin-10 gene transfer induces apoptosis of alloreactive T cells via Fas/FasL pathway, improves function, and prolongs survival of cardiac allograft. *Transplantation,* 73, 1019–1026.

Ott, M. G., Schmidt, M., Schwarzwaelder, K., Stein, S., Siler, U., Koehl, U., Glimm, H., Kuhlcke, K., Schilz, A., Kunkel, H., Naundorf, S., Brinkmann, A., Deichmann, A., Fischer, M., Ball, C., Pilz, I., Dunbar, C., DU, Y., Jenkins, N. A., Copeland, N. G., Luthi, U., Hassan, M., Thrasher, A. J., Hoelzer, D., Von Kalle, C.,

Seger, R., and Grez, M. 2006. Correction of X-linked chronic granulomatous disease by gene therapy, augmented by insertional activation of Mds1-Evi1, Prdm16 or Setbp1. *Nature Medicine,* 12, 401–409.

Ozer, H., Wiernik, P. H., Giles, F., and Tendler, C. 1998. Recombinant interferon-alpha therapy in patients with follicular lymphoma. *Cancer,* 82, 1821–1830.

Pandit, A. S., Wilson, D. J., Feldman, D. S., and Thompson, J. A. 2000. Fibrin scaffold as an effective vehicle for the delivery of acidic fibroblast growth factor (Fgf-1). *Journal of Biomaterials Applications,* 14, 229–242.

Pearson, S., Jia, H., Kandachi, K. 2004. China approves first gene therapy. *Nature Biotechnology,* 22(1), 3–4.

Peer, D., Park, E. J., Morishita, Y., Carman, C. V., and Shimaoka, M. 2008. Systemic leukocyte-directed sirna delivery revealing cyclin D1 as an anti-inflammatory target. *Science,* 319, 627–630.

Pelisek, J., Fuchs, A., Engelmann, M. G., Shimizu, M., Golda, A., Mekkaoui, C., Rolland, P. H., and Nikol, S. 2003. Vascular endothelial growth factor response in porcine coronary and peripheral arteries using nonsurgical occlusion model, local delivery, and liposome-mediated gene transfer. *Endothelium-Journal of Endothelial Cell Research,* 10, 247–255.

Peng, L., Cheng, X., Zhuo, R., Lan, J., Wang, Y., Shi, B., and Li, S. 2009. Novel gene-activated matrix with embedded chitosan/plasmid Dna nanoparticles encoding Pdgf for periodontal tissue engineering. *Journal of Biomedical Material Research A,* 90, 564–576.

Pleger, S. T., Boucher, M., Most, P., and Koch, W. J. 2007. Targeting myocardial beta-adrenergic receptor signaling and calcium cycling for heart failure gene therapy. *Journal of Cardiac Failure,* 13, 401–414.

Pollner, F. 2000. Gene therapy trial and errors raise scientific, ethical, and oversite questions. *The Nih Catalyst,* 8, 1–1a.

Pons, J., Huang, Y., Takagawa, J., Arakawa-Hoyt, J., Ye, J., Grossman, W., Kan, Y. W., and SU, H. 2009. Combining angiogenic gene and stem cell therapies for myocardial infarction. *The Journal of Gene Medicine,* 11, 743–753.

Porteus, M. H., Connelly, J. P., and Pruett, S. M. 2006. A look to future directions in gene therapy research for monogenic diseases. *PLoS Genetics,* 2, e133.

Potapova, I., Plotnikov, A., Lu, Z. J., Danilo, P., Valiunas, V., Qu, J. H., Doronin, S., Zuckerman, J., Shlapakova, I. N., Gao, J. Y., Pan, Z. M., Herron, A. J., Robinson, R. B., Brink, P. R., Rosen, M. R., and Cohen, I. S. 2004. Human mesenchymal stem cells as a gene delivery system to create cardiac pacemakers. *Circulation Research,* 94, 952–959.

Potapova, I. A., Doronin, S. V., Kelly, D. J., Rosen, A. B., Schuldt, A. J. T., Lu, Z. J., Kochupura, P. V., Robinson, R. B., Rosen, M. R., Brink, P. R., Gaudette, G. R., and Cohen, I. S. 2008. Enhanced recovery of mechanical function in the canine heart by seeding an extracellular matrix patch with mesenchymal stem cells committed to a cardiac lineage. *American Journal of Physiology—Heart and Circulatory Physiology,* 295, H2257–H2263.

Prunier, F., Kawase, Y., Gianni, D., Scapin, C., Danik, S. B., Ellinor, P. T., Hajjar, R. J., and Del Monte, F. 2008. Prevention of ventricular arrhythmias with sarcoplasmic reticulum Ca2+ ATPase pump overexpression in a porcine model of ischemia reperfusion. *Circulation,* 118, 614–624.

Rajagopalan, S., Shah, M., Luciano, A., Crystal, R., and Nabel, E. G. 2001. Adenovirus-mediated gene transfer of Vegf121 improves lower-extremity endothelial function and flow reserve. *Circulation,* 104, 753–755.

Ripa, R. S., Wang, Y., Jorgensen, E., Johnsen, H. E., Hesse, B., and Kastrup, J. 2006. Intramyocardial injection of vascular endothelial growth factor-A(165) plasmid followed by granulocyte-colony stimulating factor to induce angiogenesis in patients with severe chronic ischaemic heart disease. *European Heart Journal,* 27, 1785–1792.

Rivard, C. H., Chaput, C. J., Desrosiers, E. A., Yahia, L. H., and Selmani, A. 1995. Fibroblast seeding and culture in biodegradable porous substrates. *Journal of Applied Biomaterials,* 6, 65–68.

Roncal, C., Buysschaert, I., Chorianopoulos, E. K., Georgiadou, M., Meilhac, O., Demol, M., Michel, J. B., Vinckier, S., Moons, L., and Carmeliet, P. 2008. Beneficial effects of prolonged systemic administration of Pigf on late outcome of post-ischaemic myocardial performance. *Journal of Pathology,* 216, 236–244.

Rosengart, T. K., Lee, L. Y., Patel, S. R., Sanborn, T. A., Parikh, M., Bergman, G. W., Hachamovitch, R., Szulc, M., Kligfield, P. D., Okin, P. M., Hahn, R. T., Devereux, R. B., Post, M. R., Hackett, N. R., Foster, T., Grasso, T. M., Lesser, M. L., Isom, O. W., and Crystal, R. G. 1999. Angiogenesis gene therapy—Phase I assessment of direct intramyocardial administration of an adenovirus vector expressing Vegf121 cdna to individuals with clinically significant severe coronary artery disease. *Circulation,* 100, 468–474.

Rubin, G. M. and Spradling, A. C. 1982. Genetic transformation of Drosophila with transposable element vectors. *Science,* 218, 348–353.

Saba, A. A., Freedman, B. M., Gaffield, J. W., Mackay, D. R., and Ehrlich, H. P. 2002. Topical platelet-derived growth factor enhances wound closure in the absence of wound contraction: an experimental and clinical study. *Annals of Plastic Surgery,* 49, 62–66; discussion 66.

Sabbah, H. N., Sharov, V. G., Gupta, R. C., Mishra, S., Rastogi, S., Undrovinas, A. I., Chaudhry, P. A., Todor, A., Mishima, T., Tanhehco, E. J., and Suzuki, G. 2003. Reversal of chronic molecular and cellular abnormalities due to heart failure by passive mechanical ventricular containment. *Circulation Research,* 93, 1095–1101.

Saghizadeh, M., Kramerov, A. A., Yu, F. S., Castro, M. G., and Ljubimov, A. V. 2010. Normalization of wound healing and diabetic markers in organ cultured human diabetic corneas by adenoviral delivery of c-Met gene. *Investigative Ophthalmology and Visual Science,* 51, 1970–1980.

Sales, V. L., Mettler, B. A., Lopez-Ilasaca, M., Johnson, J. A., and Mayer, J. E. 2007. Endothelial progenitor and mesenchymal stem cell-derived cells persist in tissue-engineered patch in vivo: Application of green and red fluorescent protein-expressing retroviral vector. *Tissue Engineering,* 13, 525–535.

Sangadala, S., Titus, L., Viggeswarapu, M., Liu, Y., Hair, G. A., Gibson, E., Oliver, C., and Boden, S. D. 2003. Use of Lmp-1 fusion protein to induce bone formation without risks of gene therapy. *Journal of Bone and Mineral Research,* 18, S185–S185.

Sarkissian, S. D., Grobe, J. L., Yuan, L., Narielwala, D. R., Walter, G. A., Katovich, M. J., and Raizada, M. K. 2008. Cardiac overexpression of angiotensin converting enzyme 2 protects the heart from ischemia-induced pathophysiology. *Hypertension,* 51, 712–718.

Sawa, Y., Morishita, R., Suzuki, K., Kagisaki, K., Kaneda, Y., Maeda, R., Kadoba, K., and Matsuda, H. 1997. A novel strategy for myocardial protection using *in vivo* transfection of cis element 'decoy' against NFkB binding site—Evidence for a role of NFkB in ischemia – reperfusion injury. *Circulation,* 96, 280–284.

Schmidt, U., Del Monte, F., Miyamoto, M. I., Matsui, T., Gwathmey, J. K., Rosenzweig, A., and Hajjar, R. J. 2000. Restoration of diastolic function in senescent rat hearts through adenoviral gene transfer of sarcoplasmic reticulum Ca2 + -ATPase. *Circulation,* 101, 790–796.

Schwarz, E. R., Speakman, M. T., Patterson, M., Hale, S. S., Isner, J. M., Kedes, L. H., and Kloner, R. A. 2000. Evaluation of the effects of intramyocardial injection of Dna expressing vascular endothelial growth factor (Vegf) in a myocardial infarction model in the rat—Angiogenesis and angioma formation. *Journal of the American College of Cardiology,* 35, 1323–1330.

Schwarzwaelder, K., Schmidt, M., Deichmann, A., Ott, M. G., Stein, S., Glimm, H., Siler, U., Hoelzer, D., Seger, R., Grez, M., and Von Kalle, C. 2006. Insertional activation of Mds1/Evi1, Prdm16 and Setbp1 in a successful chronic granulomatous disease (Cgd) gene therapy trial. *Blood,* 108, 3274.

Selvin, E. and Erlinger, T. P. 2004. Prevalence of and risk factors for peripheral arterial disease in the United States: Results from the National Health and Nutrition Examination Survey, 1999–2000. *Circulation,* 110, 738–743.

Sen, L., Hong, Y. S., Luo, H. M., Cui, G. G., and Laks, H. 2001. Efficiency, efficacy, and adverse effects of adenovirus- vs. liposome-mediated gene therapy in cardiac allografts. *American Journal of Physiology-Heart and Circulatory Physiology,* 281, H1433–H1441.

Shah, A. S., White, D. C., Emani, S., Kypson, A. P., Lilly, R. E., Wilson, K., Glower, D. D., Lefkowitz, R. J., and Koch, W. J. 2001. *In vivo* ventricular gene delivery of a {beta}-adrenergic receptor kinase inhibitor to the failing heart reverses cardiac dysfunction. *Circulation,* 103, 1311–1316.

Shau, H., Isacescu, V., Ibayashi, Y., Tokuda, Y., Golub, S. H., Fahey, J. L., and Sarna, G. P. 1990. A pilot study of intralymphatic interleukin-2. I. Cytotoxic and surface marker changes of peripheral blood lymphocytes. *J Biological Response Model,* 9, 71–80.

Shayakhmetov, D. M., DI Paolo, N. C., and Mossman, K. L. 2010. Recognition of virus infection and innate host responses to viral gene therapy vectors. *Molecular Therapy,* 18, 1422–1429.

Shi, W. F., Arnold, G. S., and Bartlett, J. S. 2001. Insertional mutagenesis of the adeno-associated virus type 2 (Aav2) capsid gene and generation of Aav2 vectors targeted to alternative cell-surface receptors. *Human Gene Therapy,* 12, 1697–1711.

Shigematsu, H., Yasuda, K., Iwai, T., Sasajima, T., Ishimaru, S., Ohashi, Y., Yamaguchi, T., Ogihara, T., and Morishita, R. 2010. Randomized, double-blind, placebo-controlled clinical trial of hepatocyte growth factor plasmid for critical limb ischemia. *Gene Therapy,* 17, 1152–1161.

Shyu, K. G., Chang, H., Wang, B. W., and Kuan, P. 2003. Intramuscular vascular endothelial growth factor gene therapy in patients with chronic critical leg ischemia. *American Journal of Medicine,* 114, 85–92.

Simpson, D., Liu, H., Fan, T. H. M., Nerem, R., and Dudley, S. C. 2007. A tissue engineering approach to progenitor cell delivery results in significant cell engraftment and improved myocardial remodeling. *Stem Cells,* 25, 2350–2357.

Song, Y., Hahn, T., Thompson, I. P., Mason, T. J., Preston, G. M., LI, G., Paniwnyk, L., and Huang, W. E. 2007. Ultrasound-mediated DNA transfer for bacteria. *Nucleic Acids Research,* 35, e129.

Spradling, A. C. and Rubin, G. M. 1982. Transposition of cloned P elements into Drosophila germ line chromosomes. *Science,* 218, 341–347.

Steed, D. L. 1998. Modifying the wound healing response with exogenous growth factors. *Clinical and Plastic Surgery,* 25, 397–405.

Stewart, A. K., Lassam, N. J., Quirt, I. C., Bailey, D. J., Rotstein, L. E., Krajden, M., Dessureault, S., Gallinger, S., Cappe, D., Wan, Y., Addison, C. L., Moen, R. C., Gauldie, J., and Graham, F. L. 1999. Adenovector-mediated gene delivery of interleukin-2 in metastatic breast cancer and melanoma: Results of a phase 1 clinical trial. *Gene Therapy,* 6, 350–363.

Sun, L., XU, L., Chang, H., Henry, F. A., Miller, R. M., Harmon, J. M., and Nielsen, T. B. 1997. Transfection with aFGF cDNA improves wound healing. *Journal of Investigative Dermatology,* 108, 313–318.

Supp, D. M. and Boyce, S. T. 2005. Engineered skin substitutes: Practices and potentials. *Clinical Dermatology,* 23, 403–412.

Suzuki, K., Murtuza, B., Smolenski, R. T., Sammut, I. A., Suzuki, N., Kaneda, Y., and Yacoub, M. H. 2001. Cell transplantation for the treatment of acute myocardial infarction using vascular endothelial growth factor-expressing skeletal myoblasts. *Circulation,* 104, I207–I212.

Suzuki, K., Sawa, Y., Kaneda, Y., Ichikawa, H., Shirakura, R., and Matsuda, H. 1997. *In vivo* gene transfection with heat shock protein 70 enhances myocardial tolerance to ischemia – reperfusion injury in rat. *Journal of Clinical Investigation,* 99, 1645–1650.

Symes, J. F., Losordo, D. W., Vale, P. R., Lathi, K. G., Esakof, D. D., Mayskiy, M., and Isner, J. M. Year. Gene therapy with vascular endothelial growth factor for inoperable coronary artery disease. In: *35th Annual Meeting of the Society-of-Thoracic-Surgeons,* Jan 24–29 1999 San Antonio, TX. 830–836.

Tadic, D. and Epple, M. 2004. A thorough physicochemical characterisation of 14 calcium phosphate-based bone substitution materials in comparison to natural bone. *Biomaterials,* 25, 987–994.

Tan, P. H., Xue, S. A., Wei, B., Holler, A., Voss, R. H., and George, A. J. 2007. Changing viral tropism using immunoliposomes alters the stability of gene expression: Implications for viral vector design. *Molecular Medicine,* 13, 216–226.

Tani, K., Azuma, M., Nakazaki, Y., Oyaizu, N., Hase, H., Ohata, J., Takahashi, K., Oiwamonna, M., Hanazawa, K., Wakumoto, Y., Kawai, K., Noguchi, M., Soda, Y., Kunisaki, R., Watari, K., Takahashi, S., Machida, U., Satoh, N., Tojo, A., Maekawa, T., Eriguchi, M., Tomikawa, S., Tahara, H., Inoue, Y., Yoshikawa, H., Yamada, Y., Iwamoto, A., Hamada, H., Yamashita, N., Okumura, K., Kakizoe, T., Akaza, H., Fujime, M., Clift, S., Ando, D., Mulligan, R., and Asano, S. 2004. Phase I study of autologous tumor vaccines transduced with the GM-Csf gene in four patients with stage IV renal cell cancer in Japan: Clinical and immunological findings. *Molecular Therapy,* 10, 799–816.

Taniyama, Y., Morishita, R., Hiraoka, K., Aoki, M., Nakagami, H., Yamasaki, K., Matsumoto, K., Nakamura, T., Kaneda, Y., and Ogihara, T. 2001. Therapeutic angiogenesis induced by human hepatocyte growth factor gene in rat diabetic hind limb ischemia model: Molecular mechanisms of delayed angiogenesis in diabetes. *Circulation,* 104, 2344–2350.

Themis, M., May, D., Coutelle, C., and Newbold, R. F. 2003. Mutational effects of retrovirus insertion on the genome of V79 cells by an attenuated retrovirus vector: Implications for gene therapy. *Gene Therapy,* 10, 1703–1711.

Trudel, S., Trachtenberg, J., Toi, A., Sweet, J., LI, Z. H., Jewett, M., Tshilias, J., Zhuang, L. H., Hitt, M., Wan, Y., Gauldie, J., Graham, F. L., Dancey, J., and Stewart, A. K. 2003. A phase I trial of adenovector-mediated delivery of interleukin-2 (AdIL-2) in high-risk localized prostate cancer. *Cancer Gene Therapy,* 10, 755–763.

Uemura, H., Fujimoto, K., Tanaka, M., Yoshikawa, M., Hirao, Y., Uejima, S., Yoshikawa, K., and Itoh, K. 2006. A phase I trial of vaccination of Ca9-derived peptides for Hla-A24-positive patients with cytokine-refractory metastatic renal cell carcinoma. *Clinical Cancer Research,* 12, 1768–1775.

Vale, P. R., Losordo, D. W., Milliken, C. E., Mcdonald, M. C., Gravelin, L. M., Curry, C. M., Esakof, D. D., Maysky, M., Symes, J. F., and Isner, J. M. 2001. Randomized, single-blind, placebo-controlled pilot study of catheter-based myocardial gene transfer for therapeutic angiogenesis using left ventricular electromechanical mapping in patients with chronic myocardial ischemia. *Circulation,* 103, 2138–2143.

Veves, A., Falanga, V., Armstrong, D. G., and Sabolinski, M. L. 2001. Graftskin, a human skin equivalent, is effective in the management of noninfected neuropathic diabetic foot ulcers: A prospective randomized multicenter clinical trial. *Diabetes Care,* 24, 290–295.

Viggeswarapu, M., Bargouti, M., Teklemariam, M., Baker, N., Rogers, C., Zhu, L., Titus, L., and Boden, S. D. 2005. Increasing Bmp responsiveness in human mesenchymal stem cells *in vitro* by addition of the osteoinductive Lmp-1 gene. *Journal of Bone and Mineral Research,* 20, S359–S359.

Viggeswarapu, M., Boden, S. D., Liu, Y. S., Hair, G. A., Louis-Ugbo, J., Murakami, H., Kim, H. S., Mayr, M. T., Hutton, W. C., and Titus, L. 2001. Adenoviral delivery of Lim mineralization protein-1 induces new-bone formation *in vitro* and in vivo. *Journal of Bone and Joint Surgery-American Volume,* 83A, 364–376.

Viggeswarapu, M., Kim, H., Boden, S. D., Hair, G. A., Oliver, C., and Titus, L. 2002. Overcoming the immune response to permit ex vivo gene therapy for spine fusion using human type 5 adenovirus to deliver Lim mineralization protein-1 (Lmp-1) cdna. *Journal of Bone and Mineral Research,* 17, M45.

Vinge, L. E., Raake, P. W., and Koch, W. J. 2008. Gene therapy in heart failure. *Circulation Research,* 102, 1458–1470.

Wang, J. C., Kanim, L. E. A., Yoo, S., Campbell, P. A., Berk, A. J., and Lieberman, J. R. 2003. Effect of regional gene therapy with bone morphogenetic protein-2-producing bone marrow cells on spinal fusion in rats. *Journal of Bone and Joint Surgery-American Volume,* 85A, 905–911.

Wang, W., LI, W., Ong, L. L., Lutzow, K., Lendlein, A., Furlani, D., Gabel, R., Kong, D., Wang, J., LI, R. K., Steinhoff, G., and MA, N. 2009. Localized and sustained Sdf-1 gene release mediated by fibronectin films: A potential method for recruiting stem cells. *International Journal of Artificial Organs,* 32, 141–149.

Wang, Y. Z., Ripa, R. S., Jorgensen, E., Hesse, B., Mortensen, S., and Kastrup, J. 2007. Mobilization of haematopoietic and non-haematopoietic cells by granulocyte-colony stimulating factor and vascular endothelial growth factor gene therapy in patients with stable severe coronary artery disease. *Scandinavian Cardiovascular Journal,* 41, 397–404.

Wang, Z. and Li, L. 2009. The plasmid encoding Hsp47 enhances collagen expression and promotes skin wound healing in an alloxan-induced diabetic model. *Cell Biology International,* 33, 705–710.

Wang, Z. G., Ling, Z. Y., Ran, H. T., Hong, R., Zhang, Q. X., Huang, A. L., QI, L., Zhao, C. J., Tang, H. L., Lin, G., Peng, M. L., and PU, S. Y. 2004. Ultrasound-mediated microbubble destruction enhances Vegf gene delivery to the infarcted myocardium in rats. *Clinical Imaging,* 28, 395–398.

Wei, H. J., Chen, C. H., Lee, W. Y., Chiu, I., Hwang, S. M., Lin, W. W., Huang, C. C., Yeh, Y. C., Chang, Y., and Sung, H. W. 2008. Bioengineered cardiac patch constructed from multilayered mesenchymal stem cells for myocardial repair. *Biomaterials,* 29, 3547–3556.

Werner, S. and Grose, R. 2003. Regulation of wound healing by growth factors and cytokines. *Physiology Reviews,* 83, 835–870.

White, D. C., Hata, J. A., Shah, A. S., Glower, D. D., Lefkowitz, R. J., and Koch, W. J. 2000. Preservation of myocardial beta-adrenergic receptor signaling delays the development of heart failure after myocardial infarction. *Proceedings of the National Academy of Sciences of the United States of America,* 97, 5428–5433.

Winn, S. R., Chen, J. C., Gong, X., Bartholomew, S. V., Shreenivas, S., and Ozaki, W. 2005a. Non-viral-mediated gene therapy approaches for bone repair. *Orthodontics and Craniofacial Research,* 8, 183–190.

Winn, S. R., Chen, J. C., Gong, X., Bartholomew, S. V., Shreenivas, S., and Ozaki, W. 2005b. Non-viral-mediated gene therapy approaches for bone repair. *Orthodontics and Craniofacial Research,* 8, 183–190.

Woo, C. Y., Osada, T., Clay, T. M., Lyerly, H. K., and Morse, M. A. 2006. Recent clinical progress in virus-based therapies for cancer. *Expert Opinion in Biological Therapy,* 6, 1123–1134.

Wu, X., Gao, H., Pasupathy, S., Tan, P. H., Ooi, L. L., and Hui, K. M. 2005. Systemic administration of naked Dna with targeting specificity to mammalian kidneys. *Gene Therapy,* 12, 477–486.

Wukich, D. K. 2010. Current concepts review: diabetic foot ulcers. *Foot and Ankle International,* 31, 460–467.

Xiang, Z., Liao, R. L., Kelly, M. S., and Spector, M. 2006. Collagen-Gag scaffolds grafted onto myocardial infarcts in a rat model: A delivery vehicle for mesenchymal stem cells. *Tissue Engineering,* 12, 2467–2478.

Xie, Y. B., Yang, S. T., and Kniss, D. A. 2001. Three-dimensional cell-scaffold constructs promote efficient gene transfection: Implications for cell-based gene therapy. *Tissue Engineering,* 7, 585–598.

Yang, J. F., Zhou, W. W., Zheng, W., Ma, Y. L., Lin, L., Tang, T., Liu, J. X., Yu, J. F., Zhou, X. M., and Hu, J. G. 2007. Effects of myocardial transplantation of marrow mesenchymal stem cells transfected with vascular endothelial growth factor for the improvement of heart function and angiogenesis after myocardial infarction. *Cardiology,* 107, 17–29.

Yang, L., Jiang, J., Drouin, L. M., Agbandje-Mckenna, M., Chen, C., Qiao, C., Pu, D., Hu, X., Wang, D. Z., Li, J., and Xiao, X. 2009. A myocardium tropic adeno-associated virus (Aav) evolved by Dna shuffling and *in vivo* selection. *Proceedings of the National Academy of Sciences USA,* 106, 3946–3951.

Ye, L., Haider, H. K., Jiang, S., Tan, R. S., GE, R. W., Law, P. K., and Sim, E. K. W. 2007. Improved angiogenic response in pig heart following ischaemic injury using human skeletal myoblast simultaneously expressing Vegf(165) and angiopoietin-1. *European Journal of Heart Failure,* 9, 15–22.

Ylosmaki, E., Hakkarainen, T., Hemminki, A., Visakorpi, T., Andino, R., and Saksela, K. 2008. Generation of a conditionally replicating adenovirus based on targeted destruction of E1A mrna by a cell type-specific Microrna. *Journal of Virology,* 82, 11009–11015.

Yoon, C. S., Jung, H. S., Kwon, M. J., Lee, S. H., Kim, C. W., Kim, M. K., Lee, M., and Park, J. H. 2009. Sonoporation of the minicircle-Vegf(165) for wound healing of diabetic mice. *Pharmaceutical Research,* 26, 794–801.

Yoon, S. T. and Boden, S. D. 2004. Spine fusion by gene therapy. *Gene Therapy,* 11, 360–367.

Yoon, Y. S., Uchida, S., Masuo, O., Cejna, M., Park, J. S., Gwon, H. C., Kirchmair, R., Bahlman, F., Walter, D., Curry, C., Hanley, A., Isner, J. M., and Losordo, D. W. 2005. Progressive attenuation of myocardial vascular endothelial growth factor expression is a seminal event in diabetic cardiomyopathy—Restoration of microvascular homeostasis and recovery of cardiac function in diabetic cardiomyopathy after replenishment of local vascular endothelial growth factor. *Circulation,* 111, 2073–2085.

Yuan, B., Zhang, Y. R., Zhao, Z., Wu, D. L., Yuan, L. Z., Wu, B., Wang, L. S., and Huang, J. 2008a. Treatment of chronical myocardial ischemia by adenovirus-mediated hepatocyte growth factor gene transfer in minipigs. *Science in China Series C-Life Sciences,* 51, 537–543.

Yuan, B., Zhao, Z., Zhang, Y. R., Wu, C. T., Jin, W. G., Zhao, S., Wang, W., Zhang, Y. Y., Zhu, X. L., Wang, L. S., and Huang, J. 2008b. Short-term safety and curative effect of recombinant adenovirus carrying hepatocyte growth factor gene on ischemic cardiac disease. *In Vivo*, 22, 629–632.

Zagon, I. S., Sassani, J. W., Malefyt, K. J., and Mclaughlin, P. J. 2006. Regulation of corneal repair by particle-mediated gene transfer of opioid growth factor receptor complementary DNA. *Archives in Ophthalmology*, 124, 1620–1624.

Zhang, G., Wang, X., Wang, Z., Zhang, J., and Suggs, L. 2006. A PEGylated fibrin patch for mesenchymal stem cell delivery. *Tissue Engineering*, 12, 9–19.

Zhang, H., Kusunose, J., Kheirolomoom, A., Seo, J. W., QI, J., Watson, K. D., Lindfors, H. A., Ruoslahti, E., Sutcliffe, J. L., and Ferrara, K. W. 2008a. Dynamic imaging of arginine-rich heart-targeted vehicles in a mouse model. *Biomaterials*, 29, 1976–1988.

Zhang, Y., Wang, Y., Boado, R. J., and Pardridge, W. M. 2008b. Lysosomal enzyme replacement of the brain with intravenous non-viral gene transfer. *Pharmaceutical Research*, 25, 400–406.

Zhao, X. Y., HU, S. J., LI, J., Mou, Y., Bian, K., Sun, J., and Zhu, Z. H. 2008. raav-asplb transfer attenuates abnormal sarcoplasmic reticulum Ca2+ -ATPase activity and cardiac dysfunction in rats with myocardial infarction. *European Journal of Heart Failure*, 10, 47–54.

Zimmermann, W. H., Melnychenko, I., and Eschenhagen, T. 2004. Engineered heart tissue for regeneration of diseased hearts. *Biomaterials*, 25, 1639–1647.

# 19

# Nanotechnology-Based Cell Engineering Strategies for Tissue Engineering and Regenerative Medicine Applications

Joaquim Miguel
Oliveira
*University of Minho*
*ICVS/3B's*

João Filipe Mano
*University of Minho*
*ICVS/3B's*

Rui Luís Reis
*University of Minho*
*ICVS/3B's*

19.1   Introduction ...................................................................................19-1
19.2   Cell Engineering Strategies.........................................................19-2
       Intracellular Delivery • Nanoparticles in Cell Engineering
       and Cellular Responses
19.3   Concluding Remarks....................................................................19-7
References....................................................................................................19-7

## 19.1 Introduction

We have been assisting a multitude of scientific achievements in the merging fields of cell- and tissue engineering and regenerative medicine (TERM), and thus there is a need to highlight the most recent and relevant works in these particular areas of research. Owing to the multidisciplinary nature of these fields, we were encouraged to briefly overview other important issues namely, those related with the application of nanotechnology principles in regenerative medicine. This particular topic is appealing since there is the need for developing more effective treatments to cure the several spontaneous and injuries-related diseases. Owing to the limited regenerative capacity of the body, scientists envision for example, nanoparticle systems for efficiently delivering specific drugs, bioactive agents, and genetic material, and to target-specific cells or even cellular compartments. In this chapter, the regenerative potential of different cells (and its sources), and their responsiveness to modulators are succinctly addressed. The cell engineering strategies that have been designed for targeting the regeneration or repair of specific body parts is also discussed herein. Focus is placed on the research dealing with new promising strategies, namely the use of nanocarriers, polymeric, and ceramic, for the control delivery of biomolecules intracellularly. These vehicles are aimed at modulating cell functions such as, adhesion, proliferation, and differentiation of cells. If this strategy on one side, allowed our group to envision regenerate bone by means of controlling stem cells differentiation *in vitro* while maintaining their cellular phenotype *in vivo* upon reimplantation, whereas on the other, we were able to apply the developed nanocarriers to cross other biological barriers such as the blood–brain barrier, opening up new possibilities for targeting the central nervous system (CNS).

## 19.2 Cell Engineering Strategies

In our body there are different cell types, which can be classified as: (i) germ cells, (ii) somatic cells, and (iii) stem cells. Germ cells are cells that give rise to gametes, both male and female. Somatic cells are the specialized ones and makeup the adult body. In their differentiated state they may possess one or more copies of the genome, with the exception of erythrocytes which do not possess. Finally, stem cells can be defined as cells that possess the capacity to divide indefinitely, that is, proliferate in culture and potentially may also differentiate into functionally distinct cellular phenotypes (Spangrude 2003). Stem cells can be grouped according to the source or tissue of origin. Alternatively, they can also be classified for their capacity of differentiation as follows: (i) totipotent, that is, the cells can differentiate in all types of specialized cells of the body, including the entire fetus and placenta; (ii) pluripotent, it means that cells can differentiate in all cells constituting the three germ layers (ectoderm, mesoderm, and endoderm), but not the whole organism; (iii) multipotent, that is, the cells can only differentiate in a limited type of specialized cells; and (iv) unipotent, that is, these cells can only give rise to one differential cell lineage.

It is well-known that the identification of several stem cell sources and their isolation promise to revolutionize the concept of regenerative medicine (Conrad and Huss 2005), allowed us to develop numerous cell-based therapies. For cell therapy, either differentiated (e.g., autologous chondrocytes) (Risbud and Sittinger 2002) or undifferentiated (e.g., stem cells) cells (Spangrude 2003, Zeng and Rao 2007) can be used. An implantation at the injury site of freshly isolated cells (e.g., own-patient cells) or cultured cells (differentiated cells alone or in combination with stem cells, and with or without the presence of bioactive molecules) is a possibility.

Despite, the use of stem cells in clinical practice being limited it raises many problems and concerns, especially a subtype of stem cells, the embryonic stem (ES) cells. This problem is not only due to ethical/religious issues (McKay 2000, McLaren 2001), safety (Dawson et al. 2003, Rando 2006) or technical limitations, but also to the legislative/regulatory constraints (Spangrude 2003). Adult stem cells are seen as an alternative to ES cells, as their clinical use seems to be safe, without complications and major ethical issues (Pountos and Giannoudis 2005, Verfaillie 2002). Stem cells can proliferate and differentiate beyond the tissues in which they normally reside or may be artificially placed (Wright et al. 2001). In fact, it has been shown that bone marrow-derived stem cells can not only reconstitute the bone marrow but also are capable of forming several types of mesenchymal tissues, including bone (Trojani et al. 2006), muscle cells (Dezawa et al. 2004), lung and gut (Jiang et al. 2002). For example, cell-sheet transplantation has been proving to be a breakthrough therapeutic strategy for the treatment of myocardial infarction (Miyahara et al. 2006), among others. The intensive research efforts and technological advances allowed to identify and isolate different types of stem cells from germ cells, embryo, fetus (e.g., fetal blood, placenta, and umbilical cord blood), and adult tissues and organs (Anker et al. 2003, Barry and Murphy 2004, Bongso and Richards 2004, Fraser et al. 2006, Loebel et al. 2003, Romanov et al. 2003). In addition, it was reported that the isolation of stem cells derived from amniotic fluid that express embryonic and adult stem cell markers (De Coppi et al. 2007). The amniotic fluid-derived stem cells were found to be pluripotent, meaning that they have the potential to differentiate into cell types representing each embryonic germ layer, including cells of adipogenic, osteogenic, myogenic, endothelial, neuronal, and hepatic lineages.

Interestingly, differentiated cells can be reprogrammed to a pluripotent state by transfer of nuclear contents into oocytes, by fusion with ES cells, and for male germ cells by cell culture alone. Quite recently, Takahashi et al. (Takahashi et al. 2007, Takahashi and Yamanaka 2006) demonstrated that pluripotent stem cells can be directly generated from fibroblast cultures, the so-called induced pluripotent stem (iPs) cells by retrovirus-mediated transfection with four transcription factors, namely Oct3/4, Sox2, c–Myc, and Klf4, under ES cell culture conditions. The four factors, however, cannot fully explain iPs cell induction (Yamanaka 2008). Though, this step further has major implications in regenerative medicine as for the first time, it was possible to create pluripotent cells directly from the somatic cells of humans (Park et al. 2008).

Growth factors and other bioactive molecules may be provided to control cell's fate either from cultural media (Heng et al. 2004, Zhang and Li 2005) or simply by incorporating into the scaffold (Hosseinkhani et al. 2006, Kato et al. 2006), a temporary three-dimensional matrix (3D), which can be more advantageous from a practical point of view. Often, this process may take days or weeks until it forms a tissue similar to that which is aimed at repair or regeneration. With simple tissues, only one cell type may be required (e.g., chondrocytes in cartilage repair), but in other cases, more than one cell type is a must, as the tissue to be regenerated consists of multiple structures (e.g., osteochondral tissues) (Wendt et al. 2005, Mano and Reis 2007). Thus, this will require considerable sophistication with respect to the therapeutic strategy itself, and tissue-engineering (TE) solutions seem to be the most adequate ones. In the following subsections, we review the advances resulting from targeting therapeutics and intracellular delivery, and the benefits to therapies associated with this type of approach. The advantages of using nanocarriers to accomplish the site-directed manner of drug delivery aimed at controlling different cellular functions will be also addressed.

## 19.2.1 Intracellular Delivery

Intracellular delivery is now a commonplace subject in the advanced regenerative strategies and it is gaining a clinical significance. In particular, the current work is investigating the synthesis of smart nanocarriers for delivering drugs (Breunig et al. 2008, Faraji and Wipf 2009, Nishiyama and Kataoka 2006) as an alternative to traditional drug regimens. These have been designed not only to allow drug molecules or a genetic material to be attached or loaded within the nanocarriers but also to incorporate different functionalities for cellular and subcellular targetability, traceability, and stimuli-responsiveness (Oh et al. 2009, Onaca et al. 2009). These nanocarriers can reduce the uptake of toxic agents, avoid the secondary effects of certain drugs, and improve its bioavailability, that is, these systems allow for enhancing drug accumulation and solubility at the target site and decrease their clearance by the body, thus decreasing the dosage needs. Certain biological barriers such as cell membrane and blood–brain barrier are impermeable to biomolecules larger than 1 kDa (Bareford and Swaan 2007). Therefore, nanocarriers exhibiting high permeability may accommodate these macromolecules and improve the transport across these barriers (Allard et al. 2009, Smith and Gumbleton 2006).

Cellular internalization mechanism can be grouped as follows: (i) phagocytosis, that is, uptake of large particles (in the order of a few micrometers), which is restricted to specialized cells (e.g., macrophages) and (ii) pinocytosis, that is, molecules are taken up by cells by means of fluid-phase endocytosis, clathrin-assisted and receptor-mediated endocytosis (~120 nm), caveolin-assisted and receptor-mediated endocytosis (~60 nm), and clathrin and caveolin-independent endocytosis (~90 nm) (Alberola and Radler 2009, Bareford and Swaan 2007, Conner and Schmid 2003).

At the present moment, researchers are able to bioengineer the macromolecular complexes using the ability of all cells of our body toward internalizing certain macromolecules by means of endocytosis, a mechanism which retains them in transporting vesicles within the cell. Despite, there is a possibility of lysosomal degradation (e.g., hydrolytic and enzymatic degradation) of the drug delivery complexes upon internalization, thus most strategies should bear in mind this premise. In other cases, such a deleterious possibility can be advantageous namely, those involving an enzymatic release of therapeutics which are aimed at treating lysosomal storage diseases (e.g., Gaucher's disease), cancer, and Alzheimer's disease.

Another reported possibility is the lipid-raft endocytic internalization, which opens up the possibility of avoiding the degradative intracellular drug delivery route. By means of surface engineering of macromolecules with lipid-raft-associated ligands, cellular internalization and vesicular trafficking to nonlysosomal subcellular compartments became possible. Further details on the endocytic mechanisms for the targeted delivery of macromolecules and its intracellular fate can be found elsewhere (Bareford and Swaan 2007).

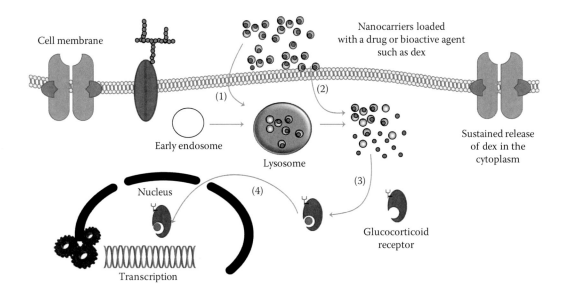

**FIGURE 19.1**   Scheme of the nanoparticles' intracellular reservoir for the sustained release of Dex aimed at modulating the osteogenic differentiation of stem cells. (1 and 2) Indicate the internalization contact and crossing of the cell membrane through different mechanisms; (2) dex release from nanoparticles into the cytoplasm; (3) interaction of dex with the glucocorticoid receptor in the cytoplasm; and (4) translocation of the complex receptor/drug into the nucleus, and mRNA transcription followed by protein translation from mRNA. (Adapted from Oliveira J. M. et al. 2010b. *Prog Polym Sci* 35:1163–94.)

Interestingly, our first study (Oliveira et al. 2008) on the surface engineering of macromolecules reported the modification of poly(amidoamine) dendrimers (PAMAM) with the water-soluble carboxymethylchitosan (CMCht), the so-called CMCht/PAMAM dendrimer nanoparticles. The developed nanoparticles were aimed at finding application as intracellular carriers to deliver bioactive molecules for controlling the fate of stem cells, namely their proliferation and differentiation. Figure 19.1 shows a scheme of the rationale proposed by our group for the intracellular drug delivery of dexamethasone (Dex) by means of using the CMCht/PAMAM dendrimer nanoparticles.

Our data showed that the dex-loaded CMCht/PAMAM dendrimer nanoparticles can be internalized by different cell types and play a crucial role in the regulation of osteogenesis *in vitro*, both in 2D and 3D culturing conditions (Oliveira et al. 2008, 2009). Applying the cell- and TE principles, we have demonstrated that the dex-loaded CMCht/PAMAM dendrimer nanoparticles may be beneficial as an intracellular nanocarrier, which supplied dex in a regimented manner *ex vivo* and promoted a superior ectopic *de novo* bone formation *in vivo* (Oliveira et al. 2010a). So far, this new approach evidenced the usefulness of the intracellular drug delivery for controlling the behavior of stem cells. The exceptional properties of the dendrimer nanoparticles, namely its biocompatibility and internalization efficiency, triggered their potential use for not only, producing the living tissues *in vitro* but also, for finding a wider application in CNS and gene therapy strategies (Oliveira 2010b), despite the need of conducting further fundamental studies.

## 19.2.2  Nanoparticles in Cell Engineering and Cellular Responses

The physicochemical properties of the nanoparticles can affect the internalization efficiency and cellular responses (Alberola and Radler 2009, Clift et al. 2010). Size, concentration, $M_w$ and surface properties are some features of the nanocarriers that will dictate its ability for being taken up by the living cells (Allard et al. 2009, Cho et al. 2009, Chung et al. 2007, Lu et al. 2010, Oliveira et al. 2008, Pedraza et al. 2008). The shape of the nanoparticles has been shown to affect its cellular uptake and their functions (Huang et al. 2010). In turn, the zeta potential of the cerium oxide nanoparticles also modulates its internalization ability by adenocarcinoma lung cells (A549) (Patil et al. 2007). However, the first step for optimizing drug delivery and targeting is to understand the mechanism of drug release from nanoparticles and its route of internalization by the cells. There are different techniques that allow us to study the targeting of nanoparticles to cells and their intracellular fate (Huth et al. 2006, Mady et al. 2009, Richardson et al. 2008, Torchilin 2005).

The genetically modified cells opened new possibilities in the field of TERM (Sheyn et al. 2010). In fact, the ability of small molecules to regulate the gene expression has potential therapeutic applications namely interfering RNA (siRNA), but its use is limited by inefficient delivery. Several solutions have been advanced to circumvent this problem, such as the use of stimuli-responsive nanocarriers which can improve their delivery efficiency. Many examples of pH-responsive systems are provided in literature (Checot et al. 2007, Hatakeyama et al. 2009, Schmaljohann 2006, Simões et al. 2001, Wang et al. 2005, Xu et al. 2010). An interesting work is related with the triggered release of adsorbed poly(ethylene glycol) (PEG)-b-polycation polymers from pH-dependent (PD) liposomes (Auguste et al. 2008). These were found to possibly protect from immune recognition (pH 7.4) and subsequent intracellular delivery of siRNA within the endosome (pH ~5.5). In this work, the polycationic blocks, based on either poly[2-(dimethylamino)ethyl methacrylate] or polylysine enabled the anchoring of the PEG protective block. By encapsulating siRNA, the authors have shown green fluorescent protein (GFP) silencing in the genetically modified, GFP-expressing human cervical epithelioid carcinoma (HeLa) cells and glyceraldehyde-3-phosphate dehydrogenase (GAPD) knockdown in the human umbilical vein endothelial cells (HUVEC). Akita and coworkers (Akita et al. 2010) reported on the *ex vivo* siRNA delivery to the primary mouse bone marrow-derived dendritic cells for finding applications as a cancer vaccine. In their studies, a successful endosomal escape was achieved by using a PD fusogenic peptide (GALA) modified on a lipid mixture that was optimized for endosomal fusion. Results showed that siRNA loaded in nanocarirers efficiently suppresses the endogenous gene expression and enhanced the dendritic cell-based vaccine potency *in vivo*. In turn, Potineni et al. (2003) reported on poly(ethylene oxide)-modified poly(b-amino ester) nanoparticles as a pH-sensitive biodegradable carrier for paclitaxel delivery. Pluronic/poly(ethylenimine) nanocapsules, which are cationic and thermally sensitive, have also been proposed as an siRNA delivery nanocarrier (Lee et al. 2008).

As previously discussed herein, the intracellular fate of macromolecular complexes is determined by the internalization mechanism and consequently by the intracellular trafficking. For targetability, caveolae-dependent endocytic route seems to be most promising since it does not transport the internalized material to endosomes and lysosomes where the internalized material can undergo degradation. Lee et al. (2007) revealed that the hyaluronic acid (HA) nanogels were selectively internalized by colorectal carcinoma cell line (HCT-116 cells) via the receptor-mediated endocytosis. In this work, siRNA was encapsulated into HA nanogels by means of using an inverse water-in-oil emulsion route. Their studies demonstrated that the HA/siRNA nanogels were up taken by HA receptor-positive cells (HCT-116 cells) having HA-specific CD44 receptors on the surface. The *in vitro* studies using glutathione (GSH) showed that the degradation/erosion of the disulfide-crosslinked HA nanogels, triggered by an intracellular reductive agent, controlled the release pattern of siRNA, which evidences the target-specific intracellular delivery of siRNA using degradable hyaluronic acid nanogels. The linking of different targeting ligands to nanocarriers have also been used for this purpose (Nakase et al. 2008, Santos et al. 2010, Shao et al. 2006).

For traceability, nanocarriers can be labeled by linking or encapsulating a probe. Several molecules can be used as markers or probes, namely histological and fluorescent dyes, radiotracers, and contrast agents (Burks et al. 2009, Domanski et al. 2004, Fretz et al. 2004, Huth et al. 2006, Straubinger et al. 1983, Sun et al. 2008). Our group followed a similar strategy and linked fluorescein isothiocyanate (FITC) to CMCht/PAMAM dendrimer nanoparticles to investigate the uptake and the mechanism of internalization by rat bone marrow stromal cells (Oliveira et al. 2008). To gain further insight into the internalization mechanism, it was used colchicine, an endocytic inhibitor that binds tightly to microtubules and causes microtubule depolymerization. This assay suggested that nanoparticles were taken up by cells through a mechanism that is not exclusively endocytic.

Succinctly, research dealing with the uptake and the intracellular behavior of stimuli-sensitive nano-carriers can be investigated by means of: (i) combining different inhibitors aimed at selectively block-ing different pathways, (ii) using different permeabilizing agents, (iii) using fluorescent probes, which should be specific for the different endocytic routes, and (iv) using different types of cells, which inter-nalize the stimuli-sensitive nanocarriers by means of different mechanisms (Douglas et al. 2008).

Now, let us focus on the cellular responses to different nanoparticles upon its internalization, namely dendrimers, quantum dots (QDs), core–shell cationic nanoparticles, liposomes, and magnetic nanopar-ticles (MNPs). For example, the cytoxicity screening and applicability of CMCht/PAMAM dendrimer nanoparticles for CNS applications have been recently assessed using neurons, astrocytes, and oligo-dendrocytes (Salgado et al. 2010). Post-natal hippocampal neurons and cortical glial cells were able to internalize the FITC-labeled CMCht/PAMAM dendrimer nanoparticles with high efficiency. This work revealed that the binding of these nanoparticles to fluorescent probes for tracing purposes was also pos-sible. We have found that cell viability was not significantly affected upon exposure to these nanopar-ticles. Moreover, it was possible to observe that neurons, astrocytes, oligodendrocytes, and microglial cells were able to internalize the CMCht/PAMAM dendrimer nanoparticles at different rates. The ongo-ing studies are focused on loading relevant drugs (e.g., methylprednisolone) for CNS-related applica-tions into the CMCht/PAMAM dendrimer nanoparticles.

Shieh et al. (2008) reported a controllable and nontoxic gene transfection method, the photochemical internalization (PCI)-mediated gene delivery, by means of using polyamidoamine (PAMAM, G4) den-drimers surface modified with 5,10,15-tri(4-acetamidophenyl)-20-mono(4-carboxyl-phenyl) porphyrin (TAMCPP) as intracellular nanocarriers. TAMCPP conjugation do not increase the cytotoxicity of the PAMAM dendrimer below 20 μm, but significantly induced cell death after suitable irradiation. Under almost nontoxic PAMAM G4-TAMCPP-mediated PCI treatment, the expression of GFP could be mark-edly enhanced in HeLa cells. Therefore, the conjugate showed the potential as a nanocarrier for PCI-mediated gene therapy. For further details on the current state and achievements on the development of nanocarriers for light-induced gene transfection may be found elsewhere (Nishiyama and Kataoka 2006).

QDs have been proposed as ideal candidates for innumerous biological applications, including imag-ing and labeling of cells (Howarth et al. 2005, Prinzen et al. 2007, Smith et al. 2008, Xing et al. 2006). Since they provide outstanding features such as a small and uniform size and unique optical properties, they are powerful nanotools for the investigation of distinct cellular processes, like uptake, receptor trafficking, and intracellular delivery (Hild et al. 2008). Despite, there is a need to surface and modify the QDs, as they often present a certain degree of toxicity (Hezinger et al. 2008). For example, Chang et al. (2008) labeled the human bone mesenchymal stem cells (hADAS) with CdSe/ZnS QDs. In this study, cell proliferation assays demonstrated that peptide-1-labeled QD delivery protects hADAS from the damage caused by the internalization of QDs. They also concluded that the endo-/lysosome degra-dation of QDs may depend on different surface coatings and critically influence the differentiation of hADAS. Iron oxide ($Fe_2O_3$) nanoparticles, with different sizes and surface potentials, have also been proposed for labeling bone marrow-derived mesenchymal stem cells (Jo et al. 2010). This group has demonstrated that $Fe_2O_3$-pullulan nanoparticles may be a promising nanotool for the magnetic reso-nance imaging (MRI) labeling of stem cells.

Genetic vaccination using core–shell cationic nanoparticles have been proposed (Castaldello et al. 2006). In this work, a hydrophilic tentacular shell bearing positively charged groups and PEG chains were covalently linked to a poly(methylmethacrylate) (PMMA) core by means of following an emul-sion polymerization method. The *in vitro* studies demonstrated that nanoparticles reversibly adsorbed large amounts of DNA, preserved its functional structure, and were efficiently taken up by cells. *In vivo* studies revealed that nanoparticles were non toxic. In turn, intramuscular immunization using the nanoparticle loaded with a plasmid (pCV-tat), promoted significant antigen-specific humoral and long-lasting cellular responses, and significantly improved Th1-type T cell responses and cytotoxic T lymphocytes against human immunodeficiency virus (HIV)-1 Tat.

Thompson and coworkers (Thompson and Gross 1988) reported a system for efficiently packaging antibodies and other macromolecules into liposomes. The strategy was based on delivering the encapsulated molecules into living cells through liposome-cell fusion. Results have shown that antibodies maintained their ability to recognize and bind to their specific antigens. To determine if the antibodies were capable of interfering with cellular processes *in vivo*, the group measured the effects of liposome-introduced antiribosome antibodies on translation and antitubulin antibodies on mitosis. Their data demonstrated a significant inhibition and the antibodies could in fact, be used to interfere with specific functions at specific times. Other liposomal formulations namely Doxil® and Visudyne®, have been approved for clinical use. Nevertheless, the aforementioned polymeric micelles have been attracting much attention as compared to stealth liposomes. This is mainly due to the secondary effects associated with the administration of PEG-liposome formulations, which often requires the preadministration of anti-histamine and anti-inflammatory drugs. In turn, it is believed that polymeric micelles might not cause toxicity problems such as those observed for stealth liposomes (Nishiyama and Kataoka 2006). In turn, Ito et al. (2005) showed that cell attachment can be stimulated by means of linking an Arg-Gly-Asp (RGD)-motif-containing peptide to magnetite cationic liposomes (MCLs).

MNPs have been shown as promising for finding an application for intracellular delivery, diagnostics, and therapy purposes (Shubayev et al. 2009). Despite, Pisanic Ii et al. (2007) reported that the intracellular delivery of moderate levels of $Fe_2O_3$ nanoparticles may adversely affect cell functioning. Actually, their cytotoxicity experiments demonstrated that an exposure to the increasing concentrations of anionic MNPs, from 0.15 to 15 mm of iron, resulted in a dose-dependent diminishing viability and capacity of rat pheochromocytoma (PC12) cells to extend neurites. They have concluded that more studies on $Fe_2O_3$ internalization are needed, to screen its biocompatibility.

## 19.3 Concluding Remarks

Nanotechnology has been showing great promise in intracellular drug delivery and human therapeutics and diagnose. A wide variety of nanotools exists already, and have been explored in cell- and TE strategies. Different materials, formulations, and methods of synthesis have been put forward. Despite, careful use a comprehensive research to understand better and assess their effects on cells, and assess its bio-safety prior administration to humans must be considered. We can envision particularly interesting applications of nanoparticles in drug delivery, namely those that relate to the central nervous system. Since many neuropharmacologic agents do not reach the brain due to the blood–brain barrier, it can be expected that the use of nanotools allow us to overcome these barrier challenges and establish new therapeutic possibilities, in the near future.

## References

Akita, H., Kogure, K., Moriguchi, R. et al. 2010. Nanoparticles for ex vivo siRNA delivery to dendritic cells for cancer vaccines: Programmed endosomal escape and dissociation. *J Control Release* 143:311–17.

Alberola, A. P. and Radler, J. O. 2009. The defined presentation of nanoparticles to cells and their surface controlled uptake. *Biomaterials* 30:3766–70.

Allard, E., Passirani, C., and Benoit, J.P. 2009. Convection-enhanced delivery of nanocarriers for the treatment of brain tumors. *Biomaterials* 30:2302–18.

Anker, P. S., Noort, W. A., Scherjon, S. A. et al. 2003. Mesenchymal stem cells in human second-trimester bone marrow, liver, lung, and spleen exhibit a similar immunophenotype but a heterogeneous multilineage differentiation potential. *Haematologica* 88:845–52.

Auguste, D. T., Furman, K., Wong, A. et al. 2008. Triggered release of siRNA from poly(ethylene glycol)-protected, pH-dependent liposomes. *J Control Release* 130:266–74.

Bareford, L. M. and Swaan, P. M. 2007. Endocytic mechanisms for targeted drug delivery. *Adv Drug Deliv Rev* 59:748–58.

Barry, F. P. and Murphy, J. M. 2004. Mesenchymal stem cells: Clinical applications and biological characterization. *Int J Biochem Cell Biol* 36:568–84.

Bongso, A. and Richards, M. 2004. History and perspective of stem cell research. *Best Pract Res Clin Obstet Gynaecol* 18:827–42.

Breunig, M., Bauer, S., and Goepferich, A. 2008. Polymers and nanoparticles: Intelligent tools for intracellular targeting? *Eur J Pharm Biopharm* 68:112–28.

Burks, S. R., Barth, E. D., Halpern, H. J., Rosen, G. M., and Kao, J. P. Y. 2009. Cellular uptake of electron paramagnetic resonance imaging probes through endocytosis of liposomes. *Biochim Biophys Acta (BBA)—Biomembranes* 1788:2301–8.

Castaldello, A., Brocca-Cofano, E., Voltan, R. et al. 2006. DNA prime and protein boost immunization with innovative polymeric cationic core-shell nanoparticles elicits broad immune responses and strongly enhance cellular responses of HIV-1 tat DNA vaccination. *Vaccine* 24:5655–69.

Chang, J.C., Su, H.L., and Hsu, S.H. 2008. The use of peptide-delivery to protect human adipose-derived adult stem cells from damage caused by the internalization of quantum dots. *Biomaterials* 29:925–36.

Checot, F., Rodriguez-Hernandez, J., Gnanou, Y., and Lecommandoux, S. 2007. pH-responsive micelles and vesicles nanocapsules based on polypeptide diblock copolymers. *Biomol Eng* 24:81–5.

Cho, M., Cho, W.S., Choi, M. et al. 2009. The impact of size on tissue distribution and elimination by single intravenous injection of silica nanoparticles. *Toxicol Lett* 189:177–83.

Chung, T.H., Wu, S.H., Yao, M. et al. 2007. The effect of surface charge on the uptake and biological function of mesoporous silica nanoparticles in 3T3-L1 cells and human mesenchymal stem cells. *Biomaterials* 28:2959–66.

Clift, M. J. D., Rothen-Rutishauser, B., Brown, D. M. et al. 2010. The impact of different nanoparticle surface chemistry and size on uptake and toxicity in a murine macrophage cell line. *Toxicol Appl Pharmacol* 232:418–27.

Conner, S. D. and Schmid, S. L. 2003. Regulated portals of entry into the cell. *Nature* 422:37–44.

Conrad, C. and Huss, R. 2005. Adult stem cell lines in regenerative medicine and reconstructive surgery. *J Surgical Res* 124:201–08.

Dawson, L., Bateman-House, A. S., Agnew, D. M. et al. 2003. Safety issues in cell-based intervention trials. *Fertil Steril* 80:1077–85.

De Coppi, P., Bartsch, J. G., Siddiqui, M. M. et al. 2007. Isolation of amniotic stem cell lines with potential for therapy. *Nature Biotechnol* 25:100–6.

Dezawa, M., Kanno, H., Hoshino, M. et al. 2004. Specific induction of neuronal cells from bone marrow stromal cells and application for autologous transplantation. *J Clin Invest* 113:1701–10.

Domanski, D. M., Klajnert, B., and Bryszewska, M. 2004. Incorporation of fluorescent probes into PAMAM dendrimers. *Bioelectrochemistry* 63:193–7.

Douglas, K. L., Piccirillo, C. A., and Tabrizian, M. 2008. Cell line-dependent internalization pathways and intracellular trafficking determine transfection efficiency of nanoparticle vectors. *Eur J Pharm Biopharm* 68:676–87.

Faraji, A. H. and Wipf, P. 2009. Nanoparticles in cellular drug delivery. *Bioorg Med Che* 17:2950–62.

Fraser, J. K., Wulur, I., Alfonso, Z., and Hedrick, M. H. 2006. Fat tissue: An underappreciated source of stem cells for biotechnology. *Trends Biotechnol* 24:150–4.

Fretz, M. M., Koning, G. A., Mastrobattista, E., Jiskoot, W., and Storm, G. 2004. OVCAR-3 cells internalize TAT-peptide modified liposomes by endocytosis. *Biochim Biophys Acta (BBA)—Biomembranes* 1665:48–56.

Hatakeyama, H., Ito, E., Akita, H. et al. 2009. A pH-sensitive fusogenic peptide facilitates endosomal escape and greatly enhances the gene silencing of siRNA-containing nanoparticles in vitro and in vivo. *J Control Release* 139:127–32.

Heng, B. C., Haider, H. K., Sim, E. K.W., Tong Cao, T., and Ng, S. C. 2004. Strategies for directing the differentiation of stem cells into the cardiomyogenic lineage in vitro. *Cardiovasc Res* 62:34–42.

Hezinger, A. F. E., Tessmar, J., and Göpferich, A. 2008. Polymer coating of quantum dots—A powerful tool toward diagnostics and sensorics. *Eur J Pharm Biopharm* 68:138–52.

Hild, W. A., Breunig, M., and Goepferich, A. 2008. Quantum dots—Nano-sized probes for the exploration of cellular and intracellular targeting. *Eur J Pharm Biopharm* 68:153–68.

Hosseinkhani, H., Yamamoto, M., Inatsugu, Y. et al. 2006. Enhanced ectopic bone formation using a combination of plasmid DNA impregnation into 3-D scaffold and bioreactor perfusion culture. *Biomaterials* 27:1387–98.

Howarth, M., Takao, K., Hayashi, Y., and Ting, A. Y. 2005. Targeting quantum dots to surface proteins in living cells with biotin ligase. *Proc Natl Acad Sci USA* 102:7583–8.

Huang, X., Teng, X., Chen, D., Tang, F., and He, J. 2010. The effect of the shape of mesoporous silica nanoparticles on cellular uptake and cell function. *Biomaterials* 31:438–48.

Huth, U. S., Schubert, R., and Peschka-Süss, R. 2006. Investigating the uptake and intracellular fate of pH-sensitive liposomes by flow cytometry and spectral bio-imaging. *J Control Release* 110:490–504.

Ito, A., Ino, K., Kobayashi, T., and Honda, H. 2005. The effect of RGD peptide-conjugated magnetite cationic liposomes on cell growth and cell sheet harvesting. *Biomaterials* 26:6185–93.

Jiang, Y., Jahagirdar, B. N., Reinhardt, R. L. et al. 2002. Pluripotency of mesenchymal stem cells derived from adult marrow. *Nature* 418:41–9.

Jo, J.I., Aoki, I. and Tabata, Y. 2010. Design of iron oxide nanoparticles with different sizes and surface charges for simple and efficient labeling of mesenchymal stem cells. *J Control Release* 142:465–73.

Kato, M., Namikawa, T., Terai, H. et al. 2006. Ectopic bone formation in mice associated with a lactic acid/dioxanone/ethylene glycol copolymer–tricalcium phosphate composite with added recombinant human bone morphogenetic protein-2. *Biomaterials* 27:3927–33.

Lee, H., Mok, H., Lee, S., Oh, Y.K., and Park, T. G. 2007. Target-specific intracellular delivery of siRNA using degradable hyaluronic acid nanogels. *J Control Release* 119:245.

Lee, S. H., Choi, S. H., Kim, S. H., and Park, T. G. 2008. Thermally sensitive cationic polymer nanocapsules for specific cytosolic delivery and efficient gene silencing of siRNA: Swelling induced physical disruption of endosome by cold shock. *J Control Release* 125:25–32.

Loebel, D. A. F., Watson, C. M., De Young, R. A., and Tam, P. P. L. 2003. Lineage choice and differentiation in mouse embryos and embryonic stem cells. *Dev Biol* 264:1–14.

Lu, S., Xia, D., Huang, G. et al. 2010. Concentration effect of gold nanoparticles on proliferation of keratinocytes. *Colloids Surf B: Biointerfaces* 81:406–11.

Mady, M. M., Ghannam, M. M., Khalil, W. A., Müller, R., and Fahr, A. 2009. Efficiency of cytoplasmic delivery by non-cationic liposomes to cells in vitro: A confocal laser scanning microscopy study. *Phys Med* 25:88–93.

Mano, J. F. and Reis, R. L. 2007. Osteochondral defects: Present situation and tissue engineering approaches. *J Tissue Eng Reg Med* 1: 261–73.

McKay, R. 2000. Stem cells—Hype and hope. *Nature* 406:361–64.

McLaren, A. 2001. Ethical and social considerations of stem cell research. *Nature* 414:129–31.

Miyahara, Y., Nagaya, N., Kataoka, M. et al. 2006. Monolayered mesenchymal stem cells repair scarred myocardium after myocardial infarction. *Nat Med* 12:459–65.

Nakase, I., Takeuchi, T., Tanaka, G., and Futaki, S. 2008. Methodological and cellular aspects that govern the internalization mechanisms of arginine-rich cell-penetrating peptides. *Adv Drug Deliv Rev* 60:598.

Nishiyama, N. and Kataoka, K. 2006. Current state, achievements, and future prospects of polymeric micelles as nanocarriers for drug and gene delivery. *Pharmacol Ther* 112:630–48.

Oh, J. K., Lee, D. I., and Park, J. M. 2009. Biopolymer-based microgels/nanogels for drug delivery applications. *Prog Polym Sci* 34:1261–82.

Oliveira, J. M., Kotobuki, N., Marques, A. P. et al. 2008. Surface engineered carboxymethylchitosan/poly(amidoamine) dendrimer nanoparticles for intracellular targeting. *Adv Funct Mater* 18:1840–53.

Oliveira, J. M., Kotobuki, N., Tadokoro, M. et al. 2010a. Ex vivo culturing of stromal cells with dexametha-sone-loaded carboxymethylchitosan/poly(amidoamine) dendrimer nanoparticles promotes ectopic bone formation. *Bone* 46:1424–35.

Oliveira, J. M., Salgado, A. J., Sousa, N., Mano, J. F., and Reis, R. L. 2010b. Dendrimers and derivatives as a potential therapeutic tool in regenerative medicine strategies—A review. *Prog Polym Sci* 35:1163–94.

Oliveira, J. M., Sousa, R. A., Kotobuki, N. et al. 2009. The osteogenic differentiation of rat bone marrow stromal cells cultured with dexamethasone-loaded carboxymethylchitosan/poly(amidoamine) dendrimer nanoparticles. *Biomaterials* 30:804–13.

Onaca, O., Ramona, E., Hughes, D. W., and Meier, W. 2009. Stimuli-responsive polymersomes as nanocar-riers for drug and gene delivery. *Macromol Biosci* 9:129–39.

Park, I.H., Zhao, R., West, J. A. et al. 2008. Reprogramming of human somatic cells to pluripotency with defined factors. *Nature* 451:141–6.

Patil, S., Sandberg, A., Heckert, E., Self, W., and Seal, S. 2007. Protein adsorption and cellular uptake of cerium oxide nanoparticles as a function of zeta potential. *Biomaterials* 28:4600–7.

Pedraza, C. E., Bassett, D. C., McKee, M. D. et al. 2008. The importance of particle size and DNA condensa-tion salt for calcium phosphate nanoparticle transfection. *Biomaterials* 29:3384–92.

Pisanic Ii, T. R., Blackwell, J. D., Shubayev, V. I., Fiñones, R. R., and Jin, S. 2007. Nanotoxicity of iron oxide nanoparticle internalization in growing neurons. *Biomaterials* 28:2572–81.

Potineni, A., Lynn, D. M., Langer, R., and Amiji, M. M. 2003. Poly(ethylene oxide)-modified poly([beta]-amino ester) nanoparticles as a pH-sensitive biodegradable system for paclitaxel delivery. *J Control Release* 86:223–34.

Pountos, I. and Giannoudis, P. V. 2005. Biology of mesenchymal stem cells. *Injury, Int J Care Injured* 365: S8–S12.

Prinzen, L., Miserus, R.J. J. H. M., Dirksen, A. et al. 2007. Optical and magnetic resonance imaging of cell death and platelet activation using annexin A5-functionalized quantum dots. *Nano Lett* 7:93–100.

Rando, T. A. 2006. Stem cells, ageing and the quest for immortality. *Nature* 441:1080–6.

Richardson, S. C. W., Wallom, K.L., Ferguson, E. L. et al. 2008. The use of fluorescence microscopy to define polymer localisation to the late endocytic compartments in cells that are targets for drug delivery. *J Control Release* 127:1–11.

Risbud, M. V. and Sittinger, M. 2002. Tissue engineering: Advances in in vitro cartilage generation. *Trends Biotechnol* 20:351–6.

Romanov, Y. A., Svintsitskaya, V. A., and Smirnov, V. N. 2003. Searching for alternative sources of post-natal human mesenchymal stem cells: Candidate MSC-like cells from umbilical cord. *Stem Cells* 21:105–10.

Salgado, A. J., Oliveira, J. M., Pirraco, R. P. et al. 2010. Carboxymethylchitosan/poly(amidoamine) den-drimer nanoparticles in central nervous systems-regenerative medicine: Effects on neuron/glial cell viability and internalization efficiency. *Macromol Biosci* 10:1130–40.

Santos, A. O., da Silva, L. C. G., Bimbo, L. M. et al. 2010. Design of peptide-targeted liposomes containing nucleic acids. *Biochim Biophys Acta (BBA)—Biomembranes* 978:56–64.

Schmaljohann, D. 2006. Thermo- and pH-responsive polymers in drug delivery. *Adv Drug Deliv Rev* 58:1655–70.

Shao, K., Hou, Q., Duan, W. et al. 2006. Intracellular drug delivery by sulfatide-mediated liposomes to gliomas. *J Control Release* 115:150–7.

Sheyn, D., Mizrahi, O., Benjamin, S. et al. 2010. Genetically modified cells in regenerative medicine and tissue engineering. *Adv Drug Deliv Rev* 62:683–98.

Shieh, M.J., Peng, C.L., Lou, P.J. et al. 2008. Non-toxic phototriggered gene transfection by PAMAM-porphyrin conjugates. *J Control Release* 129:200–6.

Shubayev, V. I., Pisanic Ii, T. R., and Jin, S. 2009. Magnetic nanoparticles for theragnostics. *Adv Drug Deliv Rev* 61:467–77.

Simões, S., Slepushkin, V., Düzgünes, N., and Pedroso de Lima, M. C. 2001. On the mechanisms of internalization and intracellular delivery mediated by pH-sensitive liposomes. *Biochim Biophys Acta (BBA)—Biomembranes* 1515:23–37.

Smith, A. M., Duan, H., Mohs, A. M., and Nie, S. 2008. Bioconjugated quantum dots for in vivo molecular and cellular imaging. *Adv Drug Deliv Rev* 60:1226–40.

Smith, M. W. and Gumbleton, M. 2006. Endocytosis at the blood brain barrier: From basic understanding to drug delivery strategies. *J Drug Target* 14:191–214.

Spangrude, G. J. 2003. Stem cells and tissue regeneration: When is a stem cell really a stem cell? *Bone Marrow Transplant* 32: S7–S11.

Straubinger, R. M., Hong, K., Friend, D. S., and Papahadjopoulos, D. 1983. Endocytosis of liposomes and intracellular fate of encapsulated molecules: Encounter with a low pH compartment after internalization in coated vesicles. *Cell* 32:1069–79.

Sun, C., Lee, J. S. H., and Zhang, M. 2008. Magnetic nanoparticles in MR imaging and drug delivery. *Adv Drug Deliv Rev* 60:1252–65.

Takahashi, K., Okita, K., Nakagawa, M., and Yamanaka, S. 2007. Induction of pluripotent stem cells from fibroblast cultures. *Nat Protoc* 2:3081–9.

Takahashi, K. and Yamanaka, S. 2006. Induction of pluripotent stem cells from mouse embryonic and adult fibroblast cultures by defined factors. *Cell* 126:663–76.

Thompson, W. S. and Gross, R. H. 1988. Antibodies introduced into living cells with liposomes localize specifically and inhibit specific intracellular processes. *Gene Anal Tech* 5:73–9.

Torchilin, V. P. 2005. Fluorescence microscopy to follow the targeting of liposomes and micelles to cells and their intracellular fate. *Adv Drug Deliv Rev* 57:95–109.

Trojani, C., Boukhechba, F., Scimeca, J.C. et al. 2006. Ectopic bone formation using an injectable biphasic calcium phosphate/Si-HPMC hydrogel composite loaded with undifferentiated bone marrow stromal cells. *Biomaterials* 27:3256–64.

Verfaillie, C. M. 2002. Adult stem cells: Assessing the case for pluripotency. *Trends in Cell Biol* 12:502–8.

Wang, C.H., Wang, C.H., and Hsiue, G.H. 2005. Polymeric micelles with a pH-responsive structure as intracellular drug carriers. *J Control Release* 108:140–9.

Wendt, D., Jakob, M., and Martin, I. 2005. Bioreactor-based engineering of osteochondral grafts: From model systems to tissue manufacturing. *J Biosci Bioeng* 100:489–94.

Wright, D. E., Wagers, A. J., Gulati, A. P., Johnson, F. L., and Weissman, I. L. 2001. Physiological migration of hematopoietic stem and progenitor cells. *Science* 294:1933–6.

Xing, Y., Smith, A. M., Agrawal, A., Ruan, G., and Nie, S. M. 2006. Molecular profiling of single cancer cells and clinical tissue specimens with semiconductor quantum dots. *Int. J. Nanomed* 1:473–81.

Xu, S., Luo, Y., Graeser, R. et al. 2010. Development of pH-responsive core-shell nanocarriers for delivery of therapeutic and diagnostic agents. *Bioorg Med Chem Lett* 198:73.

Yamanaka, S. 2008. Induction of pluripotent stem cells from mouse fibroblasts by four transcription factors. *Cell Prolif* 41:51–6.

Zhang, J. and Li, L. 2005. BMP signaling and stem cell regulation. *Dev Biol* 284:1–11.

Zeng, X. and Rao, M. S. 2007. Human embryonic stem cells: Long term stability, absence of senescence and a potential cell source for neural replacement. *Neuroscience* 145:1348–58.

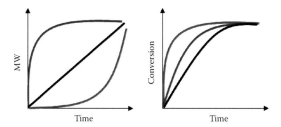

**FIGURE 5.3** Progression of polymer molecular weight and monomer conversion with time for step growth (red), chain growth (blue), and living (black) polymerizations.

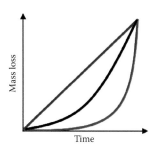

**FIGURE 5.4** Mass loss profile for idealized bulk eroding (red) and surface eroding (blue) polymeric materials. The actual mass loss profile is a hybrid of the two profiles, shown in black.

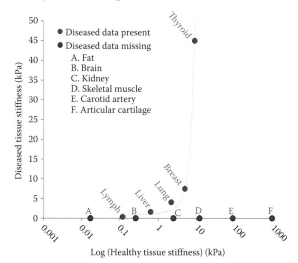

**FIGURE 14.1** Stiffness (Young's modulus) of diseased tissue versus the log10 of healthy tissue. Blue data points indicate tissues for which the stiffnesses of both the healthy and diseased conditions are known. These points seem to follow an exponential trend, with equation $E_{dis} = 755e^{-0.0005}E_{healthy}$. This trend suggests that there exists an underlying mechanism which regulates tissue biomechanics during disease development. Diseases of the tissues shown include lymph containing metastases, fibrotic liver, lung fibrosis, breast tumor, and thyroid cancer. Red data points indicate tissues for which the stiffness of only the healthy condition is known. Further work is necessary to fill in the stiffnesses of diseased conditions for these tissues. (This data was pooled from the following sources: Dolhnikoff, M., T. Mauad, and M.S. Ludwig. 1999. *American Journal of Respiratory and Critical Care Medicine* 160(5): 1750–7; Engler, A.J. et al. 2004b. *Journal of Cell Biology* 166(6): 877–87; Freed, L.E. et al. 1997. *Proceedings of the National Academy of Sciences of the United States of America* 94(25): 13885–90; Guo, X.M. et al. 2006b. *American Journal of Physiology-Heart and Circulatory Physiology* 290(5): H1788–97; Lyshchik, A. et al. 2005. *Ultrasonic Imaging* 27(2): 101–10; Miller, K. et al. 2000b. *Journal of Biomechanics* 33(11): 1369–76; Miyaji, K. et al. 1997. *Cancer* 80(10): 1920–5; Nasseri, S., L.E. Bilston, and N. Phan-Thien. 2002. *Rheologica Acta* 41(1–2): 180–92; Norman, L.L. and H. Aranda-Espinoza. 2010. *Cellular and Molecular Bioengineering* (accepted); Paszek, M.J. et al. 2005b. *Cancer Cell* 8(3): 241–54; Wellman, P. et al. 1999. Harvard Biorobotics Laboratory Technical Report; Yeh, W.C. et al. 2002. *Ultrasound in Medicine and Biology* 28(4): 467–74; Yuan, H.C. et al. 2000. *Journal of Applied Physiology* 89(1): 3–14.)

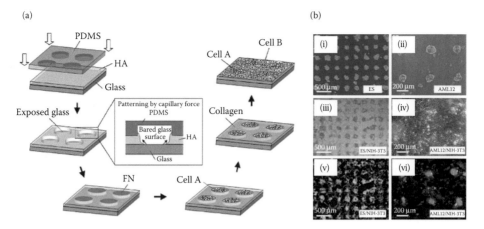

**FIGURE 16.2** (a) The scheme for patterning of cellular cocultures by using capillary force lithography and layer-by-layer deposition. A few drops of HA solution were spun coated onto a glass slide, and a PDMS mold was immediately placed on the thin layer of HA. HA under the void space of the PDMS mold receded until the glass surface became exposed. The exposed region of a glass substrate was coated with FN, where primary cells could be selectively adhered. Subsequently, the HA surface was complexed with collagen, allowing for the subsequent adhesion of secondary cells. (b) Images of patterned cells and patterned cell cocultures on HA/collagen surfaces. (i) Murine ES cells and (ii) AML12 murine hepatocytes selectively adhered to the FN-coated region on HA-patterned surface after an 8 h incubation. The HA surface including the primary cells was treated with collagen and seeded with NIH-3T3 fibroblasts. After 3 days of culture, ES cells formed dense spherical aggregates and were clearly distinct from the surrounding fibroblasts monolayer. (iii) The coculture of AML12 hepatocytes and NIH-3T3 fibroblasts was difficult to distinguish under a light microscope. (iv) Fluorescently stained primary cells (green) and secondary cells (red) were visualized for ES/NIH-3T3 (v) and AML12/NIH-3T3. (vi) Cocultures at 3 days of culture. (Adapted with permission from Fukuda, J. et al. 2006. *Biomaterials* **27**(8): 1479–1486.)

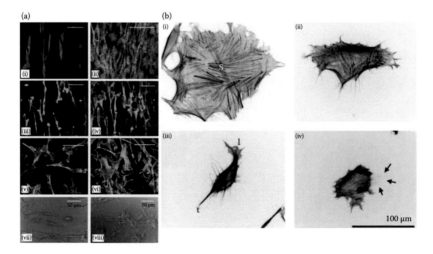

**FIGURE 16.3** (a) Confocal micrographs of F-actin stained SMCs on (i) nano-imprinted PMMA at a low cell density, (ii) nano-imprinted PMMA at a high cell density, (iii) nanopatterned PDMS at a low cell density, (iv) nanopatterned PDMS at a high cell density, (v) nonpatterned PMMA, and (vi) glass cover slip. SEM micrographs of SMC cultured on (vii) nano-imprinted gratings on PMMA coated on $SiO_2$ wafer and (viii) nonpatterned PMMA coated on $SiO_2$ wafer. Bar = 50 µm for all except (ii) Bar = 100 µm. (b) Fluorescent actin staining (images inverted to show filopodia more clearly). (i and ii) Fibroblasts on control, (iii and iv) fibroblasts on nano-columns. (i) A well-spread cell with many stress fibers (s); (ii) cells becoming well-spread, but still with a polarized morphology; (iii) a rounded cell that is clearly polarized with lamellipodia at the leading edge (l) and a trailing tail (t); (iv) spreading cell, which is still notably smaller, and has fewer stress fibers than the cells seen in (i and ii) (arrows point to faint filopodia). (Figure 16.3a is adapted with permission from Yim E. K. F. et al. 2005. *Biomaterials* **26**(26): 5405–5413; Figure 16.3b is adapted with permission from Dalby, M. J. et al. 2004b. *Biomaterials* **25**(23): 5415–5422.)

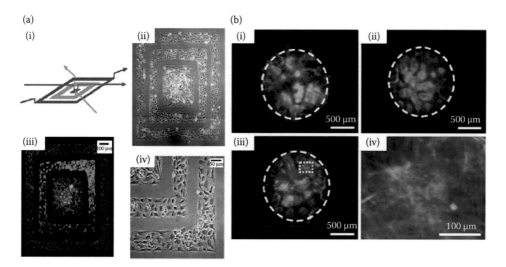

**FIGURE 16.5** (i) Fluorescence (ii) and phase-contrast (iii and iv) pictures of two cell types deposited on a tissue culture dish in a concentric square pattern by using the 3D stamp depicted in (a). The cells that appear green are (ECVs) labeled with 5-chloromethylfluorescein diacetate (CMFDA); the cells that appear red are BCEs labeled with DiI-conjugated acetylated low density lipoprotein. Suspensions of cells were introduced into the three sets of channels and were allowed to sediment and attach to the surface of the tissue-culture dish. These cells were cultured with the stamp in place for ≈24 h to grow and spread into a confluent layer. An expanded view of the lower right corner of (iii) is shown in (iv). (b) Different regions of a hydroxyapatite scaffold patterned with osteoblasts using a single agarose stamp with 1000 μm diameter circular features. Images (i through iii) show an area on the top surface of the same scaffold that was patterned during the same stamping event. The dashed white lines indicate the areas patterned with cells. (iv) Higher magnification of the area within the white box in (iii). Actin was stained bright green with phalloidin and DNA stained bright blue with Hoescht 33342. The dark blue/gray features in the unpatterned background of the images in (i through iii) are artifacts of fluorescence microscopy, resulting from the light reflected from the white hydroxyapatite scaffolds. The images were acquired 24 h after patterning. (Figure 16.5a is adapted with permission from Chiu D. T. et al. 2000. *Proceedings of the National Academy of Sciences of the United States of America* **97**(6): 2408–2413; Figure 16.5b is adapted with permission from Stevens, M. M. et al. 2005. *Biomaterials* **26**(36): 7636–7641.)

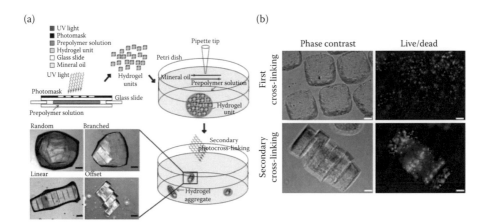

**FIGURE 16.6** (a) Schematic diagram of microgel (micron-sized hydrogel) self-assembly process. Microgel units were synthesized by photolithography, transferred into a dish containing mineral oil, and subjected to mechanical agitation applied by manually manipulating a pipette-tip in a back-and-forth manner. Four structural types of microgel assemblies were observed: linear, branched, random, and offset. Secondary cross-linking was achieved by exposing the microgel assemblies to UV light. (Scale bars, 200 μm.) (b) Phase-contrast and fluorescence images of cell-laden (NIH 3T3) microgel assemblies. (Adapted with permission from Du, Y. A. et al. 2008. *Proceedings of the National Academy of Sciences of the United States of America* **105**(28): 9522–9527.)

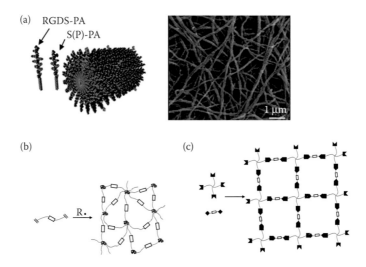

**FIGURE 20.1** Examples of gelation mechanisms that have been successfully employed in cell encapsulation strategies: (a) self-assembling peptides that assemble via noncovalent interactions into cylindrical, micellar structures, and subsequently into nanofibers that form a macroscopic hydrogel, (b) radical chain polymerization whereby in this example a radical initiates polymerization of a divinyl macromolecular monomer leading to a covalently cross-linked network, and (c) step growth polymerization whereby in this example two distinctly different macromolecular monomers form a homogeneous crosslinked network. (Panel (a) is reprinted from *Biomaterials*, 31, Mata, A. et al. Bone regeneration mediated by biomimetic mineralization of a nanofiber matrix, 6004–12. Copyright 2010, with permission from Elsevier.)

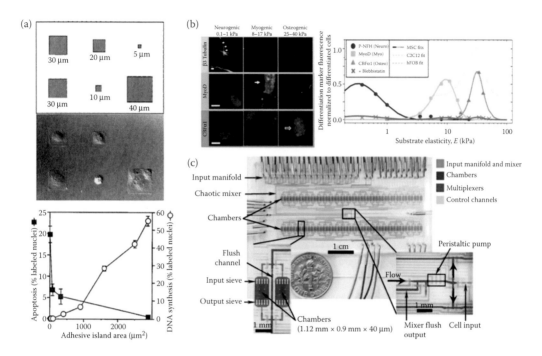

**FIGURE 22.1** Substrate geometry and stiffness influence cell responses. (a) Effect of spreading on cell growth and apoptosis. Schematic diagram showing the initial pattern design containing different-sized square adhesive islands and images of the final shapes of bovine endothelial cells adherent to the fabricated substrate. Distances indicate lengths of the square's sides. The graph plots the apoptotic index and DNA synthesis index after 24 h, plotted as a function of the projected cell area. Data were obtained only from islands that contained single adherent cells; similar results were obtained with circular or square islands and with human or bovine endothelial cells. (From Chen, C. S. et al. 1997. *Science* **276**: 1425–28.) (b) Protein and transcript profiles are elasticity dependent under identical media conditions. The neuronal cytoskeletal marker b3 tubulin is expressed in branches (arrows) of initially naive MSCs (>75%) and only on the soft, neurogenic matrices. The muscle transcription factor MyoD1 is upregulated and nuclear localized (arrow) only in MSCs on myogenic matrices. The osteoblast transcription factor CBFa1 (arrow) is likewise expressed only on stiff, osteogenic gels. Scale bar is 5 μm. The graph represents fluorescent intensity of differentiation markers versus substrate elasticity, revealing maximal lineage specification at the E typical of each tissue type. (From Engler, A. J. et al. 2006. *Cell* **126**: 677–89.) Panel (c) Design of an integrated cell culture chip. Annotated photograph of a chip with the channels filled with colored water to indicate different parts of the device. The left inset gives a closer view of two culture chambers, with the multiplexer flush channel in between them. The right inset shows the root of the input multiplexer, with the peristaltic pump, a waste output for flushing the mixer, and the cell input line. (From Gomez-Sjoberg, R. et al. 2007. *Anal Chem* **79**: 8557–63.)

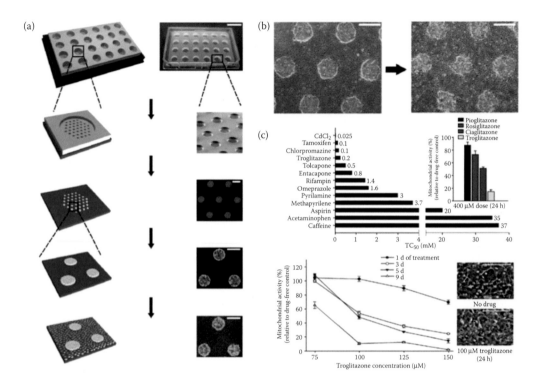

**FIGURE 22.2** Micropatterned cell co-culture maintains hepatocyte function. (a) Schematic representations and photomicrographs of the steps of the soft lithographic process to fabricate microscale liver hepatocyte cultures in a multiwell format. A reusable PDMS stencil consists of membranes with through-holes at the bottom of each well in a 24-well mold. Each well is incubated with a solution of ECM protein to allow protein to selectively adsorb to the substrate via the through-holes (fluorescently labeled collagen pattern). Primary hepatocytes selectively adhere to matrix-coated domains, allowing supportive stromal cells to be seeded into the remaining bare areas (hepatocytes labeled green and fibroblasts orange; scale bar is 500 μm). (b) Phase-contrast micrographs of micropatterned co-cultures. Primary human hepatocytes are spatially arranged in 500 μm collagen coated islands with 1200 μm center-to-center spacing, surrounded by 3T3-J2 fibroblasts. Images depict pattern fidelity over several weeks of culture. Scale bars, 500 μm. (c) Cellular response to exposure to hepatotoxins by TC50; (Top) shows the rank ordering of the compounds tested. Inset classifies relative toxicity of structurally related PPARg agonists in the thiazolidinediones class (24 h exposure at 400 mM). (Bottom) proves the time and dose-dependent chronic toxicity of Troglitazone in micropatterned cocultures (2–3 weeks old) dosed repeatedly every 48 h. Phase-contrast micrographs show human hepatocyte morphology under untreated conditions and after treatment with 100 mM of Troglitazone for 24 h (scale bars are 100 μm).

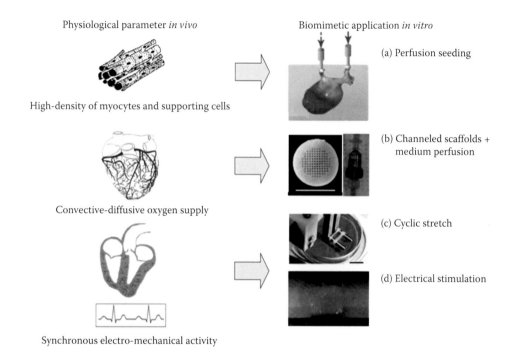

Physiological parameter *in vivo*

High-density of myocytes and supporting cells

Convective-diffusive oxygen supply

Synchronous electro-mechanical activity

Biomimetic application *in vitro*

(a) Perfusion seeding

(b) Channeled scaffolds + medium perfusion

(c) Cyclic stretch

(d) Electrical stimulation

**FIGURE 22.4** Biomimetic paradigm for cardiac tissue engineering bioreactors. Important cardiac physiological parameters (e.g., high density of tissue, convective–diffusive oxygen supply, and electro-mechanical coupling) are emulated for *in vitro* application via bioreactors. Example bioreactor systems incorporating these parameters are shown to the right. (a) Schematic of working heart bioreactor showing cannulation of left atrium and ascending aorta in order to repopulate decellularized rat hearts with neonatal cardiac cells. (b) Left: Light image of channeled PGS scaffold (channels 250 μm diameter, 250 μm wall-to-wall spacing, space bar indicates 10 mm). Right: A perfusion bioreactor for cultivation of cardiac tissue constructs under culture medium flow, in which the chamber is connected to inlet/outlet extension tubing. (c) Close-up view of ring-shaped engineered cardiac tissue constructs placed in a bioreactor employing a stretch apparatus that applies unidirectional cyclic stretch. (d) Close-up view of rectangular-shaped engineered cardiac tissue construct positioned in a bioreactor between two carbon rod electrodes that apply pulsatile electrical field stimulation (scale bar corresponds to 3 mm).

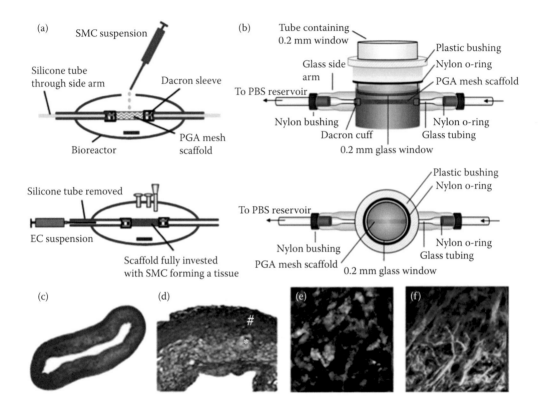

**FIGURE 22.5** Bioreactor for cultivation of functional tissue-engineered arteries. (a) Schematic of cell-seeding. (Upper): A suspension of smooth muscle cells (SMC) is seeded unto the outer surface of the tubular mesh scaffold and cultured for an extended period. (Lower): Endothelial cells are seeded on the luminal surface of the scaffold by injection of a cell suspension while turning the scaffold to facilitate even distribution of the cells. (b) Bioreactor design showing the engineered vessel submerged in a reservoir of cultivation medium. At the same time, medium is pumped through the tubing using a pulsatile flow to stimulate radial distension of the vessel. This bioreactor is designed with a glass window to enable imaging in situ. (c) Histological cross-section of the engineered vessel stained with H&E. (d) Trichrome staining at higher magnification shows collagen deposition (#) in blue and the original scaffold (*). (e, f) Nonlinear optical microscopy images of the engineered construct in the bioreactor at 30 μm depth into the vessel wall after 6 weeks of cultivation. (e) Scaffold and cellular material. (f) Deposited collagen fibrils.

**TABLE 22.1** Overview of Key Features for the Representative Bioreactor Systems Outlined in This Chapter

| Bioreactor Type | Key Features | Example System |
|---|---|---|
| Micro-bioreactor | • Decoupled spatio-temporal control of soluble factors<br>• Microscale control of tissue architecture<br>• Local control of soluble factors<br>• Compatibility with integrated microdevices<br>• High-throughput data acquisition | • Hui et al., 2007<br><br>• Khetani et al., 2008<br>• Lutolf et al., 2005<br>• Gomez-Sjoberg et al., 2007<br>• Figallo et al., 2007 |
| Cardiac | • Increased cell density and uniformity via perfusion seeding<br>• Convective-diffusion oxygen supply<br>• Induction of synchronous electro-mechanical activity via:<br>  • Electrical stimulation, and/or<br>  • Cyclic mechanical stretch | • Taylor et al., 2008<br>• Maidhof et al., 2010<br>• Radisic et al., 2008<br><br><br>• Tandon et al., 2009<br>• Eschenhagen et al., 2006 |
| Vascular | • Application of shear and radial strain via pulsatile flow<br>• Separated media compartments to support layered structure of vessel wall<br>• Lengthened cultivation times for cellular differentiation | • Niklason et al., 2001<br><br>• Gong et al., 2008<br><br>• McKee et al., 2003 |
| Bone | • Homogeneous cell distribution via perfusion<br>• Application of physiologic flow/shear for enhanced matrix deposition<br>• 3-dimensional support of geometrically-complex anatomically-shaped grafts<br>• Application of mechanical loading via:<br>  • Cyclic stretching, and/or<br>  • Compression | • Bancroft et al., 2002<br>• Sikavitsas et al., 2003<br><br>• Grayson et al., 2010<br><br><br>• Neiglinger-Wilke, 1994<br>• Orr and Burg, 2008 |
| Cartilage | • Application of physiologic shear via:<br>  • Spinner flasks<br>  • Rotating wall vessels<br>  • Perfusion<br>  • Parallel plates<br>• Physiologic compression via:<br>  • Dynamic deformational loading, and/or<br>  • Hydrostatic pressure | <br>• Gooch et al., 2001<br>• Saini et al., 2003<br>• Razzano et al., 2000<br>• Gemmiti et al., 2009<br><br>• Lima et al., 2006<br>• Elder et al., 2009 |
| Tendon/Ligament | • Stretching stimulation on<br>  • MSCs-seeded collagen type I gel<br>  • Fibroblasts-seeded collagen matrix<br>  • Tenocytes-seeded decellularized tendon | <br>• Altman et al., 2002<br>• Garvin et al., 2003<br>• Saber et al., 2010 |

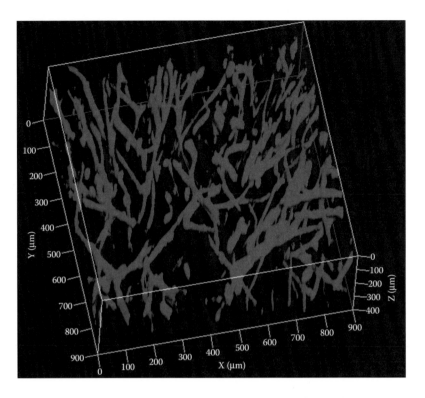

**FIGURE 24.3** Three-dimensional confocal microscopy image of vascular networks formed in collagen gels.

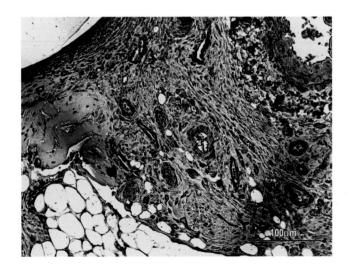

**FIGURE 24.4** Immunohistochemical stain showing vessels formed in response to the sustained delivery of FGF-1. The brown stain indicates the presence of smooth muscle alpha actin-positive mural cells coating the vessels after 3 weeks of stimulation.

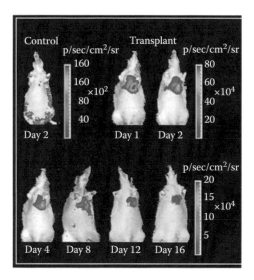

**FIGURE 25.2** Bioluminescent imaging of cardiac cell transplantation in living animals. Shown is a representative rat transplanted with embryonic cardiomyoblasts expressing Fluc imaged on days 1, 2, 4, 8, 12, and 16 postimplantation. The control rat shows background signal only. (Reproduced with permission from Wu, J. C., I. Y. Chen et al. 2003. *Circulation* 108(11): 1302–1305.)

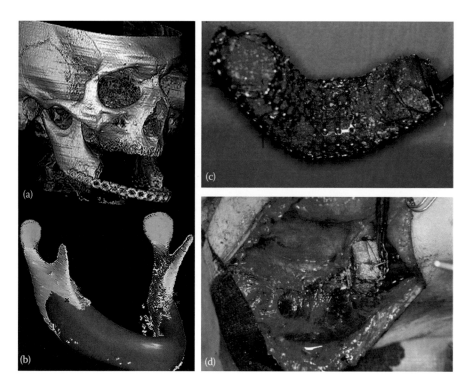

**FIGURE 28.1** Three-dimensional CT scan of size defect (a) CAD plan of an ideal mandibular transplant (b) titanium mesh cage filled with bone mineral blocks infiltrated with recombinant human BMP7 and bone-marrow mixture (c) and implantation into right latissimus dorsi muscle (d).

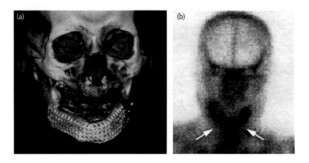

**FIGURE 28.2** Three-dimensional CT scans (a) after transplantation of bone replacement with the enhancement of soft tissue (red) and repeated skeletal scintigraphy (b) with the tracer enhancement showing continued bone remodeling and mineralization (arrows).

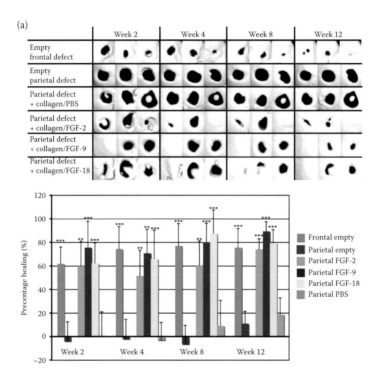

**FIGURE 28.4** FGF-ligands accelerate calvarial healing. (a) Healing in CD1 p7 mice: CT images of the defects of p7 mice at 2, 4, 8, and 12 weeks. In addition to the frontal defects (top row), parietal defects, and parietal defects treated with PBS are presented (second and third row). The frontal defects healed significantly better than the parietal defects. The FGF-treated parietal defects are shown in the lower three rows. By adding FGF-ligands to parietal defects, the parietal bone healed like the frontal bone. The graph represents the quantification of calvarial healing in p7 mice over the course of time. (b) Healing in CD1 p60 mice: CT images of p60 mice revealed an increased healing capacity of the frontal bone compared to the parietal bone. FGF-ligands enhanced the healing of parietal defects, however only FGF-18 could mimic the healing capacity of the frontal bone. The graph represents the quantification of calvarial healing in p60 mice. The asterisks indicate the significant levels of the Student $t$-test frontal versus parietal defects (left bars) and FGF-treated versus controls (right bars): $*p < 0.05$, $**p < 0.005$, and $***p < 0.0005$. (c) CT-scans and corresponding Pentachrome staining of calvaria 12 weeks postoperatively: For each calvaria, the top section (F) represents the frontal defect and the bottom section the parietal defect (P). The yellow color indicates the mature bone. The dashed arrows highlight the defects and the osteogenic fronts are lateral of these markings. At the top row, the superior healing potential of the untreated frontal defect as compared to the parietal defect can be appreciated. The application of FGF-2 to parietal defects led to increased healing in p7 and p60 mice (middle row). FGF-18 substantially increased healing in p60 parietal defects (bottom row). The arrowheads indicate the dura mater. Abbreviation: F, frontal; P, parietal (scale bar: 200 μm).

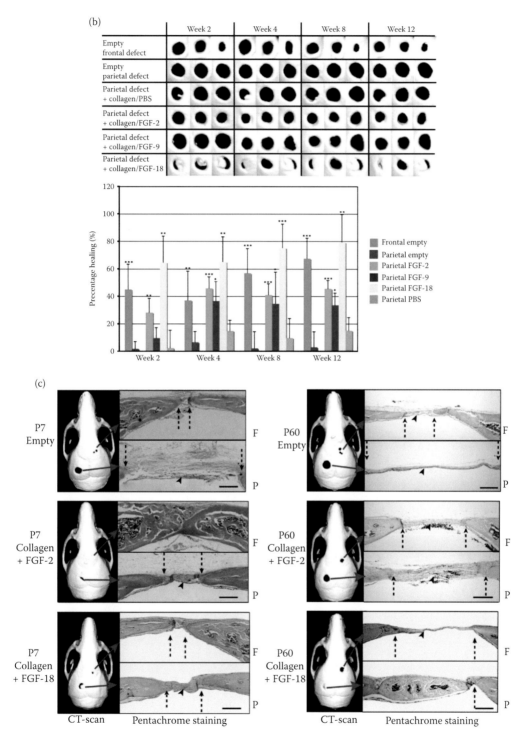

**FIGURE 28.4** (Continued.)

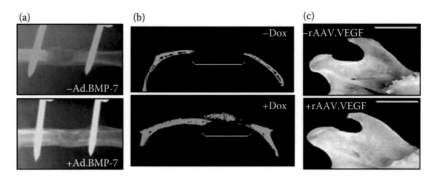

**FIGURE 28.6** Gene therapy for bone regeneration. (a) An "expedited *ex vivo*" bone regeneration strategy has recently been proposed in which explants of adipose tissue or muscle can be directly transduced with Ad.BMP-2 without culture. This has shown promising results in the regeneration of critical-sized rat femoral defects. (From Betz, V. M. et al. 2008. *Front Biosci* 13: 833–841.) (b) A vector for rAAV-based BMP-2 gene delivery regulated by the TetON has been generated. (Adapted from Gafni, Y., Pelled, G., Zilberman, Y. et al. 2004. *Mol Ther* 9(4): 587–595.). Calvarial defect bone formation was noted in mice only after the administration of Doxycycline via drinking water to induce BMP-2 expression. This represents a novel strategy for localized inducible gene expression. (c) Local injection of rAAV-VEGF to the mandibular condyle of rats results in increased condylar growth after 60 days, as demonstrated by increased condyle width and length.

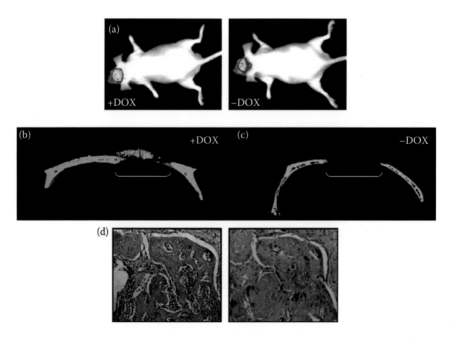

**FIGURE 28.7** *In vivo* transduction of hMSCs in an orthotopic site (critically sized calvarial defect). Human AMSC Retro-Luc was transplanted into a critically sized calvarial defect and transduced with a viral mixture of AAV-BMP-2 at 4 days postimplantation. (a) CCCD images of +Dox and −Dox mice indicate cell localization and survival at 8 days postimplantation. The experiment was terminated on day 28 and the dissected calvaria was analyzed with micro-CT imaging. (b) In the +Dox group rAAV-BMP-2 activity is apparent, resulting in the regeneration of bone within the defect on day 28. (c) In the −Dox group, no regeneration of bone is evident on day 28. (d) Histological sections stained with H&E and Masson trichrome showing the presence of new bone in the calvarial defect in animals treated with Dox (original magnification ×20.)

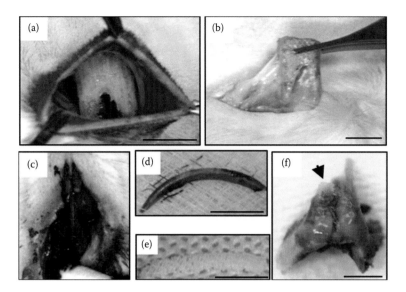

**FIGURE 28.8** *In vivo* orthotopic and ectopic implantation of anatomically shaped tooth scaffolds. (a) *In vivo* implantation of human mandibular molar scaffold into the rat's dorsum constitutes an ectopic model for tooth regeneration. (b) Harvest of human molar scaffold showing integration and tissue ingrowth. (c) Extraction of the right rat's mandibular central incisor. (d) The extracted rat's mandibular central incisor. (e) The fabricated rat's mandibular central incisor scaffold. (f) Harvest of *in vivo*-implanted rat's mandibular central incisor scaffold orthotopically in the extraction socket showing integration of the implanted scaffold. Scale: 5 mm.

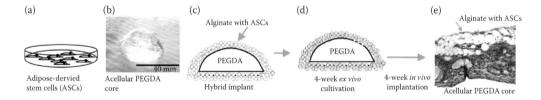

**FIGURE 28.9** Fabrication of the hybrid soft tissue implant. (a) Human ASCs were culture expanded for 3 weeks. (b) PEGDA hydrogel was photopolymerized in breast shape (diameter 40 mm) without any cells. (c) ASCs were seeded in alginate solution and painted on PEDGA surface to form a hybrid construct. (d) After 4-week *ex vitro* cultivation, alginate-PEGDA hybrid construct showed no delamination, with or without ASCs. (e) After 4-week *in vivo* implantation, the adipose tissue formed in ASC-seeded alginate later encapsulating an acellular PEGDA core.

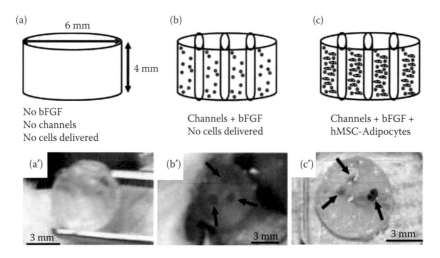

**FIGURE 28.10** *In vivo* implantation of bFGF and microchanneled PEG hydrogel loaded with adipogenic cells derived from hMSCs. The diagrams (top row) correspond to the representative photographs at the time of harvest of *in vivo* samples. (a) PEG hydrogel molded into $6 \times 4$ mm (width × height) cylinder (without either bFGF or microchannels). (b) PEG hydrogel cylinder loaded with both 0.5 mg/mL bFGF and three microchannels, but without the delivery of cells. (c) PEG hydrogel cylinder loaded with both 0.5 mg/mL bFGF and three microchannels, in addition to the encapsulation of adipogenic cells that have been derived from human mesenchymal stem cells at a cell-seeding density of $3 \times 10^6$ cells/mL. Following *in vivo* implantation subcutaneously in the dorsum of immunodeficient mice, the harvested PEG hydrogel samples showed distinct histological features. (a′) PEG hydrogel cylinder without either microchannels or bFGF showed somewhat transparent appearance. (b′) PEGhydrogel cylinder with both bFGF and three microchannels, but without delivered cells, showed darker color and a total of three openings of microchannels (arrows). (c′) PEG hydrogel cylinder with both microchannels and bFGF in addition to the encapsulated hMSC-derived adipogenic cells showed the opening of microchannels (red color and pointed with arrows).

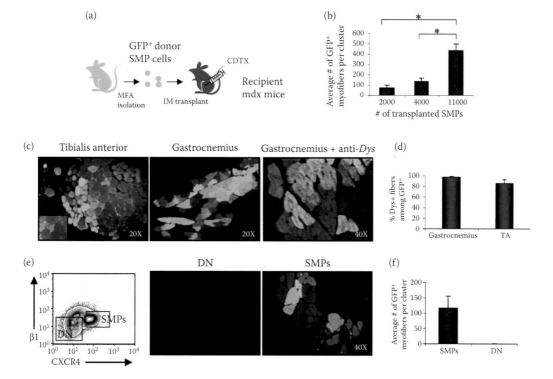

**FIGURE 28.11** SMPs robustly engraft skeletal muscle *in vivo* (a) experimental design. Double-sorted GFP⁺ SMPs were injected intramuscularly into the recipient *mdx* mice injured 1 day previously by injection of cardiotoxin (CDTX) into the same muscle. (b) Quantitative analysis of donor-derived (GFP⁺) myofibers in TA muscles injected with 2000 (*n* = 3), 4000 (*n* = 3), or 11,000 (*n* = 3) SMPs. The recipient muscles were harvested 4 weeks after transplantation and analyzed for GFP expression by direct epifluorescence microscopy of the transverse muscle sections. The total number of GFP⁺ myofibers per section was determined for 100–300 sections taken throughout the muscle, to determine the maximal number of donor-derived fibers generated in each muscle. The data are plotted as the mean (±SEM) number of GFP⁺ myofibers detected in the section of each engrafted muscle that contained the most GFP⁺ myofibers. *$p < 0.01$. (c) Transverse frozen sections of TA (left panel) and gastrocnemius (middle and right panels) muscles obtained from *mdx* mice transplanted 4 weeks previously with 11,000 GFP⁺ SMPs showed large clusters of regenerating donor-derived myofibers (GFP⁺, shown in green) with characteristics of the centrally localized nuclei (inset) and the restored dystrophin expression (shown in red; dystrophin staining is shown on the right image only). GFP detection by epifluorescence (as in c) was confirmed by indirect immunofluorescence and immunohistochemistry using anti-GFP antibodies. (d) Quantification of the frequency (mean ± SD) of dystrophin⁺ myofibers among GFP⁺ donor-derived myofibers in the TA or gastrocnemius of *mdx* mice transplanted with 11,000 SMP cells per muscle revealed that the majority (85–100%) of GFP⁺ myofibers contained dystrophin protein (red), which normally is lacking on most *mdx* myofibers. (e and f) Myofiber-associated cells lacking SMP markers do not generate myofibers when transplanted *in vivo*. CD45⁻Sca-1⁻Mac-1⁻CXCR4⁻β1-integrin⁻ (double negative, DN) cells or CD45⁻Sca-1⁻Mac-1⁻CXCR4⁺β1-integrin⁺ SMPs were twice-sorted (to ensure purity) from β-actin/GFP mice and then transferred at equal cell number (4000 per muscle) into separate preinjured *mdx* recipients. Four weeks after transplant, the injected muscles were harvested and sectioned. No GFP⁺ myofibers were found in muscles transplanted with DN cells (*n* = 3), while muscles receiving GFP⁺ SMPs showed an efficient contribution of GFP⁺ myofibers (*n* = 3).

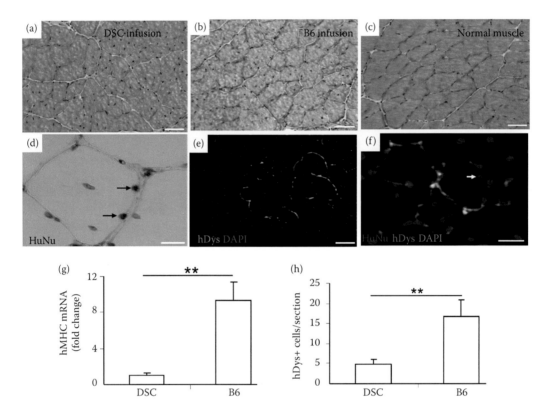

**FIGURE 28.12** Engraftment of the undifferentiated ectopic stem cell clone in the damaged muscle. The TA muscles in NOD/SCID mice were injured by multipoint CTX injection. 24 h following CTX injections, dental stem cells (DSC) and a tested clone (B6) were separately infused in CTX-injured TA muscles with contralateral TA muscles as controls. (a) H&E staining shows the presence of centralized nuclei in the representative DSC-infused sample. (b) The representative B6-infused sample showed an abundant centralized nuclei. In contrast, the representative normal TA muscle has peripheral nuclei (c). The immunohistochemistry staining (brown) of the human-specific nuclei (d) and immunefluorescent staining of the human-specific dystrophin (green) and the human nuclei (red) (e,f) indicates the presence of transplanted human cells in the host TA muscle in the representative B6-infused group. We then harvested *in vivo* muscle samples, isolated RNA for real-time PCR analysis of myogenic differentiation *in vivo*. The quantitative RT-PCR assay revealed that human MHC gene expression in the B6 infusion group after 4 weeks of injection is ~8 times greater than DSC infusion group ($N = 3$, **$p < 0.01$) (g). The quantification of human dystrophin positive cells present in the TA muscle shows that the expression of human dystrophin mRNA was ~3 times greater following B6 infusion than DSC infusion ($N = 3$, **$p < 0.01$) (h). In (d) and (f), the arrows indicate the human nuclei. In (g), the $y$ axis represents a fold-change relative to the heterogeneous DSC. Scale bars: A–C, E, F: 50 μm; D: 20 μm.

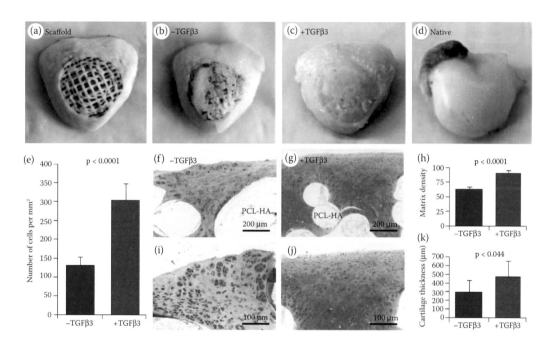

**FIGURE 28.13** Articular cartilage regeneration. Indian ink staining of (a) unimplanted bioscaffold, (b) TGFβ3-free and (c) TGFβ3-infused bioscaffolds after 4 months of implantation, and (d) native cartilage. (e) Number of chondrocytes present in TGFβ3-infused and TGFβ3-free regenerated articular cartilage samples ($n = 8$ per group). Safranin O-staining of TGFβ3-free (f,i) and TGFβ3-infused (g,j) articular cartilage. The matrix density (h) and cartilage thickness (k) of TGFβ3-infused and TGFβ3-free samples ($n = 8$ per group for both comparisons).

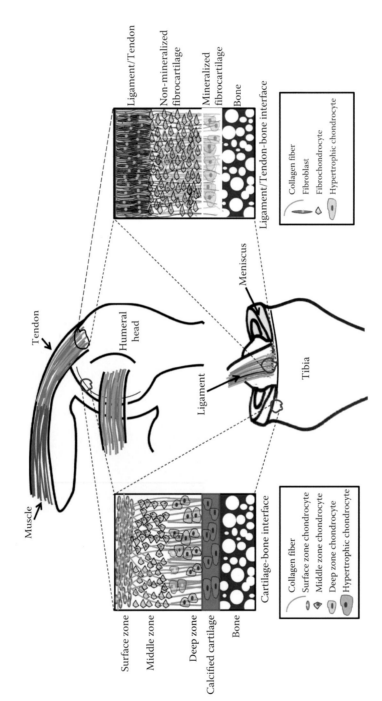

**FIGURE 32.1** Schematic of soft-to-hard tissue interfaces.

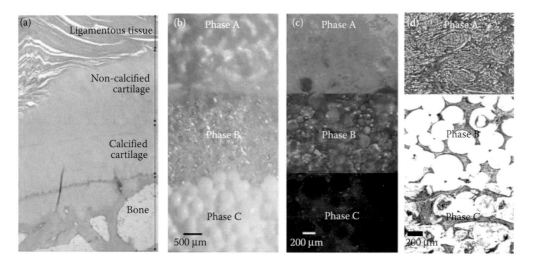

**FIGURE 32.2** Scaffold design for ligament-to-bone interface tissue engineering. (a) Histologic image of human ACL insertion showing the three main tissue types found at the ACL-bone interface: ligament, fibrocartilage (FC), and bone. (b) A tri-phasic stratified scaffold designed to mimic the three interface regions (bar = 200 μm). (c) *In vitro* co-culture of fibroblasts and osteoblasts on the tri-phasic scaffold resulted in region-specific cell distribution and cell-specific matrix deposition. Fibroblasts (Calcein AM, green) were localized in Phase A and osteoblasts (CM-DiI, red) in Phase C, and both osteoblasts and fibroblasts migrated into Phase B over time (bar = 200 μm). (d) *In vivo* evaluation of the tri-phasic scaffold tri-cultured with fibroblasts (Phase A), chondrocytes (Phase B), and osteoblasts (Phase C) showed abundant host tissue infiltration and matrix production (week 4, Modified Goldner Masson Trichrome Stain, bar = 500 μm). (Modified from Iwahashi et al. 2010. *Arthroscopy.* 26(9 Suppl):S13–S20; Spalazzi, J. P. et al. 2006a. *Tissue Eng.* 12:3497–3508; Spalazzi, J. P. et al. 2008a. *J. Biomed. Mater. Res. Part A.* 86A:1–12; Lu et al. 2010. *Ann. Biomed. Eng.* 38(6):2142–2154.)

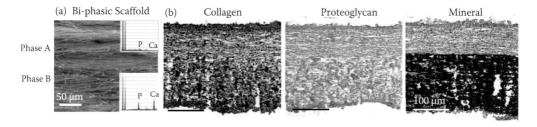

**FIGURE 32.3** Bi-phasic nanofiber scaffold for tendon-to-bone integration. (a) Cross-section of the bi-phasic scaffold (1000×, bar = 50 μm), Insert: Elemental composition of the two phases, calcium (Ca) and phosphorous (P) present only in Phase B. (b) Matrix deposition on bi-phasic scaffold after 3 weeks of subcutaneous implantation in athymic rats (Collagen—picrosirius red, Proteoglycan—Alcian blue, Mineral—Von Kossa; 20×, bar = 100 μm). (From Moffat, K. L. et al. 2010. *Transactions of the 56th Orthopaedic Research Society.* New Orleans, LA.)

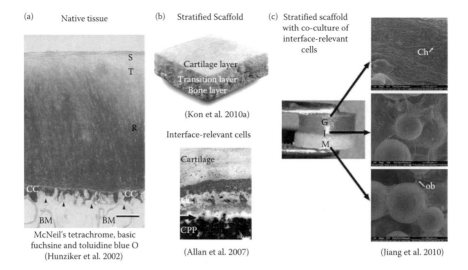

**FIGURE 32.4** Osteochondral tissue engineering. (a) Stratified organization of the human cartilage and the osteo-chondral junction. (b) Stratified scaffold designed to mimic zonal organization regions and cell-based approaches for cartilage-to-bone integration. (c) *In vitro* co-culture of chondrocytes and osteoblasts on a stratified scaffold. (Modified from Hunziker et al. 2002. *Osteoarthritis Cartilage.* 10(7):564–572; Kon et al. 2010a. *Injury.* 41:778–786; Allan, K. S. et al. 2007. *Tissue Eng.* 13:167–177; Jiang et al. 2010. *Ann. Biomed. Eng.* 38(6):2183–2196.)

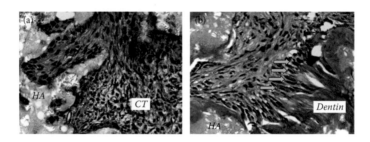

**FIGURE 33.3** Hematoxylin and eosin staining of representative DPSC transplants. (a) After 1 week posttransplantation, DPSC transplants contain connective tissue (*CT*) around HA/TCP carrier (*HA*), without any sign of dentin formation. (b) After 6 weeks posttransplantation, DPSCs differentiate into odontoblasts (arrows) that are responsible for the dentin formation on the surface of HA/TCP (*HA*). Original magnification: 40×.

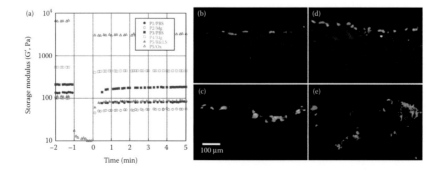

**FIGURE 33.5** Mechanical strength of peptides prepared with different solutions. (a) A time sweep experiment showing shear recovery properties of nanofibrous scaffolds. After application of a high load, the hydrogels returned to the original storage modulus (*G′*) within 1 min. (b) Green-fluorescent cells were seeded on top of hydrogels without cleavage site (b, c) and hydrogels where the cleavage motif is present (d, e). Both peptides carry the cell adhesion motif RGD. Images show cells after 1 day (b, d) and after 5 days (c, e) in culture. Cells remain as a monolayer on top of hydrogels without a cleavage site (c), they migrate and spread into hydrogels with a cleavage motif (e).

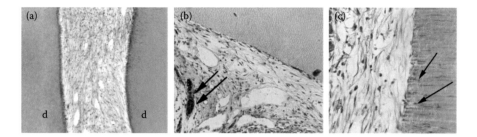

**FIGURE 33.6** *In vivo* culture of MDP nanofibers. (a) and (b) show the formation of vascularized pulp-like soft connective tissue with blood formation (arrows). (c) DPSC seem to have extended their processes into the dentin tubules (arrows), which is suggestive of DPSC differentiation into odontoblasts in the presence of hydrogels containing growth factors.

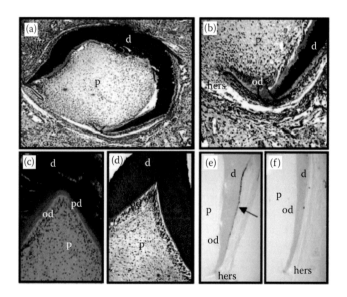

**FIGURE 33.7** Histology and immunohistochemistry of a 20-week implant. (a) Von Kossa stain for calcified mineralization in bioengineered tooth crown (50× magnification). Dark brown stain is positive for mineralized tissues. (b) A high-magnification (400×) photomicrograph of the Hertwig's epithelial root sheath is shown, stained by the Von Kossa method to detect calcified mineralization. (c) High-magnification (200×) photomicrograph of cuspal region in bioengineered tooth crown. The tissue was stained by the Von Kossa method. (d) Hematoxylin and eosin (H&E) stain of a positive control porcine third molar cuspal region demonstrates morphology similar to that of the bioengineered tooth structure (200×). (e) BSP immunostain of 20-week-old bioengineered tooth crown (100×). Positive BSP expression is indicated by the arrow. (f) Negative preimmune control immunostain for BSP in bioengineered tooth crown (100×). Abbreviations: d, dentin; od, odontoblasts; p, pulp; pd, predentin, hers, Hertwig's epithelial root sheath. (Reproduced with permission from Young CS et al. 2002. *J Dent Res* 81(10): 695–700.)

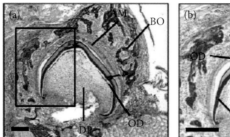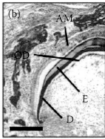

**FIGURE 33.8** Recombinant explant between bone marrow-derived cells and oral epithelium following 12 days of development in a renal capsule. All the tissues visible are donor-derived, since the host kidney makes no cellular contribution to the tissue. Where epithelium in the recombinations was from GFP mice, *in situ* hybridization of sections of these tissues confirmed that all mesenchyme-derived cells were of wildtype origin (not shown). Scale bar: 80 μm. (a) Bioengineered tooth organ showing normal morphogenesis, cell differentiation and matrix deposition, BO: bone; DP: dental pulp. (b) High magnification view of boxed area showing functional ameloblasts (AM), odontoblasts (OD) and normal deposition of enamel (E), dentin (D) matrices. (Reproduced with permission from Ohazama A et al. 2004. *J Dent Res* 83(7): 518–522.)

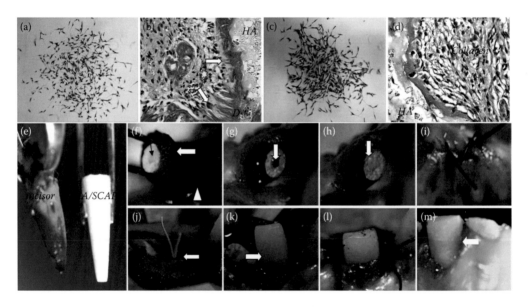

**FIGURE 33.9** SCAP/PDLSC-mediated root/periodontal structure as an artificial crown support for the restoration of tooth function in swine. (a) SCAP isolated from swine were capable of forming a single colony cluster when plated at a low cell density. (b) When transplanted into immunocompromised mice for 8 weeks, swine SCAP differentiate into odontoblasts (open arrows) to regenerate dentin (*D*) on the surface of the hydroxyapatite carrier (*HA*). (c) Swine PDLSCs were capable of forming a single colony cluster. (d) After transplantation into immunocompromised mice, PDLSCs formed cementum (*C*) on the surface of hydroxyapatite carrier (*HA*). Collagen fibers were found to connect to newly formed cementum. (e) Extracted minipig lower incisor and root-shaped HA/TCP carrier loaded with SCAP. (f) Gelfoam containing $10 \times 10^6$ PDLSCs (open arrow) was used to cover the HA/SCAP (black arrow) and implanted into the lower incisor socket (open triangle). (g) HA/SCAP-Gelfoam/PDLSCs were implanted into a newly extracted incisor socket. A post channel was created inside the root shape HA carrier (open arrow). (h) The post channel was sealed with a temporary post for affixing a crown in the next step. (i) The HA/SCAP-Gelfoam/PDLSC implant was sutured for 3 months. (j) The HA/SCAP-Gelfoam/PDLSC implant (open arrow) was reexposed and the temporary post was removed to expose the post channel. (k) A premade porcelain crown was cemented to the HA/SCAP-Gelfoam/PDLSC structure. (l) The exposed section was sutured. (m) After 4 weeks' fixation, the porcelain crown was retained in the swine for exertion of masticatory function as shown by open arrows. (Reproduced with permission from Sonoyama W et al. 2006. *PLoS ONE* 20(1): e79.)

# 20

# Cell Encapsulation

20.1 Introduction ...................................................................20-1
20.2 Gelation Mechanisms Employed in Cell Encapsulation ..........20-2
    Gelation via Noncovalent Interactions • Gelation via Covalent
    Crosslinking: Radical Chain Polymerization • Gelation via
    Covalent Crosslinking: Step Growth Polymerization
20.3 Hydrogel Structure and Degradation.........................................20-8
    The Role of Hydrogel Structure in Tissue Development • Modes of
    Degradation
20.4 Concluding Remarks.................................................................20-11
References.........................................................................................20-12

Stephanie J. Bryant
*University of Colorado*

## 20.1 Introduction

The general approach in tissue engineering is to culture cells in 3D scaffolds that serve as temporary cell supports for guiding new tissue growth. The scaffold may be prefabricated with high porosity whereby cells are seeded into the pores or the scaffold may be formed in the presence of cells thus directly encapsulating cells. In the former strategy, the size of the pores is generally much larger (~10–50 times) than that of a cell effectively presenting a 2D surface onto which cells adhere. However, cells interacting with surfaces in two dimensions is generally an unnatural interaction that can ultimately affect the fate of the cell (Gieni and Hendzel 2008). Rather, cells in their native environment are surrounded in *three* dimensions by an extracellular matrix with which to interact (Cukierman et al. 2001). Therefore, in the latter scaffold strategy, encapsulating cells in 3D scaffolds creates microenvironments that more closely resemble the architecture and mechanics of native tissues (Saha et al. 2007; Tibbitt and Anseth 2009). How cells interact with their extracellular environment influences many cellular functions such as proliferation, differentiation, and matrix synthesis, which are important for engineering living and functional tissues.

From a practical perspective, cell encapsulation strategies offer several additional advantages. For example, by suspending cells in a solution prior to solidification, cells can be uniformly distributed throughout the scaffold (Bryant and Anseth 2001b). Since the process of encapsulating cells is inherently mild and cell-friendly, it often can be employed as a means to deliver cells *in vivo* and minimally invasively whereby cells suspended in a liquid precursor solution are injected to the site of interest and cured *in situ* (Atala et al. 1993; Elisseeff et al. 1999a; Passaretti et al. 2001). By curing the scaffold directly at the site of interest, the precursors are able to diffuse into the neighboring tissue and upon gelation create a bond between the scaffold and the tissue without the need for external fixatives. With these many advantages, it is not surprising that cell encapsulation strategies have received significant attention in recent years. However, developing scaffolds for cell encapsulation comes with stringent requirements, thus limiting the range of suitable precursors and processes by which scaffolds are formed.

The materials most commonly employed to encapsulate cells are hydrogels. Hydrogels are water swellable, yet water insoluble crosslinked polymeric networks that imbibe large amounts of water and exhibit tissue-like elastic properties making them ideal candidates as scaffolds for tissue engineering. The earliest hydrogels used for cell encapsulations were naturally forming hydrogels based on proteins, such as collagen (Elsdale and Bard 1972) and fibrin (Sims et al. 1998), and polysaccharides, such as alginate (Lim and Sun 1980) and agarose (Dupuy et al. 1988). These early and seminal contributions demonstrated both the importance of culturing cells in a 3D environment over traditional 2D culture platforms and the ability for hydrogels to serve as suitable platforms for regenerating new tissue.

The advantages of natural hydrogels include their inherent biocompatibility, their ability to form via benign processes, and for those prepared from proteins the presentation of biological cues that promote cellular interactions with the hydrogel. However, natural hydrogels inherently suffer from batch-to-batch variations and a greater potential for contamination and are generally more difficult to control and tune. To overcome these shortcomings, synthetic hydrogels have become more widely studied for cell encapsulation. Synthetic hydrogels can be formed from synthetic polymers, providing purely 3D structural support for cells and tissue deposition, or from natural polymers, proteins, or peptides, which have been modified in such a way as to impart both biological functionality as well as control over the 3D environment. Strategies that combine synthetic polymers with natural polymers or their derivatives offer an ideal platform for tuning many of the macroscopic properties while simultaneously presenting biological cues in a controlled manner. The level of control afforded by synthetic hydrogels continues to increase as new chemistries *and* new strategies for hydrogel formation are developed and being designed with cell encapsulation in mind.

The following sections highlight (i) different gelation mechanisms and hydrogel chemistries, which have been successfully employed to encapsulate cells for a variety of tissue engineering applications and (ii) the role that hydrogel structure and the different modes of degradation have on directing cellular behavior in 3D.

## 20.2 Gelation Mechanisms Employed in Cell Encapsulation

Regardless of the gelation mechanism employed to encapsulate cells, the liquid precursors and gelation mechanisms must be suitable for cells. Since cells are suspended in the liquid precursor solution, there are several requirements. The precursors must be water-soluble and cyto-compatible. In general, hydrogel precursors are comprised of macromolecular monomers or macromers derived from biocompatible polymers instead of low molecular monomers, which are often cytotoxic (Schweikl et al. 2006). As a general rule, designing macromers with molecular weights that are 3000 Da or greater will minimize their cyto-toxicity. Finally, the aqueous solution must be buffered to a physiological osmolarity to prevent cell lysis.

The two primary mechanisms by which gelation occurs and are through noncovalent interactions, such as hydrophobic or ionic interactions, and through covalent crosslinking via chain or step growth polymerization. Examples of each gelation mechanism are shown in Figure 20.1. Noncovalent interactions can be reversible or irreversible, while covalent crosslinks are generally irreversible. While gelation mechanisms via noncovalent interactions are typically benign, they often result in hydrogels with weak mechanical properties limiting their applications to areas where high stresses are not prevalent. On the other hand, hydrogels formed from covalent crosslinks cover a wide range of macroscopic properties making them highly tunable for tissue engineering applications. However, their gelation mechanisms require additional components that may introduce cyto-toxic species if the polymerization conditions are not carefully selected. Each gelation mechanism has its advantages and limitations. Therefore, choosing a cell encapsulation strategy will depend on a number of factors including, but not limited to, the type(s) of cells to be encapsulated, the tissue to be engineered, if cells are to be delivered *in vivo*, the clinical application, the ease of use, and of course, user preference. The following sections give several examples of cell encapsulation strategies that have successfully employed gelation mechanisms via noncovalent interactions with a specific focus on self-assembling polymers, covalent crosslinking via radical chain polymerization, and covalent crosslinking via step

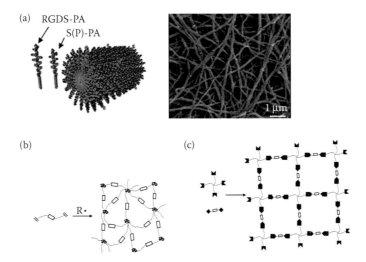

**FIGURE 20.1**  (**See color insert**.) Examples of gelation mechanisms that have been successfully employed in cell encapsulation strategies: (a) self-assembling peptides that assemble via noncovalent interactions into cylindrical, micellar structures, and subsequently into nanofibers that form a macroscopic hydrogel, (b) radical chain polymerization whereby in this example a radical initiates polymerization of a divinyl macromolecular monomer leading to a covalently crosslinked network, and (c) step growth polymerization whereby in this example two distinctly different macromolecular monomers form a homogeneous crosslinked network. (Panel (a) is reprinted from *Biomaterials*, 31, Mata, A. et al. Bone regeneration mediated by biomimetic mineralization of a nanofiber matrix, 6004–12. Copyright 2010, with permission from Elsevier.)

growth polymerizations. While not comprehensive, references are provided to direct the reader to more complete reviews.

## 20.2.1  Gelation via Noncovalent Interactions

An interesting subset of hydrogels are those which self-assemble in aqueous solutions either spontaneously or in response to a stimuli, such as temperature. In general, these polymers are comprised of hydrophobic and hydrophilic segments that give rise to their unique behaviors in aqueous solutions. When designed properly, these amphiphilic polymers undergo a transition from a soluble polymer solution to a semisolid gel capable of entrapping large amounts of water and living cells. Two types of self-assembling hydrogels which are attractive for cell encapsulation are those formed from thermoresponsive polymers and self-assembling peptides.

Thermoresponsive hydrogels are one type of stimuli responsive hydrogel which when designed to undergo a sol–gel transition near body temperature, are particularly attractive for delivering cells *in vivo* and minimally invasively (Ruel-Gariepy and Leroux 2004; Klouda and Mikos 2008). In general, thermoresponsive polymers in aqueous solutions respond to changes in temperature because of a decrease in their overall hydrophilicity that leads to a decrease in the solubility of the polymer chains. This transition leads to unfavorable water–polymer interactions and thus thermodynamically promotes polymer–polymer and water–water interactions. For cell encapsulations and tissue engineering, designing thermoresponsive polymers that undergo a sol–gel transition when temperature is increased from ambient to physiological is most desirable.

Several polymers have been designed to exhibit thermoresponsive behavior near physiological temperatures with demonstrated suitability for cell encapsulation and tissue engineering. Two examples of common polymers are the triblock copolymer, poly(ethylene glycol)-*b*-poly(propylene)-*b*-poly(ethylene glycol), commercially known as Pluronics® and poly(*N*-isopropylacrylamide) (pNiPAAm). Specifically,

Pluronic F-127 at a concentration above its critical micelle concentration forms a micellar liquid at room temperature but transforms to a macroscopic hydrogel near physiological temperature (Wanka et al. 1994) enabling *in vivo* delivery of cells (Saim et al. 2000). Hydrogels formed from Pluronics® have been successfully used to encapsulate several different cell types including chondrocytes (i.e., cartilage cells) (Cao et al. 1998), osteoblasts (i.e., bone cells) (Lippens et al. 2009), human mesenchymal stem cells (hMSCs) (Dang et al. 2006), intervertebral disc cells (Dang et al. 2006), and hepatocytes (Khattak et al. 2005). PNiPAAm, on the other hand, contains a hydrophilic amide bond and a hydrophobic isopropyl group within each repeat unit, which gives the polymer its remarkable ability to respond to changes in temperature, with a lower critical solution temperature (LCST) near physiological temperature (Schild 1992). However, in its collapsed form, much of the water is excluded from the pNiPAAm making it unsuitable for encapsulating cells. In addition, PNiPAAm forms a stable crosslinked polymer making it undesirable for applications in tissue engineering. To overcome these shortcomings, copolymers have been designed where NiPAAm is copolymerized with chemistries that impart hydrophilicity to enhance water retention and chemistries that are susceptible to degradation. This strategy offers a highly flexible platform from which to design polymers that self-assemble into hydrogels with tunable properties. For example, copolymers have been designed with a LCST near body temperature, enabling gelation upon injection into the body, but as the polymer degrades to a certain composition and molecular weight its LCST decreases to below body temperature inducing reverse gelation and solubilizing the hydrogel (Fujimoto et al. 2009). Copolymers containing pNiPAAm have been successfully employed to encapsulate hMSCs while maintaining their viability and multipotency (Pollock and Healy 2010; Wang et al. 2010).

A different subset of hydrogels which are formed from noncovalent interactions and which have been successfully employed in cell encapsulation is self-assembling polypeptides. In general, peptides are designed to contain hydrophobic and hydrophilic amino acids, which through noncovalent interactions facilitate self-assembly into higher order structures (Branco and Schneider 2009). The choice of amino acids and the length of the polypeptide dictate the self-assembly process. In addition, the mechanical properties and speed of self-assembly can be enhanced by increasing the degree of hydrophobicity (Caplan et al. 2002). Peptides have been designed with hydrophobic and ionic amino acids that self-assemble in physiological medium making them particularly attractive for encapsulating cells (Gelain et al. 2007; Cui et al. 2010). Self-assembly occurs because the charges on the polypeptide become shielded when placed in a physiological medium leading to an increase in the overall hydrophobicity of the peptide driving it to self-assemble. One example is a peptide containing a periodic repetition of alternating hydrophobic and ionic hydrophilic amino acids (i.e., lysine-leucine-aspartic acid-leucine (KLDL)...), which self-assemble into β-sheets and subsequently into nanofibers that form a macroscopic hydrogel (Gelain et al. 2007; Yang et al. 2010). These structures imbibe large amounts of water (>99% water) and are supportive of cell encapsulation and tissue growth as demonstrated by encapsulating chondrocytes and adult equine progenitor cells for cartilage tissue engineering (Kisiday et al. 2002, 2008). Another example is polypeptides comprised of hydrophobic alkyl chains and ionic peptides, which self-assemble into cylindrical, micellar structures in physiological medium (e.g., Figure 20.1a) (Mata et al. 2010) and which are also supportive of cell encapsulation (Cui et al. 2010). While these polypeptides are unnatural, they may be further modified with peptide sequences that are recognizable by cells (Gelain et al. 2006). For example, when the laminin epitope, isoleucine-lysine-valine-alanine-valine (IKVAV), was incorporated into the polypeptide, encapsulated neural progenitor cells rapidly differentiated into neurons (Silva et al. 2004). Peptide sequences that are susceptible to enzymatic cleavage have also been engineered into the polypeptides without sacrificing self-assembly processes, thus enabling cell migration (Galler et al. 2010).

Another class of self-assembling polypeptides that have been employed in cell encapsulation strategies is elastin-like-polypeptide (ELP) (MacEwan and Chilkoti 2010). This polypeptide is different from the aforementioned polypeptides in that it undergoes self-assembly in response to changes in temperature forming micelle-like structures. Its transition temperature can be tuned by varying the guest amino acid residue, $X$, within the repeating amino acid sequence, $(VPGXG)_m$ and by the length of the polypeptide (Meyer and Chilkoti 2002). Further functionalization of the polypeptide via side groups is possible without adversely affecting its thermal responsiveness. ELPs have been used to encapsulate chondrocytes leading to cartilage-like matrix deposition (Betre et al. 2002) and human adipose derived adult stem cells where the ELP hydrogel provided an environment that promoted chondrogenesis in the absence of chondrogenic factors (Betre et al. 2006).

Taken together, self-assembling polymers and polypeptides that form hydrogels have many advantages with respect to encapsulating cells, delivering cells *in vivo*, and recovering cells for further manipulation due to their reversible gelation (Huang et al. 2007). Their main shortcoming, however, is insufficient mechanical properties and lack stability for many tissue engineering applications (Klouda and Mikos 2008). To overcome this limitation, thermogelling polymers have been modified to contain reactive groups, such as acrylates or methacrylates, to permit subsequent chemical crosslinking (Hacker et al. 2008; Lee and Park 2009). In self-assembling peptides, the mechanical properties have been improved similarly by incorporating chemical crosslinks. For example, reacting a lysine-containing ELP with an organophosphorous crosslinker facilitated covalent crosslinking without adversely affecting cell viability during encapsulation (Lim et al. 2007). From a clinical perspective, the advantage of a dual gelation system is that immediately upon injection solidification occurs rapidly, thus entrapping the cells in place and which is then followed by chemical crosslinking to impart stability and mechanical integrity. The latter process may be designed to occur more slowly thus minimizing the potential cytotoxic effects of chemical crosslinking (described in more detail in the following sections). Nonetheless, self-assembling polymers and peptides offer an attractive platform for encapsulating cells under gentle gelation conditions.

## 20.2.2  Gelation via Covalent Crosslinking: Radical Chain Polymerization

Radical chain polymerizations are attractive for cell encapsulations because they are rapid, occurring on clinically relevant time scales, can be performed under mild conditions at physiological pH and temperature, and polymerized *in vivo* using minimally invasive procedures. Radical chain polymerization involves the polymerization of vinyl macromers through initiation, propagation, and termination to create crosslinked polymer networks (i.e., Figure 20.1b). For cell encapsulation strategies, macromers are typically comprised of biocompatible polymers that have been modified with two or more vinyl groups to enable crosslinking. The most common vinyl groups are acrylates, methacrylates, and fumarates. Initiation of the polymerization reaction requires an initiator molecule(s) and in certain instances an initiating signal such as temperature or exposure to light. The two most common initiating systems employed in cell encapsulations are redox initiating systems and photoinitiating systems.

Redox initiating systems are comprised of two components typically a peroxide oxidizing agent and an amine reducing agent, which react together to form active centers (e.g., radical anions) that initiate the polymerization reaction. The cytotoxicity of redox initiating systems has been primarily linked to changes in the pH of the initiators and to a lesser extent on the active centers, but is dependent on both initiator concentration and chemistry (Temenoff et al. 2003, 2004a). The cytotoxicity can be minimized by using low initiator concentrations and initiators dissolved in cell culture medium, which acts as a buffer to maintain a neutral pH, while still permitting polymerization (Temenoff et al. 2003, 2004a). The most common redox initiating system is ammonium persulfate and $N,N,N',N'$-tetramethylethylenediamine and which has been shown to lead to gelation times on clinically relevant times scales, <10 min (Temenoff et al. 2004a).

Photoinitiating systems are comprised of photoinitiator molecules and initiating light. Upon exposure to light, photoinitiator molecules absorb photons of light energy and dissociate into radicals that initiate the polymerization. The reaction conditions can be quite harsh on cells if not carefully chosen. Therefore, photoinitiators are typically selected based on their ability to dissociate into radicals by either long-wave ultraviolet light (~365 nm) or visible light (~400–700 nm). In addition, photoinitiator concentration, photoinitiator efficiency (a measure of the ability of a photoinitiator to dissociate into radicals), radical chemistry, and exposure time will affect cell viability during encapsulation (Bryant et al. 2000; Williams et al. 2005). The most common UV photoinitiator used in cell encapsulations is the water soluble photoinitiator, 2-hydroxy-1-[4-(hydroxyethoxy)phenyl]-2-methyl-1-propanone also referred to as Irgacure® 2959, a registered trademark name of Ciba Specialty Chemical, for its cytocompatibility (Bryant et al. 2000). Other UV photoinitiators (e.g., 2,2-dimethoxy-2-phenylacetophenone) have been successfully employed in cell encapsulations but typically require low initiator concentrations and/or short polymerization times to minimize their cytotoxic effects (Bryant et al. 2000; Mann et al. 2001). One primary concern with using ultraviolet light in cell encapsulations is its potential adverse affects on DNA. DNA damage was reported in ~10% of cells immediately following their encapsulation by a UV photoinitiating system, but the damage appeared to be repaired within a few days postencapsulation (Fedorovich et al. 2009). An alterative is visible light photoinitiating systems, which are attractive for several reasons. Visible light is known to be less damaging to cells than UV light and visible light penetrates deeper through thick and dense materials, such as human tissue, making it possible to cure through tissues, for example, transdermally (Elisseeff et al. 1999a). Examples of visible light photoinitiators, which have been used in cell encapsulations are eosin-Y and triethanolamine and camphorquinone (Cruise et al. 1998; Cruise et al. 1999; Ahmed et al. 2007). However, the shortcoming of visible light photoinitiators is their low photoinitiator efficiency; often requiring longer polymerization times. Because of these limitations, UV photoinitiating systems remain the most widely used in photopolymerizations involving cell encapsulations despite their potential drawbacks.

Numerous chemistries have been modified with acrylates and methacrylates to produce macromers suitable for cell encapsulations. Acrylates are known to have increased cyto-toxicity over methacrylates, when small monomers are employed (Yoshii 1997). However, the author is not aware of any reports indicating differences in cytotoxicity between acrylates and methacrylates when macromolecular monomers are employed for cell encapsulations. Another main difference between acrylates and methacrylates is the methyl group on the methacrylate helps to stabilize the propagating radical resulting in generally slower rates of polymerization (Jager et al. 1997). However, reaction times for both acrylate- and methacrylate-based macromers can occur on clinically relevant timescales, on the order of seconds to several minutes. One of the most widely employed macromers for cell encapsulations is poly(ethylene glycol) diacrylate or dimethacrylate and its degradable form poly($\alpha$-hydroxy ester)-_b_-poly(ethylene glycol)-_b_-poly($\alpha$-hydroxy ester) di(meth)acrylate (Sawhney et al. 1993), which have been used to encapsulate numerous types of cells including islets (Hill et al. 1997; Weber et al. 2006), smooth muscle cells (Mann and West 2002), chondrocytes (Elisseeff et al. 1999b; Bryant and Anseth 2003), osteoblasts (Burdick and Anseth 2002), neural precursor cells (Mahoney and Anseth 2006), hepatocytes (Tsang et al. 2007), and mesenchymal stem cells (Williams et al. 2003; Nuttelman et al. 2005). Other chemistries such as poly(vinyl alcohol), poly(2-hydroxyethyl methacrylate), and polysaccharides (e.g., hyaluronan, chondroitin sulfate, chitosan, etc.) enable functionalization with multiple (meth)acrylates offering an additional mechanism by which to control the resulting hydrogel properties (Martens and Anseth 2000; Smeds and Grinstaff 2001; Bryant et al. 2004b). For example, when neural progenitor cells were encapsulated in hydrogels containing the same concentration of hyaluronic acid, but which were prepared with varying degrees of methacrylate substitution, the differentiation of the progenitor cells was significantly impacted (Seidlits et al. 2010). A lower methacrylate substitution led to soft hydrogels, which promoted differentiation into neurons while higher methacrylate substitution led to stiffer hydrogels and differentiation into the undesirable cell type, astrocytes.

An alternative to using (meth)acrylate functionalized polymers for cell encapsulation is macromers containing fumarate (Yaszemski et al. 1996). Fumarate is a natural compound that contains a polymerizable vinyl group and an ester linkage that imparts degradability. The most common strategy has been to incorporate a single fumarate moiety into the backbone of a synthetic polymer, namely poly(ethylene glycol), which when reacted with a divinyl crosslinker (e.g., poly(ethylene glycol) diacrylate) leads to a crosslinked and biodegradable hydrogel. Fumarate-based macromers have been successfully used to encapsulate several types of cells including chondrocytes (Park et al. 2005) and marrow stromal cells for chondrogenesis (Park et al. 2009) and osteogenesis (Temenoff et al. 2004b).

## 20.2.3 Gelation via Covalent Crosslinking: Step Growth Polymerization

More recently, there have been significant efforts to design hydrogels that form via step growth polymerization (i.e., Figure 20.1c). One of the main advantages of a step growth polymerization is that the resulting hydrogel forms a homogeneous network structure, which is in contrast to the inhomogeneous structure formed by radical chain polymerization. These well-defined networks lead to improved mechanical properties and higher degrees of swelling over hydrogels formed from similar macromers under radical chain polymerization (Malkoch et al. 2006). Cell encapsulations have been successful in such hydrogels synthesized by Michael-type addition reactions (Lutolf et al. 2003; Shu et al. 2004), radical mediated thiol-ene photopolymerizations, a type of click reaction (Fairbanks et al. 2009), and copper-free "click" reactions (DeForest et al. 2009).

In Michael-type addition, the reaction occurs between thiols and unsaturated groups (e.g., vinyl sulfones and acrylates) under slightly basic conditions. While the basic environment does not adversely affect cells during encapsulation, the reactivity of thiolates (i.e., the reactive form of thiols) can be increased at neutral pH by altering the chemistry adjacent to the thiol (Lutolf et al. 2001; Shu et al. 2004). In cell encapsulation it is common to employ two distinct macromolecular monomers where one macromer contains three or more functional groups to enable crosslinking and the second macromer contains two functional groups. For example, synthetic extracellular matrix (sECM) including polysaccharides (e.g., hyaluronan and chondroitin sulfate) and proteins (e.g., gelatin) have been modified with multiple thiol groups and subsequently reacted with poly(ethylene glycol) diacrylate to create 3D environments with tunable chemistry (Serban and Prestwich 2008). For example, a hyaluronan sECM hydrogel containing encapsulated human adipose-derived stem cells supported their maturation into mature adipocytes *in vivo* (Flynn et al. 2009) while a hyaluronan and gelatin sECM hydrogel supported *in situ* delivery of mesenchymal stem cells for osteochondral repair (Liu et al. 2006). One of the attractive features of the Michael-type addition reaction is the ease with which peptides can be incorporated into the hydrogel. By simply functionalizing peptides with one or more cysteines (the amino acid containing a thiol side group) the peptide is readily incorporated into a network. Mono-cysteine peptides enable proteins to be tethered to the hydrogel backbone, while di-cysteine peptides become incorporated into the crosslinks of the network. This strategy has enabled facile fabrication of hydrogels comprised of cell adhesion ligands to permit cell attachment and of peptide crosslinks that are sensitive to matrix metalloproteinases (MMPs) (i.e., matrix-degrading enzymes) to enable cell-mediated degradation and migration (Lutolf et al. 2003).

Click reactions are highly selective and highly efficient orthogonal reactions that offer a reliable and modular platform for designing new chemistries (Kolb et al. 2001). Thiol-ene polymerizations are considered to be one type of click reaction (Hoyle and Bowman 2010) and offer an alternative to the base-catalyzed Michael-type addition reaction. The reaction undergoes a step-growth mechanism by altering between propagation, where a thiyl radical propagates across the alkene, and chain transfer reactions that leads to the formation of a thioether linkages while simultaneously producing a thiyl radical (Cramer and Bowman 2001; Fairbanks et al. 2009). When a photoinitiator is employed, the reaction can be both spatially and temporally controlled (Fairbanks et al. 2009), while simultaneously forming a near ideal hydrogel network. By reacting –ene functionalized (e.g., norobornene) and thiol functionalized (e.g., peptides) *macromolecular* monomers with a cytocompatible photoinitiator and concentration, thiol-ene click reactions are suitable for encapsulating cells (Benton et al. 2009). For copper-free click reactions between azides and alkynes (Baskin et al. 2007), the development of a difluorinated cyclooctyne as the alkyne has enabled the reaction to proceed without the need for the cytotoxic metal catalyst making it possible to perform these types of click reactions *in vivo* (Agard et al. 2004; Baskin et al. 2007) and in the presence of cells (DeForest et al. 2009). For cell encapsulations, high molecular weight macromers have been designed to contain tetra-azides which when reacted with bis(cyclooctyne)-functionalized peptides within physiological medium enable encapsulation of cells. The reaction, however, was reported to take ~1 h, which is significantly slower than that reported for radical initiated polymerizations (~10 min). Nonetheless, no additional components are required for this click reaction and high cell viability can be achieved after encapsulation.

Overall, a variety of strategies have been developed from which to create covalently crosslinked hydrogels for cell encapsulation. The strategies range from simple and versatile platforms for delivering cells *in situ* to complex 3D environments that are spatially and/or temporally controlled towards recapitulating the complex architecture of native tissues. While the polymerization and/or crosslinking reactions require additional components, utilizing macromolecular monomers and selecting appropriate reaction conditions has enabled cells to be encapsulated through a variety of gelation mechanisms without adversely affecting their viability.

## 20.3 Hydrogel Structure and Degradation

The molecular structure of the hydrogel controls many of the macroscopic properties important in developing a tissue engineering strategy including water content, mesh size (i.e., pore structure), mechanical properties, and degradation behavior. Because these properties are closely linked through the crosslinking density of the hydrogel, careful consideration of all properties must be taken into account when optimizing a hydrogel for a given application. For example, high mechanical strength is critical when designing a hydrogel for *in situ* placement within an articulating joint that is subjected to large stresses, however, the water content and diffusional capabilities are sacrificed. Incorporating degradation into the hydrogel allows for temporal changes to the hydrogel structure, but the rate of degradation must be tuned with elaboration of new tissue. This requirement is in contrast to prefabricated porous scaffolds where large pores (~200 μm) provide ample space for new tissue to be deposited prior to scaffold degradation. Therefore, an understanding of how the hydrogel structure impacts tissue development is critical to optimizing a hydrogel formulation for tissue engineering.

### 20.3.1 The Role of Hydrogel Structure in Tissue Development

The act of encapsulating and retaining cells within a 3D hydrogel requires that the mesh size of the hydrogel be sufficiently smaller than that of a cell. A typical mesh size or the average distance between crosslinks for poly(ethylene glycol)(PEG) hydrogels formed from di(meth)acrylate macromers ranges from ~4 to 20 nm (Bryant and Anseth 2001a). The relatively *small* dimensions of the polymer mesh impact a number of critical factors important to a successful tissue engineering strategy including morphology of the cells, the ability to form cell–cell contacts, diffusion of nutrients to the cells, and diffusion of extracellular matrix molecules for macroscopic tissue evolution. Since degradation directly impacts mesh size, engineering in degradable linkages is often necessary to support many of these critical factors, which would otherwise be hindered by a tight crosslinked network.

When cells are suspended in a liquid precursor solution prior to encapsulation, they naturally exhibit a round morphology. Upon encapsulation, the hydrogel network essentially surrounds each cell, entrapping them as single cells in a relatively tight mesh, and acting as a physical restraint that forces the cells to retain a round morphology. This round morphology can be observed in the examples in Figure 20.2. For cells such as chondrocytes, a round morphology is essential to retaining their differentiated phenotype making hydrogels an ideal platform for culturing chondrocytes. However, for many types of cells the ability for a cell to spread (Chen et al. 1997) and/or form cell–cell contacts (Hosokawa et al. 2010) is critical to its survival and/or function. Therefore, tuning the hydrogel chemistry with proteins and/or peptides to promote cell attachment *and* to facilitate degradation are critical design features for many applications.

In addition to influencing the morphology of the encapsulated cells, the mesh size also impacts diffusion of molecules through the hydrogel. The mesh size is generally sufficiently large as to not hinder diffusion of small nutrients such as glucose and oxygen, but may impact diffusion of large growth factors and other important signaling factors especially when designing high moduli hydrogels. However,

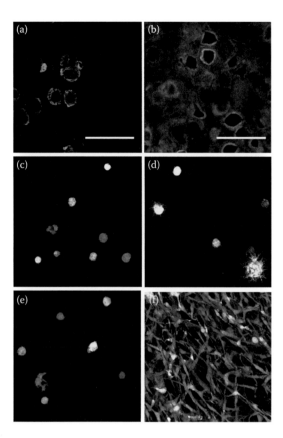

**FIGURE 20.2** The impact of temporal changes in hydrogel structure via degradation in hydrolytically labile hydrogels (a,b) and enzymatically labile hydrogels (c–f). In panels a and b, bovine articular cartilage cells (i.e., chondrocytes) were encapsulated in hydrogels formed from poly(ethylene glycol) dimethacrylate macromers, which did not exhibit signs of degradation (a) and encapsulated in hydrogels formed from poly(lactic acid)-*b*-poly(ethylene glycol)-*b*-poly(lactic acid) dimethacrylate, which were completed degraded within 2 weeks (b). After 25 days, collagen type II deposited by the cartilage cells (gray) is localized to the pericellular region in nondegrading hydrogels (a), but is deposited throughout the extracellular matrix in degrading hydrogels (b). In panels c–f, murine myofibroblasts were encapsulated in poly(ethylene glycol) hydrogels formed from a step-growth polymerization containing either highly sensitive (c,d) or moderately sensitive (e,f) crosslinkers to MMPs. Panels c,e are three days postencapsulation and panels d,f are 21 days postencapsulation. Cells were transfected with a fluorescent protein for visualization. (Panals c–f are reprinted from *Biomaterials*, Patterson, J. and Hubbell, J. A. Enhanced proteolytic degradation of molecuarly engineered PEG hydrogels in response to mmp-1 and mmp-2, doi:10.1016/j.biomaterials.2010.06.061. Copyright 2010, with permission from Elsevier.)

it is thought that a 3D culture system with some hindrances to diffusion is representative of the native tissue environment. Equally important is the impact that the mesh size will have on diffusion of newly synthesized tissue macromolecules. The extracellular matrix that makes up tissues is comprised of large macromolecules that can reach dimensions on nanometer length scales. For example, collagen, which is one of the most abundant extracellular matrix proteins found in the body, can reach dimensions up to several hundred nanometers in diameter (Svoboda et al. 1983; Moeller et al. 1995). In nondegrading hydrogels, many extracellular matrix molecules are restricted to regions immediately surrounding the cell. For example, collagen type II deposited by chondrocytes or chondrogenically differentiated mesenchymal stem cells was localized to the pericellular matrix throughout the course of culture (Bryant and Anseth 2003; Bryant et al. 2003; Sontjens et al. 2006). Similar findings were reported for collagen type I and elastin deposited by vocal fold fibroblasts (Liao et al. 2008). The incorporation of degradable linkages into the hydrogel enables temporal increases in the gel mesh size permitting the deposition of these large matrix molecules into the extracellular space of the hydrogels (Bryant and Anseth 2003). For example, when chondrocytes were encapsulated in biodegradable poly(ethylene glycol) hydrogels, a macroscopic tissue developed. Figure 20.2a,b illustrates the impact that temporal changes in the gel structure have on a developing tissue. However, for many of the very large matrix macromolecules, the hydrogel must reach near complete degradation for macroscopic tissue development (Bryant et al. 2004a).

## 20.3.2 Modes of Degradation

The primary mechanisms by which hydrogels are designed to degrade is through hydrolysis, enzyme-mediated, or a combination. In enzyme mediated degradation schemes, degradation may occur through exogenous delivery of enzymes or through enzymes secreted by the cell. By explicitly programming degradable linkages into the polymer network and through careful selection of the chemistry, degradation can often be controlled and tuned to match tissue evolution. If degradation is too slow, tissue growth may be retarded as the extracellular matrix that is deposited by the cell quickly fills the pericellular space. If degradation is too fast, dissolution of the hydrogel may occur leading to a loss of cells and/or defects in the engineered tissue. Additionally, environmental factors should be taken into account as they may impact degradation kinetics (e.g., the *in vivo* environment).

The majority of hydrolytically labile hydrogels are designed to degrade through ester linkages that are located in the crosslink or backbone of the hydrogel. Examples of ester linkages which have been successfully employed in cell encapsulation include α-hydroxy esters (e.g., lactic acid and ε-caprolactone) (Bryant et al. 2003; Benoit et al. 2006), fumarates (Fisher et al. 2004; Temenoff et al. 2004b), and phosphoesters (Wang et al. 2003, 2005). For these hydrogels, degradation begins immediately upon exposing the hydrogel to an aqueous environment. Therefore, the rate of degradation and overall timing of degradation must be tuned for each cell type and tissue application. The degradation rate can be controlled through the chemistry of the degradable linker. For example, the ester linkage in poly(lactic acid) will have a higher degradation rate than the ester linkage in poly(caprolactone) resulting in degradation times that can vary substantially from days to months (Sawhney et al. 1993). Bimodal degradation schemes have also been investigated in an effort to temporally tune degradation for enhanced tissue deposition (Martens et al. 2003; Rice and Anseth 2004). For example, fast degrading linkages may allow for immediate tissue deposition, while slower degrading crosslinks may help to maintain mechanical integrity and a 3D structure during tissue maturation (Bryant et al. 2004a). Alternatively, hydrogels have been engineered with degradable linkages that are sensitive to enzymes not typically produced by cells enabling the user to define degradation. For example, caprolactone linkages, which degrade slowly via hydrolysis, may also degrade by the enzyme lipase at a much faster rate under appropriate enzyme concentrations. This strategy offers the ability to *turn on* and *turn off* degradation at defined periods of time. This temporal control over degradation has led to enhanced macroscopic tissue development for cartilage tissue engineering (Rice and Anseth 2007).

Alternatively, cell-mediated degrading hydrogels have been engineered as a mechanism where cells dictate degradation rather than the user setting *a priori* a fixed degradation rate. Hydrogels designed from natural biopolymers, such as hyaluronic acid (Smeds and Grinstaff 2001; Shu et al. 2004; Burdick et al. 2005; Masters et al. 2005) and chondroitin sulfate (Li et al. 2004; Bryant et al. 2005; Shu et al. 2006) can be degraded by cell-secreted hyaluronidases and chondroitinases, respectively. Another attractive strategy is to incorporate into the crosslinks of synthetic hydrogels short peptide sequences that represent the enzyme substrate site within a protein (Lutolf et al. 2003). Peptides that are collagen-based are the most widely investigated and are recognized by a number of MMPs, which are secreted by a variety of cell types. This strategy leads to local degradation (Lee et al. 2007), providing a mechanism by which to maintain mechanical integrity during hydrogel degradation. While many MMPs will degrade multiple substrates, the rate of degradation can vary dramatically (Turk et al. 2001). Therefore, it is possible to select for a sequence that leads to fast or slow degradation (Patterson and Hubbell 2010). An example of a poly(ethylene glycol) hydrogel comprised of two different peptide substrates both of which are cleavable by MMPs secreted by cells, but which exhibit different degradation rates is shown in Figure 20.2c,f. These figures clearly demonstrate the impact that temporal differences in degradation can have on cellular behavior. Cells encapsulated in a hydrogel containing crosslinks that are highly susceptible to MMPs leads to cell proliferation, cell spreading, and the formation of cell–cell connections whereas crosslinks with low susceptibility essentially retain the cells in a rounded and isolated state.

In addition to controlling degradation via the choice of degradable linker, and so on, the presence of cells, as well as, the *in vivo* environment may also impact hydrogel degradation. While many ester linkages degrade via hydrolysis, they are also susceptible to cleavage by enzymes, that is, esterases, present in serum containing culture medium and the *in vivo* environment. For example, the overall degradation time was significantly reduced when poly(ethylene glycol) hydrogels containing poly(lactic acid) degradable linkages were degraded in cell culture medium containing serum compared to a phosphate buffered saline solution (Martens et al. 2003). However, degradation of poly(ethylene glycol)-based hydrogels containing fumarate as the degradable linker, was not enhanced in serum-containing medium suggesting the fumarate ester linkage may not be as susceptible to serum containing proteases (Temenoff et al. 2004a). The presence of cells and developing tissue *in vitro* has also been shown to affect the degradation behavior of hydrolytically labile hydrogels (Bryant et al. 2003). This observation is attributed to the fact that when tissue is deposited the hydrogel does not undergo large degrees of swelling and hence degradation is not as fast. The *in vivo* environment is also known to accelerate cleavage of ester linkages (Kurono et al. 1979; Catiker et al. 2000) enhancing degradation of many hydrolytically labile hydrogels. Furthermore, the act of implanting a material in the body will lead to some degree of inflammation of which MMPs are known to be involved (Parks et al. 2004) and hence may affect the degradation behavior of MMP-susceptible hydrogels. Taken together, a better understanding of how the environment impacts the degradation behavior of a hydrogel will help to design strategies that are in tune with tissue development.

## 20.4 Concluding Remarks

Cell encapsulation strategies are an enabling technology for tissue engineering where cells are combined with a precursor solution prior to gelation offering ease of handling and facilitating minimally invasive delivery of cells *in situ*. In addition, there are numerous synthetic and natural chemistries from which to choose and/or combine enabling the fabrication of tailor made hydrogels that recapitulate many of the mechanical and biochemical characteristics of native tissue. As we gain better understandings of the native niche surrounding cells *in vivo*, there has been a paradigm shift from designing permissive environments from purely synthetic hydrogels to designing promoting environments that give cells biological cues to direct their fate and function. For example, biomimetic hydrogels offer a platform from which to fine-tune the macroscopic properties through manipulations in the bioinert and synthetic chemistry independently from the incorporation of biological recognition sites. In addition to creating a 3D environment suitable for cell and tissue growth, there are several practical aspects that need to be considered when developing a clinically relevant cell encapsulation strategy and which are worth noting. These considerations include an easily scalable process for manufacturing, the marketability, the acceptance by surgeons, patients, and health care providers, and the ability to receive food and drug administration (FDA) approval. Although there are stringent requirements to develop a successful strategy for encapsulating cells, there have been significant advances in cell encapsulations for a variety of cell types and tissues with many successes reported *in vitro* and *in vivo*. In summary, cell encapsulation holds great promise as an enabling technology for regenerating tissues.

# References

Agard, N. J., Prescher, J. A., and Bertozzi, C. R. 2004. A strain-promoted [3 + 2] azide-alkyne cycloaddition for covalent modification of blo molecules in living systems. *J Am Chem Soc* 126: 15046–47.

Ahmed, T. A. E., Griffith, M., and Hincke, M. 2007. Characterization and inhibition of fibrin hydrogel-degrading enzymes during development of tissue engineering scaffolds. *Tissue Eng* 13: 1469–77.

Atala, A., Cima, L. G., Kim, W. et al. 1993. Injectable alginate seeded with chondrocytes as a potential treatment for vesicoureteral reflux. *J Urol* 150: 745–47.

Baskin, J. M., Prescher, J. A., Laughlin, S. T. et al. 2007. Copper-free click chemistry for dynamic *in vivo* imaging. *Proc Natl Acad Sci U S A* 104: 16793–97.

Benoit, D. S. W., Durney, A. R., and Anseth, K. S. 2006. Manipulations in hydrogel degradation behavior enhance osteoblast function and mineralized tissue formation. *Tissue Eng* 12: 1663–73.

Benton, J. A., Fairbanks, B. D., and Anseth, K. S. 2009. Characterization of valvular interstitial cell function in three dimensional matrix metalloproteinase degradable PEG hydrogels. *Biomaterials* 30: 6593–603.

Betre, H., Ong, S. R., Guilak, F. et al. 2006. Chondrocytic differentiation of human adipose-derived adult stem cells in elastin-like polypeptide. *Biomaterials* 27: 91–99.

Betre, H., Setton, L. A., Meyer, D. E., and Chilkoti, A. 2002. Characterization of a genetically engineered elastin-like polypeptide for cartilaginous tissue repair. *Biomacromolecules* 3: 910–16.

Branco, M. C. and Schneider, J. P. 2009. Self-assembling materials for therapeutic delivery. *Acta Biomater* 5: 817–31.

Bryant, S. J. and Anseth, K. S. 2001a. Hydrogel properties influence ecm production by chondrocyte photoencapsulated in poly(ethylene glycol) hydrogels. *J Biomed Mater Res* 59: 63–72.

Bryant, S. J. and Anseth, K. S. 2001b. The effects of scaffold thickness on tissue engineered cartilage in photocrosslinked poly(ethylene oxide) hydrogels. *Biomaterials* 22: 619–26.

Bryant, S. J. and Anseth, K. S. 2003. Controlling the spatial distribution of ECM components in degradable PEG hydrogels for tissue engineering cartilage. *J Biomed Mater Res* 64A: 70–79.

Bryant, S. J., Arthur, J. A., and Anseth, K. S. 2005. Incorporation of tissue-specific molecules alters chondrocyte metabolism and gene expression in photocrosslinked hydrogels. *Acta Biomater* 1: 243–52.

Bryant, S. J., Bender, R. J., Durand, K. L., and Anseth, K. S. 2004a. Encapsulating chondrocytes in degrading PEG hydrogels with high modulus: Engineering gel structural changes to facilitate cartilaginous tissue production. *Biotechnol Bioeng* 86: 747–55.

Bryant, S. J., Davis-Arehart, K. A., Luo, N. et al. 2004b. Synthesis and characterization of photopolymerized multifunctional hydrogels: Water-soluble poly(vinyl alcohol) and chondroitin sulfate macromers for chondrocyte encapsulation. *Macromolecules* 37: 6726–33.

Bryant, S. J., Durand, K. L., and Anseth, K. S. 2003. Manipulations in hydrogel chemistry control photoencapsulated chondrocyte behavior and their extracellular matrix production. *J Biomed Mater Res* 67A: 1430–36.

Bryant, S. J., Nuttelman, C. R., and Anseth, K. S. 2000. Cytocompatibility of ultraviolet and visible light photoinitiating systems on cultured nih/3t3 fibroblasts *in vitro*. *J Biomater Sci Polym Ed* 11: 439–57.

Burdick, J. A. and Anseth, K. S. 2002. Photoencapsulation of osteoblasts in injectable rgd-modified PEG hydrogels for bone tissue engineering. *Biomaterials* 23: 4315–23.

Burdick, J. A., Chung, C., Jia, X. Q., Randolph, M. A., and Langer, R. 2005. Controlled degradation and mechanical behavior of photopolymerized hyaluronic acid networks. *Biomacromolecules* 6: 386–91.

Cao, Y. L., Rodriguez, A., Vacanti, M. et al. 1998. Comparative study of the use of poly(glycolic acid), calcium alginate and pluronics in the engineering of autologous porcine cartilage. *J Biomater Sci-Polym Ed* 9: 475–87.

Caplan, M. R., Schwartzfarb, E. M., Zhang, S. G., Kamm, R. D., and Lauffenburger, D. A. 2002. Control of self-assembling oligopeptide matrix formation through systematic variation of amino acid sequence. *Biomaterials* 23: 219–27.

Catiker, E., Gumusderelioglu, M., and Guner, A. 2000. Degradation of pla, plga homo- and copolymers in the presence of serum albumin: A spectroscopic investigation. *Polym Int* 49: 728–34.

Chen, C. S., Mrksich, M., Huang, S., Whitesides, G. M., and Ingber, D. E. 1997. Geometric control of cell life and death. *Science* 276: 1425–28.

Cramer, N. B. and Bowman, C. N. 2001. Kinetics of thiol-ene and thiol-acrylate photopolymerizations with real-time fourier transform infrared. *J Polym Sci Part A-Polym Chem* 39: 3311–19.

Cruise, G. M., Hegre, O. D., Lamberti, F. V. et al. 1999. *In vitro* and *in vivo* performance of porcine islets encapsulated in interfacially photopolymerized poly(ethylene glycol) diacrylate membranes. *Cell Transplant* 8: 293–306.

Cruise, G. M., Scharp, D. S., and Hubbell, J. A. 1998. Characterization of permeability and network structure of interfacially photopolymerized poly(ethylene glycol) diacrylate hydrogels. *Biomaterials* 19: 1287–94.

Cui, H. G., Webber, M. J., and Stupp, S. I. 2010. Self-assembly of peptide amphiphiles: From molecules to nanostructures to biomaterials. *Biopolymers* 94: 1–18.

Cukierman, E., Pankov, R., Stevens, D. R., and Yamada, K. M. 2001. Taking cell-matrix adhesions to the third dimension. *Science* 294: 1708–12.

Dang, J. M., Sun, D. D. N., Shin-Ya, Y. et al. 2006. Temperature-responsive hydroxybutyl chitosan for the culture of mesenchymal stem cells and intervertebral disk cells. *Biomaterials* 27: 406–18.

Deforest, C. A., Polizzotti, B. D., and Anseth, K. S. 2009. Sequential click reactions for synthesizing and patterning three-dimensional cell microenvironments. *Nat Mater* 8: 659–64.

Dupuy, B., Gin, H., Baquey, C., and Ducassou, D. 1988. Insitu polymerization of a microencapsulating medium round living cells. *J Biomed Mater Res* 22: 1061–70.

Elisseeff, J., Anseth, K., Sims, D. et al. 1999a. Transdermal photopolymerization for minimally invasive implantation. *Proc Natl Acad Sci USA* 96: 3104–07.

Elisseeff, J., Anseth, K., Sims, D. et al. 1999b. Transdermal photopolymerization of poly(ethylene oxide)-based injectable hydrogels for tissue-engineered cartilage. *Plast Reconstr Surg* 104: 1014–22.

Elsdale, T. and Bard, J. 1972. Collagen substrata for studies on cell behavior. *J Cell Biol* 54: 626.

Fairbanks, B. D., Schwartz, M. P., Halevi, A. E. et al. 2009. A versatile synthetic extracellular matrix mimic via thiol-norbornene photopolymerization. *Adv Mater (Weinheim, Ger)* 21: 5005–10.

Fedorovich, N. E., Oudshoorn, M. H., Van Geemen, D. et al. 2009. The effect of photopolymerization on stem cells embedded in hydrogels. *Biomaterials* 30: 344–53.

Fisher, J. P., Jo, S., Mikos, A. G., and Reddi, A. H. 2004. Thermoreversible hydrogel scaffolds for articular cartilage engineering. *Journal of Biomedical Materials Research Part A* 71A: 268–74.

Flynn, L., Prestwich, G. D., Semple, J. L., and Woodhouse, K. A. 2009. Adipose tissue engineering *in vivo* with adipose-derived stem cells on naturally derived scaffolds. *Journal of Biomedical Materials Research Part A* 89A: 929–41.

Fujimoto, K. L., Ma, Z. W., Nelson, D. M. et al. 2009. Synthesis, characterization and therapeutic efficacy of a biodegradable, thermoresponsive hydrogel designed for application in chronic infarcted myocardium. *Biomaterials* 30: 4357–68.

Galler, K. M., Aulisa, L., Regan, K. R., D'souza, R. N., and Hartgerink, J. D. 2010. Self-assembling multidomain peptide hydrogels: Designed susceptibility to enzymatic cleavage allows enhanced cell migration and spreading. *J Am Chem Soc* 132: 3217–23.

Gelain, F., Bottai, D., Vescovi, A., and Zhang, S. G. 2006. Designer self-assembling peptide nanofiber scaffolds for adult mouse neural stem cell 3-dimensional cultures. *PLoS ONE* 1: e119.

Gelain, F., Horii, A., and Zhang, S. G. 2007. Designer self-assembling peptide scaffolds for 3-d tissue cell cultures and regenerative medicine. *Macromol Biosci* 7: 544–51.

Gieni, R. S. and Hendzel, M. J. 2008. Mechanotransduction from the ECM to the genome: Are the pieces now in place? *J Cell Biochem* 104: 1964–87.

Hacker, M. C., Klouda, L., Ma, B. B., Kretlow, J. D., and Mikos, A. G. 2008. Synthesis and characterization of injectable, thermally and chemically gelable, amphiphilic poly($n$-isopropylacrylamide)-based macromers. *Biomacromolecules* 9: 1558–70.

Hill, R. S., Cruise, G. M., Hager, S. R. et al. 1997. Immunoisolation of adult porcine islets for the treatment of diabetes mellitus. The use of photopolymerizable polyethylene glycol in the conformal coating of mass-isolated porcine islets. *Ann NY Acad Sci* 831: 332–43.

Hosokawa, K., Arai, F., Yoshihara, H. et al. 2010. Cadherin-based adhesion is a potential target for niche manipulation to protect hematopoietic stem cells in adult bone marrow. *Cell Stem Cell* 6: 194–98.

Hoyle, C. E. and Bowman, C. N. 2010. Thiol-ene click chemistry. *Angew. Chem.-Int Ed* 49: 1540–73.

Huang, X., Zhang, Y., Donahue, H. J., and Lowe, T. L. 2007. Porous thermoresponsive-co-biodegradable hydrogels as tissue-engineering scaffolds for 3-dimensional *in vitro* culture of chondrocytes. *Tissue Eng* 13: 2645–52.

Jager, W. F., Lungu, A., Chen, D. Y., and Neckers, D. C. 1997. Photopolymerization of polyfunctional acrylates and methacrylate mixtures: Characterization of polymeric networks by a combination of fluorescence spectroscopy and solid state nuclear magnetic resonance. *Macromolecules* 30: 780–91.

Khattak, S. F., Bhatia, S. R., and Roberts, S. C. 2005. Pluronic f127 as a cell encapsulation material: Utilization of membrane-stabilizing agents. *Tissue Eng* 11: 974–83.

Kisiday, J., Jin, M., Kurz, B. et al. 2002. Self-assembling peptide hydrogel fosters chondrocyte extracellular matrix production and cell division: Implications for cartilage tissue repair. *Proc Natl Acad Sci USA* 99: 9996–10001.

Kisiday, J. D., Kopesky, P. W., Evans, C. H. et al. 2008. Evaluation of adult equine bone marrow- and adipose-derived progenitor cell chondrogenesis in hydrogel cultures. *J Orthop Res* 26: 322–31.

Klouda, L. and Mikos, A. G. 2008. Thermoresponsive hydrogels in biomedical applications. *Eur J Pharm Biopharm* 68: 34–45.

Kolb, H. C., Finn, M. G., and Sharpless, K. B. 2001. Click chemistry: Diverse chemical function from a few good reactions. *Angew. Chem.-Int Ed* 40: 2004–21.

Kurono, Y., Maki, T., Yotsuyanagi, T., and Ikeda, K. 1979. Esterase-like activity of human-serum albumin—structure-activity-relationships for the reactions with phenyl acetates and para-nitrophenyl esters. *Chem Pharm Bull* 27: 2781–86.

Lee, H. and Park, T. G. 2009. Photo-crosslinkable, biomimetic, and thermo-sensitive pluronic grafted hyaluronic acid copolymers for injectable delivery of chondrocytes. *J Biomed Mater Res Part A* 88A: 797–806.

Lee, S. H., Moon, J. J., Miller, J. S., and West, J. L. 2007. Poly(ethylene glycol) hydrogels conjugated with a collagenase-sensitive fluorogenic substrate to visualize collagenase activity during three-dimensional cell migration. *Biomaterials* 28: 3163–70.

Li, Q., Williams, C. G., Sun, D. D. N. et al. 2004. Photocrosslinkable polysaccharides based on chondroitin sulfate. *J Biomed Mater Res Part A* 68A: 28–33.

Liao, H. M., Munoz-Pinto, D., Qu, X. et al. 2008. Influence of hydrogel mechanical properties and mesh size on vocal fold fibroblast extracellular matrix production and phenotype. *Acta Biomater* 4: 1161–71.

Lim, D. W., Nettles, D. L., Setton, L. A., and Chilkoti, A. 2007. Rapid cross-linking of elastin-like polypeptides with (hydroxymethyl)phosphines in aqueous solution. *Biomacromolecules* 8: 1463–70.

Lim, F. and Sun, A. M. 1980. Microencapsulated islets as bioartificial endocrine pancreas. *Science* 210: 908–10.

Lippens, E., Declercq, H., Molera, J. G. et al. 2009. Modified pluronic f127 hydrogel as a cell delivery system for bone tissue engineering. *Tissue Eng Part A* 15: 40.

Liu, Y. C., Shu, X. Z., and Prestwich, G. D. 2006. Osteochondral defect repair with autologous bone marrow-derived mesenchymal stem cells in an injectable, in situ, cross-linked synthetic extracellular matrix. *Tissue Eng* 12: 3405–16.

Lutolf, M. P., Lauer-Fields, J. L., Schmoekel, H. G. et al. 2003. Synthetic matrix metalloproteinase-sensitive hydrogels for the conduction of tissue regeneration: Engineering cell-invasion characteristics. *Proc Natl Acad Sci U S A* 100: 5413–18.

Lutolf, M. P., Tirelli, N., Cerritelli, S., Cavalli, L., and Hubbell, J. A. 2001. Systematic modulation of michael-type reactivity of thiols through the use of charged amino acids. *Bioconjug Chem* 12: 1051–56.

Macewan, S. R. and Chilkoti, A. 2010. Elastin-like polypeptides: Biomedical applications of tunable bio-polymers. *Biopolymers* 94: 60–77.

Mahoney, M. J. and Anseth, K. S. 2006. Three-dimensional growth and function of neural tissue in degrad-able polyethylene glycol hydrogels. *Biomaterials* 27: 2265–74.

Malkoch, M., Vestberg, R., Gupta, N. et al. 2006. Synthesis of well-defined hydrogel networks using click chemistry. *Chem Commun (Camb)*: 2774–76.

Mann, B. K., Gobin, A. S., Tsai, A. T., Schmedlen, R. H., and West, J. L. 2001. Smooth muscle cell growth in photopolymerized hydrogels with cell adhesive and proteolytically degradable domains: Synthetic ecm analogs for tissue engineering. *Biomaterials* 22: 3045–51.

Mann, B. K. and West, J. L. 2002. Cell adhesion peptides alter smooth muscle cell adhesion, proliferation, migration, and matrix protein synthesis on modified surfaces and in polymer scaffolds. *J Biomed Mater Res* 60: 86–93.

Martens, P. and Anseth, K. S. 2000. Characterization of hydrogels formed from acrylate modified poly(vinyl alcohol) macromers. *Polymer* 41: 7715–22.

Martens, P. J., Bryant, S. J., and Anseth, K. S. 2003. Tailoring the degradation of hydrogels formed from multivinyl poly(ethylene glycol) and poly(vinyl alcohol) macromers for cartilage tissue engineering. *Biomacromolecules* 4: 283–92.

Masters, K. S., Shah, D. N., Leinwand, L. A., and Anseth, K. S. 2005. Crosslinked hyaluronan scaffolds as a biologically active carrier for valvular interstitial cells. *Biomaterials* 26: 2517–25.

Mata, A., Geng, Y. B., Henrikson, K. J. et al. 2010. Bone regeneration mediated by biomimetic mineraliza-tion of a nanofiber matrix. *Biomaterials* 31: 6004–12.

Meyer, D. E. and Chilkoti, A. 2002. Genetically encoded synthesis of protein-based polymers with pre-cisely specified molecular weight and sequence by recursive directional ligation: Examples from the elastin-like polypeptide system. *Biomacromolecules* 3: 357–67.

Moeller, H. D., Bosch, U., and Decker, B. 1995. Collagen fibril diameter distribution in patellar tendon autografts after posterior cruciate ligament reconstruction in sheep—changes over time. *J Anat* 187: 161–67.

Nuttelman, C. R., Tripodi, M. C., and Anseth, K. S. 2005. Synthetic hydrogel niches that promote hmsc viability. *Matrix Biol* 24: 208–18.

Park, H., Guo, X., Temenoff, J. S. et al. 2009. Effect of swelling ratio of injectable hydrogel composites on chondrogenic differentiation of encapsulated rabbit marrow mesenchymal stem cells *in vitro*. *Biomacromolecules* 10: 541–46.

Park, H., Temenoff, J. S., Holland, T. A., Tabata, Y., and Mikos, A. G. 2005. Delivery of tgf-beta 1 and chondrocytes via injectable, biodegradable hydrogels for cartilage tissue engineering applications. *Biomaterials* 26: 7095–103.

Parks, W. C., Wilson, C. L., and Lopez-Boado, Y. S. 2004. Matrix metalloproteinases as modulators of inflammation and innate immunity. *Nat Rev Immunol* 4: 617–29.

Passaretti, D., Silverman, R. P., Huang, W. et al. 2001. Cultured chondrocytes produce injectable tissue-engineered cartilage in hydrogel polymer. *Tissue Eng* 7: 805–15.

Patterson, J. and Hubbell, J. A. 2010. Enhanced proteolytic degradation of molecuarly engineered PEG hydrogels in response to mmp-1 and mmp-2. *Biomaterials* doi:10.1016/j.biomaterials.2010.06.061.

Pollock, J. F. and Healy, K. E. 2010. Mechanical and swelling characterization of poly($n$-isopropyl acryl-amide-co-methoxy poly(ethylene glycol) methacrylate) sol-gels. *Acta Biomater* 6: 1307–18.

Rice, M. A. and Anseth, K. S. 2004. Encapsulating chondrocytes in copolymer gels: Bimodal degradation kinetics influence cell phenotype and extracellular matrix development. *J Biomed Mater Res Part A* 70A: 560–68.

Rice, M. A. and Anseth, K. S. 2007. Controlling cartilaginous matrix evolution in hydrogels with degrada-tion triggered by exogenous addition of an enzyme. *Tissue Eng* 13: 683–91.

Ruel-Gariepy, E. and Leroux, J. C. 2004. *In situ*-forming hydrogels—Review of temperature-sensitive sys-tems. *Eur J Pharm Biopharm* 58: 409–26.

Saha, K., Pollock, J. F., Schaffer, D. V., and Healy, K. E. 2007. Designing synthetic materials to control stem cell phenotype. *Curr Opin Chem Biol* 11: 381–87.

Saim, A. B., Cao, Y. L., Weng, Y. L. et al. 2000. Engineering autogenous cartilage in the shape of a helix using an injectable hydrogel scaffold. *Laryngoscope* 110: 1694–97.

Sawhney, A. S., Pathak, C. P., and Hubbell, J. A. 1993. Bioerodible hydrogels based on photopolymerized poly(ethylene glycol)-co-poly(alpha-hydroxy acid) diacrylate macromers. *Macromolecules* 26: 581–87.

Schild, H. G. 1992. Poly (*n*-isopropylacrylamide)—experiment, theory and application. *Prog Polym Sci* 17: 163–249.

Schweikl, H., Spagnuolo, G., and Schmalz, G. 2006. Genetic and cellular toxicology of dental resin monomers. *J Dent Res* 85: 870–77.

Seidlits, S. K., Khaing, Z. Z., Petersen, R. R. et al. 2010. The effects of hyaluronic acid hydrogels with tunable mechanical properties on neural progenitor cell differentiation. *Biomaterials* 31: 3930–40.

Serban, M. A. and Prestwich, G. D. 2008. Modular extracellular matrices: Solutions for the puzzle. *Methods* 45: 93–98.

Shu, X. Z., Ahmad, S., Liu, Y. C., and Prestwich, G. D. 2006. Synthesis and evaluation of injectable, in situ crosslinkable synthetic extracellular matrices for tissue engineering. *J Biomed Mater Res Part A* 79A: 902–12.

Shu, X. Z., Liu, Y. C., Palumbo, F. S., Lu, Y., and Prestwich, G. D. 2004. *In situ* crosslinkable hyaluronan hydrogels for tissue engineering. *Biomaterials* 25: 1339–48.

Silva, G. A., Czeisler, C., Niece, K. L. et al. 2004. Selective differentiation of neural progenitor cells by high-epitope density nanofibers. *Science* 303: 1352–55.

Sims, C. D., Butler, P. E., Cao, Y. L. et al. 1998. Tissue engineered neocartilage using plasma derived polymer substrates and chondrocytes. *Plast Reconstr Surg* 101: 1580–85.

Smeds, K. A. and Grinstaff, M. W. 2001. Photocrosslinkable polysaccharides for *in situ* hydrogel formation. *J Biomed Mater Res* 54: 115–21.

Sontjens, S. H. M., Nettles, D. L., Carnahan, M. A., Setton, L. A., and Grinstaff, M. W. 2006. Biodendrimer-based hydrogel scaffolds for cartilage tissue repair. *Biomacromolecules* 7: 310–16.

Svoboda, E. L. A., Howley, T. P., and Deporter, D. A. 1983. Collagen fibril diameter and its relation to collagen turnover in 3 soft connective tissues in the rat. *Connect Tissue Res* 12: 43–48.

Temenoff, J. S., Park, H., Jabbari, E. et al. 2004a. Thermally cross-linked oligo(poly(ethylene glycol) fumarate) hydrogels support osteogenic differentiation of encapsulated marrow stromal cells *in vitro*. *Biomacromolecules* 5: 5–10.

Temenoff, J. S., Park, H., Jabbari, E. et al. 2004b. *In vitro* osteogenic differentiation of marrow stromal cells encapsulated in biodegradable hydrogels. *J Biomed Mater Res Part A* 70A: 235–44.

Temenoff, J. S., Shin, H., Conway, D. E., Engel, P. S., and Mikos, A. G. 2003. *In vitro* cytotoxicity of redox radical initiators for cross-linking of oligo(poly(ethylene glycol) fumarate) macromers. *Biomacromolecules* 4: 1605–13.

Tibbitt, M. W. and Anseth, K. S. 2009. Hydrogels as extracellular matrix mimics for 3D cell culture. *Biotechnol Bioeng* 103: 655–63.

Tsang, V. L., Chen, A. A., Cho, L. M. et al. 2007. Fabrication of 3D hepatic tissues by additive photopatterning of cellular hydrogels. *FASEB J* 21: 790–801.

Turk, B. E., Huang, L. L., Piro, E. T., and Cantley, L. C. 2001. Determination of protease cleavage site motifs using mixture-based oriented peptide libraries. *Nat Biotechnol* 19: 661–67.

Wang, D. A., Williams, C. G., Li, Q. A., Sharma, B., and Elisseeff, J. H. 2003. Synthesis and characterization of a novel degradable phosphate-containing hydrogel. *Biomaterials* 24: 3969–80.

Wang, D. A., Williams, C. G., Yang, F. et al. 2005. Bioresponsive phosphoester hydrogels for bone tissue engineering. *Tissue Eng* 11: 201–13.

Wang, F., Li, Z. Q., Khan, M. et al. 2010. Injectable, rapid gelling and highly flexible hydrogel composites as growth factor and cell carriers. *Acta Biomater* 6: 1978–91.

Wanka, G., Hoffmann, H. and Ulbricht, W. 1994. Phase-diagrams and aggregation behavior of poly(oxyethylene)-poly(oxypropylene)-poly(oxyethylene) triblock copolymers in aqueous-solutions. *Macromolecules* 27: 4145–59.

Weber, L. M., He, J., Bradley, B., Haskins, K., and Anseth, K. S. 2006. PEG-based hydrogels as an *in vitro* encapsulation platform for testing controlled beta-cell microenvironments. *Acta Biomater* 2: 1–8.

Williams, C. G., Kim, T. K., Taboas, A. et al. 2003. *In vitro* chondrogenesis of bone marrow-derived mesenchymal stem cells in a photopolymerizing hydrogel. *Tissue Eng* 9: 679–88.

Williams, C. G., Malik, A. N., Kim, T. K., Manson, P. N., and Elisseeff, J. H. 2005. Variable cytocompatibility of six cell lines with photoinitiators used for polymerizing hydrogels and cell encapsulation. *Biomaterials* 26: 1211–18.

Yang, Y., Khoe, U., Wang, X. et al. 2010. Designer self-assembling peptide nanomaterials. *Nano Today* 4: 193–210.

Yaszemski, M. J., Payne, R. G., Hayes, W. C., Langer, R., and Mikos, A. G. 1996. *In vitro* degradation of a poly(propylene fumarate)-based composite material. *Biomaterials* 17: 2127–30.

Yoshii, E. 1997. Cytotoxic effects of acrylates and methacrylates: Relationships of monomer structures and cytotoxicity. *J Biomed Mater Res* 37: 517–24.

# 21

# Coculture Systems for Mesenchymal Stem Cells

21.1 Introduction ................................................................. 21-1
21.2 Cells of Interest ........................................................... 21-2
      Mesenchymal Stem Cells
21.3 Overview of Coculture Methods.................................. 21-3
      Two-Dimensional Coculture Systems • Three-Dimensional
      Coculture Systems
21.4 Cocultures with Chondrocytes ................................... 21-4
      MSC Differentiation into Hypertrophic Chondrocytes • Chondrocyte
      Coculture with MSCs
21.5 Osteoblast Coculture with MSCs................................ 21-6
      Indirect Osteoblast Coculture with MSCs • Direct Osteoblast
      Coculture with MSCs
21.6 Myoblast Coculture with MSCs .................................. 21-8
21.7 Communication between Mesenchymal and Endothelial
      Lineages ...................................................................... 21-8
21.8 Future Outlook............................................................ 21-9
Acknowledgments .................................................................. 21-10
References................................................................................ 21-10

Song P. Seto
*Georgia Institute of Technology*
*Emory University*

Johnna S. Temenoff
*Georgia Institute of Technology*
*Emory University*

## 21.1 Introduction

Orthopedic tissues are composed of heterogeneous populations of cells that regulate the development, repair, and adaptation of tissues in response to various environmental stimuli. Bone, muscle, cartilage, ligament, and tendon are increasingly viewed as plastic tissues that have the potential to remodel, perhaps due to interactions between various resident cells (Caplan 2007, Chargé and Rudnicki 2004). For example, it has been hypothesized that muscle satellite cells can mobilize in response to injured myofibers, endothelial cells communicate with osteoblasts in bone development and synovial lining cells can affect chondrocyte phenotype and pathology (Philippou et al. 2007, Clarkin et al. 2008, Grellier et al. 2009, Rouwkema et al. 2008, Bakker et al. 2001). Currently, *in vivo* mechanisms for these phenomena remain unclear, but advances in *in vitro* systems may elucidate important cellular interactions.

The notion that cells can communicate, either by factors that bind to cell receptors or by physical cell–cell interaction via gap junctions, tight junctions, and adhesion proteins is of great interest to regenerative medicine (Loewenstein 1981, Takeichi 1990). Paracrine and autocrine signaling can affect gene expression, protein production, proliferation, and apoptosis in the tissue microenvironment—significant issues in forming physiologically viable tissues, from development to remodeling to regeneration (Caplan 2007, Chen et al. 2008, 2010). The concept of cocultures, studies involving at least two different cell types to understand the potential cellular crosstalk effects, attempt to address the paradigm of tissues as modular systems that cannot be treated in isolation. With this perspective, crosstalk between cells affects the metabolism and fate of neighboring cells. This systems view of tissues is an important approach to orthopedic tissue engineering since many mechanisms are interrelated.

Replacement of injured orthopedic tissues is currently limited to autologous or allogenic grafts or synthetic replacements, but drawbacks include donor site morbidity, limited availability of replacement tissue, and lack of integration with surrounding tissues (Benhardt and Cosgriff-Hernandez 2009, Zhou et al. 2008). Tissue engineering has the potential to address these obstacles, but intensive research is still required to understand the *in vivo* molecular and cellular mechanisms that can ensure the long-term success of regenerated tissues. Thus, by understanding the interactions between cells *in vitro*, new strategies for regenerative medicine may become more physiologically relevant.

In addition to understanding the biological mechanisms between cells of interest, coculture systems have the potential to expand the available number of cells for clinical applications. Certain cell types have limited proliferation capacities so the ability to use signals from a small pool of primary cells to induce differentiation in a large population of stem cells may be useful for a variety of cell-based therapies (Urban and Roberts 2003). Given the importance of understanding cellular interactions for the aforementioned applications, this chapter will begin by highlighting mesenchymal stem cells (MSCs) as a cell of interest in many coculture studies. A brief overview of current two-dimensional (2D) and three-dimensional (3D) coculture techniques will be included. Soluble factor signaling and physical cell interactions between cells of interest in orthopedic tissue engineering, with a focus on chondrocytes, osteoblasts, and myoblasts, since these cell types have been intensively studied, will be discussed. Finally, future directions in the field of coculture studies that emphasize the role of vascularization and new coculture technologies will be addressed.

## 21.2 Cells of Interest

### 21.2.1 Mesenchymal Stem Cells

MSCs are adherent nonhematopoietic multipotent cells that can differentiate into cells such as osteoblasts, chondrocytes, adipocytes, and tenocytes (Prockop 1997, Chamberlain et al. 2007). MSCs can be isolated from many tissues and are currently identified by the International Society of Cellular Therapy to have the above characteristics, as well as be positive for cell markers CD73, CD90, and CD105 and negative for CD11b or CD14, CD19 or CD79α, CD34, CD45, and HLA–DR (Dominici et al. 2006). Currently, MSCs are of great interest for cell-based therapies because they can be easily isolated and expanded *in vitro* without phenotypic changes before lineage-specific differentiation (Kolf et al. 2007, Baksh et al. 2004). Additionally, they are self-renewing and can exhibit high proliferation rates, which make them attractive for clinical applications in which many cells are needed (Colter et al. 2000, Bruder et al. 1997, Chen et al. 2006, Baksh et al. 2004, Tuan et al. 2003, Tsutsumi et al. 2001). They are often considered when *ex vivo* expansion of terminally differentiated cells is not feasible or practical for clinical applications (Colter et al. 2000, Johnstone et al. 1998, Chanda et al. 2010). After expansion, MSCs can be induced into varying phenotypes by differentiation factors introduced through the culture media (Pittenger et al. 1999).

The differentiation potential of MSCs has been studied extensively (Pittenger et al. 1999). Differentiation of stem cells into phenotypes including bone, cartilage, tendon, muscle, adipose tissue, and hematopoietic-supporting stroma can be affected by biochemical factors. Biochemical influences are typically chemicals and proteins such as growth factors that can be added exogenously into cell culture media or can be produced by neighboring cells *in vivo* (Chen et al. 2010, Grassel and Ahmed 2007). For MSCs, differentiation into osteogenic and chondrogenic lineages have been the most comprehensively studied to date. Soluble factors that are often added to achieve osteogenic differentiation of MSCs are bone morphogenetic proteins (BMPs), specifically BMP-2 and BMP-6 (Hartmann 2006, Gooch et al. 2002). Similarly, members of the transforming growth factor-β (TGF-β) superfamily (often combinations of TGF-β1, TGF-β3, BMP-2, BMP-4, BMP-6, BMP-7) as well as fibroblast growth factor family-2 and insulin-like growth factor-1 (IGF-1) can be supplied to induce chondrogenic differentiation (Goepfert et al. 2010, Miljkovic et al. 2008, Thorp et al. 1992, Mohan et al. 2010, Weiss et al. 2010). The ability to differentiate MSCs *in vitro* has been an important research tool for studying lineage commitment and cell fate in different biochemical environments.

Recently, MSCs are emerging as a therapeutic tool beyond being an attractive cell source. MSCs may exert effects on other cells by releasing trophic, immunomodulatory, antiscarring, and chemoattractive factors (Caplan and Dennis 2006, da Silva Meirelles et al. 2009, Caplan 2007, Chanda et al. 2010). For example, it has been shown that MSC-conditioned media can have antiapoptotic effects on neighboring endothelial cells in an ischemic injury to the kidney. The same study showed that MSC-conditioned media contained vascular endothelial growth factor, hepatocyte growth factor, and IGF-1, factors that enhance endothelial growth and survival (Tögel et al. 2007). The secretory activity of MSCs can establish a microenvironment that supports reciprocal signaling between different cell types.

## 21.3 Overview of Coculture Methods

Cell communication can be studied between cells by direct or indirect contact. Indirect cell contact allows the study of soluble, diffusible factors to influence cell communication while direct cell contact introduces the additional factor of cell–cell contact through tight junctions, gap junctions, and adhesion proteins (Loewenstein 1981, Takeichi 1990). This section will provide a brief overview of cocultures involving both types of cell communication in the context of 2D and 3D systems. Figure 21.1 provides an overview of these coculture systems.

### 21.3.1 Two-Dimensional Coculture Systems

The 2D coculture systems of interest for this chapter involve a semipermeable membrane separating different cell types and systems that allow cell communication with direct contact between cells.

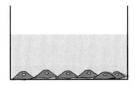

**Conditioned media**
- One-way signaling to cell of interest

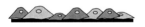

**2D Direct coculture**
- Permits soluble factor signaling and direct contact
- Need to extract cell of interest

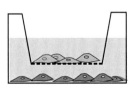

**2D Transwell system**
- Permits soluble factor signaling
- Two-way signaling between cells
- Easy to isolate cell of interest

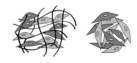

**3D Direct coculture**
- Two-way soluble factor signaling
- May permit cell contact with or without a scaffold
- Need to extract cell of interest

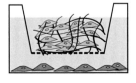

**2D/3D Transwell system**
- Two-way soluble factor signaling
- One cell type in 3D environment

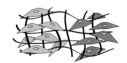

**3D Cell patterning**
- Allows spatial organization of cells
- May produce gradients of signals

**FIGURE 21.1** Coculture systems for two cell populations. Systems include indirect cell culture by use of conditioned media or semipermeable membranes. Direct coculture systems permit cell–cell contact in addition to soluble factor signaling. Patterning technologies allow control of cell placement and use of various scaffold materials.

Additional coculture systems, which will not be discussed in this section, include the use of conditioned media or conditioned extracellular matrices (ECM). Conditioned media systems, in which the cell culture medium from one cell type is used to incubate another cell type, have been useful in identifying soluble factors involved in signaling (Lacombe-Gleize et al. 1995, Ilmer et al. 2009, Bai et al. 2007, Chen et al. 2007, D'Angelo and Pacifici 1997, Walter et al. 2010).

Indirect communication between cells can be studied by physically separating cell types with a semipermeable membrane. These transwell systems allow the response of cells to be attributed to soluble signals, with signaling occurring in both directions (Domenech et al. 2009). The transwell system allows the cell type of interest to be easily isolated and analyzed. Although this transwell technique is limited to the use of just two cell types, a multitude of information has been obtained from this *in vitro* technique.

Coculturing with direct cell contact allows cells to interact with each other through gap junctions or membrane molecules such as adherens and tight junctions (Loewenstein 1981, Takeichi 1990). *In vitro* methods can be as simple as establishing cell interactions on culture dishes or glass slides (Richardson et al. 2006, Csaki et al. 2009). This system allows direct contact as well as soluble factor diffusion between cells, enabling maximal cellular interaction. It is important to be able to separate cells after coculture, for example, with the use of immunomagnetic beads or fluorescent sorting, in order to determine how coculture has affected the phenotype of the cell of interest (Guillotin et al. 2008, Wang et al. 2007).

### 21.3.2 Three-Dimensional Coculture Systems

While 2D systems can provide detailed information on cell-to-cell communication, it is generally thought that 3D systems are more representative of the architecture of native tissues (Raimondi 2006). 3D coculture systems can consist of a scaffold to support cellular adhesion, migration, and cellular contact. They may also be used to physically separate cells and allow nutrient and soluble signal diffusion without cell contact (Benoit et al. 2007, Betz et al. 2010). Scaffolds may be synthetic, naturally occurring, or a combination of the two and tailored to support specific cell-type survival. Collagen sponges and alginate beads are examples of naturally derived scaffolds commonly used (Badylak et al. 2009, Wee and Gombotz 1998). For synthetic scaffolds, adhesion peptides such as Arg–Gly–Asp (RGD) and Gly–Phe–Hyp–Gly–Glu–Arg (GFOGER) can be immobilized within by covalent linkages to facilitate a more natural environment (Zhang et al. 2003, Mann and West 2002, Nuttelman et al. 2005, Paxton et al. 2009, Salinas and Anseth 2008, Lutolf and Hubbell 2005). Additionally, enzyme-degradable peptides such matrix metalloproteinase (MMPs)-sensitive sequences may be incorporated to facilitate cell-mediated remodeling of the scaffold (Park et al. 2004, Lutolf et al. 2003, Gobin and West 2003, Raeber et al. 2005, Lee et al. 2005). Different cell types may be uniformly mixed throughout the scaffold to maximize cellular interaction, but with the advent of micropatterning techniques available for biological materials, spatial organization of cells is now feasible (Khademhosseini et al. 2006, Albrecht et al. 2006, Choi et al. 2007, Hammoudi et al. 2010).

3D cell structures can also be prepared without a scaffold in the form of a spheroid or cell pellet (Nagahata et al. 2004, Zhang et al. 2004, Rouwkema et al. 2006). Cells can be centrifuged or encouraged to aggregate in order to form a high-density cell pellet. With microfluidic systems, cell pellet cultures can become more high throughput and repeatable (Ong et al. 2008). In these micromass cultures, cellular interaction can be maximized and are suitable for cells that are not contact inhibited. Specific cell types, such as chondrocytes, exhibit a stable phenotype when cultured as a cell pellet (Zhang et al. 2004). Different cell types can be cultured together in pellet cultures, but heterokaryons may form between cells, which complicate extraction of cells of interest (Ying et al. 2002).

## 21.4 Cocultures with Chondrocytes

Intervertebral disc (IVD) injuries and articular cartilage damage incurred through injury and disease may be ameliorated by new cellular therapies designed to restore tissue and decrease pain (Elisseeff et al. 2005, Chen et al. 2006, Vats et al. 2006). One strategy is to use autologous chondrocyte (cartilage cell) implantation to support and repopulate the damaged tissue, but the relatively low *ex vivo* proliferative rates and metabolic activity of chondrocytes are a limitation to clinical application of these cells (Urban and Roberts 2003). These obstacles have encouraged the use of an alternate cell source, such as MSCs, that may be induced into the chondrogenic phenotype.

## 21.4.1 MSC Differentiation into Hypertrophic Chondrocytes

MSCs have the capacity to become chondrogenic, but the mechanism remains poorly understood. Factors such as TGF-β can be added to cell culture media to induce MSCs into a chondrogenic phenotype, but studies have shown that prolonged culture or *in vivo* implantation of these cells result in calcified cartilage, similar to that seen in growth plate chondrocytes in endochondral ossification (Pelttari et al. 2006, Mackay et al. 1999, Johnstone et al. 1998, Yoo et al. 1998). In endochondral ossification, chondrocytes proliferate until they mature into hypertrophic chondrocytes, which secrete calcified ECM and eventually undergo programmed cell death or apoptosis (Hojo et al. 2010). As a result, MSCs that are induced into the hypertrophic chondrocyte phenotype have limited regeneration capacity *in vivo* (Hojo et al. 2010).

The hallmarks of hypertrophic chondrocytes include high levels of alkaline phosphatase (ALP) activity, MMP-13 secretion, and type X collagen. While induced MSCs seem to undergo differentiation representative of endochondral ossification, the mechanism for the transitions remains unclear. *In vitro* development of a stable, noncalcified cartilage was difficult to produce until it was shown that by continuously coculturing growth plate chondrocytes with articular cartilage without cell contact, ALP activity could become inhibited (Jikko et al. 1999). The presence of differentiated articular chondrocytes seemed to prevent terminal differentiation of growth plate chondrocytes. In a similar study, coculturing differentiating sternal cells with as little as 10% articular chondrocytes impaired sternal cell maturation (D'Angelo and Pacifici 1997). The factors involved in producing a stable chondrocyte phenotype are still being investigated.

## 21.4.2 Chondrocyte Coculture with MSCs

Soluble factor diffusion in 2D transwell systems has been widely used to study how chondrocytes alter stem cell differentiation. Monolayers of articular chondrocytes cocultured with human MSCs or human embryonic stem cells showed an increased expression of Sox9, Col2A1, and aggrecan, putative markers for chondrocytes (Chen et al. 2009, Vats et al. 2006). Similar gene expression profiles were observed when rat MSCs were cultured with whole IVD tissue for 30 days (Wei et al. 2009). Expression of Col2A1, Sox9, and aggrecan reached a peak by day 14 and MSCs were observed to approach the phenotype of nucleus pulposus cells, cartilaginous cells from the interior of the IVD. Furthermore, MSCs became aggregated on the transwell membrane, forming 3D masses that immunostained for type II collagen and aggrecan. Taken together, these studies indicate that chondrocytes induce chondrogenic differentiation in MSCs. However, when nonhypertrophic chondrocytes were cocultured with C3H10T1/2 stem cells in a transwell system, elevated expressions of the bone-related markers core binding factor-1 (Cbfa1) and osteocalcin mRNA were observed (Gerstenfeld et al. 2002). The discrepancies in these results may represent the spectrum of MSC differentiation from transitional chondrocytes to hypertrophic chondrocytes. These studies also highlight the variable culture methods used, which may alter the phenotype of cells sensitive to their microenvironment.

Dedifferentiation of chondrocytes can occur when grown in monolayer and consequently alter the profile of secreted signals (Pelttari et al. 2006, Dell'Accio et al. 2001). In order to prevent dedifferentiation, chondrocytes are often cultured in 3D structures, within a scaffold or in micromass pellets (Lemare et al. 1998). For coculture, a single cell type can be cultured in a 3D scaffold and suspended over a monolayer of MSCs or a mixture of cells can be cultured together in a cell pellet. Recent results with chondrocytes cultured in 3D environments have shown that cocultured MSCs express osteogenic phenotypes. Articular chondrocytes encapsulated in alginate beads and suspended over a monolayer of bone marrow-derived MSCs (BM–MSCs) remained viable in the system for up to 21 days. ALP expression, an indicator of mineralization, was elevated in MSCs with exposure to chondrocytes. In fact, the longer the time in coculture, the more accelerated the calcium deposition and phenotypic change from spindle-shaped to osteoblast-like cuboidal-shaped (Thompson et al. 2009). An osseous phenotype could form by day 28 when both MSCs and articular chondrocytes were encapsulated in alginate and cultured in the presence of dexamethasone and ascorbic acid, suggesting that one of the cell types was maturing or differentiating (Mo et al. 2009). By utilizing cells from two different species of animals to allow specific gene probing, the cartilaginous phenotype of the coculture was shown to originate from the chondrocytes, but higher glycosaminoglycan (GAG) production and type II collagen production was seen with a greater number of MSCs in the coculture system (Mo et al. 2009). Several additional studies have utilized encapsulated MSCs cocultured with chondrocytes cultured in 3D, and have shown increased expression of chondrocyte markers such as type II collagen and aggrecan, but did not report the presence of hypertrophic markers (Li et al. 2005, Varshney et al. 2010, Yang et al. 2009).

MSCs are presumed to be more sensitive to contact-dependent signals than more differentiated cells, which may make them amenable to direct cell culture (Ball et al. 2004). In addition, the cell ratio between MSCs and chondrocytes in coculture studies may affect the phenotype observed. With MSC to chondrocyte ratios of 2:1, 1:1, and 1:2, the chondrogenic phenotype was observed in all the 3D alginate scaffolds, but greater production of GAG and expression of osteocalcin was observed in the 2:1 group (Mo et al. 2009). In a similar study, the ALP activity was measured in 1:1 and 1:2 MSC to chondrocyte pellet cocultures. Both groups suppressed ALP activity, but the 1:2 group exhibited a significantly lower ALP activity than controls (Fischer et al. 2010). Furthermore, these MSC-chondrocyte cell pellets fully inhibited mineralization when implanted subcutaneously into immunodeficient mice (Fischer et al. 2010). Conversely, the MSC-only pellet produced a calcified cartilage when implanted and exhibited the presence of collagen type X and elevated ALP levels. When rabbit MSCs were cultured with chondrocytes in hydrogels at ratios of 1:1 and 3:1, higher type II collagen and aggrecan expression was observed for the 1:1 group compared to the 3:1 group (Yang et al. 2009). Taken together, the relative amount of chondrocytes in the coculture system may affect the levels of chondrogenic expression observed as well as the degree of chondrocyte hypertrophy. MSC contact with articular chondrocytes in a 3D environment may help prevent hypertrophy, but more studies need to be conducted to examine this concept (Chen et al. 2009, Bigdeli et al. 2009).

## 21.5 Osteoblast Coculture with MSCs

Osteoblasts have been proposed to be a crucial component to the subendochondral niche, which host mesenchymal and hematopoietic stem cells (HSCs). Although much research has focused on the cooperative signaling between osteoblasts and HSCs, what remains less understood is the interaction between MSCs and osteoblasts *in vivo* (Porter and Calvi 2008, de Barros et al. 2010, Arai et al. 2004, Martinez-Agosto et al. 2007).

Mature osteoblasts are derived from precursor cells from the bone marrow, but it is not fully understood how the transition to the osteoblast stage occurs. *In vitro* studies with MSCs have shown that exogenously added morphogens such as dexamethasone and BMPs can induce osteogenesis, but the mechanism has not been elucidated (Chamberlain et al. 2007). Gene markers for osteogenesis, however, have been established for cell characterization. Expression levels of the CBFA-1/Runx2 and osterix transcription factors are typically measured as indicators of early osteogenesis (Kassem et al. 2008). Levels of lipoprotein-related receptor 5, ALP activity, bone sialoprotein-2 (BSP-2), and osteocalcin production are commonly used to mark the differentiation into more mature osteoblasts (Kassem et al. 2008, Gaur et al. 2005, Ducy et al. 1997). By evaluating gene expression changes, many cocultures studies examine whether it is possible to transform a large population of MSCs into a differentiated cell type with a small pool of osteoblasts.

## 21.5.1 Indirect Osteoblast Coculture with MSCs

Osteoblasts are derived from MSCs and are involved in the regulation of stem cells by signaling in the microenvironment, presenting an opportunity to study these two cells *in vitro*. Studies with conditioned media from osteoblasts have indicated that osteogenic genes and phenotype can be induced in stem cells, but some of these studies utilized dexamethasone, a potent glucocorticoid, which can mask signaling between cells (Heino et al. 2004, Maxson and Burg 2010). Results from these conditioned media experiments contradict another study in which mature osteoblasts were only slightly osteogenic toward C3H10T1/2 stem cells (Gerstenfeld et al. 2003), indicating that media type can affect the phenotype observed. Furthermore, the use of conditioned media is not representative of the dynamic signaling that can occur between two cell types over time.

Two-way signaling between osteoblasts and MSCs may produce a differentiation niche similar to that seen in the natural microenvironment (Ilmer et al. 2009). Murine osteoblasts cocultured with MSCs in a transwell system showed no change in proliferation or gene expression over 3 weeks in dexamethasone-free medium. The cocultured MSCs, however, showed increased expression of runx2, osterix, osteopontin, and bone sialoprotein at 3 weeks compared to MSC-only controls (Wang et al. 2007). Similarly, human MSCs cocultured with human osteoblasts in a transwell system exhibited upregulation in bone sialoprotein-2, lipoprotein receptor, ALP, and osteocalcin by day 14 when cocultured with twice the amount of osteoblasts than MSCs (Ilmer et al. 2009). The results indicate that soluble factors from osteoblasts can induce MSCs into a more osteogenic phenotype by upregulating both early and late bone markers over time.

## 21.5.2 Direct Osteoblast Coculture with MSCs

Cell-to-cell contact between MSCs and osteoblasts can enhance communication between cells. Gap junctions, transmembrane channels between neighboring cells that allow communication through the cytoplasm, are present between osteoblasts, osteoclasts, and osteocytes (Civitelli 2008). Connexin 43 is the most abundant gap junction in bone and beyond allowing cells to respond to external stimuli, has been shown to be required for osteoblast differentiation and function (Civitelli 2008, Loewenstein 1981, Schiller et al. 1992). Each gap junction is composed of a hemichannel on each cell that allows for the diffusion of ions, metabolites, and small signaling molecules. Different connexins have varying permeabilities for molecules, allowing selective cell communication. Human osteoblasts were shown to couple to bone marrow stromal cells and allow luciferase dye transfer, a phenomenon that was inhibited by the application of octanol, an inhibitor of gap junction communication (Civitelli et al. 1993). One study proposed cell-to-cell contact to be osteoinductive for MSCs, but the use of cells from different species may have prohibited ideal communication (Kim et al. 2003).

The exact mechanisms that link cell contact or soluble signaling to gene expression remain elusive, but depend on the types of signals, downstream effects, and cell contact proteins involved. The Wnt pathway was identified to play an inductive role in MSC differentiation in studies comparing indirect and direct coculture without osteogenic factors (Zhou et al. 2008, Wang et al. 2007). The increased secretion of Wnt by osteoblasts was observed with a concomitant increase in β-catenin and TCF/LEF1 levels, downstream effectors of Wnt, in MSCs cultured indirectly with osteoblasts. However, the upregulation of bone-related markers in indirect coculture were reversed when osteoblasts were cultured in direct contact with MSCs in a ratio 1:4 in a mixed monolayer (Wang et al. 2007). Direct cell culture offset the stimulatory effect of osteoblasts by crosstalk between cadherin-β-catenin pathway and the Wnt pathway. In this study, it is suggested that soluble factors can induce osteogenesis in MSCs while cell contact can reduce osteogenic differentiation potential.

## 21.6  Myoblast Coculture with MSCs

Skeletal muscles have an exceptional ability to repair after injury. Repair involves recruitment of myogenic cells to proliferate, differentiate, and fuse together to form multinucleated muscle fibers (Chargé and Rudnicki 2004). However, in certain pathologies such as muscular dystrophy, muscle regeneration is limited (Ferrari and Mavilio 2002). Thus, techniques are needed to understand the mechanisms of muscle regeneration (Quattrocelli et al. 2010). Several studies have focused on skeletal myoblasts in the context of myocardial infarction (Carvalho et al. 2006, Baffour et al. 2006, Carvalho et al. 2006). MSCs injected into an ischemic region of the heart have been shown to produce muscle-associated proteins, indicating that there is crosstalk between cell types. However, coculture systems between muscle cells and MSCs have not been widely reported in terms of soluble factor signaling. Rather, studies have been focused on the cellular fusion that occurs when MSCs are in contact with muscle.

It has been well reported that cell fusion occurs when MSCs are incorporated into myofibers (Saito et al. 1995, Lee et al. 2005, Grove et al. 2004, Shi et al. 2004). It was unknown whether this cell fusion allowed continued MSC expression, until species-specific immunofluorescence and genetic lineage tracing confirmed the incorporation and expression of donor-specific proteins by the hybrid cells. To understand whether nuclear reprogramming occurred prior to cell fusion or as a result of fusion, mouse C2C12 myoblasts were seeded with human MSCs in a 1:5 cell ratio on 2D surfaces until multinucleated myotubes formed (Lee et al. 2005). The resulting multinucleated myofibers were chimeric, with nuclei from both donor and recipient cells, and expressed human nestin after cell fusion. Nestin, a marker of regenerating skeletal muscle, was not detected in the human MSCs cultured alone, indicating that MSCs had the myogenic potential to produce nestin after cell fusion (Lee et al. 2005).

In order to identify whether all cells from the bone marrow could fuse with myotubes, various preparations of bone marrow cells were directly cocultured with C2C12 myoblasts in 1:1 ratio (Shi et al. 2004). Myotube fusion was promoted with the addition of insulin and transferrin to the culture medium. It was found that bone marrow stromal cells were able to fuse with high efficiency to myoblasts, especially when compared to hematopoietic cells. In contrast, when MSCs were cultured with C2C12 without cell contact, MSCs did not exhibit staining for myosin heavy chain or undergo fusion, while C2C12 cells underwent normal myogenesis (Shi et al. 2004). The results indicate that stromal cells require cell contact in order to contribute to myotube fusion. *In vivo* studies have been conducted to extend the potential benefit of MSC fusion to myoblasts (LaBarge and Blau 2002, Dreyfus et al. 2004). When MSCs were cocultured with myoblasts and then injected into the tibialis anterior muscle of the muscular dystrophic mice, mdx mice, a small but significant increase of muscle mass was seen in the coculture group as well as positive staining for dystrophin, the molecule necessary for muscle fiber connection to the ECM (Ferrari and Mavilio 2002). The MSCs are thought to become more myogenic after incorporation into myofibers, but more research is needed to delineate the cell expression profile of MSCs from other cells present when fused into myofibers.

## 21.7  Communication between Mesenchymal and Endothelial Lineages

Vascularization of tissues, particularly bone, is one of the main obstacles in tissue engineering (Santos and Reis 2010). Maintenance of newly formed tissue rests on proper nutrient supply provided by blood vessels from the host or implanted with the tissue engineering construct. Survival of cells require a nutrient supply located less than 200 μm away, and several strategies to improve the vascularization of tissue-engineered constructs have been described elsewhere (Rouwkema et al. 2008, Yang et al. 2001, Kaigler et al. 2006). The relationship between endothelial cells and osteoblasts has been documented for years and has provided new strategies on understanding the viability of regenerated tissues (Clarkin et al. 2008, Guillotin et al. 2008). Therefore, studying *in vitro* communication between endothelial cells and bone-forming cells, MSCs, is a fundamental approach to further understanding tissue development.

When human MSCs are cultured with human umbilical vein endothelial cells (HUVECs) in suspension, they can spontaneously form spheroids. In one particular approach, this phenomenon was used to fabricate a 3D prevascular network that could be maintained after implantation (Rouwkema et al. 2006). Direct interaction between endothelial cells and MSCs also resulted in an upregulation of osteogenic markers such as ALP and mineralization *in vivo* (Kaigler et al. 2005). For larger tissue implants, the initial stage of neovascularization by endothelial cells was implicated in greater bone regeneration in a critical-sized defect (Seebach et al. 2010). The complementary roles that endothelial cells and MSCs play may sustain viable bone formation.

Cell source and differentiation stage of endothelial cells is an important parameter to consider, since these may affect both the ability of the cells to direct differentiation of MSCs toward the osteogenic lineage, as well as the stability of any resulting vascular networks. Human primary vascular endothelial cells, including endothelial precursor cells, isolated from cord blood and the saphenous vein were able to induce higher ALP activity in osteoprogenitor cells, while a transformed cell line did not modify osteoblastic differentiation (Guillotin et al. 2004). Endothelial precursor cells have been used successfully in forming complex prevascular networks *in vitro*, but fewer tubular structures were formed compared to HUVECs or human dermal microvascular endothelial cells cultures (Rouwkema et al. 2009).

Endothelial cells have divergent roles at different levels of osteogenesis. While most 2D and 3D studies have shown that endothelial cells can be osteoinductive mediators by stimulating ALP activity, endothelial cells may also inhibit MSCs from differentiating into mature osteoblasts. HUVECs reversibly inhibited osteogenesis by interfering with osterix expression while not affecting Runx2 expression (Meury et al. 2006). Taken together, endothelial cells can participate at different levels of differentiation by releasing paracrine factors, by controlling expression of transcription factors, and by facilitating mineralized ECM production by MSCs (Grellier et al. 2009).

## 21.8 Future Outlook

The ability to regenerate functional tissue necessitates understanding the molecular and cellular interactions that occur *in vivo*. To address these questions, *in vitro* coculture methods offer the advantage that they simplify the environment to allow the study of signaling between limited numbers of cell types. To date, coculture systems have revealed that MSCs in the presence of chondrocytes are directed toward the calcified cartilage phenotype, although the mechanisms are still unclear. MSCs in the presence of osteoblasts have shown somewhat less potent interactions, unless direct cell contact is involved, and the role of MSCs in skeletal muscle regeneration has yet to be fully determined. How these cell interactions play a role in developing complex orthopedic tissues from stem cell precursors will require more sophisticated culture and analysis techniques.

Currently, many established coculture systems are relatively simple, but the ability to perform multiple-cell coculture may be achieved with the advent of new micropatterning and microfluidic strategies (Ong et al. 2008, Bhatia et al. 1997, Domenech et al. 2009, Hammoudi et al. 2010). Using these technologies, now available for cell and/or scaffold patterning, spatial organization of cells at high resolution is possible and will advance the study of soluble factor signaling between cells. Furthermore, coculture systems that can mimic *in vivo* microenvironments while allowing easy extraction of cells for analysis is desirable. While many current coculture studies isolate one cell type to study, more insights can be gained by simultaneously examining all cells involved in crosstalk, which necessitates cell extraction technologies for complex cocultures.

As the techniques for coculturing cells advance, so will the information gathered about cellular communication. The merger of developmental biology and tissue engineering will continue to produce impactful results on understanding how cell–cell signaling affects stem cell differentiation. With the development of new coculture techniques and the scrupulous use of current coculture systems, fundamental biological questions can be addressed and translated into robust engineered tissues for a variety of applications.

## Acknowledgments

This work was supported by the Center for Drug Design, Development, and Delivery (CD4) Graduate Assistance in Areas of National Need (GAANN) Fellowship awarded to S.P.S. and a National Science Foundation CAREER award to J.S.T. (CBET-0746209).

## References

Albrecht, D.R., Underhill, G.H., Wassermann, T.B. et al. 2006. Probing the role of multicellular organization in three-dimensional microenvironments. *Nat Meth* 3(5):369–75.

Arai, F., Hirao, A., Ohmura, M. et al. 2004. Tie2/angiopoietin-1 signaling regulates hematopoietic stem cell quiescence in the bone marrow niche. *Cell* 118(2):149–61.

Badylak, S.F., Freytes, D.O., and Gilbert, T.W. 2009. Extracellular matrix as a biological scaffold material: Structure and function. *Acta Biomater* 5(1):1–13.

Baffour, R., Pakala, R., Hellinga, D. et al. 2006. Bone marrow-derived stem cell interactions with adult cardiomyocytes and skeletal myoblasts in vitro. *Cardiovasc Revasc Med* 7(4):222–30.

Bai, L., Caplan, A., Lennon, D. et al. 2007. Human mesenchymal stem cells signals regulate neural stem cell fate. *Neurochem Res* 32(2):353–62.

Bakker, A.C., van de Loo, F.A., van Beuningen, H.M. et al. 2001. Overexpression of active TGF-beta-1 in the murine knee joint: Evidence for synovial-layer-dependent chondro-osteophyte formation. *Osteoarthr Cartil* 9(2):128–36.

Baksh, D., Song, L., and Tuan, R.S. 2004. Adult mesenchymal stem cells: Characterization, differentiation, and application in cell and gene therapy. *J Cell Mol Med* 8(3):301–16.

Ball, S.G., Shuttleworth, A.C., and Kielty, C.M. 2004. Direct cell contact influences bone marrow mesenchymal stem cell fate. *Int J Biochem Cell Biol* 36(4):714–27.

Benhardt, H.A. and Cosgriff-Hernandez, E.M. 2009. The role of mechanical loading in ligament tissue engineering. *Tissue Eng Part B Rev* 15(4):467–75.

Benoit, D.S.W., Collins, S.D., and Anseth, K.S. 2007. Multifunctional hydrogels that promote osteogenic hMSC differentiation through stimulation and sequestering of BMP2. *Adv Funct Mater* 17(13):2085–93.

Betz, M.W., Yeatts, A.B., Richbourg, W.J. et al. 2010. Macroporous hydrogels upregulate osteogenic signal expression and promote bone regeneration. *Biomacromolecules* 11(5):1160–8.

Bhatia, S.N., Yarmush, M.L., and Toner, M. 1997. Controlling cell interactions by micropatterning in cocultures: Hepatocytes and 3T3 fibroblasts. *J Biomed Mater Res* 34(2):189–99.

Bigdeli, N., Karlsson, C., Strehl, R. et al. 2009. Coculture of human embryonic stem cells and human articular chondrocytes results in significantly altered phenotype and improved chondrogenic differentiation. *Stem Cells* 27(8):1812–21.

Bruder, S.P., Jaiswal, N., and Haynesworth, S.E. 1997. Growth kinetics, self-renewal, and the osteogenic potential of purified human mesenchymal stem cells during extensive subcultivation and following cryopreservation. *J Cell Biochem* 64(2):278–94.

Caplan, A.I. 2007. Adult mesenchymal stem cells for tissue engineering versus regenerative medicine. *J Cell Physiol* 213(2):341–47.

Caplan, A.I. and Dennis, J.E. 2006. Mesenchymal stem cells as trophic mediators. *J Cell Biochem* 98(5):1076–84.

Carvalho, K.A.T., Guarita-Souza, L.C., Hansen, P. et al. 2006. Cell transplantation after the coculture of skeletal myoblasts and mesenchymal stem cells in the regeneration of the myocardium scar: An experimental study in rats. *Transplant Proc* 38(5):1596–602.

Carvalho, K.A.T., Guarita-Souza, L.C., Simeone, R.B. et al. 2006. Proliferation of bone marrow mesenchymal stem cells, skeletal muscle cells and co-culture of both for cell myocardium therapy in Wistar rats. *Transplant Proc* 38(6):1955–56.

Chamberlain, G., Fox, J., Ashton, B. et al. 2007. Concise review: Mesenchymal stem cells: Their phenotype, differentiation capacity, immunological features, and potential for homing. *Stem Cells* 25(11):2739–49.

Chanda, D., Kumar, S., and Ponnazhagan, S. 2010. Therapeutic potential of adult bone marrow-derived mesenchymal stem cells in diseases of the skeleton. *J Cell Biochem* 111(2):249–57.

Chargé, S.B.P. and Rudnicki, M.A. 2004. Cellular and molecular regulation of muscle regeneration. *Physiol Rev* 84(1):209–38.

Chen, F.H., Rousche, K.T., and Tuan, R.S. 2006. Technology Insight: Adult stem cells in cartilage regeneration and tissue engineering. *Nat Clin Pract Rheumatol* 2(7):373–82.

Chen, F.M., Zhang, M., and Wu, Z.F. 2010. Toward delivery of multiple growth factors in tissue engineering. *Biomaterials* 31(24):6279–308.

Chen, L., Tredget, E.E., Wu, P.Y.G. et al. 2008. Paracrine factors of mesenchymal stem cells recruit macrophages and endothelial lineage cells and enhance wound healing. *PLoS ONE* 3(4):e1886.

Chen, L., Zhang, W., Yue, H. et al. 2007. Effects of human mesenchymal stem cells on the differentiation of dendritic cells from CD34+ cells. *Stem Cells Dev* 16(5):719–31.

Chen, S., Emery, S.E., and Pei, M. 2009. Coculture of synovium-derived stem cells and nucleus pulposus cells in serum-free defined medium with supplementation of transforming growth factor-beta1: A potential application of tissue-specific stem cells in disc regeneration. *Spine* 34(12):1272–80.

Chen, W.H., Lai, M.T., Wu, A.T.H. et al. 2009. *in vitro* stage-specific chondrogenesis of mesenchymal stem cells committed to chondrocytes. *Arthritis Rheum* 60(2):450–9.

Choi, N.W., Cabodi, M., Held, B. et al. 2007. Microfluidic scaffolds for tissue engineering. *Nat Mater* 6(11):908–15.

Civitelli, R. 2008. Cell-cell communication in the osteoblast/osteocyte lineage. *Arch Biochem Biophys* 473 (2):188–92.

Civitelli, R., Beyer, E.C., Warlow, P.M. et al. 1993. Connexin43 mediates direct intercellular communication in human osteoblastic cell networks. *J Clin Invest* 91(5):1888–96.

Clarkin, C.E., Emery, R.J., Pitsillides, A.A. et al. 2008. Evaluation of VEGF-mediated signaling in primary human cells reveals a paracrine action for VEGF in osteoblast-mediated crosstalk to endothelial cells. *J Cell Physiol* 214(2):537–44.

Clarkin, C.E., Garonna, E., Pitsillides, A.A. et al. 2008. Heterotypic contact reveals a COX-2-mediated suppression of osteoblast differentiation by endothelial cells: A negative modulatory role for prostanoids in VEGF-mediated cell: Cell communication? *Exp Cell Res* 314(17):3152–61.

Colter, D.C., Class, R., DiGirolamo, C.M. et al. 2000. Rapid expansion of recycling stem cells in cultures of plastic-adherent cells from human bone marrow. *Proc Natl Acad Sci USA* 97(7):3213–18.

Csaki, C., Matis, U., Mobasheri, A. et al. 2009. Co-culture of canine mesenchymal stem cells with primary bone-derived osteoblasts promotes osteogenic differentiation. *Histochem Cell Biol* 131(2):251–66.

D'Angelo, M. and Pacifici, M. 1997. Articular chondrocytes produce factors that inhibit maturation of sternal chondrocytes in serum-free agarose cultures: A TGF-beta independent process. *J Bone Miner Res* 12 (9):1368–77.

da Silva Meirelles, L., Fontes, A.M., Covas, D.T. et al. 2009. Mechanisms involved in the therapeutic properties of mesenchymal stem cells. *Cytokine Growth Factor Rev* 20(5–6):419–27.

de Barros, A.P.D.N., Takiya, C.M., Garzoni, L.R. et al. 2010. Osteoblasts and bone marrow mesenchymal stromal cells control hematopoietic stem cell migration and proliferation in 3D *in vitro* model. *PLoS ONE* 5(2):e9093.

Dell'Accio, F., De Bari, C., and Luyten, F.P. 2001. Molecular markers predictive of the capacity of expanded human articular chondrocytes to form stable cartilage in vivo. *Arthritis Rheum* 44(7):1608–19.

Domenech, M., Yu, H., Warrick, J. et al. 2009. Cellular observations enabled by microculture: Paracrine signaling and population demographics. *Integr Biol (Camb)* 1(3):267–74.

Dominici, M., Le Blanc, K., Mueller, I. et al. 2006. Minimal criteria for defining multipotent mesenchymal stromal cells. The International Society for Cellular Therapy position statement. *Cytotherapy* 8(4):315–7.

Dreyfus, P.A., Chretien, F., Chazaud, B. et al. 2004. Adult bone marrow-derived stem cells in muscle connective tissue and satellite cell niches. *Am J Pathol* 164(3):773–79.

Ducy, P., Zhang, R., Geoffroy, V. et al. 1997. Osf2/Cbfa1: A transcriptional activator of osteoblast differentiation. *Cell* 89(5):747–54.

Elisseeff, J., Puleo, C., Yang, F. et al. 2005. Advances in skeletal tissue engineering with hydrogels. *Orthod Craniofac Res* 8(3):150–61.

Ferrari, G. and Mavilio, F. 2002. Myogenic stem cells from the bone marrow: A therapeutic alternative for muscular dystrophy? *Neuromuscul Disord* 12 Suppl 1:S7–10.

Fischer, J., Dickhut, A., Richter, W. et al. 2010. Articular chondrocytes secrete parathyroid hormone-related protein and inhibit hypertrophy of mesenchymal stem cells in coculture during chondrogenesis. *Arthritis Rheum.* 62(9):2696–706.

Gaur, T., Lengner, C.J., Hovhannisyan, H. et al. 2005. Canonical WNT signaling promotes osteogenesis by directly stimulating Runx2 gene expression. *J Biol Chem* 280(39):33132–40.

Gerstenfeld, L.C., Barnes, G.L., Shea, C.M. et al. 2003. Osteogenic differentiation is selectively promoted by morphogenetic signals from chondrocytes and synergized by a nutrient rich growth environment. *Connect Tissue Res* 44 Suppl 1:85–91.

Gerstenfeld, L.C., Cruceta, J., Shea, C.M. et al. 2002. Chondrocytes provide morphogenic signals that selectively induce osteogenic differentiation of mesenchymal stem cells. *J Bone Miner Res* 17(2):221–30.

Gobin, A.S. and West, J.L. 2003. Effects of epidermal growth factor on fibroblast migration through biomimetic hydrogels. *Biotechnol Prog* 19(6):1781–5.

Goepfert, C., Slobodianski, A., Schilling, A.F. et al. 2010. Cartilage engineering from mesenchymal stem cells. *Adv Biochem Eng Biotechnol.* 123:163–200.

Gooch, K.J., Blunk, T., Courter, D.L. et al. 2002. Bone morphogenetic proteins-2, -12, and -13 modulate *in vitro* development of engineered cartilage. *Tissue Eng* 8(4):591–601.

Grassel, S. and Ahmed, N. 2007. Influence of cellular microenvironment and paracrine signals on chondrogenic differentiation. *Front Biosci* 12:4946–56.

Grellier, M., Bordenave, L., and Amédée, J. 2009. Cell-to-cell communication between osteogenic and endothelial lineages: Implications for tissue engineering. *Trends Biotechnol* 27(10):562–71.

Grove, J.E., Bruscia, E., and Krause, D.S. 2004. Plasticity of bone marrow-derived stem cells. *Stem Cells* 22(4):487–500.

Guillotin, B., Bareille, R., Bourget, C. et al. 2008. Interaction between human umbilical vein endothelial cells and human osteoprogenitors triggers pleiotropic effect that may support osteoblastic function. *Bone* 42(6):1080–91.

Guillotin, B., Bourget, C., Remy-Zolgadri, M. et al. 2004. Human primary endothelial cells stimulate human osteoprogenitor cell differentiation. *Cell Physiol Biochem* 14(4–6):325–32.

Hammoudi, T.M., Lu, H., and Temenoff, J.S. 2010. Long-term spatially defined coculture within three-dimensional photopatterned hydrogels. *Tissue Eng Part C Methods.* 16(6):1621–8.

Hartmann, C. 2006. A Wnt canon orchestrating osteoblastogenesis. *Trends Cell Biol* 16(3):151–58.

Heino, T.J., Hentunen, T.A., and Vaananen, H.K. 2004. Conditioned medium from osteocytes stimulates the proliferation of bone marrow mesenchymal stem cells and their differentiation into osteoblasts. *Exp Cell Res* 294(2):458–68.

Hojo, H., Ohba, S., Yano, F. et al. 2010. Coordination of chondrogenesis and osteogenesis by hypertrophic chondrocytes in endochondral bone development. *J Bone Miner Metab.* 28(5):489–502.

Ilmer, M., Karow, M., Geissler, C. et al. 2009. Human osteoblast-derived factors induce early osteogenic markers in human mesenchymal stem cells. *Tissue Eng Part A* 15(9):2397–409.

Jikko, A., Kato, Y., Hiranuma, H. et al. 1999. Inhibition of chondrocyte terminal differentiation and matrix calcification by soluble factors released by articular chondrocytes. *Calcif Tissue Int* 65(4):276–9.

Johnstone, B., Hering, T.M., Caplan, A.I. et al. 1998. *in vitro* chondrogenesis of bone marrow-derived mesenchymal progenitor cells. *Exp Cell Res* 238(1):265–72.

Kaigler, D., Krebsbach, P.H., West, E.R. et al. 2005. Endothelial cell modulation of bone marrow stromal cell osteogenic potential. *FASEB J* 19(6):665–67.

Kaigler, D., Wang, Z., Horger, K. et al. 2006. VEGF scaffolds enhance angiogenesis and bone regeneration in irradiated osseous defects. *J Bone Miner Res* 21(5):735–44.

Kassem, M., Abdallah, B.M., and Saeed, H. 2008. Osteoblastic cells: Differentiation and trans-differentiation. *Arch Biochem Biophys* 473(2):183–7.

Khademhosseini, A., Langer, R., Borenstein, J. et al. 2006. Microscale technologies for tissue engineering and biology. *Proc Natl Acad Sci USA* 103(8):2480–7.

Kim, H., Lee, J.H., and Suh, H. 2003. Interaction of mesenchymal stem cells and osteoblasts for *in vitro* osteogenesis. *Yonsei Med J* 44(2):187–97.

Kolf, C.M., Cho, E., and Tuan, R.S. 2007. Mesenchymal stromal cells. Biology of adult mesenchymal stem cells: Regulation of niche, self-renewal and differentiation. *Arthritis Res Ther* 9(1):204.

LaBarge, M.A., and Blau, H.M. 2002. Biological progression from adult bone marrow to mononucleate muscle stem cell to multinucleate muscle fiber in response to injury. *Cell* 111(4):589–601.

Lacombe-Gleize, S., Grégoire, M., Demignot, S. et al. 1995. Implication of TGF beta 1 in co-culture of chondrocytes-osteoblasts. *In Vitro Cell Dev Biol Anim* 31(9):649–52.

Lee, J.H., Kosinski, P.A., and Kemp, D.M. 2005. Contribution of human bone marrow stem cells to individual skeletal myotubes followed by myogenic gene activation. *Exp Cell Res* 307(1):174–82.

Lee, S.H., Miller, J.S., Moon, J.J. et al. 2005. Proteolytically degradable hydrogels with a fluorogenic substrate for studies of cellular proteolytic activity and migration. *Biotechnol Prog* 21(6):1736–41.

Lemare, F., Steinberg, N., Le Griel, C. et al. 1998. Dedifferentiated chondrocytes cultured in alginate beads: Restoration of the differentiated phenotype and of the metabolic responses to interleukin-1beta. *J Cell Physiol* 176(2):303–13.

Li, X., Lee, J.P., Balian, G. et al. 2005. Modulation of chondrocytic properties of fat-derived mesenchymal cells in co-cultures with nucleus pulposus. *Connect Tissue Res* 46(2):75–82.

Loewenstein, W.R. 1981. Junctional intercellular communication: The cell-to-cell membrane channel. *Physiol Rev* 61(4):829–913.

Lutolf, M.P. and Hubbell, J.A. 2005. Synthetic biomaterials as instructive extracellular microenvironments for morphogenesis in tissue engineering. *Nat Biotechnol* 23(1):47–55.

Lutolf, M.P., Lauer-Fields, J.L., Schmoekel, H.G. et al. 2003. Synthetic matrix metalloproteinase-sensitive hydrogels for the conduction of tissue regeneration: Engineering cell-invasion characteristics. *Proc Natl Acad Sci USA* 100(9):5413–8.

Mackay, A.M., Beck, S.C., Murphy, J.M. et al. 1999. Chondrogenic differentiation of cultured human mesenchymal stem cells from marrow. *Tissue Eng* 4(4):415–28.

Mann, B.K. and West, J.L. 2002. Cell adhesion peptides alter smooth muscle cell adhesion, proliferation, migration, and matrix protein synthesis on modified surfaces and in polymer scaffolds. *J Biomed Mater Res* 60(1):86–93.

Martinez-Agosto, J.A., Mikkola, H.K.A., Hartenstein, V. et al. 2007. The hematopoietic stem cell and its niche: A comparative view. *Genes Dev* 21(23):3044–60.

Maxson, S. and Burg, K.J. 2010. Conditioned media enhance osteogenic differentiation on Poly(ʟ-lactide-co-epsilon-caprolactone)/hydroxyapatite scaffolds and chondrogenic differentiation in alginate. *J Biomater Sci Polym Ed* 21(11):1441–58.

Meury, T., Verrier, S., and Alini, M. 2006. Human endothelial cells inhibit BMSC differentiation into mature osteoblasts *in vitro* by interfering with osterix expression. *J Cell Biochem* 98(4):992–1006.

Miljkovic, N.D., Cooper, G.M., and Marra, K.G. 2008. Chondrogenesis, bone morphogenetic protein-4 and mesenchymal stem cells. *Osteoarthr Cartil* 16(10):1121–30.

Mo, X.T., Guo, S.C., Xie, H.Q. et al. 2009. Variations in the ratios of co-cultured mesenchymal stem cells and chondrocytes regulate the expression of cartilaginous and osseous phenotype in alginate constructs. *Bone* 45(1):42–51.

Mohan, N., Nair, P.D., and Tabata, Y. 2010. Growth factor-mediated effects on chondrogenic differentiation of mesenchymal stem cells in 3D semi-IPN poly(vinyl alcohol)-poly(caprolactone) scaffolds. *J Biomed Mater Res A* 94(1):146–59.

Nagahata, M., Tsuchiya, T., Ishiguro, T. et al. 2004. A novel function of N-cadherin and Connexin43: Marked enhancement of alkaline phosphatase activity in rat calvarial osteoblast exposed to sulfated hyaluronan. *Biochem Biophys Res Commun* 315(3):603–11.

Nuttelman, C.R., Tripodi, M.C., and Anseth, K.S. 2005. Synthetic hydrogel niches that promote hMSC viability. *Matrix Biol* 24(3):208–18.

Ong, S.M., Zhang, C., Toh, Y.C. et al. 2008. A gel-free 3D microfluidic cell culture system. *Biomaterials* 29(22):3237–44.

Park, Y., Lutolf, M.P., Hubbell, J.A. et al. 2004. Bovine primary chondrocyte culture in synthetic matrix metalloproteinase-sensitive poly(ethylene glycol)-based hydrogels as a scaffold for cartilage repair. *Tissue Eng* 10(3–4):515–22.

Paxton, J.Z., Donnelly, K., Keatch, R.P. et al. 2009. Engineering the bone-ligament interface using polyethylene glycol diacrylate incorporated with hydroxyapatite. *Tissue Eng Part A* 15(6):1201–9.

Pelttari, K., Winter, A., Steck, E. et al. 2006. Premature induction of hypertrophy during *in vitro* chondrogenesis of human mesenchymal stem cells correlates with calcification and vascular invasion after ectopic transplantation in SCID mice. *Arthritis Rheum* 54(10):3254–66.

Philippou, A., Halapas, A., Maridaki, M. et al. 2007. Type I insulin-like growth factor receptor signaling in skeletal muscle regeneration and hypertrophy. *J Musculoskelet Neuronal Interact* 7(3):208–18.

Pittenger, M.F., Mackay, A.M., Beck, S.C. et al. 1999. Multilineage potential of adult human mesenchymal stem cells. *Science* 284(5411):143–7.

Porter, R.L. and Calvi, L.M. 2008. Communications between bone cells and hematopoietic stem cells. *Arch Biochem Biophys* 473(2):193–200.

Prockop, D.J. 1997. Marrow stromal cells as stem cells for nonhematopoietic tissues. *Science* 276(5309):71–4.

Quattrocelli, M., Cassano, M., Crippa, S. et al. 2010. Cell therapy strategies and improvements for muscular dystrophy. *Cell Death Differ* 17(8):1222–9.

Raeber, G.P., Lutolf, M.P., and Hubbell, J.A. 2005. Molecularly engineered PEG hydrogels: A novel model system for proteolytically mediated cell migration. *Biophys J* 89(2):1374–88.

Raimondi, M.T. 2006. Engineered tissue as a model to study cell and tissue function from a biophysical perspective. *Curr Drug Discov Technol* 3(4):245–68.

Richardson, S.M., Walker, R.V., Parker, S. et al. 2006. Intervertebral disc cell-mediated mesenchymal stem cell differentiation. *Stem Cells* 24(3):707–16.

Rouwkema, J., de Boer, J., and van Blitterswijk, C.A. 2006. Endothelial cells assemble into a 3-dimensional prevascular network in a bone tissue engineering construct. *Tissue Eng* 12(9):2685–93.

Rouwkema, J., Rivron, N.C., and van Blitterswijk, C.A. 2008. Vascularization in tissue engineering. *Trends Biotechnol* 26(8):434–41.

Rouwkema, J., Westerweel, P.E., de Boer, J. et al. 2009. The use of endothelial progenitor cells for prevascularized bone tissue engineering. *Tissue Eng Part A* 15(8):2015–27.

Saito, T., Dennis, J.E., Lennon, D.P. et al. 1995. Myogenic expression of mesenchymal stem cells within myotubes of mdx mice *in vitro* and *in vivo*. *Tissue Eng* 1(4):327–43.

Salinas, C.N. and Anseth, K.S. 2008. The enhancement of chondrogenic differentiation of human mesenchymal stem cells by enzymatically regulated RGD functionalities. *Biomaterials* 29(15):2370–7.

Santos, M.I. and Reis, R.L. 2010. Vascularization in bone tissue engineering: Physiology, current strategies, major hurdles and future challenges. *Macromol Biosci* 10(1):12–27.

Schiller, P.C., Mehta, P.P., Roos, B.A. et al. 1992. Hormonal regulation of intercellular communication: Parathyroid hormone increases connexin 43 gene expression and gap-junctional communication in osteoblastic cells. *Mol Endocrinol* 6(9):1433–40.

Seebach, C., Henrich, D., Kähling, C. et al. 2010. Endothelial progenitor cells and mesenchymal stem cells seeded onto beta-TCP granules enhance early vascularization and bone healing in a critical-sized bone defect in rats. *Tissue Eng Part A* 16(6):1961–70.

Shi, D., Reinecke, H., Murry, C.E. et al. 2004. Myogenic fusion of human bone marrow stromal cells, but not hematopoietic cells. *Blood* 104(1):290–94.

Takeichi, M. 1990. Cadherins: A molecular family important in selective cell-cell adhesion. *Annu Rev Biochem* 59:237–52.

Thompson, A.D., Betz, M.W., Yoon, D.M. et al. 2009. Osteogenic differentiation of bone marrow stromal cells induced by coculture with chondrocytes encapsulated in three-dimensional matrices. *Tissue Eng Part A* 15 (5):1181–90.

Thorp, B.H., Anderson, I., and Jakowlew, S.B. 1992. Transforming growth factor-beta 1, -beta 2 and -beta 3 in cartilage and bone cells during endochondral ossification in the chick. *Development* 114(4):907–11.

Tögel, F., Weiss, K., Yang, Y. et al. 2007. Vasculotropic, paracrine actions of infused mesenchymal stem cells are important to the recovery from acute kidney injury. *Am J Physiol Renal Physiol* 292(5):F1626–35.

Tsutsumi, S., Shimazu, A., Miyazaki, K. et al. 2001. Retention of multilineage differentiation potential of mesenchymal cells during proliferation in response to FGF. *Biochem Biophys Res Commun* 288(2):413–19.

Tuan, R.S., Boland, G., and Tuli, R. 2003. Adult mesenchymal stem cells and cell-based tissue engineering. *Arthritis Res Ther* 5(1):32–45.

Urban, J.P.G. and Roberts, S. 2003. Degeneration of the intervertebral disc. *Arthritis Res Ther* 5(3):120–30.

Varshney, R.R., Zhou, R., Hao, J. et al. 2010. Chondrogenesis of synovium-derived mesenchymal stem cells in gene-transferred co-culture system. *Biomaterials* 31(26):6876–91.

Vats, A., Bielby, R.C., Tolley, N. et al. 2006. Chondrogenic differentiation of human embryonic stem cells: The effect of the micro-environment. *Tissue Eng* 12(6):1687–97.

Walter, M.N.M., Wright, K.T., Fuller, H.R. et al. 2010. Mesenchymal stem cell-conditioned medium accelerates skin wound healing: An *in vitro* study of fibroblast and keratinocyte scratch assays. *Exp Cell Res* 316(7):1271–81.

Wang, Y., Volloch, V., Pindrus, M.A. et al. 2007. Murine osteoblasts regulate mesenchymal stem cells via WNT and cadherin pathways: Mechanism depends on cell-cell contact mode. *J Tissue Eng Regen Med* 1(1):39–50.

Wee, S. and Gombotz, W. 1998. Protein release from alginate matrices. *Adv Drug Deliv Rev* 31(3):267–285.

Wei, A., Chung, S.A., Tao, H. et al. 2009. Differentiation of rodent bone marrow mesenchymal stem cells into intervertebral disc-like cells following coculture with rat disc tissue. *Tissue Eng Part A* 15(9):2581–95.

Weiss, S., Hennig, T., Bock, R. et al. 2010. Impact of growth factors and PTHrP on early and late chondrogenic differentiation of human mesenchymal stem cells. *J Cell Physiol* 223(1):84–93.

Yang, H.N., Park, J.S., Na, K. et al. 2009. The use of green fluorescence gene (GFP)-modified rabbit mesenchymal stem cells (rMSCs) co-cultured with chondrocytes in hydrogel constructs to reveal the chondrogenesis of MSCs. *Biomaterials* 30(31):6374–85.

Yang, S., Leong, K.F., Du, Z. et al. 2001. The design of scaffolds for use in tissue engineering. Part I. Traditional factors. *Tissue Eng* 7(6):679–89.

Ying, Q.L., Nichols, J., Evans, E.P. et al. 2002. Changing potency by spontaneous fusion. *Nature* 416(6880):545–48.

Yoo, J.U., Barthel, T.S., Nishimura, K. et al. 1998. The chondrogenic potential of human bone-marrow-derived mesenchymal progenitor cells. *J Bone Joint Surg Am* 80(12):1745–57.

Zhang, W.M., Kapyla, J., Puranen, J.S. et al. 2003. alpha 11beta 1 integrin recognizes the GFOGER sequence in interstitial collagens. *J Biol Chem* 278(9):7270–7.

Zhang, Z., McCaffery, J.M., Spencer, R.G.S. et al. 2004. Hyaline cartilage engineered by chondrocytes in pellet culture: Histological, immunohistochemical and ultrastructural analysis in comparison with cartilage explants. *J Anat* 205(3):229–37.

Zhou, H., Mak, W., Zheng, Y. et al. 2008. Osteoblasts directly control lineage commitment of mesenchymal progenitor cells through Wnt signaling. *J Biol Chem* 283(4):1936–45.

Zhou, X.Z., Leung, V.Y., Dong, Q.R. et al. 2008. Mesenchymal stem cell-based repair of articular cartilage with polyglycolic acid-hydroxyapatite biphasic scaffold. *Int J Artif Organs* 31(6):480–489.

# 22

# Tissue Engineering Bioreactors

22.1 Introduction ...........................................................22-2
22.2 Overview of the Field .............................................22-3
 Micro-Bioreactors • Cardiac Tissue Engineering
 Bioreactors • Vascular Bioreactors • Bone Tissue Engineering
 Bioreactors • Cartilage Tissue Engineering Bioreactors • Tendon
 Tissue Engineering Bioreactors • Current Trends
22.3 Principles of Bioreactor Design .............................22-6
 General Requirements • Mass Transport
 Considerations • Biochemical and Mechanical Cues • Other Types
 of Bioreactors • Key Issues in Translating to the Clinic
22.4 Microscale Technologies ........................................22-9
 Structure and Organization of the Cellular Microenvironment •
 Composition of the Cellular Microenvironment • Flow
 Conditions • Applications • Microscale Culture of Human Liver
 Cells • Expansion of Hematopoietic Stem Cells
22.5 Cardiac Tissue Engineering Bioreactors ...............22-14
 Cardiac Tissue Requirements • Cardiac Tissue Engineering Bioreactor
 Design Strategies • Perfusion Seeding Bioreactors • Perfusion
 Culture Bioreactors • Mechanical Stimulation Bioreactors • Electrical
 Stimulation Bioreactors • Cardiac Tissue Engineering Bioreactor
 Limitations and Challenges
22.6 Vascular Bioreactors ...............................................22-17
 Key Requirements • Bioreactor Design • Limitations and
 Challenges
22.7 Bone Tissue Engineering Bioreactor .....................22-19
 Spinner Flask Bioreactor • Perfusion Bioreactors for Cylindrical
 Constructs • Perfusion Bioreactors for Anatomically Shaped
 Grafts • Other Bone Bioreactors • Limitations and Challenges
22.8 Cartilage Tissue Engineering Bioreactors .............22-22
 Cartilage Tissue Engineering Bioreactor Design Strategies • Static,
 Spinner Flask, and Rotating Wall Vessel Bioreactors • Perfusion
 Bioreactors • Mechanical Loading Bioreactors • Surface Shear
 Bioreactor • Limitations and Challenges
22.9 Tendon/Ligament Tissue Engineering Bioreactors ...22-25
 Tendon/Ligament Tissue Engineering Bioreactor Design
 Principles • Tendon and Ligament Tissue Engineering Bioreactor
 Limitations and Challenges
22.10 Summary and Challenges ......................................22-26
Acknowledgment ..............................................................22-27
References ..........................................................................22-27

Sarindr
Bhumiratana
*Columbia University*

Elisa Cimetta
*Columbia University*

Nina Tandon
*Columbia University*

Warren Grayson
*Johns Hopkins University*

Milica Radisic
*University of Toronto*

Gordana
Vunjak-Novakovic
*Columbia University*

## 22.1 Introduction

The term, "bioreactor," was originally coined to describe systems regulating the bioactive processes of unicellular microbial organisms. The groundwork for their development was laid in the nineteenth century by Louis Pasteur whose pioneering studies led to the understanding that the widely used fermentation process was due to the biological activity of yeast. As the fermentation process became understood and the parameters defined, well-developed chemical engineering approaches could be utilized to regulate the biological reactions and guide specific outcomes and the field of bioreactor design was born. The bioreactor approach has significantly impacted subsequent industrialized processes, particularly those related to pharmaceutics and food technology.

With the advent of tissue engineering over a century later (Langer and Vacanti 1993), bioreactors were again needed to provide precise control of the culture microenvironment and successfully guide the growth of cells in three-dimensional (3D) scaffold systems into viable tissues. In multicellular tissues, the complexity of cell–cell interactions makes it considerably more challenging to correlate the effect of experimental parameters with any single outcome measure of "functionality" in the resulting tissue. Indeed various general criteria (e.g., cell number and viability) and tissue-specific properties (e.g., spatial organization of cells and matrix, as well as mechanical, biological, and phenotypic properties) are evaluated to determine successful tissue-engineering outcomes. As a result, the design of tissue engineering bioreactors has evolved significantly over the last 20 years, yet the guiding principles remain unchanged.

Why are bioreactors used for tissue culture? Cells within the developing embryo respond to the presence of specific biological, mechanical, and physiological cues within their immediate micro-environment. These signals arise during gestation with spatial and temporal specificity and are critical for guiding the cellular organization and extracellular matrix (ECM) structures that define each of the tissues within the body. To recapitulate these developmental and morphological events *in vitro*, it is necessary to understand and characterize these native environments and translate them into experimental parameters. This has become known as the "biomimetic" principle, and it relies on the predictability of *global* cellular responses to specific stimuli (Grayson et al. 2009). That is, cells—the building blocks of tissues and organs—orchestrate their integration into a functional whole in response to biological and biophysical cues from the environment. Bioreactors are essential for mimicking these environments and providing cell-based constructs with physiologically relevant stimuli with spatio-temporal specificity to guide their conversion into functional tissue types.

The Petri dish, invented at the end of the nineteenth century, is among the most basic of cell culture tools. It has proven invaluable for enabling experiments to probe and understand aspects of cellular biology. However, with the advent of 3D culture methods in the late 1980s, it was soon realized that static cultivation methods provided by the Petri dish gave rise to undesirable inhomogeneities within the developing 3D constructs due to nonuniform availability of nutrients and gases to cells. This led to the development of the spinner flask (Cherry and Papoutsakis 1988), and was closely followed by the rotating wall vessels (RWV) in different geometries: the slow turning lateral vessels (STLV) (Schwarz et al. 1992) and the high-aspect ratio vessel (HARV) (Prewett et al. 1993). These first-generation bioreactors improved the transfer kinetics from the bulk medium to the surface of constructs and were useful for growing various tissue types. In particular, they were used to improve the cartilage grown from isolated chondrocytes (Freed and Vunjaknovakovic 1995; Freed et al. 1998; Vunjak-Novakovic et al. 1999), but were also adopted for bone (Ishaug et al. 1997) and cardiac muscle (Bursac et al. 1999; Carrier et al. 1999) with limited success.

It was soon noted for the cartilage tissue-engineering approaches that while the cellularity and distribution of matrix proteins improved significantly in the spinner flasks and RWVs, the mechanical properties of these cartilage constructs remained orders of magnitude lower than that needed for functioning in a normal joint. The concept of "functional tissue engineering" was therefore introduced in 2000 (Butler et al. 2000; Guilak et al. 2001) to emphasize this aspect of engineered constructs, that is, not only should the cells display the relevant phenotype and express the tissue specific proteins, but the resulting construct should possess the ability to provide the same functions as the native tissue it is intended to replace. In cartilage, this function is the absorption and distribution of compressive loads. Consequently, this led to the development of a new generation of bioreactors that utilized biophysical cues in the cultivation protocol to improve tissue structure and organization. Contemporary state-of-the-art bioreactors provide tissue-specific biophysical stimulation in addition to the relevant biological signals to induce *functional* tissue formation. The following sections provide an overview of the bioreactor field, which today also includes bioreactors for expansion of nonadherent cells (e.g., hematopoietic stem cells) as well as "micro-bioreactors," which can be used to provide high-throughput screening for multifactorial experiments, and describe the features common to all tissue-engineering bioreactors. Subsequently, their use as an enabling technology for growing improved tissue grafts and facilitating their use in regenerative medicine is presented in case studies for various tissues.

## 22.2 Overview of the Field

Tissues and organs in the body are subjected to complex biomechanical environments with dynamic stresses and strains, fluid flow, and electrical signals. These biophysical signals not only play a role in cell physiology *in vivo* but also modulate the activity of cells within engineered tissues cultured *in vitro*. Since the invention of the Petri dish, and the advent of 3D culture methods in the late 1980s, bioreactor design for functional tissue engineering purposes has made many strides towards providing cells with the appropriate tissue-specific biophysical cues and stimulation. Mammalian cells, which present demanding nutrient needs, along with high sensitivity to wastes and shear stresses, present significant challenges to bioreactor design (Freshney 2000). The exact requirements with respect to nutrients, waste elimination, shear stress, and biophysical cues, however, vary widely for different types of tissues. As described in the following sections, there is a great diversity in bioreactor designs that mirrors the range of environmental and regulatory signals that need to be provided to the cells to direct their differentiation into various lineages and assembly into engineered tissues. An overview of the current state of the art for various tissues is outlined in Table 22.1 and described in this section.

When reviewing the diverse range of bioreactors currently available, it is worth revisiting the notion of biocompatibility, which is an essential prerequisite for all bioreactor components that come in contact with the cells and culture medium. Analogous to biomaterials used for clinical applications, the materials used for bioreactor chambers, gas and medium exchange and contact instruments need to be as inert and neutral as possible, so that the cells and molecular factors in culture medium are not affected. In addition, however, components of bioreactors that deliver biophysical cues must also be able to retain their biocompatibility, as much as possible, as they perform their various tasks (e.g., platens used to provide compressive forces or electrodes, which impart electrical stimuli, must not corrode during cultivation).

### 22.2.1 Micro-Bioreactors

Micro-bioreactors refer to devices that employ microfluidic and micromachining techniques to provide bioactive control of multiple molecular and physical regulatory signals of cellular microenvironments (Table 22.1). Such "living cell arrays" can offer unique advantages, including the ability to decouple multiple elements of microenvironment, as well as the ability to introduce transients in both space and time. Micro-bioreactors therefore provide high-throughput platforms that allow screening for multifactorial experiments.

### 22.2.2 Cardiac Tissue Engineering Bioreactors

Cardiac tissue's high density, with its associated high metabolic demands, combined with its high sensitivity to shear stresses and electromechanical activity, has inspired various bioreactor designs. Perfusion

**TABLE 22.1** **(See color insert.)** Overview of Key Features for the Representative Bioreactor Systems Outlined in This Chapter

| Bioreactor Type | Key Features | Example System |
| --- | --- | --- |
| Micro-bioreactor | • Decoupled spatio-temporal control of soluble factors | • Hui et al., 2007 |
| | • Microscale control of tissue architecture | • Khetani et al., 2008 |
| | • Local control of soluble factors | • Lutolf et al., 2005 |
| | • Compatibility with integrated microdevices | • Gomez-Sjoberg et al., 2007 |
| | • High-throughput data acquisition | • Figallo et al., 2007 |
| Cardiac | • Increased cell density and uniformity via perfusion seeding | • Taylor et al., 2008 |
| | | • Maidhof et al., 2010 |
| | • Convective-diffusion oxygen supply | • Radisic et al., 2008 |
| | • Induction of synchronous electro-mechanical activity via: | |
| |   • Electrical stimulation, and/or | • Tandon et al., 2009 |
| |   • Cyclic mechanical stretch | • Eschenhagen et al., 2006 |
| Vascular | • Application of shear and radial strain via pulsatile flow | • Niklason et al., 2001 |
| | • Separated media compartments to support layered structure of vessel wall | • Gong et al., 2008 |
| | • Lengthened cultivation times for cellular differentiation | • McKee et al., 2003 |
| Bone | • Homogeneous cell distribution via perfusion | • Bancroft et al., 2002 |
| | • Application of physiologic flow/shear for enhanced matrix deposition | • Sikavitsas et al., 2003 |
| | • 3-dimensional support of geometrically-complex anatomically-shaped grafts | • Grayson et al., 2010 |
| | • Application of mechanical loading via: | |
| |   • Cyclic stretching, and/or | • Neiglinger-Wilke, 1994 |
| |   • Compression | • Orr and Burg, 2008 |
| Cartilage | • Application of physiologic shear via: | |
| |   • Spinner flasks | • Gooch et al., 2001 |
| |   • Rotating wall vessels | • Saini et al., 2003 |
| |   • Perfusion | • Razzano et al., 2000 |
| |   • Parallel plates | • Gemmiti et al., 2009 |
| | • Physiologic compression via: | |
| |   • Dynamic deformational loading, and/or | • Lima et al., 2006 |
| |   • Hydrostatic pressure | • Elder et al., 2009 |
| Tendon/Ligament | • Stretching stimulation on | |
| |   • MSCs-seeded collagen type I gel | • Altman et al., 2002 |
| |   • Fibroblasts-seeded collagen matrix | • Garvin et al., 2003 |
| |   • Tenocytes-seeded decellularized tendon | • Saber et al., 2010 |

bioreactors, for example, have been employed to not only enhance the density and uniformity of cell seeding, but also have been employed to enhance the mass transport and nutrient exchange. In these cases, channeled scaffolds have also been employed to decrease shear stresses experienced by cultured cells. Various groups have outfitted cardiac tissue engineering bioreactors with mechanical and/or electrical stimulation to enhance electro-mechanical coupling of engineered tissue (Table 22.1). Current challenges in this field include the need to further optimize cell culture regime, explore the simultaneous application of biophysical cues, as well as to improve the vascularization of implanted tissue.

## 22.2.3 Vascular Bioreactors

Blood vessels are characterized mainly by the mechanical properties of the vessel walls, which are comprised of both endothelial cells lining the luminal surface, as well as smooth muscle cells, providing the structure. Vascular tissue engineering bioreactors typically employ a two-chamber design, where the vessel itself acts as an interior "chamber" that facilitates intra-luminal pulsatile flow and an external reservoir is provided for the cultivation medium, which is continuously recirculated (Table 22.1). At the same time, the container surrounding the tissue graft is filled with appropriate culture medium specific for smooth-muscle-cell growth and matrix deposition. In this design, it is possible to grow the smooth muscle layer for an extended period of time to induce maturation prior to injecting endothelial cells, which only need to form a confluent monolayer. Additionally, by providing peristaltic flow through the vessel lumen, it is possible to induce shear stress-dependent responses from the endothelium as well as impart radial stresses to the smooth muscle.

## 22.2.4 Bone Tissue Engineering Bioreactors

Although linear straining and pressure loading correlate most closely to physiological conditions, perfusion of tissue-engineered bone has shown promising results in bone tissue formation and homogeneity of bone matrix. Recent advances aim at fabricating large clinical-size anatomical-shape bone grafts and incorporating perfusion together with the other stimuli such as compression to further enhance bone formation (Table 22.1).

## 22.2.5 Cartilage Tissue Engineering Bioreactors

Cartilage tissue is characterized by its high mechanical strength, low cell density, low oxygen tension, and its negatively charged, avascular and aneural ECM. The function of cartilage relies on matrix composition and its organization. To enhance the formation of cartilage, tissue-engineering bioreactors have employed several types of forces, including hydrostatic pressure, direct compression, and shear (Table 22.1).

## 22.2.6 Tendon Tissue Engineering Bioreactors

Like cartilage, tendon and ligaments sustain quite large *in vivo* stress, strain and torsion, possess lower cell densities than many other tissues, and are practically avascular, and aneural. Bioreactors for such tissue have employed stretching devices that apply physiologic strain, as well as provide traction and torsion (Table 22.1).

## 22.2.7 Current Trends

Part of the motivation behind bioreactor development has been to create greater correlation between *in vitro* studies and *in vivo* outcomes. To date, much progress has been made: engineered "biomimetic" environments are allowing cells to be measured and physically manipulated in unprecedented ways and are now replacing the simple but deficient environments of culture dishes. In recent years, trends in bioreactor design have involved both increases and decreases in scale, as well as certain supply-chain considerations. Micro-bioreactors, for example, with volumes of the order of micro- or even nanoliters are helping open new perspectives in studying cell biology and physiology as they allow experiments conducted at the characteristic time and length scales of biological processes.

Advances have also been made to engineer more clinically sized, and even anatomically shaped grafts, which would have tremendous potential for reconstructions after congenital defects, cancer resections, and trauma. With respect to supply-chain considerations, production-sized as well as disposable bioreactors have increasingly been incorporated into biotechnological facilities at all stages of development (Eibl et al. 2010). Going forward, we may expect these advances to bring us closer to success in delivering on the promise of a "one stop shop" of engineered tissues for the entire body.

## 22.3 Principles of Bioreactor Design

### 22.3.1 General Requirements

Tissue-engineering bioreactors are designed primarily to provide precise control of the cultivation environment. Several characteristics are essential irrespective of the specific bioreactor type or design requirements. These include:

1. *Maintenance of sterility*: bioreactors should be amenable to sterilization using traditional methods (autoclaving, ethylene oxide, gamma sterilization). In cases where seeding is performed prior to cultivation, it might be necessary to reassemble their presterilized bioreactor components in the tissue culture hood together with the preseeded construct. Therefore, assembly should be relatively simple so as not to compromise the integrity of the system. To aid in the maintenance of sterility throughout culture, it is useful to minimize the number of connecting parts as this reduces the potential for leaks. Likewise, various ports for seeding, medium changes or sampling, need to be carefully monitored as they provide a potential opening for microbial contaminants.

2. *Improved mass transfer to cells*: The aforementioned spinner flasks and RWVs transport nutrients from the bulk of the medium to the surface of constructs. Perfusion systems, and in some cases compression systems, aid in transporting oxygen and nutrients to the inner regions of scaffolds as well. Improving the convective transfer of nutrients to cells is critical for maintaining uniform cell survival throughout entire tissue constructs. This has become increasingly important as tissue engineers have attempted to grow constructs of larger sizes to facilitate their clinical relevance. For example, myocardial constructs as thick as 1 cm are required to match the thickness of the native ventricular wall and engineered bone as thick as 6 cm is required as the smaller fractures generally heal spontaneously. It is challenging to grow such large constructs *in vitro* in the absence of a vascular supply.

3. *Adequate gas exchange to the bulk culture media*: Cells are constantly using $O_2$ and producing $CO_2$. Hence, it is essential to either provide active gas exchange to the culture medium, or in cases where bioreactors are in a suitable incubator environment, enable sufficient surface area for passive gas exchange between the culture medium and the prevailing atmosphere. There has been an increasing interest in the use of hypoxic conditions for the growth of stem cells. This provides a unique challenge in bioreactors, especially when they have been designed to equilibrate with the prevailing atmosphere. For such systems, it will be necessary to have them air tight with precisely regulated gas exchange loops.

4. *Temperature/pH control*: Adequate gas transfer plays a crucial role in regulating the pH of the culture medium, which is generally buffered for specific $CO_2$ concentrations. For the control of temperature, many bioreactor systems are placed within tissue culture incubators and thus maintain the ambient temperature (37°C). However, certain systems are "stand alone" and here it is important to account for heat transfer throughout the system so that cells are cultured at physiologically relevant temperatures.

5. *Replenishment of spent medium*: Bioreactors are equipped with a reservoir for medium, which may be together with or separate from the engineered constructs (or both, as in the case of vascular tissue engineering). For long-term culture, it is essential to enable the full or partial replacement of this medium using techniques that do not compromise the sterility of the system. Some bioreactor designs enable regular cell culture methods for changing medium, that is, transfer of the bioreactor to the biological hood. Bulkier systems, which cannot be easily transported to and from, may require ports for removal and replacement of culture medium.

6. *Physiological stimuli*: The type of physiological cues provided to the cells is tissue specific. However, in general, it has been realized that when physiological signals are coupled with biological factors, they work synergistically to improve construct functionality. Bioreactors may be designed to enable mechanical stimulation of tissues (compression, tension, torsion, shear-stress) or to provide specific physiological environments, such as electrical stimulation or hypoxia.

## 22.3.2 Mass Transport Considerations

Cells grown in monolayer all have equal access to oxygen and nutrients present within the culture medium. In contrast, when cells are grown in 3D scaffolds under "static" conditions, the cells in the inner regions depend on diffusion kinetics both for receiving nutrients as well as the removal of metabolic waste products. The cells on the outer regions of the constructs, which have adequate nutrient and oxygen availability, proliferate and express ECM typically form a dense outer shell of material. As such, cells in the inner regions become nutrient deprived and there are theoretical limits to the sizes of constructs that can be cultured statically, beyond which considerable cell death takes place in the central regions of the scaffolds. Bioreactors are required to grow larger constructs and achieve uniform cell viability by improving the transport of nutrients, oxygen, and regulatory molecules to the cells. Mass transfer from the bulk medium to the tissue surfaces is determined mainly by the hydrodynamic conditions in the bioreactor system, whereas both diffusion and convection (due to medium perfusion or mechanically induced scaffold deformation) regulate the transport of nutrients to cells in the inner regions.

Oxygen is generally considered more limiting than glucose and other nutrients due to its extremely low solubility in aqueous media. Hence, emphasis is generally placed on enhancing oxygen availability to cells. Oxygen concentrations in fully oxygenated culture medium at 37°C may get up to 220 μM, while the total oxygen concentration in oxyhemoglobin can reach levels as high as 8600 μM. Therefore, oxygen transfer may become limiting even in conventional monolayer tissue culture where the only barriers are the diffusion limitations through the depth of culture medium (Randers-Eichorn et al. 1996). In native tissues, the diffusional penetration depth of oxygen is in the range of 100–200 μm (Muschler et al. 2004). This is highly restrictive for growing clinically relevant sizes of tissue constructs. Thus, a major aim of tissue engineering bioreactors is to improve mass transfer of oxygen. Traditional methods of improving convection might be used to improve transfer of oxygen to the tissue surfaces. However, internal mass transfer mechanisms should reflect the particular characteristics and functions of the tissue. For example, perfusion culture works well for bone tissue where cells respond positively to shear stress. However, in cardiac constructs, perfusion may be detrimental at high flow rates, since cardiomyocytes have low tolerance for shear forces. The particular considerations for individual tissues will be discussed in more detail in the following case study sections.

## 22.3.3 Biochemical and Mechanical Cues

The biophysical cues to which tissues are exposed during development and postnatally influence their structure and organization, and ultimately, their function. Bioreactors can be custom-designed to impart these biophysical stimuli to developing tissue constructs and guide the cell–cell interactions that result in hierarchical tissue organization. Current designs may incorporate mechanical and/or electrical stimuli in order to exert greater influence over cellular differentiation (Vunjak-Novakovic et al. 1996) and development into functional tissue constructs. For example, compressive strains have been used to induce matrix organization in developing cartilage (Mauck et al. 2000; Mauck et al. 2003; Hung et al. 2004; Lima et al. 2007), shear-stress enhanced matrix deposition and calcification in engineered bone constructs (Bancroft et al. 2002; Sikavitsas et al. 2003; Grayson et al. 2008), tensile stresses stimulated fibroblastic differentiation of stem cells in engineered ligaments (Altman et al. 2002; Vunjak-Novakovic et al. 2004) as well as cardiomyocyte organization in cardiac muscle constructs (Fink et al. 2000; Zimmermann et al.

2002, 2006), radial stresses regulate smooth muscle cell organization and differentiation in vascular grafts (Niklason et al. 1999), and electrical stimulation enhances cell–cell contacts along with tissue structure and organization in engineered myocardium (Radisic et al. 2004; Tandon et al. 2009). Interestingly, in liver organization, it is the spatial orientation of the various cellular phenotypes that strongly influences its function (Albrecht et al. 2006). Bioreactor designs for all of these tissues are described in greater detail in the latter portions of this chapter.

### 22.3.4  Other Types of Bioreactors

The previous sections have described bioreactors used to engineer functional tissue constructs. However, other types of bioreactors are being utilized in the field of regenerative medicine. Two other classes of bioreactors relevant to our objectives are cell expansion bioreactors and micro-bioreactors used to screen parameters and facilitate high-throughput assays. A major consideration in stem cell-based regenerative medicine approaches is that billions of cells are required for effective treatments. Therefore, cell expansion bioreactors have been developed for both adherent mesenchymal stem cell (MSC) populations (Zhao and Ma 2005) as well as nonadherent hematopoietic stem cells (Zandstra et al. 1994) and MSC populations (Baksh et al. 2003). The unique aspect of these cases is that, unlike the bioreactors for engineered tissues, the key consideration is expanding the cells in their *undifferentiated* states. Micro-bioreactors are a relatively new addition to the family of bioreactors. They are so called because they make use of various micro-scale technologies to culture minute quantities of cells and assay specific phenotypic responses. The advantage of this technology is that the small sizes enable multifactorial analysis for testing specific growth factor combinations where the cost would otherwise be prohibitive using conventional technologies.

### 22.3.5  Key Issues in Translating to the Clinic

Bioreactors have been used predominantly to address fundamental scientific questions regarding cellular and molecular processes. However, a primary concern facing the field of tissue engineering two decades after its inception is the limited number of engineered constructs that have been translated to the clinic. If bioreactors are to play a major role in bridging the gap, there are still a number of issues that must be addressed. For example, a prerequisite for clinical products is that the tissues should be engineered with a high degree of reproducibility. To facilitate this, it may be necessary to have the process as fully automated as possible to minimize operator variability. This may require extensive use of sensor-based technologies to noninvasively monitor biochemical characteristics of the tissue and ensure minimum levels of maturation prior to harvesting (Martin et al. 2009). Additionally, or as an alternative, sample ports may be included so that various readouts could be obtained throughout culture as a form of quality control.

Quality control may also be enhanced by improving the imaging capabilities, that is, bioreactor design may have to account for the ability to noninvasively monitor the construct maturation during cultivation. Hence, the choice of materials may need to be compatible with various imaging modalities including NMR (Petersen et al. 2000; Seagle et al. 2008), MRI (Ramaswamy et al. 2009), CT ($\mu$CT) (Porter et al. 2007), and two-photon second-harmonic generation imaging (Niklason et al. 2010). Another nontrivial aspect is ensuring that the bioreactors surpass GMP standards. For this reason, single-use bioreactors, or systems where the key components required to maintain sterility are disposable, may be more practical alternatives as opposed to the reusable systems typically employed for scientific studies (Glindkamp et al. 2009).

A novel aspect of bioreactor application that is currently under consideration is the use of bioreactors as "shipping containers." That is, small, portable, battery-operated, stand-alone units capable of maintaining all key design aspects (temperature/pH control, sterility, mass transfer and physiological stimulation) over relatively short periods of time (1–2 days) to facilitate the shipment of viable tissue grafts. This would considerably improve the versatility of this approach by ameliorating the practical constraints imposed by geography and the need for technical expertise in each clinical center.

# 22.4 Microscale Technologies

It is now evident how living cell-arrays can offer unique advantages when used as the sensing element for a multiplicity of biological applications such as: drug development and differentiation studies (Flaim et al. 2005), studying tissues and diseases physiology in a controlled environment (Baar 2005) and for basic studies on tissue development and cell functions in response to genetic alterations, drugs, and physiological stimuli (Gerecht-Nir et al. 2006). From this perspective, it is becoming increasingly clear that cells are extremely sensitive to their local environments in terms of chemistry, physics and topography, on scales that differ from the sole "macro" level (Stevens and George 2005). The complexity of cellular functions and their responses to internal events and environmental perturbations or stimuli, develop in both time and space on scales characteristically spanning over several orders of magnitude (Cervinka et al. 2008; Jamshidi and Palsson 2008). Regarding scaling to the biologically relevant lengths and time scales, the conventional methodologies of the so-called "flat biology" fail, being scarcely representative of the real state of physiologic systems. Standard culture systems are typically dominated by intrinsically uncontrollable diffusive transport phenomena, thus giving rise to scarcely predictable spatial–temporal combinations of different soluble factors or and cell–cell interactions and therefore may result in unrealistic and uncontrollable biological readouts.

Taken together, these observations lead to the impelling necessity of developing novel tools capable of providing an active control over the cell microenvironment and the processes that regulate cell biology and physiology also at the microscale (Folch and Toner 2000; Kaplan et al. 2005; Albrecht et al. 2006; Jang and Schaffer 2006; Khademhosseini et al. 2006). The main aim of microscale technologies is to gain bioactive control of the microenvironment (Lutolf and Hubbel 2005; Dellatore et al. 2008), while providing more insight into the actual functionality and requirements of tissues or biological systems in general. Another advantage of microscale technologies is the possibility of acquiring vast amounts of information, thus facilitating the high-throughput characteristics of these systems.

Microscale technologies allow for a more accurate control of cell cultures both concerning the soluble (fluid compartment) and the structural components (cell adhesion, organized architecture and co-cultures, substrate development, etc.) constituting the cell microenvironment. We will now briefly review some of the most important characteristic and key components that lead to the development of micro-bioreactor, the ultimate product obtained integrating multiple microscale technologies, combining and exploiting all the above listed advantages.

## 22.4.1 Structure and Organization of the Cellular Microenvironment

Cells can be guided to adhere onto specifically developed substrates with the desired physical properties using patterning techniques (Xia and Whitesides 1998; Falconnet et al. 2006). These methods have long been used to study the effects of geometry, spatial organization and interaction with the surrounding materials on cell fate (Figure 22.1a). Microscale technologies allow exploring the underlying mechanisms through which the local microenvironment regulates cell behavior including cell migration, proliferation, differentiation (Figure 22.1b), and apoptosis (Chen et al. 1997; Discher et al. 2005; Engler et al. 2006; Guilak et al. 2009; Gao et al. 2010).

## 22.4.2 Composition of the Cellular Microenvironment

The soluble microenvironment is typically controlled via micromanipulations of fluid motion and composition in a discipline known as "microfluidics." A microfluidic device is essentially comprised of the same main components of the above-described bioreactors, and adhere to the same basic requirements;

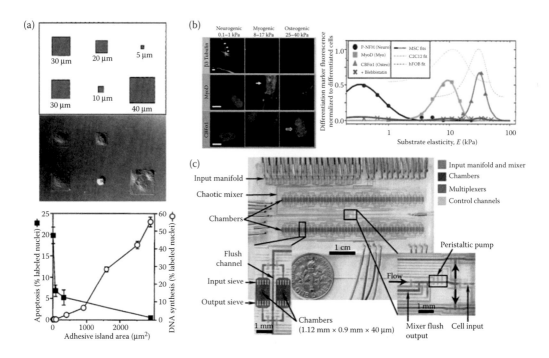

**FIGURE 22.1** (**See color insert.**) Substrate geometry and stiffness influence cell responses. (a) Effect of spreading on cell growth and apoptosis. Schematic diagram showing the initial pattern design containing different-sized square adhesive islands and images of the final shapes of bovine endothelial cells adherent to the fabricated substrate. Distances indicate lengths of the square's sides. The graph plots the apoptotic index and DNA synthesis index after 24 h, plotted as a function of the projected cell area. Data were obtained only from islands that contained single adherent cells; similar results were obtained with circular or square islands and with human or bovine endothelial cells. (From Chen, C. S. et al. 1997. *Science* **276**: 1425–28.) (b) Protein and transcript profiles are elasticity dependent under identical media conditions. The neuronal cytoskeletal marker b3 tubulin is expressed in branches (arrows) of initially naive MSCs (>75%) and only on the soft, neurogenic matrices. The muscle transcription factor MyoD1 is upregulated and nuclear localized (arrow) only in MSCs on myogenic matrices. The osteoblast transcription factor CBFa1 (arrow) is likewise expressed only on stiff, osteogenic gels. Scale bar is 5 µm. The graph represents fluorescent intensity of differentiation markers versus substrate elasticity, revealing maximal lineage specification at the E typical of each tissue type. (From Engler, A. J. et al. 2006. *Cell* **126**: 677–89.) Panel (c) Design of an integrated cell culture chip. Annotated photograph of a chip with the channels filled with colored water to indicate different parts of the device. The left inset gives a closer view of two culture chambers, with the multiplexer flush channel in between them. The right inset shows the root of the input multiplexer, with the peristaltic pump, a waste output for flushing the mixer, and the cell input line. (From Gomez-Sjoberg, R. et al. 2007. *Anal Chem* **79**: 8557–63.)

the overall dimensions of the systems, however, scale down, leading to micrometer–millimeter scale culture chambers and fluidic channels. At the relevant scale for micro-flows inside the micro-channels and culture chambers of microfluidic devices, the physics of fluids differ from the most known, macro-scale ones (Stone and Kim 2001; Beebe et al. 2002; Squires and Quake 2005; Whitesides 2006).

## 22.4.3 Flow Conditions

The first and most common feature of microfluidic devices is the fact that flow is always laminar (Reynolds numbers are well below the turbulence threshold, and in most cases Re < 10), the inertial forces are therefore dominated by viscous forces, and the transport is dominated by molecular diffusion or by convective regime of well-defined hydrodynamic profile. The laminar flow profile and exclusion of the nonlinearities and turbulence carried by inertia allow for precise calculation of mass transport and of the convective flow profiles as a function of channel geometry, pressure drops or flow rates and of the fluid properties. In addition, due to the very short transport distances, which are in turn associated with shorter time constants, biological responses are not limited by the slow kinetics of physical phenomena. As in laminar flows the streamlines remain constant over time and mixing occurs primarily by diffusion, the feasible control over the operating parameters allows a precise and localized application as well as spatially and temporally dynamic perturbations. The design principles for microscale bioreactors and microfluidic platforms must thus take into account all these phenomena, and the respect of the biological constraints dictated by the cell samples under analysis (Cimetta et al. 2009).

## 22.4.4 Applications

Since its first appearance decades ago, microfluidics has been adapted to a multiplicity of studies. Microscale technologies were designed for applications ranging from studies at a single cell level (DiCarlo et al. 2006) to the recreation of more complex 3D structures (Chiu et al. 2000; Gottwald et al. 2007; Kim et al. 2007), the development of diagnostics platforms (Toner and Irimia 2005; Linder 2007) and studies on human embryonic stem cells (Figallo et al. 2007; Zhong et al. 2008). Microfluidics has been adopted also for tissue engineering purposes, and examples exist in applications involving basal lamina, vascular tissue, liver, bone, cartilage and neurons (Andersson and van den Berg 2004). Finally, high-tech platforms involving integrated microdevices such as micro-valves, injectors, pumps, or mixers (Gomez-Sjoberg et al. 2007; Melin and Quake 2007) are also being used in live cell experimentation, fully proving the strength and efficacy of the concept of "lab-on-a-chip" (Figure 22.1c).

## 22.4.5 Microscale Culture of Human Liver Cells

Sangeeta Bhatia and collaborators have developed a miniaturized, multiwell culture system for culturing human liver cells with optimized microscale architecture that maintains phenotypic functions for several weeks (Khetani and Bhatia 2008) (Figure 22.2). With a microtechnology-based process incorporating soft lithography with reusable, elastomeric stencils of microfabricated structures, they have been able to study the effects of cell physiology when primary human hepatocytes (and other liver cells) adhered to patterned collagen islands of different diameters and in the condition of pure cultures or coculture (Figure 22.2a). After proving that hepatocyte clustering improved liver-specific functions compared with unorganized cultures, they validated their system for high-throughput toxicity screening, by successfully quantifying the acute and chronic toxicity of model hepatotoxins (Figure 22.2b,c). The combination of microtechnology and tissue engineering is thus enabling the development of integrated tissue models in form of a "human on a chip," with potential application in pharmacological screening and assessment of drug-induced liver toxicity.

Under a more conventional tissue engineering approach, but still at the microscale, Bhatia's group cultured three-dimensional photopatterned densely cellularized constructs in a continuous flow bioreactor, where they performed favorably in comparison to unpatterned, unperfused constructs (Tsang et al. 2007). Aware of the high metabolic rate of hepatocytes, they developed a system overcoming the limitations of diffusive transport that is only sufficient over short length scales. To do so, they fabricated a multilayer hepatic construct consisting of a three-layered hexagonal branching structure that minimize transport limitations, and mimic the branching architecture of the liver *in vivo*. When transferred to a perfusion bioreactor, the channels created in the multilayer structure allowed for convective flow of culture medium and relatively short distance for diffusive transport to all encapsulated cells. The levels of function achieved in the patterned, perfused constructs can be attributed to a combination of microenvironmental factors, including cell–cell interactions, adhesive peptides and improved nutrient transport. An interplay between improved microscale tissue architecture allowing

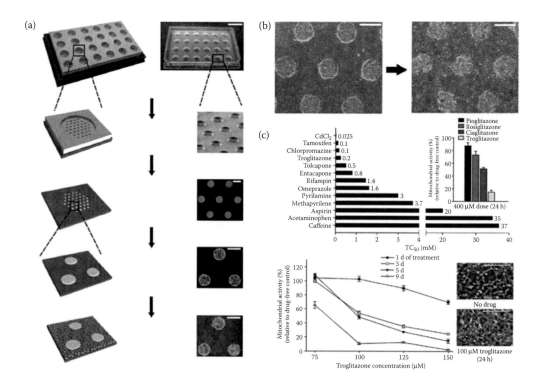

**FIGURE 22.2** (**See color insert.**) Micropatterned cell co-culture maintains hepatocyte function. (a) Schematic representations and photomicrographs of the steps of the soft lithographic process to fabricate microscale liver hepatocyte cultures in a multiwell format. A reusable PDMS stencil consists of membranes with through-holes at the bottom of each well in a 24-well mold. Each well is incubated with a solution of ECM protein to allow protein to selectively adsorb to the substrate via the through-holes (fluorescently labeled collagen pattern). Primary hepatocytes selectively adhere to matrix-coated domains, allowing supportive stromal cells to be seeded into the remaining bare areas (hepatocytes labeled green and fibroblasts orange; scale bar is 500 μm). (b) Phase-contrast micrographs of micropatterned co-cultures. Primary human hepatocytes are spatially arranged in 500 μm collagen coated islands with 1200 μm center-to-center spacing, surrounded by 3T3-J2 fibroblasts. Images depict pattern fidelity over several weeks of culture. Scale bars, 500 μm. (c) Cellular response to exposure to hepatotoxins by TC50; (Top) shows the rank ordering of the compounds tested. Inset classifies relative toxicity of structurally related PPARg agonists in the thiazolidinediones class (24 h exposure at 400 mM). (Bottom) proves the time and dose-dependent chronic toxicity of Troglitazone in micropatterned cocultures (2–3 weeks old) dosed repeatedly every 48 h. Phase-contrast micrographs show human hepatocyte morphology under untreated conditions and after treatment with 100 mM of Troglitazone for 24 h (scale bars are 100 μm).

cell organization into higher hierarchical 3D structures and the use of perfusion bioreactors matching the tissues metabolical demand, will enable the investigation of fundamental structure/function relationships in a 3D tissue context.

## 22.4.6 Expansion of Hematopoietic Stem Cells

The clinical potential of umbilical cord blood-derived stem and progenitor cells has been demonstrated, but the development and success of these therapies is limited by the need for increased cell numbers. *Ex vivo* expansion has been widely studied as a method to overcome this limitation. To be effective, cell therapy bioprocess design and optimization needs to incorporate a few basic criteria (Kirouac and Zandstra 2008): (i) assessment of relevant cell properties; (ii) measurement and control of key parameters; (iii) robust predictive strategies for interrogating and evaluating the many parameters that may

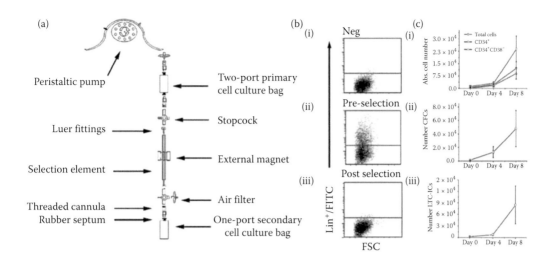

**FIGURE 22.3** Perfusion bioreactor for expansion of hematopoietic stem cells. (a) Schematic representation of the closed system bioprocess consisting of two cell culture bags joined through a subpopulation selection element removing contaminating lin+ cells from culture. A peristaltic pump controls the flow rate of cells. (b) Validation of the subpopulation selection element. Representative flow cytometric plots show the amount of lin+ cells present (ii) before and (iii) after selection. (i) The negative control was not labeled with the anti-lin+ antibody. (c) Kinetic analysis of the absolute numbers of hematopoietic cells generated and recovered from the bioprocess over the 8-day culture period. Purified UCB lin− cells ($1 \times 10^5$ cells/mL) were cultured for 8 days with subpopulation selection and media dilution/exchange at day 4. Kinetic growth profiles for (i) total cell, CD34+ cells, and CD34+ CD38− cells, (ii) colony-forming cells (CFCs), and (iii) long-term culture-initiating cells (LTC-ICs).

impact the culture output; and (iv) approaches to test such parameters in a high-throughput and scale-relevant manner. Madlambayan et al. (2006) describe a clinically relevant single-use, closed-system bioprocess capable of generating greater numbers of hematopoietic stem and progenitor cells that maintain *in vivo* and *in vitro* developmental potential. The bioreactor consists of two gas-permeable cell culture bags and a subpopulation selection element, responsible for removing lin+ cells from culture (Figure 22.3a) The design is modular such that each component can be separated without exposing cell contacting areas to environmental contaminants.

Isolated lin− cells from umbilical cord blood (UCB) were injected into the primary cell culture bag (of appropriate volume) through the free self-sealing rubber septum by using a sterile syringe attached to a threaded cannula. The bioreactor was then maintained at 37°C in a humidified atmosphere of 5% $CO_2$ in air. Subpopulation selection and media dilution/exchange were performed at day 4. Flow cytometric analysis confirmed that the subpopulation selection element was capable of efficiently removing lin+ cells from cultured cells (Figure 22.3b) without significant cell loss. This process was flow rate-dependent and a peristaltic pump was used to establish flow rates of 0.45–1.3 mL/min. All flow rates tested yielded high levels of lin− cell purity and proved that increasing flow rate significantly decreased nonspecific cell loss through the selection element.

UCB lin− cells were subjected to 8-day cultures and exposed to subpopulation selection and media dilution/exchange at day 4 to control the production of endogenous negative regulators. Input cell densities were $1 \times 105$ cells/mL, resulting in a range of culture volumes between 2.3 and 24.5 mL. Overall, the bioprocess yielded average expansions of 24.6 ± 3.6, 30.8 ± 7.2, 105.5 ± 31.6, 31.3 ± 5.8, and 32.6 ± 7.5 for total cells, CD34+ cells, CD34+ CD38− cells, CFCs, and LTC-ICs, respectively (Figure 22.3c). The authors quantitatively demonstrate that 3.3-fold more LT-SRCs were generated.

Importantly, the bioprocess-generated LT-SRCs maintained their engraftment potency, on a per-LT-SRC basis, in comparison with noncultured cells and were capable of multilineage engraftment.

In addition, cells maintained their long-term engraftment potential *in vivo* as shown by their ability to repopulate secondary recipients. By increasing cellular flow rate through the selection element, the authors eliminate nonspecific cell loss, increasing overall lin– cell recovery without decreasing purity. This may be explained by the decreased residence time of cells within the subpopulation selection element, preventing cells from contacting nonspecific binding sites. The modularity of the bioprocess may be useful to address some of this sample heterogeneity because culture volumes, medium supplementation, and other bioprocesses parameters can be modified without compromising the closed culture conditions. The bioprocess is a single-use system, which makes it attractive for clinical applications because the risk of cell contamination due to repeated use is removed.

## 22.5 Cardiac Tissue Engineering Bioreactors

Cardiac tissue engineering aims to create functional tissue constructs that can either reestablish the structure and function of injured myocardium, or serve as high-fidelity models for studies of cardiac development and disease. Cardiac tissue is a highly dense, metabolically active tissue performing high amounts of mechanical work with each heartbeat. Bioreactors implemented for engineering functional cardiac tissue must therefore be able to meet the design constraints imposed by these requirements, and various strategies, including perfusion seeding and culture, as well as the application of biophysical cues (including electrical and/or mechanical) have been successfully implemented by various groups in recent years.

### 22.5.1 Cardiac Tissue Requirements

Much effort has been made in recent years to tailor the bioreactor design principles outlined above to the specific requirements of cardiac tissue. The heart itself is an organ of marvelous structural and functional complexity: it is a highly dense tissue with high metabolic demands, it consumes large amounts of oxygen but with low tolerance to hypoxia, and it forms a three-dimensional synctium coordinating electrical and mechanical activity. The three key features of native myocardium: (i) high density of myocytes and supporting cells, (ii) convective–diffusive oxygen supply, and (iii) synchronous electro-mechanical activity, form a set of design requirements for engineering cardiac tissue (see Figure 22.4).

### 22.5.2 Cardiac Tissue Engineering Bioreactor Design Strategies

The design requirements imposed by cardiac tissue density, metabolic demands, and electromechanical activity, have inspired various bioreactor strategies. More particularly, perfusion seeding strategies have helped address the need to engineer tissues highly packed with cells, they have improved mass transport and nutrient exchange, and the incorporation of electrical and mechanical stimulation into bioreactors has resulted in more highly organized tissue.

### 22.5.3 Perfusion Seeding Bioreactors

Taylor and colleagues have recently developed a perfusion system allowing for the preparation of native decellularized ECM scaffolds supporting high densities of cells, as well as the recellularization of these scaffolds (Figure 22.4a) (Ott et al. 2008). First, they utilized a modified Langendorff apparatus to perform coronary perfusion of cadaveric rat hearts with detergents, which removed cells while preserving the underlying ECM, and producing an acellular, perfusable vascular architecture, with intact chamber geometry. For reseeding these constructs with cells, they developed a bioreactor system in which they mounted recellularized whole rat hearts by cannulating the left atrium and ascending aorta to provide coronary perfusion. They were able to generate preparations that produced macroscopic contractions, as well as some pumping function.

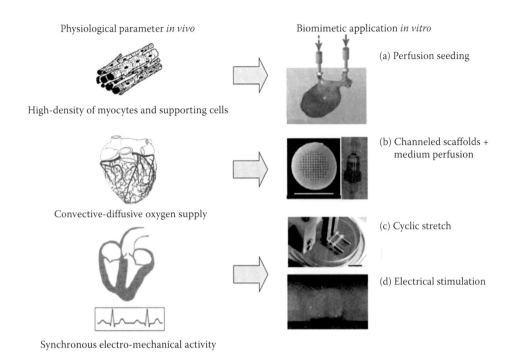

**FIGURE 22.4** (**See color insert.**) Biomimetic paradigm for cardiac tissue engineering bioreactors. Important cardiac physiological parameters (e.g., high density of tissue, convective–diffusive oxygen supply, and electro-mechanical coupling) are emulated for *in vitro* application via bioreactors. Example bioreactor systems incorporating these parameters are shown to the right. (a) Schematic of working heart bioreactor showing cannulation of left atrium and ascending aorta in order to repopulate decellularized rat hearts with neonatal cardiac cells. (b) Left: Light image of channeled PGS scaffold (channels 250 μm diameter, 250 μm wall-to-wall spacing, space bar indicates 10 mm). Right: A perfusion bioreactor for cultivation of cardiac tissue constructs under culture medium flow, in which the chamber is connected to inlet/outlet extension tubing. (c) Close-up view of ring-shaped engineered cardiac tissue constructs placed in a bioreactor employing a stretch apparatus that applies unidirectional cyclic stretch. (d) Close-up view of rectangular-shaped engineered cardiac tissue construct positioned in a bioreactor between two carbon rod electrodes that apply pulsatile electrical field stimulation (scale bar corresponds to 3 mm).

In our laboratory, we have developed perfusion bioreactors that allow rapid cell inoculation into scaffolds using forward–reverse flow (Radisic et al. 2008; Maidhof et al. 2010) (Figure 22.4b). The design of the perfusion bioreactor consists of perfusion loops comprised of tubing and perfusion cartridges (outfitted with silicone gaskets made from silicone tubing to hold scaffolds in place), maintained inside a cell culture incubator and connected to a peristaltic pump. During cell inoculation, we applied forward–reverse flow for an initial period of 1.5–4.5 h to increase the spatial uniformity of cell seeding. When applied to seeding of channeled scaffolds with neonatal rat cardiac myocytes, these conditions resulted in high efficiency (77.2% ± 23.7%) of cell seeding, and highly uniform spatial cell distributions.

## 22.5.4 Perfusion Culture Bioreactors

In addition to requiring high amounts of oxygen, in native heart muscle blood is confined within the capillary bed and is not in direct contact with cardiac myocytes, which are highly sensitive to shear stress. When designing perfusion bioreactors, therefore, the two most important parameters that we attempt to control during cultivation are oxygen supply and shear stress experienced by the cells. Overall, as the culture medium flow rate increases, so does the supply of oxygen and nutrients; however, the shear stress, which may have detrimental effects on heart cells, increases as well. In the native heart, cardiomyocytes are shielded from direct contact with blood by endothelial cells. Low values of shear stress may induce phenotypic changes in cardiac cells, including elongation. However, higher values (e.g., >2.4 dyn/cm$^2$) have detrimental effects on cardiac cells including de-differentiation, cell death, and apoptosis.

In order to reduce the exposure of cardiac myocytes to hydrodynamic shear, we have designed porous elastomer scaffolds of poly(glycerol sebacate) with arrays of channels providing a separate compartment for medium flow (Maidhof et al. 2010) (Radisic et al. 2008) (Figure 22.4b). Culture conditions are also modified by stacking scaffolds two at a time so as to "block" medium flow through channels during seeding, and subsequently separating them (so as to reveal channels) to be cultured individually (Maidhof et al. 2010).

When cultured under these conditions, after only 3 days, constructs were observed to contract synchronously in response to electrical stimulation, while channels remained open, and improved construct properties were correlated with the enhanced supply of oxygen to the cells. Notably, the final cell viability in perfused constructs cultured for 8 days was indistinguishable from the viability of the freshly isolated cells and markedly higher than the cell viability in dish-grown constructs.

## 22.5.5  Mechanical Stimulation Bioreactors

Eschenhagen and Zimmermann and colleagues hypothesized that the application of passive force in addition to active force via bioreactors could improve cell alignment and differentiation of cardiac cells (Figure 22.4c) (Fink et al. 2000; Zimmermann et al. 2002, 2006). They built bioreactors for the cultivation of neonatal rat heart cells in collagen gel and Matrigel, with the application of mechanical stretch which could accommodate five loop-shaped constructs as they fused to form a single synchronously contracting multiloop construct of ~15 mm diameter and thickness of 1–4 mm. The approach developed by Eschenhagen and colleagues has shown, in a rigorous and convincing way, that immature cardiac cell populations have remarkable ability to assemble into cardiac constructs, if subjected to mechanical signals during cultivation. Furthermore, when these constructs were grafted onto infarcted hearts, they attenuated pathological remodeling and improved the diastolic and systolic function of the heart in comparison to the untreated infarcted rat hearts.

## 22.5.6  Electrical Stimulation Bioreactors

In native heart, mechanical stretch is induced by electrical signals, and the orderly coupling between electrical pacing signals and macroscopic contractions is crucial for the development and function of native myocardium. In order to deliver electrical signals inducing synchronous contractions in cultured constructs, we designed a custom bioreactor delivering signals mimicking those in native heart (Radisic et al. 2004; Tandon et al. 2009) (Figure 22.4d). This bioreactor had several design requirements, including the maintenance of a constant position of the scaffolds with respect to direction of the electrical field gradient, while neither restricting the contractions of cells nor the ability to observe the constructs with a microscope. The bioreactor was composed of carbon rod electrodes placed lengthwise along the bottom of a Petri dish and held in place by silicone adhesive. The spacing between the electrodes accommodates the width of the constructs. The wires dangle free so as to facilitate making detachable electrical connections, which is necessary to change medium and monitor the cells in culture.

When cardiac constructs prepared by seeding neonatal rat cardiomyocytes in Matrigel onto collagen sponges were cultured for 3 days then subjected to trains of electrical pulses (5 V/cm, 1 Hz, 2 ms duration), we observed the progressive development of conductive and contractile properties, including increased expression of myosin heavy chain, Cx-43, creatine kinase-MM, and cardiac troponin-I, as well as increased cell alignment and elongation (Radisic et al. 2004).

## 22.5.7 Cardiac Tissue Engineering Bioreactor Limitations and Challenges

In recent years, much progress has been made in cardiac tissue engineering bioreactor design: engineered biomimetic environments are allowing cells to be physically manipulated in unprecedented ways and are leading to engineered tissues outperforming those that could ever be grown in static culture dishes. However, several important challenges remain to be resolved not only to engineer bioreactors producing conditions more predictive of cell behavior *in vivo*, but, perhaps just as importantly, to provide bioreactors beyond the lab bench.

Current systems still lag behind nature's ability to deliver the highly coordinated sequences of spatial and temporal gradients of regulatory factors at the level of the cell that are necessary to regulate cell function in a developing and adult organism. Along these lines, another remaining challenge is the development of bioreactors that will allow for the performance of screening studies to determine the optimal cell culture regimes, both spatially and temporally.

Even assuming the discovery of all necessary biophysical and/or molecular cues is successful, significant challenges remain in order to incorporate these cues into bioreactors, especially when this involves the combination of multiple physiologically relevant signals (such as electrical, perfusion and mechanical) simultaneously. Furthermore, some known biophysical cues, such as molecular gradients, although relatively facile to apply in microfluidic conditions, are difficult to produce in the larger-scale 3D culture settings of the bioreactor, without applying significant shear stresses or using excessive amounts of expensive culture medium. Another important challenge revolves around the performance assessment of cardiac tissue, in particular the ability to perform *on-line* assessment of the progressive development of cardiac tissue *in vitro* without having to sacrifice constructs during culture. Until these challenges are met, the speed with which culture regimes may be optimized will be impeded.

Finally, the last set of challenges revolve around the ability to provide bioreactors beyond the lab bench: bioreactors are still most often custom-designed and, even among the population of highly specialized designers and users of bioreactors, there is still a certain amount of user-dependency that is expected, impeding the ability for cardiac tissue engineering bioreactors to surpass the regulatory, logistical hurdles related to supply chain and cardiac surgery. Until these challenges are met, the bioreactor-engineered cardiac tissues will remain restricted to the research laboratory.

## 22.6 Vascular Bioreactors

### 22.6.1 Key Requirements

The blood vessel wall is comprised of three discrete layers. For arteries and arterioles, the major component is the central region (*tunica media*), with circumferentially aligned smooth muscle cells. This is flanked on the luminal surface by a monolayer lining of endothelial cells (*tunica intima*), and on the outside by fibroblasts and connective tissue (*tunica externa*). Functional engineered blood vessels should possess two key characteristics: (1) an antithrombogenic surface for blood flow and (2) high burst strengths (>2000 mmHg). Endothelial cells (ECs) are essential for providing antithrombogenic properties. It is therefore crucial that these cells achieve 100% confluence over the exposed luminal surface area of the graft. The ECs are also responsive to the flow-induced shear stress, which, in arteries, can be as high as 20 dyn/cm². ECs in blood vessels align in the direction of shear. However, ECs that have not been pre-conditioned by exposure to shear stress in bioreactor conditions, may detach after implantation in response to high levels of shear stress induced by blood flow and compromise the antithrombogenic characteristics of the graft.

The patency of the grafts is also dependent on their abilities to withstand the high pulsatile stresses, which range from 80 to 120 mmHg in arteries and result in radial distensions up to 10%. The robust mechanical properties of the graft are imparted primarily by the tunica media and rely on the alignment of the smooth muscle cells (SMCs) and their maintenance of a contractile phenotype. The spatial organization of the smooth muscle layer occurs in response to radial distension. Both the shear stress and the radial tensile forces are achieved in culture by providing pulsatile flow through the lumen of the engineered grafts.

## 22.6.2 Bioreactor Design

In general, the cultivation of tissue-engineered blood vessels begins with the cultivation of the medial layer (Niklason et al. 1999, 2001; Gong and Niklason 2006, 2008) (Figure 22.5). Smooth muscle cells or stem cells capable of smooth muscle differentiation were seeded unto a tubular scaffold (Figure 22.5a). Both ends of the tube were attached to silicon tubing within a bioreactor, immersed in a bath of medium, and exposed to pulsatile flow of cultivation medium through the lumen. Radial strains of 1.5–5% are employed at a frequency of 2–3 Hz and constructs were cultivated for up to 8 weeks (Figure 22.5b). At the end of this period, ECs were injected into the luminal space, allowed to attach under static conditions (with rotation of the tube to ensure coverage on all sides) and the flow was increased gradually over a 3-day period to minimize cell wash out due to shear (Figure 22.5a). Using these approaches, arteries

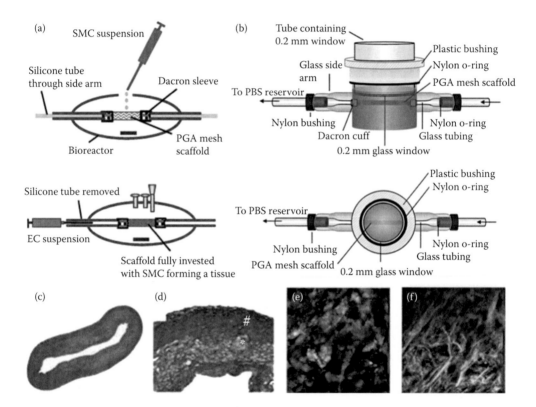

**FIGURE 22.5** (**See color insert.**) Bioreactor for cultivation of functional tissue-engineered arteries. (a) Schematic of cell-seeding. (Upper): A suspension of smooth muscle cells (SMC) is seeded unto the outer surface of the tubular mesh scaffold and cultured for an extended period. (Lower): Endothelial cells are seeded on the luminal surface of the scaffold by injection of a cell suspension while turning the scaffold to facilitate even distribution of the cells. (b) Bioreactor design showing the engineered vessel submerged in a reservoir of cultivation medium. At the same time, medium is pumped through the tubing using a pulsatile flow to stimulate radial distension of the vessel. This bioreactor is designed with a glass window to enable imaging in situ. (c) Histological cross-section of the engineered vessel stained with H&E. (d) Trichrome staining at higher magnification shows collagen deposition (#) in blue and the original scaffold (*). (e, f) Nonlinear optical microscopy images of the engineered construct in the bioreactor at 30 μm depth into the vessel wall after 6 weeks of cultivation. (e) Scaffold and cellular material. (f) Deposited collagen fibrils.

with internal diameters of 3 mm and lengths of 8 cm have been grown using cells from various mammalian species (including humans) (Niklason et al. 1999, 2001; McKee et al., 2003) (Figure 22.5c–f). Preconditioning of these grafts with pulsatile flow was essential to provide them with the functional mechanical properties, confluent, shear-resistant ECs and contractile SMCs.

### 22.6.3 Limitations and Challenges

One limitation of this approach has been the lengthy cultivation times required to condition the grafts. As such, their use is limited to cases of chronic illness, where the patients can wait 2–3 months for a replacement. Another significant consideration is the need to obtain suitable autologous SMC and EC sources. This challenge has been addressed by using mesenchymal stem cells to form the smooth muscle layer (Gong and Niklason 2008). Other potentially autologous stem and progenitor cell sources including adipose-derived stem cells (Zuk et al., 2001, 2002) or induced pluripotent stem cells (Takahashi and Yamanaka 2006), which can be directed into smooth muscle or endothelial lineages prior to graft development. Another approach has been to manipulate the telemorase activity so that cells harvested from adults can be culture expanded to achieve sufficient quantities (Fields et al. 2003).

## 22.7 Bone Tissue Engineering Bioreactor

Bone is a hard connective tissue, which continuously undergoes dynamic remodeling processes throughout a person's life. It plays various roles in mechanical, synthetic, and metabolic functions such as supports the body's framework, synthesizes most of the blood cells for the entire body and maintains mineral and fat reserves. The ability to perform several of these functions is the main consideration for a successful engineered bone tissue. In order to engineer functional bone, the bioreactor must provide 3D support, sufficient nutrient supply, and the biophysical stimulation required for the development and maintenance of active cells. Different types of bone such as craniofacial and long bones are very different in geometry, cellularity, and mechanical properties. While the bones in these different locations also form via different mechanisms during development, the fundamental principles adopted for the tissue engineering bioreactors are similar.

### 22.7.1 Spinner Flask Bioreactor

Previously, studies have shown that conventional static culture of three-dimensional bone grafts resulted in nonhomogenous cell and matrix distributions (Ishaug et al. 1997). Improvement in the development of engineered bone has been achieved with the addition of media convection. Sikavitsas et al. (2002) cultured marrow stromal cells seeded 75:25 PLGA scaffolds in three different conditions: statically, in a spinner flask and in a rotating wall vessel. The marrow stromal cell seeded PLGA constructs in the spinner flask bioreactor showed the largest number of cells and higher calcium content. However, the engineered bone cultured in the spinner flask bioreactor still lacked the uniform cell distribution. Similar results were also found with different types of cell and scaffold (Shea et al. 2000). This phenomenon is likely caused by the convection scheme of spinner flasks in which cells on the scaffold surface received more media and higher shear stress than those residing inside the scaffold.

### 22.7.2 Perfusion Bioreactors for Cylindrical Constructs

Previous studies have shown that shear loads can enhance osteocompetent cell proliferation and differentiation. In addition, osteoblasts have been found to be more responsive to fluid shear forces than mechanical strain (Owan et al. 1997). Therefore, the incorporation of fluid flow, which distributes nutrient supplies throughout the porous scaffold as well as induces shear on the cell is desired in order to enhance engineered bone formation.

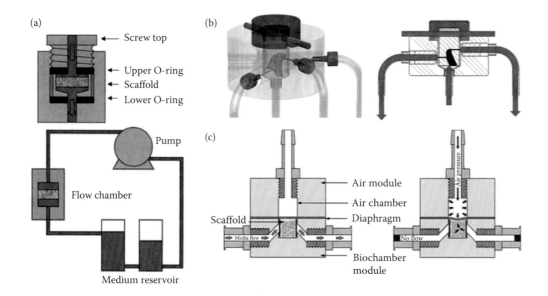

**FIGURE 22.6**  Schematics of various bioreactors for bone tissue engineering. (a) Perfusion bioreactor for cylindrical construct and its set up. The pump circulates media from medium reservoir, through the scaffold and back to the reservoir. (b) Perfusion bioreactor for anatomical TMJ graft. Medium is pumped into the TMJ scaffold from the bottom and exits on the side through needle outlet. (c) Combination of perfusion and compression bioreactor. Cells are exposed to both shear stress and pressure.

Perfusion bioreactors have been employed in many bone tissue engineering laboratories. In perfusion bioreactors, medium is pumped through the scaffold, thereby providing both mechanical stimulation of shear load and transport of nutrients inside the porous scaffold (Figure 22.6a). Perfusion bioreactors have been shown to be superior over static cultures (Bancroft et al. 2002) and spinner flask bioreactors (Meinel et al. 2004) in terms of the resulting homogeneity of cell distribution. Sikavitsas et al. (2003) further studied the direct effect of shear stress. Increasing cell culture media viscosity, which translated into greater shear stresses, resulted in a progressive increase in mineralized matrix deposition and the distribution of ECM throughout the constructs.

Grayson et al. (2008) used a perfusion bioreactor to study the combination effect of initial seeding density and fluid perfusion rate and found that effect of seeding density did not measurably influence the characteristics of tissue-engineered bone. On the other hand, the increase in perfusion rate radically improved final cell numbers, cell distributions throughout the constructs, and the amounts of bone proteins and minerals produced. Interestingly, they related the perfusion rate to the shear rate using simple tube-flow models and suggested that the approximate range of shear stress the cells encounter in the perfusion rate of 100 and 400 μm/s are 0.7–3 and 3–10 mPa, respectively. Although the model was simplified by neglecting the rational tortuosity of the flow inside bone pore space, the approximate shear stress should be a close representation of what cells actually sense. The model to accurately determine shear stress would allow researchers to compare shear stress among several studies and obtain the optimum shear stress that should be applied for certain cell types.

## 22.7.3 Perfusion Bioreactors for Anatomically Shaped Grafts

Most bone tissue engineering perfusion studies have used scaffolds of either thin disk shapes or small cylindrical blocks which allowed for the simplicity of bioreactor designs, controlled flow schemes, and minimization of material used. Recently, an attempt to tissue engineer large anatomically shaped human bone was established (Figure 22.6b). Grayson et al. engineered grafts in the shape of the temporomandibular joint condyle (TMJ) using hMSCs seeded into TMJ-shaped decellularized bovine trabecular bone scaffolds. The human mandibular structure was obtained from the clinical CT of a patient and reconstructed to include only the region that contained the TMJ condyle. The 3D geometry was imported into computer-numerical-control milling machine to grind cylindrical pieces of trabecular bone harvested from the knee joints into an exact shape of human TMJ condyle. The final scaffold's volume was approximately 1 cm$^3$. Due to the large structure and in order to convectively drive cells inside the scaffold, the constructs were seeded in spinner flask bioreactor as compared to static seeding used in small disks and cylindrical blocks bone tissue engineering studies (Grayson et al. 2010).

A specialized perfusion bioreactor was developed for culturing the TMJ condyle. The seeded scaffolds were tightly fitted into a PDMS mold of the exact shape and placed in the acrylic culture chamber. The chamber had one port along the central axis used as a medium inlet and six outlet radial cylindrical ports each serving as a guide for controlling the exact position and depth of insertion of the 23-G needle into the scaffold. In the study, the medium flow was perfused through the scaffold and equally exited out of three needle ports. In the bioreactor, the cells proliferated by approximately 2.5 folds over static culture and grew 10-fold over 4 weeks of culture reaching an average of $250 \times 10^6$ cells per construct. Bioreactor grown constructs exhibited homogenous cell distribution and osteoid formation throughout the scaffold. This system showed the very first time tissue engineering of fully cellularized large anatomical shaped human bone graft and revealed the possibility to engineer clinically-sized anatomically-shaped bone grafts.

## 22.7.4 Other Bone Bioreactors

Nutrient supplies and shear stress are the two essential components for bone tissue engineering. Other stimuli such as mechanical strain, mechanical compression and electrical current also exhibit a possibility in enhancing tissue engineer bone formation (Figure 22.6c). A bioreactor was developed that allowed the continuous exposure of cells to cyclic stretching (Neidlinger-Wilke et al. 1994). When primary osteoblast-like cells were seeded in silicone rubber and cultured under the presence of mechanical strain (1000 microstrains at 1 Hz either continuously or in periods of 60 min), cellularity and calcium deposition were enhanced (Winter et al. 2003). However, in another bioreactor configured to deliver a four-point bending regime, the mechanical stretch had a negative impact in the mineral deposition (Shimko 2003).

Tissue engineering researchers seek to emulate *in vivo* conditions by incorporating similar loading mechanisms in bioreactors. Two-dimensional *in vitro* experiments have demonstrated the positive response of bone cells to independent loading regimens of hydrostatic compression (Roelofsen et al. 1995; Nagatomi et al. 2001; Orr and Burg 2008). Based on the positive effect of both perfusion bioreactor and hydrostatic compression, Orr and Burg (2008) designed a modular bioreactor to incorporate both perfusion flow and hydrostatic compression for bone tissue engineering applications.

Electrical currents and electromagnetic fields have been shown to stimulate bone regeneration and enhance its healing (Bassett et al. 1974; Yonemori et al. 1996; Brighton et al. 2001; Supronowicz et al. 2002). Commercial stimulation systems designed to increase healing rates in fractures have shown osteogenic effects with frequencies ranging from 2 to 123 Hz (Gupta et al. 1991). In cell studies, bioreactors have been designed to electrically stimulate cells and enhanced their osteogenic expression. Applying an electric field of 10 μA and 10 Hz for 6 h/day for 21 days on calvarial osteoblasts enhanced the cell number by 46% and calcium deposition by 307% as well as upregulation of collagen type I mRNA (Supronowicz et al. 2002). In a study on stimulating adipotic stem cells with trains of square waves of 50 Hz direct current electric fields and 6 V/cm peak-to-peak amplitude, there were increase in alkaline phosphatase, collagen type I, osteopontin, and Runx2 expressions but no effect on cell number and osteocalcin expression comparing to unstimulated cells (Hammerick et al. 2010). The positive results in addition to clinical use of electrical stimulation opens up a promising venue for bone tissue engineering.

### 22.7.5 Limitations and Challenges

The application of flow perfusion through porous scaffolds greatly enhances the formation of bone matrix through mechanotransduction and nutrient supplies. There are still great challenges in understanding the actual mechanism that influence the cellular behavior. Currently, only estimates of the shear rates induced from flows through three-dimensional scaffolds have been provided. Detailed mathematical modeling is still in need in order to determine the actual values of shear rate. In addition, the experimentation and modeling to obtain an optimum flow rate to be implemented in a bioreactor is a very challenging task. The ability to predict flow condition and shear rate will offer control and reproducibility of engineered bone grafts of various size and shape.

As demonstrated, large anatomically shaped bone was successfully engineered. The future challenges lie within the survivability of the graft after implantation. The employment of pre-vascularized bone graft to rapidly enhance physiologic nutrient supply is likely to be the solution. The vascularized bone graft is a much more complex tissue and will require much more scientific understanding and creativity on how to engineer vasculatures within the engineered bone and in designing a complex bioreactor to successfully fulfill the requirements.

## 22.8 Cartilage Tissue Engineering Bioreactors

Cartilage is a stiff connective tissue found in many areas in the body including articular joints, rib cage, ear, nose, bronchial tubes, and the intervertebral discs. It has limited capabilities of regeneration when damaged due to the minimal existence of blood vessels within the tissue, hence; the tissue engineering of cartilage construct offers high clinical impact. Cartilage tissue is composed of chondrocytes that produce large amounts of ECM such as collagen type II, proteoglycan, and elastin fibers. Different types of cartilage contain different relative amount of ECM, differ in organization, and provide different function. Articular cartilage is continuously exposed to mechanical forces and needs to dissipate loads under physiological conditions. In other parts of the body, the elastic properties of the cartilage are more prominent. The bioreactor must provide the stimulations that enhance matrix production and tissue organization in addition to maintaining cell growth and survivability.

### 22.8.1 Cartilage Tissue Engineering Bioreactor Design Strategies

Cartilaginous tissue has been engineered using spinner flasks, rotating wall bioreactors, perfusion systems, and compression bioreactors that better mimic the physiological environment of the cartilage tissue (Figure 22.7). The most widely used cell types for tissue engineering cartilage are primary chondrocytes and mesenchymal stem cells. Different scaffold types were employed ranging from porous scaffold to synthetic and natural hydrogels such as agarose and α-hydroxy esters, to fibrinogen-based and glycosaminoglycan (GAG)-based matrices. Many bioreactors designed were utilized in the past decade in order to enhance nutrient transport or mimic physiologic environments.

### 22.8.2 Static, Spinner Flask, and Rotating Wall Vessel Bioreactors

The performance of different bioreactors (static, spinner flask, and rotating wall) on the formation of cartilaginous matrix were compared (Figure 22.7a,b) (Vunjak-Novakovic et al. 2002). Chondrocytes were seeded in highly porous PGA scaffolds and cultured for 6 weeks. The rotating bioreactor induced the largest production of GAGs and collagen type II followed by spinner flask. Histomorphometric studies revealed the formation of tissue in the periphery of the constructs cultured statically, while those in the spinner flask had an outer fibrous capsule in spite of the increment in mass transport. Scaffold cultured in the rotating-wall bioreactor, on the other hand, showed a better distribution of the matrix, but a gradient in concentration of GAGs was observed in all the constructs.

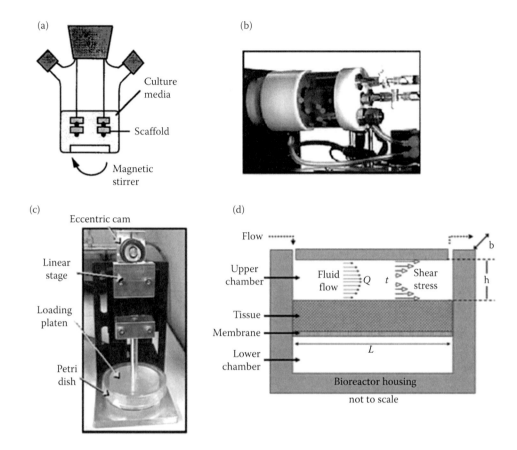

**FIGURE 22.7** Bioreactors for cartilage tissue engineering. (a) Spinner flask bioreactor for culturing engineered cartilage. The scaffolds are anchored to the rods and submerged in culture media. Convection of fluid is generated by magnetic stirrer. (b) Rotating wall vessel bioreactor. The scaffolds are left free inside media chamber which rotates in circular motion. (c) Mechanical loading bioreactor. Scaffolds are placed at the bottom of a Petri dish and are compressed by loading platen controlled by eccentric cam and linear stage. (d) Surface shear induction through fluid flow. Constructs are exposed to media from top and bottom to maximize nutrient supplies. The fluid flow only occurs at the top surface mimicking shear on cartilage surface.

The effect of shear stress on the formation of cartilage matrix in a spinner flask was compared with a static culture (Gooch et al. 2001). Chondrocytes were seeded on fibrous PGA matrices and cultured for 6 weeks at different mixing intensities. Higher mixing intensity resulted in greater GAGs production. Collagen production showed similar behavior but no significant differences. Similar study was also conducted in a rotating-wall vessel on chondrocytes seeded PLA foams (Saini and Wick 2003). As a result, the deposition of GAGs decreased at higher shear rates, whereas the collagen production showed a contrary behavior. It is important to note that the fluid flow scheme around and through the constructs between the two bioreactors were very different since the scaffolds were fixed in place in spinner flask while, in rotating-wall vessel, the scaffolds were free.

## 22.8.3 Perfusion Bioreactors

Medium perfusion was employed to produce stress stimulation at the interior of the construct. In cultivating chondrocyte-seeded PGA scaffold, the perfusion system increased the amount of GAGs by 180% compared to the static conditions with a more organized and homogenous matrix (Pazzano et al. 2000).

The chondrocytes exhibited an alignment in the flow direction creating a structure similar to some region of native articular cartilage.

## 22.8.4 Mechanical Loading Bioreactors

Bioreactors that mimic physiologic compressive mechanism of a native articular cartilage have been implemented and offered promising results. While static compressive loads (0.001–3 MPa) have been demonstrated to cause a decrease in proteoglycan synthesis as well as a decrease in protein synthesis (Jones et al. 1982; Gray et al. 1988; Guilak et al. 1994; Park et al. 2003; Hung et al. 2004), cyclical uniaxial compression has been extensively used in cartilage tissue engineering since it was considered to be the most physiologic-like compressive regime.

Hung's group (Hung et al. 2004) cultured chondrocyte-seeded agarose gel construct under dynamic unconfined compression (Figure 22.7c) with a peak-to-peak compressive strain amplitude of 10%, at a frequency of 1 Hz, three 1-h periods per day, and 5 days per week and obtained cartilage-like properties. In addition, when dynamic deformational loading were applied for an additional 4 weeks after culturing the construct with TGF-β3 supplementation for 2 weeks and discontinued, the constructs yielded increase in overall mechanical properties (Lima et al. 2006). The equilibrium modulus reached 1306 ± 79 kPa and glycosaminoglycan levels reached 8.7 ± 1.6%ww which are comparable to the host cartilage properties (994 ± 280 kPa and 6.3 ± 0.9%ww). The study showed that in addition to the direct effect of mechanical stimuli and biochemical factors, the temporal effect is also essential. Another study applied uniaxial compression on mesenchymal progenitor cells-seeded hyaluronan–gelatin composites and also found positive results in term of cartilage development (Angele et al. 2004).

One effect of the mechanism of uniaxial compression on cartilage development is an increasing internal hydrostatic pressure inside the tissue. The negative charges of the scaffold solid phase providing frictional resistance to a shifting of the fluid phase out of the tissue together with the incompressibility of the aqueous solution are the reason for high hydrostatic pressure. In addition to uniaxial compressive bioreactor, many studies look directly into the effect of hydrostatic pressure.

Elder and Athanasiou (2009) nicely summarized the studies on the effect of hydrostatic pressure in articular cartilage tissue engineering from chondrocytes. The dynamic hydrostatic pressure was applied at loads ranging from 0.8 to 10 MPa, frequency ranging from 0.1 to 1 Hz, and different temporal loading scheme on monolayer and 3-D scaffolds (Parkkinen et al. 1993; Smith et al. 1996; Carver and Heath 1999; Suh et al. 1999; Jortikka et al. 2000; Ikenoue et al. 2003; Hu and Athanasiou 2006). Studies showed positive results for cartilage development when dynamic hydrostatic was applied in term of gene expression such as aggrecan and collagen type II, sulfated GAG production, and collagen production.

The static hydrostatic pressure was studied at loads ranging from 1 to 10 MPa and loading scheme ranging from 1 h/day to 20 h on monolayer and 3-D scaffolds (Hall et al. 1991; Smith et al. 1996; Takahashi et al. 1997; Jortikka et al. 2000; Mizuno et al. 2002; Toyoda et al. 2003; Elder and Athanasiou 2008). The static hydrostatic pressure also shows positive results in term of aggregan and collagen II expression, sulfated GAG and collagen production. Both the uniaxial compression and the application of hydrostatic pressure have direct affect on cell behavior and enhance cartilage development when applied at the appropriate condition.

## 22.8.5 Surface Shear Bioreactor

Constructs grown under compressive bioreactor produce the amount of sulfate GAGs comparable to that of native tissue. However, the constructs posses inferior amount of collagen type II and improper organization. The presence of collage type II distinguishes articular cartilage from other cartilage types. Gemmiti and Guldberg employed a custom-designed parallel-plate bioreactor (Figure 22.7d) to culture 3-D scaffold-free chondrocyte constructs (Gemmiti and Guldberg 2009). The constructs were exposed to shear stress of 0.001 and 0.1 Pa after 2 weeks of static culture to allow cells to settle structurally.

This resulted in constructs with significantly higher amounts of total collagen, collagen type II, tensile Young's modulus and ultimate strength. The study demonstrated that shear stress is a potent modulator of both the amount and type of synthesized ECM constituents in engineered.

### 22.8.6 Limitations and Challenges

Cartilage differs in different locations and by zones within the same location due to its variability in the synthesis and mechanical properties. Both matrix composition and matrix organization play roles in cartilage function and are the criteria for success. Hence, engineering cartilage pieces to mimic native tissue is a very challenging task. Nevertheless, a perfectly engineered cartilage piece may not be suitable for clinical use if it does not integrate well to the host tissue. Optimization in maturity of an engineered cartilage tissue that is suitable for implantation and allows integration to the host tissue is a goal for scientists. Furthermore, most cartilage tissue engineering studies use primary chondrocytes which are not the ideal type of cells for clinical use. Progenitor cells such as MSCs, IPS cells, and embryonic stem cells should be employed as an alternative cell sources. Great challenges arise in term of how to optimally differentiate these cells to produce a cartilage construct at the same level as the chondrocytes.

## 22.9 Tendon/Ligament Tissue Engineering Bioreactors

Tendon is a band of dense connective tissue that connects to bones at both ends and is highly elastic. It plays an essential role in joint movement. There are extensive needs for tendon or ligament replacement because, once these tissues are torn, they cannot be repaired. Tissue engineering of tendon offers a great clinical potential and bioreactor has shown to be a promising instrument for producing tissue grafts. Similar to bioreactors for other tissue, tendon/ligament tissue engineering bioreactors must provide conditions and stimuli that enhance development of this elastic tissue.

### 22.9.1 Tendon/Ligament Tissue Engineering Bioreactor Design Principles

The main principle of a bioreactor that mimics the biomechanical conditions of tendons or ligaments is the mechanics of traction. In this loading scheme, a cell-seeded construct is attached between two holders in which, at least one, connect to a mechanism such as stepper motor in order to move one apart from another and back to its original location at desired frequency and length (Figure 22.8). Addition of computer control allows flexibility in designing experimental conditions of stretching.

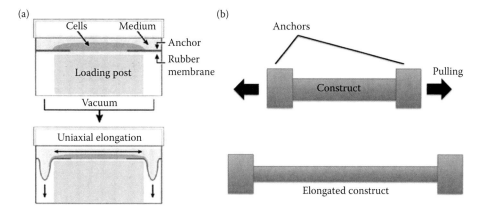

**FIGURE 22.8**  Two examples of traction mechanisms for tendon and ligament bioreactors. (a) By vacuum and (b) by mechanical pulling.

The effect of traction on tendon and ligament tissue engineering from different types of cells has shown positive results. MSCs seeded on collagen gels were cultured under translational and rotational strain concurrently. After 21 days of culture, a ligament-like morphology was observed with organization of collagen types I and III in the longitudinal direction. In addition, the mechanical strain enhanced the production of tenascin-C, a marker of ligament ECM (Altman et al. 2002). In tendon tissue engineering, avian tendon internal fibroblasts were seeded in collagen type I matrices and cultured under mechanical loading 1 h per day with 1% elongation at 1 Hz for 11 days (Garvin et al. 2003). The results showed cell alignment throughout the matrix with elongated nuclei and cytoplasmic extensions. The elastic modulus of the loaded constructs was 2.9 times greater than the nonstimulated group (Garvin et al. 2003). Saber et al. (2010) applied cyclic strain on tenocyte-seeded acellularized tendon scaffold. After 5-day cultivation, the loaded group had significantly higher ultimate tensile stress and elastic modulus than the nonloaded control. Moreover, the constructs were comparable in strength to freshly harvested tendons. The study showed that the biomechanical properties of native tendon can be accomplished *in vitro*.

### 22.9.2 Tendon and Ligament Tissue Engineering Bioreactor Limitations and Challenges

While previous studies showed that tendon and ligament can be engineered from tenocytes and that traction stimulation results in tissue organization and strength similar to native tissue, the tissues engineered from progenitor cells still have inferior properties. The use of specific growth factor combinations to initiate and enhance the differentiation may have a significant impact on the development of the engineered tissue. In addition, the optimization of the time course for growth factor application and initiation of mechanical stimulation is still to be determined.

Another requirement in engineering a clinically successful tendon or ligament graft is to have bone attachments on both ends similarly to the use of autografts. Bone physiologically integrates to the host tissue better than tendon and would result in a more promising graft. The engineering of bone–tendon–bone tissue will require much more complex bioreactors that provide stimulations and conditions needed in all three regions of this complex tissue.

## 22.10 Summary and Challenges

The field of bioreactor design emerged by using engineering principles to design cultivation vessels for fermentation of microorganisms that yield useful pharmaceuticals and food products. In the past 20 years, bioreactors aimed at cultivation of highly sensitive mammalian cells have been developed. As a general principle, these bioreactors provide spatial and temporal control of oxygen, nutrients (e.g., glucose) and pH, just as the original fermentation vessels have done. However, the bioreactors for cultivation of mammalian cells go beyond, by providing instructive stimuli that enable these cells to assemble into functional tissues and organs. For this functional assembly to occur, coordinated application of physical stimuli (electrical and mechanical), growth factors and appropriate biomaterials/ECM is required. Thus, tissue-engineering bioreactors provide inert, well-controlled environments in which the cells come in contact with appropriate biomaterials and experience physiological biophysical stimulation. Specifically, here we provided an overview of micro-bioreactors and microsystems for cultivation of liver cells and bioreactors that provide millimeter to centimeter sized tissues with focus on cardiac, vascular tissues, bone, and cartilage.

Progress in the fields of tissue engineering and regenerative medicine will certainly be accelerated by the design of new analytical techniques that allow real-time monitoring of cell and tissue function to gain insight into the complex mechanisms of tissue assembly by isolated cells and differentiation of progenitor cells as they generate functional tissues. Bioreactors that incorporate these new analytical and imaging capabilities will thus emerge. We expect that improved bioreactors capable of simultaneous application of multiple biochemical (e.g., growth factors) and physical (e.g., electrical, mechanical, perfusion) stimuli will continue to be developed. In contrast to cultivating grafts of clinical size for cardiac repair, the basic pre-requisite for developing effective, high-throughput methods for pharmacological and developmental studies is the miniaturization of engineered tissue. For these studies, we anticipate that microfluidic and BioMEMS (Micro-Electro-Mechanical Systems) techniques will be invaluable.

Bioreactors enabling tissue engineering of complete organs such as those recently demonstrated with the heart (Ott et al. 2008) and lung (Petersen et al. 2010) will probably gain a prominent place in the coming years. We anticipate that in addition to the increased complexity and multifunctionality of bioreactors there will be a trend towards making them disposable. Thus, a tissue or an organ will be cultivated in a bioreactor and transported to the end-point recipient in the same contained, sterile vessel. Finally, it has been boldly suggested that bioreactors for cultivation of mammalian cells may find their future use in the production of high-protein foods to satisfy the nutritional needs of the world's growing population (Fox 2009).

## Acknowledgment

We gratefully acknowledge the NIH support of the work described in this chapter (HL076485, DE016525, HL089913, EB002520, RR026244).

## References

Albrecht, D. R., G. H. Underhill et al. 2006. Probing the role of multicellular organization in three-dimensional microenvironments. *Nat Methods* **3**(5): 369–75.

Altman, G. H., R. L. Horan et al. 2002. Cell differentiation by mechanical stress. *FASEB J* **16**(2): 270–72.

Altman, G. H., H. H. Lu et al. 2002. Advanced bioreactor with controlled application of multi-dimensional strain for tissue engineering. *J Biomech Eng-Trans ASME* **124**(6): 742–49.

Andersson, H. and A. van den Berg 2004. Microfabrication and microfluidics for tissue engineering: State of the art and future opportunities. *Lab On a Chip* **4**(2): 98–103.

Angele, P., D. Schumann et al. 2004. Cyclic, mechanical compression enhances chondrogenesis of mesenchymal progenitor cells in tissue engineering scaffolds. *Biorheology* **41**(3–4): 335–46.

Baar, K. 2005. New dimensions in tissue engineering: Possible models for human physiology. *Exp Physiol* **90**(6): 799–806.

Baksh, D., J. E. Davies et al. 2003. Adult human bone marrow-derived mesenchymal progenitor cells are capable of adhesion-independent survival and expansion. *Exp Hematol* **31**(8): 723–32.

Bancroft, G. N., V. I. Sikavitsas et al. 2002. Fluid flow increases mineralized matrix deposition in 3D perfusion culture of marrow stromal osteoblasts in a dose-dependent manner. *Proc Natl Acad Sci USA* **99**(20): 12600–5.

Bassett, C. A., R. J. Pawluk et al. 1974. Augmentation of bone repair by inductively coupled electromagnetic fields. *Science* **184**(136): 575–77.

Beebe, D. J., G. A. Mensing, and G. M. Walker 2002. Physics and applications of microfluidics in biology. *Annu Rev Biomed Eng* 4: 261–86.

Brighton, C. T., W. Wang et al. 2001. Signal transduction in electrically stimulated bone cells. *J Bone Jt Surg Am* **83**-A(10): 1514–23.

Bursac, N., M. Papadaki et al. 1999. Cardiac muscle tissue engineering: Toward an *in vitro* model for electrophysiological studies. *Am J Physiology-Heart Circ Physiol* **277**(2): H433–H444.

Butler, D. L., S. A. Goldstein et al. 2000. Functional tissue engineering: The role of biomechanics. *J Biomech Eng-Trans ASME* **122**(6): 570–75.

Carrier, R. L., M. Papadaki et al. 1999. Cardiac tissue engineering: Cell seeding, cultivation parameters, and tissue construct characterization. *Biotechnol Bioeng* **64**(5): 580–89.

Carver, S. E. and C. A. Heath 1999. Increasing extracellular matrix production in regenerating cartilage with intermittent physiological pressure. *Biotechnol Bioeng* **62**(2): 166–74.

Cervinka, M., Z. Cervinkova et al. 2008. The role of time-lapse fluorescent microscopy in the characterization of toxic effects in cell populations cultivated *in vitro*. *Toxicology* **22**(5): 1382–86.

Chen, C. S., M. Mrksich et al. 1997. Geometric control of cell life and death. *Science* **276**: 1425–1428.

Cherry, R. S. and E. T. Papoutsakis 1988. Physical-mechanisms of cell-damage in microcarrier cell-culture bioreactors. *Biotechnol Bioeng* **32**(8): 1001–14.

Chiu, D. T., N. L. Jeon et al. 2000. Patterned deposition of cells and proteins onto surfaces by using three-dimensional microfluidic systems. *PNAS* **97**(6): 2408–13.

Cimetta, E., E. Figallo et al. 2009. Micro-bioreactor arrays for controlling cellular environments: Design principles for human embryonic stem cell applications. *Methods* **47**: 81–89.

Dellatore, S. M., A. S. Garcia et al. 2008. Mimicking stem cell niches to increase stem cell expansion. *Curr Opin Biotechnol* **19**: 534–40.

DiCarlo, D., L. Y. Wu et al. 2006. Dynamic single cell culture array. *Lab on a Chip* **6**: 1445–49.

Discher, D. E., P. Janmey et al. 2005. Tissue cells feel and respond to the stiffness of their substrate. *Science* **310**: 1139–43.

Eibl, R., S. Kaiser et al. 2010. Disposable bioreactors: The current state-of-the-art and recommended applications in biotechnology. *Appl Microbiol Biotechnol* **86**(1): 41–49.

Elder, B. D. and K. A. Athanasiou 2008. Synergistic and additive effects of hydrostatic pressure and growth factors on tissue formation. *PLoS One* **3**(6): e2341.

Elder, B. D. and K. A. Athanasiou 2009. Hydrostatic pressure in articular cartilage tissue engineering: From chondrocytes to tissue regeneration. *Tissue Eng Part B Rev* **15**(1): 43–53.

Engler, A. J., S. Sen et al. 2006. Matrix elasticity directs stem cell lineage specification. *Cell* **126**: 677–89.

Falconnet, D., G. Csucs et al. 2006. Surface engineering approaches to micropattern surfaces for cell-based assays. *Biomaterials* **27**: 3044–63.

Fields, R. C., A. Solan et al. 2003. Gene therapy in tissue-engineered blood vessels. *Tissue Eng* **9**(6): 1281–1287.

Figallo, E., C. Cannizzaro et al. 2007. Micro-bioreactor array for controlling cellular microenvironments. *Lab on a Chip* **7**: 710–19.

Fink, C., S. Ergun et al. 2000. Chronic stretch of engineered heart tissue induces hypertrophy and functional improvement. *FASEB J* **14**(5): 669–79.

Flaim, C. J., S. Chien et al. 2005. An extracellular matrix microarray for probing cellular differentiation. *Nat Methods* **2**: 119–25.

Folch, A. and M. Toner 2000. Microengineering of cellular interactions. *Annu Rev Biomed Eng* **2**: 227–56.

Fox, J. L. 2009. Test tube meat on the menu? *Nat Biotechnol* **27**(10): 873.

Freed, L. E., A. P. Hollander et al. 1998. Chondrogenesis in a cell-polymer-bioreactor system. *Exp Cell Res* **240**(1): 58–65.

Freed, L. E. and G. Vunjaknovakovic 1995. Cultivation of cell-polymer tissue constructs in simulated microgravity. *Biotechnol Bioeng* **46**(4): 306–13.

Freshney, R. 2000. *Culture of Animal Cells—A Manual of Basic Techniques*, 4th ed. New York, Wiley-Liss.

Gao, L., R. McBeath et al. 2010. Stem cell shape regulates a chondrogenic versus myogenic fate through rac1 and N-cadherin. *Stem Cells* **28**: 564–72.

Garvin, J., J. Qi et al. 2003. Novel system for engineering bioartificial tendons and application of mechanical load. *Tissue Eng* **9**(5): 967–79.

Gemmiti, C. V. and R. E. Guldberg 2009. Shear stress magnitude and duration modulates matrix composition and tensile mechanical properties in engineered cartilaginous tissue. *Biotechnol Bioeng* **104**(4): 809–20.

Gerecht-Nir, S., M. Radisic et al. 2006. Biophysical regulation during cardiac development and application to tissue engineering. *Int J Dev Biol* **50**(2–3): 233–43.

Glindkamp, A., D. Riechers et al. 2009. Sensors in disposable bioreactors status and trends. *Disposable Bioreactors* **115**: 145–69.

Gomez-Sjoberg, R., A. A. Leyrat et al. 2007. Versatile, fully automated, microfluidic cell culture system. *Anal Chem* **79**: 8557–63.

Gong, Z. D. and L. E. Niklason 2006. Blood vessels engineered from human cells. *Trends Cardiovasc Med* **16**(5): 153–56.

Gong, Z. D. and L. E. Niklason 2008. Small-diameter human vessel wall engineered from bone marrow-derived mesenchymal stem cells (hMSCs). *FASEB J* **22**(6): 1635–48.

Gooch, K. J., J. H. Kwon et al. 2001. Effects of mixing intensity on tissue-engineered cartilage. *Biotechnol Bioeng* **72**(4): 402–7.

Gottwald, E., S. Giselbrecht et al. 2007. A chip-based platform for the in vitro generation of tissues in threedimensional organization. *Lab Chip* **7**: 777–85.

Gray, M. L., A. M. Pizzanelli et al. 1988. Mechanical and physiochemical determinants of the chondrocyte biosynthetic response. *J Orthop Res* **6**(6): 777–92.

Grayson, W. L., S. Bhumiratana et al. 2008. Effects of initial seeding density and fluid perfusion rate on formation of tissue-engineered bone. *Tissue Eng A* **14**(11): 1809–20.

Grayson, W. L., M. Frohlich et al. 2010. Engineering anatomically shaped human bone grafts. *Proc Natl Acad Sci USA* **107**(8): 3299–304.

Grayson, W. L., T. P. Martens et al. 2009. Biomimetic approach to tissue engineering. *Sem Cell Dev Biol* **20**(6): 665–73.

Guilak, F., D. L. Butler et al. 2001. Functional tissue engineering—The role of biomechanics in articular cartilage repair. *Clin Orthop Relat Res* (391): S295–S305.

Guilak, F., D. M. Cohen et al. 2009. Control of stem cell fate by physical interactions with the extracellular matrix. *Cell Stem Cell* **5**: 17–26.

Guilak, F., B. C. Meyer et al. 1994. The effects of matrix compression on proteoglycan metabolism in articular cartilage explants. *Osteoarthritis Cartilage* **2**(2): 91–101.

Gupta, T. D., V. K. Jain et al. 1991. Comparative study of bone growth by pulsed electromagnetic fields. *Med Biol Eng Comput* **29**(2): 113–20.

Hall, A. C., J. P. Urban et al. 1991. The effects of hydrostatic pressure on matrix synthesis in articular cartilage. *J Orthop Res* **9**(1): 1–10.

Hammerick, K. E., A. W. James et al. 2010. Pulsed direct current electric fields enhance osteogenesis in adipose-derived stromal cells. *Tissue Eng Part A* **16**(3): 917–31.

Hu, J. C. and K. A. Athanasiou 2006. The effects of intermittent hydrostatic pressure on self-assembled articular cartilage constructs. *Tissue Eng* **12**(5): 1337–44.

Hung, C. T., R. L. Mauck et al. 2004. A paradigm for functional tissue engineering of articular cartilage via applied physiologic deformational loading. *Ann Biomed Eng* **32**(1): 35–49.

Ikenoue, T., M. C. Trindade et al. 2003. Mechanoregulation of human articular chondrocyte aggrecan and type II collagen expression by intermittent hydrostatic pressure *in vitro*. *J Orthop Res* **21**(1): 110–16.

Ishaug, S. L., G. M. Crane et al. 1997. Bone formation by three-dimensional stromal osteoblast culture in biodegradable polymer scaffolds. *J Biomed Mater Res* **36**(1): 17–28.

Jamshidi, N. and B. Ø. Palsson 2008. Top-down analysis of temporal hierarchy in biochemical reaction networks. *PLoS Comput Biol* **4**(9): e1000177.

Jang, J. H. and D. V. Schaffer 2006. Microarraying the cellular microenvironment. *Mol Syst Biol* **2**:39.

Jones, I. L., A. Klamfeldt et al. 1982. The effect of continuous mechanical pressure upon the turnover of articular cartilage proteoglycans *in vitro*. *Clin Orthop Relat Res* **165**: 283–9.

Jortikka, M. O., J. J. Parkkinen et al. 2000. The role of microtubules in the regulation of proteoglycan synthesis in chondrocytes under hydrostatic pressure. *Arch Biochem Biophys* **374**(2): 172–80.

Kaplan, D., R.T. Moon, and G. Vunjak-Novakovic 2005. It takes a village to grow a tissue. *Nat Biotechnol* **23**(10): 1237–9.

Khademhosseini, A., R. Langer et al. 2006. Microscale technologies for tissue engineering and biology. *PNAS* **103**(8): 2480–7.

Khetani, S. R. and S. N. Bhatia 2008. Microscale culture of human liver cells for drug development. *Nat Biotechnol* **26**(1): 120–26.

Kim, M. S., J. H. Yeon, and J. K. Park 2007. A microfluidic platform for 3-dimensional cell culture and cell-based assays. *Biomed Microdev* **9**: 25–34.

Kirouac, D. C. and P. W. Zandstra 2008. The systematic production of cells for cell therapies. *Cell Stem Cell* **3**(4): 369–81.

Langer, R. and J. P. Vacanti 1993. Tissue engineering. *Science* **260**(5110): 920–26.

Lima, E. G., L. Bian et al. 2006. The effect of applied compressive loading on tissue-engineered cartilage constructs cultured with TGF-beta3. *Conf Proc IEEE Eng Med Biol Soc* **1**: 779–82.

Lima, E. G., L. Bian et al. 2007. The beneficial effect of delayed compressive loading on tissue-engineered cartilage constructs cultured with TGF-beta 3. *Osteoarthritis Cartilage* **15**(9): 1025–33.

Linder, V. 2007. Microfluidics at the crossroad with point-of-care diagnostics. *The Analyst* **132**: 1186–92.

Lutolf, M. P. and J. A. Hubbel 2005. Synthetic biomaterials as instructive extracellular microenvironments for morphogenesis in tissue engineering. *Nat Biotechnol* **23**(1): 47–55.

Madlambayan, G. J., I. Rogers et al. 2006. Clinically relevant expansion of hematopoietic stem cells with conserved function in a single-use, closed-system bioprocess. *Biol Blood Marrow Transpl* **12**(10): 1020–30.

Maidhof, R., A. Marsano et al. 2010. Perfusion seeding of channeled elastomeric scaffolds with myocytes and endothelial cells for cardiac tissue engineering. *Biotechnol Progr* **26**(2): 565–72.

Martin, I., T. Smith et al. 2009. Bioreactor-based roadmap for the translation of tissue engineering strategies into clinical products. *Trends Biotechnol* **27**(9): 495–502.

Mauck, R. L., S. B. Nicoll et al. 2003. Synergistic action of growth factors and dynamic loading for articular cartilage tissue engineering. *Tissue Eng* **9**(4): 597–611.

Mauck, R. L., M. A. Soltz et al. 2000. Functional tissue engineering of articular cartilage through dynamic loading of chondrocyte-seeded agarose gels. *J Biomech Eng* **122**(3): 252–60.

McKee, J. A., S. S. Banik et al. 2003. Human arteries engineered *in vitro. EMBO Rep* **4**(6): 633–38.

Meinel, L., V. Karageorgiou et al. 2004. Bone tissue engineering using human mesenchymal stem cells: Effects of scaffold material and medium flow. *Ann Biomed Eng* **32**(1): 112–22.

Melin, J. and S. R. Quake 2007. Microfluidic large-scale integration: The evolution of design rules for biological automation. *Ann Rev Biophys Biomol Struct* **36**: 213–31.

Mizuno, S., T. Tateishi et al. 2002. Hydrostatic fluid pressure enhances matrix synthesis and accumulation by bovine chondrocytes in three-dimensional culture. *J Cell Physiol* **193**(3): 319–27.

Muschler, G. F., C. Nakamoto et al. 2004. Engineering principles of clinical cell-based tissue engineering. *J Bone Jt Surg. American Volume* **86-A**(7): 1541–58.

Nagatomi, J., B. P. Arulanandam et al. 2001. Frequency- and duration-dependent effects of cyclic pressure on select bone cell functions. *Tissue Eng* **7**(6): 717–28.

Neidlinger-Wilke, C., H. J. Wilke et al. 1994. Cyclic stretching of human osteoblasts affects proliferation and metabolism: A new experimental method and its application. *J Orthop Res* **12**(1): 70–78.

Niklason, L. E., W. Abbott et al. 2001. Morphologic and mechanical characteristics of bovine engineered arteries. *J Vasc Surg* **33**: 628–38.

Niklason, L. E., W. Abbott et al. 2001. Morphologic and mechanical characteristics of engineered bovine arteries. *J Vasc Surg* **33**(3): 628–38.

Niklason, L. E., J. Gao et al. 1999. Functional arteries grown *in vitro. Science* **284**(5413): 489–93.

Niklason, L. E., A. T. Yeh et al. 2010. Enabling tools for engineering collagenous tissues integrating bioreactors, intravital imaging, and biomechanical modeling. *Proc Natl Acad Sci USA* **107**(8): 3335–39.

Orr, D. E. and K. J. Burg 2008. Design of a modular bioreactor to incorporate both perfusion flow and hydrostatic compression for tissue engineering applications. *Ann Biomed Eng* **36**(7): 1228–41.

Ott, H. C., T. S. Matthiesen et al. 2008. Perfusion-decellularized matrix: Using nature's platform to engineer a bioartificial heart. *Nat Med* **14**(2): 213–21.

Owan, I., D. B. Burr et al. 1997. Mechanotransduction in bone: Osteoblasts are more responsive to fluid forces than mechanical strain. *Am J Physiol* **273**(3 Pt 1): C810–15.

Park, S., R. Krishnan et al. 2003. Cartilage interstitial fluid load support in unconfined compression. *J Biomech* **36**(12): 1785–96.

Parkkinen, J. J., J. Ikonen et al. 1993. Effects of cyclic hydrostatic pressure on proteoglycan synthesis in cultured chondrocytes and articular cartilage explants. *Arch Biochem Biophys* **300**(1): 458–65.

Pazzano, D., K. A. Mercier et al. 2000. Comparison of chondrogensis in static and perfused bioreactor culture. *Biotechnol Prog* **16**(5): 893–96.

Petersen, E. F., K. W. Fishbein et al. 2000. P-31 NMR spectroscopy of developing cartilage produced from chick chondrocytes in a hollow-fiber bioreactor. *Magn Reson Med* **44**(3): 367–72.

Petersen, T. H., E. A. Calle et al. 2010. Tissue-engineered lungs for *in vivo* implantation. *Science* **329**(5991): 538–41.

Porter, B. D., A. S. P. Lin et al. 2007. Noninvasive image analysis of 3D construct mineralization in a perfusion bioreactor. *Biomaterials* **28**(15): 2525–33.

Prewett, T. L., T. J. Goodwin et al. 1993. Three-dimensional modeling of T-24 human bladder carcinoma cell line: A new simulated microgravity culture system. *J Tissue Culture Methods* **15**: 29–36.

Radisic, M., A. Marsano et al. 2008. Cardiac tissue engineering using perfusion bioreactor systems. *Nat Protocols* **3**(4): 719–38.

Radisic, M., H. Park et al. 2004. Functional assembly of engineered myocardium by electrical stimulation of cardiac myocytes cultured on scaffolds. *Proc Natl Acad Sci USA* **101**(52): 18129–34.

Ramaswamy, S., J. B. Greco et al. 2009. Magnetic resonance imaging of chondrocytes labeled with superparamagnetic iron oxide nanoparticles in tissue-engineered cartilage. *Tissue Eng Part A* **15**(12): 3899–10.

Randers-Eichorn, L., R. Bartlett et al. 1996. Noninvasive oxygen measurements and mass transfer considerations in tissue culture flasks. *Biotechnol Bioeng* **51**: 466–78.

Roelofsen, J., J. Klein-Nulend et al. 1995. Mechanical stimulation by intermittent hydrostatic compression promotes bone-specific gene expression *in vitro*. *J Biomech* **28**(12): 1493–503.

Saber, S., A. Y. Zhang et al. 2010. Flexor tendon tissue engineering: Bioreactor cyclic strain increases construct strength. *Tissue Eng Part A* **16**(6): 2085–90.

Saini, S. and T. M. Wick 2003. Concentric cylinder bioreactor for production of tissue engineered cartilage: Effect of seeding density and hydrodynamic loading on construct development. *Biotechnol Prog* **19**(2): 510–21.

Schwarz, R. P., T. J. Goodwin et al. 1992. Cell culture for three-dimensional modeling in rotating-wall vessels: An application of simulated microgravity. *J Tissue Culture Methods* **14**: 51–58.

Seagle, C., M. A. Christie et al. 2008. High-throughput nuclear magnetic resonance metabolomic footprinting for tissue engineering. *Tissue Engineering Part C-Methods* **14**(2): 107–18.

Shea, L. D., D. Wang et al. 2000. Engineered bone development from a pre-osteoblast cell line on three-dimensional scaffolds. *Tissue Eng* **6**(6): 605–17.

Shimko, D. A., K. K. White et al. 2003. A device for long term, in vitro loading of three-dimensional natural and engineered tissues. *Annals of Biomed Eng* **31**(11): 1347–56.

Sikavitsas, V. I., G. N. Bancroft et al. 2002. Formation of three-dimensional cell/polymer constructs for bone tissue engineering in a spinner flask and a rotating wall vessel bioreactor. *J Biomed Mater Res* **62**(1): 136–48.

Sikavitsas, V. I., G. N. Bancroft et al. 2003. Mineralized matrix deposition by marrow stromal osteoblasts in 3D perfusion culture increases with increasing fluid shear forces. *Proc Natl Acad Sci USA* **100**(25): 14683–88.

Smith, R. L., S. F. Rusk et al. 1996. *In vitro* stimulation of articular chondrocyte mRNA and extracellular matrix synthesis by hydrostatic pressure. *J Orthop Res* **14**(1): 53–60.

Squires, T. M. and S. R. Quake 2005. Microfluidics: Fluid physics at the nanoliter scale. *Rev Modern Phys* **77**: 977–1016.

Stevens, M. M. and J. H. George 2005. Exploring and engineering the cell surface interface. *Science* **310**: 1135–38.

Stone, H. A. and S. Kim 2001. Microfluidics: Basic issues, applications, and challenges. *AIChE Journal* **47**(6): 1250–4.

Suh, J. K., G. H. Baek et al. 1999. Intermittent sub-ambient interstitial hydrostatic pressure as a potential mechanical stimulator for chondrocyte metabolism. *Osteoarthritis Cartilage* **7**(1): 71–80.

Supronowicz, P. R., P. M. Ajayan et al. 2002. Novel current-conducting composite substrates for exposing osteoblasts to alternating current stimulation. *J Biomed Mater Res* **59**(3): 499–506.

Takahashi, K., T. Kubo et al. 1997. Hydrostatic pressure influences mRNA expression of transforming growth factor-beta 1 and heat shock protein 70 in chondrocyte-like cell line. *J Orthop Res* **15**(1): 150–58.

Takahashi, K. and S. Yamanaka 2006. Induction of pluripotent stem cells from mouse embryonic and adult fibroblast cultures by defined factors. *Cell* **126**(4): 663–76.

Tandon, N., C. Cannizzaro et al. 2009. Electrical stimulation systems for cardiac tissue engineering. *Nat Protocols* **4**(2): 155–73.

Toner, M. and D. Irimia 2005. Blood-on-a-Chip. *Annu Rev Biomed Eng* **7**: 77–103.

Toyoda, T., B. B. Seedhom et al. 2003. Upregulation of aggrecan and type II collagen mRNA expression in bovine chondrocytes by the application of hydrostatic pressure. *Biorheology* **40**(1–3): 79–85.

Tsang, V. L., A. A. Chen et al. 2007. Fabrication of 3D hepatic tissues by additive photopatterning of cellular hydrogels. *FASEB J* **21**(3): 790–801.

Vunjak-Novakovic, G., G. Altman et al. 2004. Tissue engineering of ligaments. *Ann Rev Biomed Eng* **6**: 131–56.

Vunjak-Novakovic, G., L. E. Freed et al. 1996. Effects of mixing on the composition and morphology of tissue-engineered cartilage. *AIChE Journal* **42**(3): 850–60.

Vunjak-Novakovic, G., I. Martin et al. 1999. Bioreactor cultivation conditions modulate the composition and mechanical properties of tissue-engineered cartilage. *J Orthop Res* **17**(1): 130–38.

Vunjak-Novakovic, G., B. Obradovic et al. 2002. Bioreactor studies of native and tissue engineered cartilage. *Biorheology* **39**(1–2): 259–68.

Whitesides, G. M. 2006. The origins and the future of microfluidics. *Nature* **442**(27): 368–73.

Winter, L. C., X. F. Walboomers et al. 2003. Intermittent versus continuous stretching effects on osteoblast-like cells *in vitro*. *J Biomed Mater Res A* **67**(4): 1269–75.

Xia, Y. and G. M. Whitesides 1998. Soft lithography. *Angew Chem Int Ed* **37**: 550–75.

Yonemori, K., S. Matsunaga et al. 1996. Early effects of electrical stimulation on osteogenesis. *Bone* **19**(2): 173–80.

Zandstra, P. W., C. J. Eaves et al. 1994. Expansion of hematopoietic progenitor-cell populations in stirred suspension bioreactors of normal human bone-marrow cells. *Bio-Technology* **12**(9): 909–14.

Zhao, F. and T. Ma 2005. Perfusion bioreactor system for human mesenchymal stem cell tissue engineering: Dynamic cell seeding and construct development. *Biotechnol Bioeng* **91**(4): 482–93.

Zhong, J. F., Y. Chen et al. 2008. A microfluidic processor for gene expression profiling of single human embryonic stem cells. *Lab on a Chip* **8**: 68–74.

Zimmermann, W.-H., M. Didie et al. 2002. Cardiac grafting of engineered heart tissue in syngenic rats. *Circulation* **106**(90121): I-151–57.

Zimmermann, W.-H., I. Melnychenko et al. 2006. Engineered heart tissue grafts improve systolic and diastolic function in infarcted rat hearts. *Nat Med* **12**(4): 452–58.

Zuk, P. A., Ashijian, P., De Ugarte, D. A., Huang, J. I., Mizuno, H., Alfonso, Z. C., Fraser, J. K., Benhalm, P., and Hedrick, M. H. 2002. Human adipose tissue is a source of multipotent stem cells. *Mol Biol Cell* **13**(12): 4279–95.

Zuk, P. A., Zhu, M., Mizuno, H., Huang, J., Futrell, J. W., Katz, A. J., Benhaim, P., Lorenz, H. P., and Hedrick, M. H., 2001. Multilineage cells from human adipose tissue: Implications for cell-based therapies. *Tissue Eng* **7**(2): 211–28.

Jose F.
Alvarez-Barreto
*Instituto de Estudios
Avanzados*

Samuel B.
VanGordon
*University of Oklahoma*

Brandon W.
Engebretson
*University of Oklahoma*

Vasillios I.
Sikavitsas
*University of Oklahoma*

# 23

# Shear Forces

23.1 Introduction: Cells and Shear Forces .......................................... 23-1
23.2 Effect of Shear Forces on Tissue-Specific Cells ......................... 23-2
    Cartilage • Bone • Tendons • Skin • Cardiac • Vascular
    Grafts • Skeletal Muscle
References................................................................................................ 23-10

## 23.1 Introduction: Cells and Shear Forces

Modulation of cell function is a common, crucial aspect of tissue engineering approaches. It has been well understood from the very beginning that the success of tissue engineered constructs depends on the capacity of the cellular component to generate an extracellular matrix (ECM) that closely resembles the native one. This resemblance occurs at different levels; not only is it important to obtain an ECM with a molecular composition similar to that found *in vivo*, but it must also posses topographical and morphological assets that provide the cells an *in vivo*-like surface where they can properly function. Both aspects will in turn regulate cell function at the site of implantation and thereby affect tissue formation. It is therefore important to stimulate cells to generate an ECM with the aforementioned characteristics.

*In vitro* cell stimulation can be achieved through biochemical means by the use of ECM-specific molecules such as growth and differentiation factors, polysaccharides, peptides, among others (Moss et al. 2009; Chen et al. 2010; Huang and Fu 2010). However, cells not only depend on ECM biochemical cues; their microenvironment is also dominated by specific physiomechanical conditions that equally control their phenotype and function (Stoltz et al. 2000; Alvarez-Barreto and Sikavitsas 2006; Hamill and Martinac 2001). Researchers have recognized the need to imitate these mechanical environments to upregulate the molecular processes related to the production of a tissue-like matrix that can grant the construct tissue inductive properties (Alvarez-Barreto and Sikavitsas 2006; Botchwey et al. 2001; Darling and Athanasiou 2003; Engelmayr et al. 2003; Gomes et al. 2003; Martin et al. 2004). The mechanisms through which cell behavior can be altered by mechanical forces are yet to be fully elucidated, but research in cell mechanotransduction has yielded hypotheses that are worth exploring further.

It is well known that the development of human physiology is affected by mechanical forces that can act at two different but related levels: some forces are generated by contractile actions of the cellular membrane while other forces are externally exerted by the surroundings, such as shear stress due to fluid flow, compression, expansion/contraction, and other means (Bao et al. 2010). Cells are capable of sensing mechanical forces and transducing them into specific biological responses (Zhu et al. 2000). Examples of this are the ability of chondrocytes to respond to compressive forces, endothelial cells being able to reorganize the magnitude of shear stress due to blood flow, osteoblast, and osteocyte response to mechanical loading, or keratinocytes adapting to skin stretching (Lehoux et al. 2006; Sweigart and Athanasiou 2005; Riddle and Donahue 2009; Yano et al. 2004).

Researchers have reported on the existence of cell membrane-specific mechanosensors, ion channels, and hypothesized that, being activated through stretching, these channels sense changes in membrane tension due to an applied force. They can then convert the mechanical signal into a cascade of internal biochemical pathways that regulate numerous cell functions such as migration, proliferation, and even their phenotype (Matthews et al. 2006; Gautam et al. 2006; Davidson et al. 1990; Martinac 2004). However, ion channels are not the only widely considered hypothesis. Molecular membrane-specific receptors are believed to play a more crucial role in mechanotansduction mechanisms and are at the center of current research efforts.

Membrane receptors (i.e., integrins, vinculin, and talin) determine the bidirectional communication between the cell and its surroundings (Roberts and Critchley 2009; Wang and Thampatty 2006; Mofrad et al. 2004). Changes on the surface topography and cell–cell interactions and application of external forces will cause the cells to adapt its adhesions and cytoskeleton, also affecting the internal biochemical processes, and ultimately cell's function and phenotype (Chicurel et al. 1998; Chen et al. 2004). Cell–cell interactions are regulated via adherens junctions, but when attached to rigid surfaces, they develop focal adhesion (FA) (Gumbiner 1996; Burridge et al. 1988). FAs are composed of numerous signaling molecules, such as integrins, that are also involved in growth factor signaling cascades (Burridge et al. 1988; Bao et al. 2010).

Integrins are transmembrane heterodimers composed of a ligand-binding domain that specifically binds to specific ECM components, such as fibronectin and collagen. This ligand-binding head connects to the intracellular domain via a single-pass transmembrane helix. Some of integrins functions are stabilization of tissue structure and architecture, facilitating cell migration, influencing different cell processes, and bearing stress and transmitting force (Shyy and Chien 1997). Generally, cell adhesion via integrins increases tyrosine phosphorilation of FA cytoskeletal and signaling proteins, such as FA kinase (FAK) and Src protein tyrosing kinsases, among others (Numaguchi et al. 1999; Domingos et al. 2002). FAs regulate the responses achieved by a certain combination of specific ECM compositions and growth factors, and thereby represent a structural unit through which fundamental changes in cell function start (Chen et al. 2004).

FA activity is not only controlled by integrin-mediated cell–matrix interactions. Increased intracellular tension whenever external forces are applied can also affect FAs. One mechanotransduction model proposes that the first molecule affected in this mechanism is the FAK which is phosphorylated Tyr397 when stretching occurs. This leads to the mitogen activation of the extracellular signal-regulated kinase (ERK) through the Grb2–Sos–Ras pathway, and subsequent cell proliferation (Calalb et al. 1995; Schlaepfer and Hunter 1996; Numaguchi et al. 1999). Another example of a proposed FA-mediated mechanotransduction mechanism is the activation of vinculin-binding site 1 within Talin, a structural protein in the FA complex. In the last example, the signaling is independent of molecular recruitment (i.e., growth factor recruitment), but rather directly dependent on membrane tension (Bao et al. 2010; Roberts and Critchley 2009).

These are only some examples of proposed mechanotransduction mechanisms, and many authors suggest that the picture is incomplete as the actual intracellular cascades involved are still not well defined. However, it is clear that the mechanical forces exerted on a cell can cause conformational changes in membrane-specific proteins. This translates into alterations in protein–protein and protein–DNA recognitions, enzymatic activities and downstream biochemical pathways that control cell behavior (Bao et al. 2010). This is an area of ongoing research, and the complete elucidation of these mechanisms could help in the development of new cell therapy and tissue engineering alternatives by recognizing the type, intensity, and pattern of application of a given mechanical stimulus.

## 23.2 Effect of Shear Forces on Tissue-Specific Cells

Mechanotransduction studies suggest that similar patterns of mechanical stimulation exist in most cell types. However, the transduction mechanisms and their outcome vary depending on the tissue and the mechanical regime it is subjected to. In the following sections, we describe the relevance of mechanical modulation of cell activity in tissue engineering through the expression of important macromolecular, tissue-specific markers. We also provide a brief insight into the molecular mechanosensing and transduction processes that take place at the cellular level when these forces are applied.

## 23.2.1 Cartilage

Cartilage is a tissue with limited capabilities of regeneration when damaged due to low cell turnover, highly senescent chondrocytes, and limited vasculature (Yang and Elisseeff 2006). Among the two general types of cartilage, articular cartilage is continuously exposed to mechanical forces and needs to dissipate loads under physiological conditions. In contrast, in other parts of the body the elastic properties of the cartilage are more important. Cartilage being a hydrated tissue, when a compressive load is applied, the aqueous phase is responsible for absorbing it. Gradients in pressure and stress due to the nonuniformity of the load will push the water out of the tissue, and the friction between the solid and aqueous phases dissipate the load (Elder and Athanasiou 2009). Therefore, there are two main mechanical forces that cells are exposed to during this process. The most prevalent are the compression forces, but there are also shear stresses created by the internal displacement of the interstitial fluid phase. It has been estimated that typical joint loads create stresses between 3 and 10 MPa, but they can go up to 20 MPa (Elder and Athanasiou 2009; Hung et al. 2004; Afoke et al. 1987).

The recreation of both compression forces and shear stresses in chondrocyte cultures *in vitro* has led to the generation of cartilaginous matrices that resemble the structure and organization of native cartilage more closely than those obtained in nonstimulated cultures (Carver and Heath 1999; Darling and Athanasiou 2003; Grodzinsky et al. 2000; Marlovits et al. 2003). Several investigators have cultured primary chondrocytes on three-dimensional scaffolds under conditions of fluid shear to generate cartilage tissue engineered constructs. All studies show an upregulation of glycosaminoglycan (GAG) and collagen type II production, as early as 28 days. These values were significantly higher than those yielded by statically cultured chondrocytes, with an increase of up to 180% in GAG production. In addition, some studies reported an alignment of the cells in the direction of the flow-producing ECM structurally similar to some areas of native articular cartilage.

Mizuno et al. (2001) compared the application of hydrostatic pressure and shear stresses due to fluid flow on three-dimensional chondrocyte cultures. Both means of stimulation resulted in higher GAG production than the static controls; however, hydrostratic compression of 2.8 MPa resulted in greater upregulation than fluid shearing. It was also shown in this study that the pattern of application of the hydrostatic pressure is an important factor in chondrocyte stimulation, with cyclic compression with a frequency as low as 0.015 Hz yielding greater matrix production than constant compression at the same values of the applied force. In all conditions, a native-like matrix was observed, containing lacunae that entrapped the chondrocytes and a uniform spatial distribution. Carver and Heath (1999) had found similar results but reported that the combination of fluid flow and intermittent pressurization seemed to accelerate cartilaginous matrix formation. Hung et al. (2004) reported the production of cartilage-like tissue after culturing chondrocytes seeded on agarose gels for 8 weeks under physiologic deformational loading.

Hu and Athanasiou (2006b) have been able to make scaffoldless tissue engineered cartilage constructs by self assembly of articular chondrocytes. Application of hydrostatic pressure on these self-assembled constructs resulted in significant upregulation of collagen production and maintenance of GAG content, which seemed to decrease in nonstimulated samples (Hu and Athanasiou 2006a). In a later study from the same group, it was found that stimulated constructs not only showed increases on levels of ECM molecules, but also an improvement in the mechanical properties, with over 100% increase in the values of aggregate and Young's modulus. This same study also demonstrated the importance of combining mechanical stimulation via hydrostatic compression with biochemical stimulation via growth factor supplementation. It was found that hydrostatic pressure of 10 MPa combined with transforming growth factor $\beta 1$ supplementation resulted in additive effects on mechanical properties, but effects on ECM synthesis were synergistic (Elder and Athanasiou 2008). A similar effect was observed earlier by

Bonassar et al. (2001), whom also reported that combining mechanical stimulation with insulin-like growth factor resulted in additive ECM synthesis. Growth factors interact with chondrocytes via integrin receptors, which at the same time act as cell mechanosensors, as explained below (Ostergaard et al. 1998; Wright et al. 1997).

The mechanotransduction mechanisms that govern chondrocyte function are poorly understood, as it happens with most cell types of the skeletal system. Sensing of an applied mechanical load on the condrocyte's membrane seems to be carried out by stretch-activated ion channels and by integrin receptors. Natoli et al. (2010) recently demonstrated that increasing $Ca^{2+}$ and $Na^+$ outflux from the cell by using ATPase-specific inhibitors, improves the tensile properties of engineered cartilage constructs via increases in GAG and collagen production. Chondrocytes cultured in monolayers and exposed to cyclic compression exhibited hyperpolarization of their membranes due to the activation of SK, slow conductance $Ca^{2+}$ and $Na^+$ channels. Compression also seems to activate L-type stretch-activated $Ca^{2+}$ channels, which are involved in tyrosine phosphorylation of FAK and paxillin (Wright et al. 1996; Ramage et al. 2009). In addition, it has been reported that the application of mechanical loads stimulates ATP release via activation of hemichannels, in turn activating P2 receptors (Garcia and Knight 2010).

Integrin receptors also play an important role in mechanosensing. Blocking of these receptors results in unresponsiveness of chondrocytes to compression, decreasing levels of aggrecan and matrix metalloprotein (MMP) 3 mRNA expression (Kock et al. 2009). Particularly $\alpha_5\beta_1$ controls $K^+$ influx, thereby intervening in tyrosine phosphorylation of FAK and paxillin, and activation of protein kinase C (Lee et al. 2002; Wright et al. 1997). FAK phosphorylation leads to the activation of MEK–ERK–MAP kinase (MAPK) cascade, which in turn induce transcription factors AP-1 and Runx2 (Ramage et al. 2009; Papachristou et al. 2005). Furthermore, mechanical loads have been reported to stimulate Sox9, a transcription factor directly involved in aggrecan and collagen type II production (Hardingham et al. 2006).

## 23.2.2 Bone

Bone is a hard connective tissue that provides mechanical support to the human body and is a frame for locomotion. Therefore, on a macroscopic level, bone is one of the tissues most obviously exposed to mechanical, gravitational forces in the form of weight loads. Furthermore, it is well known that physical activity like exercising promotes bone growth, while extended resting and low-gravity conditions result in a loss of bone mass. Interstitial fluid flow changes depending on the different physical activities that translate into compression, bending, and resting, as well as other physiological conditions such as hypertension or increased vascularization during wound healing.

Mechanical forces stimulate bone deformation and remodeling by creating a transcortical pressure gradient and forcing the interstitial fluid to move from the bone matrix into the harvesian lumens (Piekarski and Munro 1977). Both osteocytes and osteoblasts are exposed to hydromechanical forces exerted on the membrane by interstitial fluid flow within the haversian system. It is believed that shear stresses generated by these forces regulate osteocyte and osteoblast functions and thereby bone formation and remodeling. Values of shear stresses due to interstitial fluid flow have been estimated, and they seem to be location dependent, ranging from values of 0 to 20 dyn/cm$^2$ (Hillsley and Frangos 1994; Mi et al. 2005). Researchers have been imitating these flow dynamic conditions *in vitro* to elucidate the mechanisms by which shear-induced bone cell stimulation works.

In bone tissue engineering strategies, the most obvious choice as the cellular component is the osteoblast as it is the main cell type involved in bone production. The effect of fluid flow on osteoblast function has been widely studied, and some of the findings are summarized below (Werntz et al. 1996). Nevertheless, it is important to point out that due to their advanced state of maturation, osteoblasts have limited proliferative capacity and a high senescence rate that make them poor candidates for these applications (Bruder and Fox 1999). Bone marrow mesenchymal stem cells (MSCs) are pluripotent progenitor cells whose proliferation rates are significantly higher than those of osteoblasts. In addition, they can be expanded over numerous passages without losing its differentiation potential, making then an appealing alternative (Caplan 2005). Currently, most bone tissue engineering studies that contemplate the use of cells, concentrate on MSC. In this section, we talk about the effect of fluid shear stresses (FSSs) on osteoblast function, as well as on MSCs undergoing osteoblastic differentiation.

*In vitro* studies to assess the effect of FSS have been conducted on two-dimensional surfaces, in which cells are seeded and a given flow rate is applied. Some studies have concentrated on the morphological changes of osteoblasts due to FSS by looking at the cytoskeleton. Liu et al. (2010b) were able to observe morphological changes on osteoblasts by exposing them to FSS at values of 1.2, 1.6, and 1.9 Pa for 1 h. By fluorescently tagging the cytoskeleton, they observed that, after 1.6 Pa, there was significant cell elongation and alignment along the direction of the flow. However, they demonstrated that this effect is dependent on extracellular calcium as no morphological changes took place when calcium-depleted medium was used, implying that calcium may play an important role in FSS-mediated osteoblast stimulation. The effect of shear stress on the cytoskeleton is not only morphological, there seem to be changes in its molecular composition and distribution as well. Using a parallel plate flow chamber, Jackson et al. (2008) exposed the preosteoblastic cell line MC3T3-E1 and human fetal osteoblasts to 2 Pa of fluid shear for 2 h. Western blots analyses revealed a dramatic increase in cross-linking proteins actin and filamin, as well as vimentin, after fluid flow exposure. Moreover, they were also more uniformly distributed throughout the cytoskeleton.

As mentioned earlier, changes on the cells membrane and cytoskeleton are directly related to mechanotransduction mechanisms, altering the cell's internal biochemical pathways that govern its function. In the case of osteoblasts, this fact was illustrated by Gardinier et al. (2009) when exposing mouse preosteblastic MC3T3-E1 to either FSS (12 dyn/cm$^2$) or cyclic hydrostatic pressure. Also observing cytoskeletal changes, they reported an increase in ATP and cell stiffness, when compared with static cultures, after 5 and 15 min of stimulus application, respectively. It was also reported an upregulation on the secretion of cyclooxygenase-2 after 1 h of both means of mechanical stimulation. Both cyclic hydrostatic pressure and FSS applied for 1 h increased expression of cyclooxygenase-2 (Gardinier et al. 2009). Reich and Frangos (1993) also showed FSS stimulation on osteoblast function. Nitric oxide and PGE2 production and release from osteoblasts due to fluid flow increased in a dose-dependent manner. Prostaglandin PGE2 induces accumulation of cyclic adenosine monophosphate (cAMP), and translates into osteoblast proliferation and bone formation (Reich and Frangos 1993; Riddle and Donahue 2009; Sikavitsas et al. 2001). For a more detailed review on possible mechanotransduction mechanisms related to osteoblasts, we refer the reader to the review by Sikavitsas et al. (2001).

As mentioned earlier, MSC are an appealing alternative in bone tissue engineering. Their osteoblastic differentiation when cultured in osteogenic media (supplemented with b-glycerophosphate, dexamethasone, and ascorbic acid) has been widely reported in the literature (Jaiswal et al. 1997). Even more importantly, their differentiation into the osteogenic lineage is enhanced by exposure to shear stress due to the flow of media. Bancroft et al. (2002) cultured mouse MSCs on titanium fiber meshes in a flow perfusion bioreactor a different flow rates (0.3, 1.0, and 3.0 mL/min), using osteogenic media. Increases in calcium deposition and upregulation in alkaline phosphatase (ALP) activity were under FSS, when compared with static cultures. To isolate the effect of shear forces from the improved mass transport due to the perfusion, shear forces were changed by varying the viscosity of the culture medium under a constant flow rate. An increase in viscosity, which translates into greater shear forces, was found to enhance the deposition of mineralized ECM, thus corroborating that greater MSC osteogenic differentiation was in fact a result of the shear forces exerted on the cells (Sikavitsas et al. 2003).

In addition to stimulating the generation of mineralized matrix, shear stresses induce greater functionalization of tissue engineering constructs. Gomes et al. (2006) found that MSC secreted greater levels of several growth factors (transforming growth factor-β1, fibroblast growth factor-2, vascular endothelial growth factor, and bone morphogenetic protein-2) under fluid flow than on static conditions, and was directly proportional to flow rate. This effect was even more pronounced at later time points perhaps because of a combined effect between shear forces and the already deposited growth factors, providing evidence on how the substrate may influence the extent of FSS-mediated differentiation via stimulation of integrins in FAs. This is further illustrated by the findings of Alvarez-Barreto et al. (2011), who cultured MSCs on scaffolds functionalized with the adhesion peptide Arg–Gly–Asp (RGD). It was found that the effects of shear stresses due to flow perfusion on important osteogenic markers (calcium deposition and ALP activity) were greater on RGD-modified surfaces than on plain, unmodified scaffolds. Even more interesting was the fact that there seems to be an optimal RGD surface concentration for MSC osteoblastic differentiation, and it depends on the applied flow rate.

There is tantalizing evidence on how FSS stimulate MSCs differentiation into an ostoblastic phenotype, but the exact mechanisms by which this happens are not clear. It is believed that MSC sense shear forces by different mechanisms. One of them is through stretch-activated ion channels. Unlike osteoblasts, $Ca^{2+}$ secretion by MSCs does not occur via L-type $Ca^{2+}$ channels but is rather mediated by inositol 1,4,5-trisphosphate receptors (InsP3Rs) and its entry is controlled by store-operated $Ca^{2+}$ channels (Kawano et al. 2002; Liu et al. 2010a). Integrins represent another form of MSCs mechanosensing abilities by inducing the activation of ERK1/2 that further upregulate and activate transcription factors, such as AP-1 (Kapur et al. 2003; Ward et al. 2007; Baba et al. 2003). Changes in the cytoskeleton also contribute to sensing mechanical forces in these cells, especially through actin filaments whose contraction is important in differentiation via overexpression of Rho or Rho-associated kinase (Rock) (Arnsdorf et al. 2009; Rodriguez et al. 2004).

As far as transforming the mechanical signals into biochemical signals, MMPs are believed to play an important role, particularly MMP-13, and disruption of the balance between MMPs and their inhibitors (Kasper et al. 2007). Furthermore, MMPs modulate the activity of important osseous growth factors such as transforming growth factor β1, fibroblast growth factor 2, and vascular endothelial growth factor (Scutt and Bertram 1999). The translated biochemical signals activate NO, PGE2/PKA, $Ca^{2+}$/protein kinase C and MAPK-signaling pathways that, in turn, increase the activity of transcription factors Runx2 and AP-1. These factors promote the expression of important markers such as ALP, osteocalcin, collagen I, and osteopontin (Liu et al. 2010a; Sikavitsas et al. 2001).

## 23.2.3 Tendons

Tendons connect muscle to bone and transmit forces from the former to the latter, often in a cyclical behavior. As tendons such as the Achilles tendon are needed to transmit forces up to 9 kN, the maximum tensile strength of the tendon is also required to be large, and it can vary from 60 to 100 MPa (Butler et al. 2004; Johnson et al. 1994). Unfortunately, with these stresses come routine injuries to athletes or the general population and the tendon itself does not possess strong individual healing capabilities (Åström 1998; Kannus and Jozsa 1991; Khan et al. 1999). This necessitates the research and development of tissue engineered tendon constructs.

In tendon tissue engineering, the application of cyclical stretching has shown to increase cell proliferation, alignment, and gene expression of stem cells and tenocytes (Butler et al. 2004). By applying a routine cyclical longitudinal stretching program *in vitro* to a human umbilical vein construct seeded with mesenchymal stem cells, there was an 800% increase in cell density with improved cell integration and orientation in the ECM when compared with a nonstimulated control group. This was in addition to a doubling of the original vein tensile strength, indicating remodeling and excretion of ECM due to the cellular signals from the mechanical stimulus (Abousleiman et al. 2009).

As stated, mechanical stimulation can also increase gene expression of specific tendon markers such as collagen I, insulin growth factor-1, tenascin C, decorin, matrix metalloproteinase-2 (MMP-2), MMP-3, MMP-13, and others (Chiquet et al. 1996; Chiquet-Ehrismann et al. 1994; Chokalingam et al. 2009; Eckes et al. 1993; Hatamochi et al. 1989; Lambert et al. 1992; Leigh et al. 2008; Li et al. 2008; Mauch et al. 1989; Scott et al. 2007). It has been shown that when the duration of stimulation is brief, gene expression (a decrease in MMP-3 and decorin B) is similar to gene expression when tendinosis occurs (Alfredson and Ohberg 2005). Rapid frequency of stretching for 3 days also shows decreases in tendon markers such as collagen 1, collagen 3, MMP-3, and decorin B which simulates nonhealthy tenocyte growth (Yates 2009).

These results indicate that there is a balance between the duration and frequency of mechanical stimulation that is optimal for cell differentiation (if using stem cells), proliferation, and health.

In addition to traditional unidirectional mechanical stimulation, bioreactors have been designed that can deliver both rotational and translational stimulus, which more closely simulated normal tendon use. With this technique, collagen I, collagen III, and tenascin-C all were positively expressed along with cells aligned with the collagen fibers in the direction of stretching (Altman et al. 2002a,b).

## 23.2.4 Skin

There are many tissue engineering solutions available for the replacement of damaged or lost skin (MacNeil 2007, 2008). The current gold standard for the repair of damaged or lost skin is autologous tissue grafts. The availability of autologous skin tissue for transplantation is limited and can cause necrosis at the donor site. This has brought about the need for improved skin grafts. These grafts can be composed of synthetic or natural materials and also can come in acellular and cellular varieties (Boyce et al. 2002; Dieckmann et al. 2010). There are many problems associated with these graft solutions including poor physical properties, biocompatibility, and ephemeral duration of use. The physical strength of the construct is one of the greatest concerns. Many tissue engineered grafts have been found to be much weaker than normal human skin (Agache et al. 1980; Clark et al. 1996; Khatyr et al. 2004; Lafrance et al. 1995). The inability to match the physical properties of grafts with that of native skin tissue presents major problems in their clinical use (MacNeil 2008; Harrison and MacNeil 2008).

Natural healthy skin is under constant stress and tension (Silver et al. 2003). This natural mechanical behavior of skin is dominated by the dermis under normal conditions. Passive tension created during the development of the collagen fiber network in the dermis is the major component of these internal forces. Fibroblasts present in the dermis are involved in the production of active tension though interactions with other cells and the surrounding ECM. These cell–cell and cell–ECM interactions are responsible for the contraction of wounds in the dermal layering. External forces along with transferred forces from dermal layering create loading and stress forces on the epidermis.

Stretching of the epidermis is considered to have a role in the proliferation (Gormar et al. 1990) and protein synthesis of keratinocytes (Silver et al. 2003). The application of uniaxial strain up to ~20% on constructs seeded with keratinocytes has been found to induce proliferation signaled by calcium influx and phosphorylation of epidermal growth factor receptor and ERK1/2 (Yano et al. 2004). Mechanical stretch of keratinocytes has also been linked to the remodeling of the ECM through the increased expression of MMP-1, 2, and 9 (Kippenberger et al. 2000). There have also been links found between static and cyclic straining of keratinocytes. Bhadal et al. (2008) found that 10% static uniaxial strain of normal human keratinocytes induced a reduction in the production of urokinase-type plasminogen activator which is important for the migration of keratinocytes during wound healing. This was in contrast to cyclic strain of the keratinocytes which showed an increase in the production of urokinase-type plasminogen activator. This demonstrates keratinocytes ability to sense different types of dynamic shear forces and create a distinctive biological response to the forces.

Fibroblasts contained in the dermal layer of skin have been found to be a major source of response to mechanical stimulation (Kessler et al. 2001; Silver et al. 2003). Statically stressed dermal fibroblasts have been found to produce upregulation of over 50 tension-inducible genes (Kessler et al. 2001), showing dermal fibroblast's ultimate ability to sense mechanical stress. These genes are responsible for ECM proteins, fibrogenic growth factors, protease inhibitors, components of FAs, and the cytoskeleton. Dermal fibroblast's response to mechanical forces has also been observed in the organization of cellular alignment due to the cyclic straining of fibroblast constructs. Uniaxial strain was shown to cause dermal fibroblasts to align perpendicular to the direction of applied stress (Berry et al. 2003a; Reno et al. 2009). This was contrary to the effect of biaxial strain that caused parallel alignment of fibroblasts (Grymes and Sawyer 1997) and even nonuniform arrangement (Berry et al. 2003a). Cyclic uniaxial strain of only ~15% has been found to be enough stress to align dermal fibroblasts (Wen et al. 2009).

This demonstrated that mechanosensation in dermal fibroblasts is dependent on the direction of the exerted force on the cellular construct. This has also been seen in the promotion of cellular proliferation and collagen production in neonatal fibroblastic dermal cells from uniaxial strain, whereas biaxial cyclic stress has been found to inhibit both cellular proliferation and collagen production in neonatal fibroblastic dermal cells (Berry et al. 2003a). Uniaxial cyclic stress was also found to induce the production of remodeling MMPs (Mudera et al. 2000; Berry et al. 2003b), most notably MMP 9 which helps in the migration of fibroblasts during wound healing (Reno et al. 2009). Increased amounts of preloading of tissues before cyclic stretching increased production of MMPs (Berry et al. 2003b) showing that greater amounts of shear forces influence dermal fibroblast's ability to remodel the ECM.

Although the expansion of skin tissue was linked to shear forces the implementation of shear forces to produce engineered skin tissue grafts is limited. Although *in vivo* tissue expanders can create dermal flaps for transplantation, they create tissues without the exact epidermal and dermal thickness. The creation of the expanded tissue can also create discomfort, take long a period to create, and require an extra surgical procedure. Ladd et al. (2009) has proposed a bioreactor for the expansion of skin tissue *in vitro* using uniaxial stretch as mechanical stimulus to human foreskin. By straining the tissue over a 6-day period, they were able to expand the skin explants to twice their size while maintaining the thickness of the tissue. The expanded tissue construct maintained its dermal and epidermal structure while keeping similar tensile properties to that of the native tissue. This approach demonstrated that the use of mechanical stress could provide an excellent method of creating engineered tissue constructs for skin grafts *in vitro*.

## 23.2.5 Cardiac

One of the major goals of heart tissue engineering is the creation of grafts for the repair of cardiac infarctions. This is not a trivial task due to the heart's complex structure and cellular composition. The heart is the first functionally active organ that is developed during embryogenesis and is responsible for helping in the development and maintenance of the body. Although the heart is influenced by active mechanical stimulation through striated muscle contraction, the interior of the heart is subjected to hemodynamic forces. With the understanding of the contribution of mechanical stimulation on the culture and development of cells and tissue, the use of mechanical stress in the form of mechanical stretch and fluid flow shear stress have been investigated widely in heart tissue-related cells.

Use of uniaxial stretching during culturing was proven to be an effective method in the engineering of functional cardiac tissue (Eschenhagen et al. 1997; Zimmermann et al. 2000, 2002a,b; Fink et al. 2000). Mechanical uniaxial stretch was found to promote improved organization of cardiac myocytes (Birla et al. 2007), lengthening of myofilaments (Komuro et al. 1990; Sadoshima and Izumo 1997), and improved contractual forces of constructs (Eschenhagen et al. 1997). These properties were seen to be similar to that of native working myocardium. The quite notable characteristic of vascular formation was found in implanted constructs that have been mechanically stretched *in vitro* (Zimmermann et al. 2002b). This was considered a major contributor to the survival of tissue constructs implanted onto the heart (Zimmermann et al. 2002a). Moving toward a solution to repair infarctions, stretch-stimulated grafts were implanted into heart infarctions of rats and showed not only signs of repair but also strengthening (Zimmermann et al. 2006).

The use of flow perfusion in the promotion of cardiac graft development has also shown some potential. Although fluid shear flow allowed for increased cell viability though increased oxygen and nutrient transport (Hecker et al. 2008; Radisic et al. 2006; Carrier et al. 2002), it did not demonstrate the promotion of ordered myocardiac structures. When fluid flow was coupled with electrical stimulation for the contraction of constructs, cell differentiation and myofibril-like organization were observed (Radisic et al. 2004). Cardiac cells did not show signs of differentiation and organization to cardiac tissue under FSS. Instead, differentiation and cardiac organization have only been seen with the inclusion of mechanical stretch or electrical stimulation.

## 23.2.6 Vascular Grafts

The blood vessel network's job is to perfuse blood to the body's tissues. Activation of the heart during morphogenesis produces hemodynamic forces that are exerted on endothelial cells. These forces stimulate the endothelial cells and help in the development (Dardik et al. 2005) and maintenance of the vasculature (Niklason 1999; Dahl et al. 2010). The application of pulsatile stress to vascular cells has shown to promote increase in nitric oxide production, endothelial nitric oxide synthase expression (Li et al. 2003), and the activation of ion channels (Chatterjee et al. 2003) for cell signaling. Pulsatile stresses have also been shown to promote the production collagen (Kim et al. 1999; O'Callaghan and Williams 2000) and of MMPs (Seliktar et al. 2001; Magid et al. 2003; O'Callaghan and Williams 2000) that influence ECM remodeling. The effect of hemodynamic shear forces (Groenendijk et al. 2005, 2004; Ahsan and Nerem 2010; Hahn and Schwartz 2009; Ando and Yamamoto 2009) on endothelial cells has prompted the preference of incorporating pulsatile stress in the development of vascular graft constructs (Lee et al. 2002; Ziegler and Nerem 1994; L'Heureux et al. 1998; Niklason 1999).

One of the first attempts at constructing a vascular graft was done by Weinberg and Bell (1986). They employed static culturing techniques to produce a well-differentiated arterial structure. The main problems associated with the generated graft were its low burst strength and longitudinal smooth muscle cell alignment. Incorporation of pulsatile radial stress during culturing has shown to increase wall thickness and burst pressure of smooth muscle cell-seeded grafts (Niklason 1999). These constructs exhibited alignment of the smooth muscle cells parallel to the induced radial stresses which mimics the morphology of native vascular tissue (Vorp et al. 1995). Pulsatile radial stress has also been used to produce multicellular grafts (L'Heureux et al. 1998) and small vessel grafts (Hoerstrup et al. 2001) with improved burst pressures. The improved mechanical strength and material modulus were correlated to the increasing circumferential tensile stress (Seliktar et al. 2001). Other investigations have used pulsatile stress to develop vascular grafts with improved cellular organization (Narita et al. 2004), growth (Jeong et al. 2005), and in the case of cocultures of endothelial cell and smooth muscle cells, ordered tissue formation (McFetridge et al. 2004), promotion of ECM deposition, and cellular differentiation (Williams and Wick 2004).

Other strategies utilizing shear forces have also been investigated in the production of vascular grafts. Although fluid flow has shown to be beneficial for the seeding and culturing of vascular grafts (Sodian et al. 2002; Nasseri et al. 2003; Ott and Ballermann 1995; Dardik et al. 1999), its absence has been accompanied by very poor results making the use of perfusion bioreactors a widely used tool in vascular graft tissue engineering. Bioreactors have been designed to induce not only pulsatile stress but also longitudinal strain on constructs (McCulloch et al. 2004). These have shown to produce similar cellular structural alignment to that of constructs that were only stimulated by pulsatile stresses. Although till today limited success has been demonstrated in the creation of tissue engineered vascular grafts appropriate for clinical use, further research is needed to optimize the design of the vascular graft bioreactors and the levels and types of the exerted forces on the cultured cells.

## 23.2.7 Skeletal Muscle

It is well known that skeletal muscle responds to active and passive mechanical activity *in vivo* (Goldspink et al. 1995, 1991; Gollnick et al. 1972, 1973; Ianuzzo et al. 1976; McCall et al. 1996). Normal responses of healthy skeletal muscle show increases in the number and cross sectional size of muscle fibers when increased mechanical loading is applied. In relation, atrophy of skeletal muscle tissue is observed when mechanical loading is reduced (Benjamin and Hillen 2003). It has even been hypothesized that the development of bone during embryogenesis causes muscle elongation (Stewart 1972) and myofilament organization (Goldspink 1970; Collinsworth et al. 2000). Exercise and stretching of skeletal muscle along with developmental formation create mechanical stress on the tissue which in turn stimulates the muscle.

*In vitro* experiments were designed to mimic the mechanical forces exerted on skeletal muscle *in vivo* (Vandenburgh et al. 1996, 1991, 1989; Collinsworth et al. 2000). Most *in vitro* studies have used mechanical loading of substrates to apply stimulation (Pang et al. 2010). FSS-induced though flow perfusion has shown better cell penetration of scaffolds in skeletal tissue engineering but overall did not prove to be greatly stimulatory (Chromiak et al. 1998). The use of axial stress has been shown to affect the metabolic activity (Hatfaludy et al. 1989), gene regulation (Carson and Booth 1998), and protein expression (Vandenburgh et al. 1990; Perrone et al. 1995; Kumar et al. 2002, 2004; Kumar and Boriek 2003) of primary muscle cells. Similar to studies performed on other cell types, mechanical stress has shown to increase cell proliferation (Vandenburgh et al. 1989; Kook et al. 2008) and potential ECM remodeling through collagen and MMP expression (Auluck et al. 2005; Tatsumi 2010). The most notable response to mechanical stress is the alignment of cells (Vandenburgh 1982) and ordered myofiber development (Collinsworth et al. 2000; Powell et al. 2002). Although cell alignment has been observed under static culture conditions for cells seeded onto patterned substrates (Patz et al. 2005) and natural materials (Engler et al. 2004), increased organization in the development of myofiber formation has been achieved by using axial stress stimulation (Vandenburgh et al. 1991; Okano and Matsuda 1997; Powell et al. 2002; Ahmed et al. 2010). Although stimulation by mechanical stress alone of cultured skeletal muscle cells may not be adequate for the development of higher ordered tissue, its coupling with multiple chemical, electrical, mechanical cues needs to be investigated further (Boonen and Post 2008; Vandenburgh 1987; Boonen et al. 2009).

# References

Abousleiman, R. I., Y. Reyes, P. McFetridge, and V. Sikavitsas. 2009. Tendon tissue engineering using cell-seeded umbilical veins cultured in a mechanical stimulator. *Tissue Eng Part A* 15(4):787–95.

Afoke, N. Y., P. D. Byers, and W. C. Hutton. 1987. Contact pressures in the human hip joint. *J Bone Joint Surg Br* 69(4):536–41.

Agache, P. G., C. Monneur, J. L. Leveque, and J. De Rigal. 1980. Mechanical properties and Young's modulus of human skin in vivo. *Arch Dermatol Res* 269(3):221–32.

Ahmed, W. W., T. Wolfram, A. M. Goldyn et al. 2010. Myoblast morphology and organization on biochemically micro-patterned hydrogel coatings under cyclic mechanical strain. *Biomaterials* 31(2):250–8.

Ahsan, T. and R. M. Nerem. 2010. Fluid shear stress promotes an endothelial-like phenotype during the early differentiation of embryonic stem sells. *Tissue Eng Part A* 16(11):3547–53.

Alfredson, H. and L. Ohberg. 2005. Neovascularisation in chronic painful patellar tendinosis—promising results after sclerosing neovessels outside the tendon challenge the need for surgery. *Knee Surg Sports Traumatol Arthrosc* 13(2):74–80.

Altman, G. H., R. L. Horan, I. Martin et al. 2002a. Cell differentiation by mechanical stress. *FASEB J* 16(2):270–2.

Altman, G. H., H. H. Lu, R. L. Horan et al. 2002b. Advanced bioreactor with controlled application of multidimensional strain for tissue engineering. *J Biomech Eng* 124(6):742–9.

Alvarez-Barreto, J. F., L. Bonnie, S. VanGordon et al. 2011. Enhanced osteoblastic differentiation of mesenchymal stem cells seeded in RGD functionalized PLLA scaffolds and cultured in a flow perfusion bioreactor. *J Tissue Eng Regen Med* 5(6):464–75.

Alvarez-Barreto, J. and V. I. Sikavitsas. 2006. Tissue engineering bioreactors. In *Tissue Engineering and Artificial Organs*, edited by J. D. Bronzino. Boca Raton: Taylor & Francis Group.

Ando, J. and K. Yamamoto. 2009. Vascular mechanobiology: Endothelial cell responses to fluid shear stress. *Circ J* 73(11):1983–92.

Arnsdorf, E. J., P. Tummala, R. Y. Kwon, and C. R. Jacobs. 2009. Mechanically induced osteogenic differentiation—the role of RhoA, ROCKII and cytoskeletal dynamics. *J Cell Sci* 122(Pt 4):546–53.

Åström, M. 1998. Partial rupture in chronic achilles tendinopathy: A retrospective analysis of 342 cases. *Acta Orthopaedica* 69:404–407.

Auluck, A., V. Mudera, N. P. Hunt, and M. P. Lewis. 2005. A three-dimensional *in vitro* model system to study the adaptation of craniofacial skeletal muscle following mechanostimulation. *Eur J Oral Sci* 113(3):218–24.

Baba, H. A., J. Stypmann, F. Grabellus et al. 2003. Dynamic regulation of MEK/Erks and Akt/GSK-3beta in human end-stage heart failure after left ventricular mechanical support: Myocardial mechanotransduction-sensitivity as a possible molecular mechanism. *Cardiovasc Res* 59(2):390–9.

Bancroft, G. N., V. I. Sikavitsas, J. van den Dolder et al. 2002. Fluid flow increases mineralized matrix deposition in 3D perfusion culture of marrow stromal osteoblasts in a dose-dependent manner. *Proc Natl Acad Sci USA* 99(20):12600–5.

Bao, G., R. D. Kamm, W. Thomas et al. 2010. Molecular biomechanics: The molecular basis of how forces regulate cellular function. *Mol Cell Biomech* 3(2):91–105.

Benjamin, M. and B. Hillen. 2003. Mechanical influences on cells, tissues and organs—"Mechanical Morphogenesis". *Eur J Morphol* 41(1):3–7.

Berry, C. C., C. Cacou, D. A. Lee, D. L. Bader, and J. C. Shelton. 2003a. Dermal fibroblasts respond to mechanical conditioning in a strain profile dependent manner. *Biorheology* 40(1–3):337–45.

Berry, C. C., J. C. Shelton, D. L. Bader, and D. A. Lee. 2003b. Influence of external uniaxial cyclic strain on oriented fibroblast-seeded collagen gels. *Tissue Eng* 9(4):613–24.

Bhadal, N., I. B. Wall, S. R. Porter et al. 2008. The effect of mechanical strain on protease production by keratinocytes. *Br J Dermatol* 158(2):396–8.

Birla, R. K., Y. C. Huang, and R. G. Dennis. 2007. Development of a novel bioreactor for the mechanical loading of tissue-engineered heart muscle. *Tissue Eng* 13(9):2239–48.

Bonassar, L. J., A. J. Grodzinsky, E. H. Frank et al. 2001. The effect of dynamic compression on the response of articular cartilage to insulin-like growth factor-I. *J Orthop Res* 19(1):11–7.

Boonen, K. J. and M. J. Post. 2008. The muscle stem cell niche: Regulation of satellite cells during regeneration. *Tissue Eng Part B Rev* 14(4):419–31.

Boonen, K. J., K. Y. Rosaria-Chak, F. P. Baaijens, D. W. van der Schaft, and M. J. Post. 2009. Essential environmental cues from the satellite cell niche: Optimizing proliferation and differentiation. *Am J Physiol Cell Physiol* 296(6):C1338–45.

Botchwey, E. A., S. R. Pollack, E. M. Levine, and C. T. Laurencin. 2001. Bone tissue engineering in a rotating bioreactor using a microcarrier matrix system. *J Biomed Mater Res* 55(2):242–53.

Boyce, S. T., R. J. Kagan, K. P. Yakuboff et al. 2002. Cultured skin substitutes reduce donor skin harvesting for closure of excised, full-thickness burns. *Ann Surg* 235(2):269–79.

Bruder, S. P. and B. S. Fox. 1999. Tissue engineering of bone—Cell based strategies. *Clin Orthop Relat Res* 367(Suppl):S68–83.

Burridge, K., K. Fath, T. Kelly, G. Nuckolls, and C. Turner. 1988. Focal adhesions: Transmembrane junctions between the extracellular matrix and the cytoskeleton. *Annu Rev Cell Biol* 4:487–525.

Butler, D. L., N. Juncosa, and M. R. Dressler. 2004. Functional efficacy of tendon repair processes. *Annu Rev Biomed Eng* 6:303–29.

Calalb, M. B., T. R. Polte, and S. K. Hanks. 1995. Tyrosine phosphorylation of focal adhesion kinase at sites in the catalytic domain regulates kinase activity: A role for Src family kinases. *Mol Cell Biol* 15(2):954–63.

Caplan, A. I. 2005. Review: Mesenchymal stem cells: Cell-based reconstructive therapy in orthopedics. *Tissue Eng* 11(7–8):1198–211.

Carrier, R. L., M. Rupnick, R. Langer et al. 2002. Perfusion improves tissue architecture of engineered cardiac muscle. *Tissue Eng* 8(2):175–88.

Carson, J. A. and F. W. Booth. 1998. Effect of serum and mechanical stretch on skeletal alpha-actin gene regulation in cultured primary muscle cells. *Am J Physiol* 275(6 Pt 1):C1438–48.

Carver, S. E. and C. A. Heath. 1999. Influence of intermittent pressure, fluid flow, and mixing on the regenerative properties of articular chondrocytes. *Biotechnol Bioeng* 65(3):274–81.

Chatterjee, S., A. B. Al-Mehdi, I. Levitan, T. Stevens, and A. B. Fisher. 2003. Shear stress increases expression of a KATP channel in rat and bovine pulmonary vascular endothelial cells. *Am J Physiol Cell Physiol* 285(4):C959–67.

Chen, C. S., J. Tan, and J. Tien. 2004. Mechanotransduction at cell-matrix and cell-cell contacts. *Annu Rev Biomed Eng* 6:275–302.

Chen, F. M., M. Zhang, and Z. F. Wu. 2010. Toward delivery of multiple growth factors in tissue engineering. *Biomaterials* 31(24):6279–308.

Chicurel, M. E., C. S. Chen, and D. E. Ingber. 1998. Cellular control lies in the balance of forces. *Curr Opin Cell Biol* 10(2):232–9.

Chiquet, M., M. Matthisson, M. Koch, M. Tannheimer, and R. Chiquet-Ehrismann. 1996. Regulation of extracellular matrix synthesis by mechanical stress. *Biochem Cell Biol* 74(6):737–44.

Chiquet-Ehrismann, R., M. Tannheimer, M. Koch et al. 1994. Tenascin-C expression by fibroblasts is elevated in stressed collagen gels. *J Cell Biol* 127(6 Pt 2):2093–101.

Chokalingam, K., N. Juncosa-Melvin, S. A. Hunter et al. 2009. Tensile stimulation of murine stem cell-collagen sponge constructs increases collagen type I gene expression and linear stiffness. *Tissue Eng Part A* 15(9):2561–70.

Chromiak, J. A., J. Shansky, C. Perrone, and H. H. Vandenburgh. 1998. Bioreactor perfusion system for the long-term maintenance of tissue-engineered skeletal muscle organoids. *In vitro Cell Dev Biol Anim* 34(9):694–703.

Clark, J. A., J. C. Cheng, and K. S. Leung. 1996. Mechanical properties of normal skin and hypertrophic scars. *Burns* 22(6):443–6.

Collinsworth, A. M., C. E. Torgan, S. N. Nagda et al. 2000. Orientation and length of mammalian skeletal myocytes in response to a unidirectional stretch. *Cell Tissue Res* 302(2):243–51.

Dahl, K. N., A. Kalinowski, and K. Pekkan. 2010. Mechanobiology and the microcirculation: Cellular, nuclear and fluid mechanics. *Microcirculation* 17(3):179–91.

Dardik, A., A. Liu, and B. J. Ballermann. 1999. Chronic *in vitro* shear stress stimulates endothelial cell retention on prosthetic vascular grafts and reduces subsequent *in vivo* neointimal thickness. *J Vasc Surg* 29(1):157–67.

Dardik, A., A. Yamashita, F. Aziz, H. Asada, and B. E. Sumpio. 2005. Shear stress-stimulated endothelial cells induce smooth muscle cell chemotaxis via platelet-derived growth factor-BB and interleukin-1alpha. *J Vasc Surg* 41(2):321–31.

Darling, E. M. and K. A. Athanasiou. 2003. Articular cartilage bioreactors and bioprocesses. *Tissue Eng* 9(1):9–26.

Davidson, R. M., D. W. Tatakis, and A. L. Auerbach. 1990. Multiple forms of mechanosensitive ion channels in osteoblast-like cells. *Pflugers Arch* 416(6):646–51.

Dieckmann, C., R. Renner, L. Milkova, and J. C. Simon. 2010. Regenerative medicine in dermatology: Biomaterials, tissue engineering, stem cells, gene transfer and beyond. *Exp Dermatol* 19(8):697–706.

Domingos, P. P., P. M. Fonseca, W. Nadruz, Jr., and K. G. Franchini. 2002. Load-induced focal adhesion kinase activation in the myocardium: Role of stretch and contractile activity. *Am J Physiol Heart Circ Physiol* 282(2):H556–64.

Eckes, B., C. Mauch, G. Huppe, and T. Krieg. 1993. Downregulation of collagen synthesis in fibroblasts within three-dimensional collagen lattices involves transcriptional and posttranscriptional mechanisms. *FEBS Lett* 318(2):129–33.

Elder, B. D. and K. A. Athanasiou. 2008. Synergistic and additive effects of hydrostatic pressure and growth factors on tissue formation. *PLoS One* 3(6):e2341.

Elder, B. D. and K. A. Athanasiou. 2009. Hydrostatic pressure in articular cartilage tissue engineering: From chondrocytes to tissue regeneration. *Tissue Eng Part B Rev* 15(1):43–53.

Engelmayr, G. C. Jr, D. K. Hildebrand, F. W. Sutherland, J. E. Jr Mayer, and M. S. Sacks. 2003. A novel bioreactor for the dynamic flexural stimulation of tissue engineered heart valve biomaterials. *Biomaterials* 24(14):2523–32.

Engler, A. J., M. A. Griffin, S. Sen et al. 2004. Myotubes differentiate optimally on substrates with tissue-like stiffness: Pathological implications for soft or stiff microenvironments. *J Cell Biol* 166(6):877–87.

Eschenhagen, T., C. Fink, U. Remmers et al. 1997. Three-dimensional reconstitution of embryonic cardio-myocytes in a collagen matrix: A new heart muscle model system. *FASEB J* 11(8):683–94.

Fink, C., S. Ergun, D. Kralisch et al. 2000. Chronic stretch of engineered heart tissue induces hypertrophy and functional improvement. *FASEB J* 14(5):669–79.

Garcia, M. and M. M. Knight. 2010. Cyclic loading opens hemichannels to release ATP as part of a chon-drocyte mechanotransduction pathway. *J Orthop Res* 28(4):510–5.

Gardinier, J. D., S. Majumdar, R. L. Duncan, and L. Wang. 2009. Cyclic hydraulic pressure and fluid flow differentially modulate cytoskeleton re-organization in MC3T3 osteoblasts. *Cell Mol Bioeng* 2(1):133–43.

Gautam, M., A. Gojova, and A. I. Barakat. 2006. Flow-activated ion channels in vascular endothelium. *Cell Biochem Biophys* 46(3):277–84.

Goldspink, G. 1970. Morphological adaptation due to growth and activity. In *The Physiology and Biochemistry of Muscle as a Food, 2*, edited by Briskey, E. J., Cassens, R. G., and Trautman, J. C. University of Wisconsin. Madison: University of Wisconsin Press.

Goldspink, D. F., V. M. Cox, S. K. Smith et al. 1995. Muscle growth in response to mechanical stimuli. *Am J Physiol* 268(2 Pt 1):E288–97.

Goldspink, D. F., J. Easton, S. K. Winterburn, P. E. Williams, and G. E. Goldspink. 1991. The role of passive stretch and repetitive electrical stimulation in preventing skeletal muscle atrophy while reprogram-ming gene expression to improve fatigue resistance. *J Card Surg* 6(1 Suppl):218–24.

Gollnick, P. D., R. B. Armstrong, B. Saltin et al. 1973. Effect of training on enzyme activity and fiber com-position of human skeletal muscle. *J Appl Physiol* 34(1):107–11.

Gollnick, P. D., R. B. Armstrong, C. W. th Saubert, K. Piehl, and B. Saltin. 1972. Enzyme activity and fiber composition in skeletal muscle of untrained and trained men. *J Appl Physiol* 33(3):312–9.

Gomes, M. E., C. M. Bossano, C. M. Johnston, R. L. Reis, and A. G. Mikos. 2006. *In vitro* localization of bone growth factors in constructs of biodegradable scaffolds seeded with marrow stromal cells and cultured in a flow perfusion bioreactor. *Tissue Eng* 12(1):177–88.

Gomes, M. E., V. I. Sikavitsas, E. Behravesh, R. L. Reis, and A. G. Mikos. 2003. Effect of flow perfusion on the osteogenic differentiation of bone marrow stromal cells cultured on starch-based three-dimensional scaffolds. *J Biomed Mater Res* 67A(1):87–95.

Gormar, F. E., A. Bernd, J. Bereiter-Hahn, and H. Holzmann. 1990. A new model of epidermal differentia-tion: Induction by mechanical stimulation. *Arch Dermatol Res* 282(1):22–32.

Grodzinsky, A. J., M. E. Levenston, M. Jin, and E. H. Frank. 2000. Cartilage tissue remodeling in response to mechanical forces. *Annu Rev Biomed Eng* 2:691–713.

Groenendijk, B. C., B. P. Hierck, A. C. Gittenberger-De Groot, and R. E. Poelmann. 2004. Development-related changes in the expression of shear stress responsive genes KLF-2, ET-1, and NOS-3 in the developing cardiovascular system of chicken embryos. *Dev Dyn* 230(1):57–68.

Groenendijk, B. C., B. P. Hierck, J. Vrolijk et al. 2005. Changes in shear stress-related gene expression after experimentally altered venous return in the chicken embryo. *Circ Res* 96(12):1291–8.

Grymes, R. A. and C. Sawyer. 1997. A novel culture morphology resulting from applied mechanical strain. *In vitro Cell Dev Biol Anim* 33(5):392–7.

Gumbiner, B. M. 1996. Cell adhesion: The molecular basis of tissue architecture and morphogenesis. *Cell* 84(3):345–57.

Hahn, C. and M. A. Schwartz. 2009. Mechanotransduction in vascular physiology and atherogenesis. *Nat Rev Mol Cell Biol* 10(1):53–62.

Hamill, O. P., and B. Martinac. 2001. Molecular basis of mechanotransduction in living cells. *Physiol Rev* 81(2):685–740.

Hardingham, T. E., R. A. Oldershaw, and S. R. Tew. 2006. Cartilage, SOX9 and Notch signals in chondro-genesis. *J Anat* 209(4):469–80.

Harrison, C. A. and S. MacNeil. 2008. The mechanism of skin graft contraction: An update on current research and potential future therapies. *Burns* 34(2):153–63.

Hatamochi, A., M. Aumailley, C. Mauch et al. 1989. Regulation of collagen VI expression in fibroblasts. Effects of cell density, cell-matrix interactions, and chemical transformation. *J Biol Chem* 264(6):3494–9.

Hatfaludy, S., J. Shansky, and H. H. Vandenburgh. 1989. Metabolic alterations induced in cultured skeletal muscle by stretch-relaxation activity. *Am J Physiol* 256(1 Pt 1):C175–81.

Hecker, L., L. Khait, D. Radnoti, and R. Birla. 2008. Development of a microperfusion system for the culture of bioengineered heart muscle. *ASAIO J* 54(3):284–94.

Hillsley, M. V. and J. A. Frangos. 1994. Bone tissue engineering: The role of interstitial fluid flow. *Biotechnol Bioeng* 43(7):573–81.

Hoerstrup, S. P., G. Zund, R. Sodian et al. 2001. Tissue engineering of small caliber vascular grafts. *Eur J Cardiothorac Surg* 20(1):164–9.

Hu, J. C. and K. A. Athanasiou. 2006a. The effects of intermittent hydrostatic pressure on self-assembled articular cartilage constructs. *Tissue Eng* 12(5):1337–44.

Hu, J. C. and K. A. Athanasiou. 2006b. A self-assembling process in articular cartilage tissue engineering. *Tissue Eng* 12(4):969–79.

Huang, S. and X. Fu. 2010. Naturally derived materials-based cell and drug delivery systems in skin regeneration. *J Control Release* 142(2):149–59.

Hung, C. T., R. L. Mauck, C. C. Wang, E. G. Lima, and G. A. Ateshian. 2004. A paradigm for functional tissue engineering of articular cartilage via applied physiologic deformational loading. *Ann Biomed Eng* 32(1):35–49.

Ianuzzo, C. D., P. D. Gollnick, and R. B. Armstrong. 1976. Compensatory adaptations of skeletal muscle fiber types to a long-term functional overload. *Life Sci* 19(10):1517–23.

Jackson, W. M., M. J. Jaasma, R. Y. Tang, and T. M. Keaveny. 2008. Mechanical loading by fluid shear is sufficient to alter the cytoskeletal composition of osteoblastic cells. *Am J Physiol Cell Physiol* 295(4):C1007–15.

Jaiswal, N., S. E. Haynesworth, A. I. Caplan, and S. P. Bruder. 1997. Osteogenic differentiation of purified, culture-expanded human mesenchymal stem cells in vitro. *J Cell Biochem* 64(2):295–312.

Jeong, S. I., J. H. Kwon, J. I. Lim et al. 2005. Mechano-active tissue engineering of vascular smooth muscle using pulsatile perfusion bioreactors and elastic PLCL scaffolds. *Biomaterials* 26(12):1405–11.

Johnson, G. A., D. M. Tramaglini, R. E. Levine et al. 1994. Tensile and viscoelastic properties of human patellar tendon. *J Orthop Res* 12(6):796–803.

Kannus, P. and L. Jozsa. 1991. Histopathological changes preceding spontaneous rupture of a tendon. A controlled study of 891 patients. *J Bone Joint Surg Am* 73(10):1507–25.

Kapur, S., D. J. Baylink, and K. H. Lau. 2003. Fluid flow shear stress stimulates human osteoblast proliferation and differentiation through multiple interacting and competing signal transduction pathways. *Bone* 32(3):241–51.

Kasper, G., J. D. Glaeser, S. Geissler et al. 2007. Matrix metalloprotease activity is an essential link between mechanical stimulus and mesenchymal stem cell behavior. *Stem Cells* 25(8):1985–94.

Kawano, S., S. Shoji, S. Ichinose et al. 2002. Characterization of Ca(2+) signaling pathways in human mesenchymal stem cells. *Cell Calcium* 32(4):165–74.

Kessler, D., S. Dethlefsen, I. Haase et al. 2001. Fibroblasts in mechanically stressed collagen lattices assume a "synthetic" phenotype. *J Biol Chem* 276(39):36575–85.

Khan, K. M., J. L. Cook, F. Bonar, P. Harcourt, and M. Astrom. 1999. Histopathology of common tendinopathies. Update and implications for clinical management. *Sports Med* 27(6):393–408.

Khatyr, F., C. Imberdis, P. Vescovo, D. Varchon, and J. M. Lagarde. 2004. Model of the viscoelastic behaviour of skin *in vivo* and study of anisotropy. *Skin Res Technol* 10(2):96–103.

Kim, B. S., J. Nikolovski, J. Bonadio, and D. J. Mooney. 1999. Cyclic mechanical strain regulates the development of engineered smooth muscle tissue. *Nat Biotechnol* 17(10):979–83.

Kippenberger, S., A. Bernd, S. Loitsch et al. 2000. Signaling of mechanical stretch in human keratinocytes via MAP kinases. *J Invest Dermatol* 114(3):408–12.

Kock, L. M., R. M. Schulz, C. C. van Donkelaar et al. 2009. RGD-dependent integrins are mechanotransducers in dynamically compressed tissue-engineered cartilage constructs. *J Biomech* 42(13):2177–82.

Komuro, I., T. Kaida, Y. Shibazaki et al. 1990. Stretching cardiac myocytes stimulates protooncogene expression. *J Biol Chem* 265(7):3595–8.

Kook, S. H., H. J. Lee, W. T. Chung et al. 2008. Cyclic mechanical stretch stimulates the proliferation of C2C12 myoblasts and inhibits their differentiation via prolonged activation of p38 MAPK. *Mol Cells* 25(4):479–86.

Kumar, A. and A. M. Boriek. 2003. Mechanical stress activates the nuclear factor-kappaB pathway in skeletal muscle fibers: A possible role in Duchenne muscular dystrophy. *FASEB J* 17(3):386–96.

Kumar, A., I. Chaudhry, M. B. Reid, and A. M. Boriek. 2002. Distinct signaling pathways are activated in response to mechanical stress applied axially and transversely to skeletal muscle fibers. *J Biol Chem* 277(48):46493–503.

Kumar, A., R. Murphy, P. Robinson, L. Wei, and A. M. Boriek. 2004. Cyclic mechanical strain inhibits skeletal myogenesis through activation of focal adhesion kinase, Rac-1 GTPase, and NF-kappaB transcription factor. *FASEB J* 18(13):1524–35.

L'Heureux, N., S. Paquet, R. Labbe, L. Germain, and F. A. Auger. 1998. A completely biological tissue-engineered human blood vessel. *FASEB J* 12(1):47–56.

Ladd, M. R., S. J. Lee, A. Atala, and J. J. Yoo. 2009. Bioreactor maintained living skin matrix. *Tissue Eng Part A* 15(4):861–8.

Lafrance, H., L. Yahia, L. Germain, M. Guillot, and F. A. Auger. 1995. Study of the tensile properties of living skin equivalents. *Biomed Mater Eng* 5(4):195–208.

Lambert, C. A., E. P. Soudant, B. V. Nusgens, and C. M. Lapiere. 1992. Pretranslational regulation of extracellular matrix macromolecules and collagenase expression in fibroblasts by mechanical forces. *Lab Invest* 66(4):444–51.

Lee, A. A., D. A. Graham, S. Dela Cruz, A. Ratcliffe, and W. J. Karlon. 2002. Fluid shear stress-induced alignment of cultured vascular smooth muscle cells. *J Biomech Eng* 124(1):37–43.

Lee, H. S., S. J. Millward-Sadler, M. O. Wright et al. 2002. Activation of Integrin-RACK1/PKCalpha signalling in human articular chondrocyte mechanotransduction. *Osteoarthritis Cartilage* 10(11):890–7.

Lehoux, S., Y. Castier, and A. Tedgui. 2006. Molecular mechanisms of the vascular responses to haemodynamic forces. *J Intern Med* 259(4):381–92.

Leigh, D. R., E. L. Abreu, and K. A. Derwin. 2008. Changes in gene expression of individual matrix metalloproteinases differ in response to mechanical unloading of tendon fascicles in explant culture. *J Orthop Res* 26(10):1306–12.

Li, F., B. Li, Q. M. Wang, and J. H. Wang. 2008. Cell shape regulates collagen type I expression in human tendon fibroblasts. *Cell Motil Cytoskeleton* 65(4):332–41.

Li, Y., J. Zheng, I. M. Bird, and R. R. Magness. 2003. Effects of pulsatile shear stress on nitric oxide production and endothelial cell nitric oxide synthase expression by ovine fetoplacental artery endothelial cells. *Biol Reprod* 69(3):1053–9.

Liu, L., W. Yuan, and J. Wang. 2010a. Mechanisms for osteogenic differentiation of human mesenchymal stem cells induced by fluid shear stress. *Biomech Model Mechanobiol* 9(6):659–70.

Liu, X., X. Zhang, and I. Lee. 2010b. A quantitative study on morphological responses of osteoblastic cells to fluid shear stress. *Acta Biochim Biophys Sin (Shanghai)* 42(3):195–201.

MacNeil, S. 2007. Progress and opportunities for tissue-engineered skin. *Nature* 445(7130):874–80.

MacNeil, S. 2008. Biomaterials for tissue engineering of skin. *Materials Today* 11(5):26–35.

Magid, R., T. J. Murphy, and Z. S. Galis. 2003. Expression of matrix metalloproteinase-9 in endothelial cells is differentially regulated by shear stress. Role of c-Myc. *J Biol Chem* 278(35):32994–9.

Marlovits, S., B. Tichy, M. Truppe, D. Gruber, and V. Vecsei. 2003. Chondrogenesis of aged human articular cartilage in a scaffold-free bioreactor. *Tissue Eng* 9(6):1215–26.

Martin, I., D. Wendt, and M. Heberer. 2004. The role of bioreactors in tissue engineering. *Trends Biotechnol* 22(2):80–6.

Martinac, B. 2004. Mechanosensitive ion channels: Molecules of mechanotransduction. *J Cell Sci* 117(Pt 12):2449–60.

Matthews, B. D., D. R. Overby, R. Mannix, and D. E. Ingber. 2006. Cellular adaptation to mechanical stress: Role of integrins, Rho, cytoskeletal tension and mechanosensitive ion channels. *J Cell Sci* 119(Pt 3):508–18.

Mauch, C., B. Adelmann-Grill, A. Hatamochi, and T. Krieg. 1989. Collagenase gene expression in fibroblasts is regulated by a three-dimensional contact with collagen. *FEBS Lett* 250(2):301–5.

McCall, G. E., W. C. Byrnes, A. Dickinson, P. M. Pattany, and S. J. Fleck. 1996. Muscle fiber hypertrophy, hyperplasia, and capillary density in college men after resistance training. *J Appl Physiol* 81(5):2004–12.

McCulloch, A. D., A. B. Harris, C. E. Sarraf, and M. Eastwood. 2004. New multi-cue bioreactor for tissue engineering of tubular cardiovascular samples under physiological conditions. *Tissue Eng* 10(3–4):565–73.

McFetridge, P. S., T. Bodamyali, M. Horrocks, and J. B. Chaudhuri. 2004. Endothelial and smooth muscle cell seeding onto processed ex vivo arterial scaffolds using 3D vascular bioreactors. *ASAIO J* 50(6):591–600.

Mi, L. Y., M. Basu, S. P. Fritton, and S. C. Cowin. 2005. Analysis of avian bone response to mechanical loading. Part two: Development of a computational connected cellular network to study bone intercellular communication. *Biomech Model Mechanobiol* 4(2–3):132–46.

Mizuno, S., F. Allemann, and J. Glowacki. 2001. Effects of medium perfusion on matrix production by bovine chondrocytes in three-dimensional collagen sponges. *J Biomed Mater Res* 56(3):368–75.

Mofrad, M. R., J. Golji, N. A. Abdul Rahim, and R. D. Kamm. 2004. Force-induced unfolding of the focal adhesion targeting domain and the influence of paxillin binding. *Mech Chem Biosyst* 1(4):253–65.

Moss, A. J., S. Sharma, and N. P. Brindle. 2009. Rational design and protein engineering of growth factors for regenerative medicine and tissue engineering. *Biochem Soc Trans* 37(Pt 4):717–21.

Mudera, V. C., R. Pleass, M. Eastwood et al. 2000. Molecular responses of human dermal fibroblasts to dual cues: Contact guidance and mechanical load. *Cell Motil Cytoskeleton* 45(1):1–9.

Narita, Y., K. Hata, H. Kagami et al. 2004. Novel pulse duplicating bioreactor system for tissue-engineered vascular construct. *Tissue Eng* 10(7–8):1224–33.

Nasseri, B. A., I. Pomerantseva, M. R. Kaazempur-Mofrad et al. 2003. Dynamic rotational seeding and cell culture system for vascular tube formation. *Tissue Eng* 9(2):291–9.

Natoli, R. M., S. Skaalure, S. Bijlani et al. 2010. Intracellular Na(+) and Ca(2+) modulation increases the tensile properties of developing engineered articular cartilage. *Arthritis Rheum* 62(4):1097–107.

Niklason, L. E. 1999. Techview: Medical technology. Replacement arteries made to order. *Science* 286(5444):1493–4.

Numaguchi, K., S. Eguchi, T. Yamakawa, E. D. Motley, and T. Inagami. 1999. Mechanotransduction of rat aortic vascular smooth muscle cells requires RhoA and intact actin filaments. *Circ Res* 85(1):5–11.

O'Callaghan, C. J., and B. Williams. 2000. Mechanical strain-induced extracellular matrix production by human vascular smooth muscle cells: Role of TGF-beta(1). *Hypertension* 36(3):319–24.

Okano, T. and T. Matsuda. 1997. Hybrid muscular tissues: Preparation of skeletal muscle cell-incorporated collagen gels. *Cell Transplant* 6(2):109–18.

Ostergaard, K., D. M. Salter, J. Petersen et al. 1998. Expression of alpha and beta subunits of the integrin superfamily in articular cartilage from macroscopically normal and osteoarthritic human femoral heads. *Ann Rheum Dis* 57(5):303–8.

Ott, M. J. and B. J. Ballermann. 1995. Shear stress-conditioned, endothelial cell-seeded vascular grafts: Improved cell adherence in response to *in vitro* shear stress. *Surgery* 117(3):334–9.

Pang, Q., J. W. Zu, G. M. Siu, and R. K. Li. 2010. Design and development of a novel biostretch apparatus for tissue engineering. *J Biomech Eng* 132(1):014503.

Papachristou, D. J., P. Pirttiniemi, T. Kantomaa, A. G. Papavassiliou, and E. K. Basdra. 2005. JNK/ERK-AP-1/Runx2 induction "paves the way" to cartilage load-ignited chondroblastic differentiation. *Histochem Cell Biol* 124(3–4):215–23.

Patz, T. M., A. Doraiswamy, R. J. Narayan, R. Modi, and D. B. Chrisey. 2005. Two-dimensional differential adherence and alignment of C2C12 myoblasts. *Mater Sci Eng B, Solid State Mater Adv Technol* 123(3):242–7.

Perrone, C. E., D. Fenwick-Smith, and H. H. Vandenburgh. 1995. Collagen and stretch modulate autocrine secretion of insulin-like growth factor-1 and insulin-like growth factor binding proteins from differentiated skeletal muscle cells. *J Biol Chem* 270(5):2099–106.

Piekarski, K. and M. Munro. 1977. Transport mechanism operating between blood supply and osteocytes in long bones. *Nature* 269(5623):80–2.

Powell, C. A., B. L. Smiley, J. Mills, and H. H. Vandenburgh. 2002. Mechanical stimulation improves tissue-engineered human skeletal muscle. *Am J Physiol Cell Physiol* 283(5):C1557–65.

Radisic, M., H. Park, F. Chen et al. 2006. Biomimetic approach to cardiac tissue engineering: Oxygen carriers and channeled scaffolds. *Tissue Eng* 12(8):2077–91.

Radisic, M., H. Park, H. Shing et al. 2004. Functional assembly of engineered myocardium by electrical stimulation of cardiac myocytes cultured on scaffolds. *Proc Natl Acad Sci USA* 101(52):18129–34.

Ramage, L., G. Nuki, and D. M. Salter. 2009. Signalling cascades in mechanotransduction: Cell-matrix interactions and mechanical loading. *Scand J Med Sci Sports* 19(4):457–69.

Reich, K. M. and J. A. Frangos. 1993. Protein kinase C mediates flow-induced prostaglandin E2 production in osteoblasts. *Calcif Tissue Int* 52(1):62–6.

Reno, F., V. Traina, and M. Cannas. 2009. Mechanical stretching modulates growth direction and MMP-9 release in human keratinocyte monolayer. *Cell Adh Migr* 3(3):239–42.

Riddle, R. C. and H. J. Donahue. 2009. From streaming-potentials to shear stress: 25 years of bone cell mechanotransduction. *J Orthop Res* 27(2):143–9.

Roberts, G. C. and D. R. Critchley. 2009. Structural and biophysical properties of the integrin-associated cytoskeletal protein talin. *Biophys Rev* 1(2):61–9.

Rodriguez, J. P., M. Gonzalez, S. Rios, and V. Cambiazo. 2004. Cytoskeletal organization of human mesenchymal stem cells (MSC) changes during their osteogenic differentiation. *J Cell Biochem* 93(4):721–31.

Sadoshima, J. and S. Izumo. 1997. The cellular and molecular response of cardiac myocytes to mechanical stress. *Annu Rev Physiol* 59:551–71.

Schlaepfer, D. D., and T. Hunter. 1996. Evidence for *in vivo* phosphorylation of the Grb2 SH2-domain binding site on focal adhesion kinase by Src-family protein-tyrosine kinases. *Mol Cell Biol* 16(10):5623–33.

Scott, A., J. L. Cook, D. A. Hart et al. 2007. Tenocyte responses to mechanical loading in vivo: A role for local insulin-like growth factor 1 signaling in early tendinosis in rats. *Arthritis Rheum* 56(3):871–81.

Scutt, A. and P. Bertram. 1999. Basic fibroblast growth factor in the presence of dexamethasone stimulates colony formation, expansion, and osteoblastic differentiation by rat bone marrow stromal cells. *Calcif Tissue Int* 64(1):69–77.

Seliktar, D., R. M. Nerem, and Z. S. Galis. 2001. The role of matrix metalloproteinase-2 in the remodeling of cell-seeded vascular constructs subjected to cyclic strain. *Ann Biomed Eng* 29(11):923–34.

Shyy, J. Y. and S. Chien. 1997. Role of integrins in cellular responses to mechanical stress and adhesion. *Curr Opin Cell Biol* 9(5):707–13.

Sikavitsas, V. I., G. N. Bancroft, H. L. Holtorf, J. A. Jansen, and A. G. Mikos. 2003. Mineralized matrix deposition by marrow stromal osteoblasts in 3D perfusion culture increases with increasing fluid shear forces. *Proc Natl Acad Sci USA* 100(25):14683–8.

Sikavitsas, V. I., J. S. Temenoff, and A. G. Mikos. 2001. Biomaterials and bone mechanotransduction. *Biomaterials* 22(19):2581–93.

Silver, F. H., L. M. Siperko, and G. P. Seehra. 2003. Mechanobiology of force transduction in dermal tissue. *Skin Res Technol* 9(1):3–23.

Sodian, R., T. Lemke, C. Fritsche et al. 2002. Tissue-engineering bioreactors: A new combined cell-seeding and perfusion system for vascular tissue engineering. *Tissue Eng* 8(5):863–70.

Stewart, D M. 1972. The role of tension in muscle growth. In *Regulation of Organ and Tissue Growth*, edited by Goss, R. J. New York: Academic Press.

Stoltz, J. F., D. Dumas, X. Wang et al. 2000. Influence of mechanical forces on cells and tissues. *Biorheology* 37(1–2):3–14.

Sweigart, M. A. and K. A. Athanasiou. 2005. Tensile and compressive properties of the medial rabbit meniscus. *Proc Inst Mech Eng H* 219(5):337–47.

Tatsumi, R. 2010. Mechano-biology of skeletal muscle hypertrophy and regeneration: Possible mechanism of stretch-induced activation of resident myogenic stem cells. *Anim Sci J* 81(1):11–20.

Vandenburgh, H., M. Del Tatto, J. Shansky et al. 1996. Tissue-engineered skeletal muscle organoids for reversible gene therapy. *Hum Gene Ther* 7(17):2195–200.

Vandenburgh, H. H. 1982. Dynamic mechanical orientation of skeletal myofibers in vitro. *Dev Biol* 93(2):438–43.

Vandenburgh, H. H. 1987. Motion into mass: How does tension stimulate muscle growth? *Med Sci Sports Exerc* 19(5 Suppl):S142–9.

Vandenburgh, H. H., S. Hatfaludy, P. Karlisch, and J. Shansky. 1989. Skeletal muscle growth is stimulated by intermittent stretch-relaxation in tissue culture. *Am J Physiol* 256(3 Pt 1):C674–82.

Vandenburgh, H. H., S. Hatfaludy, I. Sohar, and J. Shansky. 1990. Stretch-induced prostaglandins and protein turnover in cultured skeletal muscle. *Am J Physiol* 259(2 Pt 1):C232–40.

Vandenburgh, H. H., S. Swasdison, and P. Karlisch. 1991. Computer-aided mechanogenesis of skeletal muscle organs from single cells in vitro. *FASEB J* 5(13):2860–7.

Vorp, D. A., K. R. Rajagopal, P. J. Smolinski, and H. S. Borovetz. 1995. Identification of elastic properties of homogeneous, orthotropic vascular segments in distension. *J Biomech* 28(5):501–12.

Wang, J. H. and B. P. Thampatty. 2006. An introductory review of cell mechanobiology. *Biomech Model Mechanobiol* 5(1):1–16.

Ward, D. F., Jr., W. A. Williams, N. E. Schapiro et al. 2007. Focal adhesion kinase signaling controls cyclic tensile strain enhanced collagen I-induced osteogenic differentiation of human mesenchymal stem cells. *Mol Cell Biomech* 4(4):177–88.

Weinberg, C. B., and E. Bell. 1986. A blood vessel model constructed from collagen and cultured vascular cells. *Science* 231(4736):397–400.

Wen, H., P. A. Blume, and B. E. Sumpio. 2009. Role of integrins and focal adhesion kinase in the orientation of dermal fibroblasts exposed to cyclic strain. *Int Wound J* 6(2):149–58.

Werntz, J. R., J. M. Lane, A. H. Burstein et al. 1996. Qualitative and quantitative analysis of orthotopic bone regeneration by marrow. *J Orthop Res* 14(1):85–93.

Williams, C., and T. M. Wick. 2004. Perfusion bioreactor for small diameter tissue-engineered arteries. *Tissue Eng* 10(5–6):930–41.

Wright, M., P. Jobanputra, C. Bavington, D. M. Salter, and G. Nuki. 1996. Effects of intermittent pressure-induced strain on the electrophysiology of cultured human chondrocytes: Evidence for the presence of stretch-activated membrane ion channels. *Clin Sci (Lond)* 90(1):61–71.

Wright, M. O., K. Nishida, C. Bavington et al. 1997. Hyperpolarisation of cultured human chondrocytes following cyclical pressure-induced strain: Evidence of a role for alpha 5 beta 1 integrin as a chondrocyte mechanoreceptor. *J Orthop Res* 15(5):742–7.

Yang, F. and J. Elisseeff. 2006. Cartilage Tissue Engineering. In *Tissue Engineering and Artificial Organs*, edited by Bronzino, J. Bocan Raton: Taylor & Francis Group.

Yano, S., M. Komine, M. Fujimoto, H. Okochi, and K. Tamaki. 2004. Mechanical stretching *in vitro* regulates signal transduction pathways and cellular proliferation in human epidermal keratinocytes. *J Invest Dermatol* 122(3):783–90.

Yates, W. 2009. *Mechanostimulated Wharton's Jelly Stem Cells Seeded into Human Umbilical Veins for Tendon Tissue Engineering*. Chemical, Biological, and Materials Engineering. Norman: University of Oklahoma.

Zhu, C., G. Bao, and N. Wang. 2000. Cell mechanics: Mechanical response, cell adhesion, and molecular deformation. *Annu Rev Biomed Eng* 2:189–226.

Ziegler, T. and R. M. Nerem. 1994. Tissue engineering a blood vessel: Regulation of vascular biology by mechanical stresses. *J Cell Biochem* 56(2):204–9.

Zimmermann, W. H., M. Didie, G. H. Wasmeier et al. 2002a. Cardiac grafting of engineered heart tissue in syngenic rats. *Circulation* 106(12 Suppl 1):I151–7.

Zimmermann, W. H., C. Fink, D. Kralisch et al. 2000. Three-dimensional engineered heart tissue from neonatal rat cardiac myocytes. *Biotechnol Bioeng* 68(1):106–14.

Zimmermann, W. H., I. Melnychenko, G. Wasmeier et al. 2006. Engineered heart tissue grafts improve systolic and diastolic function in infarcted rat hearts. *Nat Med* 12(4):452–8.

Zimmermann, W. H., K. Schneiderbanger, P. Schubert et al. 2002b. Tissue engineering of a differentiated cardiac muscle construct. *Circ Res* 90(2):223–30.

# 24

# Vascularization of Engineered Tissues

Monica L. Moya
*University of California, Irvine*

Eric M. Brey
*Illinois Institute of Technology*

*Hines Veterans Hospital*

24.1 Introduction .......................................................................... 24-1
24.2 Neovascularization ............................................................. 24-1
    Angiogenesis • Vasculogenesis • Arteriogenesis
24.3 Strategies for Vascularizing Engineered Tissues ....................... 24-4
    Prevascularized Constructs • Inducing Vascularization upon Implantation • Surgical Approaches
24.4 Conclusions.......................................................................... 24-11
References.................................................................................. 24-11

## 24.1 Introduction

Tissue engineering has received significant attention due to its potential to provide alternatives to traditional clinical options for organ replacement and tissue reconstruction. Although success has been achieved for some clinical applications, the ability to engineer tissues of sufficient size and complexity for many applications is limited by the ability to control vascularization. The specific dimensions depend on the metabolic needs of a given tissue, but tissues are generally limited to a few 100 μm in thickness in the absence of a blood supply. Currently most successful engineered tissues are thin (Griffith and Naughton, 2002, Morrison, 2009). Although neovascularization (new blood vessel formation) occurs in these tissues the extent would be insufficient to vascularize materials of large volumes. Engineering large, complex tissues requires the ability to stimulate extensive neovascularization in sufficient time to avoid necrosis. In addition, the presence of vessels within the scaffolds is not likely to be sufficient. The structure, functionality, and stability of the resultant vascular networks must be appropriate to support tissue function.

Neovascularization limitations in tissue engineering are well established and have been an active area of research over the last decade (Skalak et al., 2002). People have investigated a number of different approaches for enhancing network formation in engineered tissues, including using cells, growth factors, prevascularizing by cell self-assembly, material patterning, and surgical techniques (Figure 24.1). Despite this attention, the ability to rapidly and appropriately assemble networks in engineered tissues remains a significant challenge. In this chapter we will describe the state of the art in vascularizing engineered tissues, identifying recent advances and challenges yet to be addressed.

## 24.2 Neovascularization

Neovascularization can occur through three mechanisms that will be described in the following sections: vasculogenesis, angiogenesis, and arteriogenesis (Figure 24.2). These processes often do not occur independently *in vivo* and many signaling events are common to more than one mechanism (Cao et al.,

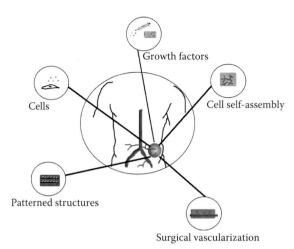

**FIGURE 24.1** Approaches investigated for promoting vascularization of engineered tissues, includes patterning vessels into the polymer scaffold, seeding cells into the scaffolds that incorporate into new vessels and/or provide signals to induce vascularization, adding growth factors or growth factor delivery systems in the scaffold to promote vessel ingrowth, inducing cells to assemble into networks prior to implantation, and surgically implanting the materials in a location that optimizes vascularization.

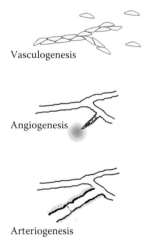

**FIGURE 24.2** Neovascularization can occur via three mechanisms: vasculogenesis, angiogenesis, and arteriogenesis. Vasculogenesis is the organization of new vessels from precursor cells. Angiogenesis is the formation of new vessels from pre-existing vessels, typically occurring by sprouting of new vessels up a gradient of soluble factors. Arteriogenesis is the process by which arteries or arterioles are remodeled into larger vessels.

2005a). It is possible that all three modes of vascularization will need to be considered when developing strategies for vascularizing engineered tissues.

## 24.2.1 Angiogenesis

Angiogenesis, the predominant mechanism of neovascularization in adults, refers to the formation of new vessels from pre-existing vessels. In this section, the primary mechanisms of angiogenesis, the sprouting of new vessels from the existing vessels, is described. However, other mechanisms of angiogenesis can occur, such as intussusception where an existing vessel is divided into two. Angiogenesis occurs during normal physiological processes, such as wound healing and the female reproductive cycle, and in disease states such as tumor growth and retinopathy (Nomi et al., 2002). Angiogenesis is initiated by soluble factors expressed by cells in response to a wide range of stimuli including hypoxia, mechanical stress, metabolic stress, and immune or inflammatory signals (Carmeliet and Jaine, 2000, Montesano et al., 1986). Endothelial cells (ECs) are normally in a quiescent or nonproliferative state with a balance of both proangiogenic and antiangiogenic signals in the environment. The cells are activated when there is a shift in the balance toward factors that promote angiogenesis (Carmeliet and Jaine, 2000).

A number of proangiogenic factors have been identified that contribute to this process, but members of the vascular endothelial growth factor (VEGF) and fibroblast growth factor (FGF) families have received the most attention. Receptors present on ECs are activated by interaction with these factors, resulting in the upregulation of proteases that degrade the underlying basement membrane (BM) and surrounding extracellular matrix (ECM). A change in the shape of ECs allows them to migrate into the surrounding matrix forming sprouts from the existing vessel (Nomi et al., 2002). Cells at the tips of the sprout migrate while cells behind the tip proliferate, allowing the sprout to elongate. For obvious reasons, angiogenesis research has primarily focused on ECs, but the initial stages of angiogenesis are a multiceullar process. Mural cells are reduced relative to the amount found in stable vessels but are still present during the initial stages and may be involved in initiating microvascular development (Brey et al., 2004, Ozerdem and Stallcup, 2003, Yana et al., 2007, Gerhardt and Betsholtz, 2003). Other cells, such as macrophages and fibroblasts, may facilitate vessel invasion by breaking down the ECM ahead of the sprout (Anghelina et al., 2004, 2006, Sunderkotter et al., 1994).

Depending on the distribution of soluble (proteins) and insoluble (ECM/biomaterials) factors in the environment, a new branch may form from the sprouting vessel or the vessel can continue to elongate. The choice between elongation and sprouting appears to depend, at least in part, on the concentration gradient of VEGF (Gerhardt et al., 2003). The sprouts eventually join up with other sprouts to form a closed loop through which blood can flow. Under physiological angiogenesis, the newly formed vasculature is remodeled into a stable network tailored to the specific metabolic demands of the local tissue. During this time some of the vessels formed become mature and stable while other regress (Francis et al., 2008). Vessel maturation involves the production of new BM and an increase in the number of mural cells surrounding the tubes. These cells are recruited, in part, by the secretion of platelet-derived growth factor-BB (PDGF-BB) (Darland and D'Amore, 1999, Nomi et al., 2002, Gaengel et al., 2009) and angiopoietin-1 (Ang-1) (Aplin et al., 2009, Hoffmann et al., 2005). Mature vessels are less dependent on angiogenic factors for survival and are required for proper vascular network function (Abramsson et al., 2002). Once vessels are matured, the ECs return to their quiescent state. Currently a significant amount of research is focused on the role of soluble factors as well as insoluble factors in the extracellular microenvironment on neovascularization (Francis et al., 2008).

## 24.2.2 Vasculogenesis

Vasculogenesis, the process of vessel development primarily occurring during embryogenesis, is the formation of new blood vessels by progenitor cells. In adults, vasculogenesis occurs when angioblasts, or endothelial precursor cells (EPCs), home to tissues from the bone marrow or circulating blood. Stromal cell-derived factor-1 is a primary mediator involved in EPC trafficking to these tissues. The EPCs differentiate into ECs and organize into nascent endothelial tubes. The ECs then secrete signals similar to those involved in the maturation stage of angiogenesis to recruit mural cells for stabilization (Nomi et al., 2002, Carmeliet, 2003). Although vasculogenesis can occur in adults, the level of its contribution remains unclear (Carmeliet, 2000, van Weel et al., 2008). Results suggest that less than 5% of ECs in newly formed vessels result from the differentiation of circulating precursor cells (Cao et al., 2005a). Although the contribution of EPCs to neovascularization in adults appears low, studies suggest that increasing the homing and recruitment of EPCs to a given tissue can enhance neovascularization (Yamaguchi et al., 2003).

### 24.2.3 Arteriogenesis

Arteriogenesis is the process by which arteries or arterioles are remodeled into larger vessels. Although arteriogenesis is the process of remodeling existing vessels and there is no formation of new vessels, it is a process that may be essential for proper vascularization of engineered tissues. This process, also known as collateralization, occurs when ECs and smooth muscle cells (SMCs) are activated (due to increased shear stress or cytokines) and upregulate growth factors that stimulate SMC proliferation and recruitment of mononuclear cells. Cell proliferation leads to an increase in the thickness of the vessel wall (Carmeliet, 2000, van Weel et al., 2008). This process is more efficient at increasing blood flow in ischemic tissues due to the formation of high-conductance vessels rather than neovascularization which primarily produces capillaries with low volumetric flow (Scholz et al., 2002, Brey et al., 2005).

## 24.3 Strategies for Vascularizing Engineered Tissues

### 24.3.1 Prevascularized Constructs

One strategy that has been explored to vascularize engineered tissues is to produce a vascular network within the construct prior to implantation. The presence of the vascular network could accelerate tissue perfusion by inosculating with host vessels that invade the scaffold from the surrounding tissue. Prevascularized tissue may allow for the construction of larger tissues and has the potential to improve the survival and function of other cells present in the scaffold that may be especially sensitive to low oxygen concentration. Critical to this approach, however, is the rate of inosculation with the host vasculature and the stability and function of the preformed vascular networks. In the following sections, methods of constructing prevascularized tissues are discussed.

#### 24.3.1.1 Cell Self-Assembly

It is well established that in the presence of appropriate soluble factors and scaffolds tuned to the correct stiffness, ECs seeded on, or in, the scaffolds will self organize into network structures (Figure 24.3). This phenomenon has been explored as an approach to create materials with vascular networks that inosculate with host vasculature to rapidly establish perfusion upon implantation. Although ECs alone were initially used in the early self-assembly systems (Montesano et al., 1983, Folkman and Haudenschild, 1980), a number of studies have shown the importance of additional cell types to the formation, stability, and function of the resultant networks. Often, mural cells are combined with ECs which are then cultured *in vitro* to allow three-dimensional (3D) capillary-like assembly via a vasculogenic-like process. This process has been applied to a number of scaffold materials, including collagen (Koike et al., 2004), fibrin (Chen et al., 2009, 2010), and poly(ethylene glycol) (PEG)-based hydrogels (Moon et al., 2010).

Materials containing self-assembled vessels consisting of ECs and mural cells have even been shown to establish connections with host vasculature that are stable for up to 1 year *in vivo* (Koike et al., 2004). Inosculation of prevascularized scaffolds has also been shown with synthetic gels but extremely small material volumes were used (5 μl) (Moon et al., 2010). Researchers have demonstrated that this approach can be used to generate specific vascularized tissues with the addition of a third cell type, including skeletal (Levenberg et al., 2005) and cardiac muscles (Caspi et al., 2007). Others have combined ECs with a cell type other than mural cells to create vascularized skin (Gibot et al., Black et al., 1998) and bone (Unger et al., 2010) *in vitro* and demonstrated successful anastamosis of the vessels in these constructs upon implantation *in vivo*. These studies show that a nonvascular cell can provide signals essential to vascular stability.

Although promising, this strategy is highly dependent on the cell source and its feasibility for routine application relies on the availability of cells that can be easily harvested, cultured, and applied. A variety of ECs have been used in these self-assembly strategies, including mature and progenitor ECs, arterial and venous cells, and cells harvested from both macro and micro vessels. Differences in cell source used can significantly influence the results. Chen et al. (2010) compared prevascularized constructs formed

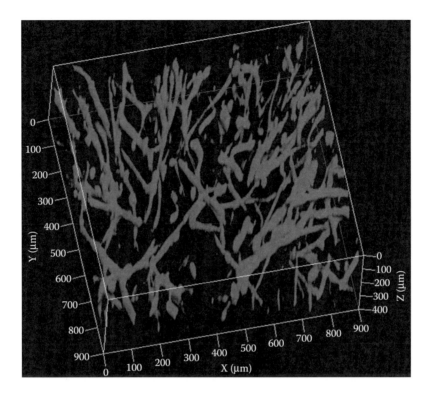

**FIGURE 24.3** (**See color insert.**) Three-dimensional confocal microscopy image of vascular networks formed in collagen gels.

using human umbilical vein EC and EPCs isolated from cord blood. In both cases the ECs were interdispersed with fibroblasts in a fibrin matrix. Although the ECs formed vessel networks at a similar rate *in vitro*, *in vivo* the EPCs outperformed constructs made with human umbilical vein ECs by anastomosing with host vasculature at a faster rate. As anastomosis rate appears to vary between cell types, the success of these approaches will require an understanding of how efficiently the cell type used in a given application inosculates with host vessels.

As for any tissue engineering application, autologous cells would be the ideal source for these strategies. They would limit the immune response to prevascularized tissue constructs on implantation. However, this may pose an additional challenge as, outside of congenital defects and trauma patients, most of the individuals in the targeted population for these vascularization therapies are older with a variety of comorbidities, including diabetes, hypertension, a history of smoking, etc. These conditions are associated with a reduced capacity for vessel assembly (Francis-Sedlak et al., 2010), which may hinder the successful application of these approaches to the patient population in most need of interventions. Studies are needed that address the capabilities of cells from these specific patient populations to form networks and inosculate with host vasculature. Vascularization of scaffolds through self-assembly of ECs is a promising strategy, but requires significantly more research before clinical application. Regardless of clinical success, these cell-based constructs serve as an environment for controlled study of the complex interaction between cells and the ECM during vessel formation.

### 24.3.1.2 Patterned Structures

The techniques described above exploit the ability of ECs to assemble into networks on their own based on soluble and insoluble factors in the culture or bioreactor environment. At best, these networks can be described as immature vessels and their 3D complexity is primarily limited to interconnected small vessels. Material and cell patterning technologies have been explored in an effort to engineer polymer scaffolds that mimic the complexity and microarchitecture of biological tissues.

Early efforts in vessel patterning focused on two-dimensional (2D) patterning on rigid substrates such as gold (Chen et al., 1998, Dike et al., 1999, Kaihara et al., 2000). Using microcontact printing, adhesive patterns of fibronectin could be created on the surface of gold (Chen et al., 1998). The spreading and proliferation of ECs were found to depend on the size and geometry of the adhesive patterns. Using this technique ECs cultured on 10-μm wide lines of fibronectin formed capillary tubular structures with a central lumen, whereas cells adhered to 30-μm lines of fibronectin formed monolayers (Dike et al., 1999). This study showed how patterning ECM proteins can be used to generate vascular structures in precise locations. However, the 2D nature of this approach and the materials used are not appropriate for tissue engineering applications.

Capillary networks consisting of vessels with diameters approaching 10 μm were etched into silicon and Pyrex surfaces using micromachining techniques (Kaihara et al., 2000). ECs and hepatocytes cultured on these 2D branched structures could be lifted off as cell monolayers and implanted. Although the hepatocytes survived following implantation, it is not clear how well the patterned vascular microstructure was maintained. Silicon wafers etched in this manner have been used as molds for the creation of vascular patterns within biodegradable cell adhesive poly(glycerol sebacate) elastomers (Fidkowski et al., 2005) and poly(lactic-*co*-glycolic acid) (PLGA) scaffolds (King et al., 2004). These networks contained inlet and outlet ports enabling perfusion. When the poly(glycerol sebacate) devices were seeded with ECs and perfused at physiological flow rates complete endothelialization was accomplished after 14 days and remained stable for 4 weeks in culture. This technique can be used to produce complex, high-resolution 2D patterns. However, their application is limited to patterning 2D with extension to 3D resulting from multilayer replication of the 2D patterns (Borenstein et al., 2007). Melt micromolding with thermal fusion bonding has been shown to enable fusion of patterned PLGA layers generated using the silicon molds (King et al., 2004).

Three-dimensional printing technologies have been used to create a vascularized "mini-liver" *in vitro* (Griffith et al., 1997). Using this approach 200-μm channels were created within biodegradable polymer scaffolds of poly(L-lactic acid) and PLGA. ECs attached and filled the channels after 5 weeks in static culture. When seeding mixed populations of hepatocytes and ECs into these scaffolds, the cells reorganized into structures that appeared similar to sinusoids. This approach provides an interesting example of generating 3D networks within a tissue parenchyma. Recently, this work has been combined with advanced bioreactor technologies to perfuse the tissue units with cell culture media (Domansky et al., 2010). Although complex 3D models of small vascularized tissues were created, research has not been performed to show how these vessels would interact with host tissue following implantation.

Micromolding has been used to generate channels within collagen gels by patterning a material that can be selectively degraded away from the bulk material (Chrobak et al., 2006). When lined with a monolayer of ECs, the channels served as functional, perfusable microvascular tubes with diameters between 75 and 150 μm after maturation and lengths spanning the entire collagen gel (5–7 mm), have been generated. These capillaries exhibited barrier function and resistance to leukocyte adhesion similar to capillaries *in vivo*. This technique of molding selectively degradable, or "sacrificial," regions within materials has been used to generate channels with complex 3D geometries (Golden and Tien, 2007), but it is not clear how these complex geometries could be seeded with ECs.

Other approaches for creating microvascular patterns within scaffolds with high resolution have focused on laser-based patterning. Laser-guided direct writing was used to deposit multiple cells on various surfaces including biological gels with micron accuracy (Nahmias et al., 2005). This approach was used to pattern ECs on mulitlayers of Matrigel (a mouse tumor extract consisting of BM proteins) to generate 3D structures. The ECs elongated and formed tube-like structures along the patterns in a self-assembly process. Laser printing has also been used to directly deposit patterns of ECs onto Matrigel (Chen et al., 2006). Again, these initially unconnected EC patterns assembled into interconnected patterns.

Photopolymerizable polymers, such as many PEG-based hydrogels, can be easily patterned using non-contact photolithography. Interfacial photopolymerization of PEG has been shown to allow production of microvascular patterns within multilayered PEG hydrogels with feature sizes between 50 and 70 μm using simple photomasks (Papavasiliou et al., 2008). When using interfacial photopolymerization, the thickness of each layer can be controlled by polymerization conditions without the need of spacers or molds. This approach could be exploited to allow formation of 3D multilayered structures with distinct pattern formation in each layer. Microchannels have also been created within PEG hydrogels by patterning degradable polymers (Chiu et al., 2009a). The patterned region can be selectively degraded away due to the greater susceptibility of the patterned material to hydrolysis than the bulk hydrogel, resulting in channel formation. Using this approach, multilayered interconnected channels were fabricated through hydrolytic degradation of the patterned regions within distinct layers. The channels can be functionalized with cell adhesion sequences to support EC growth to form capillary-like channels (Chiu et al., 2011).

Patterning technologies are far from clinical application, but have been shown to allow precise control over the generation of vascular-like structures and microchannels within polymer scaffolds commonly used in tissue engineering. The majority of the research has used these structures as model networks for the study of vessel assembly or microfluidics. Questions remains as to how well these structures will function on the inevitable remodeling encountered following implantation. In addition, cell-sourcing issues described in the previous section are not avoided with these techniques.

## 24.3.2 Inducing Vascularization upon Implantation

Another approach relies on stimulating and guiding the body to provide the vasculature. Stimuli are delivered from the polymer scaffold to accelerate the invasion and organization of vessels. Prevascularized tissues may also benefit from such approaches as preformed vessel networks would still require that the host vasculature invades the scaffold and inosculates with the scaffold network. Strategies of inducing vascularization on implantation may prove to be more practical than creating a network within each construct prior to implantation. Although this approach is likely to prolong the time required for perfusion of the entire construct *in vivo*, it will likely reduce the *in vitro* construction phase.

### 24.3.2.1 Growth Factors

The process of neovascularization is an intricate temporal and spatial orchestration of many growth factors. Understanding their involvement in the processes of vessel formation, maturation, regression, and remodeling is crucial to designing optimized therapeutics strategies for inducing blood vessel growth. Several growth factors including, but not limited to, FGF-1, FGF-2, VEGF, and PDGF have demonstrated the ability to stimulate vessel formation in both clinical and basic research (Udelson et al., 2000, Hendel et al., 2000, Benjamin et al., 1998, Lokmic and Mitchell, 2008, Schumacher et al., 1998, Nikol et al., 2008). Methods currently used in clinical trials in which angiogenic proteins are under investigation as a treatment of ischemic tissues, primarily use large bolus injections which are not optimally effective. The short half lives of proteins *in vivo* mean these methods must rely on high levels of injected proteins which may lead to abnormal vasculature and severe side effects (Gu et al., 2004, August et al., 2006).

The success of growth factor-based strategies depends significantly on the method and timing of delivery. Several studies have indicated that a timeframe may exist for which these growth factors have an optimal effect (Cao and Mooney, 2007). The untimely removal of VEGF from a vascularizing tissue, prior to the formation of a mural cell coat, caused EC detachment from the vessel wall and vessel regression (Benjamin and Keshet, 1997). Administering PDGF-BB can disrupt EC-mural cell interactions but only when administered to immature vessels (Benjamin et al., 1998). These results indicate that the timing of both growth factor addition and removal may be critical to success.

In addition to timing, growth factor dose is important for stimulating the proper response. VEGF administered at high dosages can lead tovessels with chaotic structure and hyperpermeability (Ozawa et al., 2004). Continuous low levels of FGF-1 have been shown to promote vessel growth and, more importantly, stabilize and prevent regression of vessels, a problem that may occur when delivering high concentrations of FGF-1 (Uriel et al., 2006). These studies suggest that low levels are optimal, but the actual dosage for each protein is likely to depend on the site of implantation, the presence of other angiogenic molecules, and the method of delivery (Lokmic and Mitchell, 2008).

One approach for overcoming the transient nature of proteins is to use gene therapies to prolong the duration of increased growth factor levels. Naked FGF-1 plasmid has been explored as a treatment for patients with critical limb ischemia and gave favorable results with regard to limb salvage (Nikol et al., 2008). Similarly, local intramuscular injection of naked VEGF plasmid in an animal limb ischemia model was demonstrated to increase tissue perfusion (Tsurumi et al., 1996). Incorporation of genes into polymer scaffolds can further prolong the effect, reducing the need for repeated application. Plasmid DNA encoding for VEGF delivered from PLGA scaffolds implanted subcutaneously into mice was found to be more effective at increasing blood vessel density than empty scaffolds (Jang et al., 2005). Hypoxia-inducible factor-1$\alpha$, a factor that indirectly stimulates angiogenesis by inducing the expression of VEGF, has been delivered *in vivo* by entrapment of peptide–DNA nanoparticles in a fibrin matrix (Trentin et al., 2006). This approach proved to be more efficient at stimulating angiogenesis than VEGF delivered in fibrin. Furthermore, the gene transfer of hypoxia-inducible factor-$\alpha$ increased the number of mature vessels formed.

Proteins have also been incorporated directly into polymer scaffolds to stimulate neovascularization. Growth factors have been added to both natural and synthetic polymers to generate vascularized tissues. As with other tissue engineering applications, poly(l-lactic acid), PLGA, and PEG have received significant attention (Takahiro et al., 2000). A variety of polymer properties (cross-linking, molecular weight, hydrophobicity, charge, etc.) can be modified to influence release kinetics (Pitt, 1990, Amsden and Turner, 1999). However, sometimes the fabrication process can interfere with the functionality of the proteins (Zisch et al., 2003). Natural polymers for delivery include alginate (Moya et al., 2009b, 2010), fibrin, collagen, chitosan, and gelatin (Young et al., 2005). Some ECM-based materials, such as fibrin, have both a natural ability to stimulate neovascularization and demonstrated success in delivering active biological molecules (Fasol et al., 1994, Pandit et al., 1998, 2000). To allow for better control of delivery of protein from fibrin matrices some researchers have focused on improving the retention of proteins through heparin adsorption (Pike et al., 2006, Sakiyama-Elbert and Hubbell, 2000) or covalent incorporation (Zisch et al., 2001). Proteins are typically incorporated in a form in which they readily diffuse from the scaffolds stimulating local vessels to sprout toward the implanted material. This leads to similar issues of transience seen in direct injection methods. When VEGF is covalently attached to the scaffolds its release is delayed, prolonging its biological function and reducing the risk of ectopic effects (Zisch et al., 2001). Scaffold-anchored VEGF has been shown to have improved activity and promote more extensive neovascularization relative to freely diffusing VEGF (Ehrbar et al., 2005). Covalent attachment to PEG-based hydrogels has shown similar improvements in vascularization (Seliktar et al., 2004). Collagen, which is normally not a very effective delivery conduit, modified with heparan sulfate demonstrates an ability to deliver FGF-2 and promote stable vascularization *in vivo* (Pieper et al., 2002). By attaching the protein of interest to a degradable scaffold the protein is prevented from being rapidly cleared from the body and local release can be controlled based on material degradation and tissue invasion.

Covalent attachment to the scaffold is not the only method for improving results. Sustained levels of proteins can also be attained by delivery from polymer microparticles. Delivery of FGF-1 from alginate microbeads results in both an increase in initial vessel invasion and a greater persistence of the vascularization in collagen scaffolds then a single-dose suspended within the material (Moya et al., 2009a,b, 2010) (Figure 24.4). In addition, by delivering FGF-1 from alginate the dose required to achieve vascularization is lower than what is required when the protein is suspended in the scaffold (Uriel et al., 2006, Moya et al., 2010). The FGF-1 studies described here and the VEGF studies in the previous section indicate that by control of growth factor transport in a polymer scaffold, a single growth factor can have a dramatic effect on neovascularization.

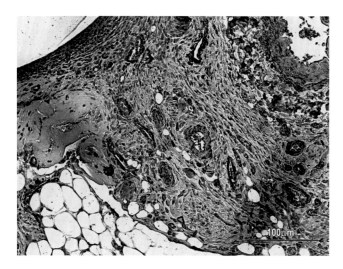

**FIGURE 24.4** (**See color insert.**) Immunohistochemical stain showing vessels formed in response to the sustained delivery of FGF-1. The brown stain indicates the presence of smooth muscle alpha actin-positive mural cells coating the vessels after 3 weeks of stimulation.

Although a single protein has been shown to enhance neovascularization when delivered appropriately, one growth factor may not be sufficient for the task of generating a stable, mature microvascular network in a large engineered tissue. Dual protein strategies have been developed to investigate whether temporally controlled delivery of two growth factors can further improve the response (Richardson et al., 2001, Peirce et al., 2004, Mandal and Kundu, 2009). Most research has focused on the sequential delivery of a protein that stimulates vessel sprouting and invasion followed by a factor involved in the recruitment of mural cells. Under some conditions vessels formed in response to VEGF alone may regress, but this regression can be inhibited by following VEGF delivery with angiopoietin-1 (Ang-1) (Peirce et al., 2004). Rapid release of VEGF followed by PDGF-BB leads to larger vessels and greater mural cell interactions in polymer scaffolds (Richardson et al., 2001). The combination of PDGF-BB with FGF-2 can increase arteriogenesis in models of tissue ischemia (Cao et al., 2003). Dual growth factor delivery approaches can also be combined with a cell-based strategy to improve results (Jay et al., 2010). Alginate microbeads containing VEGF and monocyte chemotactic protein-1 (MCP-1) dispersed in a collagen/fibronectin scaffold along with human umbilical vein ECs were found to be an improvement over ECs alone. The addition of MCP-1 was incorporated due to its documented arteriogenic properties. However, MCP improved functional vessel formation as well as increased the number of SMC-coated vessels. This research shows that controlled delivery of multiple growth factors may enhance neovascularization over a single factor. However, the delivery methods still need to be optimized. In addition, it is not clear how many growth factors need to be delivered or which combinations should be used. Polymer systems that deliver multiple proteins with different release kinetics present a significant optimization challenge.

## 24.3.2.2 Cells

In Section 24.3.1, strategies for assembling networks of ECs in polymer scaffolds before implantation were described. However, the distribution of ECs throughout the scaffold without any particular structure can also accelerate vessel assembly. Cell-based strategies have been investigated clinically for the treatment of ischemic tissues (Amrani and Port, 2003). In both research and clinical trials, these cells have exhibited regenerative potential, but it is not clear how much this potential comes from the transplanted cells forming networks or if parcrine signals from the cells accelerate host neovascularization.

Stem cells are especially attractive for vascularization strategies because of their regenerative properties, expandability and potential to differentiate into multiple cell types. In one study, both endothelial-like and smooth muscle-like vascular progenitor cells were differentiated from human embryonic bodies by exposure to PDGF or VEGF (Ferreira et al., 2007). When these cells were implanted in nude mice using Matrigel as a scaffold, microvessels formed and appeared to anastomose with the host vasculature. Similarly, ECs derived from human embryonic stem cells transplanted with a mouse mesenchymal precursor cell line in a fibronectin–collagen gel contributed to functional blood vessels formed *in vivo* that integrated with the host circulatory system (Wang et al., 2007). Transplanted stem cells may be more effective at promoting angiogenesis than injection of genes for ANG-1 and VEGF (Shyu et al., 2006).

Success for forming vessel networks *in vivo* has also been demonstrated using EPCs from human peripheral blood (Fuchs et al., 2009) particularly to address ischemia (Kawamoto et al., 2001, Kalka et al., 2000). Another source of adult stem cells that has similar proliferative potential but requires less invasive harvesting methods are adipose-derived stem cells from adipose stroma. These cells have demonstrated promising preclinical potential by differentiating into ECs and contributing to neovascularization upon implantation for the treatment of ischemia (Cao et al., 2005b, Miranville et al., 2004).

To further improve on the use of stem cells for inducing vascularization, stem cells transfected to secrete factors have also been examined for their ability to stimulate vascularization *in vivo*. In some of these studies, transfecting stem cells with growth factor genes for VEGF (Yang et al., 2010, Geiger et al., 2007) or FGF-2 (Guo et al., 2006) showed marked improvement over control groups using non-gene-transfected stem cells. This approach is attractive because it not only exploits the regenerative properties of stem cells but produces growth factors for targeted local delivery of angiogenic proteins. In combination with other vascularization strategies transfected cells have also demonstrated success at increasing vessel density (Yu et al., 2009). This method of using gene therapy to get cells to secrete angiogenic factors has also been used with other cell types such as islets to improve engraftment by overexpressing angiogenic factors to stimulate revascularization upon implantation (Su et al., 2007, Cheng et al., 2005b). To address the issue of heterogeneous expression levels in transduced cells, some researchers are focusing on developing methods for selecting out cells expressing desired levels (Misteli et al., 2010). Although gene modification of cells is a promising solution to integrate growth factors and cell delivery, long-term studies are needed to examine the effect of these cells actively remaining and secreting factors after desired vessel formation.

### 24.3.3 Surgical Approaches

Whether using growth factors, cells, or combinations of the two to promote neovascularization, the approaches can be very successful at generating microvascular networks in small volume scaffolds. Clinical application for the treatment of large defects requires a more complex vessel hierarchy within larger scaffold volumes. Techniques developed in the surgical sciences can be used to improve vascularization on implantation.

Prefabrication approaches developed in the field of reconstructive microsurgery can be exploited to enhance neovascularization (Uriel et al., 2008, Cheng et al., 2005a, 2006, 2009, 2010, Brey et al., 2007, Moya et al., 2010). In these approaches, the scaffolds are implanted in a "donor" tissue location that would promote greater neovascularization than the defect location. After a period of prefabrication time, the vascularized tissue can then be transferred to a recipient site. In one embodiment, scaffolds are implanted around a vascular pedicle. The pedicle allows *de novo* vascularization of the scaffolds that provides an option for transfer to the recipient defect with or without microsurgical techniques. Using a rodent vascular pedicle model, the alginate FGF-1 delivery strategy described in Section 24.3.2.1 greater overall vascularization is achieved when the beads are implanted around a vascular pedicle (Moya et al., 2010) than other vascularized beds (Moya et al., 2009a,b). These vascularized scaffolds along with the pedicle may be transferred to the recipient site and connected to host vessels using microsurgical techniques. It may be difficult to translate the pedicle model to clinical application, but large volumes of vascularized tissues can be created by implantation of materials around microsurgically created vessel loops (Hofer et al., 2003, Mian et al., 2000, 2001, Tanaka et al., 2003, Staudenmaier et al., 2004, Demirtas et al., 2010).

Implantation of a tissue engineering construct into a highly vascularized donor location can be used to guide fabrication of large volumes of vascularized tissues with complex 3D shape (Cheng et al., 2009). The application of prefabricated or prelaminated flap has been widely applied in clinical cases (Guo and Pribaz, 2009, Mathy and Pribaz, 2009, Pribaz and Fine, 2001). This approach has been successfully applied clinically where the prefabricated vascularized tissue was easily transferred to the recipient location (Cheng et al., 2006). The use of established surgical approaches to enhance vascularization in large volume scaffolds has received little attention for applications in tissue engineering. When combined with a novel growth factor and/or cell strategy, surgical techniques may help optimize the volumes of scaffolds vascularized.

## 24.4 Conclusions

In order for tissue engineering to approach its vast clinical potential, researchers must continue to develop new and innovative methods for controlling neovascularization. This issue has received significant attention in recent years, and the studies in this chapter describe some of the progress that has been made. However, the challenge of generating stable, extensive, microvascular networks in large volumes of tissues still remains. Research up to this point has primarily resulted in vascularization of small volume scaffolds, which do not approach the clinical volumes needed. The continued development of novel approaches that consider specifically the issue of vascularizing large, complex tissues will lead to new tissue engineering interventions.

## References

Abramsson, A., Berlin, O., Papayan, H., Paulin, D., Shani, M., and Betsholtz, C. 2002. Analysis of mural cell recruitment to tumor vessels. *Circulation,* 105, 112–7.

Amrani, D. L. and Port, S. 2003. Cardiovascular disease: Potential impact of stem cell therapy. *Expert Rev Cardiovasc Ther,* 1, 453–61.

Amsden, B. and Turner, N. 1999. Diffusion characteristics of calcium alginate gels. *Biotechnol Bioeng,* 65, 605–10.

Anghelina, M., Krishnan, P., Moldovan, L., and Moldovan, N. I. 2004. Monocytes and macrophages form branched cell columns in matrigel: Implications for a role in neovascularization. *Stem Cells Dev,* 13, 665–76.

Anghelina, M., Krishnan, P., Moldovan, L., and Moldovan, N. I. 2006. Monocytes/macrophages cooperate with progenitor cells during neovascularization and tissue repair: Conversion of cell columns into fibrovascular bundles. *Am J Pathol,* 168, 529–41.

Aplin, A. C., Fogel, E., and Nicosia, R. F. 2009. Ang-1 and MCP-1 cooperate in pericyte recruitment during angiogenesis. *FASEB J,* 23, 116.6.

August, A. D., Kong, H. J., and Mooney, D. J. 2006. Alginate hydrogels as biomaterials. *Macromol Biosci,* 6, 623–33.

Benjamin, L. E. and Keshet, E. 1997. Conditional switching of vascular endothelial growth factor (VEGF) expression in tumors: Induction of endothelial cell shedding and regression of hemangioblastoma-like vessels by VEGF withdrawal. *Proc Natl Acad Sci USA,* 94, 8761–6.

Benjamin, L. E., Hemo, I., and Keshet, E. 1998. A plasticity window for blood vessel remodelling is defined by pericyte coverage of the preformed endothelial network and is regulated by PDGF-B and VEGF. *Development,* 125, 1591–8.

Black, A. F., Berthod, F., L'heureux, N., Germain, L., and Auger, F. A. 1998. *In vitro* reconstruction of a human capillary-like network in a tissue-engineered skin equivalent. *FASEB J,* 12, 1331–40.

Borenstein, J. T., Weinberg, E. J., Orrick, B. K., Sundback, C., Kaazempur-Mofrad, M. R., and Vacanti, J. P. 2007. Microfabrication of three-dimensional engineered scaffolds. *Tissue Eng,* 13, 1837–44.

Brey, E. M., Cheng, M. H., Allori, A., Satterfield, W., Chang, D. W., Patrick, C. W., Jr., and Miller, M. J. 2007. Comparison of guided bone formation from periosteum and muscle fascia. *Plast Reconstr Surg,* 119, 1216–22.

Brey, E. M., Mcintire, L. V., Johnston, C. M., Reece, G. P., and Patrick, C. W., Jr. 2004. Three-dimensional, quantitative analysis of desmin and smooth muscle alpha actin expression during angiogenesis. *Ann Biomed Eng,* 32, 1100–7.

Brey, E. M., Uriel, S., Greisler, H. P., and Mcintire, L. V. 2005. Therapeutic neovascularization: Contributions from bioengineering. *Tissue Eng,* 11, 567–84.

Cao, L. and Mooney, D. J. 2007. Spatiotemporal control over growth factor signaling for therapeutic neovascularization. *Adv Drug Deliv Rev,* 59, 1340–50.

Cao, R., Brakenhielm, E., Pawliuk, R., Wariaro, D., Post, M. J., Wahlberg, E., Leboulch, P., and Cao, Y. 2003. Angiogenic synergism, vascular stability and improvement of hind-limb ischemia by a combination of PDGF-BB and FGF-2. *Nat Med,* 9, 604–13.

Cao, Y., Hong, A., Schulten, H., and Post, M. J. 2005a. Update on therapeutic neovascularization. *Cardiovasc Res,* 65, 639–48.

Cao, Y., Sun, Z., Liao, L., Meng, Y., Han, Q., and Zhao, R. C. 2005b. Human adipose tissue-derived stem cells differentiate into endothelial cells *in vitro* and improve postnatal neovascularization in vivo. *Biochem Biophys Res Commun,* 332, 370–9.

Carmeliet, P. 2000. Mechanisms of angiogenesis and arteriogenesis. *Nat Med,* 6, 389–95.

Carmeliet, P. 2003. Angiogenesis in health and disease. *Nat Med,* 9, 653–60.

Carmeliet, P. and Jaine, R. K. 2000. Angiogenesis in cancer and other disease. *Nature,* 407, 249.

Caspi, O., Lesman, A., Basevitch, Y., Gepstein, A., Arbel, G., Habib, I. H. M., Gepstein, L., and Levenberg, S. 2007. Tissue engineering of vascularized cardiac muscle from human embryonic stem cells. *Circ Res,* 100, 263–72.

Chen, C. S., Mrksich, M., Huang, S., Whitesides, G. M., and Ingber, D. E. 1998. Micropatterned surfaces for control of cell shape, position, and function. *Biotechnol Prog,* 14, 356–63.

Chen, C. Y., Barron, J. A., and Ringeisen, B. R. 2006. Cell patterning without chemical surface modification: Cell-cell interactions between printed bovine aortic endothelial cells (BAEC) on a homogeneous cell-adherent hydrogel. *Appl Surf Sci,* 252, 8641–5.

Chen, X., Aledia, A. S., Ghajar, C. M., Griffith, C. K., Putnam, A. J., Hughes, C. C., and George, S. C. 2009. Prevascularization of a fibrin-based tissue construct accelerates the formation of functional anastomosis with host vasculature. *Tissue Eng A,* 15, 1363–71.

Chen, X., Aledia, A. S., Popson, S. A., Him, L. K., Hughes, C. C., and George, S. 2010. Rapid anastomosis of endothelial precursor cell-derived vessels with host vasculature is promoted by a high density of co-transplanted fibroblasts. *Tissue Eng,* 16(2), 585–94.

Cheng, M. H., Brey, E. M., Allori, A., Satterfield, W. C., Chang, D. W., Patrick, C. W., Jr., and Miller, M. J. 2005a. Ovine model for engineering bone segments. *Tissue Eng,* 11, 214–25.

Cheng, M. H., Brey, E. M., Allori, A. C., Gassman, A., Chang, D. W., Patrick, C. W., Jr., and Miller, M. J. 2009. Periosteum-guided prefabrication of vascularized bone of clinical shape and volume. *Plast Reconstr Surg,* 124, 787–95.

Cheng, M. H., Brey, E. M., Ulusal, B. G., and Wei, F. C. 2006. Mandible augmentation for osseointegrated implants using tissue engineering strategies. *Plast Reconstr Surg,* 118, 1e–4e.

Cheng, M. H., Uriel, S., Moya, M. L., Francis-Sedlak, M., Wang, R., Huang, J. J., Chang, S. Y., and Brey, E. M. 2010. Dermis-derived hydrogels support adipogenesis in vivo. *J Biomed Mater Res,* 92(3), 852–8.

Cheng, Y., Zhang, J. L., Liu, Y. F., Li, T. M., and Zhao, N. 2005b. Islet transplantation for diabetic rats through the spleen. *Hepatobiliary Pancreat Dis Int,* 4, 203–6.

Chiu, Y. C., Cheng, M. H., Uriel, S., and Brey, E. M. 2011. Materials for engineering vascularized adipose tissue. *J Tissue Viability,* 20(2), 37–48.

Chiu, Y.-C., Larson, J. C., Perez-Luna, V. H., and Brey, E. M. 2009. Formation of microchannels in poly(ethylene glycol) hydrogels by selective degradation of patterned microstructures. *Chem Mater,* 21, 1677–82.

Chrobak, K. M., Potter, D. R., and Tien, J. 2006. Formation of perfused, functional microvascular tubes in vitro. *Microvasc Res,* 71, 185–96.

Darland, D. C. and D'amore, P. A. 1999. Blood vessel maturation: Vascular development comes of age. *J Clin Invest,* 103, 157–8.

Demirtas, Y., Engin, M. S., Aslan, O., Ayas, B., and Karacalar, A. 2010. The effect of "minimally invasive transfer of angiosomes" on vascularization of prefabricated/prelaminated tissues. *Ann Plast Surg,* 64, 491–5 10.1097/SAP.0b013e31819b6c6e.

Dike, L., Chen, C., Mrksich, M., Tien, J., Whitesides, G., and Ingber, D. 1999. Geometric control of switching between growth, apoptosis, and differentiation during angiogenesis using micropatterned substrates. *In Vitro Cell Dev Biol Anim,* 35, 441–8.

Domansky, K., Inman, W., Serdy, J., Dash, A., Lim, M. H., and Griffith, L. G. 2010. Perfused multiwell plate for 3D liver tissue engineering. *Lab Chip,* 10, 51–8.

Ehrbar, M., Metters, A., Zammaretti, P., Hubbell, J. A., and Zisch, A. H. 2005. Endothelial cell proliferation and progenitor maturation by fibrin-bound VEGF variants with differential susceptibilities to local cellular activity. *J Control Release,* 101, 93–109.

Fasol, R., Schumacher, B., Schlaudraff, K., Hauenstein, K.-H., and Seitelberger, R. 1994. Experimental use of a modified fibrin glue to induce site-directed angiogenesis from the aorta to the heart. *J Thorac Cardiovasc Surg,* 107, 1432–9.

Ferreira, L. S., Gerecht, S., Shieh, H. F., Watson, N., Rupnick, M. A., Dallabrida, S. M., Vunjak-Novakovic, G., and Langer, R. 2007. Vascular progenitor cells isolated from human embryonic stem cells give rise to endothelial and smooth muscle like cells and form vascular networks in vivo. *Circ Res,* 101, 286–94.

Fidkowski, C., Kaazempur-Mofrad, M. R., Borenstein, J., Vacanti, J. P., Langer, R., and Wang, Y. 2005. Endothelialized microvasculature based on a biodegradable elastomer. *Tissue Eng,* 11, 302–9.

Folkman, J. and Haudenschild, C. 1980. Angiogenesis in vitro. *Nature,* 288, 551–6.

Francis, M. E., Uriel, S., and Brey, E. M. 2008. Endothelial cell-matrix interactions in neovascularization. *Tissue Eng B Rev,* 14, 19–32.

Francis-Sedlak, M. E., Moya, M. L., Huang, J.-J., Lucas, S. A., Chandrasekharan, N., Larson, J. C., Cheng, M.-H., and Brey, E. M. 2010. Collagen glycation alters neovascularization *in vitro* and *in vivo*. *Microvasc Res,* 80, 3–9.

Fuchs, S., Ghanaati, S., Orth, C., Barbeck, M., Kolbe, M., Hofmann, A., Eblenkamp, M., Gomes, M., Reis, R. L., and Kirkpatrick, C. J. 2009. Contribution of outgrowth endothelial cells from human peripheral blood on *in vivo* vascularization of bone tissue engineered constructs based on starch polycaprolactone scaffolds. *Biomaterials,* 30, 526–34.

Gaengel, K., Genove, G., Armulik, A., and Betsholtz, C. 2009. Endothelial-mural cell signaling in vascular development and angiogenesis. *Arterioscler Thromb Vasc Biol,* 29, 630–38.

Geiger, F., Lorenz, H., Xu, W., Szalay, K., Kasten, P., Claes, L., Augat, P., and Richter, W. 2007. VEGF producing bone marrow stromal cells (BMSC) enhance vascularization and resorption of a natural coral bone substitute. *Bone,* 41, 516–22.

Gerhardt, H. and Betsholtz, C. 2003. Endothelial-pericyte interactions in angiogenesis. *Cell Tissue Res,* 314, 15–23.

Gerhardt, H. et al 2003. VEGF guides angiogenic sprouting utilizing endothelial tip cell filopodia. *J Cell Biol,* 161, 1163–77.

Gibot, L., Galbraith, T., Huot, J., and Auger, F. A. 2010. A Preexisting microvascular network Benefits *in vivo* Revascularization of a microvascularized tissue-engineered skin substitute. *Tissue Eng A,* 16(10), 3199–206.

Golden, A. P. and Tien, J. 2007. Fabrication of microfluidic hydrogels using molded gelatin as a sacrificial element. *Lab Chip,* 7, 720–5.

Griffith, L. G. and Naughton, G. 2002. Tissue engineering—current challenges and expanding opportunities. *Science,* 295, 1009–14.

Griffith, L. G., Wu, B., Cima, M. J., Powers, M. J., Chaignaud, B., and Vacanti, J. P. 1997. *In vitro* organogenesis of liver tissue. *Ann N Y Acad Sci,* 831, 382–97.

Gu, F., Amsden, B., and Neufield, R. 2004. Sustained delivery of vascular endothelial growth factor with alginate beads. *J Control Release,* 96, 463–72.

Guo, L. and Pribaz, J. J. 2009. Clinical flap prefabrication. *Plast Reconstr Surg,* 124, e340–50.

Guo, X., Zheng, Q., Kulbatski, I., Yuan, Q., Yang, S., Shao, Z., Wang, H., Xiao, B., Pan, Z., and Tang, S. 2006. Bone regeneration with active angiogenesis by basic fibroblast growth factor gene transfected mesenchymal stem cells seeded on porous beta-TCP ceramic scaffolds. *Biomed Mater,* 1, 93–9.

Hendel, R. C., Henry, T. D., Rocha-Singh, K., Isner, J. M., Kereiakes, D. J., Giordano, F. J., Simons, M., and Bonow, R. O. 2000. Effect of intracoronary recombinant human vascular endothelial growth factor on myocardial perfusion: Evidence for a dose-dependent effect. *Circulation,* 101, 118–21.

Hofer, S. O., Knight, K. M., Cooper-White, J. J., O'connor, A. J., Perera, J. M., Romeo-Meeuw, R., Penington, A. J., Knight, K. R., Morrison, W. A., and Messina, A. 2003. Increasing the volume of vascularized tissue formation in engineered constructs: An experimental study in rats. *Plast Reconstr Surg,* 111, 1186–92; discussion 1193–4.

Hoffmann, J. et al. 2005. Endothelial survival factors and spatial completion, but not pericyte coverage of retinal capillaries determine vessel plasticity. *FASEB J,* 19, 2035–6.

Jang, J. H., Rives, C. B., and Shea, L. D. 2005. Plasmid delivery *in vivo* from porous tissue-engineering scaffolds: Transgene expression and cellular transfection. *Mol Ther,* 12, 475–83.

Jay, S. M., Shepherd, B. R., Andrejecsk, J. W., Kyriakides, T. R., Pober, J. S., and Saltzman, W. M. 2010. Dual delivery of VEGF and MCP-1 to support endothelial cell transplantation for therapeutic vascularization. *Biomaterials,* 31, 3054–62.

Kaihara, S., Borenstein, J., Koka, R., Lalan, S., Ochoa, E. R., Ravens, M., Pien, H., Cunningham, B., and Vacanti, J. P. 2000. Silicon micromachining to tissue engineer branched vascular channels for liver fabrication. *Tissue Eng,* 6, 105–17.

Kalka, C., Masuda, H., Takahashi, T., Kalka-Moll, W. M., Silver, M., Kearney, M., Li, T., Isner, J. M., and Asahara, T. 2000. Transplantation of ex vivo expanded endothelial progenitor cells for therapeutic neovascularization. *Proc Natl Acad Sci USA,* 97, 3422–7.

Kawamoto, A. et al. 2001. Therapeutic potential of ex vivo expanded endothelial progenitor cells for myocardial ischemia. *Circulation,* 103, 634–7.

King, K., Wang, C., Kaazempur-Mofrad, M., Vacanti, J., and Borenstein, J. 2004. Biodegradable microfluidics. *Adv Mater,* 16, 2007–12.

Koike, N., Fukumura, D., Gralla, O., Au, P., Schechner, J. S., and Jain, R. K. 2004. Tissue engineering: Creation of long-lasting blood vessels. *Nature,* 428, 138–9.

Levenberg, S. et al. 2005. Engineering vascularized skeletal muscle tissue. *Nat Biotech,* 23, 879–84.

Lokmic, Z. and Mitchell, G. M. 2008. Engineering the microcirculation. *Tissue Eng B Rev,* 14, 87–103.

Mandal, B. B. and Kundu, S. C. 2009. Calcium alginate beads embedded in silk fibroin as 3D dual drug releasing scaffolds. *Biomaterials,* 30, 5170–7.

Mathy, J. A. and Pribaz, J. J. 2009. Prefabrication and prelamination applications in current aesthetic facial reconstruction. *Clin Plast Surg,* 36, 493–505.

Mian, R., Morrison, W. A., Hurley, J. V., Penington, A. J., Romeo, R., Tanaka, Y., and Knight, K. R. 2000. Formation of new tissue from an arteriovenous loop in the absence of added extracellular matrix. *Tissue Eng,* 6, 595–603.

Mian, R. A., Knight, K. R., Penington, A. J., Hurley, J. V., Messina, A., Romeo, R., and Morrison, W. A. 2001. Stimulating effect of an arteriovenous shunt on the *in vivo* growth of isografted fibroblasts: A preliminary report. *Tissue Eng,* 7, 73–80.

Miranville, A., Heeschen, C., Sengenes, C., Curat, C. A., Busse, R., and Bouloumie, A. 2004. Improvement of postnatal neovascularization by human adipose tissue-derived stem cells. *Circulation,* 110, 349–55.

Misteli, H., Wolff, T., Fuglistaler, P., Gianni-Barrera, R., Gurke, L., Heberer, M., and Banfi, A. 2010. High-throughput flow cytometry purification of transduced progenitors expressing defined levels of vascular endothelial growth factor induces controlled angiogenesis in vivo. *Stem Cells,* 28, 611–9.

Montesano, R., Orci, L., and Vassalli, P. 1983. *in vitro* rapid organization of endothelial cells into capillary-like networks is promoted by collagen matrices. *J Cell Biol,* 97, 1648–52.

Montesano, R., Vassalli, J. D., Baird, A., Guillemin, R., and Orci, L. 1986. Basic fibroblast growth factor induces angiogenesis in vitro. *Proc Natl Acad Sci,* 83, 7297–301.

Moon, J. J., Saik, J. E., Poche, R. A., Leslie-Barbick, J. E., Lee, S. H., Smith, A. A., Dickinson, M. E., and West, J. L. 2010. Biomimetic hydrogels with pro-angiogenic properties. *Biomaterials,* 31, 3840–7.

Morrison, W. A. 2009. Progress in tissue engineering of soft tissue and organs. *Surgery,* 145, 127–30.

Moya, M. L., Cheng, M. H., Huang, J. J., Francis-Sedlak, M. E., Kao, S. W., Opara, E. C., and Brey, E. M. 2010. The effect of FGF-1 loaded alginate microbeads on neovascularization and adipogenesis in a vascular pedicle model of adipose tissue engineering. *Biomaterials,* 31, 2816–26.

Moya, M. L., Garfinkel, M. R., Liu, X., Lucas, S., Opara, E. C., Greisler, H. P., and Brey, E. M. 2009a. Fibroblast growth factor-1 (FGF-1) loaded microbeads enhance local capillary neovascularization. *J Surg Res,* 160, 208–12.

Moya, M. L., Lucas, S., Francis-Sedlak, M., Liu, X., Garfinkel, M. R., Huang, J. J., Cheng, M. H., Opara, E. C., and Brey, E. M. 2009b. Sustained delivery of FGF-1 increases vascular density in comparison to bolus administration. *Microvasc Res,* 78, 142–7.

Nahmias, Y., Schwartz, R. E., Verfaillie, C. M., and Odde, D. J. 2005. Laser-guided direct writing for three-dimensional tissue engineering. *Biotechnol Bioeng,* 92, 129–36.

Nikol, S. et al. 2008. Therapeutic angiogenesis with intramuscular NV1FGF improves amputation-free survival in patients with critical limb ischemia. *Mol Ther,* 16, 972–8.

Nomi, M., Atala, A., Coppi, P. D., and Soker, S. 2002. Principals of neovascularization for tissue engineering. *Mol Aspects Med,* 23, 463–83.

Ozawa, C. R., Banfi, A., Glazer, N. L., Thurston, G., Springer, M. L., Kraft, P. E., Mcdonald, D. M., and Blau, H. M. 2004. Microenvironmental VEGF concentration, not total dose, determines a threshold between normal and aberrant angiogenesis. *J Clin Invest,* 113, 516–27.

Ozerdem, U. and Stallcup, W. B. 2003. Early contribution of pericytes to angiogenic sprouting and tube formation. *Angiogenesis,* 6, 241–9.

Pandit, A., Ashar, R., Feldman, D., and Thompson, A. 1998. Investigation of acidic fibroblast growth factor delivered through a collagen scaffold for the treatment of full-thickness skin defects in a rabbit model. *Plast Reconstr Surg,* 101, 766–75.

Pandit, A. S., Wilson, D. J., and Feldman, D. S. 2000. Fibrin scaffold as an effective vehicle for the delivery of acidic fibroblast growth factor (FGF-1). *J Biomater Appl,* 14, 229–42.

Papavasiliou, G., Songprawat, P., Perez-Luna, V., Hammes, E., Morris, M., Chiu, Y. C., and Brey, E. 2008. Three-dimensional pattering of poly (ethylene Glycol) hydrogels through surface-initiated photopolymerization. *Tissue Eng C Methods,* 14, 129–40.

Peirce, S. M., Price, R. J., and Skalak, T. C. 2004. Spatial and temporal control of angiogenesis and arterialization using focal applications of VEGF164 and Ang-1. *Am J Physiol Heart Circ Physiol,* 286, H918–25.

Pieper, J. S., Hafmans, T., Van Wachem, P. B., Van Luyn, M. J., Brouwer, L. A., Veerkamp, J. H., and Van Kuppevelt, T. H. 2002. Loading of collagen-heparan sulfate matrices with bFGF promotes angiogenesis and tissue generation in rats. *J Biomed Mater Res,* 62, 185–94.

Pike, D. B., Cai, S., Pomraning, K. R., Firpo, M. A., Fisher, R. J., Shu, X. Z., Prestwich, G. D., and Peattie, R. A. 2006. Heparin-regulated release of growth factors *in vitro* and angiogenic response *in vivo* to implanted hyaluronan hydrogels containing VEGF and bFGF. *Biomaterials,* 27, 5242–51.

Pitt, C. G. 1990. The controlled parenteral delivery of polypeptides and proteins. *Int J Pharm,* 59, 173–96.

Pribaz, J. J. and Fine, N. A. 2001. Prefabricated and prelaminated flaps for head and neck reconstruction. *Clin Plast Surg,* 28, 261–72, vii.

Richardson, T. P., Peters, M. C., Ennett, A. B., and Mooney, D. J. 2001. Polymeric system for dual growth factor delivery. *Nat Biotechnol*, 19, 1029–34.

Sakiyama-Elbert, S. E., and Hubbell, J. A. 2000. Development of fibrin derivatives for controlled release of heparin-binding growth factors. *J Control Release*, 65, 389–402.

Scholz, D., Ziegelhoeffer, T., Helisch, A., Wagner, S., Friedrich, C., Podzuweit, T., and Schaper, W. 2002. Contribution of arteriogenesis and angiogenesis to postocclusive hindlimb perfusion in mice. *J Mol Cell Cardiol*, 34, 775–87.

Schumacher, B., Pecher, P., Von Specht, B. U., and Stegmann, T. 1998. Induction of neoangiogenesis in ischemic myocardium by human growth factors: First clinical results of a new treatment of coronary heart disease. *Circulation*, 97, 645–50.

Seliktar, D., Zisch, A. H., Lutolf, M. P., Wrana, J. L., and Hubbell, J. A. 2004. MMP-2 sensitive, VEGF-bearing bioactive hydrogels for promotion of vascular healing. *J Biomed Mater Res A*, 68, 704–16.

Shyu, K. G., Wang, B. W., Hung, H. F., Chang, C. C., and Shih, D. T. 2006. Mesenchymal stem cells are superior to angiogenic growth factor genes for improving myocardial performance in the mouse model of acute myocardial infarction. *J Biomed Sci*, 13, 47–58.

Skalak, T. C., Little, C. D., Mcintire, L. V., Hirschi, K. K., Tranquillo, R. T., Post, M., and Ranieri, J. 2002. Vascular assembly in engineered and natural tissues. *Ann NY Acad Sci*, 961, 255–7.

Staudenmaier, R., Hoang, T. N., Kleinsasser, N., Schurr, C., Frolich, K., Wenzel, M. M., and Aigner, J. 2004. Flap prefabrication and prelamination with tissue-engineered cartilage. *J Reconstr Microsurg*, 20, 555–64.

Su, D., Zhang, N., He, J., Qu, S., Slusher, S., Bottino, R., Bertera, S., Bromberg, J., and Dong, H. H. 2007. Angiopoietin-1 production in islets improves islet engraftment and protects islets from cytokine-induced apoptosis. *Diabetes*, 56, 2274–83.

Sunderkotter, C., Steinbrink, K., Goebeler, M., Bhardwaj, R., and Sorg, C. 1994. Macrophages and angiogenesis. *J Leukoc Biol*, 55, 410–22.

Takahiro, M., Yumi, S., Yuji, H., Takehiko, S., and Yoshino, H. 2000. Protein encapsulation into biodegradable microspheres by a novel S/O/W emulsion method using poly(ethylene glycol) as a protein micronization adjuvant. *J Control Release*, 69, 435–44.

Tanaka, Y., Sung, K. C., Tsutsumi, A., Ohba, S., Ueda, K., and Morrison, W. A. 2003. Tissue engineering skin flaps: Which vascular carrier, arteriovenous shunt loop or arteriovenous bundle, has more potential for angiogenesis and tissue generation? *Plast Reconstr Surg*, 112, 1636–44.

Trentin, D., Hall, H., Wechsler, S., and Hubbell, J. A. 2006. Peptide-matrix-mediated gene transfer of an oxygen-insensitive hypoxia-inducible factor-1alpha variant for local induction of angiogenesis. *Proc Natl Acad Sci USA*, 103, 2506–11.

Tsurumi, Y., Takeshita, S., Chen, D., Kearney, M., Rossow, S. T., Passeri, J., Horowitz, J. R., Symes, J. F., and Isner, J. M. 1996. Direct intramuscular gene transfer of naked DNA encoding vascular endothelial growth factor augments collateral development and tissue perfusion. *Circulation*, 94, 3281–90.

Udelson, J. E., Dilsizian, V., Laham, R. J., Chronos, N., Vansant, J., Blais, M., Galt, J. R., Pike, M., Yoshizawa, C., and Simons, M. 2000. Therapeutic angiogenesis with recombinant fibroblast growth factor-2 improves stress and rest myocardial perfusion abnormalities in patients with severe symptomatic chronic coronary artery disease. *Circulation*, 102, 1605–10.

Unger, R. E., Ghanaati, S., Orth, C., Sartoris, A., Barbeck, M., Halstenberg, S., Motta, A., Migliaresi, C., and Kirkpatrick, C. J. 2010. The rapid anastomosis between prevascularized networks on silk fibroin scaffolds generated *in vitro* with cocultures of human microvascular endothelial and osteoblast cells and the host vasculature. *Biomaterials*, 31, 6959–67.

Uriel, S., Brey, E. M., and Greisler, H. P. 2006. Sustained low levels of fibroblast growth factor-1 promote persistent microvascular network formation. *Am J Surg*, 192, 604–9.

Uriel, S., Huang, J. J., Moya, M. L., Francis, M. E., Wang, R., Chang, S. Y., Cheng, M. H., and Brey, E. M. 2008. The role of adipose protein derived hydrogels in adipogenesis. *Biomaterials*, 29, 3712–9.

Van Weel, V., Van Tongeren, R. B., Van Hinsbergh, V. W., Van Bockel, J. H., and Quax, P. H. 2008. Vascular growth in ischemic limbs: A review of mechanisms and possible therapeutic stimulation. *Ann Vasc Surg,* 22, 582–97.

Wang, Z. Z., Au, P., Chen, T., Shao, Y., Daheron, L. M., Bai, H., Arzigian, M., Fukumura, D., Jain, R. K., and Scadden, D. T. 2007. Endothelial cells derived from human embryonic stem cells form durable blood vessels in vivo. *Nat Biotech,* 25, 317–8.

Yamaguchi, J. et al. 2003. Stromal cell-derived factor-1 effects on ex vivo expanded endothelial progenitor cell recruitment for ischemic neovascularization. *Circulation,* 107, 1322–8.

Yana, I. et al. 2007. Crosstalk between neovessels and mural cells directs the site-specific expression of MT1-MMP to endothelial tip cells. *J Cell Sci,* 120, 1607–14.

Yang, F. et al. 2010. Genetic engineering of human stem cells for enhanced angiogenesis using biodegradable polymeric nanoparticles. *Proc Natl Acad Sci USA,* 107, 3317–22.

Young, S., Wong, M., Tabata, Y., and Mikos, A. G. 2005. Gelatin as a delivery vehicle for the controlled release of bioactive molecules. *J Control Release,* 109, 256–74.

Yu, J. X., Huang, X. F., Lv, W. M., Ye, C. S., Peng, X. Z., Zhang, H., Xiao, L. B., and Wang, S. M. 2009. Combination of stromal-derived factor-1alpha and vascular endothelial growth factor gene-modified endothelial progenitor cells is more effective for ischemic neovascularization. *J Vasc Surg,* 50, 608–16.

Zisch, A. H., Lutolf, M. P., and Hubbell, J. A. 2003. Biopolymeric delivery matrices for angiogenic growth factors. *Cardiovasc Pathol,* 12, 295–310.

Zisch, A. H., Schenk, U., Schense, J. C., Sakiyama-Elbert, S. E., and Hubbell, J. A. 2001. Covalently conjugated VEGF—fibrin matrices for endothelialization. *J Control Release,* 72, 101–13.

# 25

# Biomedical Imaging of Engineered Tissues

Nicholas E.
Simpson
*University of Florida*

Athanassios
Sambanis
*Georgia Institute of
Technology*

| 25.1 | Introduction | 25-1 |
| 25.2 | Optical Imaging | 25-2 |
| 25.3 | Radiation-Based Imaging | 25-4 |
| 25.4 | Ultrasound | 25-5 |
| 25.5 | Infrared Imaging | 25-6 |
| 25.6 | Nuclear Magnetic Resonance | 25-6 |
| | Principles of NMR • MRI and Spectroscopy • Contrast Agents and Techniques • Implantable Coils • Examples | |
| 25.7 | Conclusion | 25-12 |
| | Acknowledgments | 25-12 |
| | References | 25-13 |

## 25.1 Introduction

Readers of this book are well aware that tissue engineering is a vibrant field that aims to develop biological substitutes that can replace, repair, or enhance lost tissue or organ function. As this field comes to the forefront of medicine, it becomes critical for basic and clinical researchers to understand some of the methods that can be employed to study engineered constructs and tissues under development *in vitro*, or while functioning *in vivo*. Methods designed to image tissues can greatly aid in the advancement of tissue engineering. Today's imaging techniques, such as x-ray, computed tomography (CT), ultrasound, positron emission tomography (PET), single photon emission computed tomography, and magnetic resonance imaging (MRI), can allow for more than just mere pictures of the tissues of interest. Indeed, even optical techniques have progressed significantly, and can generate images of exquisite detail and clarity. These modern biomedical imaging techniques can see into objects without physically peeling through the interposing layers. They also have the desired ability to yield information related to many physical and physiological characteristics important to the study of engineered tissues. Among these characteristics are the structural integrity and physical attributes of the scaffolding; the perfusion/diffusion of blood and nutrients into the tissue; the distribution of oxygen within the tissue; and changes in the cellular function and remodeling of engineered tissue over time. These critical data can be collected and used to optimize design, monitor function, and observe, predict and possibly also prevent failure of engineered tissues.

The subject of biomedical imaging is far too vast to be comprehensive in this short chapter. Therefore, it is the purpose of this chapter to briefly touch upon some of the important imaging techniques that are appropriate for observing engineered tissues. To this end, this chapter will discuss a number of current imaging techniques that have been or can be applied to the study of cells and tissue engineered substitutes, with a more extensive description of magnetic resonance techniques. Strengths and weaknesses of each of these methods will be pointed out. The overarching goal of this chapter is to give the reader a brief view into the imaging toolbox that is presently at our disposal, and thus a greater insight into the imaging methods that can enhance the experimental design, characterization, and functional assessment of tissue constructs *in vitro* and, primarily, *in vivo*. It should be noted that these techniques often provide complementary information, and no one imaging modality is appropriate for all applications. Rather, the choice of imaging technique depends on the information desired.

## 25.2 Optical Imaging

Optical techniques are highly sensitive and can generate images with subcellular resolution. Although excellent for *in vitro* applications, they are limited by the short transmission length of light through tissue. *In vivo* optical imaging is noninvasive, unless catheter-based probes are used to image deeper tissues. Optical methods underwent a revolution when fluorescent (Chalfie et al. 1994; Gee et al. 2002; Hadjantonakis et al. 2003) and luminescent (Greer III and Szalay 2002) reporter proteins were incorporated into cells, and newer detection techniques were developed (Piston 1999). The method typically utilizes fluorescent or bioluminescent endogenous reporters or exogenous probes to monitor biological processes (Choy et al. 2003; Hickson 2009), or optical techniques to study tissue structure *in vivo*. These methods are further described below, along with specific examples.

Both bioluminescence and fluorescence involve emission and detection of visible light which, however, is produced by different mechanisms. Bioluminescence produces light of 550–650-nm wavelength via an enzymatically catalyzed chemical reaction, such as the reaction of luciferin by the enzyme firefly luciferase (Fluc). Its principal advantage is the minimal background signal emitted by natural tissues, resulting in high signal-to-noise ratio and high sensitivity of detection. In contrast, fluorescence involves absorption of a photon of 400–600-nm wavelength by a fluorescent reporter, which triggers the emission of another photon of a longer wavelength (450–650 nm). Fluorescent reporters come in a variety of forms. They include expressed proteins, such as green and red fluorescent proteins, dyes, microspheres, and nanoparticles used to tag tissues or cells. The major disadvantage of fluorescence is the higher autofluorescent background signal emitted by tissues *in vivo*. For both bioluminescent and fluorescent modalities, the emitted visible light is attenuated approximately 10-fold for each centimeter of tissue depth due to absorption and scattering. The development of probes that fluoresce at the near infrared region (NIR) (650–850 nm) may partially solve this problem, as NIR light has significantly longer tissue penetration lengths. An added benefit of NIR is the minimal natural tissue autofluorescence at NIR wavelengths (Hickson 2009).

Emitted light is usually detected by a charged-couple device camera. Besides the camera, an imaging setup typically includes a light-proof enclosure, animal support devices, and necessary optical software and hardware, such as emission and excitation filters and imaging algorithms (Figure 25.1). The development of three-dimensional (3D) tomographic reconstructions, along with integrated multimodal imaging, has allowed the acquisition with a single instrument of both functional and structural information from the same animal whether a bioluminescence or fluorescence modality is employed (Choy et al. 2003; Brindle 2008; Hickson 2009).

One promising application of optical imaging is tracking implanted cells. Indeed, a critical challenge in cell-based therapies is the low engraftment efficiency of delivered cells because of extensive cell death and/or cell entrainment or migration to nontarget tissues. Cells are engineered to express luciferase, or a fluorescent protein, then the animal is imaged periodically to assess the location and viability of the implanted cells. Examples include the *in vivo* bioluminescent imaging of human cord blood-derived mesenchymal stem cells engineered to express Fluc and injected intramyocardially in rats: in these studies bioluminescence decreased with time, but was detectable 6 days posttransplantation (Min et al. 2006). Also, bioluminescence from embryonic rat cardiomyoblasts engineered to express Fluc and injected intramyocardially in rats was detected for more than 2 weeks *in vivo* (Figure 25.2) (Wu et al. 2003). In similar applications with pancreatic islets, islets retrieved from a transgenic mouse strain

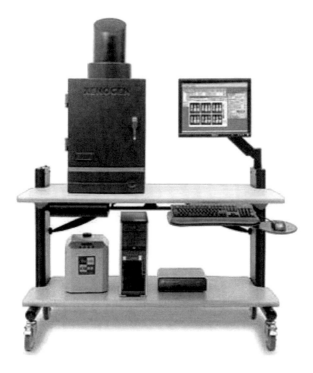

**FIGURE 25.1**  Typical fluorescence/bioluminescence small animal imaging system.

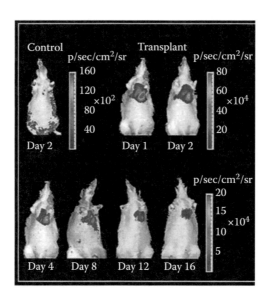

**FIGURE 25.2**  (**See color insert.**) Bioluminescent imaging of cardiac cell transplantation in living animals. Shown is a representative rat transplanted with embryonic cardiomyoblasts expressing Fluc imaged on days 1, 2, 4, 8, 12, and 16 postimplantation. The control rat shows background signal only. (Reproduced with permission from Wu, J. C. et al. 2003. *Circulation* 108(11): 1302–1305.)

constitutively expressing Fluc were implanted as syngeneic or allogeneic grafts at various anatomic sites in diabetic mouse recipients. Bioluminescence imaging allowed tracking of the fate of the islets with high sensitivity (as few as 10 islets could be detected) and over long time periods (18 months) posttransplantation (Chen et al. 2006; Chen and Kaufman 2009). These studies clearly demonstrate the utility of optical imaging approaches for temporal *in vivo* studies.

Optical imaging has been used successfully for the *in vivo* tracking of transgenes expression. One possibility is to fuse the coding region of the transgene with a fluorescent protein or luciferase (Golzio et al. 2004). Alternatively, if the expressed protein alters the fluorescence of a substrate, then it can be detected through its activity (Mahmood and Weissleder 2003; Tung et al. 2004). Immunodetection techniques using quantum dots (QDs) may offer another promising approach (West and Halas 2003).

Of significance is the use of optical methods in cancer research. For tumor detection, QDs have been successfully implemented. These are 10–15-nm sized semiconductor nanocrystals that exhibit stable fluorescence and can be covalently linked to biorecognition molecules, including antibodies, nucleic acids, or ligands. QDs target and accumulate in tumors because of the enhanced permeability and retention of tumor sites (passive targeting) and by being conjugated with antibodies against cancer-specific cell surface antigens (active targeting) (Gao et al. 2004). QDs have been used to detect human prostate cancer growths in nude mice (Gao et al. 2004) and to manage brain tumors, where in the latter case the QDs were delivered through macrophages that phagocytized the particles and infiltrated the tumors (Popescu and Toms 2006). Delivery of antibody conjugated, PEGylated gold nanoparticles, followed by detection with optical coherence tomography, has also been reported for detection of oral dysplasia in a hamster model (Kim et al. 2009). Malignant cells engineering to express luciferase or a fluorescent protein and injected in animals to induce tumor formation can be used to track tumor growth kinetics, metastasis, and response to treatment (Choy et al. 2003). For example, human multiple myeloma cells stably transfected to express green fluorescent protein and injected in mice were imaged to monitor the development and progression of tumors (Mitsiades et al. 2003).

For structural studies, various optical imaging methods have been used *in vivo* to study tissues in experimental animals and humans. For studies on tissue structure with micron scale resolution, optical coherence tomography, whose principle is similar to ultrasound except that light instead of acoustic waves are used, has been successfully applied *in vivo* to image tissues, such as the bladder and trachea (Zagaynova et al. 2002; Fujimoto 2003; Han et al. 2005). Other examples include *in vivo* optical brain imaging using techniques including, but not limited to, two-photon microscopy and near infrared imaging (Hillman 2007); studies on embryonic heart microstructure with a combination of optical imaging techniques (Yelin et al. 2007); and confocal and multiphoton imaging for *in vivo* microendoscopy (Kim et al. 2008). For engineered tissues, structural studies with optical imaging have been limited; however, the use of optical coherence tomography to measure flow in a blood vessel substitute in a bioreactor *in vitro* has been reported (Mason et al. 2004).

In summary, optical methods have been successfully used to study biological function and tissue structure *in vivo*, including engraftment of implanted cells, gene expression, tumor detection, growth and metastasis, and natural tissue structure. These methods could be easily translated to implanted tissue substitutes comprised of cells associated with biomaterials in functional 3D configurations. *In vivo* applications in tissue engineering have been very limited; however, they are well poised to provide significant novel contributions in the not so distant future.

## 25.3 Radiation-Based Imaging

Radiation-based imaging techniques can be broken into two sections: imaging methods that detect radionuclides coming from within the sample, and methods that irradiate the sample with ionizing radiation and measure the radiation that passes through the sample. The two chief imaging techniques using radionuclide detection are PET, which detects positrons, and single photon emission tomography, which detects gamma radiation. These are highly sensitive techniques capable of detecting trace amounts of a radiolabel. However, both suffer from low spatial resolution, though microPET systems provide improved resolution of about 1 mm (Cherry et al. 1997; Correia et al. 1999; Tai et al. 2003). Irradiating methods include x-ray and CT, and more recently, microCT (Schambach et al. 2010). These methods are ideal for studying dense radio-opaque tissues, and excel in providing structural information. Consequently, a number of quantitative analyses of tissue engineered constructs, many involving bone and cartilage and vascularization of implanted scaffolds (Young et al. 2008), have been pursued using microCT imaging analysis. Some of these are highlighted here. One study used microCT to view dense polymeric casts of embryonic bird hearts toward studying cardiovascular developmental changes (Butcher et al. 2007). Although invasive and destructive, this approach can be used to quantify temporal changes in tissue. MicroCT was also used to observe collateral blood vessel formation in mice, and measure the effect of osteopontin on vascular growth and recovery from limb ischemia (Duvall et al. 2008). One proponent of the microCT imaging approach for bone studies (Guldberg et al. 2004, 2008) uses the technique to analyze mineralization of 3D bone scaffolds (Cartmell et al. 2004), and has looked at the effect of osteoblastic transcription factor expression on the repair of bone defects in 3-D scaffolds (Byers et al. 2006). Finally, machines that are capable of performing combinations of PET/microPET, CT/microCT, and MRI have been developed to take advantage of their complementary strengths (Beyer et al. 2000; Catana et al. 2008; Goetz et al. 2008; Pichler et al. 2008). Although often employed in small animal research, such machines can be valuable in studying engineered tissues, both *in vitro* and *in vivo*.

## 25.4 Ultrasound

Ultrasound imaging, or ultrasonography, is a commonly encountered clinical technique that can create images by measuring the reflection of high-frequency sound waves to obtain structural information from within tissues. Ultrasonic waves can penetrate deeply, thus this method is appropriate for studying implanted tissues, or tissues within bioreactors. It is useful for real-time biopsy or other real-time intervention. In addition, the technique is relatively inexpensive, noninvasive (or minimally invasive), and repeatable. Thus, ultrasound is an excellent method for temporal studies. A disadvantage is that a skilled sonographer is key to obtaining useful images, and ultrasound findings can be operator dependent. In addition, deeply embedded tissues may be difficult to study if there are interposing obstructions. However, this is a versatile technique can yield more than just static images. Applying ultrasonic techniques to measure blood flow to tissues is now a standard clinical procedure. If the engineered tissue is connected to the vasculature, key perfusion information can be obtained through application of this technique. The use of contrast agents in ultrasound is also making inroads. By encapsulating microbubbles (in the micron diameter range), enhancement of microvasculature can be attained (Hope Simpson et al. 1999, 2001). Recent contrast innovations include perfluorocarbon nanoparticles (Stride and Saffari 2004) and microtubules (Bekeredian et al. 2002) that may be synthesized with antibodies for targeted ultrasonic contrast. Another ultrasound technique that is presently mature enough to be exploited in the field of tissue engineering is elasticity imaging (Doyley et al. 2005; Righetti et al. 2005). This approach uses ultrasound to determine critical tissue properties such as viscosity, and elasticity, the latter measured through Young's modulus, a measure of material stiffness, and Poisson's ratio, a measure of perpendicular expansion or contraction resulting from an applied compression or decompression. In temporal studies, changes in these measures in the tissue engineered construct may indicate cellular growth, remodeling, or changes in the structural integrity of the engineered device. For example, immunoreaction to the implant by the host may be detected through changes in measures values due to increased stiffness from fibrotic overgrowth of the implant. Such techniques could also indicate changes in the materials used to create the implanted constructs, for instance, a softening (or hardening) of a biomaterial that may indicate impending failure. The field of ultrasound is continually growing, and new techniques are being steadily advanced that may prove beneficial to the study of implanted engineered devices.

# 25.5  Infrared Imaging

Molecules can absorb energy from the infrared region of the electromagnetic spectrum. In the mid-infrared band, this resonant frequency absorption is dictated by the vibrational frequency of the chemical bonds within the substance under study. Sophisticated machines dedicated to perform this analysis are required. Fourier transform infrared (FT-IR) analysis of the absorption by a material yields information related to the rotation and vibration of the molecules under study. FT-IR techniques have been used in tissue engineering, predominantly in the study of cartilage and bone, as these materials contain many bonds that resonate in the mid-infrared region (Carden and Morris 2000; Boskey and Mendelsohn 2005). Strengths of the method include the ability to measure a number of important properties of bone such as mineralization, carbonate/phosphate ratio, crystallinity, and acid phosphate content. FT-IR imaging studies have been performed on cartilage to study composition, including collagen (Kim et al. 2005) and proteoglycan content, and collagen orientation (Bi et al. 2005). The technique is amenable to temporal studies aimed to investigate tissue degeneration, growth, and composition of engineered tissues, and efficacy of repair strategies. A recent review of this technique highlights applications of FT-IR imaging to bone and cartilage (Boskey and Camacho 2007). FT-IR has also been used to study vascular changes to tissue due to tumor angiogenesis, as both protein content and protein secondary structure (beta sheets, alpha helices, etc.) can be determined (Wehbe et al. 2008). A major weakness of the FT-IR technique is that the procedure is invasive. Biological samples contain water, and effective analysis is often done on dehydrated tissue samples embedded in a hard resin. Therefore, *in vivo* analysis is not presently done. However, for analysis of the molecular structure and composition of bone, cartilage, or vasculature, it is an effective method that can be included in the tissue engineer's toolbox.

# 25.6  Nuclear Magnetic Resonance

Nuclear magnetic resonance (NMR) was first demonstrated in 1946 (Bloch et al. 1946; Purcell et al. 1946). NMR techniques include MRI and spectroscopic methods. Although the concepts of NMR and MRI are too complex to be given justice in a few short paragraphs, rudimentary "classical" descriptions of the phenomenon and imaging technique are offered here to give the reader a cursory understanding. Imaging and spectroscopic applications are then discussed.

## 25.6.1  Principles of NMR

The term NMR fairly well describes the phenomenon: it is a magnetic component of the nucleus that resonates (and can absorb electromagnetic energy) at a certain frequency. This resonance occurs because the components of the nucleus, protons, and neutrons, possess a physical property termed angular momentum, or spin. Because these fundamental particles try to pair up and cancel out their individual angular momentum, not all nuclei have a net spin; therefore, not all nuclei can be observed with NMR techniques. For example, the net nuclear angular momentum is zero if the nuclei contain an even number of both protons and neutrons (i.e., nuclei with an even atomic mass and number). However, nuclei with odd atomic mass or odd atomic number possess nuclear spin. Because nuclei have a positive electric charge, those nuclei that have angular momentum can be considered as tiny spinning charges which generate small magnetic fields. When placed in an external magnetic field, these nuclei try to align with it, not all in the same orientation (energy state), but with a preference toward the lower energy state, resulting in a net magnetization vector. This energy state preference is magnetic field strength dependent, which is why magnets of increasing strength are used in NMR/MRI. Importantly, these spins can be considered to wobble, or precess, at a frequency that is dependent on the nuclei and the strength of the magnetic field to which the nuclei are exposed, though other factors influence this frequency.

The NMR experiment requires the following: a sample containing NMR-observable nuclei in sufficient abundance (often in millimolar concentrations); a strong homogeneous magnetic field; and a

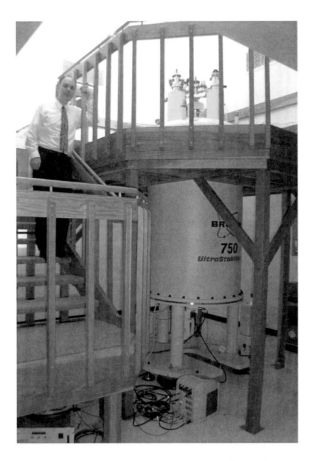

**FIGURE 25.3** Image of a 17.6-Tesla vertical bore magnet housed in the advanced magnetic resonance imaging and spectroscopy facility in the McKnight Brain Institute of the University of Florida, Gainesville, Florida. This magnet is ideal for *in vitro* perfusion studies and small animal work. An author (N.E.S.) of this chapter is depicted for scale.

radiofrequency (RF) coil to both apply the electromagnetic pulses that the nuclei absorb, and measure the return of the nuclei to their equilibrium state after these pulses. Typical NMR/MRI machines (which are specialized and expensive) have a powerful magnet, gradient coil systems that influence the magnetic field, RF amplifiers, and other equipment that allow for data collection and analysis. Figure 25.3 depicts a high magnetic field research machine well suited for many tissue engineering studies. In essence, the NMR measurement occurs thusly. The sample is placed in the homogeneous magnetic field, causing the nuclei of interest to resonate at some given frequency. RF pulses are applied at this resonant frequency causing the nuclei to absorb the energy, and moving their net magnetization vector. After the pulse, the net magnetization vector returns to equilibrium, and analysis of this decaying signal yields information about the nuclei of interest (e.g., the frequencies and amplitudes of the nuclei under study).

## 25.6.2 MRI and Spectroscopy

Obtaining images by exploitation of the NMR phenomenon is commonly termed MRI. In most cases, these images arise from the signals of hydrogen nuclei of water. The technique of MRI was first proposed and developed in the early 1970s by Paul Lauterbur (1973), with critical early advances made by Peter Mansfield (Mansfield and Grannell 1973). The process is somewhat complex, and a detailed description is beyond the scope of this chapter, but the method can be thought of as using magnetic fields and

RF waves to identify the spatial location of nuclear spins within the sample. In very simplistic terms, the position of each small volume element within an image, called a voxel, is defined by the distinctive resonance frequency, or phase, of the spins the pixel contains. These distinct differences are achieved through the use of three orthogonal electromagnet coils, called gradients. Each coil imposes small changes in the magnetic field (thus the name gradient) throughout the sample (in Cartesian terms, along the x, y, and z directions). Through the timing and application of these gradients and RF pulses, spins within individual voxels can be identified by frequency and phase, and an image reconstructed. Tissue images of high resolution are possible due to the high concentration of water and the high sensitivity of the hydrogen nuclei. Simple NMR images yielding anatomical information based on the local water concentrations are termed proton-density weighted images, though additional RF pulses and gradients can be applied to the process to manipulate the spins and achieve various types of contrast, described below. Full descriptions of the principles of NMR and MRI are available in a number of excellent books of varying detail (Abragam 1961; Farrar and Becker 1971; Smith and Ranallo 1989).

NMR/MRI has become a valued tool in the study of engineered tissues because of its many positive attributes. A distinct advantages NMR holds over other imaging techniques is its ability to acquire structural as well as chemical, metabolic, and physiologic information. There are a number of powerful techniques that allow for the discrimination of tissues in images based on physical characteristics. Among these are methods to determine diffusion, relaxation parameters, and elasticity, each of which is described below. One can even combine the imaging and spectroscopy so that chemical information from specific locations of the sample can be obtained. MRI is a noninvasive technique well suited for surface or deep tissue investigation. It is ideal for studying soft tissues, and it can be applied *in vitro* or *in vivo* repeatedly, making it a useful technique for long-term studies. NMR is not without its disadvantages, though. One disadvantage of the method is the relative insensitivity of the NMR phenomenon, particularly when trying to study nuclei other than hydrogen in water. Another disadvantage is the expense of performing NMR/MRI studies and the necessity to have skilled operators available to obtain the information.

### 25.6.3  Contrast Agents and Techniques

As mentioned above, the ability to discriminate tissue and tissue characteristics is an advantage of the NMR method. One approach is to obtain contrast by introducing a compound, termed a contrast agent, which enhances physical differences between tissues due to their paramagnetic properties. This approach is called enhanced contrast, and the added contrast agent often works by altering the relaxation, or return to equilibrium, of the net magnetization vector. Commonly used contrast agents include transition metals, in the form of iron oxide, and lanthanide series metals, particularly gadolinium complexes. These are described in more detail below. Other NMR contrast techniques use what is termed native contrast, or contrast derived from the intrinsic characteristics of the nuclei within the tissues. The more commonly encountered techniques such as $T_1$, $T_2$, $T_2^*$, diffusion or magnetization transfer enhancement are described in brief here. Exploiting differences in relaxation of the net magnetization vectors is possible because the local environment can have a profound effect on the relaxation rate. Two processes describe this return to equilibrium of the magnetization vector: longitudinal and transverse relaxation. If the magnetization vector at equilibrium is considered to be on the Cartesian coordinate's z-axis, longitudinal relaxation refers to the restoration of the net magnetization along the z-axis after an RF pulse. The return occurs as individual spins go from an excited energy state to the lower energy state, transferring energy to surrounding areas. Spins do not lose their energy simultaneously: the z-component of the magnetization vector recovers in a time-dependent manner that can be fitted to an exponential equation with a time constant ($T_1$); thus the name $T_1$ relaxation. Images exploiting $T_1$ differences are considered $T_1$-weighted. Transverse relaxation describes loss of the net magnetization vector in the x–y plane due to small local magnetic field interactions between the nuclei, and is also called spin–spin relaxation. The local magnetic field inhomogeneities (both internal and external) make the spins precess at different frequencies, causing the net magnetization vector to vanish in a time-dependent manner that can be fitted to an exponential equation with a time constant ($T_2$), giving the process the name $T_2$ relaxation. Images taking advantage of $T_2$ differences are termed $T_2$-weighted. Because NMR image signal is dominated by water, compartmented regions of tissues will have restricted water exchange. A method to measure and map this restriction is through diffusion-weighted imaging. Here, magnetic gradients of varying time and magnitude are imposed onto the sample after the RF pulse, differentiating tissues based on their local diffusive character. In essence, spins that are restricted cannot diffuse away from a region; spins that are not restricted will diffuse out of an area. The direction of the diffusion can also yield important information on structure; this approach is termed diffusion tensor imaging. Magnetization transfer is another NMR technique that distinguishes the structural integrity of tissues based on the rotational freedom of the water molecules in the sample. Water molecules that are free (i.e., not bound or hydrated to other molecules such as proteins) tumble faster, and have a narrow resonance frequency band; bound molecules have a broader band. By exciting the restricted water nuclei, and allowing them to transfer their energy to free water, a measure of the structural integrity of the tissues can be estimated. Although adding native contrast methods to an imaging sequence can lead to signal loss, a balance between signal, spatial resolution, and total imaging time can usually be achieved.

Methods to enhance the NMR signal from implanted tissues often involve adding contrast agents to label the cells or the biomaterials. The goal is to better visualize cells, biological processes, or construct characteristics with NMR techniques. For extensive information on MRI contrast agents, the reader can refer to a number of reviews (Gupta and Gupta 2005; Gupta et al. 2007; Strijkers et al. 2007; Sun et al. 2008). Novel gadolinium nanoparticles have been used to successfully track stem cells with MRI (Tseng et al. 2010). Karfeld-Sulzer et al. (2011) have included protein polymer contrast agents into their constructs to enhance the presence, degradation, and change of the implant as a function of time. A commonly encountered NMR contrast agent used to track cells are iron-oxide based (Modo et al. 2005). As a result of their paramagnetic (or superparamagnetic) properties, these agents affect NMR relaxation times. NMR imaging has been used to monitor a number of different types of labeled cells (Dodd et al. 1999; Foster-Gareau et al. 2003; Cahill et al. 2004; Kriz et al. 2005; Evgenov et al. 2006), a subject reviewed by Gupta (Gupta and Gupta 2005; Gupta et al. 2007). Their use as an MRI enhancer in tissue engineered devices is limited (Terrivitis et al. 2006; Constantinidis et al. 2009), but 3D constructs have been generated by guiding cells containing these agents with magnetic fields (Ito et al. 2005; Dobson et al. 2006; Ino et al. 2007).

## 25.6.4 Implantable Coils

Another approach to enhance the NMR signal and quantitatively analyze the structure and function of implanted bioartificial organs is to implant the RF coil with the engineered tissue (Volland et al. 2010). Early studies connected the implanted coil with a wire through the skin (Arnder et al. 1996), but later approaches use inductive coupling to link the implanted coil to an external surface coil (Schnall et al. 1986; Wirth et al. 1993; Silver et al. 2001; Hoult and Tomanek 2002) both avoiding intrusive wires and reducing potential for infection. The approach by Volland et al. (2010) uses an inductively coupled method to obtain signal from essentially only the tissue the implanted coil surrounds. This approach results in a 2-fold sensitivity improvement over that obtainable with a surface coil, allowing for significant gain in information obtained from an implanted construct (e.g., images with higher contrast-to-noise ratio; spectroscopy with greater SNR; potential detection of less-sensitive nuclei). Figure 25.4 shows a cross-sectional MRI of a mouse which has been implanted with an alginate-bead containing construct that houses a coil. The reader is referred to Volland et al. (2010) for details concerning the implantable coil. Although an implantable coil approach is currently used to monitor bioartificial pancreatic constructs *in vitro* and *in vivo*, it could certainly be applied to a number of implantable tissue engineered products. The results establish that large gains in signal-to-noise can be obtained with this coil system. Work to expand the capabilities of NMR detection includes creating a wireless multiple-frequency capable circuitry system. This system uses a "single-resonant" approach, where an array of

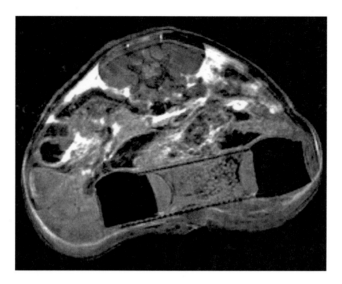

**FIGURE 25.4** Cross-sectional MRI (spin-echo) of a mouse implanted intraperitoneally with an alginate-bead containing construct. The construct contains an RF coil that can be used to acquire spectroscopic or imaging data from only the beads/tissue housed within the construct, as described in the chapter. This image was obtained in a horizontal bore 11.1-Tesla magnet by Nelly A. Volland, PhD, when she was a graduate student of N.E.S.

capacitors (here, varactors on a microchip) is remotely switched by a digital controller to tune and match the coil to any desired frequency. The coil behaves as a single-resonant frequency coil thus providing optimal signal sensitivity.

## 25.6.5 Examples

Noninvasive monitoring of tissue-engineered constructs, both those in development *in vitro*, and those implanted *in vivo*, is important to optimize design, assess structural attributes, evaluate and predict cellular efficacy, and observe changes in these components (cellular and noncellular) over time. To this end, because of its diverse applications and strengths, NMR/MRI has been integrated into a number of studies in the field of tissue engineering. Some of these studies have been aimed to evaluate the biomaterials. For example, NMR microimaging studies determined NMR properties of alginate (a polysaccharide biomaterial commonly used in tissue engineering) microbeads (Simpson et al. 2003; Grant et al. 2005; Constantinidis et al. 2007). Because changes in the relaxation values and diffusion characteristics are related to the gelation and structural integrity of the biomaterial, noninvasive *in vivo* monitoring of the biomaterials can assist in determining the state of an implanted construct. Also, a recent *in vivo* imaging study evaluated the efficacy of tissue engineered heart patches, and demonstrated the utility of MRI in evaluating engineered scaffolds (Stuckey et al. 2010). Other studies have been interested in monitoring the growth and development of tissues *in vitro*, though advances to enhance the capability to monitor engineered tissues *in vivo* have also been pursued. Below are some examples of how researchers are implementing NMR/MRI to address aspects of tissue engineering, both *in vitro* and *in vivo*. Keep in mind that the examples given are far from exhaustive, and merely scratch the surface of what has and can be performed with these powerful techniques.

Because NMR is an inherently weak signal, as discussed earlier, high cell densities are helpful when obtaining cellular information. To create these high cell densities *in vitro*, bioreactors have been used in tissue engineering to develop and study bioartificial organs and tissues. The use of NMR in these bioreactor studies has been extensive, and encompasses biochemistry, physiology, cellular growth and remodeling, and cell and biomaterial tracking. Many *in vitro* bioreactor studies are aimed toward elucidating NMR parameters so that similar NMR studies can be extended *in vivo*. Bioreactor studies are predominantly spectroscopic studies aimed to measure metabolism through analysis of $^{1}H$, $^{31}P$, or $^{13}C$ NMR spectra, though imaging studies to monitor construct architecture, tissue remodeling, tracking agents, or flow patterns through the bioreactor have also been performed. Varieties of bioreactors have been studied, each dependent on the type of tissue under study. Two common perfused bioreactors are the hollow fiber (Mancuso and Fernandez 1990; Gillies et al. 1993) and fixed bed reactors (Constantinidis and Sambanis 1995; Papas et al. 1999a,b; Thelwall and Brindle 1999). By including perfusion loops and replenishment capabilities, these bioreactor systems can maintain nutrient delivery to tissues. Early studies with perfused hollow fiber systems were used to study hybridoma metabolism with $^{31}P$ and $^{13}C$ NMR spectroscopy (Mancuso and Fernandez 1990; Gillies et al. 1991; Mancuso et al. 1994, 1998). Hollow fiber bioreactors seeded with rat hepatocytes were used to study the transport of hepatobiliary contrast agents by MRI (Planchamp et al. 2004a,b). Fixed bed bioreactor studies of Chinese hamster ovary cells seeded onto microcarriers used diffusion-weighted $^{1}H$ MRI and NMR spectroscopy to evaluate the cellular distribution and assess the bioreactor cellular fraction, respectively (Thelwall and Brindle 1999). The same study showed that maximal cell growth occurred at the periphery of the microcarriers. These bioreactor systems are appropriate for long-term *in vitro* studies and can and have been adapted to tissue engineering.

Tissue engineering of bone as a substitute for bone grafts is of high interest due to the lack of graft availability and the difficulty in native tissue regeneration. Although NMR is better suited for soft tissues, approaches to study bone and engineered constructs have been exploited. Magnetic resonance microscopy (MRM) studies found the NMR signal decreasing over time as the scaffold fills with bone due to osteogenic processes (Wahburn et al. 2004; Xu et al. 2006). Another study used MRM to track tissue growth and mineralization of hollow fiber bioreactors seeded with primary osteoblasts over a 9-week period (Chesnick et al. 2007), and found that the MRM measurements were comparable to the spatial mapping by FTIR microspectroscopy, indicating that MRM is well suited to monitor bone formation *in vitro*. And a study by Buschmann et al. (2011) used gadolinium and MRI techniques to determine relaxation parameters toward quantitating perfusion capability during the early stages of bone formation in constructs with mixed cell cultures. To monitor changes in bone formation over time *in vivo*, MRI has shown its value (Hartman et al. 2002; Potter et al. 2006). MRI was used to monitor bone formation in a rat model over 7 weeks, and identified small changes in size, as well as the 3D shape of the new bone (Hartman et al. 2002). In a mouse model, MRM was used to noninvasively visualize tissue engineered phalange constructs and identified changes in size and mineralization (Potter et al. 2006).

NMR studies on chondrocytes have been implemented to assess cells that can repair and replace articular cartilage (Potter et al. 1998; Chen et al. 2003; Ramaswamy et al. 2009; Irrechukwu et al. 2010; Nugent et al. 2010). In hollow fiber systems seeded with chondrocytes, neocartilage formation was followed by $^{1}H$ MR microimaging, and the fixed charge tissue density was evaluated by gadolinium exclusion (Potter et al. 1998; Chen et al. 2003). The MR methods were able to track increases in tissue volume, cellularity and macromolecular content, and reveal regional variations in cell size and sulfated glycosaminoglycan content. Labeling chondrocytes with iron oxide nanoparticles also allowed for effective tracking of these cells in tissue engineered cartilage (Ramaswamy et al. 2009). MRI was also effectively used to temporally study isolated chondrocytes cultured in a collagen scaffold, and demonstrated the ability to apply NMR endpoints for comparing cultured tissue to native cartilage (Nugent et al. 2010). A recent study used MRI to monitor changes in the development of cartilage constructs, and found that MRI was sensitive to compositional changes in the collagen and sulfated glycosaminoglycan content due to a treatment by pulsed low-intensity ultrasound (Irrechukwu et al. 2010), and may be a useful technique to evaluate cartilage and repair processes *in situ*.

Bladder tissue engineering is another field that has used MRI methods to study the development of viable tissues grown on collagen scaffolds or previously acellularized matrices. Early studies used MRI with gadolinium contrast agents to observe the effect of vascular endothelial growth factor on the vascularization of bladder constructs (Cheng et al. 2005). Later, these MRI-observable effects were correlated to vascular endothelial growth factor dose and quantified using vascular bed contrast agents of differing molecular weights (Cheng et al. 2007). Recent studies by this same group used MRI to determine the effect adding hyaluronic acid to the matrix. The addition of hyaluronic acid to the matrix enhanced the cellular development, strength, and hydration of the engineered bladder, and altered the $T_2^*$ relaxation rate of the tissue, allowing for MRI methods to noninvasively monitor and track changes to the developing bladder (Cheng et al. 2010).

Our laboratories have been interested in the bioartificial pancreas toward the treatment of type 1 diabetes, and to this end, have studied encapsulated systems of insulin-secreting cells in fixed bed reactors by $^1$H MRI, $^{31}$P, and $^1$H MR spectroscopy, and $^{19}$F MR spectroscopy of perfluorocarbons in the encapsulation matrix. We also have observed the encapsulated tissues *in vivo* with mouse models. Initial studies used NMR to study alginate-encapsulated, insulin-secreting recombinant murine pituitary AtT-20 cells in a perfused fixed bed bioreactor for more than 60 days (Constantinidis and Sambanis 1995). $^{31}$P NMR measured high energy phosphate levels (e.g., phosphocreatine and nucleotide triphosphates) and $^1$H NMR imaging verified uniform bed packing, visualized flow, and ensured no significant flow channeling occurred across the bed. Papas et al. (1999a,b) used a similar setup to study effects of glucose and oxygen concentrations on the bioenergetics of alginate-encapsulated murine insulinoma βTC3 cells. These and subsequent (Gross et al. 2007a) studies indicated that the number of metabolically active cells supported in a given bead volume is mainly determined by available oxygen in the surrounding medium. NMR studies on perfused and encapsulated βTC3 cells correlated the total $^1$H choline (TCho) resonance to the number of metabolically active cells toward estimating the viable cell number in a volume of interest (Long et al. 2000). This work was successfully applied *in vivo* by collecting localized NMR spectra from an implanted disk-shaped agarose construct housing encapsulated βTC3 cells (Stabler et al. 2005a). Although the glucose resonance interferes with the TCho signal, a glucose-corrected TCho area (Stabler et al. 2005a) from constructs implanted in live animals had a strong positive correlation with an MTT viability assay performed on the same explanted constructs. Therefore, NMR techniques can be used to select a volume from which to collect spectroscopic signal, determine viable cell numbers within the implanted construct, and assess the structural integrity of the constructs *in vitro* (Stabler et al. 2005b) and *in vivo* (Stabler et al. 2005a). Recent *in vitro* (Gross et al. 2007b; Goh et al. 2010) and *in vivo* (Goh et al. 2011) studies incorporating $^{19}$F compounds into the encapsulating hydrogel have been successfully used to monitor the dissolved oxygen concentration in the cellular constructs, thus providing another means to measure metabolism and viability.

## 25.7 Conclusion

It is hoped that this chapter provided the reader with a good cross-section of the imaging techniques at the tissue engineer's disposal, as well as a hint of the breadth and depth of information that can now be gleaned from these powerful techniques. The present imaging tool-box seems full, but there are undoubtedly many new advances that will occur to improve current technologies and unveil new as of yet unimagined methods with which to obtain structural and metabolic information on tissue implants. Although this short chapter cannot be comprehensive on current technologies (entire books have been written on the many different imaging approaches), the reader should have little trouble realizing the many ways these tools can be integrated into studies in the field of tissue engineering. In closing, though the imaging techniques described here arise from vastly different fundamental principles, in the end, they each provide us with visual information that is both satisfying to look at and instructive toward our scientific goals.

## Acknowledgments

The studies in the authors' laboratories referenced in this article have been supported by grants from the National Institutes of Health, the Juvenile Diabetes Research Foundation, and the Georgia Tech/Emory Center for the Engineering of Living Tissues (GTEC). This support is gratefully acknowledged.

# References

Abragam, A. 1961. *Principles of Nuclear Magnetism.* Oxford, England, Oxford University Press.

Arnder, L., M. D. Shattuck. et al. 1996. Signal-to-noise ratio comparison between surface coils and implanted coils. *Magn Reson Med* 35: 727–733.

Bekeredian, R., S. Behrens. et al. 2002. Potential of gold-bound microtubules as a new ultrasound contrast agent. *Ultrasound Med Biol* 28: 691–695.

Beyer, T., D. W. Townsend. et al. 2000. A combined PET/CT scanner for clinical oncology. *J Nucl Med* 41(8): 1369–1379.

Bi, X., G. Li. et al. 2005. A novel method for determination of collagen orientation in cartilage by Fourier transform imaging spectroscopy (FT-IRIS). *Osteoarthritis Cartilage* 13: 1050–1058.

Bloch, F., W. W. Hansen. et al. 1946. The nuclear induction experiment. *Phys Rev* 70: 460–474.

Boskey, A. and N. P. Camacho 2007. FT-IR imaging of native and tissue-engineered bone and cartilage. *Biomaterials* 28: 2465–2478.

Boskey, A. and R. Mendelsohn 2005. Infrared analysis of bone in health and disease. *J Biomed Opt* 10: 31102–31106.

Brindle, K. 2008. New approaches for imaging tumour responses to treatment. *Nat Rev Cancer* 8(2): 94–107.

Buschmann, J., M. Welti. et al. 2011. 3D co-cultures of osteoblasts and endothelial cells in DegraPol foam: Histological and high field MRI analysis of pre-engineered capillary networks in bone grafts. *Tissue Eng Part A*: 17(3–4): 291–299.

Butcher, J. T., D. Sedmera. et al. 2007. Quantitative volumetric analysis of cardiac morphogenesis assessed through micro-computed tomography. *Dev Dyn* 236(3): 802–809.

Byers, B. A., R. E. Guldberg. et al. 2006. Effects of Runx2 genetic engineering and *in vitro* maturation of tissue-engineered constructs on the repair of critical size bone defects. *J Biomed Mater Res A* 76(3): 646–655.

Cahill, K. S., G. Gaidosh. et al. 2004. Noninvasive monitoring and tracking of muscle stem cell transplants. *Transplantation* 78: 1626–1633.

Carden, A. and M. D. Morris. 2000. Application of vibrational spectroscopy to the study of mineralized tissues. *J Biomed Opt* 5: 259–268.

Cartmell, S. H., K. Huynh. et al. 2004. Quantitative microcomputed tomography analysis of mineralization within three-dimensional scaffolds in vitro. *J Biomed Mater Res A* 69(1): 97–104.

Catana, C., D. Procissi. et al. 2008. Simultaneous *in vivo* positron emission tomography and magnetic resonance imaging. *Proc Natl Acad Sci* 105(10): 3705–3710.

Chalfie, M., Y. Tu. et al. 1994. Green fluorescent protein as a marker for gene expression. *Science* 263: 802–805.

Chen, C. T., K. W. Fishbein. et al. 2003. Matrix fixed-charge density as determined by magnetic resonance microscopy of bioreactor-derived hyaline cartilage correlates with biochemical and biomechanical properties. *Arthritis Rheum* 48: 1047–1056.

Chen, X. and D. B. Kaufman 2009. Bioluminescent imaging of transplanted islets. *Methods Mol Biol* 574: 75–85.

Chen, X., X. Zhang. et al. 2006. In vivo bioluminescence imaging of transplanted islets and early detection of graft rejection. *Transplantation* 81(10): 1421–1427.

Cheng, H. L., J. Chen. et al. 2005. Dynamic Gd-DTPA enhanced MRI as a surrogate marker of angiogenesis in tissue-engineered bladder constructs: A feasibility study in rabbits. *J Magn Reson Imaging* 21: 415–423.

Cheng, H. L., Y. Loai. et al. 2010. The acellular matrix (ACM) for bladder tissue engineering: A quantitative magnetic resonance imaging study. *Magn Reson Med* 64: 341–348.

Cheng, H. L., C. Wallis. et al. 2007. Quantifying angiogenesis in VEGF-enhanced tissue-engineered bladder constructs by dynamic contrast-enhanced MRI using contrast agents of different molecular weights. *J Magn Reson Imaging* 25: 137–145.

Cherry, S. R., Y. Shao. et al. 1997. MicroPET: A high resolution PET scanner for imaging small animals. *IEEE Trans Nucl Sci* 44: 1161–1166.

Chesnick, I. E., F. A. Avallone. et al. 2007. Evaluation of bioreactor-cultivated bone by magnetic resonance microscopy and FTIR microspectroscopy. *Bone* 40(4): 904–912.

Choy, G., P. Choyke. et al. 2003. Current advances in molecular imaging: Noninvasive *in vivo* bioluminescent and fluorescent optical imaging in cancer research. *Mol Imaging* 2(4): 303–312.

Constantinidis, I., S. C. Grant. et al. 2007. Non-invasive evaluation of alginate/poly-L-lysine/alginate microcapsules by magnetic resonance microscopy. *Biomaterials* 28: 2438–2445.

Constantinidis, I., S. C. Grant. et al. 2009. Use of magnetic nanoparticles to monitor alginate-encapsulated bTC-tet cells. *Magn Reson Med* 61: 282–290.

Constantinidis, I. and A. Sambanis 1995. Towards the development of artificial endocrine tissues: 31P NMR spectroscopic studies of immunoisolated, insulin-secreting AtT-20 cells. *Biotechnol Bioeng* 47: 431–443.

Correia, J. A., C. A. Burnham. et al. 1999. Development of a small animal PET imaging device with resolution approaching 1 mm. *IEEE Trans Nucl Sci* 46(3): 631–635.

Dobson, J., S. H. Cartmell. et al. 2006. Principles and design of a novel magnetic force mechanical conditioning bioreactor for tissue engineering, stem cell conditioning, and dynamic *in vitro* screening. *IEEE Trans Nanobiosci* 5: 173–177.

Dodd, S. J., M. Williams. et al. 1999. Detection of single mammalian cells by high-resolution magnetic resonance imaging. *Biophys J* 76: 103–109.

Doyley, M. M., S. Srinivasa. et al. 2005. Comparative evaluation of strain-based and model-based modulus elastography. *Ultrasound Med Biol* 31: 787–802.

Duvall, C. L., D. Weiss. et al. 2008. The role of osteopontin in recovery from hind limb ischemia. *Arterioscler Thromb Vasc Biol* 28(2): 290–295.

Evgenov, N. V., Z. Medarova. et al. 2006. In vivo imaging of islet transplantation. *Nat Med* 12: 144–148.

Farrar, T. C. and E. D. Becker 1971. *Pulse and Fourier Transform NMR: Introduction to Theory and Methods.* New York, NY, Academic Press.

Foster-Gareau, P., C. Heyn. et al. 2003. Imaging single cells with a 1.5T clinical MRI scanner. *Magn Reson Med* 49: 968–971.

Fujimoto, J. G. 2003. Optical coherence tomography for ultrahigh resolution *in vivo* imaging. *Nat Biotechnol* 21(11): 1361–1367.

Gao, X., Y. Cui. et al. 2004. In vivo cancer targeting and imaging with semiconductor quantum dots. *Nat Biotechnol* 22(8): 969–976.

Gee, K. R., Z.-L. Zhou. et al. 2002. Detection and imaging of zinc secretion from pancreatic b-cells using a new fluorescent zinc indicator. *J Am Chem Soc Comm* 124: 776–778.

Gillies, R. J., J. P. Galons. et al. 1993. Design and application of NMR-compatible bioreactor circuits for extended perfusion of high-density mammalian cell cultures. *NMR Biomed* 6(1): 95–104.

Gillies, R. J., P. G. Scherer. et al. 1991. Iteration of hybridoma growth and productivity in hollow fiber bioreactors using 31P NMR. *Magn Reson Med* 18(1): 181–192.

Goetz, C., E. Breton. et al. 2008. SPECT low-field MRI system for small-animal imaging. *J Nucl Med* 49(1): 88–93.

Goh, F., J. D. Gross. et al. 2010. Limited beneficial effects of perfluorocarbon emulsions on encapsulated cells in culture: Experimental and modeling studies. *J Biotechnol* 150(2): 232–239.

Goh, F., R. C. Long Jr. et al. 2011. Dual perfluorocarbon method to noninvasively monitor dissolved oxygen concentration in tissue constructs *in vitro* and in vivo. *Biotechnol Prog* 27(4): 1115–1125.

Golzio, M., M. P. Rols. et al. 2004. Optical imaging of *in vivo* gene expression: A critical assessment of the methodology and associated technologies. *Gene Ther* 11(Suppl 1): S85–S91.

Grant, S. C., S. Celper. et al. 2005. Alginate assessment by NMR microscopy. *J Mater Sci* 16: 511–514.

Greer III, L. F. and A. A. Szalay 2002. Imaging of light emission from the expression of luciferases in living cells and organisms: A review. *Luminescence* 17: 43–74.

Gross, J. D., I. Constantinidis. et al. 2007a. Modeling of encapsulated cell systems. *J Theor Biol* 244(3): 500–510.

Gross, J. D., R. C. Long Jr. et al. 2007b. Monitoring of dissolved oxygen and cellular bioenergetics within a pancreatic substitute. *Biotechnol Bioeng* 98(1): 261–270.

Guldberg, R. E., C. L. Duvall. et al. 2008. 3-D imaging of tissue integration with porous biomaterials. *Biomaterials* 29(28): 3757–3761.

Guldberg, R. E., A. S. Lin. et al. 2004. Microcomputed tomography imaging of skeletal development and growth. *Birth Defects Res C Embryo Today* 72(3): 250–259.

Gupta, A. K. and M. Gupta 2005. Synthesis and surface engineering of iron oxide nanoparticles for biomedical applications. *Biomaterials* 26: 3995–4021.

Gupta, A. K., R. R. Naragelkar. et al. 2007. Recent advances on surface engineering of magnetic iron oxide nanoparticles and their biomedical applications. *Nanomedicine* 2: 23–39.

Hadjantonakis, A.-K., M. E. Dickinson. et al. 2003. Technicolour transgenics: Imaging tools for functional genomics in the mouse. *Nat Genet* 4: 613–625.

Han, S., N. H. El-Abbadi. et al. 2005. Evaluation of tracheal imaging by optical coherence tomography. *Respiration* 72(5): 537–541.

Hartman, E. H. M., J. A. Pikkemmat. et al. 2002. In vivo magnetic resonance imaging explorative study of ectopic bone formation in the rat. *Tissue Eng* 8: 1029–1036.

Hickson, J. 2009. In vivo optical imaging: Preclinical applications and considerations. *Uro Oncol* 27(3): 295–297.

Hillman, E. M. 2007. Optical brain imaging in vivo: Techniques and applications from animal to man. *J Biomed Opt* 12(5): 051402.

Hope Simpson, D., P. N. Burns. et al. 2001. Techniques for perfusion imaging with microbubble contrast agents. *IEEE Trans Ultrason Ferroelectr Freq Control* 48: 1483–1494.

Hope Simpson, D., C. T. Chin. et al. 1999. Pulse inversion Doppler: A new method for detecting nonlinear echoes from microbubble contrast agents. *IEEE Trans Ultras Ferroelectr Freq Control* 46: 372–382.

Hoult, D. I. and B. Tomanek 2002. Use of mutually inductive coupling in probe design. *Concepts Magn Reson* 15(4): 262–285.

Ino, K., A. Ito. et al. 2007. Cell patterning using magnetite nanoparticles and magnetic force. *Biotechnol Bioeng* 97: 1309–1317.

Irrechukwu, O. N., P.-C. Lin. et al. 2010. Magnetic resonance studies of macromolecular content in engineered cartilage treated with pulsed low-intensity ultrasound. *Tissue Eng Part A* 17(3–4): 407–415.

Ito, A., M. Shinkai. et al. 2005. Medical application of functionalized magnetic nanoparticles. *J Biosci Bioeng* 100: 1–11.

Karfeld-Sulzer, L. S., E. A. Waters. et al. 2011. Protein polymer MRI contrast agents: Longitudinal analysis of biomaterials in vivo. *Magn Reson Med* 65(1): 220–228.

Kim, C. S., P. Wilder-Smith. et al. 2009. Enhanced detection of early-stage oral cancer *in vivo* by optical coherence tomography using multimodal delivery of gold nanoparticles. *Biomed Opt* 14(3): 034008.

Kim, M., X. Bi. et al. 2005. Fourier transform infrared imaging spectroscopic analysis of tissue engineered cartilage: Histologic and biochemical correlations. *J Biomed Opt* 10: 31105.

Kim, P., M. Puoris'haag. et al. 2008. In vivo confocal and multiphoton microendoscopy. *Biomed Opt* 13(1): 010501.

Kriz, J., D. Jirak. et al. 2005. Magnetic resonance imaging of pancreatic islets in tolerance and rejection. *Transplantation* 80: 1596–1603.

Lauterbur, P. C. 1973. Image formation by induced local interactions: Examples employing nuclear magnetic resonance. *Nature* 242: 190–191.

Long Jr, R. C., K. K. Papas. et al. 2000. In vitro monitoring of total choline levels in a bioartificial pancreas: (1)H NMR spectroscopic studies of the effects of oxygen level. *J Magn Reson* 146(1): 49–57.

Mahmood, U. and R. Weissleder 2003. Near-infrared optical imaging of proteases in cancer. *Mol Cancer Ther* 2(5): 489–496.

Mancuso, A. and E. J. Fernandez 1990. A nuclear magnetic resonance technique for determining hybridoma cell concentration in hollow fiber bioreactors. *Biotechnology* 8(12): 1282–1285.

Mancuso, A., S. T. Sharfstein. et al. 1994. Examination of primary metabolic pathways in a murine hybridoma with carbon-13 nuclear magnetic resonance spectroscopy. *Biotechnol Bioeng* 44(5): 563–585.

Mancuso, A., S. T. Sharfstein. et al. 1998. Effect of extracellular glutamine concentration on primary and secondary metabolism of a murine hybridoma: An *in vivo* 13C nuclear magnetic resonance study. *Biotechnol Bioeng* 57(2): 172–186.

Mansfield, P. and P. K. Grannell 1973. NMR diffraction in solids. *J Phys C* 6: L422–L426.

Mason, C., J. F. Markusen. et al. 2004. Doppler optical coherence tomography for measuring flow in engineered tissue. *Biosens Bioelectron* 20(3): 414–423.

Min, J. J., Y. Ahn. et al. 2006. In vivo bioluminescence imaging of cord blood derived mesenchymal stem cell transplantation into rat myocardium. *Ann Nucl Med* 20(3): 165–170.

Mitsiades, C. S., N. S. Mitsiades. et al. 2003. Fluorescence imaging of multiple myeloma cells in a clinically relevant SCID/NOD *in vivo* model: Biologic and clinical implications. *Cancer Res* 63(20): 6689–6696.

Modo, M., M. Hoehn. et al. 2005. Cellular MR imaging. *Mol Imaging* 4: 143–164.

Nugent, A. E., D. A. Reiter. et al. 2010. Characterization of ex-vivo-generated bovine and human cartilage by immunohistochemical, biochemical, and magnetic resonance imaging analysis. *Tissue Eng Part A* 16(7): 2183–2196.

Papas, K. K., R. C. Long Jr. et al. 1999a. Development of a bioartificial pancreas: I. long-term propagation and basal and induced secretion from entrapped betaTC3 cell cultures. *Biotechnol Bioeng* 66(4): 219–230.

Papas, K. K., R. C. Long Jr. et al. 1999b. Development of a bioartificial pancreas: II. Effects of oxygen on long- term entrapped betaTC3 cell cultures. *Biotechnol Bioeng* 66(4): 231–237.

Pichler, B. J., M. S. Judenhofer. et al. 2008. Multimodal imaging approaches: PET/CT and PET/MRI. *Handb Exp Pharmacol* 185: 109–132.

Piston, D. W. 1999. Imaging living cells by two-photon excitation microscopy. *Trends Cell Biol* 9: 66–69.

Planchamp, C., M. Gex-Fabry. et al. 2004a. Gd-BOPTA transport into rat hepatocytes: Pharmacokinetic analysis of dynamic magnetic resonance images using a hollow-fiber bioreactor. *Invest Radiol* 39(8): 506–515.

Planchamp, C., M. K. Ivancevic. et al. 2004b. Hollow fiber bioreactor: New development for the study of contrast agent transport into hepatocytes by magnetic resonance imaging. *Biotechnol Bioeng* 85(6): 656–665.

Popescu, M. A. and S. A. Toms 2006. In vivo optical imaging using quantum dots for the management of brain tumors. *Expert Rev Mol Diagn* 6(6): 879–890.

Potter, K., J. J. Butler. et al. 1998. Cartilage formation in a hollow fiber bioreactor studied by proton magnetic resonance microscopy. *Matrix Biol* 17(7): 513–523.

Potter, K., D. E. Sweet. et al. 2006. Non-destructive studies of tissue-engineered phalanges by magnetic resonance microscopy and X-ray microtomography. *Bone* 38: 350–358.

Purcell, E. M., H. C. Torrey. et al. 1946. Resonance absorption by nuclear magnetic moments in a solid. *Phys Rev* 69: 37–38.

Ramaswamy, S., J. B. Greco. et al. 2009. Magnetic resonance imaging of chondrocytes labeled with superparamagnetic iron oxide nanoparticles in tissue-engineered cartilage. *Tissue Eng Part A* 15(12): 3899–3910.

Righetti, R., J. Ophir. et al. 2005. A method for generating permeability elastograms and Poisson's ratio time-constant elastograms. *Ultrasound Med Biol* 31: 803–816.

Schambach, S. J., S. Bag. et al. 2010. Applications of micro-CT in small animal imaging. *Methods* 50(1): 2–13.

Schnall, M. D., C. Barlow. et al. 1986. Wireless implanted magnetic resonance probes for *in vivo* NMR. *J Magn Reson* 68: 161–167.

Silver, X., W. X. Ni. et al. 2001. In vivo 1H magnetic resonance imaging and spectroscopy of the rat spinal cord using an inductively-coupled chronically implanted RF coil. *Magn Reson Med* 46: 1216–1222.

Simpson, N. E., S. C. Grant. et al. 2003. NMR properties of alginate microbeads. *Biomaterials* 24: 4941–4948.

Smith, H.-J. and F. N. Ranallo 1989. *A Non-Mathematical Approach to Basic MRI.* Madison, WI, Medical Physics Publishing.

Stabler, C. L., R. C. Long Jr. et al. 2005a. In vivo noninvasive monitoring of a tissue engineered construct using 1H NMR spectroscopy. *Cell Transplant* 14(2–3): 139–149.

Stabler, C. L., R. C. Long Jr. et al. 2005b. Noninvasive measurement of viable cell number in tissue-engineered constructs in vitro, using 1H nuclear magnetic resonance spectroscopy. *Tissue Eng* 11(3–4): 404–414.

Stride, E. and N. Saffari 2004. Theoretical and experimental investigation of the behaviour of ultrasound contrast agent particles in whole blood. *Ultrasound Med Biol* 30: 1495–1509.

Strijkers, G. J., W. J. M. Mulder. et al. 2007. MRI contrast agents: Current status and future perspectives. *Anticancer Agents Med Chem* 7(3): 291–305.

Stuckey, D. J., H. Ishii. et al. 2010. Magnetic resonance imaging evaluation of remodeling by cardiac elastomeric tissue scaffold biomaterials in a rat model of myocardial infarction. *Tissue Eng A* 16(11): 3395–3402.

Sun, C., J. S. H. Lee. et al. 2008. Magnetic nanoparticles in MR imaging and drug delivery. *Adv Drug Deliv Rev* 60: 1252–1265.

Tai, Y. C., A. F. Chatziioannou. et al. 2003. MicroPET II: Design, development and initial performance of an improved microPET scanner for small-animal imaging. *Phys Med Biol* 48(11): 1519–1537.

Terrivitis, J. V., J. W. Bulte. et al. 2006. Magnetic resonance imaging of ferumoxide-labeled mesenchymal stem cells seeded on collagen scaffolds- relevance to tissue engineering. *Tissue Eng* 12: 2765–2775.

Thelwall, P. E. and K. M. Brindle 1999. Analysis of CHO-K1 cell growth in a fixed bed bioreactor using magnetic resonance spectroscopy and imaging. *Cytotechnology* 30(1–3): 121–132.

Tseng, C. L., I. L. Shih. et al. 2010. Gadolinium hexanedione nanoparticles for stem cell labeling and tracking via magnetic resonance imaging. *Biomaterials* 31: 5427–5435.

Tung, C. H., Q. Zeng. et al. 2004. In vivo imaging of beta-galactosidase activity using far red fluorescent switch. *Cancer Res* 64(5): 1579–1583.

Volland, N. A., T. H. Mareci. et al. 2010. Development of an inductively-coupled MR system for imaging and spectroscopic analysis of an implantable bioartificial construct at 11.1T. *Magn Reson Med* 63: 998–1006.

Wahburn, N. R., M. Weir. et al. 2004. Bone formation in polymeric scaffolds evaluated by proton magnetic resonance microscopy and X-ray microtomography. *J Biomed Mater Res A* 69(4): 738–747.

Wehbe, K., R. Pinneau. et al. 2008. FT-IR spectral imaging of blood vessels reveals protein secondary structure deviations induced by tumor growth. *Anal Bioanal Chem* 392: 129–135.

West, J. L. and N. J. Halas 2003. Engineered nanomaterials for biophotonics applications improving sensing, imaging, and therapeutics. *Annu Rev Biomed Eng* 5: 285–292.

Wirth, E. D. I., T. H. Mareci. et al. 1993. A comparison of an inductively coupled implanted coil with optimized surface coils for *in vivo* NMR imaging of the spinal cord. *Magn Reson Med* 30: 626–633.

Wu, J. C., I. Y. Chen. et al. 2003. Molecular imaging of cardiac cell transplantation in living animals using optical bioluminescence and positron emission tomography. *Circulation* 108(11): 1302–1305.

Xu, H., S. F. Othman. et al. 2006. Magnetic resonance microscopy for monitoring osteogenesis in tissue-engineered construct in vitro. *Phys Med Biol* 51: 719–732.

Yelin, R., D. Yelin. et al. 2007. Multimodality optical imaging of embryonic heart microstructure. *J Biomed Opt* 12(6): 064021.

Young, S., J. D. Kretlow. et al. 2008. Microcomputed tomography characterization of neovascularization in bone tissue engineering applications. *Tissue Eng Part B Rev* 14(3): 295–306.

Zagaynova, E. V., O. S. Streltsova. et al. 2002. In vivo optical coherence tomography feasibility for bladder disease. *J Urol* 167(3): 1492–1496.

# 26

# Multiscale Modeling of *In Vitro* Tissue Cultivation

26.1 Introduction ..................................................................26-1
26.2 Model Detail and Abstraction .....................................26-3
26.3 Cell Proliferation and Migration................................26-3
26.4 Cell Population Dynamics and Mass Transport .....................26-4
26.5 Continuous, Discrete, and Hybrid Models
for Tissue Growth................................................26-4
26.6 A Modeling Framework for *In Vitro* Tissue Cultivation..........26-5
26.7 Components of the Hybrid Multiscale Model .........................26-6
Discrete Model for Cell Population Dynamics • Continuous Model
for Mass Transport Dynamics • Coupling of Mass Transport
Dynamics and Cellular Functions • Experimental Protocols: Cell
Seeding and Bioreactor Configuration
26.8 Results and Discussion .............................................26-9
Internal and External Mass Transport Modulates Tissue Growth
and Structure • Differential Effects of Migration Speeds and
Initial Conditions • Cell Population Heterogeneity and Nutrient
Limitations Lead to Emergent Behavior
References...................................................................26-13

Kyriacos
Zygourakis
*Rice University*

## 26.1 Introduction

Recent advances in molecular biology have provided us with powerful experimental tools for studying individual processes at the molecular and cellular levels. However, the complexity of biological behavior is the result of dynamic interactions occurring not only among the various components of a cell, but also among the populations of cells that form human tissues. As shown schematically in Figure 26.1, biological processes and interactions occur across a $10^9$ range of spatial scales: from the nanometer scale at the molecular level to the meter scale at the human tissue and organ system level. The time scales encountered are even broader. Molecular interactions occur at the $10^{-9}$ or $10^{-6}$ scale, whereas human life spans a period of $10^9$ s. An impressive array of experimental techniques has been developed to acquire data across the spectrum of spatial scales: from protein biochemistry and other proteomic techniques at the molecular level, to sophisticated microscopy techniques at the cell level and magnetic resonance imaging or computed tomography diagnostic imaging at the human level.

However, our ability to integrate our rapidly expanding knowledge base across these spatial and time scales is still limited [1]. It is not always clear, for example, how to use information about specific protein interactions or other intracellular processes to guide the development of bioartificial tissues. This has been one of the main challenges of tissue engineering, a discipline that seeks to integrate the knowledge gained in biochemistry, biology, medical sciences, and engineering to develop bioartificial implants or

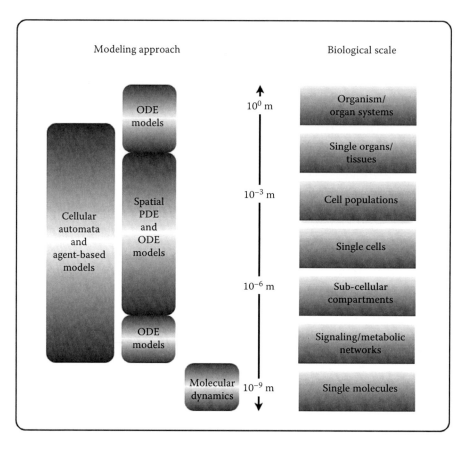

**FIGURE 26.1** Biological spatial scales and modeling approaches that may be used to describe processes that occur at each scale.

to induce tissue remodeling to replace, repair, or enhance the function of a particular tissue or organ [2–4]. One of the main approaches to the development of bioartificial implants and tissue remodeling involves the use of three-dimensional (3D) scaffolds made from suitable biomaterials. Scaffolds can be made either from natural proteins (like collagen gels) or from biodegradable polymers [5]. Besides serving as the structural component, the scaffolds provide the proper shape of the bioartificial construct and a 3D matrix for guided cell migration and proliferation [4]. Scaffolds may also be used to promote wound healing, a serious problem with patients suffering from many debilitating diseases [6].

Tissue growth in a 3D scaffold is a complex process that spans the entire spectrum of spatial and time scales described above. Both the structure and the growth rate of tissues are affected by a multitude of system parameters that range from the intracellular signaling mechanisms and molecules that regulate key cellular functions [7], to the complex cell–cell or cell–scaffold interactions that determine cell differentiation or sorting [8] and a large number of engineering system parameters that include the density and spatial distribution of seed cells, the culture conditions, and the configuration of the bioreactor [9–15]. All these factors act simultaneously to directly or indirectly modulate basic cell functions like adhesion, migration, proliferation, and differentiation.

System-based approaches and computational models can provide powerful frameworks for studying biocomplexity across multiple spatial and time scales. Even simple models can improve our understanding of fundamental biological processes by helping us interpret experimental data or by suggesting new ways of conducting experiments. More sophisticated multiscale and mechanistic models can be used to elucidate the biological mechanisms responsible for the observed behavior and assess the effect of modifying these mechanisms on system behavior. Thus, such models will help tissue engineers predict the dynamic response of cell populations to external stimuli, enabling them to quickly evaluate the potential effects of various system parameters on the structure, quality, and growth rates of bioartificial tissues.

## 26.2 Model Detail and Abstraction

To cultivate bioartificial tissues *in vitro*, the appropriate type(s) of cells may first be seeded into a highly porous scaffold made from natural materials such as fibrin, collagen, and chitosan [16–19], biocompatible synthetic polymers such as polylactic acid, polyglycolic acid, poly-lactic-glycolic acid, and poly(propylene fumarate-co-ethylene glycol) [20–25], or a combination of both [26–29]. The cell–scaffold construct is then cultured in bioreactors where appropriate conditions (temperature, pH, nutrient concentration, etc.) are maintained to promote cell migration, proliferation, and differentiation. There are many obstacles to overcome before clinically useful bioartificial tissues can be readily made in laboratories [30]. In particular, the identification of the optimal conditions for *in vitro* or *in vivo* cultivation of bioartificial tissues requires a better understanding of the complex interactions between fundamental intracellular processes and the constantly changing extracellular environment.

Therefore, a multiscale model for *in vitro* tissue cultivation must consider the following:

1. *Essential cellular processes*: Cells migrate in the scaffold by constantly forming and breaking bonds with the substrate and by actively altering their cytoskeleton. They also go through a cell cycle that involves growth, DNA duplication, division, and apoptosis.
2. *Interactions between cells and extracellular environment*: Key cellular processes (like migration, proliferation, apoptosis, or necrosis) are regulated by the extracellular concentrations of nutrients or growth factors (GFs). In addition, cells may receive signals from neighboring cells (through gap junctions or active binding), form distant cells (via diffusion of soluble agents), or from the substrate.
3. *Cell population heterogeneity*: Even isogenic populations exhibit significant phenotype heterogeneity, like differences in migration speed or division time. The heterogeneity of a population is enhanced by the presence of multiple phenotypes, cell differentiation, and mass transport limitations that affect the extracellular concentrations of molecules that regulate intracellular functions.
4. *Effects of experimental protocol*: By altering the initial and boundary conditions of the mathematical problems, different experimental protocols (e.g., different cell seeding patterns, culture conditions, or bioreactor configurations) can have a strong influence on the structure and function of the final construct. Thus, the multiscale model must be flexible enough to handle such differences.
5. *Emergent behavior*: The multiscale model must be able to predict self-assembly of cells in structures that lead to tissues with desired function.

## 26.3 Cell Proliferation and Migration

Cell proliferation is central to tissue-regeneration and wound-healing processes. Rigorous mathematical models have been developed to describe the cellular rhythms generated by complex interactions among genes, proteins, and metabolites [31–34]. Such detailed cell cycle models, however, have not been yet incorporated into multiscale tissue growth models. To simplify things, multiscale models usually assume either that measurements of cell proliferation rates are available for the conditions of interest, or that proliferation is regulated according to a known function by the extracellular concentration of a key nutrient of GF [35].

Cell migration is another essential part of tissue regeneration and wound healing. The movement of a mammalian cell on a substrate requires at least three structural elements: an extracellular matrix (ECM) ligand on the substrate, its cell surface receptor, and the intracellular cytoskeleton [36]. The receptors that play key roles for cell movement belong to a large family of transmembrane proteins called *integrins* [37].

Migration is a cyclic process consisting of four steps that are regulated by the binding of ECM ligands to the extracellular domains of the integrins and by soluble polypeptide factors [38–40]. Elegant mathematical models have been developed to relate cell migration speed to surface adhesiveness [41] and asymmetry in bond affinity defined by differences in the dissociation rate constants between the front and the rear of the migrating cell [42,43]. Many multiscale models, however, account for the influence of cell migration on tissue development by assuming that the migration speed has been measured for the specific cell lines and substrates considered [35,44]. Migration speeds can be measured by several well-established two-dimensional (2D) and 3D assays [45–51].

## 26.4 Cell Population Dynamics and Mass Transport

It is known for a long time that cell population dynamics play an important role in tissue development. For example, it has been demonstrated experimentally and computationally [44,52] that the speed and persistence of cell locomotion modulate the rates of tissue regeneration by overcoming the adverse effects of contact inhibition, a process that characterizes the proliferation of anchorage-dependent mammalian cells cultured either on flat surfaces or 3D scaffolds [53–62]. Cheng et al. [44] and Lee et al. [52] based their 2D and 3D models on cellular automata (CA) [63,64] and also found that the magnitude of the observed effects strongly depend on the spatial distribution of seed cells and the geometry of the scaffold, a conclusion that has significant implications for the design of experiments that test the efficacy of biomimetical surface modifications designed to enhance cell migration speeds [65–71].

However, tissue growth is also affected by the availability of nutrients and GFs. As cells proliferate in the scaffold interior, the total demand for nutrients and GFs increases and may outstrip the ability of the system to transport these compounds from the culture media to the scaffold interior. Such mass transport limitations decrease the availability of nutrients and GFs in the scaffold and limit the viable size of bioartificial constructs. Several studies have shown that the formation of engineered tissues in bioreactors was limited to a thin peripheral layer (less than a few hundred microns deep) surrounding a relatively cell-free scaffold interior [10,12,72,73]. Mass transport limitations become even more severe for tissues that normally have high metabolic demands. Only very thin peripheral layers ranging from 50 to 180 μm have been reported for engineered cardiac tissues when passive diffusion was the only mass transport mode inside the scaffolds [72]. Similar transport limitations appear during the wound healing of corneal epithelium, a process that is modulated by the local concentration of the epidermal growth factor and the cell density [74–76].

## 26.5 Continuous, Discrete, and Hybrid Models for Tissue Growth

Over the past 40 years, numerous modeling studies have focused on the cellular slime mold *Dictyostelium discoideum*. This is because *D. discoideum* provides an experimentally accessible and relatively simple system for studying key developmental processes like chemotaxis, cell sorting, and complex pattern formation. Early studies adopted continuous models [77–80]. More recent studies used elegant hybrid approaches that combined CA models and partial differential equations to model 2D and 3D problems involving aggregation and self-organization of *D. discoideum* [81–84].

The cellular Potts model (CPM) is another well-known computational approach for modeling of biological systems [85]. An extension of the classical Ising model [86], the CPM model was developed to describe the sorting of an aggregate of cells due to their different adhesivities to a surface. The original model describes cells as a connected set of lattice sites and updates the lattice one site at a time by minimizing a Hamiltonian function that describes the effective energy of the system [85,87]. The CPM model has evolved into a 3D simulation framework that has been used to model development of multicellular organisms, tumor growth, and blood vessel formation [88–92]. An open-source software package implementing this framework for study cellular behavior is freely available (http://www.com-pucell3d.org/).

In an effort to address the specific issues encountered in tissue engineering, several research groups have focused on the development of theoretical models that can predict the steady-state distribution of key nutrients (such as oxygen or glucose) inside bioartificial tissues (see, e.g., [93–98]). Although these modeling studies provide valuable insights into the interplay between transport and nutrient consumption in tissues, they cannot elucidate the dynamics of tissue development in the 3D scaffolds or describe emergent behavior where cells self-assemble in structures that lead to tissues with desired function.

Galban and Locke [99] proposed a dynamic model for the *in vitro* growth of cartilage tissues based on species continuity equations and the volume-averaging method. The volume-averaging method, how-ever, removes the spatial dependence from the diffusion-reaction equations for nutrients, thus ignor-ing the spatial heterogeneity that is a very important characteristic of bioartificial tissue growth. Also, proliferation is the only cellular function considered in their model while it has been shown that low-passage primary chondrocytes not only migrate in some biomaterial scaffolds, but also form aggregates from cell–cell collisions [100–103]. Chung et al. [104] developed a similar volume-averaging model with cell migration added as another important cellular function. By describing cell migration as a diffusion-like process, this model requires the estimation of the key motility parameter, the cell "diffusion" coef-ficient, from population measurements and the solution of an inverse problem for each system studied. Moreover, this approach does not allow us to study how tissue growth is affected by migration speed and persistence, cell collision frequency and other important single-cell properties that can be measured directly [44]. Similar limitations can be found in another continuous modeling approach [105].

A better alternative for tissue growth modeling is the hybrid discrete-continuous approach. Hybrid discrete-continuous models employ a discrete algorithm to simulate the dynamics of a cell population, while processes such as diffusion and consumption of GFs or nutrients are described with a continuous, deterministic component usually based on partial differential equations.

In addition to the previously mentioned models describing aggregation and self-organization of *D. discoideum* [81–84], hybrid approaches have been used to model transient 2D and 3D problems involv-ing the interactions between ECM and fibroblasts [106] and tumor development. Chaplain et al. [107–111] used 2D and 3D models to describe angiogenesis and tumor growth, Patel et al. [112] used a 2D model to study acidosis, whereas Jiang et al. [113] employed a 3D model to investigate avascular tumor growth. The CA component of these models only considered proliferation, adhesion, and viability of individual cells. The migration of individual tumor cells was incorporated in 2D models developed by Anderson et al. [111,114,115] to study tumor morphology and phenotypic evolution. Several other inves-tigators have also used multiscale hybrid approaches with *agent-based models* to describe the dynamics of tumor growth in various cancers [116–119].

## 26.6 A Modeling Framework for *In Vitro* Tissue Cultivation

This section will outline the development of a hybrid and multiscale modeling framework that addresses the problems encountered during *in vitro* cultivation of tissue constructs in bioreactors [35,44,120]. It is well known that tissue growth in biomimetic scaffolds is strongly influenced by the dynamics and the heterogeneity of cell populations. A significant source of heterogeneity is the depletion of nutrients and GFs due to transport limitations (see, e.g., [9,10,15]). Cells slow down, stop dividing, or even die when the concentrations of key nutrients and GFs drop below certain levels in the scaffold interior. As a result, we have not yet been able to grow *in vitro* tissue samples thicker than a few millimeters for metabolically active cells.

To address some of these issues, Cheng et al. [35,44,120] followed a hybrid approach that uses a dis-crete, stochastic model based on CA to describe the population dynamics of migrating, interacting, and proliferating cells. The diffusion and consumption of a key nutrient or GF can be modeled by a partial differential equation (PDE) (see, e.g., Equation 26.1 or 26.4 below) subject to boundary conditions appropriate for the bioreactor used in each case. This PDE is solved numerically and the computed concentration profiles are fed to receptor-mediated binding/trafficking models or simplified kinetic expressions to modulate cell proliferation rates and migration speeds (see also [52]). To meet the significant computational requirements of this model, its algorithms have been parallelized for execution on distributed-memory multicomputers [120]. Simulations on grids corresponding to tissue constructs with sizes as large as $6 \times 6 \times 6$ mm and spatial resolution of 20 μm have been run on parallel clusters [120].

# 26.7 Components of the Hybrid Multiscale Model

## 26.7.1 Discrete Model for Cell Population Dynamics

The CA model assumes that the scaffold provides an isotropic structure that allows cells to move freely in all directions while going through their division cycles. It is also assumed that the degradation of scaffold material does not affect tissue growth. The behavior of individual cells and cell–cell interaction are then simulated with a cellular automaton consisting of a 3D array with cubic computational sites [44,52,63,64]. Every site is "connected" to six neighbors (von Neumann neighborhood) and its state evolves at discrete time steps through interactions with the neighbors [44,120]. These interactions are governed by a set of "rules" that simulate cell migration and proliferation, as well as cell–cell collisions. Other cellular activities such as differentiation is currently not considered, but can be easily incorporated when necessary.

In accordance with experimental observations, the model assumes that cells migrate by executing persistent random walks [49,121,122] as they go through their division cycle. In a uniform environment, the direction after each turn is randomly selected. However, cell movement can be biased to simulate chemotaxis or haptotaxis. If the cell does not collide with another cell, this persistent random movement continues until the end of the cell's current division cycle upon which the cell stops and divides into two daughter cells. Cell division is asynchronous and the distribution of cell division time $t_d$ is a measurable characteristic of each cell phenotype.

Even though this CA model does not employ any of the previously presented mathematical descriptions of cell cycle or adhesion/migration, it must be noted that migration speeds, persistence of movement, and division times can be measured directly through time-lapse observation of cell migration [123–125]. In addition to the average values, these time-lapse techniques measure the distributions of these important parameters and, thus, provide a measure of the heterogeneity of the specific cell populations.

## 26.7.2 Continuous Model for Mass Transport Dynamics

Several experimental studies have shown that concentration gradients of glucose or oxygen, two key nutrients for cellular functions, exist in bioartificial scaffolds and affect tissue growth [93,126,127]. To demonstrate the importance of mass transport dynamics, Cheng et al. [35] assumed that glucose is the single limiting nutrient. However, more than one nutrient can be modeled by introducing additional partial differential equations.

As cells are much smaller than the size of the scaffold, we can employ a continuous formulation to describe nutrient or GF transport in the scaffold/tissue scale. In the presence of forced convection (i.e., unidirectional fluid flow through the scaffold or perfusion [9]), the spatiotemporal evolution of the extracellular concentration $C(x,y,z,t)$ can be computed by solving a convection-diffusion-reaction problem described by the following partial differential equation:

$$\frac{\partial C}{\partial t} + v_z \frac{\partial C}{\partial z} = \frac{\partial}{\partial x}\left(D_e \frac{\partial C}{\partial x}\right) + \frac{\partial}{\partial y}\left(D_e \frac{\partial C}{\partial y}\right) + \frac{\partial}{\partial z}\left(D_e \frac{\partial C}{\partial z}\right) - R(\rho_{cell}, C) + S(\rho_{cell}, C) + D(C) \quad \text{in } \Omega \quad (26.1)$$

where $\Omega$ denotes the scaffold, $v_z$ is the velocity of the media perfusing the scaffold in one direction, $D_e$ is the effective diffusion coefficient of the molecule that depends on the local cell density $\rho_{cell}$ [35], $R(\rho_{cell}, C)$ is the cell uptake (consumption) rate, $S(\rho_{cell}, C)$ is the rate at which cells secrete the molecule, and $D(C)$ is the rate of natural degradation.

The continuous PDE of Equation 26.1 must be coupled and solved together with the CA model that treats cells as discrete entities. Thus, the migrating and proliferating cells must be considered as moving sinks (and/or sources) for the convection-diffusion-reaction problem and the cell density $\rho_{cell}$ is actually a discontinuous function that is nonzero only in lattice sites occupied by cells:

$$\rho_{cell} = \gamma(x, y, z, t)\rho_{cell}^*$$

where $\rho_{cell}^*$ is the cell density at confluence and

$$\gamma(x, y, z, t) = \begin{cases} 1 & \text{if there is a cell at } (x, y, z) \text{ at time } t \\ 0 & \text{if there is no cell at } (x, y, z) \text{ at time } t \end{cases}$$

To integrate Equation 26.1, we must define boundary conditions consistent with the experimental protocol used for *in vitro* tissue cultivation. The following boundary condition can be adapted to handle most bioreactor configurations and construct positioning [35]:

$$D_e \frac{\partial C}{\partial n} = k_g (C_b - C) \quad \text{on } \partial\Omega \quad (26.2)$$

where $\partial\Omega$ refers to the external surface of the scaffold, $\partial C/\partial n$ denotes the derivative with respect to the normal to the scaffold surface, $k_g$ is the mass transfer coefficient at the media-scaffold interface, and $C_b$ is the bulk nutrient concentration in culture media. Finally, we must know the initial concentration profile $C_0(x, y, z)$ in the scaffold:

$$C(x, y, z, 0) = C_0(x, y, z) \quad (26.3)$$

where $C_0(x, y, z)$ is the known initial concentration profile.

Depending on the actual problem, Equation 26.1 may be simplified by dropping some of the terms. The convection term may be ignored, for example, if the scaffold is not perfused. If Equation 26.1 describes the mass balance of a small molecule like glucose that can pass directly across the cell membrane, the kinetics of uptake and metabolism will generally lead to a Michaelis–Menten-type dependence for the cell uptake rate $R(\rho_{cell}, C)$ [128] and the secretion term $S(\rho_{cell}, C)$ will be zero since the cells do not produce glucose. In the case of glucose, therefore, the following diffusion-reaction PDE is obtained:

$$\frac{\partial C}{\partial t} = \frac{\partial}{\partial x}\left(D_e \frac{\partial C}{\partial x}\right) + \frac{\partial}{\partial y}\left(D_e \frac{\partial C}{\partial y}\right) + \frac{\partial}{\partial z}\left(D_e \frac{\partial C}{\partial z}\right) - \rho_{cell} \frac{V_{max} \cdot C}{K_m + C} \quad (26.4)$$

where $V_{\max}$ is the maximum cell-uptake rate, $K_m$ is the saturation constant and we have also assumed that the natural degradation term $D(C)$ is ignored because it is insignificant compared to diffusion and cell-uptake. Both $V_{\max}$ and $K_m$ can be measured experimentally [129,130].

By transforming Equation 26.4 and its boundary conditions into their dimensionless forms (see [35] for details), we arrive at one of the most powerful theoretical results of reaction engineering [131]. Namely, that we can estimate the extent of mass transport limitations (or, equivalently, the severity of nutrient depletion in the scaffold) by just calculating the magnitude of two dimensionless numbers generated in the nondimensionalization process:

1. Thiele modulus

$$\phi = L\sqrt{\frac{\rho_{cell}^* V_{\max}}{D_e^* C_b}}$$

This dimensionless number indicates the relative magnitude of the nutrient uptake rate over the nutrient diffusion rate. For this definition, $L$ is the characteristic length of the scaffold [35,131], $D_e^*$ is the effective diffusion coefficient of the molecule in the _tissue-filled_ scaffold, and $C_b$ is a reference concentration of the molecule (depends on problem formulation).

2. Biot number

$$Bi = \frac{k_g L}{D_e^*}$$

This dimensionless number indicates the relative magnitude of the external nutrient transport rate (from the media to the surface of the scaffold) over the nutrient diffusion rate in the interior of the scaffold. Again, $L$ is the characteristic length of the scaffold, $D_e^*$ is the effective diffusion coefficient of the molecule in the _tissue-filled_ scaffold, and $k_g$ is the external mass transfer coefficient. This coefficient is strongly influenced by the shape of the scaffold, the stirring or flow of the media around the scaffold, etc.

An additional dimensionless number becomes important in the case of perfusion bioreactors [9,10,12]:

3. Peclet number

$$Pe_z = \frac{v_z L}{D_e^*}$$

The dimensionless Peclet number indicates the relative magnitude of mass transfer rate due to convection (i.e., flow of media through the scaffold) over the diffusion rate in the interior of the scaffold. Again, $L$ is the characteristic length of the scaffold, $D_e^*$ is the effective diffusion coefficient of the molecule in the _tissue-filled_ scaffold, and $v_z$ is the flow velocity.

## 26.7.3 Coupling of Mass Transport Dynamics and Cellular Functions

Several experimental studies have established that extracellular glucose concentration modulates both cell division times and migration speeds [132–134]. Cheng et al. [35] used a Monod-type expression to describe the dependence of cell-doubling rates on extracellular nutrient concentration:

$$r_g = \frac{r_{g,\max} C}{K + C}$$

Values for the maximum cell-doubling rate $r_{g,\max}$ and the saturation constant $K$ can be measured experimentally [129,135,136].

The energy required to maintain cell migration is provided from either glycolysis or oxidative phosphorylation. Kouvroukoglou et al. [134] reported that the speed of cell migration decreased significantly when cells were transferred from glucose-containing to glucose-free media. Accordingly, Cheng et al. assumed that the cell migration speed $S$ is modulated by the extracellular glucose concentration according to the following rules:

$$\begin{cases} \text{If } C \leq C_{\text{low}}, & S = 0 \\ \text{If } C_{\text{low}} < C < C^{\text{high}}, & S = S_{\max}\left[\dfrac{C - C_{\text{low}}}{C^{\text{high}} - C_{\text{low}}}\right] \\ \text{If } C \geq C^{\text{high}} & S = S_{\max} \end{cases}$$

## 26.7.4 Experimental Protocols: Cell Seeding and Bioreactor Configuration

The configuration of the tissue engineering bioreactor and the culturing conditions can vary widely. One example is the "well-stirred bioreactor" where several scaffolds seeded with cells are fixed on needles and cultured in continuously stirred media. This is the so-called "dynamic tissue culture" method that has been shown to promote both cell proliferation and ECM component deposition in bioartificial tissues [137–139]. However, the aforementioned multiscale model can handle other reactor configurations by appropriately changing the boundary condition [2] of the diffusion-reaction problem.

This model also allows the user to tailor the spatial distributions of seed cells (i.e., the initial conditions of the simulations) so that they match actual experimental protocols. A dynamic seeding method has been developed in which mixing or stirring was employed to promote the penetration of cells into the scaffold interior and achieve a "uniform" initial distribution of cells [11,140]. Other investigators, however, seeded the cells by simply immersing an empty scaffold into a static cell solution for a certain period of time. As a result, the seed cells were placed in a thin layer next to the scaffold surface, resulting in what is referred to as "surface" seeding mode. This is likely the case when the scaffold is big or its pore structure is too tortuous for cells to penetrate deeply. These and other seeding modes can be easily specified as initial conditions for the simulations. The same is true for the seeding densities that ranged from 0.37% to 1.33% and the various combinations of cell type and scaffold materials used in experimental studies [141–147].

# 26.8 Results and Discussion

## 26.8.1 Internal and External Mass Transport Modulates Tissue Growth and Structure

The diffusion-reaction problem in a scaffold that progressively fills with cells is mathematically more challenging than the classical isothermal diffusion-reaction problem that has been extensively studied in the engineering literature [131]. Similar to the active sites in a catalyst particle, cells act as "sinks" for the nutrient that is transported into the scaffold. In the case of a cellularized scaffold, however, these "sinks" move constantly, multiply and may even die by apoptosis or necrosis. At first, this problem may seem intractable because of the complex interplay between mass transport and cell population dynamics induced by the temporal and spatial variations of the cell distribution function $\gamma$.

However, the dimensionless numbers defined in the previous section allow us to quickly make qualitative predictions about the relative effect of system parameters on the severity of transport limitations that may appear in a scaffold and the appearance or size of necrotic zones in the scaffold interior [11,12,72,148,149]. This is a testament to the power of the mathematical theory on diffusion and reaction that was introduced more than 50 years ago and has led to significant advances in reaction engineering [131]. For example, the Thiele modulus allows us to predict the conditions that will cause severe nutrient transport limitations inside the scaffold. These are

- Large scaffold (tissue) size $L$;
- High final cell density $\rho^*_{cell}$ and high values of the nutrient consumption rate $V_{max}$;
- Low nutrient diffusivity $D_{e,s}$; and
- Low nutrient concentration on the scaffold surface $C_b$.

Moreover, we can now predict that to overcome a doubling of the characteristic length $L$ (which is linked to the thickness of the construct) we must be able to decrease by a factor of four the value of the ratio $(\rho^*_{cell} V_{max}/D^*_e C_b)$, which may or may not be possible.

Figure 26.2 shows how increasing values of the Thiele modulus lead to the appearance and growth of a necrotic zone in the scaffold interior as the values of the Thiele modulus progressively increase over two orders of magnitude from $\phi = 1.15$ to 115. For small values of the Thiele modulus, the nutrient uptake rate and the mass transport rate are closely matched. As a result, the nutrient quickly diffuses into the scaffold and allows the cells to proliferate and reach confluence. As $\phi$ increases, the nutrient transport rate becomes significantly slower than the nutrient uptake rate and concentration gradients develop in the scaffold interior, decreasing the availability of nutrient [35]. At very high values of the Thiele modulus, diffusion can no longer meet the cell uptake requirements and very sharp nutrient concentration gradients appear soon after the culture begins. As a result, only a thin layer of cells is able to form just below the surface of the scaffold [35]. This enhances even more the "bottleneck effect" of diffusional limitations and increases the size of the necrotic zone. As seen in Figure 26.2, simulations predict that less than 40% of the scaffold is filled with cells when $\phi = 115$. Simulations with very high $\phi$ values predict that the dense peripheral tissue layer formed just below the surface of the scaffold has a thickness of about 100 μm [35]. This is similar to what has been observed when bioartificial tissues with high metabolic demand (e.g., cardiac tissues) are cultured in bioreactors [11,12,72,148,149].

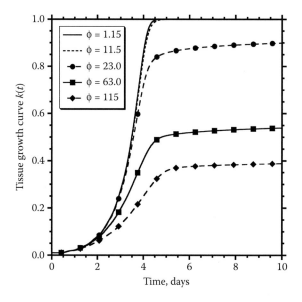

**FIGURE 26.2** Effect of the Thiele modulus $\phi = L\sqrt{(\rho^*_{cell} V_{max}/D_{e,t} C_b)}$ on tissue growth rates. Multiple combinations of parameter values can be used to produce the values of $\phi$ listed in the legend. See Reference 35 for full list of parameter values used. (Adapted from Cheng, G., P. Markenscoff, and K. Zygourakis. 2009. _Biophys J_ 97:401–414.)

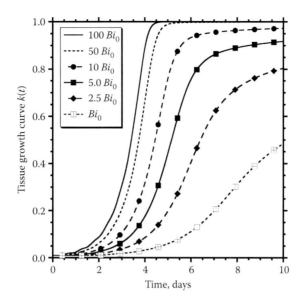

**FIGURE 26.3** Effect of the Biot number $Bi = (k_g L/D_e')$ on tissue growth rates. Here, the base case value is $Bi_0 = 7.41 \times 10^{-4}$ and the mass transfer coefficient $k_g$ is varied to obtain the other values of Bi listed in the legend. See Reference 35 for full list of parameter values. (Adapted from Cheng, G., P. Markenscoff, and K. Zygourakis. 2009. *Biophys J* 97:401–414.)

For the simulations discussed in this section, Cheng et al. [35] assumed that there was no cell death due to necrosis when the nutrient level drops to low values. Cells would just stop migrating and dividing when the extracellular concentration of the nutrient dropped to near-zero levels. The differential effects of cell death due to necrosis will be discussed in a subsequent section.

When the tissue culture medium in the bioreactor is vigorously stirred, external mass transport rates (from the medium to the scaffold surface) are fast and one can safely assume that the concentration of the nutrient on the surface of the scaffold is equal to its concentration in the bulk of the medium. The Dirichlet boundary conditions can then be used to solve Equation 26.4. When the medium is not vigorously stirred, however, external mass transport rates may become comparable to internal transport rates. This effect can be explored by varying the dimensionless Biot number Bi, which (as mentioned earlier) provides a measure of the relative magnitude of the external and internal resistances to mass transport. Figure 26.3 shows the effect of Bi on tissue growth. Large values of the Biot number (achieved, for example, by vigorously stirring the tissue culture medium) clearly promote tissue growth, but this beneficial effect gradually diminishes.

## 26.8.2 Differential Effects of Migration Speeds and Initial Conditions

Simulations of tissue growth in the presence or absence of transport limitations revealed a complicated interplay between cell migration speeds and the initial distributions of seed cells in the scaffold. When seed cells were uniformly distributed in the scaffold and in the absence of transport limitations, simulations showed that increasing migration speeds initially enhanced tissue growth rates. When migration speeds were raised above 2 μm/h, however, the beneficial effect of enhanced migration diminished rapidly and disappeared completely for migration speeds above 10 μm/h. Simulations with the "wound" seeding mode, however, predicted that the wound healing times would continue to decrease as migration speeds on the biomaterial filling the wound increased to 60 μm/h [44]. This conclusion has significant implications for the design of experiments that seek to test the efficacy of biomimetic surface modifications designed to enhance cell migration speeds. To study how surface modifications and the resulting changes of migration speeds affect tissue growth rates, assays based on the "wound"-seeding

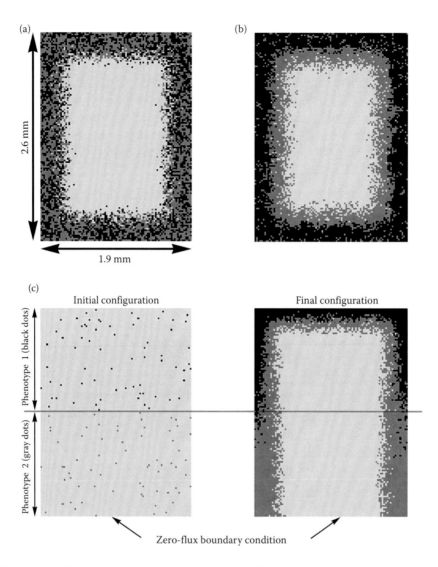

**FIGURE 26.4** (a and b) Cross-sections through the middle of a 3D scaffold showing the final spatial distributions of cells belonging to two phenotypes (black and dark gray dots). Both simulations started by uniformly distributing throughout the scaffold an equal number of cells from the two phenotypes. Constant concentration (Dirichlet) boundary conditions were applied to all the external surfaces. See the text for further details and an explanation of the differences in the final structures of the constructs. (c) This simulation started by uniformly distributing cells of phenotype 1 (black dots) in the top half of the scaffold and cells of phenotype 2 (dark gray dots) in the bottom half of the scaffold. The two cell phenotypes had the same characteristics as in the simulation of (b). Phenotypic differences of the two cell populations, the segregated initial distribution of seed cells, and the zero-flux boundary condition applied to the bottom of the scaffold influenced the segregated organization of the final structure of the construct. All three simulations were carried out in a domain shaped like a rectangular prism corresponding to a scaffold with dimensions 1.9 mm × 1.9 mm × 2.6 mm and the cross-sections were taken through the middle of the scaffold and parallel to the two larger sides.

mode [150] must be adopted. Experiments that begin by uniformly distributing seed cells in modified scaffolds may not be sensitive enough to elucidate these effects.

Cell migration was also shown to be very important for tissue growth under conditions that lead to significant transport limitations both because enhanced migration (a) helps diminish contact inhibition effects and (b) increases the dispersion of the cells and alleviates a "bottleneck effect" that dense peripheral cell layers have on nutrient transport into the scaffold [35]. In fact, high cell migration speeds are more beneficial if cells are initially seeded close to the scaffold surface versus if they are uniformly distributed throughout the entire scaffold. The recent study by Cheng et al. [35] offers interesting insights on the interplay of cell population dynamics, the diffusion and uptake rates of nutrients (or GFs), and the spatial distribution of seed cells.

## 26.8.3 Cell Population Heterogeneity and Nutrient Limitations Lead to Emergent Behavior

The hybrid multiscale model of Cheng et al. [35] has been extended to model tissue growth from populations with two phenotypes exhibiting widely different motility or proliferation characteristics [151]. The extended model can handle differential cell death by nutrient depletion (necrosis) when the nutrient extracellular concentration drops below the critical levels $C_1^*$ for cells of phenotype 1 and $C_2^*$ for cells of phenotype 2. When the two cell phenotypes consume nutrient at the same rate and have equal critical nutrient concentrations for cell necrosis ($C_2^* = C_1^*$), a simulation with a uniform distribution of seed cells leads to a tissue with the structure shown in Figure 26.4a. Nutrient depletion leads to the formation of a necrotic zone in the middle of the scaffold. The cell layer, however, consists of almost equal fractions of layers belonging to the two phenotypes, even though the two phenotypes had widely different distributions of cell migration speeds. This simulation was carried out in a domain shaped like a rectangular prism corresponding to a scaffold with dimensions 1.9 mm × 1.9 mm × 2.6 mm and Dirichlet boundary conditions on all the external surfaces.

Emergent behavior is observed, however, when the two phenotypes exhibit different uptake rates ($V_{max,1} = 2V_{max,2}$), as well as different critical nutrient concentrations for cell necrosis ($C_1^* = 2 \cdot C_2^*$). Again, the simulation starts with a uniform distribution of seed cells. As their nutrient uptake rate is larger and they need higher nutrient concentrations to survive, cells of phenotype 1 rapidly migrate toward the external surfaces of the scaffold as nutrient gradients appear and form a dense peripheral layer. Phenotype 2 cells, in contrast, have a lower extracellular critical nutrient concentration. Some of them survive in the scaffold interior and then move slowly toward the exterior of the scaffold forming a second layer that contains exclusively cells of phenotype 2 (see Figure 26.4b). Simulations with surface-seeding modes and different boundary conditions (e.g., Neumann or zero flux condition on the bottom surface) lead to even more interesting structures (see Figure 26.4c).

Clearly, this multiscale model can predict self-assembly of heterogeneous cell populations into structures that mimic the stratified structure of several tissues. It is also important to note that self-assembly is not a result of some "programmed" behavior of the two cell phenotypes. The two cell subpopulations self-assemble in structures like those of Figures 26.4b and 26.4c as a result of the interplay between mass transport dynamics (nutrient depletion) and differential effects of essential cellular functions (different nutrient uptake rates and resistance to necrosis).

# References

1. Hunter, P. J., E. J. Crampin, and P. M. F. Nielsen. 2008. Bioinformatics, multiscale modeling and the IUPS Physiome Project. *Brief Bionform* 9:333–343.
2. Langer, R. and J. P. Vacanti. 1993. Tissue engineering. *Science* 260:920–926.
3. Mooney, D. J. and A. G. Mikos. 1999. Growing new organs. *Sci Am* 280:60–65.
4. Nerem, R. M. and A. Sambanis. 1995. Tissue engineering: From biology to biological substitutes. *Tissue Eng* 1:3–13.

5. Pachence, J. M. and J. Kohn. 1997. Biodegradable polymers for tissue engineering. In *Principles of Tissue Engineering*. R. P. Lanza, R. L. Langer, and E. W. L. Chick, eds. Academic Press, San Diego, CA.

6. Clark, R. A. F. 1997. Wound healing: Lessons for tissue engineering. In *Principles of Tissue Engineering*. R. P. Lanza, R. L. Langer, and W. L. Chick, eds. Academic Press, San Diego, CA.

7. Lauffenburger, D. A. and J. J. Linderman. 1993. *Receptors: Models for Binding Trafficking and Signaling*. Oxford University Press, New York, NY.

8. Palsson, B. O. and S. N. Bhatia. 2004. *Tissue Engineering*. Pearson Prentice Hall, Upper Saddle River, NJ.

9. Bancroft, G. N., V. I. Sikavitsas, and A. G. Mikos. 2003. Design of a flow perfusion bioreactor system for bone tissue-engineering applications. *Tissue Eng* 9:549–554.

10. Bancroft, G. N., V. I. Sikavitsas, J. van den Dolder, T. L. Sheffield, C. G. Ambrose, J. A. Jansen, and A. G. Mikos. 2002. Fluid flow increases mineralized matrix deposition in 3D perfusion culture of marrow stromal osteoblasts in a dose-dependent manner. *PNAS* 99:12600–12605.

11. Carrier, R. L., M. Papadaki, M. Rupnick, F. J. Schoen, N. Bursac, R. Langer, L. E. Freed, and G. Vunjak-Novakovic. 1999. Cardiac tissue engineering: Cell seeding, cultivation parameters, and tissue construct characterization. *Biotechnol Bioeng* 64:580–589.

12. Carrier, R. L., M. Rupnick, R. Langer, F. J. Schoen, L. E. Freed, and G. Vunjak-Novakovic. 2002. Perfusion improves tissue architecture of engineered cardiac muscle. *Tissue Eng* 8:175–188.

13. Radisic, M., L. Yang, J. Boublik, R. J. Cohen, R. Langer, L. E. Freed, and G. Vunjak-Novakovic. 2004. Medium perfusion enables engineering of compact and contractile cardiac tissue. *Am J Physiol Heart Circ Physiol* 286:H507–H516.

14. Ratcliffe, A. and L. E. Niklason. 2002. Bioreactors and bioprocessing for tissue engineering. *Ann N Y Acad Sci* 961:210–215.

15. Sikavitsas, V. I., G. N. Bancroft, and A. G. Mikos. 2002. Formation of three-dimensional cell/polymer constructs for bone tissue engineering in a spinner flask and a rotating wall vessel bioreactor. *J Biomed Mater Res* 62:136–148.

16. Dang, J. M. and K. W. Leong. 2006. Natural polymers for gene delivery and tissue engineering. *Adv Drug Deliv Rev* 58:487–499.

17. Eyrich, D., F. Brandl, B. Appel, H. Wiese, G. Maier, M. Wenzel, R. Staudenmaier, A. Goepferich, and T. Blunk. 2007. Long-term stable fibrin gels for cartilage engineering. *Biomaterials* 28:55–65.

18. Helm, C. L., A. Zisch, and M. A. Swartz. 2007. Engineered blood and lymphatic capillaries in 3-D VEGF-fibrin-collagen matrices with interstitial flow. *Biotechnol Bioeng* 96:167–176.

19. Wu, X., L. Black, G. Santacana-Laffitte, and C. W. Patrick, Jr. 2006. Preparation and assessment of glutaraldehyde-crosslinked collagen-chitosan hydrogels for adipose tissue engineering. *J Biomed Mater Res A* 81:59–65.

20. Cao, D., W. Liu, X. Wei, F. Xu, L. Cui, and Y. Cao. 2006. *In vitro* tendon engineering with avian tenocytes and polyglycolic acids: A preliminary report. *Tissue Eng* 12:1369–1377.

21. Fisher, J. P., S. Jo, A. G. Mikos, and A. H. Reddi. 2004. Thermoreversible hydrogel scaffolds for articular cartilage engineering. *J Biomed Mater Res* 71A:268–274.

22. Georgiou, G., L. Mathieu, D. P. Pioletti, P. E. Bourban, J. A. Manson, J. C. Knowles, and S. N. Nazhat. 2006. Polylactic acid-phosphate glass composite foams as scaffolds for bone tissue engineering. *J Biomed Mater Res B Appl Biomater* 80:322–331.

23. Sedrakyan, S., Z. Y. Zhou, L. Perin, K. Leach, D. Mooney, and T. H. Kim. 2006. Tissue engineering of a small hand phalanx with a porously casted polylactic acid-polyglycolic acid copolymer. *Tissue Eng* 12:2675–2683.

24. Shin, H., J. S. Temenoff, G. C. Bowden, K. Zygourakis, M. C. Farach-Carson, M. J. Yaszemski, and A. G. Mikos. 2005. Osteogenic differentiation of rat bone marrow stromal cells cultured on Arg–Gly–Asp modified hydrogels without dexamethasone and β-glycerol phosphate. *Biomaterials* 26:3645–3654.

25. Xin, X., M. Hussain, and J. J. Mao. 2007. Continuing differentiation of human mesenchymal stem cells and induced chondrogenic and osteogenic lineages in electrospun PLGA nanofiber scaffold. *Biomaterials* 28:316–325.

26. Fujita, M., Y. Kinoshita, E. Sato, H. Maeda, S. Ozono, H. Negishi, T. Kawase, Y. Hiraoka, T. Takamoto, Y. Tabata, and Y. Kameyama. 2005. Proliferation and differentiation of rat bone marrow stromal cells on poly(glycolic acid)-collagen sponge. *Tissue Eng* 11:1346–1355.

27. Hiraoka, Y., Y. Kimura, H. Ueda, and Y. Tabata. 2003. Fabrication and biocompatibility of collagen sponge reinforced with poly(glycolic acid) fiber. *Tissue Eng* 9:1101–1112.

28. Hosseinkhani, H., M. Hosseinkhani, F. Tian, H. Kobayashi, and Y. Tabata. 2007. Bone regeneration on a collagen sponge self-assembled peptide-amphiphile nanofiber hybrid scaffold. *Tissue Eng* 13:11–19.

29. Ito, T., T. Nakamura, T. Takagi, T. Toba, A. Hagiwara, H. Yamagishi, and Y. Shimizu. 2003. Biodegradation of polyglycolic acid-collagen composite tubes for nerve guide in the peritoneal cavity. *ASAIO J* 49:417–421.

30. McIntire, L. V. 2002. World technology panel report on tissue engineering. *Ann Biomed Eng* 30: 1216–1220.

31. Csikasz-Nagy, A., O. Kapuy, A. Toth, C. Pal, L. J. Jensen, F. Uhlmann, J. J. Tyson, and B. Novak. 2009. Cell cycle regulation by feed-forward loops coupling transcription and phosphorylation. *Mol Syst Biol* 5:236.

32. Kapuy, O., E. He, S. Lopez-Aviles, F. Uhlmann, J. J. Tyson, and B. Novak. 2009. System-level feedbacks control cell cycle progression. *FEBS Lett* 583:3992–3998.

33. Novak, B. and J. J. Tyson. 2008. Design principles of biochemical oscillators. *Nat Rev Mol Cell Biol* 9:981–991.

34. Tyson, J. J. and B. Novak. 2008. Temporal organization of the cell cycle. *Curr Biol* 18:R759–R768.

35. Cheng, G., P. Markenscoff, and K. Zygourakis. 2009. A 3D Hybrid model for tissue growth: The interplay between cell population and mass transport dynamics. *Biophys J* 97:401–414.

36. Lackie, J. M. 1986. *Cell Movement and Cell Behaviour*. Allen and Unwin, London.

37. Hynes, R. O. 1987. Integrins: A family of cell surface receptors. *Cell* 48:549–554.

38. Bell, G. I. 1978. Models for the specific adhesion of cells to cells. *Science* 200:618–627.

39. Lauffenburger, D. A. 1989. A simple model for the effects of receptor-mediated cell-substratuum adhesion on cellmigration. *Chem. Eng. Sci.* 44:1903–1914.

40. Lauffenburger, D. A. 1991. Models for receptor-mediated cell phenomena: adhesion and migration. *Annu Rev Biophys Biophys Chem* 20:387–414.

41. DiMilla, P. A., K. Barbee, and D. A. Lauffenburger. 1991. Mathematical model for the effects of adhesion and mechanics on cell migration speed. *Biophys J* 60:15–37.

42. Schmidt, C. E., A. F. Horwitz, D. A. Lauffenburger, and M. P. Sheetz. 1993. Integrin-cytoskeletal interactions in migrating fibroblasts are dynamic, asymmetric, and regulated. *J Cell Biol* 123:977–991.

43. Ward, M. D. and D. A. Hammer. 1993. A theoretical analysis for the effect of focal contact formation on cell-substrate attachment strength. *Biophys J* 64:936–959.

44. Cheng, G., B. B. Youssef, P. Markenscoff, and K. Zygourakis. 2006. Cell population dynamics modulate the rates of tissue growth processes. *Biophys J* 90:713–724.

45. Friedl, P. and E. B. Bröcker. 2004. Reconstructing leukocyte migration in 3D extracellular matrix by time-lapse videomicroscopy and computer-assisted tracking. *Methods Mol Biol* 239:77–90.

46. Kim, H. D., T. W. Guo, A. P. Wu, A. Wells, F. B. Gertler, and D. A. Lauffenburger. 2008. Epidermal growth factor-induced enhancement of glioblastoma cell migration in 3D arises from an intrinsic increase in speed but an extrinsic matrix- and proteolysis-dependent increase in persistence. *Mol Biol Cell* 19:4249–4259.

47. Niggemann, B., T. L. t. Drell, J. Joseph, C. Weidt, K. Lang, K. S. Zaenker, and F. Entschladen. 2004. Tumor cell locomotion: differential dynamics of spontaneous and induced migration in a 3D collagen matrix. *Exp Cell Res* 298:178–187.

48. Zaman, M. H., L. M. Trapani, A. L. Sieminski, D. Mackellar, H. Gong, R. D. Kamm, A. Wells, D. A. Lauffenburger, and P. Matsudaira. 2006. Migration of tumor cells in 3D matrices is governed by matrix stiffness along with cell-matrix adhesion and proteolysis. *Proc Natl Acad Sci U S A* 103:10889–10894.

49. Burgess, B. T., J. L. Myles, and R. B. Dickinson. 2000. Quantitative analysis of adhesion-mediated cell migration in three-dimensional gels of RGD-grafted collagen. *Ann Biomed Eng* 28:110–118.

50. Lee, Y. 1994. Computer-Assisted Analysis of Endothelial Cell Migration and Proliferation. Ph.D. Dissertation. Rice University.

51. Levine, M. D., Y. M. Youssef, P. B. Noble, and A. Boyarsky. 1980. The quantification of blood cell motion by a method of automatic digital picture processing. *IEEE Trans Pattern Anal Mach Intell* PAMI-2:444–450.

52. Lee, Y., S. Kouvroukoglou, L. V. McIntire, and K. Zygourakis. 1995. A cellular automaton model for the proliferation of migrating contact-inhibited cells. *Biophys J* 69:1284–1298.

53. Aoki, J., M. Umeda, K. Takio, K. Titani, H. Utsumi, M. Sasaki, and K. Inoue. 1991. Neural cell adhesion molecule mediates contact-dependent inhibition of growth of near-diploid mouse fibroblast cell line m5S/1M. *J Cell Biol* 115:1751–1761.

54. Folkman, J. and A. Moscona. 1978. Role of cell shape in growth control. *Nature* 273:345–349.

55. Gotlieb, A. I., W. Spector, M. K. K. Wong, and C. Lancey. 1984. *In vitro* reendothelialization: Microfilament bundle reorganization in migrating porcine endothelial cells. *Arteriosclerosis* 4:91–96.

56. Kandikonda, S., D. Oda, R. Niederman, and B. C. Sorkin. 1996. Cadherin-mediated adhesion is required for normal growth regulation of human gingival epithelial cells. *Cell Adhes Commun* 4:13–24.

57. Misago, N., S. Toda, H. Sugihara, H. Kohda, and Y. Narisawa. 1998. Proliferation and differentiation of organoid hair follicle cells co-cultured with fat cells in collagen gel matrix culture. *Br J Dermatol* 139:40–48.

58. Nehls, V., R. Herrmann, M. Hühnken, and A. Palmetshofer. 1998. Contact-dependent inhibition of angiogenesis by cardiac fibroblasts in three-dimensional fibrin gels in vitro: implications for microvascular network remodeling and coronary collateral formation. *Cell Tissue Res* 293:479–488.

59. Risbud, M. V., E. Karamuk, R. Moser, and J. Mayer. 2002. Hydrogel-coated textile scaffolds as three-dimensional growth support for human umbilical vein endothelial cells (HUVECs): possibilities as coculture system in liver tissue engineering. *Cell Transplant* 11:369–377.

60. Schmialek, P., A. Geyer, V. Miosga, M. Nu?ndel, and B. Zapf. 1977. The kinetics of contact inhibition in mammalian cells. *Cell Tissue Kinet* 10:195–202.

61. Shigematsu, M., H. Watanabe, and H. Sugihara. 1999. Proliferation and differentiation of unilocular fat cells in the bone marrow. *Cell Struct Funct* 24:89–100.

62. Takahashi, K. and K. Suzuki. 1996. Density-dependent inhibition of growth involves prevention of EGF receptor activation by E-cadherin-mediated cell-cell adhesion. *Exp Cell Res* 226:214–222.

63. Tchuente, M. 1987. Computation on automata networks. In *Automata Networks in Computer Science. Theory and Applications*. F. Fogelman-Soulie, Y. Robert, and M. Tchuente, eds. Princeton University Press, Princeton, NJ. pp. 101–129.

64. Toffoli, T. and N. Margolus. 1987. *Cellular Automata Machines. A New Environment for Modeling.* MIT Press, Cambridge, MA.

65. Barber, T. A., S. L. Golledge, D. G. Castner, and K. E. Healy. 2003. Peptide-modified p(AAm-co-EG/AAc) IPNs grafted to bulk titanium modulate osteoblast behavior in vitro. *J Biomed Mater Res* 64A:38–47.

66. Hench, L. L. and J. M. Polak. 2002. Third-generation biomedical materials. *Science* 295:1014–1017.

67. Liu, X. and P. X. Ma. 2004. Polymeric scaffolds for bone tissue engineering. *Ann Biomed Eng* 32:477–486.

68. Shin, H., S. Jo, and A. G. Mikos. 2003. Biomimetic materials for tissue engineering. *Biomaterials* 24:4353–4364.

69. Shin, H., K. Zygourakis, M. C. Farach-Carson, M. J. Yaszemski, and A. G. Mikos. 2004. Attachment, proliferation, and migration of marrow stromal osteoblasts cultured on biomimetic hydrogels modified with an osteopontin-derived peptide. *Biomaterials* 25:895–906.

70. Shin, H., K. Zygourakis, M. C. Farach-Carson, M. J. Yaszemski, and A. G. Mikos. 2004. Modulation of differentiation and mineralization of marrow stromal cells cultured on biomimetic hydrogels modified with Arg-Gly-Asp containing peptides. *J Biomed Mater Res* 69A:535–543.

71. Yang, X. B., R. S. Bhatnagar, S. Li, and R. O. Oreffo. 2004. Biomimetic collagen scaffolds for human bone cell growth and differentiation. *Tissue Eng* 10:1148–1159.

72. Bursac, N., M. Papadaki, R. J. Cohen, F. J. Schoen, S. R. Eisenberg, R. Carrier, G. Vunjak-Novakovic, and L. E. Freed. 1999. Cardiac muscle tissue engineering: toward an *in vitro* model for electrophysiological studies. *Am J Physiol* 277:H433–H444.

73. Kim, B. S., A. J. Putnam, T. J. Kulik, and D. J. Mooney. 1998. Optimizing seeding and culture methods to engineer smooth muscle tissue on biodegradable polymer matrices. *Biotechnol Bioeng* 57:46–54.

74. Dale, P. D., P. K. Maini, and J. A. Sherratt. 1994. Mathematical modeling of corneal epithelial wound healing. *Math Biosci* 124:127–147.

75. Gaffney, E. A., P. K. Maini, J. A. Sherratt, and S. Tuft. 1999. The mathematical modelling of cell kinetics in corneal epithelial wound healing. *J Theor Biol* 197:15–40.

76. Olsen, L., J. A. Sherratt, and P. K. Maini. 1995. A mechanochemical model for adult dermal wound contraction and the permanence of the contracted tissue displacement profile. *J Theor Biol* 177:113–128.

77. Keller, E. F. and L. A. Segel. 1971. Model for chemotaxis. *J Theor Biol* 30:225–234.

78. Levine, H. and W. Reynolds. 1991. Streaming instability of aggregating slime mold amoebae. *Phys Rev Lett* 66:2400–2403.

79. MacKay, S. A. 1978. Computer simulation of aggregation in *Dictyostelium discoideum. J Cell Sci* 33:1–16.

80. Parnas, H. and L. A. Segel. 1978. A computer simulation of pulsatile aggregation in *Dictyostelium discoideum. J Theor Biol* 71:185–207.

81. Hogeweg, P. 2000. Evolving mechanisms of morphogenesis: on the interplay between differential adhesion and cell differentiation. *J Theor Biol* 203:317–333.

82. Marée, A. F. and P. Hogeweg. 2001. How amoeboids self-organize into a fruiting body: Multicellular coordination in *Dictyostelium discoideum. Proc Natl Acad Sci USA* 98:3879–3883.

83. Palsson, E. and H. G. Othmer. 2000. A model for individual and collective cell movement in *Dictyostelium discoideum. Proc Natl Acad Sci USA* 97:10448–10453.

84. Savill, N. J. and P. Hogeweg. 1997. Modelling morphogenesis: From single cells to crawling slugs. *J Theor Biol* 184:229–235.

85. Graner, F. and J. A. Glazier. 1992. Simulation of biological cell sorting using a two-dimensional extended Potts model. *Phys Rev Lett* 69:2013–2016.

86. Onsager, L. 1944. Crystal statistics I A two-dimensional model with an order-disorder transition. *Phys Rev* 65:117–149.

87. Glazier, J. A. and F. Graner. 1993. Simulation of the differential adhesion driven rearrangement of biological cells. *Phys Rev E Stat Phys Plasmas Fluids Relat Interdisc Top* 47:2128–2154.

88. Merks, R. M. H., E. D. Perryn, A. Shirinifard, and J. A. Glazier. 2008. Contact-inhibited chemotaxis in De Novo and sprouting blood-vessel growth. *PLoS Comput Biol* 4[9]: Article Number: e1000163.

89. Cickovski, T., K. Aras, M. S. Alber, J. A. Izaguirre, M. Swat, J. A. Glazier, R. M. H. Merks, T. Glimm, H. G. E. Hentschel, and S. A. Newman. 2007. From genes to organisms via the cell—A problem-solving environment for multicellular development. *Comput Sci Eng* 9:50–60.

90. Merks, R. M. H. and J. A. Glazier. 2006. Dynamic mechanisms of blood vessel growth. *Nonlinearity* 19:C1–C10.

91. Merks, R. M. H., S. V. Brodsky, M. S. Goligorksy, S. A. Newman, and J. A. Glazier. 2006. Cell elongation is key to in silico replication of *in vitro* vasculogenesis and subsequent remodeling. *Dev Biol* 289:44–54.

92. Merks, R. M. H. and J. A. Glazier. 2005. A cell-centered approach to developmental biology. *Phys a, Stat Mech Its Appl* 352:113–130.

93. Botchwey, E. A., M. A. Dupree, S. R. Pollack, E. M. Levine, and C. T. Laurencin. 2003. Tissue engineered bone: Measurement of nutrient transport in three-dimensional matrices. *J Biomed Mater Res A* 67:357–367.

94. Malda, J., J. Rouwkema, D. E. Martens, E. P. Le Comte, F. K. Kooy, J. Tramper, C. A. van Blitterswijk, and J. Riesle. 2004. Oxygen gradients in tissue-engineered PEGT/PBT cartilaginous constructs: Measurement and modeling. *Biotechnol Bioeng* 86:9–18.

95. McClelland, R. E., J. M. MacDonald, and R. N. Coger. 2003. Modeling O2 transport within engineered hepatic devices. *Biotechnol Bioeng* 82:12–27.

96. Radisic, M., W. Deen, R. Langer, and G. Vunjak-Novakovic. 2005. Mathematical model of oxygen distribution in engineered cardiac tissue with parallel channel array perfused with culture medium containing oxygen carriers. *Am J Physiol Heart Circ Physiol* 288:H1278–H1289.

97. Radisic, M., J. Malda, E. Epping, W. Geng, R. Langer, and G. Vunjak-Novakovic. 2006. Oxygen gradients correlate with cell density and cell viability in engineered cardiac tissue. *Biotechnol Bioeng* 93:332–343.

98. Williams, K. A., S. Saini, and T. M. Wick. 2002. Computational fluid dynamics modeling of steady-state momentum and mass transport in a bioreactor for cartilage tissue engineering. *Biotechnol Prog* 18:951–963.

99. Galban, C. J. and B. R. Locke. 1999. Analysis of cell growth kinetics and substrate diffusion in a polymer scaffold. *Biotechnol Bioeng* 65:121–132.

100. Chang, C., D. A. Lauffenburger, and T. I. Morales. 2003. Motile chondrocytes from newborn calf: Migration properties and synthesis of collagen II. *Osteoarthritis Cartilage* 11:603–612.

101. Hamilton, D. W., M. O. Riehle, W. Monaghan, and A. S. Curtis. 2005. Articular chondrocyte passage number: influence on adhesion, migration, cytoskeletal organisation and phenotype in response to nano- and micro-metric topography. *Cell Biol Int* 29:408–421.

102. Hamilton, D. W., M. O. Riehle, W. Monaghan, and A. S. Curtis. 2006. Chondrocyte aggregation on micrometric surface topography: A time-lapse study. *Tissue Eng* 12:189–199.

103. Hamilton, D. W., M. O. Riehle, R. Rappuoli, W. Monaghan, R. Barbucci, and A. S. Curtis. 2005. The response of primary articular chondrocytes to micrometric surface topography and sulphated hyaluronic acid-based matrices. *Cell Biol Int* 29:605–615.

104. Chung, C. A., C. W. Yang, and C. W. Chen. 2006. Analysis of cell growth and diffusion in a scaffold for cartilage tissue engineering. *Biotechnol Bioeng* 94:1138–1146.

105. Pisu, M., N. Lai, A. Concas, and G. Cao. 2006. A novel simulation model for engineered cartilage growth in static systems. *Tissue Eng* 12:2311–2320.

106. Dallon, J. C., J. A. Sherratt, and P. K. Maini. 1999. Mathematical modelling of extracellular matrix dynamics using discrete cells: Fiber orientation and tissue regeneration. *J Theor Biol* 199:449–471.

107. Chaplain, M. A., S. R. McDougall, and A. R. Anderson. 2006. Mathematical modeling of tumor-induced angiogenesis. *Annu Rev Biomed Eng* 8:233–257.

108. McDougall, S. R., A. R. Anderson, and M. A. Chaplain. 2006. Mathematical modelling of dynamic adaptive tumour-induced angiogenesis: Clinical implications and therapeutic targeting strategies. *J Theor Biol* 241:564–589.

109. McDougall, S. R., A. R. Anderson, M. A. Chaplain, and J. A. Sherratt. 2002. Mathematical modelling of flow through vascular networks: implications for tumour-induced angiogenesis and chemotherapy strategies. *Bull Math Biol* 64:673–702.

110. Chaplain, M. A. 2000. Mathematical modelling of angiogenesis. *J Neurooncol* 50:37–51.

111. Anderson, A. R. and M. A. Chaplain. 1998. Continuous and discrete mathematical models of tumor-induced angiogenesis. *Bull Math Biol* 60:857–899.

112. Patel, A. A., E. T. Gawlinski, S. K. Lemieux, and R. A. Gatenby. 2001. A cellular automaton model of early tumor growth and invasion. *J Theor Biol* 213:315–331.

113. Jiang, Y., J. Pjesivac-Grbovic, C. Cantrell, and J. P. Freyer. 2005. A multiscale model for avascular tumor growth. *Biophys J* 89:3884–3894.

114. Anderson, A. R., M. Hassanein, K. M. Branch, J. Lu, N. A. Lobdell, J. Maier, D. Basanta, B. Weidow, A. Narasanna, C. L. Arteaga, A. B. Reynolds, V. Quaranta, L. Estrada, and A. M. Weaver. 2009. Microenvironmental independence associated with tumor progression. *Cancer Res* 69:8797–8806.

115. Anderson, A. R., A. M. Weaver, P. T. Cummings, and V. Quaranta. 2006. Tumor morphology and phenotypic evolution driven by selective pressure from the microenvironment. *Cell* 127:905–915.

116. Zhang, L., C. A. Athale, and T. S. Deisboeck. 2007. Development of a three-dimensional multiscale agent-based tumor model: simulating gene-protein interaction profiles, cell phenotypes and multicellular patterns in brain cancer. *J Theor Biol* 244:96–107.

117. Athale, C. A. and T. S. Deisboeck. 2006. The effects of EGF-receptor density on multiscale tumor growth patterns. *J Theor Biol* 238:771–779.

118. Athale, C., Y. Mansury, and T. S. Deisboeck. 2005. Simulating the impact of a molecular "decision-process" on cellular phenotype and multicellular patterns in brain tumors. *J Theor Biol* 233:469–481.

119. Deisboeck, T. S., M. E. Berens, A. R. Kansal, S. Torquato, A. O. Stemmer-Rachamimov, and E. A. Chiocca. 2001. Pattern of self-organization in tumour systems: complex growth dynamics in a novel brain tumour spheroid model. *Cell Prolif* 34:115–134.

120. Youssef, B. B., G. Cheng, K. Zygourakis, and P. Markenscoff. 2007. Parallel Implementation of a cellular automaton modeling the growth of three-dimensional tissues. *J High Perf Comp Appl* 21:196–209.

121. Shields, E. D. and P. B. Noble. 1987. Methodology for detection of heterogeneity of cell locomotory phenotypes in three-dimensional gels. *Exp Cell Biol* 55:250–256.

122. Weidt, C., B. Niggemann, W. Hatzmann, K. S. Zänker, and T. Dittmar. 2004. Differential effects of culture conditions on the migration pattern of stromal cell-derived factor-stimulated hematopoietic stem cells. *Stem Cells* 22:890–896.

123. Bergman, A. J. and K. Zygourakis. 1999. Migration of lymphocytes on fibronectin-coated surfaces: Temporal evolution of migratory parameters. *Biomaterials* 20:2235–2244.

124. Lee, Y., P. Markenscoff, L. V. McIntire, and K. Zygourakis. 1996. Characterization of endothelial cell locomotion using a markov chain model. *Biochem Cell Biol* 73:461–472.

125. Lee, Y., L. V. McIntire, and K. Zygourakis. 1994. Analysis of endothelial cell locomotion: Differential effects of motility and contact inhibition. *Biotechnol Bioeng* 43:622–634.

126. Malda, J., D. E. Martens, J. Tramper, C. A. van Blitterswijk, and J. Riesle. 2003. Cartilage tissue engineering: Controversy in the effect of oxygen. *Crit Rev Biotechnol* 23:175–194.

127. Obradovic, B., R. L. Carrier, G. Vunjak-Novakovic, and L. E. Freed. 1999. Gas exchange is essential for bioreactor cultivation of tissue engineered cartilage. *Biotechnol Bioeng* 63:197–205.

128. Murray, J. D. 1989. *Mathematical Biology*. Springer-Verlag, New York, NY.

129. McKeehan, W. L. and K. A. McKeehan. 1981. Extracellular regulation of fibroblast multiplication: A direct kinetic approach to analysis of the role of low molecular weight nutrients and serum growth factors. *J Supramol Struct Cell Biochem* 15:83–110.

130. McKeehan, W. L., K. A. McKeehan, and D. Calkins. 1981. Extracellular regulation of fibroblast multiplication. Quantitative differences in nutrient and serum factor requirements for multiplication of normal and SV40 virus-transformed human lung cells. *J Biol Chem* 256:2973–2981.

131. Aris, R. 1975. *The Mathematical Theory of Diffusion and Reaction in Permeable Catalysts: Questions of Uniqueness, Stability and Transient Behaviour*. Clarendon Press, Oxford, UK.

132. Cedrola, S., R. Cardani, and C. A. La Porta. 2004. Effect of glucose stress conditions in BL6T murine melanoma cells. *Melanoma Res* 14:345–351.

133. Hwang, S. O. and G. M. Lee. 2008. Nutrient deprivation induces autophagy as well as apoptosis in Chinese hamster ovary cell culture. *Biotechnol Bioeng* 99:678–685.

134. Kouvroukoglou, S., C. L. Lakkis, J. D. Wallace, K. Zygourakis, and D. E. Epner. 1998. Bioenergetics of rat prostate cancer cell migration. *Prostate* 34:137–144.

135. Cheng, G. 2005. Hybrid Computational Modeling of Cell Population and Mass Transfer Dynamics in Tissue Growth Processes. Ph.D. Dissertation. Rice University.

136. McKeehan, W. L. and K. A. McKeehan. 1981. Extracellular regulation of fibroblast multiplication: a direct kinetic approach to analysis of role of low molecular weight nutrients and serum growth factors. *J Supramol Struct Cell Biochem* 15:83–110.

137. Neves, A. A., N. Medcalf, and K. M. Brindle. 2005. Influence of stirring-induced mixing on cell proliferation and extracellular matrix deposition in meniscal cartilage constructs based on polyethylene terephthalate scaffolds. *Biomaterials* 26:4828–4836.

138. Shangkai, C., T. Naohide, Y. Koji, H. Yasuji, N. Masaaki, T. Tomohiro, and T. Yasushi. 2006. Transplantation of allogeneic chondrocytes cultured in fibroin sponge and stirring chamber to promote cartilage regeneration. *Tissue Eng* 13:483–492.

139. Wang, H. J., M. Bertrand-de Haas, C. A. van Blitterswijk, and E. N. Lamme. 2003. Engineering of a dermal equivalent: Seeding and culturing fibroblasts in PEGT/PBT copolymer scaffolds. *Tissue Eng* 9:909–917.

140. Vunjak-Novakovic, G., B. Obradovic, I. Martin, P. M. Bursac, R. Langer, and L. E. Freed. 1998. Dynamic cell seeding of polymer scaffolds for cartilage tissue engineering. *Biotechnol Prog* 14:193–202.

141. Dar, A., M. Shachar, J. Leor, and S. Cohen. 2002. Optimization of cardiac cell seeding and distribution in 3D porous alginate scaffolds. *Biotechnol Bioeng* 80:305–312.

142. Dvir-Ginzberg, M., I. Gamlieli-Bonshtein, R. Agbaria, and S. Cohen. 2003. Liver tissue engineering within alginate scaffolds: Effects of cell-seeding density on hepatocyte viability, morphology, and function. *Tissue Eng* 9:757–766.

143. Holy, C. E., M. S. Shoichet, and J. E. Davies. 2000. Engineering three-dimensional bone tissue *in vitro* using biodegradable scaffolds: investigating initial cell-seeding density and culture period. *J Biomed Mater Res* 51:376–382.

144. Kim, B. S., J. P. Andrew, J. K. Thomas, and D. J. Mooney. 1998. Optimizing seeding and culture methods to engineer smooth muscle tissue on biodegradable polymer matrices. *Biotechnol Bioeng* 57:46–54.

145. Mauck, R. L., C. C. Wang, E. S. Oswald, G. A. Ateshian, and C. T. Hung. 2003. The role of cell seeding density and nutrient supply for articular cartilage tissue engineering with deformational loading. *Osteoarthritis Cartilage/OARS, Osteoarthritis Res Soc* 11:879–890.

146. Saini, S. and T. M. Wick. 2003. Concentric cylinder bioreactor for production of tissue engineered cartilage: Effect of seeding density and hydrodynamic loading on construct development. *Biotechnol Prog* 19:510–521.

147. Wiedmann-Al-Ahmad, M., R. Gutwald, G. Lauer, U. Hübner, and R. Schmelzeisen. 2002. How to optimize seeding and culturing of human osteoblast-like cells on various biomaterials. *Biomaterials* 23:3319–3328.

148. Akins, R. E., R. A. Boyce, M. L. Madonna, N. A. Schroedl, S. R. Gonda, T. A. McLaughlin, and C. R. Hartzell. 1999. Cardiac organogenesis in vitro: Reestablishment of three-dimensional tissue architecture by dissociated neonatal rat ventricular cells. *Tissue Eng* 5:103–118.

149. Papadaki, M., N. Bursac, R. Langer, J. Merok, G. Vunjak-Novakovic, and L. E. Freed. 2001. Tissue engineering of functional cardiac muscle: molecular, structural, and electrophysiological studies. *Am J Physiol Heart Circ Physiol* 280:H168–H178.

150. Gosiewska, A., A. Rezania, S. Dhanaraj, M. Vyakarnam, J. Zhou, D. Burtis, L. Brown, W. Kong, M. Zimmerman, and J. C. Geesin. 2001. Development of a three-dimensional transmigration assay for testing cell—polymer interactions for tissue engineering applications. *Tissue Eng* 7:267–277.

151. Markenscoff, P., J. Feng, and K. Zygourakis. 2010. Cell Population Heterogeneity and Mass Transport Dynamics Modulate Tissue Regeneration Processes. In 2010 Anual Meeting of the AIChE, Salt Lake City, UT.

# III

# Applications

**27 Bone Engineering** *Lucas A. Kinard, Antonios G. Mikos, and F. Kurtis Kasper*............**27**-1
Introduction • References

**28 Dental and Craniofacial Bioengineering** *Hemin Nie and Jeremy J. Mao*..................**28**-1
Introduction • Clinical Challenges of Dental, Oral, and Craniofacial
Bioengineering • Bone Regeneration • Tooth Regeneration • Soft-Tissue
Regeneration • Concluding Remarks • Acknowledgments • References

**29 Tendon and Ligament Engineering** *Nicholas Sears, Tyler Touchet, Hugh
Benhardt, and Elizabeth Cosgriff-Hernández*.....................................................................**29**-1
Introduction • Structure of Fibrous Connective Tissues • Current Ligament
Reconstructive Techniques • Engineered Tendon and Ligament Grafts • Mechanical
Stimulation • *In Vivo* Models to Demonstrate Efficacy • Key Challenges and Critical
Issues • References

**30 Cartilage Tissue Engineering** *Emily E. Coates and John P. Fisher*...............................**30**-1
Cartilage Tissue: Composition, Function, and Disease • Cartilage
Tissue Engineering • Zonal Cartilage Engineering • Stem Cells in
Cartilage Tissue Engineering • Dynamic Culture Systems for Cartilage
Engineering • Acknowledgments • References

**31 TMJ Engineering** *Michael S. Detamore* ............................................................................**31**-1
Introduction • Structure and Function of TMJ Tissues • Tissue Engineering
Approaches • Looking to the Future in TMJ Tissue Engineering • References

**32 Interface Tissue Engineering** *Helen H. Lu, Nora Khanarian, Kristen Moffat, and
Siddarth Subramony*..........................................................................................................**32**-1
Introduction • Interface Scaffold Design for Ligament-to-Bone Interface Tissue
Engineering • Interface Scaffold Design for Tendon-to-Bone Interface Tissue
Engineering • Stratified Scaffold Design for Cartilage-to-Bone Interface Tissue
Engineering • Summary and Future Directions • References

**33 The Bioengineering of Dental Tissues** *Rena N. D'Souza, Katherine R. Regan,
Kerstin M. Galler, and Songtao Shi*..................................................................................**33**-1
Introduction • The Tooth and Its Supporting Structures • Genetic
Control of Tooth Development • Tooth Regenerative
Strategies • Conclusion • Acknowledgments • References

**34 Tissue Engineering of the Urogenital System** *In Kap Ko, Anthony Atala, and
James J. Yoo*......................................................................................................................**34**-1
Introduction • Fundamental Components of Urogenital Tissue Engineering • Engineering
Specific Urogenital Structures • Perspective • Acknowledgment • References

**35  Vascular Tissue Engineering** *Laura J. Suggs*.................................................... **35**-1
Introduction • Cell Source • Scaffolds/Extracellular Matrix • Growth Factor
Signaling • Vascular Grafts and Medial Equivalents • Engineered Vascular
Networks • Conclusions • References

**36  Neural Engineering** *Yen-Chih Lin and Kacey G. Marra*.................................... **36**-1
Overview of the Anatomy of the Nervous System • Peripheral Nerve Repair • CNS
Repair • Animal Models of Nervous System Injury Research • Overall Summary of
Neural Tissue Engineering • References

**37  Tumor Engineering: Applications for Cancer Biology and Drug
Development** *Joseph A. Ludwig and Emily Burdett*...........................................**37**-1
Introduction • Cancer Fundamentals and Relationship to Tissue
Engineering • Preclinical Drug Evaluation • Advanced 3D Models of Cancer • Tools
for Creation of a Bioengineered Tumor Model • Applications of Advanced 3D Cancer
Models • Conclusions • References

# 27

# Bone Engineering

Lucas A. Kinard
*Rice University*

Antonios G. Mikos
*Rice University*

F. Kurtis Kasper
*Rice University*

27.1 Introduction ................................................................. 27-1
  Bone Biology • Bone Engineering Paradigm • Recent
  Developments • Clinical Translation • Conclusion
References............................................................................ 27-13

## 27.1 Introduction

Bone engineering is a heavily investigated area of tissue engineering due to the importance of bone to the overall function of the body and the aesthetic importance of bone for human appearance and social interaction. Significant strides have been made in tissue engineering since its inception, and many of the developments in this field have found their impetus in the design of novel strategies for bone engineering applications. Bone engineering is an area that is expected to flourish in terms of new discoveries and clinical translation, making tissue engineering a clinical reality in the years ahead. The text that follows will lay out the basic structure of a complete bone engineering strategy from a fundamental understanding of bone biology, to a description of the research efforts developing each part of the bone engineering paradigm, to an update on topics of recent focus, and concluding with a description of the challenges of clinical translation.

### 27.1.1 Bone Biology

The following will explain the aspects of bone biology that are most important to bone engineering. Bone biology in this context is divided into the areas of shape, structure, composition, and their variation with skeletal location and with time.

#### 27.1.1.1 Shape

Bone shape is governed by genetically indicated patterns, mechanical forces, and movement. During initial skeletal modeling, the formation of the organic matrix and its subsequent replacement by immature bone is directed by sequential gene expression (Murray and Huxley 1925). Mechanical forces and movement have a role in later stages of bone development influencing maturation, remodeling, and refinement (Carter 1987, Robling and Turner 2009). The bone engineer should be cognizant of the stochastic influence of the factors governing bone shape. Bone shape is altered by the process known as modeling, which functions by combination of periosteal and endosteal apposition and resorption. By either carving out or adding to the different dimensions of the bone, the shape can be formed into a wide range of complex morphologies.

#### 27.1.1.2 Structure

The structure of the bone is built upon three tissue types: marrow, bone tissue, and periosteum. A biomimetic engineered bone in its final form must incorporate these tissues in the correct anatomical position and composition. Marrow is a fatty substance located in the central regions of bone that supplies bone and blood forming cells, and its vasculature is important to the overall blood supply to bone. Bone itself has two forms: cortical (compact) and cancellous (trabecular) (Singh 1978, Buckwalter and Cooper 1987). Cortical bone is located on the periphery, has only 10% porosity, and makes up 80% of the skeleton (Buckwalter et al. 1995). Cancellous bone is located interiorly and has 50–90% porosity and 20 times more surface area than cortical bone. This difference enables cancellous bone to have an increased response rate to mechanical loading or unloading and a higher rate of metabolic activity and remodeling due to the higher cell-covered surface area. The two maturation levels of bone are woven and lamellar. As cortical and cancellous bones mature, the initial woven state is an immature, less rigid, and more isotropic form, which by remodeling gives way to a mature, highly rigid, and anisotropic structure known as lamellar bone. Remodeling is, therefore, defined as bone turnover without changing bone shape. Woven bone is considered as such due to its irregular arrangement of collagen fibers and woven microscopic appearance. Lamellar bone, on the other hand, takes its name from the structural bone unit lamella, which consists of parallel and directionally oriented collagen fibers. Lamellae are stacked upon one another in the radial direction and are distinguishable due to the alternating direction of collagen fibers from one to the next. The interconnections between these highly oriented regions contribute strength to lamellar bone. Woven and lamellar bone can be distinguished radiographically due to the irregular mineralization of woven bone and the tightly organized and uniform mineralization of lamellar bone allowing the bone engineer to use radiographs of *in vivo* bone formation as a measure of bone maturation. The periosteum, like the marrow, supplies cells necessary for bone remodeling, serves as a second blood supply to bone, and has numerous metabolic effects. The periosteum has two distinct layers: an outer dense and fibrous layer and an inner cellular and vascular region known as the cambium due to the presence of osteoprogenitor cells (Buckwalter and Cooper 1987, Buckwalter et al. 1995, Allen et al. 2004).

### 27.1.1.3 Composition

The composition of bone can be divided into the basic areas of matrix, cells, and bioactive factors. Bone matrix is composed of an inorganic mineral phase and an organic protein-rich phase. By wet weight, bone consists of approximately 65% inorganic phase, over 20% organic phase, and approximately 10% water (Buckwalter et al. 1995). The inorganic phase serves as an ion reservoir for predominately Ca, P, Na, and Mg and contributes stiffness and strength in the form of apatite, carbonate, acid phosphate, and brushite. The organic phase provides bone form and helps resist tension. It consists primarily of collagen type I with small amounts of collagen type V and XII composing 90% of the organic phase and noncollagenous glycoproteins and proteoglycans contributing the remaining 10%. Additional proteins prevalent in bone include osteocalcin, osteonectin, bone sialoprotein, bone phosphoproteins, and small proteoglycans (Boskey 1989). Mineralization of bone occurs within the existing organic matrix with only slight changes to the organic phase. Mineralization progresses quickly with 60% of the total mineral phase formed within the first hours of the process. As mineralization progresses further, the water and noncollagenous protein contents decrease and the collagen content and organization remain essentially the same (Buckwalter et al. 1995).

Bone consists of cells from two cell lines. The mesenchymal stem cell (MSC) line gives rise to undifferentiated osteoblast progenitors (preosteoblasts), osteoblasts, bone-lining cells, and osteocytes (fully differentiated osteoblasts). The hematopoietic stem cell (HSC) line gives rise to monocytes, preosteoclasts, and osteoclasts. MSCs are located in bone canals, endosteum, periosteum, and marrow (Cooper et al. 1966, Buckwalter and Cooper 1987, Beresford 1989), and preosteoblasts can also derive from vascular pericytes (Brighton et al. 1992, Diazflores et al. 1992). Osteoblasts line the bone surface throughout the matrix, synthesize and secrete organic matrix, play a role in electrolyte flux, and produce matrix vesicles (Raisz and Kream 1983, Buckwalter and Cooper 1987). Osteocytes are primarily mechanosensors and modulators of cell activity and compose 90% of bone cells at maturity (Buckwalter and Cooper 1987, Buckwalter et al. 1995). Bone-lining cells are also referred to as resting osteoblasts or surface osteocytes owing to their origin or morphology and function, respectively. Bone-lining cells are able to release enzymes to remove the layer of osteoid that covers mineralized matrix allowing osteoclasts to attach and begin resorption. Osteoclasts destroy bone by using proton pumps to secrete protons to an isolated area of bone, lowering the pH and solubilizing the mineral phase. Osteoclasts use acid proteases to degrade the organic phase (Blair et al. 1989, Buckwalter et al. 1995). The listed cell types create an intricate balance between formation and destruction of bone, and their activity is critically influenced by numerous factors to be introduced next.

Numerous systemic hormones, cytokines, and mechanical factors affect the activities of bone cells. These factors are used by physicians and bone engineers to achieve proper bone growth and remodeling, and the bone engineer should have an understanding of the effect of various factors in order to develop useful strategies. For instance, parathyroid hormone (PTH) increases resorption by stimulating differentiation of osteoclast precursors (Raisz 1965) as does vitamin D, and calcitonin exhibits the opposite effect by inhibiting osteoclast precursor differentiation and proliferation (Karachalios et al. 1992). Growth factors control cell growth (mitogenesis), differentiation (morphogenesis), and extracellular matrix (ECM) synthesis. They work by one of the three types of action: autocrine, paracrine, or endocrine. The initial interaction between growth factors and cells is via redundant and highly specific cell binding receptors, and the final effect of this binding is transcription factor activation, binding of nuclear DNA, and modulation of gene expression. The details of numerous growth factors will be delineated in subsequent sections. The briefness of this chapter prevents describing in detail the importance of mechanical forces to bone engineering, but they are associated with bone remodeling in numerous ways. Those most related to initiation of remodeling include strain energy density, longitudinal shear stress, and tensile stress–strain (Brown et al. 1990).

### 27.1.1.4 Dynamics

Dynamics of mature bone are divided between modeling, which alters shape, and remodeling, which changes structure and composition. However, preceding both of these is the process of bone formation, which occurs by two mechanisms termed intramembranous and endochondral ossification. In intramembranous ossification, MSCs aggregate and synthesize a loose collagenous matrix (Tortelli et al. 2010). Osteoprogenitors present in the preliminary matrix differentiate to osteoblasts which deposit additional bone matrix and become osteocytes (Buckwalter and Cooper 1987). This type of bone formation is responsible for forming the flat bones of the face, vault of the skull, pelvis, and the clavicle (Buckwalter et al. 1996). In endochondral ossification, MSCs condense and become resting chondrocytes, which then proliferate and differentiate to hypertrophic chondrocytes. Hypertrophic chondrocytes produce a hyaline cartilage model of the bone, which soon becomes calcified. Vascular buds invade delivering chondroclast and osteoclast precursors that differentiate and resorb the calcified cartilage. Osteoblasts then deposit bony matrix in the form of woven bone, which is subsequently remodeled to mature lamellar bone (Figure 27.1) (Buckwalter and Cooper 1987, Goltzman 2002). This type of bone formation is responsible for forming the short and long bones of the appendicular skeleton, vertebral column, and base of the skull. Evidence of endochondral ossification can be detected by observing the common indicator of hypertrophic chondrocytes, collagen type X, followed by localized bone and blood vessel formation. Bone modeling and remodeling of the mature skeleton occur by appositional formation in which osteoblasts align along the bone surface and synthesize osteoid in successive layers forming lamellae (Buckwalter et al. 1996). This mechanism is much more similar to intramembranous than endochondral ossification. Bone engineering methods that implant osteoblasts use the model of appositional bone formation since this type is exclusive to osteoblasts. Methods that implant stem cells employ either the intramembranous or endochondral ossification model (Jo et al. 2007). Most examples in the bone engineering literature employ intramembranous ossification due to the presence of an implanted material template, osteogenic signals, and in some cases, the flat-bone-like size and shape of bone defects in small animal models; however, there are some recent examples in the literature employing the mechanism of endochondral ossification as an advantageous alternative (Jukes et al. 2008a, Farrell et al. 2009, Doan et al. 2010, Scotti et al. 2010, Tortelli et al. 2010).

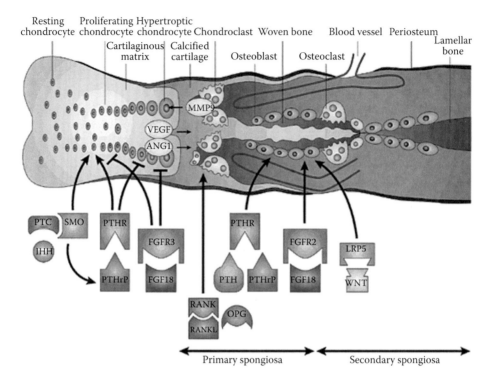

**FIGURE 27.1** Model of endochondral bone formation demonstrating the stochastic influence of numerous molecular regulators. Employing endochondral ossification as part of a bone engineering strategy presents certain advantages compared to conventional methods, including the enhanced ability of embryonic stem cells to form bone through this mechanism. (Adapted from Jukes, J. M. et al. 2008b. *Regen Med* 3: 783–85; Reprinted by permission from Macmillan Publishers Ltd: *Nat Rev Drug Discov*, Goltzman, D, Discoveries, drugs and skeletal disorders. 1: 784–96, Copyright 2002.)

Knowledge of the shape, structure, and composition of bone and their variation with position and time is critically important to the ability of the bone engineer to conceptualize and optimize potential regeneration strategies. These aspects of bone biology have natural corollaries seen in the various components involved in bone engineering design. First, the shape of a construct is determined by properties of the materials used and their ability to be molded on the macroscale. Second, the structure is determined by material choice, aspects involved in the fabrication of the construct such as spatial orientation and porosity, and particular guidance or induction of different tissue types. Third, the composition is determined by the biomimetic behavior of materials constituting the matrix, incorporation of various cell types, and release of bioactive factors. The variation of these aspects with respect to location in bone is controlled by the biological mechanisms already described; however, mimicking the temporal variation of bone biology introduces additional challenges. Modeling and remodeling of the construct depends on the degradation mechanism, degradation rate, and interaction between the material and native tissue among other factors. It is with knowledge of these corollaries that the bone engineer designs biomimetic constructs by employing the bone engineering paradigm and combinations of the various components, which will be described in detail in the following section.

## 27.1.2 Bone Engineering Paradigm

The tissue engineering paradigm was outlined near the outset of the field, and it has guided bone engineering research for nearly two decades. The components of the paradigm are matrices for cell attachment, isolated cells, and tissue-inducing substances, commonly called bioactive factors (Langer and Vacanti 1993). The importance of these aspects has been established through numerous investigations, and although bone engineering is possible without inclusion of all components, the task is often accomplished by using this strategy. Each component plays a unique role in mimicking native tissue, and omitting any one of the combination necessitates inducing the body to provide the missing item. Additional challenges are introduced toward the goal of bone engineering by attempting to manipulate the body to provide a component with temporal and quantitative specificity, therefore, making it advantageous to provide all necessary components as part of the original design. In order to understand how the bone engineer applies the paradigm, the following describes the current research in each area with respect to bone engineering, including numerous examples of their combination for evaluation in animal models and human trials.

### 27.1.2.1 Materials

When choosing a material to serve as a tissue engineering scaffold or drug delivery vehicle, the main characteristics to be considered are availability, cost, adjustable properties, crosslinking, degradation, mechanical properties, cell interactions, and covalent and noncovalent interactions with other materials and factors such as electrostatic complexation. The advantage or disadvantage of a certain characteristic is never absolute but instead depends on the application and its relation to other characteristics. Material composites are generally used to create micropores (less than 2 nm), mesopores (2–50 nm), or macropores (greater than 50 nm) (Rouquerol et al. 1994), to provide the capability of growth factor delivery, to vary mechanical characteristics, and/or to vary the degradation time. The primary materials used for current bone engineering strategies include inorganics and natural and synthetic polymers. The choice of material for bone engineering is carefully considered based upon the criteria listed above and the particular advantages relevant to the application, which is described below.

Inorganic materials provide a suitable replica of the natural mineral matrix of bone, while brittle in certain formulations normally exceed the mechanical strength of other biomaterials used in bone engineering, interact favorably with bone cells, and promote direct integration between implant and bone. Evidence has shown the promise of using inorganic materials that have osteoconductive (facilitates bone formation) and possibly osteoinductive (stimulates or induces bone formation) properties alone or in composites with other inorganic materials or synthetic or natural polymers. Inorganic materials for bone engineering can be divided generally into calcium phosphate (Ca–P)-based (bioceramics), bioactive glasses, and glass ceramics. Bioceramics are the most commonly employed type of inorganic material in bone engineering due to their prevalence in natural bone, positive bone tissue response, and injectable *in situ* setting formulations (Ruhé et al. 2006). Ca–P exists in numerous phases (Guda et al. 2008) and is used in porous formulations (Hertz and Bruce 2007). Composites of commercial Ca–P cement with primary and secondary macroporosity produced by $CO_2$ foaming and PLGA microspheres, respectively, showed an intrinsic osteoinductive response in rat subcutaneous implantation and subcritical cranial defects presenting evidence for the ability of bioceramics to act osteoinductively (Ruhé et al. 2006). Alternatively, bioactive glasses, formed by either melt processing at high temperature or sol–gel processing at ambient temperature, are made by combination of $SiO_2$ with CaO, $Na_2O$, $K_2O$, and/or $P_2O_5$. Bioactive glass in composite with a collagen sponge promoted angiogenesis in an irradiated calvarial defect model, a characteristic useful to bone engineering to be described later in this chapter (Leu et al. 2009). Although promising, the bioactive glasses have displayed problems with biocompatibility (Arcos and Vallet-Regí 2010). Glass ceramics, which are partially crystallized bioactive glasses, have been developed to overcome this limitation. A strontium and zinc incorporating calcium-silicate material was constructed with high porosity and relatively high compressive strength (2.16 MPa) for load-bearing applications. The construct formed more bone than TCP after 3 weeks when implanted into rat tibial bone defects (Zreiqat et al. 2010). As noted, the composition of bone is approximately 65% inorganic and over 20% organic. Combining materials in this proportion would be a logical strategy for bone engineering; therefore, the bone engineer should be aware of the properties of natural and synthetic polymers described next.

Natural and synthetic polymers offer an alternative to inorganic materials for bone engineering in their ability to replicate the organic matrix of bone, aptitude for controlled delivery, capacity for cell encapsulation, and availability of injectable formulations. Natural protein-based materials used commonly in bone engineering include collagen, gelatin, silk fibroin, and fibrin. Collagen type I is the most common natural material for bone engineering applications due to its high content in natural bone organic matrix. Collagen exhibits biocompatibility, crosslinking, and tunable degradation. Various forms of collagen have been tested extensively for bone engineering applications, and collagen sponges are used clinically as part of a product regulated for spinal fusion. Similarly, gelatin, which is derived from collagen, exhibits less potential for antigenicity due to its denatured form. Gelatin is capable of electrostatic complexation with proteins, which has resulted in the use of gelatin most often as a drug delivery vehicle for bone engineering in the form of microspheres or hydrogels. Implantation of Ca–P cement discs incorporating acidic or basic gelatin microspheres that undergo *in vivo* degradation at varying rates created void space for bone formation in rat critical-sized cranial defects (Link et al. 2009). Furthermore, gelatin hydrogels made by glutaraldehyde crosslinking (Tabata and Ikada 1999) impregnated with rhFGF-2 and implanted into mice maxillae increased bone augmentation volume and upregulated the expression of osteogenic markers (Kodama et al. 2009). Alternatively, silk fibroin, produced commercially using silkworms, is advantageous for its high strength and elasticity while also being lightweight. Silk fibroin has been tested in the form of a fibrous scaffold and as a hydrogel and has shown promising results for promoting bone formation (Fini et al. 2005, Li et al. 2006a, Jiang et al. 2009). In addition, porous silk fibroin scaffolds prepared by solvent evaporation and particulate leaching supported bone growth *in vivo* (Karageorgiou et al. 2006). Finally, fibrin is a protein matrix produced during the clotting cascade and contains cell binding sites that can be advantageous for bone engineering. Fibrin is also useful for its capacity to expedite cell invasion and remodeling (Schmoekel et al. 2004, Malafaya et al. 2007, Liu et al. 2009, Cui et al. 2010), and fibrin glue has been used as a cell carrier to promote bone formation *in vivo* (Kretlow et al. 2010).

In addition to the protein-based materials, there are many options of natural polysaccharide-based materials that are commonly employed in bone engineering. Alginate is commercially extracted from brown algae, readily available, and inexpensive. Since it is a block copolymer, its properties can be controlled by the relative amount of $\alpha$-L-guluronic acid (G) and $\beta$-D-mannuronic acid (M) subunits. Alginate can be reversibly crosslinked in aqueous solution by complexation with divalent cations, normally $Ca^{2+}$. However, alginate has a tendency to undergo uncontrollable degradation due to the loss of cations in solution (Shoichet et al. 1996). Alginate hydrogels shrink at low pH making them useful for drug delivery applications (Malafaya et al. 2007). Its high water content and relatively weak mechanical properties make alginate most useful for cartilage applications; however, alginate has shown positive results for the promotion of osteogenic differentiation of MSCs (Simmons et al. 2004). Nevertheless, direct comparison demonstrates the general inferiority of alginate to the bone conductive performance of more common materials such as collagen (Chang et al. 2010). Alternatively, chitosan is a fairly inexpensive material derived from chitin sourced from crustaceans, insects, and fungi. It contains amino and hydroxyl groups that can be chemically modified and chitosan can be chemically crosslinked in aqueous solution with dialdehydes such as glutaraldehyde. Chitosan is degraded by lysozyme, and its cationic nature makes it useful for complexation to negatively charged molecules and for bioadhesive purposes (Malafaya et al. 2007). Chitosan has been tested for bone applications in granular form, as freeze-dried porous scaffolds, and as pH-responsive, *in situ* forming preparations (Lee et al. 2002a, Cho et al. 2008, Martins et al. 2010). In contrast, starch is an abundant polymer that is difficult to process and brittle in its natural state. For this reason, it is often blended with other polymers or with inorganic materials for bone engineering applications (Salgado et al. 2007). Starch undergoes degradation by amylases and has been tested mostly in microparticle formulations (Silva et al. 2007a, 2007b). Finally, hyaluronan and chondroitin sulfate are two polymers that are naturally present as glycosaminoglycans (GAGs) and proteoglycans in bone ECM, respectively. Both hyaluronan and chondroitin sulfate are commercially produced by microbial fermentation and are negatively charged and nonimmunogenic.

They have seen limited use in bone engineering applications, and chondroitin sulfate is either used in composites or crosslinked to render it less water-soluble (Malafaya et al. 2007).

A unique group of natural materials gaining popularity are the polyhydroxyalkanoates (Chen and Wu 2005, Jung et al. 2005, Zhao et al. 2007). They have displayed advantageous biocompatibility and degradation following implantation. As an illustration of their use, three-dimensional poly(3-hydroxy-butyrate) (PHB) fibrous scaffolds coated with collagen I and chondroitin sulfate, seeded with hMSCs, and implanted subcutaneously displayed positive osteogenic differentiation and osteogenic matrix in close contact with PHB fibers (Rentsch et al. 2010).

In addition to the advantages shared with natural polymers, synthetic polymers offer optimal control of degradation and mechanical properties and modulation of cell interactions and surface properties. The most common synthetic polymers for bone engineering are the poly($\alpha$-hydroxy esters), including poly(glycolic acid) (PGA), poly(lactic acid) (PLA), and poly($\varepsilon$-caprolactone) (PCL). These polymers are known for biocompatibility, controlled degradation by hydrolytic cleavage, and hydrophobicity, and they are regulated by the FDA in products for numerous clinical indications. PGA has a higher modulus (12.5 GPa) than PLA due to its increased crystallinity and undergoes much faster degradation on the order of months when evaluated *in vitro*. PLA has two enantiomers, L-lactide (PLLA), which is more common, and D-lactide (PDLA). PLLA maintains a relatively high modulus (4.8 GPa) compared to other degradable polymeric constructs. Copolymers of lactic and glycolic acid, poly(lactic-*co*-glycolic acid) (PLGA), can be amorphous due to the presence of two monomer types and have lower moduli than their crystalline counterparts; however, copolymers are useful as their degradation can be controlled by the proportion of different monomers (Li et al. 1990). Finally, the poly($\alpha$-hydroxy esters) have been tested for numerous applications in bone engineering, including electrospun and nanofibrous forms, as coatings, and in composites with other natural and synthetic materials (Kim et al. 2006, Li et al. 2006b, Woo et al. 2007, Miao et al. 2008, Venugopal et al. 2008).

Poly(propylene fumarate) (PPF) consists of alternating propylene glycol and fumaric acid units enabling degradation by ester hydrolysis of the fumarate groups. As a primary advantage, PPF exhibits mechanical strength capable of bearing physiologically relevant loads. These properties are adjustable according to the molecular weight of the synthesized PPF or the crosslinking extent (Puppi et al. 2010). PPF constructs have a long established history of testing both *in vitro* and *in vivo*, and the material exhibits properties conducive to bone engineering applications, especially when paired with growth factor delivery (Peter et al. 2000, Vehof et al. 2002). More recent testing of PPF/CaSO$_4$/$\beta$-TCP composites allowed control of compressive strength and modulus and degradation by varying molecular weight, proportion of crosslinker, and CaSO$_4$/$\beta$-TCP ratio (Cai et al. 2009). This example shows the potential of PPF to be modified to suit numerous bone engineering applications. The strategies for modulating the properties of poly($\alpha$-hydroxy esters) and PPF alone or in composites apply to numerous synthetic polymers making them some of the most useful tissue engineering materials.

Other synthetic polymers commonly employed in bone engineering research include poly(ethylene glycol) (PEG)-based polymers, polyurethanes, polyanhydrides, poly(ortho esters), poly(amino acids), and polyphosphazenes; unfortunately, the conciseness of this text does not allow for a complete description of their application. Considering the scaffold materials discussed, they are often tissue conductive but lack intrinsic osteoinductivity. Osteoinductivity offers the advantage of achieving bone regeneration with limited or no cell implantation and would result in an increased rate of bone growth in cell-based strategies since this mechanism promotes cell proliferation, differentiation, and migration from existing tissue. Implanted cells can act osteoinductively by releasing bioactive factors that provide a bone forming stimulus to the native tissue. Therefore, the regenerative capacity of these materials can be increased through cell implantation and/or bioactive factor delivery, which will be discussed next.

### 27.1.2.2 Cells

In the earliest stages of bone engineering, osteoblasts were used to prove the concept of bone regeneration in two ways: osteoblasts cultured *in vitro* on scaffold materials produced bone-like matrix, and osteoblasts implanted subcutaneously resulted in ectopic bone formation. Recent studies employing osteoblasts or osteoblast-like cells most often did so for the purpose of evaluating the ability of material/material and/or material/growth factor combinations to induce bone formation _in vitro_ (Chesnutt et al. 2009, Yuan et al. 2009). Subsequent _in vivo_ testing of the system is normally carried out in the absence of transplanted cells.

Osteoblasts have the ability to form mineralized ECM at an increased rate compared to undifferentiated cells. However, osteoblasts have limited proliferative potential _in vivo_ and _ex vivo_ making expansion and production in high quantities a challenge. Furthermore, the osteoblasts of aging patients have an attenuated proliferative response. This drawback has turned investigators to the promise of using multi- or pluripotent stem cells with high proliferative potential.

MSCs are a distinct multipotent progenitor cell present in numerous tissues, including bone marrow, periosteum, muscle, peripheral blood, adipose tissue, and periodontal ligament. MSCs are present in these tissues in extremely limited amounts; for example, bone marrow consists of MSCs in the amount of 1 in 100,000 nucleated cells (El Tamer and Reis 2009). MSCs naturally differentiate into cell types of mesodermal origin such as osteoblasts, chondrocytes, adipocytes, and skeletal myocytes. MSCs are currently the most commonly investigated cells for tissue engineering purposes, including bone regeneration. Many are seeking to understand the complex interactions of signals that affect MSC differentiation for bone engineering purposes. In this way, investigations are ongoing to study the effect on bone forming potential of MSC preculture period and conditions (Castano-Izquierdo et al. 2007), initial cell phenotype (Holtorf et al. 2005), seeding density (Kim et al. 2009), coculture with other cell types (Seebach et al. 2010), and comparison of sources such as marrow or adipose tissue (Niemeyer et al. 2010). In addition, effects of scaffolds (Gomes et al. 2006, Nakamura et al. 2010), scaffold degradation (Martins et al. 2009), and growth factors (Burastero et al. 2010) are intensely studied to optimize the implementation of MSC-based bone engineering strategies. As an example, differentiated MSCs were used to synthesize an osteoinductive ECM _in vitro_, which, following decellularization, stimulated bone mineralization during subsequent culture of MSCs (Datta et al. 2005).

There are two categories of stem cells derived from adipose tissue, including the adipose tissue-derived MSCs (ATSCs) and the completely distinct adipose stem cells (ASCs). ATSCs are advantageous since they can be easily extracted in large numbers and are similar to bone-marrow-derived MSCs except demonstrating an altered bone morphogenetic protein (BMP) release profile (Hennig et al. 2007). The overall usefulness of adipose tissue as an MSC source compared to bone marrow is debated. ASCs on the other hand are a distinct multipotent cell type showing potential for osteogenic, chondrogenic, adipogenic, myogenic, and neuronal differentiation (Cowan et al. 2004, El Tamer and Reis 2009). Examples of ASC bone forming potential include numerous studies of implantation with a scaffold carrier in multiple animal models and _in vitro_ demonstration using bioreactors (Cowan et al. 2004, Froehlich et al. 2010, Pieri et al. 2010). ASCs demonstrate much promise for bone engineering; however, comparison with MSCs is difficult due to the discrepancies in culture conditions, animal source, and other factors relevant to a specific application.

Embryonic stem cells (ESCs), aside from ethical and political debate, remain under scrutiny for the tendency of these cells to form teratomas upon implantation. However, this has not prevented the study of nonhuman ESCs for bone engineering in a limited scope. Recently, increased expression of osteogenic markers was observed for human ESCs (hESCs) predifferentiated to osteoprogenitor cells and cultured on both 2D and 3D PLLA nanofibrous scaffolds. This indicates the potential of nanofibrous architecture to induce further osteogenic differentiation of hESCs (Smith et al. 2010).

Periosteal-derived progenitor cells are defined as those isolated from periosteal tissue by ECM digestion, filtration, and centrifugation. Periosteal cells can be sourced from bone surfaces throughout the body allowing cells from the region of interest to be used. Periosteal cells have displayed improved bone growth (Perka et al. 2000), similar osteogenic potential as MSCs (Park et al. 2007), osteogenic differentiation in response to genetic alteration to produce BMP-2 and vascular endothelial growth factor (VEGF) (Samee et al. 2008), and improved results in spinal fusion procedures (Putzier et al. 2008).

These results make periosteal cells a promising alternative source of postnatal multipotent cells for bone engineering.

Muscle-derived stem cells (MDSCs) are multipotential, producing cells of the myogenic and mesenchymal lineage. MDSCs are predecessors of satellite cells, which are monopotential for the myogenic lineage. MDSCs are easily harvested by muscle biopsy, tolerate *ex vivo* manipulation, and are easily transduced with viral vectors. Furthermore, MDSCs have shown capacity for self-renewal, long-term proliferation, immune-privileged behavior (Usas and Huard 2007), and significant bone growth in subcutaneous (Kim et al. 2008) and calvarial implants (Lee et al. 2002b).

The brevity of this text precludes a complete description of each of the numerous cell sources for bone engineering, allowing only a brief mention of the following. Perinatal stem cells, from cord blood, umbilical vein, amniotic fluid, and Wharton's jelly, if used autologously, must be sourced early in life and preserved until use, presenting a host of clinical challenges. Other cell types could be transdifferentiated to the osteogenic lineage, including human skin fibroblasts; however, this research remains in the early stages (El Tamer and Reis 2009). Implantation of the described cell types, or induction of their differentiation and proliferation to form bone, continues to represent an important aspect of many bone engineering strategies.

The final contributors to the current concept of the bone engineering paradigm are tissue-inducing substances, otherwise known as bioactive or growth factors. Their role can be partially or fully replaced by inclusion of the proper cell phenotype; however, their addition has enhanced bone regeneration in numerous investigations. The bone engineer, aware of the many bioactive factors described below, studies their incorporation into and delivery from biomaterials to optimize bone regeneration.

### 27.1.2.3 Bioactive Factors

There are numerous bioactive factors important to bone engineering, including systemic hormones and other cellular cues in addition to numerous growth hormones or cytokines. The usefulness of each factor individually and when delivered in a cocktail with other factors remains under investigation, but biological details have and should continue to help optimize combination and dosing for bone formation.

The transforming growth factor-β (TGF-β) superfamily consists of numerous subgroups that affect osteogenesis. Proteins of the TGF-β subgroup, including TGF-β1-5, play a role in all stages of fracture healing as evidenced by their presence at early stages and during chondrocyte proliferation and endochondral ossification and the presence of TGF-β receptors in both osteoblasts (Robey et al. 1987) and chondrocytes (Bourque et al. 1993). Each of the TGF-β proteins exhibits the same functional effect but differ in potency (Allori et al. 2008). This may explain the presence of TGF-β throughout fracture healing as unique TGF-β proteins are present in higher amounts during each stage. TGF-β1 is increased during osteogenesis while TGF-β2 and TGF-β3 are increased during chondrogenesis (Schmid et al. 1991). TGF-β1 stimulates MSCs of the periosteum to differentiate and contribute to intramembranous bone and cartilage formation. Lower doses of TGF-β1 and TGF-β2 resulted in a lower ratio of cartilage to intramembranous bone formation during fracture healing (Joyce et al. 1990, Lind et al. 1993). Although TGF-β administration promotes cellular proliferation and differentiation advantageous for bone formation, evidence indicates that positive effects require frequent and high dosing, which is difficult to achieve clinically (Lieberman et al. 2002).

BMPs from the TGF-β superfamily contribute greatly to current bone engineering strategies. BMPs regulate cell proliferation, differentiation, and tissue growth depending highly on dose and duration of exposure. High levels of BMP can promote differentiation while low levels promote proliferation of MSCs (Hogan 1996). The BMPs in total are a 30-member family with a multitude of cellular effects. Bone-inducing BMPs include BMP-2, -4, -6, -7, and -9 as evidenced by their capacity to induce mineralization and increase osteocalcin production in osteoblast cell line and to promote orthotopic ossification in mice (Kang et al. 2004). Interestingly, BMP-3 inhibits bone formation originally induced by BMP-2, -6, and -7 but not bone formation induced by BMP-9. BMP-4 may promote bone growth but has achieved contradictory results. BMPs function as either homodimers or heterodimers bound by disulfide bridges, and evidence suggests that heterodimers may better induce osteogenesis (Aono et al. 1995). Recent interest and uncertainty in the long-term bioactivity of BMP-2 released *in vivo* has motivated work to test bioactivity from controlled release composites. Notably, BMP-2 released *in vitro* maintained bioactivity in culture with preosteoblasts for 12 weeks in composites incorporating PLGA microspheres in gelatin, PPF, or PPF and gelatin and 6 weeks for gelatin hydrogels alone (Kempen et al. 2008). These results suggest the presence of clinically relevant levels of BMP-2 bioactivity in studies demonstrating linear BMP-2 release from gelatin microparticles over 4 weeks *in vivo* (Patel et al. 2008b).

The fibroblast growth factors (FGFs) are monomeric peptides that affect cell migration, angiogenesis, bone development, and epithelial–mesenchymal interactions. Basic FGF (FGF-2 or β-FGF) is the most abundant type and the most potent stimulator of osteoblast proliferation. Studies have shown enhancement of osteogenic differentiation by sequential delivery of FGF-2 and BMP-2 to MSC culture (Maegawa et al. 2007) demonstrating the temporal dependence of growth factor supplementation on bone induction.

Insulin-like growth factor 1 (IGF-1) is a 70-amino-acid single-chain polypeptide released both systemically by the liver and locally by muscle and bone (Allori et al. 2008). IGF-1 stimulates cortical and trabecular bone formation (Spencer et al. 1991). Furthermore, IGF-1 administered systemically over 2 weeks stimulated bone formation in rat calvarial defects (Thaller et al. 1993). Despite the potential bone-inducing benefits of IGF-1 administration, its use is limited in bone engineering strategies.

The platelet-derived growth factors (PDGFs) consist of multiple isoforms made by homodimeric or heterodimeric disulfide-bridged polypeptides. PDGFs are produced by platelets and MSCs and have strong chemotactic and mitogenic effects on osteoblasts and their precursors (Allori et al. 2008). PDGF stimulates osteogenic differentiation and enhancement of bone formation *in vivo* (Vikjaer et al. 1997, Schwarz et al. 2009), but much like IGF-1 its use in bone engineering strategies is limited.

The VEGF family consists of glycosylated homodimers between 121 and 206 amino acids in length. It is undetermined whether VEGF has a direct osteogenic effect; however, it directly increases endothelial cell and endothelial progenitor cell chemotaxis and mitogenesis. This action contributes to angiogenesis and vasculogenesis, which have important effects on bone growth (Allori et al. 2008). Osteoblasts secrete VEGF and have VEGF receptors (Deckers et al. 2000), and VEGF production is increased in response to hypoxia via action of hypoxia-inducible transcription factors (HIFs) (Dery et al. 2005). Invasion of vascular supply in response to VEGF promotes bone formation due to delivery of systemic growth factors, circulating stem cells, and growth-limiting nutrients and removal of metabolic waste and material degradation products. In order to evaluate the advantages of VEGF in bone engineering applications, a controlled release system for VEGF from gelatin microparticles alone and in porous PPF composites was developed, and greater than 90% of expected VEGF bioactivity was maintained over 14 days (Patel et al. 2008a).

A growing area of interest in bone engineering is the effect of delivering combinations, or cocktails, of growth factors to the site of interest simultaneously or sequentially. The main goal is to recapitulate either the local embryonic bone-forming environment or the fracture repair environment. It is difficult to assess the effect of delivering growth factor combinations in a systematic manner due to the amount of additional variables introduced; however, this type of analysis must be present for the optimization of this strategy. Several strategies for delivery of multiple growth factors are envisioned (Figure 27.2). One such investigation used two different types of submicron particles, PLGA and poly(3-hydroxybutyrate-co-3-hydroxyvalerate) (PHBV), to release BMP-2 and BMP-7, respectively. Fibrous scaffolds incorporating particles designed to release BMP-2 and BMP-7 sequentially achieved better MSC differentiation than simultaneous delivery of growth factors or delivery of each growth factor independently (Yilgor et al. 2009). Another group of studies tested the delivery of BMP-2 and VEGF simultaneously from gelatin microparticles suspended in Pluronic F-127, which was injected into porous PPF before implantation into rat critical-sized calvarial defects. The investigators found that the release of both growth factors or BMP-2 alone resulted in the same amount of bone formation at 12 weeks. The bone formation was BMP-2 dose-dependent, and increasing the amount of VEGF could not recover bone growth. Dual

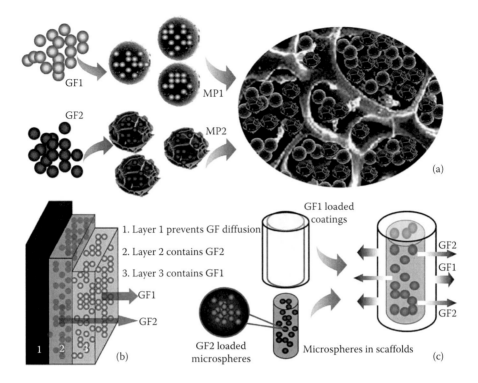

**FIGURE 27.2** Model systems for multiple growth factor (GF) delivery. (a) GF1 and GF2 are encapsulated separately into microspheres, which are entrapped in a scaffold for simultaneous or sequential delivery dependent primarily on microsphere properties. (b) A diffusive barrier (layer 1) serves as support for the layering of a material incorporating GF2 (layer 2) and GF1 (layer 3). Delivery is controlled primarily by diffusive distance caused by layering. (c) GF2 loaded microspheres are entrapped in a material core while GF1 is directly incorporated into a hydrogel shell. (Reprinted from *Biomaterials*, 31, Chen, F. M., Zhang, M. and Wu, Z. F. Toward delivery of multiple growth factors in tissue engineering, 6279–308. Copyright 2010, with permission from Elsevier.)

delivery did however increase the amount of bone formation after 4 weeks, suggesting a synergistic effect on early bone formation (Patel et al. 2008c, Young et al. 2009). Other studies delivering BMP-2 and VEGF simultaneously to an orthotopic site were not able to show increased total bone formation after 8 weeks (Kempen et al. 2009). Increased bone formation after 4 weeks has been demonstrated due to simultaneous delivery of VEGF and PDGF, but bone formation at later time points was not assessed (De La Riva et al. 2010). Overall, the strategy of delivering multiple growth factors is promising; however, the complexity of this endeavor has made proving its potential somewhat difficult.

## 27.1.3 Recent Developments

### 27.1.3.1 Nanoscale Features

In the context of this discussion, the nanoscale regime includes those constituent elements with size smaller than 100 nm in any dimension. Structural elements of this size range are relevant to bone engineering in two primary ways. First, nanoscale features impart unique surface properties such as surface topography, chemistry, wettability, and energy and in general, a higher surface area to volume ratio. Second, the natural bone ECM is nanostructured consisting of 70% nanocrystalline hydroxyapatite (HA), which is 20–80 nm long and 2–5 nm thick, and a protein-based organic phase with structural components on the same scale. Inclusion of nanoscale features in bone engineering materials has several basic advantages: increased protein adsorption leading to better cell attachment and spreading, a biomimetic 3D environment leading to enhancement of osteogenic differentiation, and doping with stronger materials without compromising the underlying structure leading to improved mechanical strength. Nanophase HA (67 nm), alumina (24 nm), and titania (39 nm) demonstrated better osteoblast adhesion and reduced fibroblast adhesion than conventional formulations of HA (179 nm), alumina (167 nm), and titania (4520 nm) with larger grains, and the effect is presumed to result from increased vitronectin adsorption on materials of smaller grain size (Webster et al. 2000). Nanophase zinc oxide (23 nm) and titania (23 nm) increased matrix mineralization by osteoblasts compared to microphase zinc oxide (4900 nm) and titania (4100 nm) (Colon et al. 2006). An upregulation of osteogenic differentiation occurred for rat MSCs seeded on peptide amphiphile (PA)-based nanofibrous scaffolds compared to cells cultured on conventional plates (Hosseinkhani et al. 2006). Incorporation of ultra-short single-walled carbon nanotubes into porous PPF constructs resulted in a threefold increase in bone ingrowth compared to the polymer alone in defects of the rabbit femoral condyle at 12 weeks (Sitharaman et al. 2008). HA nanoparticles were combined with poly(ε-caprolactone fumarate) of both amorphous and semicrystalline forms to observe the effect on mechanical properties. As HA concentration was increased, the tensile modulus increased and tensile strain at break decreased for both groups, and the compressive modulus increased for the amorphous group displaying a general increase in mechanical rigidity with nanoparticle addition (Wang et al. 2009). Fibrous scaffolds have been heavily investigated on the nanoscale, including those fabricated by templating, electrospinning, phase separation, particulate leaching, chemical etching, and 3D printing (Pham et al. 2006, Zhang and Webster 2009). Fibrin-based scaffolds with a Ca–P phase were created by sphere-templating with fibrin fiber diameter of 40–80 nm. Scaffolds with solution-deposited Ca–P stimulated osteogenic gene expression and calcium deposition by osteoblasts to a higher degree than scaffolds with a Ca–P phase created through direct incorporation of nanocrystalline HA. The two groups performed comparably in terms of *in vivo* bone regeneration (Osathanon et al. 2008). These studies demonstrate some of the unique effects of nanoscale features on bone cells and bone formation. Innovative areas of study such as nanoscale features will continue to be investigated in combination with the traditional bone engineering paradigm in order to increase the rate at which technologies are brought to the clinic. Some of the challenges and examples associated with the process of clinical translation are described next.

## 27.1.4 Clinical Translation

There are currently no cell-based bone engineering products regulated by the FDA, although several preclinical studies have been carried out. The cell-based approach has been described as isolation of MSCs from the patient, *ex vivo* expansion, and implantation into the same patient in a manner ensuring differentiation and growth of the desired tissue (Caplan 1991). In some cases, besides the implantation of adequate osteogenic cells, scaffold, and bioactive factors, the remaining necessity for a successful cell-based approach is the presence of a vascular supply at an early stage following implantation. Careful evaluation of the animal model should always be made since direct contact with vascularized tissues in small animals sometimes enhances bone regeneration more than if the same implant were used in a similar location in a human subject. Methods of vascularizing bone engineering materials are currently under intense investigation with several basic strategies. Researchers attempt to stimulate vessel growth with angiogenic factors and/or endothelial cells, engineer bone constructs *in vivo* and transplant a bone flap, or wait to apply cells to the scaffold up to a week after implantation to allow the body's healing response to invade the area with a vascular supply (Meijer et al. 2007). Additionally, many investigations attempt to guide vessel growth by using templating or 3D printing to form the structure of a vascular network within the scaffold before cell seeding and implantation.

Preclinical evaluation of cell-based approaches to bone engineering has been carried out on a limited number of patients with various bone defects. Three patients with segmental defects of the tibia (4 cm), ulna (4 cm), and humerus (7 cm) were implanted with macroporous HA scaffolds seeded with *ex vivo* expanded MSCs and externally fixated for 6.5, 6, and 13 months, respectively. The defects were repaired with clinically adequate integration at 2 months as determined radiographically and with no reports of problems between 15 and 27 months; however, the primary evaluation was performed using radiographs, and the radiopacity of the HA made this difficult (Quarto et al. 2001). The patient treated for the tibial defect showed complete healing at 7 years with the nonresorbable HA scaffold still present (Cancedda et al. 2007). Another study testing implantation of *ex vivo* expanded MSCs for mandibular augmentation resulted in bone formation by the implanted cells in only one of six patients (Meijer et al. 2008). Although human evaluation of cell-based bone engineering constructs has been limited during the early development of the discipline, results indicate that achieving successful clinical outcomes using cell-based strategies is not only highly likely at some point in the future but could occur as soon as the current decade.

## 27.1.5 Conclusion

While tissue engineering remains a relatively new field, observation indicates that collaboration between various disciplines should greatly enhance innovation and advancement due to the common use of multifaceted strategies. In order to facilitate this collaboration, the bone engineer should have a thorough understanding of bone biology and associations between the biology and various components incorporated into the design of a bone engineering construct, in addition to exhaustive knowledge of fundamental engineering principles. Bone shape, structure, composition, and the changes in these properties with position and time have corollaries in the design of constructs incorporating materials, cells, and bioactive factors, which constitute the tissue engineering paradigm. It follows that the tissue engineering paradigm influenced biomimetic strategies that have guided numerous successful experimental efforts for over two decades and continues to define bone engineering research. Many complex and unique interactions result from the combination of a variety of inorganic materials and natural and synthetic polymers, cells from numerous sources, and a multitude of bioactive factors. Much anticipated growth is expected to occur in the next few years in terms of research effort committed to studying sequential or simultaneous delivery of growth factors from a single construct and the design of materials with nanoscale features that provide unique biomimetic cell–matrix interactions. Finally, the challenges associated with clinical translation of the discussed technologies are vast and mostly unexplored. However, historical evidence of preclinical trials evaluating cell-based technologies should help direct future translational efforts. Following recent trends, investigators should continue to focus on expediting the translation of technologies to the clinic that will benefit large patient populations in need of bone healing.

## References

Allen, M. R., Hock, J. M., and Burr, D. B. 2004. Periosteum: Biology, regulation, and response to osteoporosis therapies. *Bone* 35: 1003–12.

Allori, A. C., Sailon, A. M., and Warren, S. M. 2008. Biological basis of bone formation, remodeling, and repair—Part I: Biochemical signaling molecules. *Tissue Eng Pt B-Rev* 14: 259–73.

Aono, A., Hazama, M., Notoya, K. et al. 1995. Potent ectopic bone-inducing activity of bone morphogenetic protein-4/7 heterodimer. *Biochem Bioph Res Co* 210: 670–7.

Arcos, D. and Vallet-Regí, M. 2010. Sol-gel silica-based biomaterials and bone tissue regeneration. *Acta Biomater* 6: 2874–88.

Beresford, J. 1989. Osteogenic stem cells and the stromal system of bone and marrow. *Clin Orthop Relat R* 270–80.

Blair, H., Teitelbaum, S., Ghiselli, R., and Gluck, S. 1989. Osteoclastic bone resorption by a polarized vacuolar proton pump. *Science* 245: 855–7.

Boskey, A. 1989. Noncollagenous matrix proteins and their role in mineralization. *Bone Miner* 6: 111–23.

Bourque, W. T., Gross, M., and Hall, B. K. 1993. Expression of four growth factors during fracture repair. *Int J Dev Biol* 37: 573–9.

Brighton, C., Lorich, D., Kupcha, R., Reilly, T., Jones, A., and Woodbury, R. 1992. The pericyte as a possible osteoblast progenitor cell. *Clin Orthop Relat R* 287–99.

Brown, T., Pedersen, D., Gray, M., Brand, R., and Rubin, C. 1990. Toward an identification of mechanical parameters initiating periosteal remodeling—A combined experimental and analytic approach. *J Biomech* 23: 893–905.

Buckwalter, J., Glimcher, M., Cooper, R., and Recker, R. 1995. Bone biology. I: Structure, blood supply, cells, matrix, and mineralization. *J Bone Joint Surg Am* 77A: 1256–75.

Buckwalter, J. A. and Cooper, R. R. 1987. Bone structure and function. *Instr Course Lect* 36: 27–48.

Buckwalter, J. A., Glimcher, M. J., Cooper, R. R., and Recker, R. 1996. Bone biology. II: Formation, form, modeling, remodeling, and regulation of cell function. *Instr Course Lect* 45: 387–99.

Burastero, G., Scarfi, S., Ferraris, C. et al. 2010. The association of human mesenchymal stem cells with bmp-7 improves bone regeneration of critical-size segmental bone defects in athymic rats. *Bone* 47: 117–26.

Cai, Z. Y., Yang, D. A., Zhang, N., Ji, C. G., Zhu, L., and Zhang, T. 2009. Poly(propylene fumarate)/(calcium sulphate/β-tricalcium phosphate) composites: Preparation, characterization and *in vitro* degradation. *Acta Biomater* 5: 628–35.

Cancedda, R., Giannoni, P., and Mastrogiacomo, M. 2007. A tissue engineering approach to bone repair in large animal models and in clinical practice. *Biomaterials* 28: 4240–50.

Caplan, A. 1991. Mesenchymal stem cells. *J Orthopaed Res* 9: 641–50.

Carter, D. 1987. Mechanical loading history and skeletal biology. *J Biomech* 20: 1095–109.

Castano-Izquierdo, H., Alvarez-Barreto, J., Van Den Dolder, J., Jansen, J. A., Mikos, A. G., and Sikavitsas, V. I. 2007. Pre-culture period of mesenchymal stem cells in osteogenic media influences their *in vivo* bone forming potential. *J Biomed Mater Res A* 82A: 129–38.

Chang, S. C. N., Chung, H. Y., Tai, C. L., Chen, P. K. T., Lin, T. M., and Jeng, L. B. 2010. Repair of large cranial defects by hbmp-2 expressing bone marrow stromal cells: Comparison between alginate and collagen type i systems. *J Biomed Mater Res A* 94: 433–41.

Chen, F. M., Zhang, M., and Wu, Z. F. 2010. Toward delivery of multiple growth factors in tissue engineering. *Biomaterials* 31: 6279–308.

Chen, G. and Wu, Q. 2005. The application of polyhydroxyalkanoates as tissue engineering materials. *Biomaterials* 26: 6565–78.

Chesnutt, B. M., Yuan, Y., Buddington, K., Haggard, W. O., and Bumgardner, J. D. 2009. Composite chitosan/nano-hydroxyapatite scaffolds induce osteocalcin production by osteoblasts *in vitro* and support bone formation in vivo. *Tissue Eng Pt A* 15: 2571–9.

Cho, M. H., Kim, K. S., Ahn, H. H. et al. 2008. Chitosan gel as an in situ-forming scaffold for rat bone marrow mesenchymal stem cells in vivo. *Tissue Eng Pt A* 14: 1099–108.

Colon, G., Ward, B. C., and Webster, T. J. 2006. Increased osteoblast and decreased staphylococcus epidermidis functions on nanophase zno and tio2. *J Biomed Mater Res A* 78A: 595–604.

Cooper, R., Milgram, J., and Robinson, R. 1966. Morphology of the osteon: An electron microscopic study. *J Bone Joint Surg Am A* 48: 1239–71.

Cowan, C., Shi, Y., Aalami, O. et al. 2004. Adipose-derived adult stromal cells heal critical-size mouse calvarial defects. *Nat Biotechnol* 22: 560–7.

Cui, G., Li, J., Lei, W. et al. 2010. The mechanical and biological properties of an injectable calcium phosphate cement-fibrin glue composite for bone regeneration. *J Biomed Mater Res B* 92B: 377–85.

Datta, N., Holtorf, H. L., Sikavitsas, V. I., Jansen, J. A., and Mikos, A. G. 2005. Effect of bone extracellular matrix synthesized *in vitro* on the osteoblastic differentiation of marrow stromal cells. *Biomaterials* 26: 971–7.

De La Riva, B., Sanchez, E., Hernandez, A. et al. 2010. Local controlled release of vegf and pdgf from a combined brushite-chitosan system enhances bone regeneration. *J Control Release* 143: 45–52.

Deckers, M., Karperien, M., Van Der Bent, C., Yamashita, T., Papapoulos, S., and Lowik, C. 2000. Expression of vascular endothelial growth factors and their receptors during osteoblast differentiation. *Endocrinology* 141: 1667–74.

Dery, M., Michaud, M., and Richard, D. 2005. Hypoxia-inducible factor 1: Regulation by hypoxic and non-hypoxic activators. *Int J Biochem Cell B* 37: 535–40.

Diazflores, L., Gutierrez, R., Lopezalonso, A., Gonzalez, R., and Varela, H. 1992. Pericytes as a supplementary source of osteoblasts in periosteal osteogenesis. *Clin Orthop Relat R* 280-6.

Doan, L., Kelley, C., Luong, H. et al. 2010. Engineered cartilage heals skull defects. *Am J Orthod Dentofacial Orthop* 137: 162.e1-.e9.

El Tamer, M. K., and Reis, R. L. 2009. Progenitor and stem cells for bone and cartilage regeneration. *J Tissue Eng Regen Med* 3: 327–37.

Farrell, E., Van Der Jagt, O. P., Koevoet, W. et al. 2009. Chondrogenic priming of human bone marrow stromal cells: A better route to bone repair? *Tissue Eng Pt C, Meth* 15: 285–95.

Fini, M., Motta, A., Torricelli, P. et al. 2005. The healing of confined critical size cancellous defects in the presence of silk fibroin hydrogel. *Biomaterials* 26: 3527–36.

Froehlich, M., Grayson, W. L., Marolt, D., Gimble, J. M., Kregar-Velikonja, N., and Vunjak-Novakovic, G. 2010. Bone grafts engineered from human adipose-derived stem cells in perfusion bioreactor culture. *Tissue Eng Pt A* 16: 179–89.

Goltzman, D. 2002. Discoveries, drugs and skeletal disorders. *Nat Rev Drug Discov* 1: 784–96.

Gomes, M. E., Holtorf, H. L., Reis, R. L., and Mikos, A. G. 2006. Influence of the porosity of starch-based fiber mesh scaffolds on the proliferation and osteogenic differentiation of bone marrow stromal cells cultured in a flow perfusion bioreactor. *Tissue Eng* 12: 801–9.

Guda, T., Appleford, M., Oh, S., and Ong, J. L. 2008. A cellular perspective to bioceramic scaffolds for bone tissue engineering: The state of the art. *Curr Top Med Chem* 8: 290–9.

Hennig, T., Lorenz, H., Thiel, A. et al. 2007. Reduced chondrogenic potential of adipose tissue derived stromal cells correlates with an altered TGF beta receptor and bmp profile and is overcome by bmp-6. *J Cell Physiol* 211: 682–91.

Hertz, A. and Bruce, I. J. 2007. Inorganic materials for bone repair or replacement applications. *Nanomedicine-UK* 2: 899–918.

Hogan, B. 1996. Bone morphogenetic proteins: Multifunctional regulators of vertebrate development. *Gene Dev* 10: 1580–94.

Holtorf, H., Jansen, J., and Mikos, A. 2005. Ectopic bone formation in rat marrow stromal cell/titanium fiber mesh scaffold constructs: Effect of initial cell phenotype. *Biomaterials* 26: 6208–16.

Hosseinkhani, H., Hosseinkhani, M., Tian, F., Kobayashi, H., and Tabata, Y. 2006. Osteogenic differentiation of mesenchymal stem cells in self-assembled peptide-amphiphile nanofibers. *Biomaterials* 27: 4079–86.

Jiang, X., Zhao, J., Wang, S. et al. 2009. Mandibular repair in rats with premineralized silk scaffolds and bmp-2-modified bmscs. *Biomaterials* 30: 4522–32.

Jo, I., Lee, J. M., Suh, H., and Kim, H. 2007. Bone tissue engineering using marrow stromal cells. *Biotechnol Bioproc E* 12: 48–53.

Joyce, M. E., Roberts, A. B., Sporn, M. B., and Bolander, M. E. 1990. Transforming growth factor-beta and the initiation of chondrogenesis and osteogenesis in the rat femur. *J Cell Biol* 110: 2195–207.

Jukes, J. M., Both, S. K., Leusink, A., Sterk, L. M. T., Van Blitterswijk, C. A., and De Boer, J. 2008a. Endochondral bone tissue engineering using embryonic stem cells. *Proc Natl Acad Sci USA* 105: 6840–5.

Jukes, J. M., Both, S. K., Van Blitterswijk, C. A., and De Boer, J. 2008b. Potential of embryonic stem cells for *in vivo* bone regeneration. *Regen Med* 3: 783–85.

Jung, I., Phyo, K., Kim, K., Park, H., and Kim, I. 2005. Spontaneous liberation of intracellular polyhydroxybutyrate granules in *Escherichia coli*. *Res Microbiol* 156: 865–73.

Kang, Q., Sun, M., Cheng, H. et al. 2004. Characterization of the distinct orthotopic bone-forming activity of 14 bmps using recombinant adenovirus-mediated gene delivery. *Gene Ther* 11: 1312–20.

Karachalios, T., Lyritis, G., Giannarakos, D., Papanicolaou, G., and Sotopoulos, K. 1992. Calcitonin effects on rabbit bone—Bending tests on ulnar osteotomies. *Acta Orthop Scand* 63: 615–8.

Karageorgiou, V., Tomkins, M., Fajardo, R. et al. 2006. Porous silk fibroin 3-d scaffolds for delivery of bone morphogenetic protein-2 *in vitro* and in vivo. *J Biomed Mater Res A* 78A: 324–34.

Kempen, D. H. R., Lu, L., Hefferan, T. E. et al. 2008. Retention of *in vitro* and *in vivo* bmp-2 bioactivities in sustained delivery vehicles for bone tissue engineering. *Biomaterials* 29: 3245–52.

Kempen, D. H. R., Lu, L., Heijink, A. et al. 2009. Effect of local sequential vegf and bmp-2 delivery on ectopic and orthotopic bone regeneration. *Biomaterials* 30: 2816–25.

Kim, K., Dean, D., Mikos, A. G., and Fisher, J. P. 2009. Effect of initial cell seeding density on early osteogenic signal expression of rat bone marrow stromal cells cultured on cross-linked poly(propylene fumarate) disks. *Biomacromolecules* 10: 1810–7.

Kim, K. S., Lee, J. H., Ahn, H. H. et al. 2008. The osteogenic differentiation of rat muscle-derived stem cells *in vivo* within in situ-forming chitosan scaffolds. *Biomaterials* 29: 4420–8.

Kim, S. S., Sun Park, M., Jeon, O., Yong Choi, C., and Kim, B. S. 2006. Poly(lactide-co-glycolide)/hydroxy-apatite composite scaffolds for bone tissue engineering. *Biomaterials* 27: 1399–409.

Kodama, N., Nagata, M., Tabata, Y., Ozeki, M., Ninomiya, T., and Takagi, R. 2009. A local bone anabolic effect of rhfgf2-impregnated gelatin hydrogel by promoting cell proliferation and coordinating osteoblastic differentiation. *Bone* 44: 699–707.

Kretlow, J. D., Spicer, P. P., Jansen, J., Vacanti, C. A., Kasper, F. K., and Mikos, A. G. 2010. Uncultured marrow mononuclear cells delivered within fibrin glue hydrogels to porous scaffolds enhance bone regeneration within critical size rat cranial defects. *Tissue Eng Pt A* 16: 3555–68.

Langer, R. and Vacanti, J. P. 1993. Tissue engineering. *Science* 260: 920–6.

Lee, J., Nam, S., Im, S. et al. 2002a. Enhanced bone formation by controlled growth factor delivery from chitosan-based biomaterials. *J Cont Rel* 78: 187–97.

Lee, J., Peng, H., Usas, A. et al. 2002b. Enhancement of bone healing based on ex vivo gene therapy using human muscle-derived cells expressing bone morphogenetic protein 2. *Hum Gene Ther* 13: 1201–11.

Leu, A., Stieger, S. M., Dayton, P., Ferrara, K. W., and Leach, J. K. 2009. Angiogenic response to bioactive glass promotes bone healing in an irradiated calvarial defect. *Tissue Eng Pt A* 15: 877–85.

Li, C., Vepari, C., Jin, H., Kim, H., and Kaplan, D. 2006a. Electrospun silk-bmp-2 scaffolds for bone tissue engineering. *Biomaterials* 27: 3115–24.

Li, S., Garreau, H., and Vert, M. 1990. Structure-property relationships in the case of the degradation of massive poly(alpha-hydroxy acids) in aqueous media. 2. Degradation of lactide-glycolide copolymers: Pla37.5ga25 and pla75ga25. *J Mater Sci-Mater M* 1: 131–9.

Li, W. J., Cooper, J. A., Mauck, R. L., and Tuan, R. S. 2006b. Fabrication and characterization of six electrospun poly(alpha-hydroxy ester)-based fibrous scaffolds for tissue engineering applications. *Acta Biomater* 2: 377–85.

Lieberman, J., Daluiski, A., and Einhorn, T. 2002. The role of growth factors in the repair of bone—Biology and clinical applications. *J Bone Joint Surg Am* 84A: 1032–44.

Lind, M., Schumacker, B., Søballe, K., Keller, J., Melsen, F., and Bünger, C. 1993. Transforming growth factor-β enhances fracture healing in rabbit tibiae. *Acta Orthop* 64: 553–6.

Link, D. P., Van Den Dolder, J., Van Den Beucken, J. J. J. P. et al. 2009. Evaluation of an orthotopically implanted calcium phosphate cement containing gelatin microparticles. *J Biomed Mater Res A* 90A: 372–9.

Liu, Y., Lu, Y., Tian, X. et al. 2009. Segmental bone regeneration using an rhbmp-2-loaded gelatin/nanohy-droxyapatite/fibrin scaffold in a rabbit model. *Biomaterials* 30: 6276–85.

Maegawa, N., Kawamura, K., Hirose, M., Yajima, H., Takakura, Y., and Ohgushi, H. 2007. Enhancement of osteoblastic differentiation of mesenchymal stromal cells cultured by selective combination of bone morphogenetic protein-2 (bmp-2) and fibroblast growth factor-2 (fgf-2). *J Tissue Eng Regen Med* 1: 306–13.

Malafaya, P. B., Silva, G. A., and Reis, R. L. 2007. Natural-origin polymers as carriers and scaffolds for bio-molecules and cell delivery in tissue engineering applications. *Adv Drug Deliv Rev* 59: 207–33.

Martins, A. M., Alves, C. M., Kasper, F. K., Mikos, A. G., and Reis, R. L. 2010. Responsive and in situ-forming chitosan scaffolds for bone tissue engineering applications: An overview of the last decade. *J Mater Chem* 20: 1638–45.

Martins, A. M., Pham, Q. P., Malafaya, P. B. et al. 2009. Natural stimulus responsive scaffolds/cells for bone tissue engineering: Influence of lysozyme upon scaffold degradation and osteogenic differentiation of cultured marrow stromal cells induced by cap coatings. *Tissue Eng Pt A* 15: 1953–63.

Meijer, G. J., De Bruijn, J. D., Koole, R., and Van Blitterswijk, C. A. 2007. Cell-based bone tissue engineering. *PLoS Med* 4: 260–4.

Meijer, G. J., De Bruijn, J. D., Koole, R., and Van Blitterswijk, C. A. 2008. Cell based bone tissue engineering in jaw defects. *Biomaterials* 29: 3053–61.

Miao, X., Tan, D. M., Li, J., Xiao, Y., and Crawford, R. 2008. Mechanical and biological properties of hydroxyapatite/tricalcium phosphate scaffolds coated with poly(lactic-co-glycolic acid). *Acta Biomater* 4: 638–45.

Murray, P. and Huxley, J. 1925. Self-differentiation in the grafted limb-bud of the chick. *J Anat* 59: 379–84.

Nakamura, A., Akahane, M., Shigematsu, H. et al. 2010. Cell sheet transplantation of cultured mesenchymal stem cells enhances bone formation in a rat nonunion model. *Bone* 46: 418–24.

Niemeyer, P., Fechner, K., Milz, S. et al. 2010. Comparison of mesenchymal stem cells from bone marrow and adipose tissue for bone regeneration in a critical size defect of the sheep tibia and the influence of platelet-rich plasma. *Biomaterials* 31: 3572–9.

Osathanon, T., Linnes, M. L., Rajachar, R. M., Ratner, B. D., Somerman, M. J., and Giachelli, C. M. 2008. Microporous nanofibrous fibrin-based scaffolds for bone tissue engineering. *Biomaterials* 29: 4091–9.

Park, B. W., Hah, Y. S., Kim, D. R., Kim, J. R., and Byun, J. H. 2007. Osteogenic phenotypes and mineralization of cultured human periosteal-derived cells. *Arch Oral Biol* 52: 983–9.

Patel, Z. S., Ueda, H., Yamamoto, M., Tabata, Y., and Mikos, A. G. 2008a. *In vitro* and *in vivo* release of vascular endothelial growth factor from gelatin microparticles and biodegradable composite scaffolds. *Pharm Res* 25: 2370–8.

Patel, Z. S., Yamamoto, M., Ueda, H., Tabata, Y., and Mikos, A. G. 2008b. Biodegradable gelatin microparticles as delivery systems for the controlled release of bone morphogenetic protein-2. *Acta Biomater* 4: 1126–38.

Patel, Z. S., Young, S., Tabata, Y., Jansen, J. A., Wong, M. E. K., and Mikos, A. G. 2008c. Dual delivery of an angiogenic and an osteogenic growth factor for bone regeneration in a critical size defect model. *Bone* 43: 931–40.

Perka, C., Schultz, O., Spitzer, R., Lindenhayn, K., Burmester, G., and Sittinger, M. 2000. Segmental bone repair by tissue-engineered periosteal cell transplants with bioresorbable fleece and fibrin scaffolds in rabbits. *Biomaterials* 21: 1145–53.

Peter, S., Lu, L., Kim, D. et al. 2000. Effects of transforming growth factor beta 1 released from biodegradable polymer microparticles on marrow stromal osteoblasts cultured on poly(propylene fumarate) substrates. *J Biomed Mater Res* 50: 452–62.

Pham, Q., Sharma, U., and Mikos, A. 2006. Electrospinning of polymeric nanofibers for tissue engineering applications: A review. *Tissue Eng* 12: 1197–211.

Pieri, F., Lucarelli, E., Corinaldesi, G. et al. 2010. Dose-dependent effect of adipose-derived adult stem cells on vertical bone regeneration in rabbit calvarium. *Biomaterials* 31: 3527–35.

Puppi, D., Chiellini, F., Piras, A. M., and Chiellini, E. 2010. Polymeric materials for bone and cartilage repair. *Prog Polym Sci* 35: 403–40.

Putzier, M., Strube, P., Funk, J., Gross, C., and Perka, C. 2008. Periosteal cells compared with autologous cancellous bone in lumbar segmental fusion. *J Neurosurg-Spine* 8: 536–43.

Quarto, R., Mastrogiacomo, M., Cancedda, R. et al. 2001. Repair of large bone defects with the use of autologous bone marrow stromal cells. *New Engl J Med* 344: 385–6.

Raisz, L. 1965. Bone resorption in tissue culture. Factors influencing the response to parathyroid hormone. *J Clin Invest* 44: 103–16.

Raisz, L. and Kream, B. 1983. Regulation of bone formation. 1. *New Engl J Med* 309: 29–35.

Rentsch, C., Rentsch, B., Breier, A. et al. 2010. Evaluation of the osteogenic potential and vascularization of 3d poly(3)hydroxybutyrate scaffolds subcutaneously implanted in nude rats. *J Biomed Mater Res A* 92A: 185–95.

Robey, P., Young, M., Flanders, K. et al. 1987. Osteoblasts synthesize and respond to transforming growth factor-type-beta (tgf-beta) in vitro. *J Cell Biol* 105: 457–63.

Robling, A. G. and Turner, C. H. 2009. Mechanical signaling for bone modeling and remodeling. *Crit Rev Eukar Gene* 19: 319–38.

Rouquerol, J., Avnir, D., Fairbridge, C. et al. 1994. Recommendations for the characterization of porous solids. *Pure Appl Chem* 66: 1739–58.

Ruhé, P. Q., Hedberg-Dirk, E. L., Padron, N. T., Spauwen, P. H. M., Jansen, J. A., and Mikos, A. G. 2006. Porous poly(dl-lactic-co-glycolic acid)/calcium phosphate cement composite for reconstruction of bone defects. *Tissue Eng* 12: 789–800.

Salgado, A. J., Coutinho, O. P., Reis, R. L., and Davies, J. E. 2007. *In vivo* response to starch-based scaffolds designed for bone tissue engineering applications. *J Biomed Mater Res A* 80A: 983–9.

Samee, M., Kasugai, S., Kondo, H., Ohya, K., Shimokawa, H., and Kuroda, S. 2008. Bone morphogenetic protein-2 (bmp-2) and vascular endothelial growth factor (vegf) transfection to human periosteal cells enhances osteoblast differentiation and bone formation. *J Pharmacol Sci* 108: 18–31.

Schmid, P., Cox, D., Bilbe, G., Maier, R., and Mcmaster, G. 1991. Differential expression of tgf beta-1, beta-2, and beta-3 genes during mouse embryogenesis. *Development* 111: 117–30.

Schmoekel, H., Schense, J., Weber, F. et al. 2004. Bone healing in the rat and dog with nonglycosylated bmp-2 demonstrating low solubility in fibrin matrices. *J Orthopaed Res* 22: 376–81.

Schwarz, F., Sager, M., Ferrari, D., Mihatovic, I., and Becker, J. 2009. Influence of recombinant human platelet-derived growth factor on lateral ridge augmentation using biphasic calcium phosphate and guided bone regeneration: A histomorphometric study in dogs. *J Periodontol* 80: 1315–23.

Scotti, C., Tonnarelli, B., Papadimitropoulos, A. et al. 2010. Recapitulation of endochondral bone formation using human adult mesenchymal stem cells as a paradigm for developmental engineering. *Proc Natl Acad Sci* 107: 7251–6.

Seebach, C., Henrich, D., Kaehling, C. et al. 2010. Endothelial progenitor cells and mesenchymal stem cells seeded onto beta-tcp granules enhance early vascularization and bone healing in a critical-sized bone defect in rats. *Tissue Eng Pt A* 16: 1961–70.

Shoichet, M., Li, R., White, M., and Winn, S. 1996. Stability of hydrogels used in cell encapsulation: An *in vitro* comparison of alginate and agarose. *Biotechnol Bioeng* 50: 374–81.

Silva, G. A., Coutinho, O. P., Ducheyne, P., Shapiro, I. M., and Reis, R. L. 2007a. Starch-based microparticles as vehicles for the delivery of active platelet-derived growth factor. *Tissue Eng* 13: 1259–68.

Silva, G. A., Coutinho, O. P., Ducheyne, P., Shapiro, I. M., and Reis, R. L. 2007b. The effect of starch and starch-bioactive glass composite microparticles on the adhesion and expression of the osteoblastic phenotype of a bone cell line. *Biomaterials* 28: 326–34.

Simmons, C., Alsberg, E., Hsiong, S., Kim, W., and Mooney, D. 2004. Dual growth factor delivery and controlled scaffold degradation enhance *in vivo* bone formation by transplanted bone marrow stromal cells. *Bone* 35: 562–9.

Singh, I. 1978. The architecture of cancellous bone. *J Anat* 127: 305–10.

Sitharaman, B., Shi, X., Walboomers, X. F. et al. 2008. *In vivo* biocompatibility of ultra-short single-walled carbon nanotube/biodegradable polymer nanocomposites for bone tissue engineering. *Bone* 43: 362–70.

Smith, L. A., Liu, X., Hu, J., and Ma, P. X. 2010. The enhancement of human embryonic stem cell osteogenic differentiation with nano-fibrous scaffolding. *Biomaterials* 31: 5526–35.

Spencer, E., Liu, C., Si, E., and Howard, G. 1991. *In vivo* actions of insulin-like growth factor-i (igf-i) on bone formation and resorption in rats. *Bone* 12: 21–6.

Tabata, Y. and Ikada, Y. 1999. Vascularization effect of basic fibroblast growth factor released from gelatin hydrogels with different biodegradabilities. *Biomaterials* 20: 2169–75.

Thaller, S., Dart, A., and Tesluk, H. 1993. The effects of insulin-like growth factor-1 on critical-size calvarial defects in sprague-dawley rats. *Ann Plas Surg* 31: 429–33.

Tortelli, F., Tasso, R., Loiacono, F., and Cancedda, R. 2010. The development of tissue-engineered bone of different origin through endochondral and intramembranous ossification following the implantation of mesenchymal stem cells and osteoblasts in a murine model. *Biomaterials* 31: 242–9.

Usas, A. and Huard, J. 2007. Muscle-derived stem cells for tissue engineering and regenerative therapy. *Biomaterials* 28: 5401–6.

Vehof, J., Fisher, J., Dean, D. et al. 2002. Bone formation in transforming growth factor beta-1-coated porous poly(propylene fumarate) scaffolds. *J Biomed Mater Res* 60: 241–51.

Venugopal, J. R., Low, S., Choon, A. T., Kumar, A. B., and Ramakrishna, S. 2008. Nanobioengineered electrospun composite nanofibers and osteoblasts for bone regeneration. *Artif Organs* 32: 388–97.

Vikjaer, D., Blom, S., Hjortinghansen, E., and Pinholt, E. 1997. Effect of platelet-derived growth factor-bb on bone formation in calvarial defects: An experimental study in rabbits. *Eur J Oral Sci* 105: 59–66.

Wang, S., Kempen, D. H. R., Yaszemski, M. J., and Lu, L. 2009. The roles of matrix polymer crystallinity and hydroxyapatite nanoparticles in modulating material properties of photo-crosslinked composites and bone marrow stromal cell responses. *Biomaterials* 30: 3359–70.

Webster, T., Ergun, C., Doremus, R., Siegel, R., and Bizios, R. 2000. Specific proteins mediate enhanced osteoblast adhesion on nanophase ceramics. *J Biomed Mater Res* 51: 475–83.

Woo, K. M., Jun, J. H., Chen, V. J. et al. 2007. Nano-fibrous scaffolding promotes osteoblast differentiation and biomineralization. *Biomaterials* 28: 335–43.

Yilgor, P., Tuzlakoglu, K., Reis, R. L., Hasirci, N., and Hasirci, V. 2009. Incorporation of a sequential bmp-2/bmp-7 delivery system into chitosan-based scaffolds for bone tissue engineering. *Biomaterials* 30: 3551–9.

Young, S., Patel, Z. S., Kretlow, J. D. et al. 2009. Dose effect of dual delivery of vascular endothelial growth factor and bone morphogenetic protein-2 on bone regeneration in a rat critical-size defect model. *Tissue Eng Pt A* 15: 2347–62.

Yuan, Q., Kubo, T., Doi, K. et al. 2009. Effect of combined application of bfgf and inorganic polyphosphate on bioactivities of osteoblasts and initial bone regeneration. *Acta Biomater* 5: 1716–24.

Zhang, L. and Webster, T. J. 2009. Nanotechnology and nanomaterials: Promises for improved tissue regeneration. *Nano Today* 4: 66–80.

Zhao, Y., Zou, B., Shi, Z., Wu, Q., and Chen, G. Q. 2007. The effect of 3-hydroxybutyrate on the *in vitro* differentiation of murine osteoblast mcm-e1 and *in vivo* bone formation in ovariectomized rats. *Biomaterials* 28: 3063–73.

Zreiqat, H., Ramaswamy, Y., Wu, C. et al. 2010. The incorporation of strontium and zinc into a calcium-silicon ceramic for bone tissue engineering. *Biomaterials* 31: 3175–84.

# 28

# Dental and Craniofacial Bioengineering

28.1 Introduction ........................................................................28-1
28.2 Clinical Challenges of Dental, Oral, and Craniofacial
Bioengineering........................................................................28-1
28.3 Bone Regeneration................................................................28-2
28.4 Tooth Regeneration ..............................................................28-9
28.5 Soft-Tissue Regeneration ....................................................28-11
28.6 Concluding Remarks............................................................28-16
Acknowledgments............................................................................28-17
References........................................................................................28-17

Hemin Nie
*Columbia University
Medical Center*

Jeremy J. Mao
*Columbia University
Medical Center*

## 28.1 Introduction

There are strong, unmet clinical needs for biological restoration of dental, oral, and craniofacial structures lost to congenital malformations, trauma, chronic diseases, and postneoplastic surgeries (Mao et al. 2006; Miura et al. 2006). Bioengineering offers important opportunities for the regeneration of dental, oral, and craniofacial tissues and organs. Conventionally, dental, oral, and craniofacial defects are treated with tissue grafting or durable materials such as amalgam or titanium dental implants (Zaky and Cancedda 2009). However, tissue grafting is associated with intrinsic drawbacks including donor-site trauma, tissue mismatch, and potential immune rejection, and pathogen transmission (Bhatt and Le Anh 2009). The durable materials do not necessarily translate into long-term cure. For example, both amalgam and titanium dental implants are not permanent solutions. Tissue engineering has been developed over the past two decades and promises to regenerate the native tissue analogs from biological approaches. Biomedical engineering research has been an important element of tissue engineering.

## 28.2 Clinical Challenges of Dental, Oral, and Craniofacial Bioengineering

When shifting rehabilitation strategies from prosthetic to regenerative, the unique and unusual features of dental, oral, and craniofacial tissues are of paramount importance. First, when the appendicular skeleton is derived from the mesoderm and forms bone through endochondral ossification, most of the craniofacial structures are a mixture of cranial–neural crest and the paraxial mesoderm (Akintoye et al. 2006). During facial development, the neural crest cells migrate, differentiate, and subsequently participate in the morphogenesis of virtually all craniofacial structures, including cartilage (condyles and nasal septum), bone, nerves, salivary glands, ligaments, cranial sutures, musculature, tendons, the periodontium, and teeth (Mao et al. 2006; Bhatt and Le Anh 2009). Second, most dental, oral, and craniofacial structures are richly supplied with blood vessels. This is considered highly advantageous when regenerative approaches are attempted. Third, many dental and oral structures commute with the external environment, which offers advantages for easy access and typically less surgical trauma when regenerative technologies are applied, but nonetheless present as microbial and potentially infectious environment for the survival of regenerating tissues (Bhatt and Le Anh 2009). Fourth, the restoration of dental, oral, and craniofacial tissues not only needs to consider functional outcome, but also esthetics (Zaky and Cancedda 2009). Fifth, multiple tissue phenotypes are adjacent in many of dental, oral, and craniofacial structures, presenting additional challenges for biological restoration of tissue defects. Sixth, scar formation in the oral cavity is not nearly extensive as in the skin. Seventh, cells with properties of stem/progenitor cells have been identified in dental, oral, and craniofacial structures (Miura et al. 2006; Zhao et al. 2006; Mao 2008). The dental, oral, and craniofacial stem/progenitor cells are being explored for their potential in the healing of tissues they natively develop into, as well as nondental tissues (Mao et al. 2006; Miura et al. 2006; Zhao et al. 2006; Mao 2008; Yang et al. 2010).

## 28.3 Bone Regeneration

Bone defects are one of the most commonly missing tissues among dental, oral, and craniofacial structures. Over the past decade, different biomaterials and engineering strategies have been applied for reconstructive indications. However, autologous bone grafts are still considered as the gold standard for the reconstruction of extended bone defects. While reconstruction of small to moderate-sized bone defects using engineered bone tissues is technically feasible, and some of the currently developed concepts may represent alternatives to autologous bone grafts for certain clinical conditions, the reconstruction of large volume defects remains challenging (Kneser et al. 2006). The core issue is vascularization. Adequate vascularization is a prerequisite for the formation of functional bone. Diffusion is the initial process involved in the early phase of regeneration, but can only provide for cell support within a maximum range of 200 μm into the matrix (Folkman and Hochberg 1973; Goldstein et al. 2001). The survival of cells in the center of large cell-containing constructs is therefore often limited by suboptimal initial vascularization (Kneser et al. 1999). The cell-labeling experiments disclosed a considerable loss of osteoblasts within the first week following transplantation in porous cancellous bone matrices (Kneser et al. 2006). This limitation in the size of the regenerating bone applies to soft tissues as well. For example, periodontal ligament (PDL) with direct insertions into the teeth and gingival bone exhibit a multitissue transition. Therefore, the development of integrated craniofacial tissue systems will require not only the mimicking of "isolated" structures, such as bone and muscle, but also the concurrent regeneration of the complex *tissue-to-tissue* interfaces to reestablish the systemic functions. The long-term clinical outcome of the orofacial reconstruction relies on the ability to drive local cells, stem cells, or committed progenitor cells, to completely regenerate the defect, which would not repair on its own (Bhatt and Le Anh 2009).

A major goal of research in bone transplantation is the ability to avoid the creation of secondary bone defects. For example, an important study showed the repair of an extended mandibular discontinuity defect by growing a custom bone transplant inside the latissimus dorsi muscle of an adult male patient (Warnke et al. 2004). Three-dimensional (3D) computed tomography (CT) scanning and computer-aided design techniques were used to produce a custom-made model for the mandibular defect (Figure 28.1). A titanium mesh cage was filled with bone mineral blocks and infiltrated with 7 mg recombinant human bone morphogenetic protein 7 and 20 mL of the patient's bone marrow. The transplant was then placed into the latissimus dorsi muscle for 7 weeks before it was transplanted as a free bone–muscle flap to repair a mandibular defect in a patient (Figure 28.1). The results of *in vivo* skeletal scintigraphy showed bone remodelling and mineralization inside the mandibular transplant both before and after transplantation. The radiological evidence of new bone formation (Figure 28.2) indicates heterotopic bone induction to form a mandibular replacement inside the latissimus dorsi muscle in a human patient (Warnke et al. 2004).

Large cranial defects do not spontaneously heal and pose specific health burden. A study carried out by Cowan et al. (2004) showed the *in vivo* osteogenic capability of adipose-derived adult stromal (ADAS) cells, bone marrow stromal (BMS) cells, calvarial-derived osteoblasts, and dura mater cells

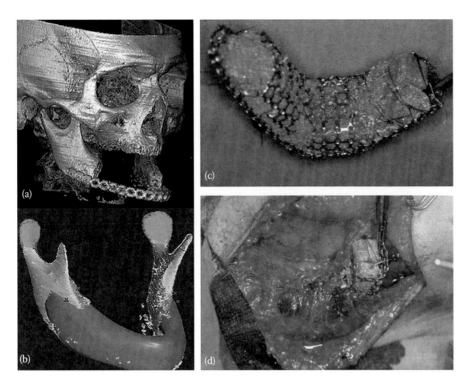

**FIGURE 28.1** **(See color insert.)** Three-dimensional CT scan of size defect (a) CAD plan of an ideal mandibular transplant (b) titanium mesh cage filled with bone mineral blocks infiltrated with recombinant human BMP7 and bone-marrow mixture (c) and implantation into right latissimus dorsi muscle (d).

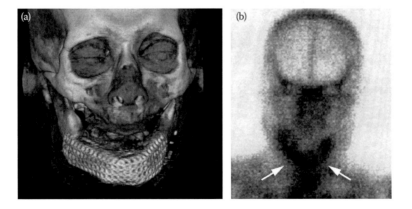

**FIGURE 28.2** **(See color insert.)** Three-dimensional CT scans (a) after transplantation of bone replacement with the enhancement of soft tissue (red) and repeated skeletal scintigraphy (b) with the tracer enhancement showing continued bone remodeling and mineralization (arrows).

to heal the critical-sized mouse calvarial defects (Cowan et al. 2004). The implanted, apatite-coated, poly(D-L-lactic-*co*-glycolic acid) (PLGA) scaffolds seeded with ADAS or BMS cells produced significant intramembranous bone formation by 2 weeks with complete bony bridging by 12 weeks as shown by x-ray analysis, histology, and live micromolecular imaging (Figure 28.3). The contribution of implanted cells to new bone formation was 84–99% by chromosomal detection. These data show that ADAS cells

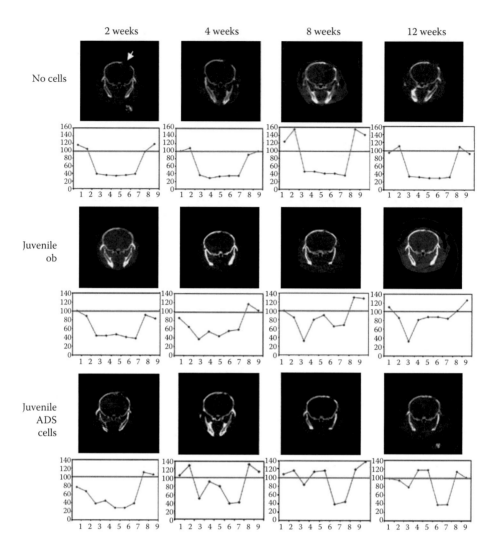

**FIGURE 28.3** Individual animals from control (no cell), juvenile calvarial-derived osteoblasts, and juvenile ADS cell-seeded scaffolds were anesthetized and imaged at 2, 4, 8, and 12 weeks after implantation. The images are a posterior view of a coronal-sliced CT. Note that the defects in the parietal bone are visible on the right side of the image. The area of the defect is indicated on the top left panel with a white arrow; defects are in a similar location in all the remaining specimens. Below each image is a graph demonstrating the location on the *x* axis and the percent density on the *y* axis as compared to the uninjured left parietal bone of each animal. The densities were measured from left to right with two points outside the defect medially, five points inside the defect, and two points outside the defect laterally. The solid line at 100% represents the density of the corresponding uninjured left parietal bone.

heal the critical-sized skeletal defects without genetic manipulation or the addition of exogenous growth factors (Cowan et al. 2004).

As mentioned in the previous section, the site-specific differences complicate the regeneration of craniofacial damages. In the skull vault, the neural crest-derived frontal bones have an increased healing capacity and higher expression levels of fibroblast growth factor-ligands as compared to mesoderm-derived parietal bones. Behr et al. studied whether fibroblast growth factor-ligands are responsible for the superior healing potential of the frontal bones (Behr et al. 2010). The parietal defects in juvenile and adult mice treated with fibroblast growth factor-2, -9 and -18 showed increased bone regeneration, comparable to frontal defects (Figure 28.4). The immunohistochemistry revealed an increased recruitment of osteoprogenitors and activation of fibroblast growth factor (FGF)-signaling pathways in FGF-treated parietal defects. Conversely, calvarial defects in *Fgf-9*[+/−] and *Fgf-18*[+/−] mice showed impaired calvarial healing which could be rescued by exogenous fibroblast growth factor ligands. Moreover, by utilizing *Wnt1Cre/R26R* mice, the migration and contribution of dura mater and pericranium cells to calvarial healing could be demonstrated. Taken together, the results demonstrated that different

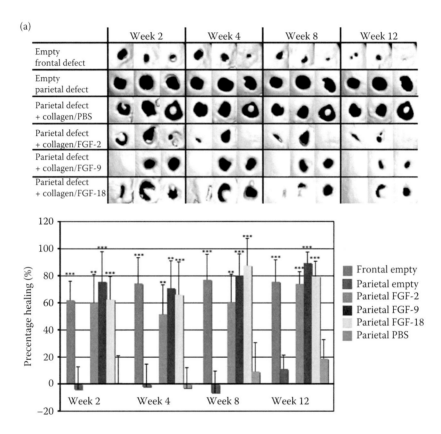

**FIGURE 28.4** (**See color insert.**) FGF-ligands accelerate calvarial healing. (a) Healing in CD1 p7 mice: CT images of the defects of p7 mice at 2, 4, 8, and 12 weeks. In addition to the frontal defects (top row), parietal defects, and parietal defects treated with PBS are presented (second and third row). The frontal defects healed significantly better than the parietal defects. The FGF-treated parietal defects are shown in the lower three rows. By adding FGF-ligands to parietal defects, the parietal bone healed like the frontal bone. The graph represents the quantification of calvarial healing in p7 mice over the course of time. (b) Healing in CD1 p60 mice: CT images of p60 mice revealed an increased healing capacity of the frontal bone compared to the parietal bone. FGF-ligands enhanced the healing of parietal defects, however only FGF-18 could mimic the healing capacity of the frontal bone. The graph represents the quantification of calvarial healing in p60 mice. The asterisks indicate the significant levels of the Student *t*-test frontal versus parietal defects (left bars) and FGF-treated versus controls (right bars): *$p < 0.05$, **$p < 0.005$, and ***$p < 0.0005$. (c) CT-scans and corresponding Pentachrome staining of calvaria 12 weeks postoperatively: For each calvaria, the top section (F) represents the frontal defect and the bottom section the parietal defect (P). The yellow color indicates the mature bone. The dashed arrows highlight the defects and the osteogenic fronts are lateral of these markings. At the top row, the superior healing potential of the untreated frontal defect as compared to the parietal defect can be appreciated. The application of FGF-2 to parietal defects led to increased healing in p7 and p60 mice (middle row). FGF-18 substantially increased healing in p60 parietal defects (bottom row). The arrowheads indicate the dura mater. Abbreviation: F, frontal; P, parietal (scale bar: 200 μm).

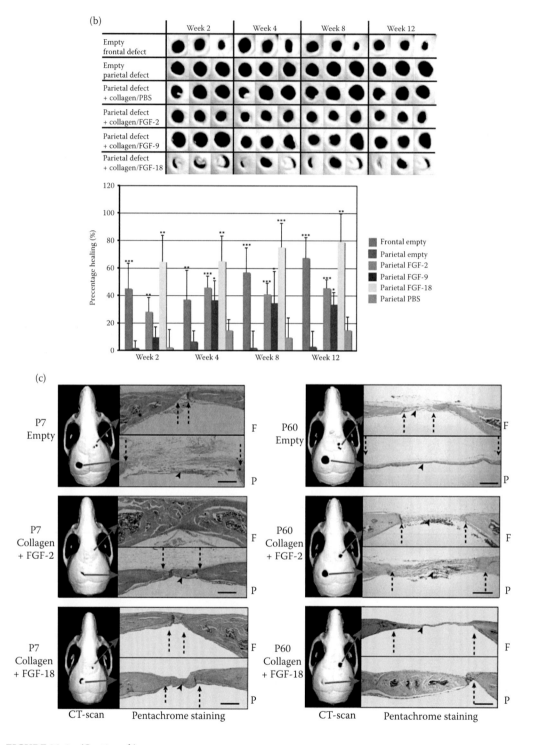

**FIGURE 28.4** (Continued.)

endogenous threshold levels of fibroblast growth factor-ligands in frontal and parietal bones have a profound impact on calvarial regeneration (Behr et al. 2010).

A controlled release technology has been successfully incorporated into wound healing and craniofacial regeneration. Moioli et al. reported the microencapsulation of TGFbeta3 in poly(D-L-lactic-*co*-glycolic acid) (PLGA) microspheres and determined its bioactivity (Moioli et al. 2006). The release profiles of PLGA-encapsulated TGFbeta3 with 50:50 and 75:25 PLA:PGA ratios differed throughout the experimental period. To compare sterilization modalities of microspheres, bFGF was encapsulated in 50:50 PLGA microspheres and subjected to ethylene oxide (EO) gas, radio-frequency glow discharge (RFGD), or ultraviolet (UV) light. The release of bFGF was significantly attenuated by UV light, but not significantly altered by either EO or RFGD. To verify its bioactivity, TGFbeta3 (1.35 ng/mL) was control-released to the culture of human mesenchymal stem cells (hMSC) under induced osteogenic differentiation. The alkaline–phosphatase-staining intensity was markedly reduced 1 week after exposing hMSC-derived osteogenic cells to TGFbeta3. This was confirmed by the lower alkaline–phosphatase activity ($2.25 \pm 0.57$ mU/mL/ng DNA) than controls (TGFbeta3- free) at $5.8 \pm 0.9$ mU/mL/ng DNA ($p < 0.05$). A control-released TGFbeta3 bioactivity was further confirmed by lack of significant differences in alkaline–phosphatase upon direct addition of 1.35 ng/mL TGFbeta3 to cell culture ($p > 0.05$). These findings provide a baseline data for the potential uses of microencapsulated TGFbeta3 in wound healing and tissue-engineering applications. Specifically, the advantages of this technology were manifested in healing craniosynostosis defects. It was demonstrated that autologous mesenchymal stem cells (MSCs) and controlled-released TGFβ3 reduced surgical trauma to the localized osteotomy and minimized osteogenesis in a rat craniosynostosis model (Moioli et al. 2008). Approximately, 0.5 mL tibial marrow content was aspirated to isolate mononucleated and adherent cells that were characterized as MSCs. Upon resecting the synostosed suture, autologous MSCs in collagen carriers with microencapsulated TGFβ3 (1 ng/mL) generated cranial suture analogs characterized as bone–soft tissue–bone interface by quantitative histomorphometric and μCT analyses (Figure 28.5). Thus, surgical trauma in craniosynostosis can be minimized by a biologically viable implant. They speculated that the proportionally larger amounts of human marrow aspirates participate in the healing of craniosynostosis

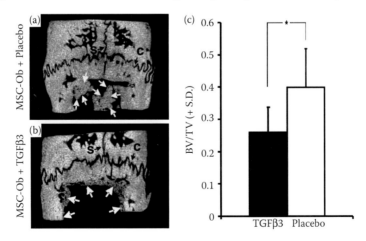

**FIGURE 28.5** Regulation of postsurgical synostosis in the engineered cranial suture. (a) Microcomputed tomography (μCT) showing substantial progression of resynostosis characterized as newly formed bone and mineralization (white arrows) in the resected cranial suture osteotomy site implanted with a placebo PLGA carrier after 4 weeks (c: coronal suture; s: sagittal suture). (b) Secondary synostosis was substantially curbed upon the implantation of autologous MSCs and control-released TGFβ3 in a collagen carrier after 4 weeks. (c) Quantification of new bone volume over total tissue volume (BV/TV) by computerized histomorphometric analysis showed significantly more mineralization in osteotomized synostosis suture healed with autologous MSCs and placebo collagen carriers than autologous MSCs and control-released TGFβ3 collagen carriers ($p < 0.05$).

defects in patients. The engineered soft tissue–bone interface may have implications in the repair of tendons, ligaments, periosteum, and periodontal ligaments.

Gene therapy is defined as the treatment of disease by transfer of genetic material into cells. Scheller et al. summarized the methods available for gene transfer as well as the current and potential applications for craniofacial regeneration, with an emphasis on future development and design (Scheller and Krebsbach 2009). Although nonviral gene delivery methods are limited by low gene transfer efficiency, they benefit from relative safety, low immunogenicity, ease of manufacture, and lack of DNA which insert size limitation. In contrast, viral vectors are nature's gene delivery machines that can be optimized to allow for tissue-specific targeting, site-specific chromosomal integration, and efficient long-term infection of dividing and nondividing cells. In contrast to traditional replacement gene therapy, craniofacial regeneration seeks to use genetic vectors as supplemental building blocks for tissue growth and repair. A synergistic combination of viral gene therapy with craniofacial tissue engineering will significantly enhance our ability to repair and replace tissues *in vivo* (Figure 28.6).

Viral delivery of the therapeutic gene bone morphogenetic protein-2 (BMP-2) is a promising approach for bone regeneration. The human parvovirus adeno-associated virus (AAV) type 2 is considered one of the most encouraging viral-vector systems because of its high transduction rates and biosafety ratings. BMP-2 is a highly potent osteoinductive protein, which induces bone formation *in vivo* and osteogenic differentiation *in vitro*. The exogenous regulation of BMP-2 expression in bone-regenerating sites is required to control BMP-2 protein secretion, thus promoting safe and controlled bone formation and regeneration. Therefore, Gafni et al. constructed a dual-construct vector for the recombinant AAV (rAAV)-based recombinant human BMP-2 (rhBMP-2) gene delivery system, which is regulated by the tetracycline-sensitive promoter (TetON) (Gafni et al. 2004). Each vector was encapsidated separately, yielding two recombinant viruses. Then they proceed to evaluate the efficiency of rAAV-hBMP-2 to induce bone formation in ectopic and orthotopic sites (Figure 28.7). Doxycycline (Dox), an analog of tetracycline, was orally administered to mice via their drinking water to induce rhBMP-2 expression. Bone formation was measured using quantitative imaging-microcomputerized tomography and cooled charge-coupled device imagingto detect osteogenic activity at the cellular level, detecting osteocalcin expression. The rAAV-hBMP-2-treated mice that were given Dox demonstrated bone formation in both *in vivo* models compared to none in mice prevented from receiving

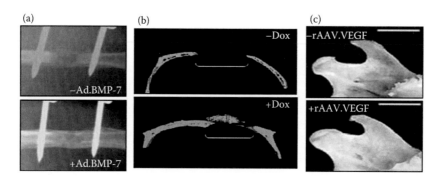

**FIGURE 28.6 (See color insert.)** Gene therapy for bone regeneration. (a) An "expedited *ex vivo*" bone regeneration strategy has recently been proposed in which explants of adipose tissue or muscle can be directly transduced with Ad.BMP-2 without culture. This has shown promising results in the regeneration of critical-sized rat femoral defects. (From Betz, V. M. et al. 2008. *Front Biosci* 13: 833–841.) (b) A vector for rAAV-based BMP-2 gene delivery regulated by the TetON has been generated. (Adapted from Gafni, Y. et al. 2004. *Mol Ther* 9(4): 587–595.) Calvarial defect bone formation was noted in mice only after the administration of Doxycycline via drinking water to induce BMP-2 expression. This represents a novel strategy for localized inducible gene expression. (c) Local injection of rAAV-VEGF to the mandibular condyle of rats results in increased condylar growth after 60 days, as demonstrated by increased condyle width and length.

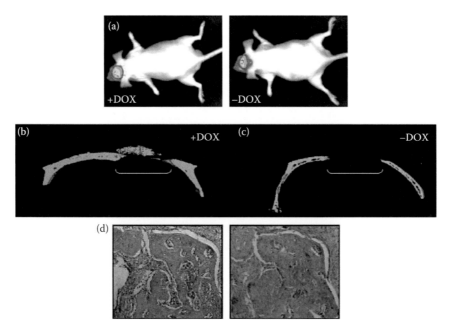

**FIGURE 28.7** **(See color insert.)** *In vivo* transduction of hMSCs in an orthotopic site (critically sized calvarial defect). Human AMSC Retro-Luc was transplanted into a critically sized calvarial defect and transduced with a viral mixture of AAV-BMP-2 at 4 days postimplantation. (a) CCCD images of +Dox and −Dox mice indicate cell localization and survival at 8 days postimplantation. The experiment was terminated on day 28 and the dissected calvaria was analyzed with micro-CT imaging. (b) In the +Dox group rAAV-BMP-2 activity is apparent, resulting in the regeneration of bone within the defect on day 28. (c) In the −Dox group, no regeneration of bone is evident on day 28. (d) Histological sections stained with H&E and Masson trichrome showing the presence of new bone in the calvarial defect in animals treated with Dox (original magnification ×20).

Dox. Thus, the Tet-regulated rAAV-hBMP-2 vector is an effective means of induction and regulation of bone regeneration and repair.

## 28.4 Tooth Regeneration

Regeneration of teeth can be broadly divided into several areas as listed below. It is impossible to cover, in one article, of the rapidly developing field of tooth regeneration in breadth or complexity

- Regeneration or de novo formation of the entire, anatomically correct teeth (discussed at length below);
- Regeneration of the dental pulp (discussed at length below);
- Regeneration of dentin based on biological approaches and potentially as biological fillers that may replace the current synthetic materials for restorative dentistry (Shi et al. 2005; Thesleff et al. 2007; Golub 2009; Huang 2009);
- Regeneration of cementum as part of periodontium regeneration or for loss of cementum and/ or dentin resulting from orthodontic tooth movement (Zeichner-David 2006; Foster et al. 2007);
- Regeneration of periodontium including cementum, PDL, and alveolar bone (Cooke et al. 2006; Lin et al. 2009; Pellegrini et al. 2009);
- Regeneration or synthesis of enamel-like structures that may be used as a biological substitute for the lost enamel (Huang et al. 2008; Palmer et al. 2008; Zhang et al. 2010);
- Remineralization of enamel and dentin (Huang et al. 2008; Palmer et al. 2008; Zhang et al. 2010).

A multiscale computational design and fabrication of composite hybrid polymeric scaffolds was used for the targeted cell transplantation of the genetically modified human cells for the formation of human tooth dentin–ligament–bone complexes *in vivo* (Park et al. 2010). The newly formed tissues demonstrate the interfacial generation of parallel- and obliquely oriented fibers that grow and traverse within the polycaprolactone (PCL)-poly(glycolic acid) (PGA)- designed constructs forming tooth cementum-like tissue, ligament, and bone structures (Park et al. 2010). This approach offers a potential for the clinical implementation of the customized periodontal scaffolds that may enable regeneration of multitissue interfaces required for oral, dental, and craniofacial engineering applications.

As an initial attempt to regenerate teeth, we first fabricated an anatomically shaped and dimensioned scaffold from biomaterials (Kim et al. 2010), using our previously reported approach (Lee et al. 2009; Stosich et al. 2009). The dimensions of the permanent mandibular first molar were derived from textbook averages and institutional review board (IRB) exempt. Scaffolds with the shape of the human mandibular first molar (Figure 28.8) were fabricated via 3D layer-by-layer apposition (Lee et al. 2009; Stosich et al. 2009). The composite consisted of 80 wt% PCL and 20 wt% of hydroxyapatite (HA) (Sigma, St. Louis, MO). PCL-HA was comolten at 120°C and dispensed through a 27-gauge metal nozzle to create repeating 3D microstrands (200 μm wall thickness) and interconnecting microchannels (dia: 200 μm) (Figure 28.8) (Kim et al. 2010).

All scaffolds were sterilized in EO for 24 h. A blended cocktail of SDF1 (100 ng/mL) and BMP7 (100 ng/mL) was adsorbed in 2 mg/mL neutralized type I collagen solution (all from R&D, Minneapolis, MN). SDF1 was selected for its effects to bind to CXCR4 receptors of multiple cell lineages including mesenchymal stem/progenitor cells (Belema-Bedada et al. 2008; Kitaori et al. 2009). BMP7 was selected for its effects on dental pulp cells, fibroblasts, and osteoblasts in elaborating mineralization (Goldberg et al. 2001). SDF1 and BMP7 doses were chosen from *in vivo* work (Vaccaro et al. 2008; Kitaori et al. 2009). SDF1- and BMP7-loaded collagen solution was infused in the scaffold's microchannels by micro-pippeting, and crosslinked at 37°C for 1 h. The control scaffolds were infused with the same collagen gel but without growth-factor delivery.

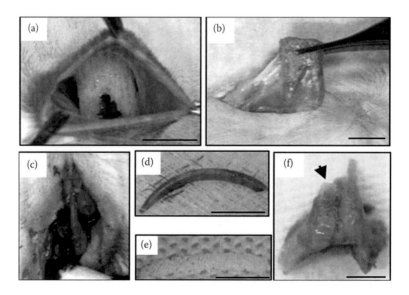

**FIGURE 28.8** **(See color insert.)** *In vivo* orthotopic and ectopic implantation of anatomically shaped tooth scaffolds. (a) *In vivo* implantation of human mandibular molar scaffold into the rat's dorsum constitutes an ectopic model for tooth regeneration. (b) Harvest of human molar scaffold showing integration and tissue ingrowth. (c) Extraction of the right rat's mandibular central incisor. (d) The extracted rat's mandibular central incisor. (e) The fabricated rat's mandibular central incisor scaffold. (f) Harvest of *in vivo*-implanted rat's mandibular central incisor scaffold orthotopically in the extraction socket showing integration of the implanted scaffold. Scale: 5 mm.

Following the Institutional Animal Care and Use Committee (IACUC) approval, a total of 22 male Sprague–Dawley rats (12-week-old) were randomly divided equally into treatment and control groups (Charles River, NY). The rat's right mandibular central incisor was extracted with periotome (data not shown but can be found in Kim et al. 2010), followed by implantation of the anatomically shaped mandibular incisor scaffold (data not shown but can be found in Kim et al. 2010) into the extraction socket. The flap was advanced for primary closure around the scaffold. Nine weeks postsurgery, all rats were euthanized by pentobarbital overdose. The dorsum scaffolds were retrieved with the surrounding fascia. The rat's incisor scaffolds were harvested with the surrounding bone and native tooth structures (Kim et al. 2010). All samples were fixed in 10% formalin, embedded in poly(methyl methacrylate) (PMMA), sectioned at 5 μm thickness for hematoxylin and eosin (H&E) and von-Kossa (VK) staining (HSRL, Jackson, VA). PMMA was used because PCL-HA scaffolds cannot be demineralized for paraffin embedding. The average areal cell density and blood vessel numbers were quantified from the coronal, middle, and apical thirds of the rat's incisor scaffolds and similarly of the human molar scaffolds by a blinded and calibrated examiner.

Microscopically, host cells populated scaffold's microchannels with growth-factor delivery (Figure 28.8). Quantitatively, the combined SDF1 and BMP7 delivery homed significantly more cells into the microchannels of the human molar scaffolds than without growth-factor delivery ($p < 0.01$) (data not shown but can be found in Kim et al. 2010). Angiogenesis took place in microchannels with growth-factor delivery as exemplified in Figure 28.8. The combined SDF1 and BMP7 delivery elaborated significantly more blood vessels than without growth-factor delivery ($p < 0.05$) (data not shown but can be found in Kim et al. 2010). Scaffolds in the shape of the rat's mandibular incisor integrated with the surrounding tissue, showed tissue ingrowth into the scaffold's microchannels (Figure 28.8). It was not possible to separate the implanted scaffolds without causing a physical damage to the surrounding tissue. Microscopically, the scaffolds within the extraction sockets clearly showed multiple tissue phenotypes including the native alveolar bone (b), newly formed bone (nb), and a fibrous tissue interface that is reminiscent of the PDL (Figure 28.8) that integrated to host the alveolar bone. Angiogenesis took place in the scaffolds' microchannels with growth-factor delivery (Figure 28.8). Quantitatively, the combined SDF1 and BMP7 delivery elaborated significantly more blood vessels than the growth-factor-free group ($p < 0.05$) (data not shown but can be found in Kim et al. 2010).

These findings are described in detail in Kim et al. (2010) representing the first report of regeneration of the anatomically shaped tooth-like structures *in vivo*, and by cell homing without cell delivery. The potency of cell homing is substantiated not only by cell recruitment into the scaffold's microchannels, but also by regeneration of a putative PDL and a newly formed alveolar bone (Kim et al. 2010). One of the pivotal issues in tooth regeneration is to devise economically viable approaches that are not cost-prohibitive and can translate into therapies for patients who cannot afford or are counter-indicated for dental implants. Cell homing-based tooth regeneration may provide a tangible pathway toward clinical translation. These two highlighted reports demonstrate the proof of concept for the potentially translatable tooth regeneration approaches (Kim et al. 2010; Park et al. 2010).

## 28.5 Soft-Tissue Regeneration

The current treatment modalities for soft-tissue defects caused by various pathologies and trauma include autologous grafting and commercially available fillers. However, these treatment methods present a number of challenges and limitations, such as donor-site morbidity and volume loss over time (Stosich et al. 2009; Choi et al. 2010; Mao et al., TE review, 2009). As such, the improved therapeutic modalities need to be developed. Tissue engineering techniques offer novel solutions to these problems through the development of bioactive tissue constructs that can regenerate adipose tissue in both structure and function. Recently, a number of studies have been designed to explore the various methods to engineer the human adipose tissue. The clinical goals for adipose tissue engineering include the regenerated tissue that both cosmetically and mechanically resembles the native tissue. This includes mechanical integrity as well as sustainability and viability of the tissue over time. Additionally, adipose tissue that possesses an active metabolic function would serve as a significant advancement over the current soft-tissue replacement strategies (Stosich et al. 2009; Choi et al. 2010; Mao et al., TE review, 2009).

A critical barrier in tissue regeneration is scale-up. The bioengineered adipose tissue implants have been limited to approximately 10 mm in diameter. Moioli et al. devised a 40 mm hybrid implant with a cellular layer encapsulating an acellular core (Moioli et al. 2010). The human adipose-derived stem cells (ASCs) were seeded in alginate. Poly(ethylene)glycol-diacrylate (PEGDA) was photopolymerized into a 40mm-diameter dome-shaped gel (Figure 28.9). Alginate-ASC suspension was painted onto PEGDA surface. The cultivation of hybrid constructs *ex vivo* in adipogenic medium for 28 days showed no delamination. Upon a 4-week *in vivo* implantation in athymic rats, hybrid implants were well-integrated with the host subcutaneous tissue and could only be surgically separated. The vascularized adipose tissue regenerated in the thin-painted alginate layer only if the ASC-derived adipogenic cells were delivered. Contrastingly, the abundant fibrous tissue-filled ASC-free alginate layer encapsulated the acellular PEGDA core in the control implants. Human-specific peroxisome proliferator-activated receptor-gamma (PPAR-gamma) was detected in human ASC-seeded implants. Interestingly, the rat-specific PPAR-gamma was absent in either human ASC-seeded or ASC-free implants. The glycerol content in the ASC-delivered implants was significantly greater than that in ASC-free implants. Remarkably, the rat-specific platelet/endothelial cell adhesion molecule (PECAM) was detected in both ASC-seeded and ASC-free implants, suggesting anastomosis of vasculature in the bioengineered tissue with the host blood vessels. Human nuclear staining revealed that a substantial number of adipocytes were of human origin, whereas endothelial cells of the vascular wall were of chemaric human and nonhuman (rat-host) origins. Together, hybrid implant appears to be a viable scale-up approach with volumetric retention attributable primarily to the acellular biomaterial core, and yet has a biologically viable cellular interface with the host. The present 40mm soft tissue implant may serve as a biomaterial tissue expander for reconstruction of lumpectomy defects.

Vascularization is critical to the survival of engineered tissues. Therefore, Stosich et al. combined the biophysical and bioactive approaches to induce neovascularization *in vivo*. They tested the effects of engineered vascularization on adipose tissue grafts. Hydrogel cylinders were fabricated from poly(ethylene glycol) diacrylate (PEG) in four configurations: PEG alone, PEG with basic fibroblast growth-factor (bFGF), microchanneled-PEG, or both bFGF-adsorbed and microchanneled-PEG (Figure 28.10). *In vivo* implantation revealed no neovascularization in PEG, but substantial angiogenesis in bFGF-adsorbed and/or microchanneled-PEG. The infiltrating host tissue consisted of erythrocyte-filled blood vessels lined by endothelial cells, and immunolocalized to vascular endothelial growth factor (VEGF). hMSC were differentiated into adipogenic cells, and encapsulated in PEG with both microchanneled- and adsorbed-bFGF. Upon *in vivo* implantation subcutaneously in immunodeficient mice, oil-red O positive adipose tissue was present and interspersed with interstitial fibrous (IF) capsules. VEGF was immunolocalized in the IF capsules surrounding the engineered adipose tissue. These findings suggest that bioactive cues and/or microchannels promote the genesis of vascularized tissue phenotypes such as the

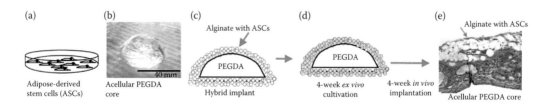

**FIGURE 28.9   (See color insert.)** Fabrication of the hybrid soft tissue implant. (a) Human ASCs were culture expanded for 3 weeks. (b) PEGDA hydrogel was photopolymerized in breast shape (diameter 40 mm) without any cells. (c) ASCs were seeded in alginate solution and painted on PEDGA surface to form a hybrid construct. (d) After 4-week *ex vitro* cultivation, alginate-PEGDA hybrid construct showed no delamination, with or without ASCs. (e) After 4-week *in vivo* implantation, the adipose tissue formed in ASC-seeded alginate later encapsulating an acellular PEGDA core.

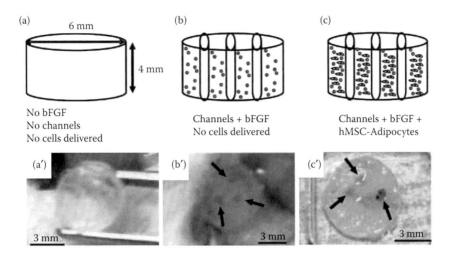

**FIGURE 28.10** (**See color insert.**) *In vivo* implantation of bFGF and microchanneled PEG hydrogel loaded with adipogenic cells derived from hMSCs. The diagrams (top row) correspond to the representative photographs at the time of harvest of *in vivo* samples. (a) PEG hydrogel molded into 6 × 4 mm (width × height) cylinder (without either bFGF or microchannels). (b) PEG hydrogel cylinder loaded with both 0.5 mg/mL bFGF and three microchannels, but without the delivery of cells. (c) PEG hydrogel cylinder loaded with both 0.5 mg/mL bFGF and three microchannels, in addition to the encapsulation of adipogenic cells that have been derived from human mesenchymal stem cells at a cell-seeding density of 3 × 10⁶ cells/mL. Following *in vivo* implantation subcutaneously in the dorsum of immuno-deficient mice, the harvested PEG hydrogel samples showed distinct histological features. (a′) PEG hydrogel cylinder without either microchannels or bFGF showed somewhat transparent appearance. (b′) PEGhydrogel cylinder with both bFGF and three microchannels, but without delivered cells, showed darker color and a total of three openings of microchannels (arrows). (c′) PEG hydrogel cylinder with both microchannels and bFGF in addition to the encapsulated hMSC-derived adipogenic cells showed the opening of microchannels (red color and pointed with arrows).

tested adipose tissue grafts. Especially, the engineered microchannels may provide a generic approach for modifying existing biomaterials by providing conduits for vascularization and/or diffusion.

Besides ASC, BMSC is another option for adipogenesis. A prerequisite to successfully engineer cell-based adipose tissue surrogates is the evaluation of *in vitro* culture conditions that facilitate the expansion of primary precursor cells under retention of their adipogenic potential and that enables a large fraction of the heterogeneous cell pool to undergo adipogenesis upon the respective stimuli. Ascorbic acid (AA) was reported to enhance differentiation of precursor cells into various mesenchymal cell types. Thus, Weiser et al. evaluated the influence of AA on hormonally induced adipogenesis of bone marrow-derived mesenchymal stromal cells (BMSCs) *in vitro* when supplemented during cell propagation and/or adipogenic differentiation (Gafni et al. 2004). BMSCs were isolated from the rat's bone marrow, propagated, and hormonally induced to undergo adipogenesis. Supplementation of AA from the time of induction increased the fraction of BMSCs differentiating into adipocytes and glycerol-3-phosphate dehydrogenase activity up to 2-fold. Furthermore, administration of AA during propagation had an even larger effect with an up to 8-fold increase in adipogenic markers. An assessment of collagen accumulation suggested that the observed effects might be attributed to an enhanced collagen synthesis during propagation. The presented results demonstrate AA as a potent medium component able to enhance adipogenic conversion of BMSCs, especially when administered during cell propagation, and one can take advantage of all the available resources related with BMSCs.

Satellite cells have been widely investigated in the interest of muscular regeneration. They reside beneath the basal lamina of skeletal muscle fibers and include cells that act as precursors for muscle growth and repair. Although they share a common anatomical localization and typically are considered a homogeneous population, satellite cells actually exhibit substantial heterogeneity. Cerletti et al.

used cell-surface marker expression to purify from the satellite cell pool a distinct population of skeletal muscle precursors (SMPs) that function as muscle stem cells (Cerletti et al. 2008). When engrafted into a muscle of dystrophin-deficient mdx mice, purified SMPs contributed up to 94% of myofibers, restoring dystrophin expression and significantly improving muscle histology and contractile function (Figure 28.11). Moreover, transplanted SMPs also entered the satellite cell compartment, renewing the

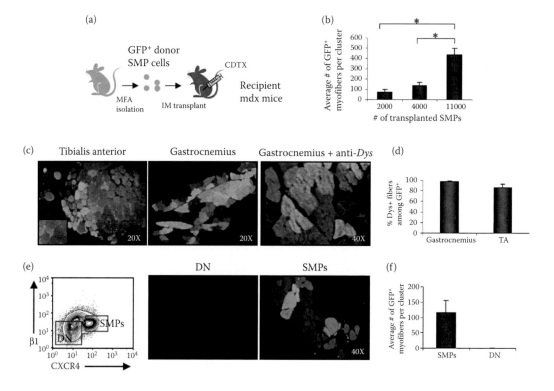

**FIGURE 28.11 (See color insert.)** SMPs robustly engraft skeletal muscle *in vivo* (a) experimental design. Double-sorted GFP+ SMPs were injected intramuscularly into the recipient *mdx* mice injured 1 day previously by injection of cardiotoxin (CDTX) into the same muscle. (b) Quantitative analysis of donor-derived (GFP+) myofibers in TA muscles injected with 2000 ($n = 3$), 4000 ($n = 3$), or 11,000 ($n = 3$) SMPs. The recipient muscles were harvested 4 weeks after transplantation and analyzed for GFP expression by direct epifluorescence microscopy of the transverse muscle sections. The total number of GFP+ myofibers per section was determined for 100–300 sections taken throughout the muscle, to determine the maximal number of donor-derived fibers generated in each muscle. The data are plotted as the mean (±SEM) number of GFP+ myofibers detected in the section of each engrafted muscle that contained the most GFP+ myofibers. *$p < 0.01$. (c) Transverse frozen sections of TA (left panel) and gastrocnemius (middle and right panels) muscles obtained from *mdx* mice transplanted 4 weeks previously with 11,000 GFP+ SMPs showed large clusters of regenerating donor-derived myofibers (GFP+, shown in green) with characteristics of the centrally localized nuclei (inset) and the restored dystrophin expression (shown in red; dystrophin staining is shown on the right image only). GFP detection by epifluorescence (as in c) was confirmed by indirect immunofluorescence and immunohistochemistry using anti-GFP antibodies. (d) Quantification of the frequency (mean ± SD) of dystrophin+ myofibers among GFP+ donor-derived myofibers in the TA or gastrocnemius of *mdx* mice transplanted with 11,000 SMP cells per muscle revealed that the majority (85–100%) of GFP+ myofibers contained dystrophin protein (red), which normally is lacking on most *mdx* myofibers. (e and f) Myofiber-associated cells lacking SMP markers do not generate myofibers when transplanted *in vivo*. CD45−Sca-1−Mac-1−CXCR4−β1-integrin− (double negative, DN) cells or CD45−Sca-1−Mac-1−CXCR4+β1-integrin+ SMPs were twice-sorted (to ensure purity) from β-actin/GFP mice and then transferred at equal cell number (4000 per muscle) into separate preinjured *mdx* recipients. Four weeks after transplant, the injected muscles were harvested and sectioned. No GFP+ myofibers were found in muscles transplanted with DN cells ($n = 3$), while muscles receiving GFP+ SMPs showed an efficient contribution of GFP+ myofibers ($n = 3$).

endogenous stem cell pool and participating in subsequent rounds of injury repair. Together, these studies indicate the presence in adult skeletal muscle of prospectively isolatable muscle-forming stem cells and directly demonstrate the efficacy of myogenic stem cell transplant for treating muscle degenerative diseases.

Little is known whether clones of ectopic, nonmuscle stem cells contribute to muscle regeneration. Stem/progenitor cells that are isolated for experimental research are typically heterogeneous. Nonmyogenic lineages in a heterogeneous population conceptually may compromise muscle repair (Yang RJ, PLoS ONE, in press). Similar to the strategy utilized by Cerletti et al., Yang et al. discovered that clones of mononucleated stem cells of the human tooth pulp fused into multinucleated myotubes that robustly expressed myosin heavy chain *in vitro* with or without coculture with mouse skeletal myoblasts (C2C12 cells). Cloned cells were sustainably Oct4+, Nanog+, and Stro1+. The fusion index of myogenic clones was approximately 16–17 folds greater than their parent, heterogeneous stem cells. Upon infusion into cardio-toxin-induced tibialis anterior (TA) muscle defects, the undifferentiated clonal progenies not only engrafted and colonized the host muscle, but also expressed human dystrophin and myosin heavy chain, more efficaciously than their parent heterogeneous stem cell populations (Figure 28.12). Strikingly, clonal progenies yielded ~9 times more human myosin heavy chain mRNA in regenerating muscles than those infused with their parent, heterogeneous stem cells. The number of human dystrophin positive cells per section in regenerating muscles infused with clonal progenies was more than 3 times greater than muscles infused with heterogeneous stem cells from which clonal progenies were derived (Figure 28.12). These findings suggest the value of myogenic clones as a therapeutic source for muscle defects (Yang RJ, PLoS ONE, in press).

Cell homing, as an alternative to cell delivery/transplantation, has drawn more and more attention due to the advantages of free immunoresponse and harness of the host's regenerative potentials. The synovial joint consists of multiple tissues including articular cartilage, subchondral bone, hematopoietic marrow, and synovium. At present, joints at later stages of osteoarthritis are treated by total joint arthroplasty using metallic and synthetic materials. The existing joint prostheses fail mainly because of aseptic loosening and infections induced by wear debris. Since the average lifespan of these prostheses is 10–15 years, total joint replacement is problematic in the substantial and increasing population of patients with arthritis who are aged 65 years or younger (Lawrence et al. 1998; Park et al. 2009). Similar to the regeneration of other tissues, cartilage regeneration is replete with examples of cell delivery (Gao et al. 2002; Jiang et al.2007; Noh et al. 2010; Scotti et al. 2010). Facing this challenge, Lee et al. tested the hypothesis that the entire articular surface of the synovial joint in a rabbit could be regenerated using a biological cue spatially embedded in an anatomically correct bioscaffold (Lee et al. 2010). In this proof of concept study, the surface morphology of a rabbit's proximal humeral joint was captured with laser scanning and reconstructed by computer-aided design. An anatomically correct bioscaffold was fabricated using a composite of poly-varepsilon-caprolactone and hydroxyapatite. The entire articular surface of unilateral proximal humeral condyles of skeletally mature rabbits was surgically excised and replaced with bioscaffolds spatially infused with the transforming growth-factor beta3 (TGFbeta3)-adsorbed or TGFbeta3-free collagen hydrogel. All animals in the TGFbeta3-delivery group fully resumed weightbearing and locomotion 3–4 weeks after surgery, more consistently than those in the TGFbeta3-free group. Defect-only rabbits limped at all times. Four months after surgery, TGFbeta3-infused bioscaffolds were fully covered with hyaline cartilage in the articular surface (Figure 28.13). TGFbeta3-free bioscaffolds had only isolated cartilage formation, and no cartilage formation occurred in defect-only rabbits. TGFbeta3 delivery yielded uniformly distributed chondrocytes in a matrix with collagen type II and aggrecan and had significantly greater thickness ($p = 0.044$) and density ($p < 0.0001$) than the cartilage formed without TGFbeta3. The compressive and shear properties of TGFbeta3-mediated articular cartilage did not differ from those of the native articular cartilage, and were significantly greater than those of the cartilage formed without TGFbeta3. The regenerated cartilage was avascular and integrated with the regenerated subchondral bone that had well-defined blood vessels. TGFbeta3 delivery recruited roughly 130% more cells in the regenerated articular cartilage

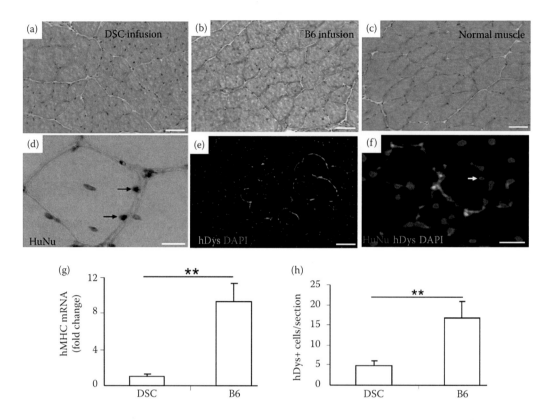

**FIGURE 28.12** **(See color insert.)** Engraftment of the undifferentiated ectopic stem cell clone in the damaged muscle. The TA muscles in NOD/SCID mice were injured by multipoint CTX injection. 24 h following CTX injections, dental stem cells (DSC) and a tested clone (B6) were separately infused in CTX-injured TA muscles with contralateral TA muscles as controls. (a) H&E staining shows the presence of centralized nuclei in the representative DSC-infused sample. (b) The representative B6-infused sample showed an abundant centralized nuclei. In contrast, the representative normal TA muscle has peripheral nuclei (c). The immunohistochemistry staining (brown) of the human-specific nuclei (d) and immunefluorescent staining of the human-specific dystrophin (green) and the human nuclei (red) (e,f) indicates the presence of transplanted human cells in the host TA muscle in the representative B6-infused group. We then harvested *in vivo* muscle samples, isolated RNA for real-time PCR analysis of myogenic differentiation *in vivo*. The quantitative RT-PCR assay revealed that human MHC gene expression in the B6 infusion group after 4 weeks of injection is ~8 times greater than DSC infusion group ($N = 3$, **$p < 0.01$) (g). The quantification of human dystrophin positive cells present in the TA muscle shows that the expression of human dystrophin mRNA was ~3 times greater following B6 infusion than DSC infusion ($N = 3$, **$p < 0.01$) (h). In (d) and (f), the arrows indicate the human nuclei. In (g), the *y* axis represents a fold-change relative to the heterogeneous DSC. Scale bars: A–C, E, F: 50 μm; D: 20 μm.

than the spontaneous cell migration without TGFbeta3. These findings suggest that the entire articular surface of the synovial joint can regenerate without cell transplantation. The regeneration of complex tissues is probable by homing of endogenous cells, as exemplified by the stratified avascular cartilage and the vascularized bone.

## 28.6 Concluding Remarks

Dental, oral, and craniofacial bioengineering continues to evolve and now has come across a pivotal point. Initially, the discovery of stem cells and development of biomaterial scaffolds were two separate fields without much interaction. Since, fundamental studies in stem cell biology and biomaterial development

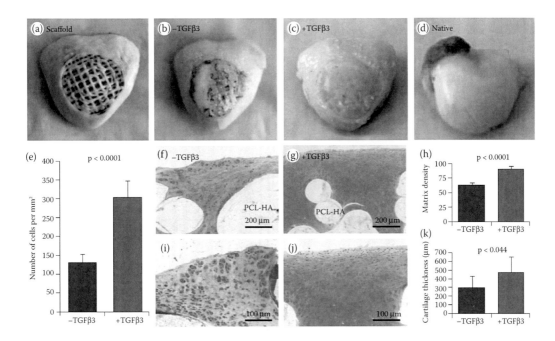

**FIGURE 28.13** (**See color insert.**) Articular cartilage regeneration. Indian ink staining of (a) unimplanted bioscaffold, (b) TGFβ3-free, (c) TGFβ3-infused bioscaffolds after 4 months of implantation, and (d) native cartilage. (e) Number of chondrocytes present in TGFβ3-infused and TGFβ3-free regenerated articular cartilage samples ($n = 8$ per group). Safranin O-staining of TGFβ3-free (f,i) and TGFβ3-infused (g,j) articular cartilage. The matrix density (h) and cartilage thickness (k) of TGFβ3-infused and TGFβ3-free samples ($n = 8$ per group for both comparisons).

undoubtedly would continue, the clinically translatable approaches are increasingly being valued. A number of original reports highlighted in this chapter serve as nonexclusive but exemplary studies illustrate tangible pathways for the translation of stem cell biology, the biomaterials' development, and *in vivo* surgical models that move dental, oral, and craniofacial bioengineering toward clinical therapies.

# Acknowledgments

We thank Michael Diggs, Qiongfen Guo, and Kening Hua for administrative and technical assistance. Some of our work described in this communication is supported by NIH grants, 5R01EB009663, 5R01DE018248, 5R01EB006261, and 1RC2DE020767.

# References

Akintoye, S. O., Lam, T., Shi, S. et al. 2006. Skeletal site-specific characterization of orofacial and iliac crest human bone marrow stromal cells in same individuals. *Bone* 38(6): 758–768.

Behr, B., Panetta, N. J., Longaker, M. T. et al. 2010. Different endogenous threshold levels of fibroblast growth factor-ligands determine the healing potential of frontal and parietal bones. *Bone* 47(2): 281–294.

Belema-Bedada, F., Uchida, S., Martire, A. et al. 2008. Efficient homing of multipotent adult mesenchymal stem cells depends on FROUNT-mediated clustering of CCR2. *Cell Stem Cell* 2(6): 566–575.

Betz, V. M., Betz, O. B., Harris, M. B. et al. 2008. Bone tissue engineering and repair by gene therapy. *Front Biosci* 13: 833–841.

Bhatt, A. and Le Anh, D. 2009. Craniofacial tissue regeneration: Where are we? *J Calif Dent Assoc* 37(11): 799–803.

Cerletti, M., Jurga, S., Witczak, C. A. et al. 2008. Highly efficient, functional engraftment of skeletal muscle stem cells in dystrophic muscles. *Cell* 134(1): 37–47.

Choi, J. H., Gimble, J. M., Lee, K. et al. 2010. Adipose tissue engineering for soft tissue regeneration. *Tissue Eng Part B Rev* 16(4): 413–426.

Cooke, J. W., Sarment, D. P., Whitesman, L. A. et al. 2006. Effect of rhPDGF-BB delivery on mediators of periodontal wound repair. *Tissue Eng* 12(6): 1441–1450.

Cowan, C. M., Shi, Y. Y., Aalami, O. O. et al. 2004. Adipose-derived adult stromal cells heal critical-size mouse calvarial defects. *Nat Biotechnol* 22(5): 560–567.

Folkman, J. and Hochberg, M. 1973. Self-regulation of growth in three dimensions. *J Exp Med* 138(4): 745–753.

Foster, B. L., Popowics, T. E., Fong, H. K. et al. 2007. Advances in defining regulators of cementum development and periodontal regeneration. *Curr Top Dev Biol* 78: 47–126.

Gafni, Y., Pelled, G., Zilberman, Y. et al. 2004. Gene therapy platform for bone regeneration using an exogenously regulated, AAV-2-based gene expression system. *Mol Ther* 9(4): 587–595.

Gao, J., Dennis, J. E., Solchaga, L. A. et al. 2002. Repair of osteochondral defect with tissue-engineered two-phase composite material of injectable calcium phosphate and hyaluronan sponge. *Tissue Eng* 8(5): 827–837.

Goldberg, M., Six, N., Decup, F. et al. 2001. Application of bioactive molecules in pulp-capping situations. *Adv Dent Res* 15: 91–95.

Goldstein, A. S., Juarez, T. M., Helmke, C. D. et al. 2001. Effect of convection on osteoblastic cell growth and function in biodegradable polymer foam scaffolds. *Biomaterials* 22(11): 1279–1288.

Golub, E. E. 2009. Role of matrix vesicles in biomineralization. *Biochim Biophys Acta* 1790(12): 1592–1598.

Huang, G. T. 2009. Pulp and dentin tissue engineering and regeneration: current progress. *Regen Med* 4(5): 697–707.

Huang, Z., Sargeant, T. D., Hulvat, J. F. et al. 2008. Bioactive nanofibers instruct cells to proliferate and differentiate during enamel regeneration. *J Bone Miner Res* 23(12): 1995–2006.

Jiang, C. C., Chiang, H., Liao, C. J. et al. 2007. Repair of porcine articular cartilage defect with a biphasic osteochondral composite. *J Orthop Res* 25(10): 1277–1290.

Kim, K., Lee, C. H., Kim, B. K., Mao, J. J. 2010. Anatomically shaped tooth and periodontal regeneration by cell homing. *J Dent Res* 89(8):842–847.

Kitaori, T., Ito, H., Schwarz, E. M. et al. 2009. Stromal cell-derived factor 1/CXCR4 signaling is critical for the recruitment of mesenchymal stem cells to the fracture site during skeletal repair in a mouse model. *Arthritis Rheum* 60(3): 813–823.

Kneser, U., Kaufmann, P. M., Fiegel, H. C. et al. 1999. Long-term differentiated function of heterotopically transplanted hepatocytes on three-dimensional polymer matrices. *J Biomed Mater Res* 47(4): 494–503.

Kneser, U., Stangenberg, L., Ohnolz, J. et al. 2006. Evaluation of processed bovine cancellous bone matrix seeded with syngenic osteoblasts in a critical size calvarial defect rat model. *J Cell Mol Med* 10(3): 695–707.

Lawrence, R. C., Helmick, C. G., Arnett, F. C. et al. 1998. Estimates of the prevalence of arthritis and selected musculoskeletal disorders in the United States. *Arthritis Rheum* 41(5): 778–799.

Lee, C. H., Cook, J. L., Mendelson, A. et al. 2010. Regeneration of the articular surface of the rabbit's synovial joint by cell homing: A proof of concept study. *Lancet* 376(9739): 440–448.

Lee, C. H., Marion, N. W., Hollister, S. et al. 2009. Tissue formation and vascularization in anatomically shaped human joint condyle ectopically in vivo. *Tissue Eng Part A* 15(12): 3923–3930.

Lin, N. H., Gronthos, S., and Mark Bartold, P. 2009. Stem cells and future periodontal regeneration. *Periodontol* 2000 51: 239–251.

Mao, J. J. 2008. Stem cells and the future of dental care. *N Y State Dent J* 74(2):20–24.

Mao, J. J., Giannobile, W. V., Helms, J. A. et al. 2006. Craniofacial tissue engineering by stem cells. *J Dent Res* 85(11): 966–979.

Miura, M., Miura, Y., Sonoyama, W. et al. 2006. Bone marrow-derived mesenchymal stem cells for regenerative medicine in craniofacial region. *Oral Dis* 12(6): 514–522.

Moioli, E. K., Chen, M., Yang, R. et al. 2010. Hybrid adipogenic implants from adipose stem cells for soft tissue reconstruction in vivo. *Tissue Eng Part A* 16(11): 3299–3307.

Moioli, E. K., Clark, P. A., Sumner, D. R. et al. 2008. Autologous stem cell regeneration in craniosynostosis. *Bone* 42(2): 332–340.

Moioli, E. K., Hong, L., Guardado, J. et al. 2006. Sustained release of TGFbeta3 from PLGA microspheres and its effect on early osteogenic differentiation of human mesenchymal stem cells. *Tissue Eng* 12(3): 537–546.

Noh, M. J., Copeland, R. O., Yi, Y. et al. 2010. Pre-clinical studies of retrovirally transduced human chondrocytes expressing transforming growth factor-beta-1 (TG-C). *Cytotherapy* 12(3): 384–393.

Palmer, L. C., Newcomb, C. J., Kaltz, S. R. et al. 2008. Biomimetic systems for hydroxyapatite mineralization inspired by bone and enamel. *Chem Rev* 108(11): 4754–4783.

Park, C. H., Rios, H. F., Jin, Q. et al. 2010. Biomimetic hybrid scaffolds for engineering human tooth-ligament interfaces. *Biomaterials* 31(23): 5945–5952.

Park, D. K., Della Valle, C. J., Quigley, L. et al. 2009. Revision of the acetabular component without cement. A concise follow-up, at twenty to twenty-four years, of a previous report. *J Bone Joint Surg Am* 91(2): 350–355.

Pellegrini, G., Seol, Y. J., Gruber, R. et al. 2009. Pre-clinical models for oral and periodontal reconstructive therapies. *J Dent Res* 88(12): 1065–1076.

Scheller, E. L. and Krebsbach, P. H. 2009. Gene therapy: Design and prospects for craniofacial regeneration. *J Dent Res* 88(7): 585–596.

Scotti, C., Tonnarelli, B., Papadimitropoulos, A. et al. 2010. Recapitulation of endochondral bone formation using human adult mesenchymal stem cells as a paradigm for developmental engineering. *Proc Natl Acad Sci U S A* 107(16): 7251–7256.

Shi, S., Bartold, P. M., Miura, M. et al. 2005. The efficacy of mesenchymal stem cells to regenerate and repair dental structures. *Orthod Craniofac Res* 8(3): 191–199.

Stosich, M. S., Moioli, E. K., Wu, J. K. et al. 2009. Bioengineering strategies to generate vascularized soft tissue grafts with sustained shape. *Methods* 47(2): 116–121.

Thesleff, I., Jarvinen, E., and Suomalainen, M. 2007. Affecting tooth morphology and renewal by fine-tuning the signals mediating cell and tissue interactions. *Novartis Found Symp* 284: 142–153; discussion 153–163.

Vaccaro, A. R., Lawrence, J. P., Patel, T. et al. 2008. The safety and efficacy of OP-1 (rhBMP-7) as a replacement for iliac crest autograft in posterolateral lumbar arthrodesis: A long-term (>4 years) pivotal study. *Spine (Phila Pa 1976)* 33(26): 2850–2862.

Warnke, P. H., Springer, I. N., Wiltfang, J. et al. 2004. Growth and transplantation of a custom vascularised bone graft in a man. *Lancet* 364(9436): 766–770.

Yang, R., Chen, M., Lee, C. H. et al. 2010. Clones of ectopic stem cells in the regeneration of muscle defects in vivo. *PLoS One* 5(10): e13547.

Zaky, S. H. and Cancedda, R. 2009. Engineering craniofacial structures: Facing the challenge. *J Dent Res* 88(12): 1077–1091.

Zeichner-David, M. 2006. Regeneration of periodontal tissues: cementogenesis revisited. *Periodontol 2000* 41: 196–217.

Zhang, J., Jiang, D., Lin, Q. et al. 2010. Synthesis of dental enamel-like hydroxyapatite through solution mediated solid-state conversion. *Langmuir* 26(5): 2989–2994.

Zhao, M., Song, B., Pu, J. et al. 2006. Electrical signals control wound healing through phosphatidylinositol-3-OH kinase-gamma and PTEN. *Nature* 442(7101): 457–460.

# 29

# Tendon and Ligament Engineering

29.1 Introduction ........................................................................29-1
    The Unmet Clinical Need • Advantages of Tissue-Engineered
    Tendons and Ligaments
29.2 Structure of Fibrous Connective Tissues ....................29-2
    Compositional Analysis • Enzymes and Growth
    Factors • Hierarchical Structure-Property Relationships
29.3 Current Ligament Reconstructive Techniques .........29-4
    Autografts • Allografts • Synthetic Prosthesis • Device Failure
    Modes
29.4 Engineered Tendon and Ligament Grafts...................29-6
    Tissue Engineering Paradigm • Cell Source • Biomaterial Scaffold
    Design • Bioreactor Systems
29.5 Mechanical Stimulation..................................................29-8
    Cellular Proliferation and Differentiation • Cellular
    Alignment • ECM Synthesis and Remodeling • Strain Magnitude
    and Rate
29.6 *In Vivo* Models to Demonstrate Efficacy...................29-11
29.7 Key Challenges and Critical Issues...........................29-11
References..................................................................................29-13

Nicholas Sears
*Texas A&M University*

Tyler Touchet
*Texas A&M University*

Hugh Benhardt
*Texas A&M University*

Elizabeth
Cosgriff-Hernández
*Texas A&M University*

## 29.1 Introduction

### 29.1.1 The Unmet Clinical Need

Overall, musculoskeletal ailments comprise more than 14% of health care expenditures in the United States. Ligament and tendon damage account for a significant portion of these ailments with over 32 million traumatic and repetitive motion injuries reported in the United States each year. Although numerous tendon injuries can be surgically repaired, large gaps and missing tendons require a graft or replacement device. Among the most common tendon injuries are traumatic and attritional tears of the rotator cuff, resulting in 4.4 million physician visits and over 50,000 repair surgeries performed each year (Praemer et al. 1999; Butler et al. 2008). However, tendons repaired in this manner are often weak and susceptible to reinjury. Excessive muscle contraction and neurovascular damage following surgical repair of rotator cuff injuries result in failure rates as high as 40%. Tendon injuries can dramatically affect a patient's quality of life; however, improving functional outcomes after tendon injury remains a significant clinical challenge.

Unlike tendons, damaged ligaments require replacement grafts after any injury regardless of severity due to their poor healing ability. The anterior cruciate ligament (ACL) is the most commonly injured ligament of the knee, with over 200,000 Americans requiring reconstructive surgery in 2002 and an associated medical cost exceeding 5 billion dollars (Albright et al. 1999; Pennisi 2002). Current standard-of-care for ligament reconstruction includes transplantation of autografts, allografts, and alloplasts (Vunjak-Novakovic et al. 2004). Despite the inherent limitations of autograft strategies, the tendon autograft remains the "gold standard" of ACL repair (Fu et al. 1999, 2000). The autograft possesses good initial mechanical strength and promotes cell proliferation and remodeling. However, there is limited availability of autografts and donor site morbidity leads to several complications including pain, muscle atrophy, and tendonitis at the donor site (Weitzel et al. 2002). Similarly, ligament allografts are limited by disease transmission, bacterial infection, unfavorable immunogenic responses, and loss of mechanical properties after sterilization. Synthetic grafts have a high percentage of implant failure due to a lack of biological incorporation that leads to stress shielding of the surrounding tissue. Woven prostheses also face the additional problems of axial splitting, low extensibility, and abrasive wear that can cause synovitis in the joint (Parsons et al. 1985; Lopez-Vazquez et al. 1991; Maletius and Gillquist 1997; Murray and Macnicol 2003; Vunjak-Novakovic et al. 2004). The limitations of current surgical techniques provide a substantial margin for improvement in the growing market of ligament and tendon reconstruction. It is expected that the number and severity of these injuries will continue to increase in our aging and active population. Given the frequency and increasing cost of these injuries, development of tissue engineered tendons and ligaments would be invaluable.

### 29.1.2 Advantages of Tissue-Engineered Tendons and Ligaments

Musculoskeletal tissue engineering has emerged as a promising alternative that circumvents the aforementioned limitations associated with biological and synthetic grafts (Kenley et al. 1993; Rose and Oreffo 2002). The traditional tissue engineering paradigm combines isolated cells with appropriate bioactive agents in a biodegradable scaffold (Bhatia and Chen 1999; Lin et al. 1999; Vunjak-Novakovic et al. 2004; Altman and Horan 2006). As the scaffold degrades, neotissue forms until the injured tissue is completely replaced by healthy tissue and functionality is restored (Vunjak-Novakovic et al. 2004; Altman and Horan 2006). Tendon and ligament reconstruction utilizing a tissue-engineered graft would: (1) eliminate donor site morbidity and increase the rate/degree of rehabilitation, (2) create a virtually unlimited supply of autologous tissue, (3) eliminate the risk of disease transmission or immunogenic responses, and (4) enhance the mechanical properties and increase the fatigue life of the graft (Vunjak-Novakovic et al. 2004; Altman and Horan 2006).

## 29.2 Structure of Fibrous Connective Tissues

### 29.2.1 Compositional Analysis

Tissue engineered graft design is naturally guided by the physiological properties of the target tissue and should build upon the successes and failures of past reconstructive approaches. Ligaments and tendons have a unique combination of molecular, structural, and mechanical properties that can be utilized to refine these design criteria. The function and material properties of various fibrous connective tissues are directly related to their composition and organization. The extracellular matrix (ECM) of fibrous connective tissue is composed of collagen, elastin, proteoglycans (PGs), and glycoproteins. The most abundant protein in fibrous connective tissue is collagen. Collagen type I forms tough, nonelastic cross-linked fibers that contribute to the tensile strength of ligaments and tendons (Neurath 1993; Riechert et al. 2001). In contrast, collagen type III forms loosely organized, thin fibrils that provide elasticity (Neurath 1993; Riechert et al. 2001). Elastin, a highly crosslinked array of tropoelastin proteins, also contributes to the elastic behavior of ligaments but is not present in tendons (Redlich et al. 2004). The collagen and elastin makeup of the connective tissue dictates its bulk mechanical properties, whereas, the PGs and glycoproteins of the ECM are involved in tissue organization. Biglycan and decorin are small leucine rich PGs that are associated with collagen fibrillogenesis and organization (Pogany and Vogel

1992; Schonherr et al. 1993). Despite their similar structure, these PGs have distinct responsibilities as evidenced by their dissimilar distribution throughout connective tissue (Bianco et al. 1990). Biglycan is associated with thick collagen fibrillogenesis and decorin binding results in the formation of thinner collagen fibrils (San Martin and Zorn 2003). Glycoproteins such as fibronectin and tenascin provide physical links between the cells and ECM. Fibronectin binds to cell surface integrins to enable cell signaling and adhesion (Neurath 1993; Tremble et al. 1994). Fibronectin also binds to other ECM proteins to control organization of the ECM network. Tenascin influences cell adhesion and migration by interacting with fibronectin and other ECM molecules (Neurath 1993). This interaction between tenascin and fibronectin also upregulates enzyme synthesis in fibroblasts (Tremble et al. 1994). Each of these ECM components plays a specific role in the maintenance of the structural integrity of connective tissue.

Fibroblast morphology, ECM composition and organization vary between ligaments and tendons based on the individual anatomy and function of the tissue. Similar to ligaments, tendons are composed of collagen fibrils that are oriented parallel to their longitudinal axis; however, tendons demonstrate distinct ECM composition and intrinsic properties that distinguish them from ligaments. For instance, tendons exhibit higher collagen content at approximately 87% of total protein synthesis, compared to 80% in ACL tissue (Amiel et al. 1984). Additionally, tendons contain fewer glycosaminoglycans than ligaments, thus indicating less PG synthesis to complement its greater collagen synthesis. Tendons also demonstrate a much higher percentage of collagen type I than ligaments with minimal expression of collagen type III. The ratio of collagen type I to collagen type III in tendons is roughly 95–5%, respectively (Amiel et al. 1984; Riechert et al. 2001). Due to its high percentage of collagen type I, the patellar tendon demonstrates sufficient mechanical strength to restore ACL function; however, its limited production of collagen type III and its lack of elastin leave it susceptible to creep prior to full restoration of damaged tissue. Overall, each component of the ECM has a specific role in the properties and remodeling of connective tissue.

## 29.2.2 Enzymes and Growth Factors

In response to injury, fibroblasts upregulate ECM proteins and proliferate to generate scar tissue. In later stages of healing, fibroblasts produce enzymes that degrade this randomly organized ECM and synthesize oriented ECM proteins with improved mechanical properties similar to healthy tissue. Fibroblasts control degradation by synthesizing enzymes that break down specific proteins in the ECM network. Common enzymes associated with the degradation of the ECM in ligament and tendons include Matrix Metalloproteinase-1 (MMP-1), MMP-2, and MMP-9. (Kerkvliet et al. 1999; Foos et al. 2001) MMP-2, a gelatinase, accounts for the most efficient degradation of collagen (Kerkvliet et al. 1999). Due to the high percentage of collagen in connective tissues, MMP-2 is often targeted as the key mediator of tendon and ligament degradation. Tissue inhibitor of metalloproteinase-1 (TIMP-1) regulates enzyme activity by interacting with MMP to prevent excessive collagen degradation. Fibroblasts also regulate ECM protein synthesis and organization by secreting growth factors that alter the structure of fibrous connective tissue. For example, transforming growth factor-β (TGF-β) induces cell proliferation and modulates the synthesis of collagen, fibronectin, biglycan, and decorin (Battegay et al. 1990; Romaris et al. 1991; Schmidt et al. 1995; Lin et al. 1999). Specifically, TGF-β upregulates the expression of collagen and biglycan while having a minimal to negative effect on the expression of decorin (Romaris et al. 1991; Westergren-Thorsson et al. 1991; Marui et al. 1997; Wegrowski et al. 2000). Thus, the production of growth factors can alter mechanical properties by modulating the synthesis of individual ECM proteins (Mann et al. 2001; Sakai et al. 2002).

## 29.2.3 Hierarchical Structure-Property Relationships

The complex organization on the cellular level accounts for a large degree of tensile strength; however, the macroscopic organization and orientation of these fibers strongly influences its behavior.

For example, fibers of the ACL are arranged in a helical fashion, which allows rotation and elongation, while retaining the ligament's isometric structure throughout the entire joint extension (Amiel et al. 1984; Vunjak-Novakovic et al. 2004; Laurencin and Freeman 2005; Altman and Horan 2006). The ACL's helical structure distributes the load equally among the fiber bundles, fully utilizing its strength (Vunjak-Novakovic et al. 2004; Altman and Horan 2006). This helical organization allows the ACL to twist 90° during knee extension while retaining structural integrity (Butler and Stouffer 1983; Vunjak-Novakovic et al. 2004; Altman and Horan 2006). This is because the rotation allows collagen bundles to unravel and become isometric at full extension, effectively distributing the applied load equally throughout the tissue. As a result, the ACL has high tensile strength throughout all degrees of motion. Additionally, collagen bundles that make up the ACL overlap in a "crimp" pattern which allows 7–16% elongation before permanent damage occurs (Vunjak-Novakovic et al. 2004; Laurencin and Freeman 2005; Altman and Horan 2006). ACL collagen bundles overlap in a crimp pattern (Laurencin and Freeman 2005) that permits 7–16% creep elongation prior to permanent deformation and ligament damage (Vunjak-Novakovic et al. 2004; Altman and Horan 2006). The complex structure–function relationships of ligaments and tendons shed some light on the difficulties creating appropriate synthetic replacements.

## 29.3 Current Ligament Reconstructive Techniques

### 29.3.1 Autografts

Current surgical techniques available for ACL reconstruction include transplantation of autografts, allografts, and synthetic grafts. Autografts are currently considered the gold standard in ACL reconstruction (Fu et al. 2000; Freeman and Kwansa 2008). Typically harvested from the inner third of the patellar tendon or hamstring tendons these grafts provide good mechanical strength as well as promote cell proliferation and differentiation (Noyes and Grood 1976; Amiel et al. 1986; Fu et al. 1999; Freeman and Kwansa 2008). The bone-patellar-bone graft incorporates bony blocks from the harvest site that allow for rigid fixation and reduce the chance of tendon creep (Amiel et al. 1986; Fu et al. 1999, 2000; Nedeff and Bach 2001; Seon et al. 2006). However, a large donor site incision and morbidity can lead to further complications such as harvest site pain, tendonitis, muscle atrophy (Seon et al. 2006). The hamstring tendon graft has gained popularity over recent years due to reduced donor site morbidity and smaller incision size compared to patellar tendon grafts. The hamstring graft is harvested by removing the semitendinosus and gracilis tendons that are then folded in half and combined to make a quadruple-strand tendon graft. The hamstring graft is a more comparable with the native intact ACL and the multiple strand graft may act as an analog to the two-bundle structure of the native ACL. Disadvantages of the hamstring tendon graft include donor site morbidity, tendon creep, and slow tendon healing due to the lack of a rigid fixation system (Fu et al. 1999, 2000; Altman and Horan 2006). The quadriceps tendon is less commonly used but allows for a larger fibrous portion that has the potential to increase mechanical properties. A bony plug for rigid fixation at one end also provides a potential for greater mechanical properties but size and location of the donor site scar along with donor site morbidity pose as serious disadvantages (Fu et al. 1999). With all autografts, the donor site morbidity and limited availability are areas of concern that have given rise into investigation for a more suitable replacement (Fu et al. 2000; Ge et al. 2005).

### 29.3.2 Allografts

Allografts typically use tendon grafts that have been harvested from cadavers and sterilized (Scheffler et al. 2005; Altman and Horan 2006). The use of allografts eliminates the need for a second surgical site and donor site morbidity (Fu et al. 1999). Typical grafts are taken from the bone-patellar tendon or the Achilles tendon (Cooper et al. 2006). Allografts are more readily available than autografts and are incorporated into the body much like autografts but at a slower rate (Fu et al. 1999). Disease transmission and bacterial infection have been a concern with the use of allografts. The chance of disease transmission from allografts is limited by harvesting grafts in sterile conditions, the use of a sterilization agent, and freezing the grafts until use (Fu et al. 1999; Lomas et al. 2004; Scheffler et al. 2005). However, sterilization methods such as ethylene oxide and gamma radiation can negatively impact the mechanical properties of the graft (Scheffler et al. 2005). Ethylene oxide gas leaves behind the toxic residues ethylene glycol and ethylene chlorohydrins that cause synovitis and dissolution of the graft. Gamma radiation is used to eliminate bacteria and viruses from the donor tissue. Radiation levels between 1 and 2 Mrad eliminate bacterial threats but radiation levels on the order of 4 Mrad radiation are required to eliminate viruses. However, above 3 Mrad has been to shown to alter the mechanical properties of the graft and change the tissue morphology (Fu et al. 1999; Scheffler et al. 2005). Dry freezing and cryofreezing bypass the sterilization process and retain the grafts original mechanical properties (Shino et al. 1984). However, the chance of disease transmission and bacterial infection remains of concern.

## 29.3.3 Synthetic Prosthesis

Synthetic prosthesis have gained wide interest recently because they provide an alternative to auto and allografts by eliminating donor site morbidity and risk of disease transmission. Current synthetic grafts include carbon fiber, polytetrafluoroethylene (Gore-Tex Ligament), polyethylene terephthalate (Leeds-Keio Ligament), and polypropylene (Kennedy Ligament Augmentation device) (Fischer and Ferkel 1988; Laurencin et al. 1999; Vunjak-Novakovic et al. 2004; Altman and Horan 2006). Synthetic prostheses allow for faster rehabilitation because they do not lose their strength during tissue remodeling and no second surgical site for harvesting tissue is required (Markolf et al. 1989). However, high linear stiffness of prostheses causes the prostheses to bare the majority of the physiological load, effectively stress shielding the surrounding tissue. Stress shielding inhibits the correct formation of collagen alignment and the hierarchical tissue organization leading to decreased mechanical properties, ligament laxity and even rupture (Moyen et al. 1992; Kumar and Maffulli 1999; Vunjak-Novakovic et al. 2004; Laurencin and Freeman 2005; Altman and Horan 2006). In addition, abrasions formed form the contact from bone tunnels can weaken the prostheses and create debris that provokes an unfavorable foreign body response (Parsons et al. 1985; Vunjak-Novakovic et al. 2004). Material fatigue is of concern as synthetic prostheses can undergo creep altering mechanical cues that can result in misalignment of new tissue formation (Lopez-Vazquez et al. 1991; Murray 2003). These mechanical mismatches due to incorrect mechanical cues provide insight into the difficulty to fabricate a prosthesis that duplicates the mechanical behavior of the native ACL. Currently synthetic prostheses lack acceptable biological incorporation, which results in high failure rates and undesirable side effects such as synovitis and osteoarthritis (Parsons et al. 1985; Lopez-Vazquez et al. 1991; Maletius and Gillquist 1997; Murray 2003; Vunjak-Novakovic et al. 2004). The manner of fabrication of these prostheses also impacts the clinical outcome of the graft. Woven prostheses, for example, are susceptible to axial splitting, have low extensibility, lack tissue infiltration, and undergo abrasive wear to different degrees based on the braid angle and thickness (Olson et al. 1988; Moyen et al. 1992; Kumar and Maffulli 1999; Vunjak-Novakovic et al. 2004; Laurencin and Freeman 2005; Altman and Horan 2006).

## 29.3.4 Device Failure Modes

Failures in ligament reconstruction can be due to surgical methods, fixation technique, and graft choice. Current surgical methods such as tunnel placement can lead to graft stretching, impingement, or over constraint of the knee. These complications result in the loss of motion and can cause graft failure by placing either too much strain on the graft or by graft abrasion leading to rupture (Fu et al. 1999, 2000). Notchplasty and Roofplasty, another current surgical method, allow for clearance when the knee is extended however, studies have shown histological changes consistent with reports found in knees with early osteoarthritis (Cushner et al. 2003; Marks et al. 2005; Seon et al. 2006). Emphasis should be placed not only on correct tunnel placement but also a conservative approach to notchplasty to avoid joint instability and abrasion between the tunnels and graft. However, surgical technique is not the only factor that can attribute to device failure in ligament reconstruction. The fixation methods have been investigated as point of failure in the system and found that fixation pull-out can occur if the surrounding bone has yet to heal (Fu et al. 1999). Placement of the fixation device can also lead to increased risk of graft failure by either allowing ligament laxity or having the ligament overly strained (Tohyama and Yasuda 1998; Fu et al. 1999, 2000). In addition, the graft itself can be susceptible to failure through many different pathways such as rejection of the biomaterial, immune response to particle debris, and abrasion causing rupture. The rejection of a biomaterial can be seen in synthetic prostheses such as the Dacron ligament and Leeds-Keio ligament which both invoke an unfavorable host response that can lead to premature graft failure as well as particle debris (Lopez-Vazquez et al. 1991; Fu et al. 1999, 2000; Murray 2003). Abrasions from tunnel placement or woven grafts can lead to graft weakening, graft rupture, and further complications such as synovitis from particle debris in the synovial environment (Lopez-Vazquez et al. 1991). Overall, the limitations of current ACL reconstruction strategies present a substantial margin for improvement in the escalating market for ACL repair.

## 29.4  Engineered Tendon and Ligament Grafts

### 29.4.1  Tissue Engineering Paradigm

Musculoskeletal tissue engineering has received growing interest throughout orthopedic medicine as a promising alternative to biologic and synthetic grafts (Kenley et al. 1993; Laurencin et al. 1999; Rose and Oreffo 2002; Laurencin and Freeman 2005). Tissue engineers attempt to harness the body's natural ability to repair and regenerate damaged tissue through the application of biological, chemical, and engineering principles. This strategy can potentially improve upon current clinical options by providing appropriate biological and mechanical properties to regenerate damaged tissue without the aforementioned limitations of other grafts (Lin et al. 1999; Vunjak-Novakovic et al. 2004; Laurencin and Freeman 2005; Altman and Horan 2006). The traditional tissue engineering paradigm combines isolated cells and bioactive factors on a biodegradable scaffold that sustains functionality during tissue regeneration and serves as a structural template for neotissue formation.

### 29.4.2  Cell Source

A fully functional tissue engineered graft requires rapid cell proliferation and differentiation into the appropriate lineage to allow for the restoration of the native tissue. To create an *ex vivo* tissue engineered graft that meets these capabilities, cells with the capacity to meet these needs can be integrated into the system (Altman and Horan 2006). The current popular cell sources under investigation include primary fibroblasts or meneschymal stem cells (MSCs). Native ACL fibroblasts have a reduced proliferative capacity, limiting their use as a cell source for ligament tissue engineering, thus alternatives for an acceptable replacement have been investigated (Bellincampi et al. 1998; Cooper Jr. et al. 2006). The use of tendon fibroblasts has been extensively studied as a suitable replacement for ACL fibroblasts. The fibroblasts found in the patellar tendon have shown to proliferate at a faster rate than fibroblasts found in ligaments and differentiate forming functional tissue (Eijk et al. 2004; Yang et al. 2004). Proliferation and differentiation of these fibroblasts can be regulated through the use of specific growth factors and dynamic mechanical stimulation such as cyclical strain (Altman et al. 2001; Hannafin et al. 2006). Although primary fibroblasts have demonstrated sufficient regenerative properties, cell harvest can lead to donor site pain, tendonitis, and prolonged recovery (Kleiner et al. 1986; Eijk et al. 2004; Altman and Horan 2006; Cooper Jr. et al. 2006). As an alternative, MSCs have gained an increasing interest for tissue engineering strategies due to their ability to rapidly proliferate and differentiate into tendon and ligament lineages through mechanical stimulation (Altman et al. 2002; Kim et al. 2002; Yang et al. 2004;

Fan et al. 2008; Liu et al. 2008). In addition, MSC allow for a plentiful supply of autologous cells without the complications from immune responses or harvest sites. Although MSC differentiation to ligament fibroblasts is established, the mechanical strength of the graft was weaker than that of the native ACL due to inconsistencies between the ECM synthesis by MSCs and the native ECM remodeling process (Chen 2006; Liu et al. 2008). Additional research is needed to identify the proper mechanical stimulation and cell culture conditions that will induce appropriate ECM synthesis and remodeling to achieve functional grafts.

## 29.4.3 Biomaterial Scaffold Design

Tissue engineers utilize a biomaterial scaffold to sustain functionality during regeneration and serve as a template for the necessary cellular interactions. The biomaterial chosen for these scaffolds must meet certain criteria to facilitate these processes including biocompatibility, biodegradability, biological integration, and mechanical integrity throughout remodeling (Langer and Vacanti 1993; Bhatia and Chen 1999; Laurencin et al. 1999; Butler et al. 2000; Freed and Vunjak-Novakovic 2000; Freyman et al. 2001; Altman and Horan 2006). Initially, the entire mechanical load is supported by the biomaterial scaffold and the graft must have sufficient mechanical strength to support physiological loading. However, the biomechanical basis for many of the synthetic graft failures has been attributed to a mismatch between the graft and native tissue (Vunjak-Novakovic et al. 2004; Altman and Horan 2006). High linear stiffness of synthetic materials causes a majority of the physiological load to be borne by the prosthesis alone and stress shields new tissue growth. Stress shielding results in nondirected collagenous organization and alignment that reduces the load-bearing capacity of the newly formed tissue. Lack of biomechanical signals can also change the natural biological state from continuous degradation and remodeling to degradation only (Altman and Horan 2006). The scaffold is then limited by its inherent fatigue properties as opposed to native ligament which is in a continuous state of remodeling and repair. In order to achieve mechanically competent tissue repair, the biomaterial scaffold must possess mechanical properties similar to native tissue to restore function and prevent stress-shielding.

Current biomaterials utilized in tissue engineering scaffolds include collagen gels, synthetic or natural fiber meshes (Vunjak-Novakovic et al. 2004; Laurencin and Freeman 2005). Collagen gels maintain the cells in a 3-D environment similar to that found in native tissue, but lack the necessary tensile properties to achieve functional ligament repair (Goulet et al. 1997; Altman et al. 2002). There has been renewed interest in silk as a biomaterial for tissue engineering due to its high tensile strength and linear stiffness, biocompatibility, and biodegradation properties (Vunjak-Novakovic et al. 2004). For ligament applications, the high linear stiffness of the silk must be reduced to prevent stress shielding of the neotissue. Silk fibroin in a wire-rope geometry has been shown to exhibit mechanical properties similar to functional ACL (Altman et al. 2002). Although the architecture may be modified to achieve a range of mechanical properties, independent control of degradation rate and mechanical properties is limited. Furthermore, concerns about mass-production, variability, and complex handling properties may limit the usefulness of natural materials (Altman and Horan 2006).

Several synthetic polymers have been investigated as potential scaffold materials for ligament repair. Polydioxanone (PDS) was investigated as a scaffold material; however, rapid loss of its mechanical strength due to degradation limits the use of PDS in ligament tissue engineering (Buma et al. 2004). A number of ligament prostheses have been made of flexible composites of woven or braided fibers including polyglycolide, polylactides, poly(lactide-*co*-glycolide), and polycaprolactone (Laurencin and Freeman 2005; Altman and Horan 2006). These scaffolds performed well during initial testing, but the long-term outcomes of these prostheses (tissue integration, nutrient diffusion, cell infiltration, abrasion resistance, fatigue) are unclear. The inherent limitation of using polymeric materials that require additional processing to achieve the necessary mechanical properties is clear. Scaffolds that derive properties from geometry and processing demand an understanding of how each structure behaves mechanically relative to each other.

Biomaterial design is further complicated by biodegradation of the scaffold which impacts both the formation of new tissue and the mechanical properties of the construct. The scaffold serves as a structural template for cell attachment/proliferation and should biodegrade at a rate matching that of new tissue deposition. It is also important that the scaffold maintain the mechanical integrity of the implant site throughout the period of repair. This is particularly important in musculoskeletal applications where mechanical stimulation is required to generate a fully functional implant. During remodeling, the loss of scaffold strength due to biodegradation is offset by the increased load bearing of the neotissue. Therefore, load-bearing of the scaffold should decrease at a rate that allows the new tissue to receive the appropriate level of load for directed collagenous organization/alignment without danger of construct rupture.

### 29.4.4 Bioreactor Systems

In order to mimic the native environments *in vitro* and provide cells with the necessary mechanical and biochemical cues to generate functional tissue, complex bioreactors have been constructed that incorporate the principles of mechanobiology (Vunjak-Novakovic and Freed 1997; Altman et al. 2002; Shi and Vesely 2005). Garvin et al. constructed a bioreactor system that applies uniaxial strains to tethered constructs of tendon fibroblasts, (Garvin et al. 2003) whereas, other studies applied multidimensional strains (axial tension/compression and torsion) that approach native ligament behavior (Altman et al. 2002; Garvin et al. 2003; Martin et al. 2004; Vunjak-Novakovic et al. 2004; Shi and Vesely 2005; Abousleiman and Sikavitsas 2006; Altman and Horan 2006; Chen 2006; Matziolis et al. 2006). Matziolis et al. showed that bioreactor systems can induce collagen type I synthesis, alkaline phosphatase activity, and calcification of ECM in mechanically loaded periosteal cells (Matziolis et al. 2006). Altman et al. reported enhanced differentiation of MSCs to ligament fibroblast phenotypes via mechanical stimulation (Altman et al. 2002). Although improved outcomes have been demonstrated with the addition of bioreactor conditioning, the mechanical properties of the constructs often fall short of native ligaments. The origin of the unique mechanical properties of connective tissues is the intricate ECM remodeling process that yields highly ordered structures. This remodeling is guided by the homeostatic tendency of soft tissues to adapt in response to mechanical stimulus via ECM reorganization. Therefore, researchers have focused on elucidating the effect of mechanical loading on ECM synthesis, degradation, and organization as a means to predict optimal loading conditions. The mechanical conditions necessary to guide the remodeling processes may then be incorporated into bioreactor design to generate improved tissue grafts.

## 29.5 Mechanical Stimulation

Mechanical stimulation of fibroblasts *in vitro* has been used to induce cell alignment and orientation of the ECM, enhance cell proliferation, increase ECM synthesis, and promote differentiation of cells to specific fibrous connective tissue lineages (Altman et al. 2001; Noth et al. 2005; Abousleiman and Sikavitsas 2006; Chen 2006; Lee et al. 2007; Fan et al. 2008) (Kim et al. 1999). Numerous studies in this area have established that mechanical stimulation is central to the successful engineering of load-bearing tissues (Lin et al. 1999; Bartold et al. 2000; Vunjak-Novakovic et al. 2004; Laurencin and Freeman 2005; Altman and Horan 2006). Without the appropriate biomechanical cues, new tissue formation lacks the necessary ECM organization for sufficient load-bearing capacity. Therefore, tissue engineers utilize mechanical conditioning to guide tissue remodeling and improve the performance of tendon and ligament grafts. Mechanotransduction refers to cellular mechanisms that convert mechanical stimuli into biochemical signals responsible for cell proliferation, differentiation, and ECM synthesis. Typical biochemical cell signaling cascades are induced by the binding of ECM proteins, growth factors, or cytokines to cell surface receptors which transmit the biochemical signals to the interior of the cell. This binding triggers intracellular messengers to phosphorylate proteins linked to specific gene expression

(Neurath 1993; Sung et al. 1996; Garrington and Johnson 1999). During mechanotransduction, the attachment of integrins to ECM proteins creates a physical link between the ECM and the interior of the cell. Mechanical signaling pathways translate physical loading of the ECM into cell signaling cascades that alter gene expression. For example, Miyaki et al. (2001) reported that mechanical stretch stimulates the extracellular signal-regulated kinase (ERK) signaling pathway that governs the expression of type I collagen and decorin in ACL-derived cells. Mechanical stimulation has been reported to induce (1) cellular proliferation and differentiation, (2) cellular alignment, and (3) ECM synthesis and remodeling (Neurath 1993; Sung et al. 1996; Giancotti 1997; Breen 2000; Miyaki et al. 2001; Arnoczky et al. 2002; Atance et al. 2004; Hannafin et al. 2006; Henshaw et al. 2006).

## 29.5.1 Cellular Proliferation and Differentiation

Several researchers have reported increased DNA synthesis of fibroblasts in response to cyclic mechanical stretch (Kletsas et al. 1998; Park et al. 2006). Mechanical stimulation was shown to increase cellular proliferation in ACL and medial collateral ligament (MCL) cell cultures (Lin et al. 1999). Studies of human tendon fibroblasts confirmed the role of mechanical stimulus on cell proliferation (Zeichen et al. 2000; Yang et al. 2004). Cyclic stretch also induces modulation of cell morphology to the elongated, spindle-like shape consistent with connective tissue phenotypes (Toyoda et al. 1998; Miyaki et al. 2001; Lee et al. 2005; Park et al. 2006). In addition to fibroblasts, mechanical stress induces the differentiation of MSCs toward the ligament lineage (Altman et al. 2001, 2002; Noth et al. 2005; Chen 2006; Lee et al. 2007; Fan et al. 2008). MSCs are of particular interest in tissue engineering because they can differentiate to multiple connective tissue cell types (Barry 2003). Isolation of MSCs from bone marrow also provides tissue engineers with an unlimited supply of autologous cells that exhibit excellent regenerative properties including superior proliferation.

## 29.5.2 Cellular Alignment

In addition to the effects on proliferation and differentiation, mechanical stretch induces actin restructuring of the cytoskeleton and cellular alignment. As a result, ECM proteins that are synthesized due to mechanical loading are also oriented. Generally, mechanical stretch of 2D monolayer cell cultures causes fibroblasts to reorganize their cytoskeleton and align perpendicular to the direction of stretch (Buck 1980; Toyoda et al. 1998; Breen 2000; Neidlinger-Wilke et al. 2001, 2002; Park et al. 2006; Lee et al. 2007). Conversely, fibroblasts that are stretched on a 3D scaffold or flexible substrate align parallel to the direction of stretch similar to actual ligament behavior (Miyaki et al. 2001; Henshaw et al. 2006; Gilbert et al. 2007). The orientation of fibroblasts to the direction of mechanical stretch influences their behavioral response (McKnight and Frangos 2003; Wang et al. 2004; Lee et al. 2005). Specifically, fibroblasts that are aligned with the direction of stretch demonstrate greater protein synthesis and the resulting tissue possesses superior tensile properties (Lee et al. 2005). Fibroblasts oriented longitudinally also generate aligned collagen matrix to further enhance mechanical properties (Wang et al. 2003). Upon mechanical stimulation, MSCs also orient parallel to the direction of stretch and form aligned collagen fibers characteristic of ligament cells (Altman et al. 2001; Noth et al. 2005; Lee et al. 2007).

## 29.5.3 ECM Synthesis and Remodeling

ECM remodeling is guided by the homeostatic tendency of soft tissues to adapt in response to mechanical stimulus. Optimally, ECM reorganization generates functional tissue with enhanced mechanical properties to withstand loading. Although the response of fibroblasts to mechanical stimuli varies among cell types, each phenotype follows a general trend. Mechanical stimulation typically increases the production of collagen as necessary for each fibroblast phenotype (Duncan et al. 1984; Howard et al. 1998; Toyoda et al. 1998; Hsieh et al. 2000; Miyaki et al. 2001; Uno et al. 2001; Kim et al. 2002; Lee et al. 2004; Ozaki et al. 2005; Gilbert et al. 2007; Juncosa-Melvin et al. 2007). Breen et al. reported that mechanical strain upregulates procollagen mRNA levels in pulmonary fibroblasts (Breen 2000). One mechanism of this increased collagen expression is the modulation of growth factor secretion (Skutek et al. 2001; Kim et al. 2002; Yang et al. 2004; Gilbert et al. 2007). As stated previously, TGF-β1 influences collagen and PG synthesis in fibroblasts. Collagen synthesis due to mechanical stress was negated in the absence of TGF-β1. Therefore, the induction of TGF-β1 expression by cyclic mechanical stretch may be linked to the observed increase in collagen production (Kim et al. 2002; Yang et al. 2004).

Despite the general increase in total collagen synthesis, mechanical stimulation can differentially affect collagen ratios of specific lineages. For example, Carver et al. discovered that cyclic mechanical stretch of cardiac fibroblasts increases mRNA levels of collagen type III but does not affect the level of collagen type I (Carver et al. 1991). In contrast, Leung et al. revealed that cyclic stretch of vascular smooth muscle cells increases the synthesis of collagen types I and III equally (Leung et al. 1976). Cyclic stretch also regulates the expression of PGs and other specialized ECM proteins characteristic of specific tissue phenotypes. PG synthesis is either upregulated or downregulated according to which collagen fibrils emerge in response to loading (Miyaki et al. 2001; Ozaki et al. 2005; Juncosa-Melvin et al. 2007). Uno et al. found that mRNA expression of collagen type XII, osteocalcin, and osteonectin increases in response to mechanical stress in periodontal ligaments (Uno et al. 2001).

In addition to structural protein expression, mechanical stimulation modulates the expression of the integrins responsible for mechanotransduction. Increased expression of these integrins amplifies the stretch-induced synthesis of ECM proteins through a positive feedback loop. Finally, cyclic stretch increases the production of MMPs to facilitate balanced ECM remodeling (Bolcato-Bellemin et al. 2000; Yang et al. 2005; Zhou et al. 2005). In this way, mechanical stretch can induce degradation of randomly oriented scar tissue and synthesis of ECM proteins that are oriented in the direction of stretch. The expression of TIMP-1 is also upregulated to counteract the synthesis of MMP-2 (Bolcato-Bellemin et al. 2000). By modulating both arms of ECM remodeling, mechanical loading can direct the composition, organization, and corollary material properties of the neotissue in tissue engineering constructs.

### 29.5.4 Strain Magnitude and Rate

There are several factors that dictate the degree of cell response to mechanical loading including the magnitude, frequency, and duration of stretch. Hsieh et al. (Hsieh et al. 2000) discovered that increasing strain magnitude provokes a time-dependent increase in collagen synthesis in the MCL. Differential magnitudes of cyclic strain also regulate the activation of mechanotransduction pathways in tendon fibroblasts (Arnoczky et al. 2002). Yang et al. confirmed that mechanically induced alterations in proliferation, collagen production, and growth factor expression of human tendon fibroblasts depend on varying magnitudes (Yang et al. 2004). In addition to ECM synthesis and cell proliferation, increasing magnitudes positively impact cell orientation. Dartsch revealed that the degree of orientation of smooth muscle cells directly relates to increasing amplitudes of mechanical stimulation (Dartsch and Hammerle 1986). Contrary to these results, Gilbert et al. deduced that changes in protein expression for fibroblasts stretched on a 3D scaffold depends on the frequency of stretch and not the magnitude .Gilbert et al. 2007). Similarly, McKnight found that the rate of mechanical strain greatly affects phosphorylation of ERK 1/2 in vascular smooth muscle cells that are oriented in the direction of uniaxial stretch (McKnight and Frangos 2003). In addition to varying degrees of magnitude and rate, modulation of the duration of stretch affects cell response. For instance, Zeichen et al. observed that the proliferative response of tendon fibroblasts to cyclic stretch fluctuates over the duration of loading (Zeichen et al. 2000). Similarly, periodontal fibroblasts demonstrate a dependency of protein synthesis on the duration of stress comparable to MCL and tendon fibroblasts (Uno et al. 2001; Redlich et al. 2004).

# 29.6 *In Vivo* Models to Demonstrate Efficacy

Many techniques have been used to mimic the native motion and forces that a reconstructed ligament will undergo. However, these *in vitro* models are not entirely representative of the multitude of factors present in the body. Therefore, various animal models have been implemented in an attempt to characterize the device function, compatibility, and mechanical viability, Table 29.1. The goat and rabbit models are the most common (Amiel et al. 1984, 1986; Chowdhury et al. 1991; Chvapil et al. 1993; Jackson et al. 1993; Dunn et al. 1994; Lee et al. 1998; Buma et al. 2004; Cooper Jr. et al. 2006; Kawai et al. 2009; Mutsuzaki et al. 2009; Tischer et al. 2009). The goat model is generally considered to be the most representative of the soft tissue healing response found in humans (Ng et al. 1996). A typical ACL reconstruction in the goat model would begin with removal of the ligament including both the tibal and femoral insertions (Ng et al. 1996). A tibial tunnel was made under the transverse ligament and the graft ligament was pulled through the tunnel. Placement is calibrated by movements of the knee, to ensure accurate range of motion. The lateral femoral side of the graft was then fixed with two stainless-steel staples (Ng et al. 1996). Evaluation of the graft success or failure includes rigorous and long term evaluation of the graft's structural and biomechanical properties (Roos et al. 1995; Ng et al. 1996; Murray 2003).

Adequate review at specific time points is critical in determination of device integration and graft success. Time points at 3, 6, and 12 months each have signified importance for graft evaluation. At 3 months the graft procedure can be deemed a technical *surgical* success or failure (initial creep, joint laxity, compromising joint function). Additionally, tissue in-growth in the bony and ligament segments should have begun by this point (Jackson et al. 1993; Ng et al. 1996). Angiogenesis and matrix abrasion should also be apparent at this point (Ng et al. 1996). At 6 months significant cellular ingrowth and vascularization should have taken place which would indicate the graft's potential for complete integration and restoration of function (Ng et al. 1996; Altman and Horan 2006). Matrix degradation and integration of viable, remodeled tissue can also be assessed. Finally, examination at 12 months or later provides evidence of a graft's potential long term strength, integration, and viability (Ng et al. 1996; Altman and Horan 2006). Although useful in preliminary assessment of safety and efficacy prior to human trials, care should always been taken in the prediction of clinical success from animal testing. Clinical failure modes can differ from animal model testing due to differences in equipment and techniques used (Altman and Horan 2006).

# 29.7 Key Challenges and Critical Issues

Musculoskeletal diseases and injuries have an enormous impact on quality of life and remain one of the leading reasons that patients seek medical care. Tissue engineering has emerged as a promising alternative that circumvents the limitations associated with biological and synthetic grafts. However, the continuing difficulty in developing suitable ligament and tendon replacements is due in part to its complex geometry and function. In addition to serving as a structural template for cell attachment/proliferation, the tissue engineered graft should restore function throughout remodeling while limiting stress-shielding effects. Development of a biomaterial scaffold that offsets the loss of mechanical properties with effective load transfer for guided tissue growth remains challenging. During remodeling, the loss of scaffold strength due to biodegradation is offset by the increased load bearing of the neotissue. Two variables must be controlled in order to maintain the mechanical integrity of the tendon or ligament: (1) neotissue formation at a complementary rate to scaffold degradation; (2) graded load transfer to the neotissue to guide orientation. Unfortunately, identifying the design criteria that meet these goals is hampered by poor understanding of the complex feedback mechanisms relating mechanical load, tissue organization and scaffold degradation. New structure-property models are required for the development of a scaffold that offsets the loss of mechanical properties with effective load transfer for guided tissue growth. Although inroads have been made in understanding the structure-property relationships

**TABLE 29.1** Animal Models Reported in the Literature

| Study Goal | Animal | Number | Graft Type | Time Period | Reference |
|---|---|---|---|---|---|
| Compare double flexor tendon graft and BPTB graft healing | Canine | 24 | FT, BPTB | 3, 6, 12 months | Tomita et al. (2001) |
| Growth factor effect on BPTB mechanical properties | Canine | 25 | 20 BPTB | 12 months | Yasuda et al. (2004) |
| Allogeneic tendon graft viability | Canine | 32 | PT (no bone) as ACL/MCL grafts | 3, 30, 52 weeks | Shino and Horibe (1991) |
| Anterior–posterior laxity effect on structural properties | Canine | 26 | 22 PT, 4 Sham | 1–2 months, 1 year | Beynnon et al. (1994) |
| Effect of graft elongation at implantation on biomechancial behavior | Canine | 12 | BPTB | 18 months | Tohyama et al. (1996) |
| Effect of nonphysiologically high initial tension on mechanical properties | Canine | 32 | Freeze dried ACL | 0, 6, 12 weeks | Katsuragi et al. (2000) |
| Effect of postoperative immobilization on reconstructed knees | Goat | 12 | PP braid | 6 months | Roth et al. (1988) |
| Comparison of ligament augmentation device and allograft | Goat | 11 | LAD and freeze dried BPTB | 3 months | Jackson et al. (1987) |
| Reaction to intraarticular allografts sterilized with ethylene oxide | Goat | 20 | PT | 2, 6, 10 weeks | Simon and Jackson (1993) |
| Biomechanics of fascia lata ligament replacements | Goat | 50 | Autogeneous Fascia Lata | 0, 2, 4, 8 weeks | Holden et al. (1988) |
| Effects of gamma irradiation on the initial mechanical properties BPTB allografts | Goat | 24 | PT bisected medial-laterally | 0 days | Gibbons et al. (1991) |
| Biomechanical evaluation of BPTB allografts | Goat | 28 | Freeze dried BPTB graft | 6, 12, 26, 52 weeks | Drez et al. (1991) |
| Viability of collagen fibers as a temporary ACL scaffold | Goat | 14 | HDI x-linked braided collagen | 4 days–6 months | Chvapil et al. (1993) |
| Biomechanics of PT autograft | Goat | 27 | PT | 0, 6, 12 weeks, 1, 3 years | Ng et al. (1995) |
| Long-term biomechanical and viscoelastic performance of ACL after hemitransection | Goat | 11 | Transected posterolateral bundle | 12, 24 weeks 1, 3 years | Ng et al. (1996) |
| Mechanical properties of BPTB ACL grafts using intraoperative force-setting | Goat | 7 | PT | 3 months | Smith et al. (1996) |
| Biomechanica/histologic study of composite collagenous prosthesis for ACL reconstruction | Rabbit | 31 | PMMA-reconstituted collagen composite | 4, 20 weeks | Dunn et al. (1992) |
| Effect of using chitin-coated fabrics ACL alloplastic grafts | Rabbit | 20 | Chitin-coated polyester, noncoated | 8 weeks | Kawai et al. (2009) |
| Effects of TGFb1 and EGF on *in situ* frozen ACL | Rabbit | 142 | Freeze-thawed ACL | 6, 12 weeks | Sakai et al. (2002) |
| Comparison of mechanical properties of MCL and ACL | Rabbit | 30 | ACL, MCL | 0 days | Woo et al. (1992) |

*Note:* FT, Flexor Tendon; BPTB, Bone-Patellar Tendon-Bone; TGFb, Tissue Growth Factor Beta; ACL, Anterior Cruciate Ligament; MCL, Medial Collateral Ligament; PP, Polypropylene; LAD, Ligament Augmentation Device; PT, Patellar Tendon; EtO, Ethylene Oxide; HDI, Hexane Diisocyanate; PMMA, Poly(methyl methacrylate); EGF, Epidermal Growth Factor.

involved in degradation and mechanical properties independently, the complexity of load transfer to new tissue and prediction of total construct properties requires a more rigorous investigation.

Furthermore, it is becoming increasingly clear that successful tissue engineering strategies are dependent on more than just mechanical or structural criteria. The complex cell-matrix interactions require the support of cell, molecular, and developmental biologists. These interdisciplinary teams are needed to elucidate complex mechanobiology mechanisms that dictate whether a tissue engineered construct expresses the correct genes and proteins for functional repair (Butler et al. 2008). This understanding can then be used to refine bioreactor design and cell culture conditions to spatially and temporally control cell phenotype and matrix production in the tissue engineering construct. Finally, the development of systems that provide accurate *in vitro* prediction of *in vivo* outcome as well as animal model prediction of clinical outcome is necessary to increase the throughput of graft assessment. These systems require quantifiable and universal benchmarks that can be used to measure success of a candidate graft and provide optimization targets (Butler et al. 2008). Substantial research efforts are still required to address these critical issues and realize the full potential of tissue engineered tendons and ligaments in clinical use. However, the tremendous rate of progress in the field and the growing need of our active and aging population ensure that tissue engineered grafts will be a clinical reality in the near future.

# References

Abousleiman, R. I. and V. I. Sikavitsas. 2006. Bioreactors for tissues of the musculoskeletal system. *Advances in Experimental Medicine and Biology* 585: 243–259.

Albright, J. C., J. E. Carpenter, B. K. Graf, and J. C. Richmond. 1999. *Knee and Leg: Soft-Tissue Trauma.* Rosemont: American Academy of Orthopaedic Surgeons.

Altman, G. H. and R. L. Horan. 2006. Tissue engineering of ligaments. In *An Introduction of Biomaterials*, Ed. S. A. Guelcher and J. O. Hollinger. Boca Raton: CRC Press, pp. 499–524.

Altman, G. H., R. L. Horan, H. H. Lu et al. 2002. Silk matrix for tissue engineered anterior cruciate ligaments. *Biomaterials* 23(20): 4131–4141.

Altman, G. H., R. L. Horan, I. Martin et al. 2001. Cell differentiation by mechanical stress. *The FASEB Journal* 16(2): 270–272.

Altman, G. H., H. H. Lu, R. L. Horan et al. 2002. Advanced bioreactor with controlled application of multi-dimensional strain for tissue engineering. *Journal of Biomechanical Engineering* 124(6): 742–749.

Amiel, D., C. Frank, F. Harwood, J. Fronek, and W. Akeson. 1984. Tendons and ligaments: A morphological and biochemical comparison. *Journal of Orthopaedic Research* 1(3): 257–265.

Amiel, D., J. B. Kleiner, R. D. Roux, F. Harwood, and W. Akeson. 1986. Phenomenon of "Ligamentization": Anterior cruciate ligament reconstruction with autogenous patellar tendon. *Journal of Orthopuedic Research* 4: 162–172.

Arnoczky, S. P., T. Tian, M. Lavagnino et al. 2002. Activation of stress-activated protein kinases (SAPK) in tendon cells following cyclic strain: The effects of strain frequency, strain magnitude, and cytosolic calcium. *Journal of Orthopaedic Research* 20(5): 947–952.

Atance, J., M. J. Yost, and W. Carver. 2004. Influence of the extracellular matrix on the regulation of cardiac fibroblast behavior by mechanical stretch. *Journal of Cellular Physiology* 200(3): 377–386.

Barry, F. P. 2003. Biology and clinical applications of mesenchymal stem cells. *Birth Defects Research* 69: 250–256.

Bartold, P. M., C. A. G. McCulloch, A. S. Narayanan, and S. Pitaru. 2000. Tissue engineering: A new paradigm for periodontal regeneration based on molecular and cell biology. *Periodontology* 24(1): 253–269.

Battegay, E. J., E. W. Raines, R. A. Seifert, D. F. Bowen-Pope, and R. Ross. 1990. TGF-β induces bimodal proliferation of connective tissue cells via complex control of an autocrine PDGF loop. *Cell* 63(3): 515–524.

Bellincampi, L. D., R. F. Closkey, R. Prasad, J. P. Zawadsky, and M. G. Dunn. 1998. Viability of fibroblast-seeded ligament analogs after autogenous implantation. *Journal of Orthopedic Research* 16(4): 414–420.

Beynnon, B., R. Johnson, H. Toyama et al. 1994. The relationship between anterior-posterior knee laxity and the structural properties of the patellar tendon graft: A study in canines. *The American Journal of Sports Medicine* 22(6):812–820.

Bhatia, S. N. and C. S. Chen. 1999. Tissue engineering at the micro-scale. *Biomedical Microdevices* 2(2): 131–144.

Bianco, P., L. W. Fisher, M. F. Young, J. D. Termine, and P. G. Robey. 1990. Expression and localization of the two small proteoglycans biglycan and decorin in developing skeletal and non-skeletal tissues. *The Journal of Histochemistry and Cytochemistry* 38(11): 1549–1563.

Bolcato-Bellemin, A. L., R. Elkaim, A. Abehsera et al. 2000. Expression of mRNAs encoding for alpha and beta integrin subunits, MMPs, and TIMPs in stretched human periodontal ligament and gingival fibroblasts. *Journal of Dental Research* 79(9): 1712–1716.

Breen, E. C. 2000. Mechanical strain increases type I collagen expression in pulmonary fibroblasts *in vitro*. *Journal of Applied Physiology* 88(1): 203–209.

Buck, R. C. 1980. Reorientation response of cells to repeated stretch and recoil of the substratum. *Experimental Cell Research* 127(2): 470–474.

Buma, P., H. J. Kok, L. Blankevoort et al. 2004. Augmentation in anterior cruciate ligament reconstruction-a histological and biomechanical study on goats. *International Orthopaedics* 28(2): 91–96.

Butler, D. L., S. A. Goldstein, and F. Guilak. 2000. Functional tissue engineering: The role of biomechanics. *Transactions of the ASME* 122: 570–575.

Butler, D. L., N. Juncosa-Melvin, G. P. Boivin et al. 2008. Functional tissue engineering for tendon repair: A multidisciplinary strategy using mesenchymal stem cells, bioscaffolds, and mechanical stimulation. *Journal of Orthopaedic Research* 26(1): 1–9.

Butler, D. L. and D. C. Stouffer. 1983. Tension-torsion characteristics of the canine anterior cruciate ligament—Part II: Experimental observations. *Journal of Biomechanical Engineering* 105(2): 6.

Carver, W., M. L. Nagpal, M. Nachtigal, T. K. Borg, and L. Terracio. 1991. Collagen expression in mechanically stimulated cardiac fibroblasts. *Circulation Research* 69(1): 116–122.

Chen, H.-C. and Y.-C. Hu. 2006. Bioreactors for tissue engineering. *Biotechnology Letters* 28(18): 1415–1423.

Chen, J., R. L. Horan, D. Bramono et al. 2006. Monitoring mesenchymal stromal cell developmental stage to apply on-time mechanical stimulation for ligament tissue engineering. *Tissue Engineering* 12(11): 3085–3095.

Chowdhury, P., J. R. Matyas, and C. B. Frank. 1991. The "epiligament" of the rabbit medial collateral ligament: A quantitative morphological study. *Connective Tissue Research* 27(1)(1?): 33–50.

Chvapil, M., D. Speer, H. Holubec, T. Chvapil, and D. King. 1993. Collagen fibers as a temporary scaffold for replacement of ACL in goats. *Journal of Biomedical Materials Research* 27(3)(3?): 313–325.

Cooper Jr., J. A., L. O. Bailey, J. N. Carter et al. 2006. Evaluation of the anterior cruciate ligament, medial collateral ligament, achilles tendon and patellar tendon as cell sources for tissue-engineered ligament. *Biomaterials* 27(13): 2747–2754.

Cushner, F. D., D. F. L. Rosa, V. J. Vigorita et al. 2003. A quantitative histologic comparison: ACL degeneration in the osteoarthritic knee. *The Journal of Arthroplasty* 18(6): 687–692.

Dartsch, P. C. and H. Hammerle. 1986. Orientation response of arterial smooth muscle cells to mechanical stimulation. *European Journal of Cell Biology* 41(2): 339–346.

Drez, D. J., J. DeLee, J. Holden et al. 1991. Anterior cruciate ligament reconstruction using bone-patellar tendon-bone allografts. A biological and biomechanical evaluation in goats. *The American Journal of Sports Medicine* 19(3): 256–263.

Duncan, G. W., E. H. K. Yen, E. T. Pritchard, and D. M. Suga. 1984. Collagen and prostaglandin synthesis in force-stressed periodontal ligament *in vitro*. *Journal of Dental Research* 63: 665–669.

Dunn, M. G., S. H. Maxian, and J. P. Zawadsky. 1994. Intraosseous incorporation of composite collagen prostheses designed for ligament reconstruction. *Journal of Orthopaedic Research* 12(1): 128–137.

Dunn, M., A. Tria, Y. Kato et al. 1992. Anterior cruciate ligament reconstruction using a composite collagenous prosthesis. A biomechanical and histologic study in rabbits. *The American Journal of Sports Medicine* 20(5)(5?): 507–515.

Eijk, F. V., D. B. F. Sris, J. Riesle, Ph.D. et al. 2004. Tissue engineering of ligaments: A comparison of bone marrow stromal cells, anterior cruciate ligament, and skin fibroblasts as cell source. *The Journal of Tissue Engineering* 10(5/6): 894–903.

Fan, H., H. Liu, S. L. Toh, and J. C. H. Goh. 2008. Enhanced differentiation of mesenchymal stem cells co-cultured with ligament fibroblasts on gelatin/silk fibroin hybrid scaffold. *Biomaterials* 29(8): 1017–1027.

Fischer, S. P. and R. D. Ferkel. 1988. *Prosthetic Ligament Reconstruction of the Knee.* Philadelphia, PA: W. B. Saunders Company.

Foos, M. J., J. R. Hickox, P. G. Mansour, J. R. Slauterbeck, and D. M. Hardy. 2001. Expression of matrix metalloprotease and tissue inhibitor of metalloprotease genes in human anterior cruciate ligament. *Journal of Orthopaedic Research* 19(4): 642–649.

Freed, L. E. and G. Vunjak-Novakovic. 2000. Tissue engineering bioreactors. In *Principles of Tissue Engineering*, Ed. R. P. Lanza, R. Langer and J. Vacanti. San Diego: Academic, pp. 143–156.

Freeman, J. W. and A. L. Kwansa. 2008. Recent advancements in ligament tissue engineering: The use of various techniques and materials for ACL repair. *Recent Patents on Biomedical Engineering* 1(1): 18–23.

Freyman, T. M., I. V. Yannas, and L. J. Gibson. 2001. Cellular materials as porous scaffolds for tissue engineering. *Progress in Materials Science* 46(3–4): 273–282.

Fu, F. H., C. H. Bennett, C. B. Ma, J. Menetrey, and C. Lattermann. 2000. Current trends in anterior cruciate ligament reconstruction part 2. Operative procedures and clinical correlations. *American Orthopaedic Society for Sports Medicine* 28(1): 124–130.

Fu, F. H., C. H. Bennett, C. Lattermann, and C. B. Ma. 1999. Current trends in anterior cruciate ligament reconstruction. *The American Journal of Sports Medicine* 27(6): 821–830.

Garrington, T. P. and G. L. Johnson. 1999. Organization and regulation of mitogen-activated protein kinase signaling pathways. *Current Opinion in Cell Biology* 11(2): 211–218.

Garvin, J., J. Qi, M. Maloney, and A. J. Banes. 2003. Novel system for engineering bioartificial tendons and application of mechanical load. *Tissue Engineering* 9(5): 967–979.

Ge, Z., J. C. H. Goh, L. Wang, E. P. S. Tan, and E. H. Lee. 2005. Characterization of knitted polymeric scaffolds for potential use in ligament tissue engineering. *Journal Biomaterial Science Polymer Edition* 16(9): 1179–1192.

Giancotti, F. G. 1997. Integrin signaling: Specificity and control of cell survival and cell cycle progression *Current Opinion in Cell Biology* 9(5): 691–700.

Gibbons, M. J., D. L. Butler, E. S. Grood et al. 1991. Effects of gamma irradiation on the initial mechanical and material properties of goat bone-patellar tendon-bone allografts. *Journal of Orthopaedic Research* 9: 209–218.

Gilbert, T. W., A. M. Stewart-Akers, J. Sydeski et al. 2007. Gene expression by fibroblasts seeded on small intentinal submucosa and subjected to cyclic stretching. *Tissue Engineering* 13(6): 1313–1323.

Goulet, F., D. Rancourt, C. Caron, A. Normand, and F. A. Auger. 1997. Tendons and ligaments. In *Principles of Tissue Engineering*, Ed. R. PLanza, R. Langer, and W. Chick. San Diego: Landes/Academic, pp. 639–645.

Hannafin, J. A., E. A. Attia, R. Henshaw, R. F. Warren, and M. M. Bhargava. 2006. Effect of cyclic strain and plating matrix on cell proliferation and integrin expression by ligament fibroblasts. *Journal of Orthopaedic Research* 24(2): 149–158.

Henshaw, D. R., E. Attia, M. Bhargava, and J. A. Hannafin. 2006. Canine ACL fibroblast integrin expression and cell alignment in response to cyclic tensile strain in three-dimensional collagen gels. *Journal of Orthopaedic Research* 24(3): 481–490.

Holden, J. P., E. S. Grood, D. L. Butler et al. 1988. Biomechanics of fascia lata ligament replacements: Early postoperative changes in the goat. *Journal of Orthopaedic Research* 6: 639–647.

Howard, P. S., U. Kucich, R. Taliwal, and J. M. Korostoff. 1998. Mechanical forces alter extracellular matrix synthesis by human periodontal ligament fibroblasts. *Journal of Periodontal Research* 33(8): 500–508.

Hsieh, A. H., C. M.-H. Tsai, Q.-J. Ma et al. 2000. Time-dependent increases in type-III collagen gene expression in medial collateral ligament fibroblasts under cyclic strains. *Journal of Orthopaedic Research* 18(2): 220–227.

Jackson, D. W., E. S. Grood, S. P. Arnoczky, D. L. Butler, and S. R. Simon. 1987 Cruciate reconstruction using freeze dried anterior cruciate ligament allograft and a ligament augmentation device (LAD). An experimental study in a goat model. *The American Journal of Sports Medicine* 15(6): 528–538.

Jackson, D. W., E. S. Grood, J. D. Goldstein, M. A. Rosen, and P. A. Kurzweil. 1993. A comparison of patellar tenon autograft and allograft used for anterior cruciate ligament reconstruction in the goat model. *The American Journal of Sports Medicine* 21(2): 176–185.

Juncosa-Melvin, N., K. S. Matlin, R. W. Holdcraft, V. S. Nirmalanandhan, and D. L. Butler. 2007. Mechanical stimulation increases collagen type I and collagen type III gene expression of stem cell—collagen sponge constructs for patellar tendon repair. *Tissue Engineering* 13(6): 1219–1226.

Katsuragi, R., K. Yasuda, J. Tsujino, M. Keira, and K. Kaneda. 2000. The effect of nonphysiologically high initial tension on the mechanical properties of *in situ* frozen anterior cruciate ligament in a canine model. *The American Journal of Sports Medicine* 28(1)(1?): 47–56.

Kawai, T., T. Yamada, A. Yasukawa et al. 2009. Anterior cruciate ligament reconstruction using chitin-coated fabrics in a rabbit model. *Artificial Organs* 34(1)(1?): 55–64.

Kenley, R., K. Yim, J. Abrams et al. 1993. Biotechnology and bone graft substitutes. *Pharmaceutical Research* 10(10): 1393–1401.

Kerkvliet, E. H. M., A. J. P. Docherty, W. Beersten, and V. Everts. 1999. Collagen breakdown in soft connective tissue explants is associated with the level of active gelatinase A (MMP-2) but not with collagenase. *Matrix Biology* 18(4): 373–380.

Kim, B.-S., J. Nikolovski, J. Bonadio, and D. J. Mooney. 1999. Cyclic mechanical strain regulates the development of engineered smooth muscle tissue. *Nature Biotechnology* 17(10): 979–983.

Kim, S.-G., T. Akaike, T. Sasagawa, Y. Atomi, and H. Kurosawa. 2002. Gene expression of type I and type III collagen by mechanical stretch in anterior cruciate ligament cells. *Cell Structure and Function* 27(3): 139–144.

Kleiner, J. B., D. Amiel, R. D. Roux, and W. H. Akeson. 1986. Origin of replacement cells for the anterior cruciate ligament autograft. *The Journal of Orthopaedic Research* 4(4): 466–474.

Kletsas, D., E. K. Basdra, and A. G. Papavassiliou. 1998. Mechanical stress induces DNA synthesis in PDL fibroblasts by a mechanism unrelated to autocrine growth factor action *FEBS Letters* 430(3): 358–362.

Kumar, K. and N. Maffulli. 1999. The ligament augmentatin device: An historical perspective. *Arthroscopy* 15(4): 422–432.

Langer, R. and J. P. Vacanti. 1993. Tissue engineering. *Science* 260(5110): 920–926.

Laurencin, C. T., A. M. A. Ambrosio, M. D. Borden, and J. A. Cooper Jr. 1999. Tissue engineering: Orthopedic applications. *Annual Review of Biomedical Engineering* 1: 19–46.

Laurencin, C. T. and J. W. Freeman. 2005. Ligament tissue engineering: An evolutionary materials science approach. *Biomaterials* 26(36): 7530–7536.

Lee, C. H., H. J. Shin, I. H. Cho et al. 2005. Nanofiber alignment and direction of mechanical strain affect the ECM production of human ACL fibroblast. *Biomaterials* 26(11): 1261–1270.

Lee, C.-Y., X. Liu, C. L. Smith et al. 2004. The combined regulation of estrogen and cyclic tension on fibroblast biosynthesis derived from anterior cruciate ligament. *Matrix Biology* 23(5): 323–329.

Lee, I.-C., J.-H. Wang, Y.-T. Lee, and T.-H. Young. 2007. The differentiation of mesenchymal stem cells by mechanical stress or/and co-culture system. *Biochemical and Biophysical Research Communications* 352(1): 147–152.

Lee, J., F. L. Harwood, W. H. Akeson, and D. Amiel. 1998. Growth factor expression in healing rabbit medial collateral and anterior cruciate ligaments. *The Iowa Orthopaedic Journal* 18: 19–25.

Leung, D. Y. M., S. Glagov, and M. B. Mathews. 1976. Cyclic stretching stimulates synthesis of matrix components by arterial smooth muscle cells *in vitro*. *Science* 191(4226): 475–477.

Lin, V. S., M. C. Lee, S. O'Neal, J. McKean, and K.-L. P. Sung. 1999. Ligament tissue engineering using synthetic biodegradable fiber scaffolds. *Tissue Engineering* 5(5): 443–451.

Lin, V. S., M. C. Lee, S. O'Neal, J. McKean, and K. L. P. Sung, 1999. Ligament tissue engineering using synthetic biodegradable fiber scaffolds. *Tissue Engineering* 5(5): 443–451.

Liu, H., H. Fan, Y. Wang, S. L. Toh, and J. C. H. Goh. 2008. The interaction between a combined knitted silk scaffold and microporous silk sponge with human mesenchymal stem cells for ligament tissue engineering. *Biomaterials* 29(6): 662–674.

Lomas, R. J., L. M. Jennings, J. Fisher, and J. N. Kearney. 2004. Effects of a peracetic acid disinfection protocol on the biocompatibility and biomechanical properties of human patellar tendon allografts. *Cell and Tissue Banking* 5(3)(3?): 149–160.

Lopez-Vazquez, E., J. A. Juan, E. Vila, and J. Debon. 1991. Reconstruction of the anterior cruciate ligament with a Dacron prosthesis. *The Journal of Bone and Joint Surgery* 73: 1294–1300.

Maletius, W. and J. Gillquist. 1997. Long-term results of anterior cruciate ligament reconstruction with a Dacron prosthesis. The frequency of osteoarthritis after seven to eleven years. *The American Journal of Sports Medicine* 25: 288–293.

Mann, B. K., R. H. Schmedlen, and J. L. West. 2001. Tethered-TGF-β increases extracellular matrix production of vascular smooth muscle cells. *Biomaterials* 22(5): 439–444.

Markolf, K., G. Pattee, G. Strum et al. 1989. Instrumented measurements of laxity in patients who have a Gore-Tex anterior cruciate-ligament substitute. *Journal of Bone and Joint Surgery* 71: 887–893.

Marks, P. H., Donaldson, F. R., and Cameron, M. L. 2005. Inflammatory cytokine profiles associated with chondral damage in the anterior cruciate ligament–deficient knee. *Arthroscopy: The Journal of Arthroscopic and Related Surgery* 21(11): 1342–1347.

Martin, I., D. Wendt, and M. Heberer. 2004. The role of bioreactors in tissue engineering. *TRENDS in Biotechnology* 22(2): 80–85.

Marui, T., C. Niyibizi, H. I. Georgescu et al. 1997. Effect of growth factors on matrix synthesis by ligament fibroblasts *Journal of Orthopaedic Research* 15(1): 18–23.

Matziolis, G., J. Tuischer, G. Kasper et al. 2006. Simulation of cell differentiatin in fracture healing: Mechanically loaded composite scaffolds in a novel bioreactor system. *Tissue Engineering* 12(1): 201–208.

McKnight, N. L. and J. A. Frangos. 2003. Strain rate mechanotransduction in aligned human vascular smooth muscle cells. *Annals of Biomedical Engineering* 31: 239–249.

Miyaki, S., T. Ushida, K. Nemoto et al. 2001. Mechanical stretch in anterior cruciate ligament derived cells regulates type I collagen and decorin expression through extracellular signal-regulated kinase 1/2 pathway. *Materials Science and Engineering* 17(1–2): 91–94.

Moyen, B. J., J. Y. Jenny, A. H. Mandrino, and J. L. Lerat. 1992. Comparison of reconstruction of the anterior cruciate ligament with and without a Kennedy ligament augmentation device. A randomized, prospective study. *The Journal of Bone and Joint Surgery* 74: 1313–1319.

Murray, A. W. and M. F. Macnicol. 2003. 10–16 year results of Leeds-Keio anterior cruciate ligament reconstruction. *The Knee* 11: 9–14.

Murray, M., K. Rice, R. J. Wright, and M. Spector. 2003. The effect of selected growth factors on human anterior cruciate ligament cell interactions with a three-dimensional collagen-GAG scaffold. *Journal of Orthopaedic Research* 21(2): 238–244.

Mutsuzaki, H., M. Sakane, S. Hattori, H. Kobayashi, and N. Ochiai. 2009. Firm anchoring between a calcium phosphate-hybridized tendon and bone for anterior cruciate ligament reconstruction in a goat model *Biomedical Materials* 4(4): 1–7.

Nedeff, D. D. and B. R. Bach. 2001. Arthroscopic anterior cruciate ligament reconstruction using patellar tendon autografts. *The American Journal of Knee Surgery* 14(4): 243–257.

Neidlinger-Wilke, C., E. Grood, L. Claes, and R. Brand. 2002. Fibroblast orientation to stretch begins within three hours. *Journal of Orthopaedic Research* 20(5): 953–956.

Neidlinger-Wilke, C., E. Grood, J. H.-C. Wang, R. Brand, and L. Claes. 2001. Cell alignment is induced by cyclic changes in cell length: Studies of cells grown in cyclically stretched substrates. *Journal of Orthopaedic Research* 19: 286–293.

Neurath, M. 1993. Structure and function of matrix components in the cruciate ligaments. An immunohistochemical, electron-microscopic, and immunoelectron-microscopic study. *Acta Anatomica* 145(4): 387–394.

Ng, G. Y., B. W. Oakes, O. W. Deacon, I. D. McLean, and D. Lampard. 1995. Biomechanics of patellar tendon autograft for reconstruction of the anterior cruciate ligament in the goat: Three-year study. *Journal of Orthopaedic Research* 13: 602–608.

Ng, G. Y., B. W. Oakes, O. W. Deacon, I. D. McLean, and D. Lampard. 1996a. Biomechanics of patellar tendon autograft for reconstruction of the anterior cruciate ligament in the goat: Three-year study. *Journal of Orthopaedic Research* 13: 602–608.

Ng, G. Y. F., B. W. Oakes, I. D. McLean, O. W. Deacon, and D. Lampard. 1996b. The long-term biomechanical and viscoelastic performance of repairing anterior cruciate ligament after hemitransection injury in a goat model. *The American Journal of Sports Medicine* 24(1): 109–117.

Noth, U., K. Schupp, A. Heymer et al. 2005. Anterior cruciate ligament constructs fabricated from human mesenchymal stem cells in a collagen type I hydrogel. *Cytotherapy* 7(5): 447–455.

Noyes, F. R. and E. S. Grood. 1976. The strength of the anterior cruciate ligament in humans and Rhesus monkeys. *Journal of Bone and Joint Surgery* 58A(8): 1074–1082.

Olson, E. J., J. D. Kang, F. H. Fu et al. 1988. The biochemical and histological effects of artificial ligament wear particales: *In vitro* and *in vivo* studies. *The American Journal of Sports Medicine* 16(6): 558–570.

Ozaki, S., S. Kaneko, K. A. Podyma-Inoue, M. Yanagishita, and K. Soma. 2005. Modulation of extracellular matrix synthesis and alkaline phosphatase activity of periodontal ligament cells by mechanical stress. *Journal of Periodontal Research* 40(2): 110–117.

Park, S. A., I. A. Kim, Y. J. Lee et al. 2006. Biological responses of ligament fibroblasts and gene expression profiling on micropatterned silicone substrates subjected to mechanical stimuli. *Journal of Bioscience and Bioengineering* 102(5): 402–412.

Parsons, J. R., S. Bhayani, H. Alexander, and A. B. Weiss. 1985. Carbon fiber debris within the synovial joint. A time-dependent mechanical and histological study. *Clinical Orthopaedics and Related Research* 196: 69–76.

Pennisi, E. 2002. Tending tender tendons. *Science* 295(5557): 1011.

Pogany, G. and K. G. Vogel. 1992. The interaction of decorin core protein fragments with type I collagen. *Biochemical and Biophysical Research Communications* 189(1): 165–172.

Praemer, A., S. Furner, and D. P. Rice (1999). Musculoskeletal condition in the United States. Parke Ridge, IL: American Academy of Orthopaedic Surgeons, 182.

Redlich, M., H. A. Roos, E. Reichenberg et al. 2004. Expression of tropoelastin in human periodontal ligament fibroblasts after simulation of orthodontic force. *Archives of Oral Biology* 49(2): 119–124.

Riechert, K., K. Labs, K. Lindenhayn, and P. Sinha. 2001. Semiquantitative analysis of types I and III collagen from tendons and ligaments in a rabbit model *Journal of Orthopaedic Science* 6(1): 68–74.

Romaris, M., A. Heredia, A. Molist, and A. Bassols. 1991. Differential effect of transforming growth factor beta on proteoglycan synthesis in human embryonic lung fibroblasts. *Biochima et Biophysica Acta* 1093: 229–233.

Roos, H., T. Adalberth, L. Dahlbeg, and L. S. Lohmander. 1995. Osteoarthritis of the knee after injury to the anterior cruciate ligament or meniscus: The influence of time and age. *Osteoarthritis and Cartilage* 3(4): 261–267.

Rose, F. R. A. J. and R. O. C. Oreffo. 2002. Bone tissue engineering: Hope vs hype. *Biochemical and Biophysical Research Communications* 292(1): 1–7.

Roth, J., H. Mendenhall, and G. McPherson. 1988. The effect of immobilization on goat knees following reconstruction of the anterior cruciate ligament. *Clinical Orthopaedics and Related Research* (229): 278–282.

Sakai, T., K. Yasuda, H. Tohyama et al. 2002. Effects of combined administration of transforming growth factor-beta1 and epidermal growth factor on properties of the *in situ* frozen anterior cruciate ligament in rabbits. *Journal of Orthopaedic Research* 20(6): 1345–1351.

San Martin, S. and T. M. T. Zorn. 2003. The small proteoglycan biglycan is associated with thick collagen fibrils in the moust decidua. *Cellular and Molecular Biology* 49(4): 673–678.

Scheffler, S., J. Scherler, A. Pruss, R. von Versen, and A. Weiler. 205. Biomechanical comparison of human bone-patellar tendon-bone grafts after sterilization with peracetic acid–ethanol. *Cell and Tissue Banking* 6: 109–115.

Scheffler, S., J. Scherler, A. Pruss, R. von Versen, and A. Weiler. 2005. Biomechanical comparison of human bone-patellar tendon-bone grafts after sterilization with peracetic acid–ethanol. *Cell and Tissue Banking* 6: 109–115.

Schmidt, C. C., H. I. Georgescu, C. K. Kwoh et al. 1995. Effect of growth factors on the proliferation of fibroblasts from the medial collateral and anterior cruciate ligaments. *Journal of Orthopaedic Research* 13(2): 184–190.

Schonherr, E., M. Winnemoller, B. Harrach, H. Robenek, and H. Kresse. 1993. Interactions of small proteoglycans with other extracellular matrix proteins. In *Dermatan Sulphate Proteoglycans*, Ed. J. E. Scott. London, UK: Portland Press, pp. 241–247.

Seon, J. K., E. K. Song, and S. J. Park. 2006. Osteoarthritis after anterior cruciate ligament reconstruction using a patellar tendon autograft. *International Orthopaedics* 30(2): 94–98.

Shi, Y. and I. Vesely. 2005. A dynamic straining bioreactor for collagen-based tissue engineering. In *Bioreactors for Tissue Engineering*, Ed. J. B. Chaudhuri and M. Al-Rubeai. Springer Dordrecht, The Netherlands, pp. 209–219.

Shino, K. and S. Horibe. 1991. Experimental ligament reconstruction by allogeneic tendon graft in a canine model. *Acta Orthopaedica Belgica* 57 Suppl 2: 44–53.

Shino, K., T. Kawasaki, H. Hirose et al. 1984. Replacement of the anterior cruciate ligament by an allogeneic tendon graft. *The Journal of Bone and Joint Surgery* 66(5): 672–681.

Simon, T. M. and D. W. Jackson. 1993. Reaction to intraarticular allografts sterilized with ethylene oxide. *Sports Medicine & Arthroscopy Review* 1(1): 61–70.

Skutek, M., M. van Griensven, J. Zeichen, N. Brauer, and U. Bosch. 2001. Cyclic mechanical stretching modulates secretion pattern of growth factors in human tendon fibroblasts. *European Journal of Applied Physiology* 86(1): 48–52.

Smith, J., J. Lewis, P. Mente et al. 1996. Intraoperative force-setting did not improve the mechanical properties of an augmented bone-tendon-bone anterior cruciate ligament graft in a goat model. *Journal of Orthopaedic Research* 14(2): 209–215.

Sung, K.-L. P., D. E. Whittemore, L. Yang, D. Amiel, and W. H. Akeson. 1996. Signal pathways and ligament cell adhesiveness. *Journal of Orthopaedic Research* 14(5): 729–735.

Tischer, T., M. Ronga, A. Tsai et al. 2009. Biomechanics of the goat three bundle anterior cruciate ligament. *Knee Surgery, Sports Traumatology, Arthroscopy* 17: 935–940.

Tohyama, H., B. D. Beynnon, R. J. Johnson, P. A. Renström, and S. W. Arms. 1996. The effect of anterior cruciate ligament graft elongation at the time of implantation on the biomechanical behavior of the graft and knee. *The American Journal of Sports Medicine* 24(5): 608–614.

Tohyama, H. and K. Yasuda. 1998. Significance of graft tension in anterior cruciate ligament reconstruction. Basic background and clinical outcome. *Knee Surgery, Sports Traumatology, Arthroscopy* 6: S30–S37.

Tomita, F., K. Yasuda, S. Mikami et al. 2001. Comparisons of intraosseous graft healing between the doubled flexor tendon graft and the bone–Patellar tendon–Bone graft in anterior cruciate ligament reconstruction. *Arthroscopy* 17(5): 461–476.

Toyoda, T., H. Matsumoto, K. Fujikawa, S. Saito, and K. Inoue. 1998. Tensile load and the metabolism of anterior cruciate ligament cells. *Clinical Orthopaedics and Related Research* 353: 247–255.

Tremble, P., R. Chiquet-Ehrismann, and Z. Werb. 1994. The extracellular matrix ligands fibronectin and tenascin collaborate in regulating collagenase gene expression in fibroblasts. *Molecular Biology of the Cell* 5(4): 439–453.

Uno, K., Y. Abiko, H. Takita et al. 2001. Effects of mechanical stress on the expression of type XII collagen mRNA in human periodontal ligament cells. *Journal of Hard Tissue Biology* 10(2): 116–122.

Vunjak-Novakovic, G., G. H. Altman, R. L. Horan, and D. L. Kaplan. 2004. Tissue engineering of ligaments. *Annual Review of Biomedical Engineering* 6: 131–156.

Vunjak-Novakovic, G. and L. E. Freed. 1997. Cell–polymer–bioreactor system for tissue engineering. *Journal of the Serbian Chemical Society* 62(2): 787–799.

Wang, J. H.-C., F. Jia, T. W. Gilbert, and S. L.-Y. Woo. 2003. Cell orientation determines the alignment of cell-produced collagenous matrix. *Journal of Biomechanics* 36(1): 97–102.

Wang, J. H.-C., G. Yang, Z. Li, and W. Shen. 2004. Fibroblast responses to cyclic mechanical stretching depend on cell orientation to the stretching direction *Biomaterials* 37(4): 573–576.

Wegrowski, Y., P. Gillery, G. Kotlarz et al. 2000. Modulation of sulfated glycosaminoglycan and small proteoglycan synthesis by the extracellular matrix. *Molecular and Cellular Biochemistry* 205: 125–131.

Weitzel, P. P., J. C. Richmond, G. A. Altman, T. Calabro, and D. L. Kaplan. 2002. Future direction of the treatment of ACL ruptures. *Orthopaedic Clinical North America* 33(4): 653–661.

Westergren-Thorsson, G., P. Antonsson, A. Malmstrom, D. Heinegard, and A. Oldberg. 1991. The synthesis of a family of structurally related proteoglycans in fibroblasts is differently regulated by TGF-beta. *Matrix* 11: 177–183.

Woo, S. L.-Y., P. O. Newton, D. A. MacKenna, and R. M. Lyon. 1992. A comparative evaluation of the mechanical properties of the rabbit medial collateral and anterior cruciate ligaments. *Journal of Biomechanics* 25(4): 377–386.

Yang, G., R. C. Crawford, and J. H.-C. Wang. 2004. Proliferation and collagen production of human patellar tendon fibroblasts in response to cyclic uniaxial stretching in serum-free conditions. *Journal of Biomechanics* 37(10): 1543–1550.

Yang, G., H.-J. Im and J. H.-C. Wang. 2005. Repetitive mechanical stretching modulates IL-1β induced COX-2, MMP-1 expression, and PGE2 production in human patellar tendon fibroblasts. *Gene* 363: 166–172.

Yasuda, K., F. Tomita, S. Yamazaki, A. Minami, and H. Tohyama. 2004. The effect of growth factors on biomechanical properties of the bone-patellar tendon-bone graft after anterior cruciate ligament reconstruction: A canine model study. *The American Journal of Sports Medicine* 32(4)(4?): 870–880.

Zeichen, J., M. van Griensven, and U. Bosch. 2000. The proliferative response of isolated human tendon fibroblasts to cyclic biaxial mechanical strain. *The American Journal of Sports Medicine* 28(6): 888–892.

Zhou, D., H. S. Lee, F. Villareal et al. 2005. Differential MMP-2 activity of ligament cells under mechanical stretch injury: An *in vitro* study on human ACL and MCL fibroblasts. *Journal of Orthopaedic Research* 23(4): 949–957.

# 30

# Cartilage Tissue Engineering

30.1 Cartilage Tissue: Composition, Function, and Disease ..........**30**-1
Cellular and Extracellular Matrix Components • Age and
Disease • Treatment
30.2 Cartilage Tissue Engineering .......................................**30**-4
Tissue Engineering Model • Challenges and Limitations
30.3 Zonal Cartilage Engineering ........................................**30**-4
Monolayer Cell Studies • Scaffold-Supported Culture • Growth
Factor Delivery • Layered Culture Systems
30.4 Stem Cells in Cartilage Tissue Engineering................**30**-7
Embryonic Stem Cells • Bone Marrow Mesenchymal
Stem Cells • Adipose-Derived Adult Stem Cells
30.5 Dynamic Culture Systems for Cartilage Engineering............**30**-16
Adult Chondrocytes • Stem Cell Differentiation • Challenges and
Limitations
Acknowledgments.......................................................**30**-19
References......................................................................**30**-19

Emily E. Coates
*University of Maryland*

John P. Fisher
*University of Maryland*

## 30.1 Cartilage Tissue: Composition, Function, and Disease

### 30.1.1 Cellular and Extracellular Matrix Components

Articular cartilage is complex in its extracellular matrix (ECM) organization in as well as cellular phenotype. The tissue is composed of predominately type II collagen, proteoglycans, and chondrocytes. However, the morphology and metabolic activity of the cells as well as the structure of the ECM vary greatly throughout the tissue depth. This intricate tissue organization allows cartilage to optimally resist loading and provide low-friction joint movement throughout a lifetime.

#### 30.1.1.1 Composition

Cartilage tissue has a low cell density, with chondrocytes comprising only 5% of the total tissue volume [1]. Furthermore, after adulthood is reached chondrocytes rarely divide to provide the tissue with a new cell population. Articular cartilage lacks both a blood supply and direct access to the lymph system; leaving nutrient, gas, and waste exchange to occur through diffusion. All of these factors contribute to the tissue's limited ability to self-heal. Cartilage defects rarely repair themselves and this often leads to complications later in life, or even disease. The most prevalent disease affecting articular cartilage is osteoarthritis (OA). The inability of cartilage to self-repair and the growing cost of OA to society (current estimates at $60 billion dollars annually in the United States [2]) have made cartilage engineering the focus of many research efforts.

Approximately 95% of cartilage tissue is composed of ECM. This matrix comprised predominately of two interconnected networks: a type II collagen network and a hyaluronic acid and proteoglycan network. Chondrocytes are linked to these networks through proteins on the cell surface which allow them to sense, and respond to, mechanical force [3]. Collagen content makes up about 10–20% of the wet weight of the tissue, and 90% of the collagen content is the type II collagen network. Type II collagen is a 300-nm long fiber with three identical polypeptide α helixes. The collagen fibers are linked by strong covalent bonds and provide much of the tensile strength to the tissue [4,5].

Aggrecan is the major proteoglycan in the tissue, and contains many branched glycosaminoglycans (GAGs) originating from a central backbone. The GAGs are predominately keratin sulfate and chondroitin sulfate, and each aggrecan molecule contains 50–100 of each. Repeating sulfate groups give the molecule a large net negative charge. Each aggrecan unit is connected via a link protein to a long, unbranched hyaluronic acid polysaccharide chain. The negative charges on the aggrecan molecules provide a high osmotic tissue pressure, which acts to resist compression during loading. Although articular cartilage has a higher osmotic pressure than many other tissues, the highly interconnected collagen network helps to maintain the integrity of the tissue by preventing tissue swelling—which in turn provides the tissue with further compressive strength [3,5–7]. However, during loading a small amount of liquid is forced out of the tissue into the synovial cavity of the joint. Here, the liquid will absorb nutrients which will be delivered to the tissue as the load is released and the liquid flows back into the cartilage. Thus, a healthy loading regime is essential for proper cartilage function [8].

### 30.1.1.2 Structure

The average height of human articular cartilage on the knee femoral condyle has been measured at 2.4 mm [9]. Below the articulating surface the tissue has been divided into three zones: the superficial or tangential zone, the middle or transitional zone, and the deep or basal zone. Each zone has distinct ECM organization, cell morphology, and metabolic activity. Many studies use slightly different definitions of zone depth. As a general rule, the superficial zone is defined as approximately the top 10–15% of the tissue and contains the articulating surface. The middle zone is the approximately the middle 60% of the tissue and the deep zone contains the remaining 30% of tissue depth. Following the deep zone is the tidemark—below which the tissue becomes calcified and eventually turns into subchondral bone. This calcified region effectively blocks any diffusion from the subchondral bone [5,10–12].

The ECM composition varies between zones. Although collagen content tends to increases with depth, it is the variation in fiber orientation which is thought to have a greater impact on tissue properties. It is hypothesized that collagen fiber orientation accounts for the differences in tensile strength and stiffness throughout the tissue depth [13,14]. The tensile strength and stiffness of the tissue are highest in the superficial zone and decrease into the middle and deep zone [14]. Collagen fibers in the superficial zone are orientated parallel to the articulating surface in tight bundles. As well as providing tensile strength these fibers are thought to block any unwanted molecules from the synovial fluid in the joint [15]. The collagen fibers of the middle zone are randomly orientated, and those of the deep zone are organized perpendicular to the articulating surface. Differences in proteoglycan content are also observed throughout the tissue depth. Proteoglycan content increases with distance from the articulating surface, and with it so does the compressive modulus of the tissue [16]. Consequently, the water content is lowest in the superficial zone, with approximately 65% of the water content of the tissue residing in the middle and deep zones. Furthermore, as a result of diffusion from the synovial fluid the oxygen concentration within the tissue is highest in the superficial zone and decreases through the middle and deep zones [3,12].

Zonal differences in matrix organization and content are largely due to variations in cellular activity [17,18]. Between zones cells display differences in morphology, density, and metabolic activity. Superficial zone cells are the smallest and the most densely populated. They are elongated, thin, and oriented parallel to the articulating surface. Middle zone cells are larger, less densely populated, and do not have a particular orientation. Deep zone cells are also larger than superficial cells and are oriented in columns perpendicular to the articulating surface which serves to anchor the articular cartilage to the calcified layer below. Although superficial and middle zone chondrocytes usually exist on their own or in pairs, deep zone cells are often found in clusters of five to eight cells [9,15].

Several secreted proteins also exist as markers for cells of various zones; however, all their functions are not fully understood. Superficial cells are the only cells which secrete the superficial zone protein (SZP), a large glycoprotein that aids in lubrication in the synovial fluid. SZP, along with similar lubricating proteins, are encoded by the proteoglycan 4 gene (PRG4) [19]. The glycoprotein clusterin has also been localized to the superficial zone; however, its exact function there is unknown [20,21]. Developmental endothelial locus-1 (Del1) protein is thought to play a role in vascularization regulation, and restricts endothelial cells during early development [22]. This protein has been reported in the cell-associated matrix of isolated superficial chondrocytes and is enriched in tissue explants from the superficial zone versus the deep zone [23]. Middle zone cells are unique in their production of cartilage intermediate layer protein. The protein's exact function is yet to be identified; however, it is thought to have a role in the progression of diseases such as OA [24]. Cartilage oligomeric matrix protein is a large extracellular glycoprotein thought to stabilize matrix bonds and found in the matrix surrounding a chondrocyte. Studies have identified its upregulation as a marker for OA and rheumatoid arthritis [25,26]; however, it is also thought to be a marker for deep zone cartilage [27,28].

## 30.1.2 Age and Disease

The natural aging process leaves cartilage less robust and with lower tensile strength as early as the third decade of life. With age the metabolic activity of the chondrocytes is altered, their ability to respond to growth factors and cytokines decreases. Compromised mechanical properties and decreased activity of the chondrocytes leave aged tissue more susceptible to damage [15,29].

Cartilage tissue can be damaged due to diseases such as arthritis or trauma which results in tissue injury. The limited cell population and reliance on diffusion for nutrients and waste exchange make it difficult for chondrocytes to restore a damaged ECM. In unhealthy tissue, the balance between matrix production and breakdown is disrupted and a cycle of tissue degradation ensues. Even minor tissue injuries cannot fully repair, as such injuries do not trigger an inflammatory and reparative response within the tissue, and leave the cartilage more susceptible to the onset of disease [3,30].

## 30.1.3 Treatment

Treating OA and cartilage injuries is challenging. It is difficult to repair a tissue lacking intrinsic repair mechanisms. Turnover in matrix proteins is relatively low even in healthy tissue, with the half life of collagen and proteoglycans approximately 100 and 3–24 years, respectively [31]. Additionally, there is no single reason or way that tissue degradation occurs—making treatment options hard to identify. Pain medication given to arthritic patients may relieve pain, but it does nothing to stop tissue erosion. Furthermore, therapies that target resident cell populations will be ineffective if cells have already become phenotypically unstable and entered hypertrophy or fibroblastic lineages [4]. Currently, engineered cartilage therapies are not standard practice in treating cartilage defects. Standard of care still involves nonsurgical interventions or traditional surgical techniques. Although these treatment methods have had some successes, they are largely inadequate for regenerating healthy tissue with functional properties similar to those of native cartilage.

Current surgical repair techniques include both joint alteration procedures, such as osteotomy, arthrodesis, and anthroplasty [32,33], as well as tissue regeneration procedure, such as bone marrow stimulation [34,35], tissue autografts and allografts [36], and autologous chondrocyte implantation (ACI) [30–32]. Joint alteration procedures are often associated with risk of infection and loss of joint mobility and function. Grafts can result in donor-site morbidity, and increase the patient's risk for the onset of OA. Bone marrow stimulation often results in poor chondrocyte phenotype retention and fibrocartilage repair tissue, and the ACI procedure includes both the drawbacks of grafts and bone marrow stimulation procedures. Owing to the many disadvantages of traditional repair strategies, tissue engineering solutions have began to make their way into clinical trials both in the United States and abroad.

## 30.2 Cartilage Tissue Engineering

### 30.2.1 Tissue Engineering Model

A tissue engineering scaffold can be seeded with a desired cell population and implanted into a defect site. The scaffold provides both mechanical support and a three-dimensional environment for cells to attach and proliferate. Signals, such as growth factors, can be delivered to the cell population to guide their activity. The cell population will produce ECM components which will infiltrate the scaffold material and surrounding tissue. Slowly the scaffold material will degrade—leaving only cells and native tissue. There are many materials used for the scaffold component of an engineered construct. Scaffolds can be made out of naturally or synthetically derived components. The majority of cartilage scaffolds contain building blocks of either proteins or polysaccharides. Scaffolds can also come in a variety of physical forms, such as foams, viscous liquids, hydrogels, and porous matrices.

### 30.2.2 Challenges and Limitations

A major obstacle in tissue engineering articular cartilage is obtaining a sufficiently large and phenotypically stable autologous cell population. Donor-site morbidity makes a large cartilage harvest impractical and even dangerous. The low number of harvested chondrocytes creates the need for expansion culture in monolayer. Although chondrocytes maintain their phenotype better in three-dimensional culture their proliferation rates are much higher in monolayer. Monolayer culture causes chondrocytes to flatten, losing their rounded morphology, and become more fibroblastic in nature. Three-dimensional culture following monolayer helps to redifferentiate the cells; however, this process is relatively inefficient and the native phenotype is never fully restored. Quality and health of the harvested chondrocytes is also an issue of concern. Currently, the mechanisms at play during chondrocyte differentiation and redifferentiation are not fully understood [31,32,37].

In addition to cell source challenges, recreating native tissue structure remains as another major challenge. Initial studies, and most currently available engineering solutions, attempt to remodel cartilage as a homogenous tissue. As the cellular and structural differences between cartilage zones are more fully understood, the need to recreate this complex tissue architecture is becoming more apparent. It is unlikely that a homogenous tissue, based on a homogenous scaffold, can functionally replace a heterogeneous tissue structure. Furthermore, it is likely that through formation of zonal organization there will be better integration with host tissue, and a more fluid transmission of stress between native and novel cartilage

## 30.3 Zonal Cartilage Engineering

Recreation of the zonal complexities of native cartilage tissue has become a focus of many cartilage engineering efforts. Although there is no current model for regenerating zonally organized tissue *in vitro*, many studies throughout the last two decades have sought to classify the differences in metabolic activity between isolated chondrocyte subpopulations from the superficial, middle, and deep zones. Monolayer studies provided initial sight to cellular differences. Three-dimensional encapsulation, growth factor delivery, and layered culture systems have all furthered this understanding and helped to achieve more stable cell populations in culture. However, comprehensive knowledge of the cellular mechanisms and developmental factors behind these differences is yet to be achieved. Here we will highlight studies which have investigated the response of chondrocytes isolated from the superficial, middle, and deep zones to *in vitro* culture.

### 30.3.1 Monolayer Cell Studies

Initial differences in culture show large variations in chondrocyte metabolism and further highlight the differences between zonal cells. However, two-dimensional culture results in a gradual trend toward homogenization of subpopulations and loss of the chondrocyte phenotype. Owing to similarities in native tissue structure and cellular activity most studies pool middle and deep zone chondrocytes and study the superficial zone separately. Cells isolated from the middle and deep zones were shown to produce significantly thicker tissue with higher compressive modulus and substantially more GAGs, large aggregating proteoglycans, and collagen than their superficial zone counterparts [38–41]. Superficial zone cells also showed weaker and slower cell attachment, and formation of clusters that were mainly cellular with little matrix [39,41]. Cells isolated from the superficial zone also demonstrated significantly higher relaxed and instantaneous moduli after an 18-h culture period [42].

With increasing culture time, these differences tend to disappear. It was demonstrated that superficial cells initially showed gene expression levels of SZP more than twice that of cells from middle/deep layers. The middle/deep zone population expressed 20 times more collagen than superficial cells. After three passages, these differences were no longer detected and after four passages gene expression of type I collagen had increased 1200-fold and 8000-fold for the superficial and middle/deep zone cells, respectively. Furthermore, suspension in alginate did not restore gene expression levels to initial values [43]. Overall, monolayer culture resulted in conversion of subpopulations to a homogenous population and rapid loss of cellular phenotype [38,41,44], demonstrating the inadequacy of this culture technique for zonal phenotype retention.

## 30.3.2 Scaffold-Supported Culture

Constructs that support chondrocytes in a three-dimensional environment have shown further success in retention of phenotype and zonal properties. In three-dimensional environments, chondrocytes are able to maintain their characteristic rounded or elongated shape, making hydrogel encapsulation a particularly popular culture method. Culture of bovine subpopulations in agarose hydrogels demonstrated deep zone cells proliferated at the greatest rate, produced the most ECM, and highest amounts of aggregating proteoglycans. Superficial zone cells produced smaller nonaggregating proteoglycans that were degraded before they could be used in matrix assembly [17,18]. Culture in an alginate hyodrogel model demonstrated retention of superficial zone markers clusterin and proteoglycan 4 [45]. Poly(ethylene glycol) (PEG)-based hydrogels have also shown success retaining populations of zonal chondrocytes [46]. Similarly, bovine chondrocytes in devitalized cartilage constructs showed increased production of PRG4 in superficial cells over middle and deep cells, a difference which was maintained throughout culture for 9 days [47]. Three-dimensional culture aids in retention of both the chondrocyte phenotype and differences between zonal populations.

## 30.3.3 Growth Factor Delivery

Major growth factrs used to stimulate *in vitro* matrix production in chondrocytes include insulin-like growth factor 1 (IGF-1), members of the transforming growth factor (TGF)-β superfamily (including TFG-βs and bone morphogenetic proteins [BMPs]), and basic fibroblast growth factor (bFGF). Although these growth factors are generally understood to stimulate synthesis of ECM proteins, the mechanisms behind their varying effects on subpopulations are not yet fully understood.

Delivery of IGF-1 (10, 100 ng/mL), bFGF (10, 100 ng/mL), and TGF-β1 (5, 30 ng/mL) over 3 weeks resulted in distinct effects on superficial versus middle/deep zone cells in monolayer. All concentrations of IGF-1 increased gene expression for aggrecan and type II collagen in the middle/deep zone populations, while all concentrations of TGF-β1 decreased expression in the same cells. The lower concentration of bFGF was found to increase aggrecan expression in the middle/deep zone, whereas the higher concentration increased type II collagen expression. Superficial zone cells displayed lower expression for matrix proteins in all conditions, and were found to increase SZP expression for both concentrations of TGF-β1 and 100 ng/mL IGF-1 [48]. Results indicate that IGF-1 may be optimal for middle and deep zone cells to promote matrix production and reduce type I collagen production, and TGF-β1 may be important for superficial cells to aid in production of SZP and matrix components. Additional studies demonstrated that TFG-β1 can stimulate production of the SZP in superficial cells [49,50].

BMPs stimulate matrix production in chondrocytes [51–53]; however, their effects on zonal cell populations are less documented. A recent study showed adenovirus-mediated delivery of both BMP 2 and 7 resulted in increased matrix accumulation in only superficial cell culture pellets [54]. These results indicate that BMPs may be more appropriate for delivery to superficial zone cell populations.

Trends in growth factor delivery indicate TGF-β1 and BMPs may be influential in stimulating superficial zone chondrocytes while IGF-1 may be important for middle/deep zone chondrocytes. Although these results provide much insight, the majority of these models have examined chondrocytes in monolayer. It has been well documented that chondrocytes and zonal phenotype are unstable in such environments. Several studies report that even with growth factor delivery morphological differences between zonal populations in two-dimensional culture are not maintained [48,55]. Further studies that utilize three-dimensional culture will provide a more accurate picture of growth factor effects on zonal chondrocytes.

## 30.3.4 Layered Culture Systems

An approach that aims to mimic the *in vivo* environment is a layered cell culture construct. These systems attempt to recreate more realistic environments by culturing chondrocytes in layers corresponding to their native arrangement. Although only a handful of such systems have attempted to classify the behavior of layered chondrocyte subpopulations, results indicate that cell activity is significantly influenced by the presence of another cell population.

An agarose system has demonstrated varying mechanical properties and cellular activity between construct layers. Constructs seeded with a mixed chondrocyte population containing a layer of 2 weight percent agarose atop of a layer of 3 weight percent agarose contained two regions with distinct mechanical properties. Initially, the 3% agarose region displayed stiffer compressive properties; however, after 28 days in culture this difference become less noticeable and the scaffold properties became more homogenous [56]. When this system was used to layer chondrocyte subpopulations modulations in cell activity depending both on weight percent agarose and the surrounding cell population were observed. After 42 days in culture it was found that superficial zone cells produced the highest levels of collagen and GAGs with higher agarose concentrations and when layered next to a population of middle/deep zone cells. Similarly, middle/deep zone cells produced more GAGs and had higher proliferation rates when layered next to a superficial zone population. Furthermore, bilayered constructs seeded with a superficial zone cell population and a middle/deep zone cell population displayed depth-dependant compressive properties similar to those of native tissue [57].

Culture systems based on photopolymerizable poly(ethylene oxide) diacrylate (PEODA) and poly(ethylene glycol) diacrylate (PEGDA) have also been used to culture layers of chondrocyte subpopulations. In PEODA hydrogels, it was reported that culturing deep zone cells next to a layer of superficial zone cells lowered their cell proliferation rate but increased production of matrix components [58]. Additionally, a PEG-based system which layered superficial, middle, and deep zone cells demonstrated histological staining similar to that of native tissue after 3 weeks in culture. Cells in the upper layer remained small and flattened, while those in the middle and deep layers were larger and more rounded. Furthermore, the upper layer contained little matrix, and collagen and proteoglycan staining increased with construct depth [59]. A layered system based on the popular hydrogel alginate has also been reported. This system has demonstrated mechanical properties similar to those of nonlayered constructs, and production of matrix components over several weeks of culture with a mixed chondrocyte population [60,61].

There are fairly limited results for layered culture systems. The few existing models demonstrate increased matrix production, especially in middle/deep zone cells, when cells are cultured in a zonally organized manner. Layered hydrogels show potential for *in vitro* production of tissue with depth-dependent mechanical properties which are on the same scale of native tissue. Current results appear promising for creating zonally organized tissue *in vitro* and it is likely that a zonally organized culture method will aid in subpopulation retention. Cell source limitations remains a challenge for regenerating zonally organized tissue. Current studies utilize primary isolated chondrocyte subpopulations. For zonal cartilage engineering to translate to clinical settings, alternate cells sources, such as stem cell populations, must be identified.

# 30.4 Stem Cells in Cartilage Tissue Engineering

Current cell-based therapies for cartilage repair have several drawbacks. Currently, the most popular cell-based cartilage repair model used is the ACI procedure. As previously mentioned, this procedure has several key disadvantages. First, harvesting the initial chondrocyte population puts the patient at higher risk for developing OA and often results in donor-site morbidity. Second, the harvested cells must be passaged in monolayer to expand cell numbers, which results in dedifferentiation. After expansion chondrocytes can be encapsulated in three-dimensional environments, which can partially restore a stable phenotype. However, these cells rarely form native-quality tissue *in vivo*. The repair tissue generated is often fibrocartilage that has decreased load-bearing capacity [62,63].

The challenges involved with generating adequate cell numbers of mature and phenotypically stable chondrocytes have driven a plethora of research investigating the use of stem and progenitor cells for cartilage tissue engineering. Stem cells have the ability to self-renew and can differentiate down multiple lineages, whereas progenitor cells have a limited ability to self-renew and are committed down a particular cellular lineage or lineages. Embryonic stem cells are pluripotent and thus have unlimited potential to both self-renew and differentiate into cells of all tissue types. However, they come with a multitude of both scientific and ethical concerns. The use of adult stem or progenitor cells avoids many of these concerns. Adult stem cells can be found in many tissues throughout the body including bone marrow, adipose tissue, lung tissue, and mammary gland. Here we highlight the popular use of stem and progenitor cells isolated from embryonic tissue, bone marrow, and adipose tissue for articular cartilage engineering.

## 30.4.1 Embryonic Stem Cells

Embryonic stem cells (ESCs) are isolated during embryonic development from the inner cell mass of the blastocyst. ESCs can differentiate into any cell lineage of the three germ layers, and can proliferate undifferentiated indefinitely *in vitro*. As a result of their limitless differentiation and proliferation capacities, ECSs are attractive for use in cartilage tissue engineering applications. However, ethical issues and scientific hurdles such as efficient differentiation of a homogenous cell population, immunorejection, and tumourigenicity have left the clinical potential of the field unrealized [64].

### 30.4.1.1 Mammalian Development

Shortly following formation of the blastocyst, at approximately day six of mouse embryogenesis, a process called gastrulation occurs. The embryo is reorganized to form the three germ layers: the ectoderm, mesoderm, and endoderm, which will later go on to form all tissue types in the body. The primitive streak is formed, and cells from the primitive streak migrate to form all three germ layers. The first mesoderm cells emerge from the posterior part of the early primitive streak and migrate anteriorly and laterally. Cardiac, cranial, and lateral plate mesoderm progenitors are formed during the mid-stage streak, and finally progenitors of muscle, bone, and cartilage cells in the late stage streak [65]. For this cell migration to occur following formation of the primitive streak, a process called epithelial mesenchymal transition (EMT) must be initiated. During EMT morphological changes occur; from epithelial cell–cell contact to the migratory mesenchymal cell–matrix phenotype [66].

### 30.4.1.2 Chondrogenesis

Development of the skeleton begins with lineage commitment of mesenchymal cells followed by migration of these cells to the site of skeletogenesis and cell condensation. Mesenchymal condensation initiates formation of chondroblasts and osteoblasts. Following mesenchymal condensation, bone development, or endothelial ossification, initiates. Chondroblasts differentiate into chondrocytes driven by expression of transcription factor SRY (sex-determining region Y)-box9 (Sox9). Chondrocytes begin producing aggrecan and type II collagen, and eventually undergo hypertrophy; producing type X collagen and expressing runt-related transcription factor 2 (Runx2) [65]. Hypertrophic chondrocytes undergo apoptosis which is followed by cartilage matrix calcification. As this happens, a vascular network is formed and osteoprogentior cells differentiate into osteoblasts and begin depositing bone on the cartilage matrix. A layer of cartilage remains on what later will become the articulating joints. Hypertrophic cells, which are positioned between this layer of remaining cartilage and the forming bone tissue, may undergo differentiation to osteoblasts capable of producing bone. This process has been termed transdifferentiation, and is sited as support that mesenchymal cells exhibit plasticity [67]. A recent study on mature chondrocytes differentiated from isolated from ESCs demonstrated such plasticity [67]. To date, it is still unclear how many parts of this complex developmental process are regulated; however, the TGF-β superfamily is known to play a critical role during many stages of cartilage development [68]. Generating stable chondrocytes that do not become hypertrophic or undergo terminal differentiation is critical for stem cell use in cartilage engineering.

### 30.4.1.3 *In Vitro* Embryonic Stem Cell Chondrogenesis

Isolation of mouse ESCs was first reported in 1981 [69]. In 1998 the first reports of human ESC isolation were published [70]. Since then researchers have been investigating chondrogenesis of ESCs and formation of cartilage tissue. Owing to their prevalence in development, members of the TGF-β superfamily, such as TGF-β1,3 and BMP 2, 4,and 6, have been widely investigated for inducing chondrogenesis. Coculture with primary chondrocytes, chondroprogenitor cells [64], or hepatic cells [71] has also shown differentiation potential. The most common markers for chondrogenesis are ECM components type II collagen and aggrecan, and transcription factor Sox9. A three-dimensional culture system, pellet or scaffold-supported, is usually considered essential due to similarity to the environment during precartilage condensation when cells adopt a spherical morphology. Pellet sizes for chondrogenesis typically range from $2 \times 10^5$ to $5 \times 10^5$. Scaffolds are often hydrogels such as alginate or agarose [72], but also include synthetic scaffolds such as polycaprolactone [73], poly(l-lactic acid) [74] and poly(lactic-co-glycolic acid) [74]. Synthetic scaffolds can be challenging to seed evenly, whereas ESCs in hydrogels often have limited viability due to lack of cell–matrix interactions. Inclusion of peptide adhesion motifs has demonstrated potential for solving this problem and resulted in production of cartilaginous tissue [75].

The majority of studies utilize ESCs to form embryoid bodies (EBs), from which cells are taken for chondrogenesis, or the entire EB is exposed to chondrogenic conditions. EBs are spontaneously forming, free-floating aggregates of ESCs that mimic the structure of developing embryos and allow many of the stages involved in germ layer formation to occur. Formation of EBs is largely uncontrolled and results in a heterogeneous combination of spontaneously differentiated cells (potentially of all three germ layers) and undifferentiated cells [68]. Cells taken from the EB, or the entire EB, are typically maintained in pellet or scaffold supported culture during chondrogenesis [64]. Spontaneous differentiation of mouse EBs in growth media has been reported to form condensed mesenchymal cells, chondroprogenitor cells, and mature and hypertrophic chondrocytes [76,77].

### 30.4.1.4 Growth Factors for ESC Chondrogenesis

Mixed results utilizing TGF-β1, 3 and BMPs indicate their effects are time dependent over the course of EB formation and chondrogenesis. Studies have shown TGF-β1 to be ineffective at inducing chondrogenesis in mouse and human ESCs [68]. However, TGF-β and parathyroid treatment following retinoic acid treatment of EBs supported chondrogenic differentiation. Exposure to BMP 2 and 4 earlier in the differentiation process (EB suspension) has upregulated chondrogenic makers as well. Success has also been reported by BMP 2 and TGF-β1 delivery during EB formation followed by insulin, ascorbic acid, and BMP 2 delivery during chondrogenesis. Furthermore, a study using human ESCs identified BMP 7 as more efficient than TGF-β1 alone, or combined treatment of both growth factors, for upregulating chondrogenic markers [78]. ESCs can be differentiated in ESC growth media with growth factors added to induce chondrogenesis, or in chondrogenic media used for adult stem cells (serum-free, insulin, transferrin, selenium [ITS], dexamethasone, proline, ascorbic acid, sodium pyruvate, and TGF-β1 or 3). However, optimal conditions are still unclear [64].

To mimic the developmental processes of EMT many studies have focused on generating mesenchymal stem cells (MSCs) from ESCs, and then inducing chondrogenesis in the MSC population. This has been achieved through culture of ESCs on a feeder later of OP9 stromal cells. Flow cytometry for MSC-positive markers showed a strong correlation, and cells differentiated down chondrogenic, osteogenic, myogenic, and adipogenic lineages [79]. Another study used monolayer culture of human ESCs in endothelial growth media to form epithelial sheet with mesodermal gene expression patterns. Upon passaging the cells formed mesenchymal-like cells which were negative for hematopoietic surface markers and positive for MSC markers by flow cytometry. The resulting population expressed chondrogenic markers under micromass culture and exposure to dexamethasone, ITS, and 10 ng/mL TGF- β3 [66]. Similarly, EB exposed to BMP 4 formed mesodermal cells expressing flk-1 and/or platelet derived growth factor receptor-α (PDGFR-α). Chondrogenesis was included in the resulting cell population by exposure to both TGF-β3 and PDGF-BB. Interestingly, noggin inhibited both the TGF-β3 and PDGF-BB induced cartilage formation, indicating that a BMP-dependent pathway is involved [80]. Mesenchymal stem growth media has also been used to induce formation of mesenchymal-like cells from EBs which exhibit both mesodermal progenitor cell markers and MSC markers. Chondrogenesis was induced in the population through exposure to TGF-β1 [75]. Table 30.1 highlights popular methods and outcomes for chondrogenesis of ESCs.

Pluripotent stem (iPS) cells have also been isolated from the primordial gonadal ridge, and are called embryonic germ cells. They also form aggregates which lead to a heterogeneous population of differentiated and undifferentiated cells. The chondrogenic potential of these cells has been demonstrated when encapsulated in PEGDA, and cultured in chondrocyte-conditioned media containing TGF-β1 [81].

### 30.4.1.5 Challenges and Limitations

Few *in vivo* studies have investigated the potential of ESCs to form cartilaginous tissue. This is in part to due to a plethora of scientific challenges. Controlled and homogenous differentiation is difficult to achieve, and producing a cell population containing only mature chondrocytes capable of producing ECM remains a challenge. Establishment and scale-up of optimal chondrogenic conditions should be established, and animal product free culture must be achieved for clinical use.

Tackling the issue of immunorejection is another major hurdle. ESCs do not exist in the body, which means they cannot be isolated from a patient. An implanted scaffold seeded with allogenic cells would result in immunorejection. ESCs would then have to be treated like organ transplants, where large banks are screened for potential human leukocyte antigen matches, and patients would have to take immunosuppressive drugs for the remainder of their lives. An alternative to this process could involve induced iPS cells. iPS cells are patient-specific somatic cells reprogramed to a pluripotent state. iPS cells have been formed from both human and mouse adult cells. Human iPS cells can form EBs containing all three germ layers and following implantation form teratomas containing many tissue types, including cartilage. However, additional research is needed to evaluate the clinical potential of these cells [64].

Another major challenge for use of ESCs in tissue engineering is their tumorigenicity, or ability to form benign tumors (teratomas) *in vivo*. Most approaches differentiate ESCs *in vitro* before implantation to avoid teratoma formation, however, even after many weeks of *in vitro* differentiation teratomas have still been observed upon implantation. Upon implantation any undifferentiated cell can potentially

**TABLE 30.1**  Chondrogenic Culture Conditions for Embryonic Stem Cells[a]

| Ref | Species | Preculture Conditions | Culture Environment | Media Additives | Key Results |
|---|---|---|---|---|---|
| [68] | Human | With and without formation of embryoid bodies: 5 days | Pellet | 10 ng/mL TGF-β1 or 1 μM SB431542 (TGF-β/activin/nodal-signaling inhibitor): 28 days | Gene and protein expression: TGF-β1 downregulated markers in all groups. SB431542 results show TGF-β inhibits early chondrogenesis, but necessary at later stages |
| [66] | Human | Monolayer: endothelial growth media to form mesoderm and mesenchymal-like cells: 30 days | Pellet | 10 ng/mL TGF-β3 | Alcian blue staining positive for proteoglycans |
| [120] | Human | Embryoid body formation: 21 days (hypoxic or normoxic) | Hypoxic (2% O₂) or normoxic (20% O₂), high density plating | Growth factor free chondrogenic media: 28 days | Hypoxic conditions resulted in: 3.4-fold increase in type II collagen and 1.9-fold increase in GAG production, 3-fold increase in tensile modulus |
| [71] | Murine | Embryoid body formation: 4 days | Bilayered PEODA hydrogel with hepatic cells | 10 ng/mL TGF-β1:21 days | Coculture: 4-fold increase in GAG production, 80-fold increase in aggrecan mRNA expression. Type II collagen mRNA and staining only in coculture groups |
| [80] | Human | Embryoid body formation: 2 days, 5% O₂ and 1.9 ng/mL BMP 4:4-6 days, sorted by flow cytometry for flk-1 or PDGFRα | Pellet | 10 ng/mL TGF-β3, 50 ng/mL PDGF-BB, 50 ng/mL BMP 4, 1 μg/mL noggin alone or in combination: 20 days | Gene and protein expression: TGF-β3 induced chondrogenesis, enhanced by PDGF-BB, noggin inhibited both; indicated BMP-dependant pathway involved in chondrogenesis |
| [74] | Human | Embryoid body formation: 9 days | Scaffolds: Matrigel and 50/50 blend PLGA/PLLA | 2 ng/mL TGF-β1, 10 ng/mL IGF-1:14 days | Immunostaining showed cartilage-like tissue with GAG present |
| [81] | Human embryonic germ cells | None | PEDGA | Chondrocytes-conditioned media + 10 ng/mL TGF-β1:21 days | Histology, gene, and protein expression: cartilage matrix formation |
| [79] | Human | Coculture with OP9 cells for mesenchymal induction: 40 days | Pellet | 10 ng/mL TGF-β3:28 days | Histology and gene expression: confirm chondrogenesis |
| [75] | Human | Embryoid body formation: 10 days, MSC growth media: up to P5 | Pellet, PEGDA, PEGDA + type I collagen (t1c), PEGDA + hyaluronic acid (HA), RGD-PEGDA | 10 ng/mL TGF-β1 or 25 ng/mL BMP 2:21 days | Histology; gene and protein expression: micromass cultures produced unorganized matrix, PEGDA, PEGDA + t1c, PEGDA + HA: no significant matrix formation, RGD-PEGDA: matrix formation upregulation of gene markers |
| [78] | Human | None | Pellet | 10 ng/mL TGF-β1 and/or 300 ng/mL BMP 7:14 days | All groups increased in size, weight, GAG content compared with no growth factor delivery, most tissue formed with both growth factors, gene expression markers highest in BMP 7 group |

[a] Methods used for inducing chondrogenesis in embryonic stem cells: popular studies and key findings.

undergo uncontrolled cell division. Therefore, it is imperative that strategies be developed in which no uncommitted cells are implanted. This can potentially be achieved by sorting for cells by negative selection of undifferentiated cells, or positive selection of mature cells. Selection of appropriate markers along the differentiation pathway, and utmost accuracy are essential for success of such strategies [64].

## 30.4.2 Bone Marrow Mesenchymal Stem Cells

MSCs are found in multiple tissues throughout the body including bone marrow, adipose tissue, the synovial membrane, and trabecular bone. They have a high proliferation rate and can be differentiated into chondrocytes, myoblasts, hepatocytes, adipocytes, and osteoblasts. The populations of MSCs derived from bone marrow are currently the best characterized and understood, here we will refer to bone marrow-derived MSCs simply as MSCs. Although no single cell surface marker has been identified for MSCs, a population should test negatively for CD 14, CD 45, and CD 34 and positively for CD 29, CD44, SH 2, SH3, CD 106, CD 120a, CD 124, CD71, and CD90. The cells can easily be isolated from bone marrow via plastic adhesion to a culture flask. Ten milliliters of human bone marrow typically results in up to 300 million cells by the second passage. Furthermore, cells can retain their multipotency for approximately 6 to 10 passages [82,83].

### 30.4.2.1 *In Vitro* Chondrogenesis of MSCs

Differentiation of MSCs to chondrocytes starts by conversion to osteochondroprogentior cells, this leads to cell condensation and finally chondrogenic differentiation. Fibronectin and members of the TGF superfamily (TFG-β1–3 and BMP 1–7) are the major proteins involved in initiating cell condensation and promoting chondrogenesis. After all cell condensation, the cells at the center of the condensation nodules first form prechondrocytes and then committed chondrocytes which produce a cartilaginous ECM rich in type II collagen and aggrecan [63,84].

Chondrogenesis is controlled by several important transcription factors, including members of the Sox and Cbfa families. As in embryonic development, Sox9 is the major transcription factor that provides essential regulation throughout the differentiation process. Sox9 is expressed in chondroprogenitor cells and chondrocytes, but not in chondrocytes which have become hypertrophic. Members of the TFB-β family are known to induce Sox9 gene expression and transcriptional activity by binding to cell surface receptors and initiating the intracellular Smad 3 signaling cascade [6,84].

Traditionally, MSCs were cultured in a pelleted micromass during chondrogenesis; however, many methods now involve culturing MSCs in a three-dimensional scaffold to promote the rounded chondrocyte phenotype. In addition, differentiating MSCs in serum-free media has also become of interest to aid clinical relevance for human use, and ensure controlled delivery of growth factors and proteins [63,82,85,86]. The most common media formulation for chondrogenesis of adult stem cells includes the media base Dulbecco's modified Eagle medium with high glucose concentration (4500 mg/L), ITS + Premix (insulin, transferring, selenium, bovine serum albumin, and linoleic acid), and often dexamethasone [72].

### 30.4.2.2 Growth Factors for MSC Chondrogenesis

As a result of their importance in cartilage development, TGF-β 1, 2, and 3 are most commonly used to induce chondrogenesis in MSCs. Delivery of TGF-β's to MSCs is characterized by an upregulation of type II collagen, aggrecan, versican, biglycan, and decorin—all components of the cartilage ECM. Terminal differentiation of MSCs to hypertrophic chondrocytes is prevented by delivery of TGF-βs. Without this delivery, uncommitted MSCs can differentiate to hypertrophic chondrocytes *in vivo*, resulting in fibrocartilage repair tissue.

TGF-β1 was first successfully used in 1998 for chondrogenesis of rabbit MSCs [87]. Since then, due to its importance in development, it has been the most widely studied growth factor for inducing chondrogenesis in adult stem cells. Media concentration of 10 ng/mL appears to be ideal for inducing chondrogenesis in MSCs. Studies using TGF- β2 and 3 indicate that, at similar concentrations, these growth factors are more efficient at inducing chondrogenesis in human MSCs than TGF-β1. Delivery of up to 500-ng/mL BMP 6 has also been shown to induce chondrogenesis in human MSCs. There is some evidence to support that BMP 6 or 2 delivered along with TGF-β further increases differentiation potential and matrix deposition in human cells, however, results remain unclear [72]. In addition, delivery of IGF-1 was shown to further increase matrix production immediately following differentiation by TGF-β [88].

Although hydrogels such as alginate, agarose, and PEG are popular for chondrogenesis differentiation, MSC chondrogenesis in a variety of culture environments has been investigated. TGF-β1 delivery to MSC on oriented polycaprolactone scaffolds reported production of the chondrocyte lineage and guidance of cell orientation [89]. Increased production of matrix components was reported in MSCs differentiated in TGF-β2 and 3 versus TGF-β1 [90]. Chondrogenesis of MSCs in a three-dimensional type I collagen and poly-l-lactate-glycolic acid copolymer has been reported via TGF-β3 delivery [91]. Production of cartilage ECM products has even been reported by MSCs plated in monolayer with TGF-β1 delivery [92]. In an *in vivo* model, it was demonstrated that incorporation of TFG-β3 into the cell scaffold was essential for MSC chondrogenesis. Addition of hyaluronic acid to the scaffold further increased cartilaginous matrix production [85].

Coculture and conditioned media models have also demonstrated success for differentiating MSCs. Cartilage chips [84], mixed micromass pellets of chondrocytes and MSCs [93], and chondrocyte-conditioned media [94] have all resulted in MSC chondrogenesis independent of TGF-β delivery. Table 30.2 lists details of these, and other popular methods, for MSC chondrogenesis.

### 30.4.2.3 Challenges and Limitations

Although methods for inducing chondrogenesis of MSCs are fairly well established, there is currently no standard or optimized protocol for differentiation. There is also no established method of producing populations of chondrocytes with varying morphologies which mimic the superficial and middle/deep zone chondrocyte cell populations. MSC-derived chondrocytes seem to display metabolic and morphologic properties similar to those of middle and deep zone cells, therefore the major unmet challenge is in differentiating a population of superficial zone chondrocytes from MSCs. A handful of studies have demonstrated the potential of infrapatellar fat pad progenitor cells, synovial progenitor cells, and a progenitor population isolated from the cartilage superficial zone to express SZP. This expression was induced by addition of BMP 7 to TGF-β1 differentiation media [98–101]. These studies indicate BMP 7 delivery as a possible mechanism for inducing SZP expression in bone marrow-derived MSCs.

Additionally, the clinical potential of MSCs in cartilage tissue engineering is largely unrealized. And while trails have demonstrated feasibility of MSCs to regenerate damaged cartilage tissue, this has not yet become a standard of care or widely used practice in clinical therapies. Bone marrow harvest is both a painful and potentially risky procedure and *in vitro* expansion and differentiation can lead to hypertrophy in the stem cell population [31,62]. As a result, current animal and human models that have used MSCs for cartilage repair have shown mixed results, often plagued by fibrocartilage formation [7,62,102].

## 30.4.3 Adipose-Derived Adult Stem Cells

Adults store excess fat not only as adipose, or fat, tissue but also as undifferentiated adipocytes whose lineage is not limited to adipogenic. The rare disorder progressive osseous heteroplasia leaves patients with ectopic bone in their subcutaneous fat layer—indicating the presence of stem or progenitor cells in the tissue [103]. In 1964 the first *in vitro* isolation of mature adipocytes and progenitor cells from fat tissue was reported [104]. The isolated tissue was minced and digested with collagenase type I and the cellular components were separated by differential centrifugation. The supernatant contained mature adipocytes that were rich in lipids and the pellet contained progenitor cells and hematopoietic lineage cells. Since then, the procedure has been adapted to isolate stem cells from liposuction aspirates, which have been

**TABLE 30.2** Chondrogenic Culture Conditions for Bone Marrow-Derived Mesenchymal Stem Cells[a]

| Ref | Species | Culture Environment | Media Additives | Key Results |
|---|---|---|---|---|
| [95] | Human | Porous silk | ITS, dexamethasone, 10 ng/mL TGF-β3:21 days | Histology, gene, and protein expression: dexamethasone and TGF-β3 essential for chondrogenesis, after 21 days tissue formed resembled native cartilage morphology |
| [90] | Human | Pellet | ITS, dexamethasone, 10 ng/mL TGF-β1, 2, or 3: 35 days | Gene and protein expression: differentiation rapidly induced by TGF-β2, 3, expression sequence of ECM components during differentiation reported |
| [86] | Human | Pellet | ITS, dexamethasone, 10 ng/mL TGF-β3:21 days | Histology and protein expression: chondrogenesis and matrix production, could induce hypertrophy by addition of thyroxine, removal of TGF-β3 and reduction of dexamethasone |
| [91] | Human | Type I collagen and PLGA mesh, pellet | Fetal calf serum, dexamethasone, 10 ng/mL TGF-β3, 100 ng/mL IGF-1: 28 days | Histology and gene expression: chondrogenic markers higher in scaffold even without growth factors than in pellets, scaffolds with growth factors significantly higher expression than pellets |
| [94] | Goat | Pellet | Bovine chondrocyte-conditioned media: 5 days | Staining, gene expression: chondrocyte-conditioned media can induce chondrogenesis |
| [84] | Rat | Alginate | Cocultured with allogenic rat articular cartilage: 21 days | Gene expression: early stage expression of sox9 and late stage repression of hypertrophic markers |
| [96] | Human | Silk fibroin, collagen, cross-liked collagen | ITS, dexamethasone, insulin, 10 ng/mL TGF-β1: 21 days | Most cell proliferation, highest GAG accumulation, upregulated chondrogenic gene expression on silk scaffolds compared with collagen, higher modulus, and homogenous distribution of matrix on silk scaffold |
| [88] | Equine | Monolayer, fibrin disks | 0.5 ng/mL TGF-β1 monolayer: 6 days, 0, 100 ng/mL IGF-1 fibrin disks: 13 days | Monolayer with TGF-β1 increased proliferation, disks with both growth factor treatments increased gene and protein expression for chondrogenic markers over controls |
| [97] | Human | Pellet: human MSCs and bovine chondrocytes mixed at varying ratios | ITS, 10 ng/mL TGF-β3: 28 days | MSC pellets alone: no cartilage tissue formation, mixed pellets: upregulation of cartilaginous markers as ratio of MSCs increased |
| [92] | Equine | Monolayer | 0,1,5,10 ng/mL TGF-β1:4 days | 5 ng/mL TGF-β1: highest cellular density, dose-dependent response of type II collagen production |

[a] Methods used for inducing chondrogenesis in bone marrow-derived mesenchymal stem cells: popular studies and key findings.

coined adipose-derived adult stem (ADAS) cells. Liposuction provides a much easier, less painful process, and results in higher cell numbers (approximately 404,000 cells/mL of lipoaspirate [105]) than bone marrow isolation, making ADAS cells attractive candidates for use in tissue engineering [72].

Immunophenotyping of ADAS cells via flow cytometry and immunohistochemistry indicates they express similar, but not identical, markers to bone marrow-derived MSCs. ADAS cells are positive for the following adhesion molecules: tetraspan protein (CD9), integrins b1 (CS29) and a4 (CD49d), intercellular adhesion molecule 1 (CD54), endoglin (CD105), vascular cell adhesion molecule (CD106), and lymphocyte cell adhesion molecule 3 (CD50). The cell surface is negative for integrins ab (CD11b) and b2 (CD18), intercellular adhesion molecule 3 (CD50), neural cell adhesion molecule (CD56), and endothelial selection (CD62) [103].

ADAS cells are also positive for receptor molecules hyaluronate (CD44) and transferrin (CD71); surface enzymes neural endopeptidase (CD10), aminopeptidase (CD13), and ecto-5-nucleotidase (CD73); and glycoproteins Thy-1 (CD90), and MUC-18(CD146). They produce ECM proteins type I and type II collagens, osteopontin, and ostenectin and are positive for complementary regulatory proteins decay accelerating factor (CD555) and complement protectin (CD59). They are negative for hematopoietic markers CD14, CD31, and CD45 [103].

ADAS cells are capable of differentiating in to chondrocytes, myocytes, cardiomyocytes, osteoblasts, adipocytes, and potentially neuronal and oligodendrocytic lineages [103,106]. A recent study published in 2010 demonstrated that by indentifying cells which were positive for CD105 via magnetic-activated cell sorting, cells with high chondrogenic potential could be enriched from isolated human ADAS cells [107]. The most widely used method of inducing chondrogenesis is through exposure to TGF-β, dexamethasone, and ascorbate in either pellet or three-dimensional scaffold culture.

### 30.4.3.1 Growth Factors for ADAS Cell Chondrogenesis

Table 30.3 highlights popular growth factors and methods for inducing chondrogenesis in ADAS cells. Similar to MSCs, 10 ng/mL TGF-β1 in combination with dexamethasone, has shown success for inducing human ADAS cell chondrogenesis [113,114]. However, results indicate TGF-β1 is more effective in MSCs than in ADAS cells. Human ADAS cells also appear to respond better to TGF-β2,3 than TGF-β1. However, higher concentrations of TGF-βs are needed in ADAS media to show similar differentiation profiles to MSCs [72].

Addition of BMP 6 at a concentration of 500 ng/mL [117] and 100 ng/mL [112] has also shown potential for inducing chondrogenesis in human ADAS cells. In an effort to mimic the transcription cascade, temporal delivery of BMP 6 following TGF-β3 has been studied in human MSCs and ADAS cells. Results showed decreased expression of chondrogenic markers in MSCs with addition of BMP 6 delivery [118], but increased expression in ADAS cells [117]. Further research showed undifferentiated human ADAS cells did not express TGF-β receptor or BMP 6, while undifferentiated human MSCs do. However, when ADAS cells were exposed to BMP 6 the TGF-β receptor was then expressed [119]. Results suggest that BMPs are necessary for chondrogenesis, and while human MSCs produce BMPs, human ADAS cells must be supplemented with exogenous delivery. BMPs delivered along with TGF-βs show greatest potential for ADAS cell differentiation. However, identification of optimal growth factor combination (BMP 2, 4, 6, TGF-β1, 2, 3) and concentrations are yet to be established for ADAS cell chondrogenesis. A 2010 publication in Nature Protocols stated for chondrogenesis of human ADAS cells they should be pelleted or encapsulated in alginate and exposed to either 10 ng/mL TGF-β1, 500 ng/mL BMP 6, or 10 ng/mL TGF-β3 and 10 ng/mL BMP 6 along with differentiation media (high glucose Dulbecco's modified Eagle medium, fetal bovine serum, ITS+, and dexamethasone) [111]. Consensus is yet to be reached on optimal and defined culture conditions.

### 30.4.3.2 Hypoxic Conditions

As cartilage is not vascularized and bone is, hypoxic conditions have been proposed as a mechanism for chondrogenic differentiation. A study using human ADAS cells cultured in either osteogenic or

**TABLE 30.3** Chondrogenic Culture Conditions for Adipose-Derived Adult Stem Cells[a]

| Ref | Species | Culture Environment | Media Additives | Key Results |
|---|---|---|---|---|
| [108] | Human | Monolayer or pellet, 5% $O_2$ or 20% $O_2$ | ITS, dexamethasone, 10 ng/mL TGF-β1:28 days | Histology; gene and protein expression: all chondrogenic markers upregulated in 5% $O_2$ |
| [109] | Human | Alginate, agarose, porous gelatin | ITS, dexamethasone, 10 ng/mL TGF-β1:28 days | All materials support chondrogenesis; gelatin scaffold culture have highest mechanical properties and GAG content, hydrogels support spherical morphology |
| [110] | Human | Cartilage-derived scaffold | FBS, ITS, dexamethasone | Histology; gene and protein expression: upregulation of matrix components and modulus on scale with native tissue |
| [111] | Human | Alginate, pellet | FBS, ITS, dexamethasone and 10 ng/mL TGF-β1, or 500 ng/mL BMP 6, or 10 ng/mL TGF-β3 + 10 ng/mL BMP 6: up to 42 days | Histology; gene and protein assays for aggrecan, type I, II, X collagen, GAG, chondroitin sulfate |
| [112] | Murine | Monolayer, pellet | 100ng/mL BMP 6: 14 days | Pellet culture induced chondrogenesis, monolayer culture osteogenesis |
| [107] | Human | Sorted by flow cytometry for CD105 positive cells; PLA-PGA scaffold | Dexamethasone, 10 ng/mL TGF-β3, 10 ng/mL BMP 6, 50 ng/mL IGF-1: 56 days | CD105+ cells higher chondrogenic potential than CD105− cells, homogenous cartilage-like tissue formed from CD105+ groups after culture time, stained positive for type II collagen and proteoglycans |
| [113] | Human | Alginate | FBS or ITS + 0,1, or 10 ng/mL TGF-β1 and or 0,10,100 ng/mL dexamethasone: 9 days | ITS + TGF-β1 increased proliferation and protein and proteoglycan synthesis, dexamethasone increased protein synthesis but decreased proteoglycan synthesis |
| [114] | Human | Alginate | FBS, ITS, dexamethasone, 10 ng/mL TGF-β1: 14 days, implanted subcutaneously in nude mice: up to 12 weeks | In vitro: significant type II collagen and GAG production, in vivo: cartilage tissue formation |
| [115] | Rabbit | Monolayer | FBS, transfected with BMP 2 and IGF-1:14 days | Immunoblotting; transfection resulted in chondrogenesis, formation of matrix proteins and lower MMP-13 levels than controls |
| [116] | Human | Pellet | TGF-β3 +/− BMP 6, 2%$O_2$ or 20%$O_2$:24 days | Gene and protein expression: TGF-β3+ BMP 6 best for inducing chondrogenesis, 2%$O_2$ downregulated markers for hypertrophic chondrocytes |
| [117] | Human | Alginate | ITS, dexamethasone, 10 ng/mL TGF-β1, 10 ng/mL TGF-β3, 100 ng/mL IGF-1, 500 ng/mL BMP 6: 7 days | Gene and protein expression: indicate BMP 6 alone significantly more efficient at upregulating chondrogenic markers than all other growth factors/combinations |

*Note:* FBS, fetal bovine serum.

[a] Methods used for inducing chondrogenesis in adipose-derived adult stem cells: popular studies and key findings.

chondrogenic conditions under 5% or 20% oxygen tension showed that hypoxic conditions upregulated chondrogenic markers and downregulated osteogenic markers [108]. A study also using human ADAS cells in various culture conditions (no growth factor, TGF-β3, BMP 2, TGF-β3 and BMP 2) under 2% or 20% oxygen tension, demonstrated hypoxic conditions reduced expression for hypertrophic markers when both growth factors were present [116]. Similar results have also been observed during ESC chondrogenesis in hypoxic conditions [120].

### 30.4.3.3 Scaffold Materials

Popular three-dimensional conditions shown to support chondrogenesis of ADAS cells include pellet culture [111,112], alginate [111,113] and agarose hydrogels, porous gelatin [109], and cartilage-derived scaffolds [110]. Use of cartilage-derived scaffolds seeded with ADAS cells have resulted in formation of cartilage tissue with an aggregate modulus of up to 150 kPa, on the same scale as native cartilage tissue at 500–900 kPa [110]. Hydrogels allow cells to take on the spherical morphology found to be important for chondrogenesis, while pellet cultures allow for increased cell–cell communication through direct contact or soluble signaling molecules.

### 30.4.3.4 Challenges and Limitations

Before ADAS can make their way into the clinical setting for cartilage engineering challenges must be overcome. Namely, protocols must be standardized and approved by the Food and Drug Administration. The tissue harvest and cell-isolation procedure must be streamlined for clinicians, any culture prior to cell use must be achieved in animal serum-free conditions, and it must be demonstrated that implantation of the isolated cells results in no adverse side effects. Although ADAS cells show great promise for cartilage tissue engineering, there are limited clinical trials to date which investigate the use of autologous ADAS.

## 30.5 Dynamic Culture Systems for Cartilage Engineering

In addition to biochemical cues from growth factors and soluble signaling molecules, physical and biomechanical stress is an integral part of cartilage tissue formation both *in vitro* and *in vivo*. Bioreactors which create dynamic culture conditions can improve mass transfer kinetics of both nutrition and waste as well as provide cellular stresses which stimulate ECM production [121]. The most common types of bioreactors for cartilage engineering include rotating wall (or vessel) bioreactors, perfusion bioreactors, spinner flasks, and unconfined and confined dynamic compression bioreactors. Bioreactors are usually loaded with cells seeded on a three-dimensional scaffold. The goal of a bioreactor system is to mimic *in vivo* conditions. Thus, bioreactor systems are used to control pH, oxygen and carbon dioxide partial pressures, temperature, nutrient supply, and mechanical environment.

A rotating wall bioreactor exposes the scaffold to low shear and high mass transfer rates. The walls of the chamber rotate and the scaffold is suspended in the enclosed media. Spinner flasks involve a flask containing media and a magnetic stir bar. They also improve mass transfer rates but impose low shear on the scaffold. Dynamic compression systems utilize a computer to apply mechanical load with controlled frequency, magnitude, and loading time. Dynamic strain is often superimposed on static strain to mimic *in vivo* loading. In cartilage studies, frequencies typically range between 0.0001 and 3 Hz, compression on the scaffold ranges from 0.1 to 24 MPa, and strain levels are between 0.1% and 25% [122].

One of the most popular bioreactors in cartilage engineering research is the perfusion system. Perfusion bioreactors pump media continuously through a porous scaffold. The scaffold is typically confined so that media must pass through it, instead of around. This results in improved mass transfer to the interior of the scaffold, and exerts shear on the scaffold and the cells. Both mass transfer and shear are dependent on the flow rate of the perfused media. Flow rates used typically range from 0.1 to 1 mL/min. Too high of a flow rate leads to removal of cells from the scaffold, and increased flow as the tissue matures is beneficial. Perfusion systems have demonstrated significant success for cartilage tissue engineering; demonstrating both increased ECM deposition and chondrogenic differentiation efficiencies compared with static controls [122].

## 30.5.1 Adult Chondrocytes

Initial bioreactor studies with chondrocyte-seeded poly(glycolic acid) scaffolds demonstrated that a rotating vessel bioreactor could upregulate cellular production of GAGs and type II collagen [123]. A similar study using bovine chondrocytes seeded in agarose hydrogels concluded that culture in a rotating bioreactor increased GAG accumulation in the cores of scaffolds when compared with static controls [124]. A recent study using human chondrocytes seeded on a hyaluronan-based hydrogel and cultured in a perfusion system (flow rate of 12 mL/min) under hypoxic conditions reported formation of homogeneous cartilage tissue with properties approaching those of native tissue and of clinically relevant size [125]. Similarly, unconfined dynamic compressive loading (1 Hz at 10% strain, 3 h/day for 28 days) of canine chondrocytes in an agarose hydrogel resulted in a significant increase in Young's modulus. The attained modulus values were on par with those of native canine cartilage [126]. A parallel plate bioreactor which flows media over fixed high-density bovine chondrocyte constructs also reported increased young's modulus and ultimate tensile strength with increasing shear stress (0, 0.001, 0.1 Pa). Higher shear conditions increased collagen expression and production [127]. Taken together, bioreactor results utilizing scaffold-seeded mature chondrocytes demonstrate increases in both modulus and ECM in response to shear and compressive loading.

## 30.5.2 Stem Cell Differentiation

Successful results using mature chondrocytes led to investigation of bioreactors for enhancing chondrogenic differentiation. A study using rabbit bone marrow MSCs in a rotating vessel bioreactor to produce allogenic cartilage grafts reported that upon implantation the grafts formed cartilage-like tissue, were well integrated, and did not form fibrous repair tissue [128]. Conversely, human MSCs seeded on silk scaffolds in a rotating bioreactor were reported to undergo slow and incomplete chondrogenesis, even when cultured in chondrogenic media containing 5 ng/mL TGF-β1 [129]. A study using human MSCs comparing a spinner flask system (rotating magnetic bar at 60 rmp), and rotating wall bioreactor (outer wall rotating at 30 rpm) reported upregulation for chondrogenic markers in the spinner system [130].

Several studies using perfusion bioreactors have reported increased chondrogenic potential due to dynamic condition. Human ADAS cells seeded in polyglycolic acid and differentiated under flow of 0.2 mL/min (with reversed flow every 3 days) produced higher levels of both GAGs and collagen than static pellet cultures [131]. Human embryoid stem cell-derived mesenchymal-like cells seeded on porous silk fibroin and differentiated in a perfusion system at a flow rate of 1 mL/min underwent more complete chondrogenesis compared with static controls. The perfusion cultured group produced more GAGs and collagen, had increased mechanical properties, and displayed elevated gene expression for chondrogenic markers compared with the control [132]. Similar results were obtained using goat bone marrow cells on starch–polycaprolactone scaffolds cultured at a flow rate of 0.1 mL/min. Groups from the perfusion system demonstrated increased gene expression and protein production of chondrogenic markers compared with static controls [133].

In addition, compression loading has been shown to be a stimulator of chondrogenesis. Rabbit bone marrow MSCs were seeded in agarose and loaded in dynamic compression (sinusoidal with 10% strain at 1 Hz for 4 h per day) both with and without TGF-β3. TGF-β3 was also delivered with no load, and a control group had no load or growth factors. Results showed that all experimental groups upregulated chondrogenic markers compared with the control. Furthermore, by the end of the culture period there were no significant differences between the groups; indicating that compressive loading alone can induce chondrogenic differentiation as effectively as growth factor treatment or growth factor treatment plus loading [134]. A similar MSC study comparing dynamic compression (continuous sinusoidal with

**TABLE 30.4**   Dynamic Culture Environments for Stem Cell Chondrogenesis: Bioreactors Systems Utilized for Stem Cell Chondrogenesis: System Details and Key Findings

| Ref | Cell Type | Bioreactor | Scaffold | Media Additives | Key Results |
|---|---|---|---|---|---|
| [131] | Human ADAS | Perfusion (flow rate 0.2 mL/min), static | PGA mesh, control: pellet | Insulin, 10 ng/mL TGF-β1, 10 ng/mL +/ − BMP 6:35 days, control media | Bioreactor groups: increased GAG and collagen than static controls, TGF-β1: increases gene expression for collagen and GAG, and GAG synthesis, BMP 6: no effect |
| [129] | Human bone marrow MSCs | Rotating vessel (16 rpm) | Porous silk | Insulin, dexamethasone, 5 ng/mL TGF-β1:36 days, control media | Chondrogenesis slow and incomplete, increased GAG and DNA over control media |
| [132] | Human embryonic stem cell-derived MSCs | Perfusion (flow rate 1 mL/min), static | Porous silk fibroin | ITS, FBS, dexamethasone, 10 ng/mL TGF-β1:28 days | Bioreactor groups: significantly higher GAG and collagen content, higher stiffness, increase gene expression for chondrogenic markers than static controls |
| [133] | Goat bone marrow stromal cells | Perfusion 0.1 ml/min, static | Starch-PCL fiber mesh | ITS, FBS, dexamethasone, 10 ng/mL β1:28 days | Bioreactor groups: significantly higher protein and gene expression for chondrogenic markers compared to static controls |
| [135] | Human bone marrow stromal cells | Perfusion (10 mL/min) and cyclic axial compression (10% strain, 0.5 Hz, sinusoidal), static | Collagen 1-bone hybrid matrix | FBS, dexamethasone, 100 ng/mL, +/ − 100 ng/mL IGF-1 and 5 ng/mL TGF-β2:28 days | No differences in matrix production between: mechanical stimulation, mechanical stimulation + IGF-1 and TGF-β2, or IGF-1 and TGF-β2 alone, similar findings: [134] |
| [130] | Human MSCs | Spinner flask (magnetic bar 60 rpm), rotating wall (30 rpm), static | Gelatin-hyaluronic acid scaffolds | FBS, ITS 10 ng/mL TGF-β: 21 days | Spinner flasks: earliest and strongest staining for type II collagen and proteoglycans |

*Note:*   FBS, fetal bovine serum.

10% strain at 0.5 Hz) and growth factor delivery concluded that compression alone produced constructs with desirable cartilage properties [135].

As cells move down a differentiation path and produce ECM, their nutrition requirements increase [122]. Therefore, bioreactors which can control nutrient delivery and applied stress are particularly advantageous for promoting chondrogenesis. Current results demonstrate significant benefits of applied shear and compressive load both for culture of mature chondrocytes and chondrogenesis of progenitor cells. Future research should establish optimal culture conditions, and parameters involved for large-scale culture methods relevant for clinical application. Table 30.4 highlights details of bioreactor systems for stem cell chondrogenesis.

## 30.5.3   Challenges and Limitations

Bioreactors have significant clinical potential as they can be used as a method to create automated, standardized, and reproducible culture methods. However, due to incomplete understanding of the role and importance of both biochemical and biomechanical clues, tissue growth in bioreactors has not yet been optimized for clinical application [121]. There remains a need for development of automated and standardized bioreactor culture methods which can easily be scaled up for clinical use. Many bioreactor models and techniques demonstrate significant potential and advantages over static culture, but a gold standard, or optimal culture method is yet to be established. Furthermore, many models, such as compression and perfusion systems, are sophisticated systems which are expensive to build and operate. Development of standardized, easy to use, scalable, and inexpensive bioreactor technologies will be necessary for translation to clinical settings.

## Acknowledgments

This work was supported by the National Science Foundation (CAREER Award to J.P.F. #0448684), Arthritis Foundation (Arthritis Investigator Award to J.P.F.), and the State of Maryland, Maryland Stem Cell Research Fund.

## References

1. McDevitt, C.A., Biochemistry of articular cartilage. Nature of proteoglycans and collagen of articular cartilage and their role in ageing and in osteoarthrosis. *Ann Rheum Dis*, 1973. **32**(4): 364–78.
2. Jackson, D.W., T.M. Simon, and H.M. Aberman, Symptomatic articular cartilage degeneration: The impact in the new millennium. *Clin Orthop Relat Res*, 2001 Oct; **391 Suppl**: S14–25.
3. Ulrich-Vinther, M. et al., Articular cartilage biology. *J Am Acad Orthop Surg*, 2003. **11**(6): 421–30.
4. Mollenhauer, J.A., Perspectives on articular cartilage biology and osteoarthritis. *Injury*, 2008. **39 Suppl 1**: S5–12.
5. Kuettner, K.E., Biochemistry of articular cartilage in health and disease. *Clin Biochem*, 1992. **25**(3): 155–63.
6. Yoon, D.M. and J.P. Fisher, Chondrocyte signaling and artificial matrices for articular cartilage engineering. *Adv Exp Med Biol*, 2006. **585**: 67–86.
7. Chen, F.H., K.T. Rousche, and R.S. Tuan, Technology Insight: Adult stem cells in cartilage regeneration and tissue engineering. *Nat Clin Pract Rheumatol*, 2006. **2**(7): 373–82.
8. Lu, X.L. and V.C. Mow, Biomechanics of articular cartilage and determination of material properties. *Med Sci Sports Exerc*, 2008. **40**(2): 193–9.
9. Hunziker, E.B., T.M. Quinn, and H.J. Hauselmann, Quantitative structural organization of normal adult human articular cartilage. *Osteoarthritis Cartilage*, 2002. **10**(7): 564–72.
10. Wong, M. et al., Zone-specific cell biosynthetic activity in mature bovine articular cartilage: A new method using confocal microscopic stereology and quantitative autoradiography. *J Orthop Res*, 1996. **14**(3): 424–32.
11. Jiang, J. et al., Interaction between zonal populations of articular chondrocytes suppresses chondrocyte mineralization and this process is mediated by PTHrP. *Osteoarthritis Cartilage*, 2008. **16**(1): 70–82.
12. Klein, T.J. et al., Tissue engineering of articular cartilage with biomimetic zones. *Tissue Eng Part B Rev*, 2009 Jun; **15**(2): 143–57.
13. Bank, R.A. et al., Ageing and zonal variation in post-translational modification of collagen in normal human articular cartilage. The age-related increase in non-enzymatic glycation affects biomechanical properties of cartilage. *Biochem J*, 1998. **330**(Pt 1): 345–51.
14. Kempson, G.E. et al., The tensile properties of the cartilage of human femoral condyles related to the content of collagen and glycosaminoglycans. *Biochim Biophys Acta*, 1973. **297**(2): 456–72.
15. Huber, M., S. Trattnig, and F. Lintner, Anatomy, biochemistry, and physiology of articular cartilage. *Invest Radiol*, 2000. **35**(10): 573–80.
16. Schinagl, R.M. et al., Depth-dependent confined compression modulus of full-thickness bovine articular cartilage. *J Orthop Res*, 1997. **15**(4): 499–506.

17. Aydelotte, M.B., R.R. Greenhill, and K.E. Kuettner, Differences between sub-populations of cultured bovine articular chondrocytes. II. Proteoglycan metabolism. *Connect Tissue Res*, 1988. **18**(3): 223–34.

18. Aydelotte, M.B. and K.E. Kuettner, Differences between sub-populations of cultured bovine articular chondrocytes. I. Morphology and cartilage matrix production. *Connect Tissue Res*, 1988. **18**(3): 205–22.

19. Khalafi, A. et al., Increased accumulation of superficial zone protein (SZP) in articular cartilage in response to bone morphogenetic protein-7 and growth factors. *J Orthop Res*, 2007. **25**(3): 293–303.

20. Yamane, S. et al., Gene expression profiling of mouse articular and growth plate cartilage. *Tissue Eng*, 2007. **13**(9): 2163–73.

21. Khan, I.M. et al., Expression of clusterin in the superficial zone of bovine articular cartilage. *Arthritis Rheum*, 2001. **44**(8): 1795–9.

22. Penta, K. et al., Del1 induces integrin signaling and angiogenesis by ligation of alphaVbeta3. *J Biol Chem*, 1999. **274**(16): 11101–9.

23. Pfister, B.E. et al., Del1: A new protein in the superficial layer of articular cartilage. *Biochem Biophys Res Commun*, 2001. **286**(2): 268–73.

24. Lorenzo, P., M.T. Bayliss, and D. Heinegard, A novel cartilage protein (CILP) present in the mid-zone of human articular cartilage increases with age. *J Biol Chem*, 1998. **273**(36): 23463–8.

25. Bjornhart, B. et al., Cartilage oligomeric matrix protein in patients with juvenile idiopathic arthritis: Relation to growth and disease activity. *J Rheumatol*, 2009. **36**(8): 1749–54.

26. Salminen, H. et al., Up-regulation of cartilage oligomeric matrix protein at the onset of articular cartilage degeneration in a transgenic mouse model of osteoarthritis. *Arthritis Rheum*, 2000. **43**(8): 1742–8.

27. Di Cesare, P.E. et al., Increased degradation and altered tissue distribution of cartilage oligomeric matrix protein in human rheumatoid and osteoarthritic cartilage. *J Orthop Res*, 1996. **14**(6): 946–55.

28. Murray, R.C. et al., The distribution of cartilage oligomeric matrix protein (COMP) in equine carpal articular cartilage and its variation with exercise and cartilage deterioration. *Vet J*, 2001. **162**(2): 121–8.

29. Abramson, S.B. and M. Attur, Developments in the scientific understanding of osteoarthritis. *Arthritis Res Ther*, 2009. **11**(3): 227.

30. Cancedda, R. et al., Tissue engineering and cell therapy of cartilage and bone. *Matrix Biol*, 2003. **22**(1): 81–91.

31. Vinatier, C. et al., Cartilage tissue engineering: Towards a biomaterial-assisted mesenchymal stem cell therapy. *Curr Stem Cell Res Ther*, 2009. **4**(4): 318–29.

32. Clouet, J. et al., From osteoarthritis treatments to future regenerative therapies for cartilage. *Drug Discov Today*, 2009. **14**(19–20): 913–25.

33. Martinez de Aragon, J.S. et al., Early outcomes of pyrolytic carbon hemiarthroplasty for the treatment of trapezial-metacarpal arthritis. *J Hand Surg Am*, 2009. **34**(2): 205–12.

34. Clair, B.L., A.R. Johnson, and T. Howard, Cartilage repair: Current and emerging options in treatment. *Foot Ankle Spec*, 2009. **2**(4): 179–88.

35. Richter, W., Mesenchymal stem cells and cartilage *in situ* regeneration. *J Intern Med*, 2009. **266**(4): 390–405.

36. Torun Kose, G. and V. Hasirci, Cartilage tissue engineering. *Adv Exp Med Biol*, 2004. **553**: 317–29.

37. Pelttari, K., A. Wixmerten, and I. Martin, Do we really need cartilage tissue engineering? *Swiss Med Wkly*, 2009. **139**(41–42): 602–9.

38. Archer, C.W. et al., Phenotypic modulation in sub-populations of human articular chondrocytes in vitro. *J Cell Sci*, 1990. **97**(Pt 2): 361–71.

39. Zanetti, M., A. Ratcliffe, and F.M. Watt, Two subpopulations of differentiated chondrocytes identified with a monoclonal antibody to keratan sulfate. *J Cell Biol*, 1985. **101**(1): 53–9.

40. Waldman, S.D. et al., The use of specific chondrocyte populations to modulate the properties of tissue-engineered cartilage. *J Orthop Res*, 2003. **21**(1): 132–8.

41. Siczkowski, M. and F.M. Watt, Subpopulations of chondrocytes from different zones of pig articular cartilage. Isolation, growth and proteoglycan synthesis in culture. *J Cell Sci*, 1990. **97**(Pt 2): 349–60.

42. Shieh, A.C. and K.A. Athanasiou, Biomechanics of single zonal chondrocytes. *J Biomech*, 2006. **39**(9): 1595–602.

43. Darling, E.M. and K.A. Athanasiou, Rapid phenotypic changes in passaged articular chondrocyte subpopulations. *J Orthop Res*, 2005. **23**(2): 425–32.

44. Schuurman, W. et al., Zonal chondrocyte subpopulations reacquire zone-specific characteristics during *in vitro* redifferentiation. *Am J Sports Med*, 2009. **37 Suppl 1**: 97S–104S.

45. Malda, J. et al., Localization of the potential zonal marker clusterin in native cartilage and in tissue-engineered constructs. *Tissue Eng Part A*, 2010 Mar; **16**(3): 897–904.

46. Hwang, N.S. et al., Response of zonal chondrocytes to extracellular matrix-hydrogels. *FEBS Lett*, 2007. **581**(22): 4172–8.

47. Schmidt, T.A. et al., Synthesis of proteoglycan 4 by chondrocyte subpopulations in cartilage explants, monolayer cultures, and resurfaced cartilage cultures. *Arthritis Rheum*, 2004. **50**(9): 2849–57.

48. Darling, E.M. and K.A. Athanasiou, Growth factor impact on articular cartilage subpopulations. *Cell Tissue Res*, 2005. **322**(3): 463–73.

49. Lee, S.Y., T. Niikura, and A.H. Reddi, Superficial zone protein (lubricin) in the different tissue compartments of the knee joint: Modulation by transforming growth factor beta 1 and interleukin-1 beta. *Tissue Eng Part A*, 2008. **14**(11): 1799–808.

50. Flannery, C.R. et al., Articular cartilage superficial zone protein (SZP) is homologous to megakaryocyte stimulating factor precursor and Is a multifunctional proteoglycan with potential growth-promoting, cytoprotective, and lubricating properties in cartilage metabolism. *Biochem Biophys Res Commun*, 1999. **254**(3): 535–41.

51. Hidaka, C. et al., Enhanced matrix synthesis and *in vitro* formation of cartilage-like tissue by genetically modified chondrocytes expressing BMP-7. *J Orthop Res*, 2001. **19**(5): 751–8.

52. Hidaka, C. et al., Acceleration of cartilage repair by genetically modified chondrocytes over expressing bone morphogenetic protein-7. *J Orthop Res*, 2003. **21**(4): 573–83.

53. Flechtenmacher, J. et al., Recombinant human osteogenic protein 1 is a potent stimulator of the synthesis of cartilage proteoglycans and collagens by human articular chondrocytes. *Arthritis Rheum*, 1996. **39**(11): 1896–904.

54. Cheng, C. et al., Differences in matrix accumulation and hypertrophy in superficial and deep zone chondrocytes are controlled by bone morphogenetic protein. *Matrix Biol*, 2007. **26**(7): 541–53.

55. Leipzig, N.D., S.V. Eleswarapu, and K.A. Athanasiou, The effects of TGF-beta1 and IGF-I on the biomechanics and cytoskeleton of single chondrocytes. *Osteoarthritis Cartilage*, 2006. **14**(12): 1227–36.

56. Ng, K.W. et al., A layered agarose approach to fabricate depth-dependent inhomogeneity in chondrocyte-seeded constructs. *J Orthop Res*, 2005. **23**(1): 134–41.

57. Ng, K.W., G.A. Ateshian, and C.T. Hung, Zonal chondrocytes seeded in a layered agarose hydrogel create engineered cartilage with depth-dependent cellular and mechanical inhomogeneity. *Tissue Eng Part A*, 2009. **15**(9): 2315–24.

58. Sharma, B. et al., Designing zonal organization into tissue-engineered cartilage. *Tissue Eng*, 2007. **13**(2): 405–14.

59. Kim, T.K. et al., Experimental model for cartilage tissue engineering to regenerate the zonal organization of articular cartilage. *Osteoarthritis Cartilage*, 2003. **11**(9): 653–64.

60. Lee, C.S. et al., Integration of layered chondrocyte-seeded alginate hydrogel scaffolds. *Biomaterials*, 2007. **28**(19): 2987–93.

61. Gleghorn, J.P. et al., Adhesive properties of laminated alginate gels for tissue engineering of layered structures. *J Biomed Mater Res A*, 2008. **85**(3): 611–8.

62. Pelttari, K., E. Steck, and W. Richter, The use of mesenchymal stem cells for chondrogenesis. *Injury*, 2008. **39 Suppl 1**: S58–65.

63. Magne, D. et al., Mesenchymal stem cell therapy to rebuild cartilage. *Trends Mol Med*, 2005. **11**(11): 519–26.

64. Jukes, J.M., C.A. van Blitterswijk, and J. de Boer, Skeletal tissue engineering using embryonic stem cells. *J Tissue Eng Regen Med*, 2010. **4**(3): 165–80.

65. Waese, E.Y. and W.L. Stanford, One-step generation of murine embryonic stem cell-derived mesoderm progenitors and chondrocytes in a serum-free monolayer differentiation system. *Stem Cell Res*, 2011. **6**(1): 34–49.

66. Boyd, N.L. et al., Human embryonic stem cell-derived mesoderm-like epithelium transitions to mesenchymal progenitor cells. *Tissue Eng Part A*, 2009. **15**(8): 1897–907.

67. Hegert, C. et al., Differentiation plasticity of chondrocytes derived from mouse embryonic stem cells. *J Cell Sci*, 2002. **115**(Pt 23): 4617–28.

68. Yang, Z. et al., Stage-dependent effect of TGF-beta1 on chondrogenic differentiation of human embryonic stem cells. *Stem Cells Dev*, 2009. **18**(6): 929–40.

69. Evans, M.J. and M.H. Kaufman, Establishment in culture of pluripotential cells from mouse embryos. *Nature*, 1981. **292**(5819): 154–6.

70. Thomson, J.A. et al., Embryonic stem cell lines derived from human blastocysts. *Science*, 1998. **282**(5391): 1145–7.

71. Lee, H.J. et al., Enhanced chondrogenic differentiation of embryonic stem cells by coculture with hepatic cells. *Stem Cells Dev*, 2008. **17**(3): 555–63.

72. Puetzer, J.L., J.N. Petitte, and E.G. Loboa, Comparative review of growth factors for induction of three-dimensional *in vitro* chondrogenesis in human mesenchymal stem cells isolated from bone marrow and adipose tissue. *Tissue Eng Part B Rev*, 2010. **16**(4): 435–44.

73. Fecek, C. et al., Chondrogenic derivatives of embryonic stem cells seeded into 3D polycaprolactone scaffolds generated cartilage tissue in vivo. *Tissue Eng Part A*, 2008. **14**(8): 1403–13.

74. Levenberg, S. et al., Differentiation of human embryonic stem cells on three-dimensional polymer scaffolds. *Proc Natl Acad Sci USA*, 2003. **100**(22): 12741–6.

75. Hwang, N.S. et al., Chondrogenic differentiation of human embryonic stem cell-derived cells in arginine-glycine-aspartate-modified hydrogels. *Tissue Eng*, 2006. **12**(9): 2695–706.

76. Kramer, J., C. Hegert, and J. Rohwedel, *in vitro* differentiation of mouse ES cells: Bone and cartilage. *Methods Enzymol*, 2003. **365**: 251–68.

77. Kramer, J. et al., Embryonic stem cell-derived chondrogenic differentiation in vitro: Activation by BMP-2 and BMP-4. *Mech Dev*, 2000. **92**(2): 193–205.

78. Nakagawa, T., S.Y. Lee, and A.H. Reddi, Induction of chondrogenesis from human embryonic stem cells without embryoid body formation by bone morphogenetic protein 7 and transforming growth factor beta1. *Arthritis Rheum*, 2009. **60**(12): 3686–92.

79. Barberi, T. et al., Derivation of multipotent mesenchymal precursors from human embryonic stem cells. *PLoS Med*, 2005. **2**(6): e161.

80. Nakayama, N. et al., Macroscopic cartilage formation with embryonic stem-cell-derived mesodermal progenitor cells. *J Cell Sci*, 2003. **116**(Pt 10): 2015–28.

81. Varghese, S. et al., Chondrogenic differentiation of human embryonic germ cell derived cells in hydrogels. *Conf Proc IEEE Eng Med Biol Soc*, 2006. **1**: 2643–6.

82. Prockop, D.J., Marrow stromal cells as stem cells for nonhematopoietic tissues. *Science*, 1997. **276**(5309): 71–4.

83. Pittenger, M.F. et al., Multilineage potential of adult human mesenchymal stem cells. *Science*, 1999. **284**(5411): 143–7.

84. Ahmed, N. et al., Soluble signalling factors derived from differentiated cartilage tissue affect chondrogenic differentiation of rat adult marrow stromal cells. *Cell Physiol Biochem*, 2007. **20**(5): 665–78.

85. Sharma, B. et al., *in vivo* chondrogenesis of mesenchymal stem cells in a photopolymerized hydrogel. *Plast Reconstr Surg*, 2007. **119**(1): 112–20.

86. Mackay, A.M. et al., Chondrogenic differentiation of cultured human mesenchymal stem cells from marrow. *Tissue Eng*, 1998. **4**(4): 415–28.

87. Johnstone, B. et al., *In vitro* chondrogenesis of bone marrow-derived mesenchymal progenitor cells. *Exp Cell Res*, 1998. **238**(1): 265–72.

88. Worster, A.A. et al., Chondrocytic differentiation of mesenchymal stem cells sequentially exposed to transforming growth factor-beta1 in monolayer and insulin-like growth factor-I in a three-dimensional matrix. *J Orthop Res*, 2001. **19**(4): 738–49.

89. Wise, J.K. et al., Chondrogenic differentiation of human mesenchymal stem cells on oriented nanofibrous scaffolds: Engineering the superficial zone of articular cartilage. *Tissue Eng Part A*, 2009. **15**(4): 913–21.

90. Barry, F. et al., Chondrogenic differentiation of mesenchymal stem cells from bone marrow: Differentiation-dependent gene expression of matrix components. *Exp Cell Res*, 2001. **268**(2): 189–200.

91. Matsuda, C. et al., Differentiation of human bone marrow mesenchymal stem cells to chondrocytes for construction of three-dimensional cartilage tissue. *Cytotechnology*, 2005. **47**(1–3): 11–7.

92. Worster, A.A. et al., Effect of transforming growth factor beta1 on chondrogenic differentiation of cultured equine mesenchymal stem cells. *Am J Vet Res*, 2000. **61**(9): 1003–10.

93. Tsuchiya, K. et al., The effect of coculture of chondrocytes with meshenchymal stem cells on their cartilaginous phenotype *in vitro*. *Mater Sci Eng C*, 2004. **24**: 391–6.

94. Hwang, N.S. et al., Morphogenetic signals from chondrocytes promote chondrogenic and osteogenic differentiation of mesenchymal stem cells. *J Cell Physiol*, 2007. **212**(2): 281–4.

95. Wang, Y. et al., *in vitro* cartilage tissue engineering with 3D porous aqueous-derived silk scaffolds and mesenchymal stem cells. *Biomaterials*, 2005. **26**(34): 7082–94.

96. Hofmann, S. et al., Cartilage-like tissue engineering using silk scaffolds and mesenchymal stem cells. *Tissue Eng*, 2006. **12**(10): 2729–38.

97. Tsuchiya, K. et al., The effect of coculture of chondrocytes with mesenchymal stem cells on their cartilaginous phenotype in vito. *Mater Sci Eng C*, 2004. **24**: 391–6.

98. Hattori, S., C. Oxford, and A.H. Reddi, Identification of superficial zone articular chondrocyte stem/progenitor cells. *Biochem Biophys Res Commun*, 2007. **358**(1): 99–103.

99. Lee, S.Y., T. Nakagawa, and A.H. Reddi, Induction of chondrogenesis and expression of superficial zone protein (SZP)/lubricin by mesenchymal progenitors in the infrapatellar fat pad of the knee joint treated with TGF-beta1 and BMP-7. *Biochem Biophys Res Commun*, 2008. **376**(1): 148–53.

100. Lee, S.Y., T. Nakagawa, and A.H. Reddi, Mesenchymal progenitor cells derived from synovium and infrapatellar fat pad as a source for superficial zone cartilage tissue engineering: Analysis of superficial zone protein/lubricin expression. *Tissue Eng Part A*. **16**(1): 317–25.

101. Yamane, S. and A.H. Reddi, Induction of chondrogenesis and superficial zone protein accumulation in synovial side population cells by BMP-7 and TGF-beta1. *J Orthop Res*, 2008. **26**(4): 485–92.

102. Hwang, N.S. and J. Elisseeff, Application of stem cells for articular cartilage regeneration. *J Knee Surg*, 2009. **22**(1): 60–71.

103. Gimble, J. and F. Guilak, Adipose-derived adult stem cells: Isolation, characterization, and differentiation potential. *Cytotherapy*, 2003. **5**(5): 362–9.

104. Rodbell, M., Metabolism of isolated fat cells. I. Effects of hormones on glucose metabolism and lipolysis. *J Biol Chem*, 1964. **239**: 375–80.

105. Aust, L. et al., Yield of human adipose-derived adult stem cells from liposuction aspirates. *Cytotherapy*, 2004. **6**(1): 7–14.

106. Guilak, F. et al., Clonal analysis of the differentiation potential of human adipose-derived adult stem cells. *J Cell Physiol*, 2006. **206**(1): 229–37.

107. Jiang, T. et al., Potent *in vitro* chondrogenesis of CD105 enriched human adipose-derived stem cells. *Biomaterials*, 2010. **31**(13): 3564–71.

108. Merceron, C. et al., Differential effects of hypoxia on osteochondrogenic potential of human adipose-derived stem cells. *Am J Physiol Cell Physiol*, 2009. **298**(2): C355–64.

109. Awad, H.A. et al., Chondrogenic differentiation of adipose-derived adult stem cells in agarose, alginate, and gelatin scaffolds. *Biomaterials*, 2004. **25**(16): 3211–22.

110. Cheng, N.C. et al., Chondrogenic differentiation of adipose-derived adult stem cells by a porous scaffold derived from native articular cartilage extracellular matrix. *Tissue Eng Part A*, 2009. **15**(2): 231–41.

111. Estes, B.T. et al., Isolation of adipose-derived stem cells and their induction to a chondrogenic phenotype. *Nat Protoc*, 2010. **5**(7): 1294–311.

112. Kemmis, C.M. et al., Bone morphogenetic protein 6 drives both osteogenesis and chondrogenesis in murine adipose-derived mesenchymal cells depending on culture conditions. *Biochem Biophys Res Commun*, 2010. **401**(1): 20–5.

113. Awad, H.A. et al., Effects of transforming growth factor beta1 and dexamethasone on the growth and chondrogenic differentiation of adipose-derived stromal cells. *Tissue Eng*, 2003. **9**(6): 1301–12.

114. Erickson, G.R. et al., Chondrogenic potential of adipose tissue-derived stromal cells *in vitro* and in vivo. *Biochem Biophys Res Commun*, 2002. **290**(2): 763–9.

115. An, C. et al., IGF-1 and BMP-2 induces differentiation of adipose-derived mesenchymal stem cells into chondrocytes-like cells. *Ann Biomed Eng*, 2010. **38**(4): 1647–54.

116. Ronziere, M.C. et al., Chondrogenic potential of bone marrow- and adipose tissue-derived adult human mesenchymal stem cells. *Biomed Mater Eng*, 2010. **20**(3): 145–58.

117. Estes, B.T., A.W. Wu, and F. Guilak, Potent induction of chondrocytic differentiation of human adipose-derived adult stem cells by bone morphogenetic protein 6. *Arthritis Rheum*, 2006. **54**(4): 1222–32.

118. Indrawattana, N. et al., Growth factor combination for chondrogenic induction from human mesenchymal stem cell. *Biochem Biophys Res Commun*, 2004. **320**(3): 914–9.

119. Hennig, T. et al., Reduced chondrogenic potential of adipose tissue derived stromal cells correlates with an altered TGFbeta receptor and BMP profile and is overcome by BMP-6. *J Cell Physiol*, 2007. **211**(3): 682–91.

120. Koay, E.J. and K.A. Athanasiou, Hypoxic chondrogenic differentiation of human embryonic stem cells enhances cartilage protein synthesis and biomechanical functionality. *Osteoarthritis Cartilage*, 2008. **16**(12): 1450–6.

121. O'Shea, T.M. and X. Miao, Bilayered scaffolds for osteochondral tissue engineering. *Tissue Eng Part B Rev*, 2008. **14**(4): 447–64.

122. Concaro, S., F. Gustavson, and P. Gatenholm, Bioreactors for tissue engineering of cartilage. *Adv Biochem Eng Biotechnol*, 2009. **112**: 125–43.

123. Freed, L.E. et al., Chondrogenesis in a cell-polymer-bioreactor system. *Exp Cell Res*, 1998. **240**(1): 58–65.

124. Buckley, C.T., S.D. Thorpe, and D.J. Kelly, Engineering of large cartilaginous tissues through the use of microchanneled hydrogels and rotational culture. *Tissue Eng Part A*, 2009. **15**(11): 3213–20.

125. Santoro, R. et al., Bioreactor based engineering of large-scale human cartilage grafts for joint resurfacing. *Biomaterials*, 2010. **31**(34): 8946–52.

126. Bian, L. et al., Dynamic mechanical loading enhances functional properties of tissue-engineered cartilage using mature canine chondrocytes. *Tissue Eng Part A*, 2010. **16**(5): 1781–90.

127. Gemmiti, C.V. and R.E. Guldberg, Shear stress magnitude and duration modulates matrix composition and tensile mechanical properties in engineered cartilaginous tissue. *Biotechnol Bioeng*, 2009. **104**(4): 809–20.

128. Yoshioka, T. et al., Repair of large osteochondral defects with allogeneic cartilaginous aggregates formed from bone marrow-derived cells using RWV bioreactor. *J Orthop Res*, 2007. **25**(10): 1291–8.

129. Marolt, D. et al., Bone and cartilage tissue constructs grown using human bone marrow stromal cells, silk scaffolds and rotating bioreactors. *Biomaterials*, 2006. **27**(36): 6138–49.

130. Wang, T.W. et al., Regulation of adult human mesenchymal stem cells into osteogenic and chondrogenic lineages by different bioreactor systems. *J Biomed Mater Res A*, 2009. **88**(4): 935–46.

131. Mahmoudifar, N. and P.M. Doran, Chondrogenic differentiation of human adipose-derived stem cells in polyglycolic acid mesh scaffolds under dynamic culture conditions. *Biomaterials*, 2010. **31**(14): 3858–67.

132. Tigli, R.S. et al., Chondrogenesis in perfusion bioreactors using porous silk scaffolds and hESC-derived MSCs. *J Biomed Mater Res A*, 2010. **96**(1): 21–8.

133. Goncalves, A. et al., Effect of flow perfusion conditions in the chondrogenic differentiation of bone marrow stromal cells cultured onto starch based biodegradable scaffolds. *Acta Biomater*, 2011 Apr; **7**(4): 1644–52.

134. Huang, C.Y. et al., Effects of cyclic compressive loading on chondrogenesis of rabbit bone-marrow derived mesenchymal stem cells. *Stem Cells*, 2004. **22**(3): 313–23.

135. Budde, S. et al., No effect in combining chondrogenic predifferentiation and mechanical cyclic compression on osteochondral constructs stimulated in a bioreactor. *Ann Anat*, 2010. **192**(4): 237–46.

# 31

# TMJ Engineering

31.1 Introduction ....................................................................... **31**-1
31.2 Structure and Function of TMJ Tissues ...................................... **31**-2
31.3 Tissue Engineering Approaches ................................................ **31**-3
    TMJ Disc Tissue Engineering • Mandibular Condyle Tissue
    Engineering
31.4 Looking to the Future in TMJ Tissue Engineering ................... **31**-6
References ................................................................................. **31**-7

Michael S.
Detamore
*University of Kansas*

## 31.1 Introduction

The temporomandibular joint (TMJ) is more colloquially known as the jaw joint, and is formed by the articulation of the condyle of the mandible over the glenoid fossa and articular eminence of the temporal bone (Figure 31.1). The TMJ disc is situated between these articulating structures, serving to provide better congruency between them, and dividing the TMJ into superior and inferior joint spaces. The TMJ is used in every day activities that most of us take for granted such as talking, laughing, chewing, and yawning.

Unfortunately for individuals who suffer from TMJ disorders, or TMDs, activities such as these can become difficult or even impossible due the pain and/or limited range of motion associated with the disorder. Speaking in a global context, there are numerous types of TMDs, each of which requires a treatment strategy tailored to the patient and the specific nature of their TMD (Tanaka et al. 2008). In many cases, TMDs are best managed, at least initially, by conservative therapy, although in some cases are best managed surgically.

TMJ tissue engineering should not be viewed as a panacea for TMDs, but rather as a category of treatments designed for a selected set of TMD patients. For example, patients with mild internal derangement (e.g., Wilkes stage I [Wilkes 1989]) would not be candidates for tissue engineering treatments, as there would be no appreciable degeneration requiring new engineered tissues. In addition, ankylosis patients could be at risk for heterotopic bone formation, and rheumatoid arthritis patients in the absence of other treatments to successfully halt the progression of their autoimmune disease would likely find new engineered tissues being attacked by their bodies. Tissue engineering instead may be better suited for conditions such as severely osteoarthritic TMJs, perhaps with advanced internal derangement (e.g., Wilkes stage IV or V), or for mandibular condylar defect repair.

A previous book chapter (Wong et al. 2006) and a book (Athanasiou et al. 2009) are suggested as further reading on the topic of TMJ tissue engineering, providing additional details on various topics not covered in this chapter. This chapter will primarily focus on establishing the need for an understanding of the structure and function of TMJ tissues, followed by an overview of progress to date in TMJ tissue engineering, and concluding with a critical look toward the future of TMJ tissue engineering.

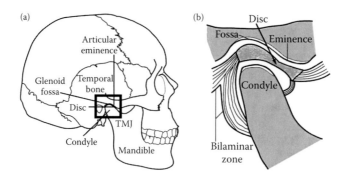

**FIGURE 31.1**   (a) Side view of the human skull. The temporomandibular joint is formed by the temporal bone and mandible. (b) The mandibular condyle is covered by a thin layer of articular cartilage. A fibrocartilaginous disc is situated between the fossa-eminence of the temporal bone and the condyle of the mandible.

## 31.2  Structure and Function of TMJ Tissues

An in-depth coverage of the biochemical content and structure, biomechanics, and cellular composition of TMJ structures will not be provided here, as this information is provided in detail elsewhere (Athanasiou et al. 2009; Detamore and Athanasiou 2003c; Singh and Detamore 2009; Wang and Detamore 2007). However, it should be emphasized that a thorough understanding of the TMJ tissues is essential for those who endeavor to engineer them. Therefore, a concise overview of salient points with regard to the TMJ disc and the mandibular condyle, the primary targets of TMJ tissue engineering, will be provided here.

With regard to the TMJ disc, it would best be described as a fibrocartilage, with perhaps more resemblance to a fibrous tissue than a cartilaginous tissue in its composition, biomechanical properties, and cell content (Johns and Athanasiou 2007a). The TMJ disc is predominately composed of type I collagen (Detamore and Athanasiou 2003b), with fibers generally oriented circumferentially around the periphery and anteroposteriorly throughout its interior (Scapino et al. 2006). This collagen fiber orientation imparts on the tissue a highly anisotropic tensile behavior (Beatty et al. 2001; Detamore and Athanasiou 2003a). Several different animal models have been investigated to elucidate the properties of the TMJ disc, and a recent study made interspecies comparisons to identify a suitable animal model for the human TMJ disc (Kalpakci et al. 2011). In this study, the mechanical properties and collagen, glycosaminoglycan and cell content were measured in rabbit, goat, human, pig, and cow TMJ discs and compared, supporting the use of the porcine TMJ disc due to its similarity to the human TMJ disc in terms of dimensions, collagen and glycosaminoglycan content, and compressive properties.

The mandibular condyle is a primarily osseous structure, with a thin layer of articular cartilage on its surface. The condylar cartilage does not resemble the hyaline cartilage found in the knee or hip, for example, but rather is organized into a fibrous zone at the surface with a more hyaline-like region below (Wang and Detamore 2007). Collagen type I predominates in the fibrous zone, whereas collagen II predominates in the underlying zones. Interestingly, the fibrous zone has a collagen fiber orientation bearing a remarkable resemblance to the TMJ disc, with anteroposteriorly oriented fibers surrounded by circumferentially oriented fibers around the periphery, although the condylar cartilage appears less anisotropic under tension than the TMJ disc (Singh and Detamore 2008).

From a validation standpoint, it is crucial to understand the composition of these tissues, to provide the design criteria with a clear endpoint in mind and basis of comparison for engineered tissues to evaluate the final product. However, engineers must not lose sight of the fact that the bottom line in evaluating success is ultimately the patient's quality of life, which relate back to pain and function. Nevertheless, it is important to understand that the TMJ cartilages are more fibrous in nature than hyaline cartilage. In fact, the most important aspect of understanding the structure and function of the TMJ tissues may lie in developing new design strategies, for example, in developing new biomaterials that can withstand the unique biomechanical environment of the TMJ and accelerate tissue regeneration.

# 31.3 Tissue Engineering Approaches

TMJ tissue engineering has made major strides in recent years. In the 1990s, there were only three TMJ tissue engineering studies published (all on the disc), whereas the following decade saw an explosion in the number of studies published. The current decade now is poised to make major strides forward in terms of *in vivo* studies and hopefully clinical studies as well. The reader is encouraged to consult resources developed by collective discussion at conferences regarding the evaluation of engineered TMJ tissues and overall directives for research needs in this field (Butler et al. 2008). In addition, a handful of reviews with broader focus have included mention of TMJ tissue engineering, with topics including nanostructured bioceramics (Adamopoulos and Papadopoulos 2007), scaffolds for drug delivery (Moioli et al. 2007) and intra-articular drug delivery (Mountziaris et al. 2009), and stem cells (Mao et al. 2006).

Heretofore, the focus of TMJ tissue engineering has been exclusively on the TMJ disc and on the mandibular condyle/ramus, and these studies have been in isolation. Therefore, the following discussion will focus on the TMJ disc and the mandibular condyle in isolation.

## 31.3.1 TMJ Disc Tissue Engineering

A number of review articles have been dedicated to the subject of TMJ disc tissue engineering (Allen and Athanasiou 2006b; Almarza and Athanasiou 2004a; Detamore and Athanasiou 2003b, c; Glowacki 2001; Johns and Athanasiou 2007a; Su and Kang 2010), detailing the emergence of early pioneering studies and offering insight on possible design strategies. TMJ disc tissue engineering appeared in the literature much earlier than mandibular condyle tissue engineering studies, which did not appear until 2000. In the 1990s, a group of three studies collectively paved the way for the field of TMJ tissue engineering in its infancy, addressing issues such as cell source, biomaterials, and shape-specific scaffolds (Girdler 1998; Puelacher et al. 1994; Springer et al. 2001; Thomas et al. 1991).

The first such study was published in 1991, at a time when many of the landmark studies characterizing the TMJ disc matrix were not yet available and tissue engineering as a field was itself in its infancy (Thomas et al. 1991). In this study, rabbit TMJ disc cells were cultured in disc-shaped collagen scaffolds, and proteoglycan synthesis and spherical cell morphology were noted. This early effort suggested that autologous TMJ disc cells for disc regeneration could be harvested during diagnostic arthroscopy. In 1994, chondrocytes were obtained from the shoulders of newborn calves, then seeded in disc-shaped PLA/polyglycolic acid (PGA) scaffolds and implanted subcutaneously in mice for 12 weeks, resulting in glycosaminoglycan and collagen II synthesis (Puelacher et al. 1994). Four years later, cells from marmoset mandibular condylar cartilage were cultured in collagen fibrinogen scaffolds, exhibiting significant proteoglycan and collagen II synthesis (Girdler 1998).

In 2001, a study compared the performance of human and porcine disc and fossa-eminence cartilage cells on different biomaterials, including expanded polytetrafluoroethylene monofilaments, PGA monofilaments, polyamide monofilaments, natural bone mineral blocks, and glass (Springer et al. 2001). Scanning electron microscopy demonstrated that cells were able to bridge the gap between monofilaments, and collagen II synthesis was observed. Two other publications emerged in 2001, one a review on strategies for TMJ tissue engineering, including cell sources and scaffolding materials (Glowacki 2001), and the other the introduction of a photopolymerization method for developing shape-specific TMJ disc scaffolds (Poshusta and Anseth 2001).

Despite the apparent generation of momentum early in the decade, it was not until 2004 that new studies appeared in the TMJ disc tissue engineering literature, where Athanasiou's group began to make what is now the most substantial contribution to date in this literature. These studies promoted the use of poly(glycolic acid) scaffolds over agarose for culturing TMJ disc cells and identified spinner flasks as the preferred seeding method for these scaffolds (Almarza and Athanasiou 2004b), then later suggested that poly(L-lactic acid) may hold advantages over poly(glycolic acid) for nonwoven mesh scaffolds in supporting TMJ disc cells (Allen and Athanasiou 2008). Athanasiou's group further promoted the use of growth factors such as insulin-like growth factor (IGF)-I and transforming growth factor (TGF)-β1 with TMJ disc cells (Allen and Athanasiou 2006a; 2008; Almarza and Athanasiou 2006a; Detamore and Athanasiou 2004, 2005a), and examined the effects of passaging, pellet culture, and culture conditions (Allen and Athanasiou 2007; Bean et al. 2006; Johns and Athanasiou 2007b), as well as the effects of hydrostatic pressure and rotating wall bioreactors (Almarza and Athanasiou 2006b; Detamore and Athanasiou 2005b).

It has been encouraging to see a number of new groups joining the field, with approaches ranging from scaffolds made by decellularizing porcine discs (Lumpkins et al. 2008), use of platelet-derived growth factor with TMJ disc cells (Hanaoka et al. 2006), finite element modeling for TMJ disc tissue engineering (Al-Sukhun et al. 2007), and incorporating adipose stem cells into nonwoven polylactide scaffolds (Maenpaa et al. 2010). Overall, the field of TMJ disc tissue engineering has emerged from its infancy, with its formative years well-established. The primary objective for TMJ disc tissue engineering in the current decade will be to advance the field to the *in vivo* stage, specifically by evaluating the performance of a tissue-engineered TMJ disc following discectomy in an animal model, and perhaps by advancing to clinical trials as well.

## 31.3.2 Mandibular Condyle Tissue Engineering

In comparison to the TMJ disc, fewer reviews have been written on tissue engineering of the mandibular condyle. However, there have been a couple of reviews (Naujoks et al. 2008; Wang and Detamore 2007), primarily focusing on the cartilage of the mandibular condyle, with a great deal of reference to strategies employed in cartilage or bone tissue engineering in general as they may pertain to the TMJ. Although mandibular condyle tissue engineering studies entered the literature much later (2000), they have been more varied in strategies and are more advanced in terms of *in vivo* trials.

In 2000, Hollister and colleagues introduced their approach of using solid free-form fabrication (SFF) to create a polymeric scaffold in the shape of the ramus and condyle of the mandibular condyle, intended to serve as a patient-specific strategy based on computed tomography (CT) and/or magnetic resonance imaging images (Hollister et al. 2000). SFF provides precise control over pore size, porosity, permeability, and mechanical integrity, made possible by its layer-by-layer printing technology. Using SFF, Hollister and colleagues engineered cylinder-shaped osteochondral constructs and condyle/ramus-shaped bone constructs using materials such as hydroxyapatite, poly(lactic acid) and polycaprolactone (Schek et al. 2004, 2005; Williams et al. 2005). Subcutaneous implantation of these constructs collectively demonstrated significant bone ingrowth and glycosaminoglycan formation (Hollister et al. 2005; Schek et al. 2004, 2005; Williams et al. 2005). These studies advanced to a TMJ reconstruction study, using a selective laser sintering method to fabricate a polycaprolactone condyle-ramus scaffold for implantation into the TMJs of 6–8-month-old Yucatan minipigs (Smith et al. 2007). The condylar heads of the scaffolds were packed with autologous iliac crest bone marrow, secured to the mandible using miniplates and screws, and evaluated after 1 and 3 months. Compared to controls, there was an increase in regenerated bone volume, and there was evidence of cartilage-like tissue as well.

Hollister later collaborated with Mao in developing a *tibial* condyle-shaped scaffold made of polycaprolactone and hydroxyapatite, with an overlying hydrogel layer, each respectively constituting an osseous and chondral region of an osteochondral construct (Lee et al. 2009). These constructs were seeded with bone marrow stem cells and implanted subcutaneously, leading to blood vessel infiltration and regional mineralized and cartilage-like tissue formation. Although the scaffold shape was based on the tibia, clearly this approach would be amenable to a mandibular condyle shape.

Prior to this collaboration with Hollister, Mao's group explored a different strategy to mandibular condyle tissue engineering based on a hydrogel-based osteochondral approach, whereby bone marrow stem cells were encapsulated in polyethylene glycol diacrylate (PEG-DA) to create stratified bone and cartilage layers in the shape of a human condyle (Alhadlaq and Mao 2003, 2005; Alhadlaq et al. 2004). In this approach, a negative mold of an adult human cadaveric condyle was created, and the stem cells were differentiated in either osteogenic or chondrogenic medium. A suspension of chondrogenic cells in liquid PEG-DA was then added to the mold, the PEG-DA was photopolymerized, then a suspension with osteogenic cells was added and polymerized as well, creating an osteochondral construct in the shape of a human condyle. After 12 weeks *in vivo*, osteopontin, osteonectin, and collagen I were observed to be localized in the osteogenic layer, and collagen II and glycosaminoglycans were localized in the chondrogenic layer (Alhadlaq and Mao 2005). A more recent approach from Mao's group was a cell-homing strategy, accomplished by adsorbing TGF-β3 to a collagen hydrogel that was infused in an anatomically-shaped polycaprolactone/hydroxyapatite composite. Although this approach was focused on rabbit shoulders, the concept of homing of endogenous cells with shape-specific scaffolds is likely to be amenable to mandibular condyle regeneration (Lee et al. 2010).

In another approach, Detamore and colleagues have focused primarily on the cell source (Bailey et al. 2007; Wang and Detamore 2009; Wang et al. 2009). For example, porcine mandibular condylar cartilage cells were compared with chondrocytes from ankle cartilage in monolayer (Wang and Detamore 2009) and on 3-D scaffolds (Wang et al. 2009). In both cases, the chondrocytes from the hyaline ankle cartilage drastically outperformed the cells from mandibular condylar cartilage in extracellular matrix production.

Beyond the three aforementioned groups, several interesting strategies have been introduced, many of which were *in vivo* studies using only histology and/or imaging as outcome measures. In the earliest of these studies, osteoblasts were seeded into condyle-shaped polyglycolic acid/polylactic acid scaffolds, with chondrocytes painted on the surface (Weng et al. 2001). These constructs were implanted subcutaneously in mice, and positive histological observations were made after 12 weeks *in vivo*. Positive histological results were also observed in a related study, where porcine mesenchymal stem cells were seeded in condyle-shaped poly(lactic-*co*-glycolic acid) (PLGA) scaffolds and cultured under osteogenic conditions in a rotating bioreactor (Abukawa et al. 2003). Two studies from another group molded coral into the shape of a human condyle and seeded them with mesenchymal stem cells, then implanted them either subcutaneously with bone morphogenetic protein (BMP)-2 in mice to demonstrate osteogenesis (Chen et al. 2002) or under blood vessels in rabbits to demonstrate construct vascularization (Chen et al. 2004). In another approach, PLGA-based constructs were implanted with growth factors in rat mandibular defects, which suggested that TGF-β1 and IGF-I were efficacious (Srouji et al. 2005), whereas BMP-2 was not (Ueki et al. 2003). In an *in vitro* study, bovine mandibular condylar cartilage cells were encapsulated in poly(ethylene glycol)-based hydrogels and compressed dynamically at a frequency of 0.3 Hz to 15% strain for 48 h (Nicodemus et al. 2007). Although gene expression did not clearly demonstrate a benefit from mechanical stimulation with these particular parameters, this important study was the first to employ mechanical stimulation for mandibular condyle tissue engineering. Recently, as an alternative strategy to Hollister and colleagues' solid free form fabrication approach, an Italian group recently reported a new approach of using CT images of a pig mandible, along with computer-aided design (CAD) and rapid prototyping to create a condyle-shaped biomaterial made of acrylonitrile butadiene styrene (ABS) plastic (Ciocca et al. 2009). The goal of this work was to move toward a perfect-fitting bone substitute model for hydroxyapatite scaffolds.

This new decade has seen the emergence of two groups new to TMJ tissue engineering, each bringing novel approaches to the field. One of these approaches was to use low-intensity pulsed ultrasound for 4 weeks to evaluate its benefits in improving results with mandibular condyle regeneration (El-Bialy et al. 2010). The left mandibular condyle in rabbits was excised and replaced by a scaffold, consisting of a chondrogenic cell-loaded collagen sponge and osteogenic cell-loaded collagen sponge folded in to a urinary bladder matrix-based pillow, which was fixed in place by suturing to surrounding muscles and using ProDense (calcium sulfate and calcium phosphate product). The results seemed to suggest that ultrasound led to better structural formation. The other approach to appear this decade was the development of a scaffold-bioreactor system (Grayson et al. 2010). Scaffolds made from decellularized trabecular bone were shaped into human-sized mandibular condyles based on digitized clinical images, and seeded with human bone marrow stem cells. These constructs were placed into a bioreactor with chambers in the shape of the mandibular condyle to provide direct perfusion of medium through the construct. Electron microscopy, histology, and microCT together suggested that constructs cultured in the bioreactor exhibited matrix deposition throughout their volume, in contrast to constructs cultured in static conditions, which had matrix primarily limited to the periphery.

To summarize mandibular condyle tissue engineering studies, a variety of approaches have been introduced to create shape-specific scaffolds, with different cell sources and bioactive signaling strategies investigated along the way. While a handful of studies have implanted scaffolds subcutaneously, only a precious few have investigated actual condylar defect repair or condyle/ramus replacement in the TMJ. The next major steps for mandibular condyle tissue engineering will be to demonstrate effective long-term defect and surface regeneration, and regeneration of an entire osteochondral mandibular condyle, in larger animals such as the pig and eventually in clinical trials.

## 31.4  Looking to the Future in TMJ Tissue Engineering

In discussions at the world's first *TMJ Bioengineering Conference* in Colorado in 2006, concerns with tissue engineering for moving toward the future were identified, including attachment, integration, metaplasia, angiogenesis, patient age, developing a marketable product, and creating a condyle-disc composite scaffold (Detamore et al. 2007). Although there have been several advances since then, as outlined in previous sections, these concerns still remain. Only through further experimentation will we begin to resolve these issues.

A major concern that lingers is the great divide between orthopedics and the TMJ, as the TMJ is unique among joints in being excluded from the orthopedic umbrella, being thrust instead under the jurisdiction of the dental community. As an example of the divide, *in vivo* studies of cartilage or osteochondral tissue regeneration in a joint such as the knee are commonplace, whereas *in vivo* regeneration studies with TMJ structures are just now emerging. Clearly, TMJ tissue regeneration as a field has fallen significantly behind its orthopedic counterpart. However, we will hopefully see the divide diminish in the coming decade with cross-pollination of experts from each respective field entering the other respective field, and with leadership from senior investigators with established reputations in both fields.

A number of considerations will be important in moving the field toward widely accepted clinical application. For example, biomechanical considerations will be crucial, ensuring that engineered tissues are able to withstand the loads placed on the TMJ. A forward-thinking group has already considered finite element modeling of an engineered TMJ disc (Al-Sukhun et al. 2007), perhaps paving the way for a new application for the burgeoning field of TMJ biomechanical modeling. Another consideration is that the ideal animal model has yet to be unequivocally identified. For tissue engineering studies with the TMJ, the rabbit is a likely starting point, although the pig may be the preferred candidate for a nonprimate large animal model as we move toward clinical studies, due to similar size and properties (Kalpakci et al. 2011), as well as a number of other reasons (Detamore et al. 2007). Another point to consider is that there really is no "one size fits all" approach to TMJ tissue engineering. Some patients may require only the regeneration of a focal defect, as opposed to others who may require a combined engineered disc-condyle unit to completely replace these structures in a ravaged joint. The disc and condyle are the only TMJ structures receiving attention in tissue engineering studies, with little clinical interest expressed in engineering other tissues in the joint at this stage. As tissue engineered products for the TMJ become a reality in clinical practice, it is possible that clinicians may express a greater interest in regeneration of surrounding structures as a means to better polish the final product, although this remains to be seen.

A major consideration with TMJ tissue engineering is the cell source. Perhaps acellular materials with homing mechanisms to attract endogenous cells are the best solution (Lee et al. 2010), or perhaps cell-seeded constructs may be the fastest and most effective route to regeneration. If a cellular strategy is selected, should those cells be autologous? Should they be stem cells? Certainly autologous cells would be better from an immune compatibility standpoint, and the field may be leaning more toward the use of stem cells. Early schools of thought were founded on the notion that the selection of a mature cell source meant that cells from the same tissue should be used (e.g., harvest TMJ disc cells from a patient to engineer a new TMJ disc). However, due to concerns such as cell numbers, donor site morbidity from a healthy(-ier) contralateral TMJ versus compromised cells from a diseased tissue, and the overall dismal performance of TMJ disc cells compared to chondrocytes from other cartilage sources in the body (Johns and Athanasiou 2008; Johns et al. 2008; Wang et al. 2009), the field is moving away from taking cells from the TMJ as a source for TMJ tissue engineering. Therefore, cells from other cartilage sources (e.g., rib) are recommended if mature cells are sought, although stem cells from bone marrow, adipose tissue, or umbilical cords, or possibly induced pluripotent stem cells, are leading candidates for cell sources in TMJ tissue engineering.

Overall, tissue engineering brings hope to the millions of people suffering from TMDs, offering the almost incomprehensible option of restoring the tissue to a "good as new" condition. We must learn from the lessons of the TMJ total joint replacement community, understanding, for example, that even in restoring function we may never be able to eliminate pain. We must further recognize that not all patients are candidates for tissue engineering treatment, but for those that are candidates, develop patient-specific approaches based on their specific condition. Building on the numerous successes over the past decade, and with cross-talk with the orthopedic community, the field of TMJ tissue engineering is poised to truly flourish in the years ahead.

# References

Abukawa, H., Terai, H., Hannouche, D., Vacanti, J. P., Kaban, L. B., Troulis, M. J. 2003. Formation of a mandibular condyle *in vitro* by tissue engineering. *J Oral Maxillofac Surg* 61(1):94–100.

Adamopoulos, O., Papadopoulos, T. 2007. Nanostructured bioceramics for maxillofacial applications. *J Mater Sci Mater Med* 18(8):1587–97.

Al-Sukhun, J., Ashammakhi, N., Penttila, H. 2007. Effects of tissue-engineered articular disc implants on the biomechanical loading of the human temporomandibular joint in a three-dimensional finite element model. *J Craniofac Surg* 18(4):781–8; discussion 789–91.

Alhadlaq, A., Elisseeff, J. H., Hong, L. et al. 2004. Adult stem cell driven genesis of human-shaped articular condyle. *Ann Biomed Eng* 32(7):911–23.

Alhadlaq, A., Mao, J. J. 2003. Tissue-engineered neogenesis of human-shaped mandibular condyle from rat mesenchymal stem cells. *J Dent Res* 82(12):951–6.

Alhadlaq, A., Mao, J. J. 2005. Tissue-engineered osteochondral constructs in the shape of an articular condyle. *J Bone Joint Surg Am* 87(5):936–44.

Allen, K. D., Athanasiou, K. A. 2006a. Growth factor effects on passaged TMJ disk cells in monolayer and pellet cultures. *Orthod Craniofac Res* 9(3):143–52.

Allen, K. D., Athanasiou, K. A. 2006b. Tissue engineering of the TMJ disc: A review. *Tissue Eng* 12(5):1183–96.

Allen, K. D., Athanasiou, K. A. 2007. Effect of passage and topography on gene expression of temporomandibular joint disc cells. *Tissue Eng* 13(1):101–10.

Allen, K. D., Athanasiou, K. A. 2008. Scaffold and growth factor selection in temporomandibular joint disc engineering. *J Dent Res* 87(2):180–5.

Almarza, A. J., Athanasiou, K. A. 2004a. Design characteristics for the tissue engineering of cartilaginous tissues. *Ann Biomed Eng* 32(1):2–17.

Almarza, A. J., Athanasiou, K. A. 2004b. Seeding techniques and scaffolding choice for tissue engineering of the temporomandibular joint disk. *Tissue Eng* 10(11–12):1787–95.

Almarza, A. J., Athanasiou, K. A. 2006a. Evaluation of three growth factors in combinations of two for temporomandibular joint disc tissue engineering. *Arch Oral Biol* 51(3):215–21.

Almarza, A. J., Athanasiou, K. A. 2006b. Effects of hydrostatic pressure on TMJ disc cells. *Tissue Eng* 12(5): 1285–94.

Athanasiou, K. A., Almarza, A. J., Detamore, M. S., Kalpacki, K. N. 2009. *Tissue Engineering of Temporomandibular Joint Cartilage*: Morgan and Claypool Publishers.

Bailey, M. M., Wang, L., Bode, C. J., Mitchell, K. E., Detamore, M. S. 2007. A comparison of human umbilical cord matrix stem cells and temporomandibular joint condylar chondrocytes for tissue engineering temporomandibular joint condylar cartilage. *Tissue Eng* 13(8):2003–10.

Bean, A. C., Almarza, A. J., Athanasiou, K. A. 2006. Effects of ascorbic acid concentration on the tissue engineering of the temporomandibular joint disc. *Proc Inst Mech Eng [H]* 220(3):439–47.

Beatty, M. W., Bruno, M. J., Iwasaki, L. R., Nickel, J. C. 2001. Strain rate dependent orthotropic properties of pristine and impulsively loaded porcine temporomandibular joint disk. *J Biomed Mater Res* 57(1): 25–34.

Butler, D. L., Lewis, J. L., Frank, C. B. 2008. Evaluation criteria for musculoskeletal and craniofacial tissue engineering constructs: A conference report 2008. *Tissue Eng Part A* 14(12):2089–104.

Chen, F., Chen, S., Tao, K. et al. 2004. Marrow-derived osteoblasts seeded into porous natural coral to prefabricate a vascularised bone graft in the shape of a human mandibular ramus: Experimental study in rabbits. *Br J Oral Maxillofac Surg* 42(6):532–7.

Chen, F., Mao, T., Tao, K., Chen, S., Ding, G., Gu, X. 2002. Bone graft in the shape of human mandibular condyle reconstruction via seeding marrow-derived osteoblasts into porous coral in a nude mice model. *J Oral Maxillofac Surg* 60(10):1155–9.

Ciocca, L., De Crescenzio, F., Fantini, M., Scotti, R. 2009. CAD/CAM and rapid prototyped scaffold construction for bone regenerative medicine and surgical transfer of virtual planning: A pilot study. *Comput Med Imaging Graph* 33(1):58–62.

Detamore, M. S., Athanasiou, K. A. 2003a. Tensile properties of the porcine temporomandibular joint disc. *J Biomech Eng* 125(4):558–65.

Detamore, M. S., Athanasiou, K. A. 2003b. Structure and function of the temporomandibular joint disc: Implications for tissue engineering. *J Oral Maxillofac Surg* 61(4):494–506.

Detamore, M. S., Athanasiou, K. A. 2003c. Motivation, characterization, and strategy for tissue engineering the temporomandibular joint disc. *Tissue Eng* 9(6):1065–87.

Detamore, M. S., Athanasiou, K. A. 2004. Effects of growth factors on temporomandibular joint disc cells. *Arch Oral Biol* 49(7):577–83.

Detamore, M. S., Athanasiou, K. A. 2005a. Evaluation of three growth factors for TMJ disc tissue engineering. *Ann Biomed Eng* 33(3):383–90.

Detamore, M. S., Athanasiou, K. A. 2005b. Use of a rotating bioreactor toward tissue engineering the temporomandibular joint disc. *Tissue Eng* 11(7–8):1188–97.

Detamore, M. S., Athanasiou, K. A., Mao, J. 2007. A call to action for bioengineers and dental professionals: Directives for the future of TMJ bioengineering. *Ann Biomed Eng* 35(8):1301–11.

El-Bialy, T., Uludag, H., Jomha, N., Badylak, S. F. 2010. *In vivo* ultrasound-assisted tissue-engineered mandibular condyle: A pilot study in rabbits. *Tissue Eng Part C Methods* 16:1315–23.

Girdler, N. M. 1998. *In vitro* synthesis and characterization of a cartilaginous meniscus grown from isolated temporomandibular chondroprogenitor cells. *Scand J Rheumatol* 27(6):446–53.

Glowacki, J. 2001. Engineered cartilage, bone, joints, and menisci. Potential for temporomandibular joint reconstruction. *Cells Tissues Organs* 169(3):302–8.

Grayson, W. L., Frohlich, M., Yeager, K. et al. 2010. Engineering anatomically shaped human bone grafts. *Proc Natl Acad Sci USA* 107(8):3299–304.

Hanaoka, K., Tanaka, E., Takata, T. et al. 2006. Platelet-derived growth factor enhances proliferation and matrix synthesis of temporomandibular joint disc-derived cells. *Angle Orthod* 76(3):486–92.

Hollister, S. J., Levy, R. A., Chu, T. M., Halloran, J. W., Feinberg, S. E. 2000. An image-based approach for designing and manufacturing craniofacial scaffolds. *Int J Oral Maxillofac Surg* 29(1):67–71.

Hollister, S. J., Lin, C. Y., Saito, E. et al. 2005. Engineering craniofacial scaffolds. *Orthod Craniofac Res* 8(3):162–73.

Johns, D. E., Athanasiou, K. A. 2007a. Design characteristics for temporomandibular joint disc tissue engineering: Learning from tendon and articular cartilage. *Proc Inst Mech Eng [H]* 221(5):509–26.

Johns, D. E., Athanasiou, K. A. 2007b. Improving culture conditions for temporomandibular joint disc tissue engineering. *Cells Tissues Organs* 185(4):246–57.

Johns, D. E., Athanasiou, K. A. 2008. Growth factor effects on costal chondrocytes for tissue engineering fibrocartilage. *Cell Tissue Res* 333(3):439–47.

Johns, D. E., Wong, M. E., Athanasiou, K. A. 2008. Clinically relevant cell sources for TMJ disc engineering. *J Dent Res* 87(6):548–52.

Kalpakci, K. N., Willard, V. P., Wong, M. E., Athanasiou, K. A. 2011. An interspecies comparison of the temporomandibular joint disc. *J Dent Res* 90:193–8.

Lee, C. H., Cook, J. L., Mendelson, A., Moioli, E. K., Yao, H., Mao, J. J. 2010. Regeneration of the articular surface of the rabbit synovial joint by cell homing: A proof of concept study. *Lancet* 376(9739):440–8.

Lee, C. H., Marion, N. W., Hollister, S., Mao, J. J. 2009. Tissue formation and vascularization in anatomically shaped human joint condyle ectopically *in vivo*. *Tissue Eng Part A* 15(12):3923–30.

Lumpkins, S. B., Pierre, N., McFetridge, P. S. 2008. A mechanical evaluation of three decellularization methods in the design of a xenogeneic scaffold for tissue engineering the temporomandibular joint disc. *Acta Biomater* 4(4):808–16.

Maenpaa, K., Ella, V., Mauno, J. et al. 2010. Use of adipose stem cells and polylactide discs for tissue engineering of the temporomandibular joint disc. *J R Soc Interface* 7(42):177–88.

Mao, J. J., Giannobile, W. V., Helms, J. A. et al. 2006. Craniofacial tissue engineering by stem cells. *J Dent Res* 85(11):966–79.

Moioli, E. K., Clark, P. A., Xin, X., Lal, S., Mao, J. J. 2007. Matrices and scaffolds for drug delivery in dental, oral and craniofacial tissue engineering. *Adv Drug Deliv Rev* 59(4–5):308–24.

Mountziaris, P. M., Kramer, P. R., Mikos, A. G. 2009. Emerging intra-articular drug delivery systems for the temporomandibular joint. *Methods* 47(2):134–40.

Naujoks, C., Meyer, U., Wiesmann, H. P. et al. 2008. Principles of cartilage tissue engineering in TMJ reconstruction. *Head Face Med* 4(3).

Nicodemus, G. D., Villanueva, I., Bryant, S. J. 2007. Mechanical stimulation of TMJ condylar chondrocytes encapsulated in PEG hydrogels. *J Biomed Mater Res A* 83(2):323–31.

Poshusta, A. K., Anseth, K. S. 2001. Photopolymerized biomaterials for application in the temporomandibular joint. *Cells Tissues Organs* 169(3):272–8.

Puelacher, W. C., Wisser, J., Vacanti, C. A., Ferraro, N. F., Jaramillo, D., Vacanti, J. P. 1994. Temporomandibular joint disc replacement made by tissue-engineered growth of cartilage. *J Oral Maxillofac Surg* 52(11):1172–7.

Scapino, R. P., Obrez, A., Greising, D. 2006. Organization and function of the collagen fiber system in the human temporomandibular joint disk and its attachments. *Cells Tissues Organs* 182(3–4):201–25.

Schek, R. M., Taboas, J. M., Hollister, S. J., Krebsbach, P. H. 2005. Tissue engineering osteochondral implants for temporomandibular joint repair. *Orthod Craniofac Res* 8(4):313–9.

Schek, R. M., Taboas, J. M., Segvich, S. J., Hollister, S. J., Krebsbach, P. H. 2004. Engineered osteochondral grafts using biphasic composite solid free-form fabricated scaffolds. *Tissue Eng* 10(9–10):1376–85.

Singh, M., Detamore, M. S. 2008. Tensile properties of the mandibular condylar cartilage. *J Biomech Eng* 130(1):011009.

Singh, M., Detamore, M. S. 2009. Biomechanical properties of the mandibular condylar cartilage and their relevance to the TMJ disc. *J Biomech* 42(4):405–17.

Smith, M. H., Flanagan, C. L., Kemppainen, J. M. et al. 2007. Computed tomography-based tissue-engineered scaffolds in craniomaxillofacial surgery. *Int J Med Robot* 3(3):207–16.

Springer, I. N., Fleiner, B., Jepsen, S., Acil, Y. 2001. Culture of cells gained from temporomandibular joint cartilage on non-absorbable scaffolds. *Biomaterials* 22(18):2569–77.

Srouji, S., Rachmiel, A., Blumenfeld, I., Livne, E. 2005. Mandibular defect repair by TGF-beta and IGF-1 released from a biodegradable osteoconductive hydrogel. *J Craniomaxillofac Surg* 33(2):79–84.

Su, X., Kang, H. 2010. Cell sources for engineered temporomandibular joint disc tissue: Present and future. *Sheng Wu Yi Xue Gong Cheng Xue Za Zhi* 27(2):463–6.

Tanaka, E., Detamore, M. S., Mercuri, L. G. 2008. Degenerative disorders of the temporomandibular joint: Etiology, diagnosis, and treatment. *J Dent Res* 87(4):296–307.

Thomas, M., Grande, D., Haug, R. H. 1991. Development of an *in vitro* temporomandibular joint cartilage analog. *J Oral Maxillofac Surg* 49(8):854–6; discussion 857.

Ueki, K., Takazakura, D., Marukawa, K. et al. 2003. The use of polylactic acid/polyglycolic acid copolymer and gelatin sponge complex containing human recombinant bone morphogenetic protein-2 following condylectomy in rabbits. *J Craniomaxillofac Surg* 31(2):107–14.

Wang, L., Detamore, M. S. 2007. Tissue engineering the mandibular condyle. *Tissue Eng* 13(8):1955–71.

Wang, L., Detamore, M. S. 2009. Effects of growth factors and glucosamine on porcine mandibular condylar cartilage cells and hyaline cartilage cells for tissue engineering applications. *Arch Oral Biol* 54(1):1–5.

Wang, L., Lazebnik, M., Detamore, M. S. 2009. Hyaline cartilage cells outperform mandibular condylar cartilage cells in a TMJ fibrocartilage tissue engineering application. *Osteoarthritis Cartilage* 17(3):346–53.

Weng, Y., Cao, Y., Silva, C. A., Vacanti, M. P., Vacanti, C. A. 2001. Tissue-engineered composites of bone and cartilage for mandible condylar reconstruction. *J Oral Maxillofac Surg* 59(2):185–90.

Wilkes, C. H. 1989. Internal derangements of the temporomandibular joint. Pathological variations. *Arch Otolaryngol Head Neck Surg* 115(4):469–77.

Williams, J. M., Adewunmi, A., Schek, R. M. et al. 2005. Bone tissue engineering using polycaprolactone scaffolds fabricated via selective laser sintering. *Biomaterials* 26(23):4817–27.

Wong, M. E. K., Allen, K. D., Athanasiou, K. A. 2006. Tissue engineering of the temporomandibular Joint. In: *Tissue Engineering and Artificial Organs*, J. D. Bronzino, editor. Boca Raton, FL: CRC Press.

# 32

# Interface Tissue Engineering

Helen H. Lu
*Columbia University*

Nora Khanarian
*Columbia University*

Kristen Moffat
*Columbia University*

Siddarth Subramony
*Columbia University*

32.1 Introduction .................................................................... 32-1
32.2 Interface Scaffold Design for Ligament-to-Bone Interface
     Tissue Engineering .................................................... 32-4
32.3 Interface Scaffold Design for Tendon-to-Bone Interface
     Tissue Engineering .................................................... 32-7
32.4 Stratified Scaffold Design for Cartilage-to-Bone Interface
     Tissue Engineering .................................................... 32-10
32.5 Summary and Future Directions ............................. 32-13
References .................................................................... 32-14

## 32.1 Introduction

Trauma and degeneration of the musculoskeletal system are commonly associated with injuries to soft tissues such as cartilage which lines the surface of articulating joints, as well as ligaments and tendons, which connect bone to bone, and muscle to bone, respectively. Interfaces or insertion sites that connect these soft tissues to bone are therefore ubiquitous in the body, and serve to facilitate synchronized joint motion and musculoskeletal function (Figure 32.1). These interfaces exhibit a gradient of structural and mechanical properties that has a number of functions, from mediating load transfer between two distinct types of tissue to sustaining the heterotypic cellular communications required for interface function and homeostasis (Benjamin et al. 1986; Lu and Jiang 2006; Woo et al. 1988). These critical junctions are however, prone to injury and unfortunately, not reestablished following standard surgical repair, and the failure to regenerate the intricate tissue-to-tissue interface has been reported to compromise graft stability and long term clinical outcome (Friedman et al. 1985; Robertson et al. 1986).

In the past decade, utilizing a combination of cells, growth factors and/or biomaterials, the principles of tissue engineering have been applied to the formation of a variety of connective tissues such as bone, cartilage, ligament, or tendon *in vitro* and *in vivo*. More recently, the emphasis in the field has shifted from tissue formation to tissue function (Butler et al. 2000), specifically on imparting biomimetic functionality to tissue engineered grafts and enabling their translation to the clinic. Presently, a significant barrier to clinical application is achieving *biological fixation* of these newly formed grafts, be it bone, ligaments, tendons, or cartilage, either with each other and/or with the body (Moffat et al. 2009b).

This chapter focuses on current biological fixation strategies aimed at engineering tissue-to-tissue interfaces, as design methodologies developed from tissue engineering can be readily applied to regenerate the critical junction between soft tissue and bone. This interface tissue engineering challenge is rooted in the complexity of the musculoskeletal system and the structural intricacy of both hard and soft tissues. These tissues, each with distinct cellular populations, must operate in unison to facilitate physiologic function and homeostasis. It is thus not surprising that the transition between various tissue types

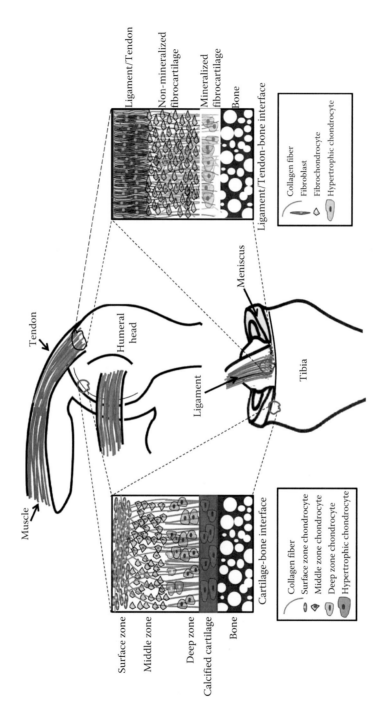

**FIGURE 32.1** **(See color insert.)** Schematic of soft-to-hard tissue interfaces.

is characterized by a high level of heterogeneous structural organization. For example, ligaments with direct insertions into subchondral bone exhibit a multitissue transition consisting of three distinct, yet continuous, regions of ligament, fibrocartilage, and bone (Benjamin et al. 1986; Cooper and Misol 1970; Wang et al. 2006). Moreover, the fibrocartilage interface is further divided into noncalcified and calcified regions. In light of this complexity, functional tissue engineering must incorporate *strategic biomimicry* in order to facilitate the formation of the tissue-to-tissue interface and effect seamless graft integration.

The detailed mechanisms that drive the formation of the soft-tissue-to-bone interface are not known. Identification of cell type and age-dependent changes in collagen fiber composition of the interface has yielded valuable clues to its development. Nawata et al. reported that at the ligament-to-bone interface, the majority of proliferating cells were near the ligament region of the insertion site at birth (Nawata et al. 2002). These cells produced type I and II collagen and slowly developed into fibrochondrocyte-like cells within 1 month, after which rapid longitudinal growth of the ligament occurred. These observations suggest that fibrochondrocytes at the ligament-to-bone interface may originate from the ligament. Moreover, studies of tendon-to-bone healing following anterior cruciate ligament (ACL) reconstruction have provided insights into the neotissue formed when soft tissue is juxtaposed against bone. Liu et al. examined the morphology and matrix composition of the interface during the early tendon-to-bone healing process (Liu et al. 1997), and found that by 2 weeks after reconstruction, the tendon attached to the bone with scar tissue filling the tendon-to-bone junction. This scar tissue had reorganized into a dense connective tissue matrix by 1 month, with predominantly fibroblasts present. After 6 weeks, contraction of the interface was prominent and significantly less type I collagen was found in the remodeling matrix, however type II collagen became detectable. As such, no well defined fibrocartilage interface was observed over time. This study correlates with the biomechanical studies of Rodeo et al. and demonstrates that surgically juxtaposing soft tissue and bone does not spontaneously result in the regeneration of the fibrocartilaginous interface (Rodeo et al. 1993). Collectively, these studies suggest that cell source is a significant consideration in interface regeneration, and moreover, the differentiation of these cells into interface-relevant populations is likely driven by both biochemical and mechanical factors during development and healing.

In additional to developmental and repair cues, studies (Benjamin et al. 1986; Bullough and Jagannath 1983; Matyas et al. 1995; Moffat et al. 2008b; Oegema, Jr. and Thompson 1992; Ralphs et al. 1998; Spalazzi et al. 2006b; Thomopoulos et al. 2003; Woo et al. 1988) characterizing the structure–function relationship inherent at the soft-tissue-to-bone insertion have revealed remarkable organizational similarities between many tissue-to-tissue interfaces, as they often consist of a multitissue, multicell transition as described above between bone and ligaments or tendons, and are associated with a controlled distribution of nonmineralized and mineralized cartilaginous interface regions which, along with other structural parameters such as collagen fiber organization, are reported to be responsible for engineering a gradient of mechanical properties progressing from soft tissue to bone. These observations have inspired the design of biomimetic scaffolds for engineering the tissue-to-tissue interface. Specifically, a stratified or multiphased scaffold will be essential for recapturing the multitissue organization observed at the soft-tissue-to-bone interface. In order to minimize the formation of stress concentrations, the scaffold should exhibit phase-specific structural and material properties, with a gradual increase in mechanical properties across the scaffold phases, similar to that of the native tissue. To this end, introducing spatial control over mineral distribution on a stratified scaffold can impart controlled mechanical heterogeneity similar to that of the native interface. Compared to a homogenous structure, a scaffold with predesigned, tissue-specific matrix inhomogeneity can better sustain and transmit the distribution of complex loads inherent at the multitissue interface. It is emphasized that while the scaffold is stratified or consists of different phases, a key criteria is that these phases must be interconnected and preintegrated with each other, thereby supporting the formation of distinct yet continuous multitissue regions. Furthermore, interactions between interface-relevant cells serve important functions in the formation, maintenance, and repair of interfacial tissue. Therefore, precise control over the spatial distribution of these cell populations is also critical for multitissue formation and interface regeneration. Consideration of these biomimetic parameters will collectively enable the design of stratified scaffolds optimized for promoting the formation and maintenance of controlled matrix heterogeneity and tissue-to-tissue integration.

This chapter will highlight current tissue engineering efforts in the regeneration of three common connective tissue interfaces, namely the ligament-to-bone, tendon-to-bone, and the cartilage-to-bone interface, focusing on biomimetic scaffold design and biomaterial- as well as cell-based strategies to engineer a functional gradient of mechanical properties that approximates that of the native interface. Each section will begin with a brief description of the current understanding of the requirements for biomimetic and functional interface scaffold design, which have been distilled through characterization and structure-function understandings of the native interface. This is followed by a brief review of stratified scaffold and gradient-based scaffold designs currently researched for soft-tissue-to-bone interface tissue engineering. Lastly, potential challenges and future directions in this rapidly expanding area of functional tissue engineering will be discussed.

## 32.2 Interface Scaffold Design for Ligament-to-Bone Interface Tissue Engineering

The site of anterior cruciate ligament (ACL) insertion into bone is a classic example of a complex soft-tissue-to-bone interface consisting of spatial variations in cell type and matrix composition resulting in three distinct yet continuous regions of ligament, fibrocartilage, and bone (Benjamin et al. 1986; Cooper et al. 1970; Wang et al. 2006), whereby the fibrocartilage region is further divided into mineralized and nonmineralized regions (Figure 32.2a). From a structure-function perspective, the complex organization of this interface is likely related to the nature and distribution of mechanical stress experienced at the region. It has been reported that matrix organization at the insertion is optimized to sustain both tensile and compressive stresses (Matyas et al. 1995; Woo et al. 1988). These region-specific mechanical properties facilitate a gradual transition in strain across the insertion and provide valuable cues for ligament-to-bone interface scaffold design.

The aforementioned multitissue transition from ligament to bone represents a significant challenge for functional ligament tissue engineering. Initial attempts to improve ligament graft to bone fixation focused on augmenting the surgical graft with a material that would encourage bone tissue ingrowth within the bone tunnel (Gulotta et al. 2008; Huangfu and Zhao 2007; Ishikawa et al. 2001; Robertson et al. 2007; Shen et al. 2010; Tien et al. 2004). For example, Tien et al. used calcium phosphate cements to fill the tendon-to-bone junction in a rabbit ACL reconstruction study and found that the addition of this ceramic helped to augment bone tissue growth and organization (Tien et al. 2004). In a similar study, the injection of tricalcium phosphate (TCP) cement into bone tunnel in a canine ACL reconstruction model resulted in more organized bone tissue formation than the uncemented control (Huangfu et al. 2007). An alternative approach to improving tendon osteointegration included soaking tendon grafts in a series of solutions which facilitated the formation of a calcium phosphate layer prior to implantation (Mutsuzaki et al. 2004). When tested in a rabbit ACL reconstruction model, the precoated tendons resulted in direct bonding between the implanted graft and the surrounding bone after 3 weeks, as opposed to the formation of fibrous tissue around control samples. Other approaches to improve bone tunnel osteointegration include the addition of periosteum wraps to the region of the graft that interacts with bone (Chen et al. 2003; Karaoglu et al. 2009; Kyung et al. 2003; Ohtera et al. 2000; Youn et al. 2004) as well as growth factors such as bone morphogenetic protein (BMP)-2 (Chen et al. 2008; Hashimoto et al. 2007; Ma et al. 2007; Martinek et al. 2002; Rodeo et al. 1999), BMP-7 (Mihelic et al. 2004), and granulocyte colony stimulating factor (Sasaki et al. 2008). Additionally, several groups have also investigated the direct application of multipotent mesenchymal stem cells (MSCs) as a method to improve graft-to-bone integration (Ju et al. 2008; Lim et al. 2004; Ouyang et al. 2004; Soon et al. 2007). While these methods have been shown to enhance both mechanically and structurally, the integration of the ACL graft within the bone tunnel, they do not result in the regeneration of the anatomic

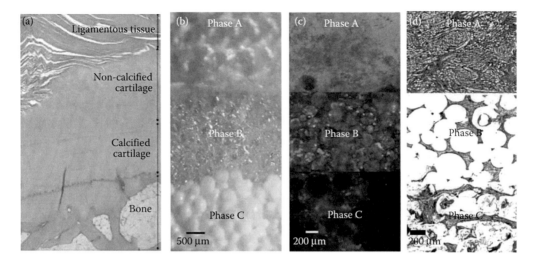

**FIGURE 32.2** (**See color insert.**) Scaffold design for ligament-to-bone interface tissue engineering. (a) Histologic image of human ACL insertion showing the three main tissue types found at the ACL-bone interface: ligament, fibrocartilage (FC), and bone. (b) A tri-phasic stratified scaffold designed to mimic the three interface regions (bar = 200 μm). (c) *In vitro* co-culture of fibroblasts and osteoblasts on the tri-phasic scaffold resulted in region-specific cell distribution and cell-specific matrix deposition. Fibroblasts (Calcein AM, green) were localized in Phase A and osteoblasts (CM-DiI, red) in Phase C, and both osteoblasts and fibroblasts migrated into Phase B over time (bar = 200 μm). (d) *In vivo* evaluation of the tri-phasic scaffold tri-cultured with fibroblasts (Phase A), chondrocytes (Phase B), and osteoblasts (Phase C) showed abundant host tissue infiltration and matrix production (week 4, Modified Goldner Masson Trichrome Stain, bar = 500 μm). (Modified from Iwahashi et al. 2010. *Arthroscopy.* 26(9 Suppl):S13–S20; Spalazzi, J. P. et al. 2006a. *Tissue Eng.* 12:3497–3508; Spalazzi, J. P. et al. 2008a. *J. Biomed. Mater. Res. Part A.* 86A:1–12; Lu et al. 2010. *Ann. Biomed. Eng.* 38(6):2142–2154.)

fibrocartilaginous interface. Moreover, the complex tendon-bone healing process involves a controlled cascade of growth factors and cytokines, thus a systematic strategy which uses a biomimetic stratified scaffold to direct the growth of the multitissue interface may overcome these shortcomings as it can be designed to recapitulate the inherent complexity of this multilayered ligament-to-bone interface while controlling the spatial and temporal distribution of growth factors for interface regeneration.

The ideal scaffold has several functions including supporting the growth and differentiation of the relevant cell populations, directing cellular interactions, and promoting the formation and maintenance of controlled matrix heterogeneity. The scaffold must also exhibit a gradation in mechanical properties, mimicking the native insertion site, with magnitudes comparable to those of the ligament-to-bone interface. Additionally, the scaffold must be biodegradable in order to be gradually replaced by living tissue. Lastly, for *in vivo* integration, the engineered graft must be easily adaptable with current ACL reconstruction grafts, or preincorporated into the design of the ligament replacement grafts.

Traditional efforts for developing tissue engineered grafts for ACL reconstruction have centered on regenerating the ligament proper (Altman et al. 2002; Dunn et al. 1992, 1995), with more recent studies (Table 32.1) focusing on the incorporation of ACL with bone (Cooper et al. 2005, 2007; Inoue et al. 2002; Lu et al. 2005a). Cooper et al. reported on a multiphased design of a synthetic ACL graft fabricated from 3-D braiding of polylactide-*co*-glycolide fibers, with a ligament proper as well as two bony regions (Cooper et al. 2005). *In vitro* (Lu et al. 2005a) and *in vivo* (Cooper et al. 2007) evaluation demonstrated scaffold biocompatibility, healing, and mechanical strength in a rabbit model. Using a cell-based approach, Ma et al. reported that it is possible to form bone-ligament-bone constructs by introducing engineered bone segments to ligament monolayers (Ma et al. 2009). The monolayer attached to bone, resulting in the self-assembly of a ligament-bone-ligament construct. Paxton et al. utilized a

**TABLE 32.1**    Scaffolds for Ligament-to-Bone Tissue Engineering

| Study | Scaffold | DesignStudy Model | Outcomes |
|---|---|---|---|
| Dunn et al. (1992) | Collagen fibers with polymethylmethacrylate (PMMA) bone fixation plugs | *In vivo*/Rabbit model | Supported the development of functional neoligament tissue |
| Bitar et al. (2005) | Phosphate-based fibers | *In vitro*/Human osteoblasts and fibroblasts | Cell differentiation maintained by both cell types and strongly related to fiber composition |
| (1) Lu et al. (2005a) (2) Cooper et al. (2007) | Multiregion knitted PLLA fiber scaffold | (1) *In vitro*/Rabbit ACL cells (2) *In vivo*/Rabbit model with primary ACL cells | (1) Supported long term matrix deposition (2) Demonstrated scaffold healing and mechanical strength *in vivo* |
| Spalazzi et al. (2006a) | Tri-phasic Phase I: PLGA mesh Phase II: PLGA (85:15) microspheres Phase III: PLGA-Bioglass composite | *In vitro*/Bovine fibroblast (phase I), osteoblast (phase III) co-culture | Scaffold supported cell proliferation and matrix production while maintaining distinct cellular regions |
| Phillips et al. (2008) | 3D poly(l-lysine) retrovirus gradient | *In vitro*/Rat dermal fibroblasts | Cells displayed spatial patterns of transcription factor expression, differentiation and matrix deposition |
| Spalazzi et al. (2008a) | Tri-phasic Phase I: PLGA mesh Phase II: PLGA (85:15) microspheres Phase III: PLGA-Bioglass composite | *In vivo*/Rat model with bovine fibroblasts, chondrocytes, osteoblasts | Interface-like matrix heterogeneity maintained *in vivo* |
| Spalazzi et al. (2008b) | Aligned PLGA (85:15) nanofibers (900 nm) PLGA (85:15) microspheres | *In vitro*/Bovine patellar tendon graft | Upregulation of fibrocartilage markers after 7 days of tendon compression |
| Ma et al. (2009) | Ligament-bone constructs from rat bone marrow-derived stromal cell (BMSC) | *In vivo*/Rat model | Engineered tissues grew and remodeled quickly with partial restoration of knee function |
| Paxton et al. (2009) | Poly(ethylene glycol) hydrogel with HA | *In vitro*/Rat Achilles tendon fibroblasts | Inclusion of HA in poly(ethylene glycol) (PEG) hydrogel enhanced mechanical strength and cell attachment |
| (1) Paxton et al. (2010a) (2) Paxton et al. (2010b) | Brushite cement anchors with cell-seeded fibrin gels | *In vitro*/Rat Achilles tendon fibroblasts | (1) Anchor shape altered longevity and strength of the bone-ligament interface (2) Scanning electron microscopy (SEM) and Raman microscopy suggested regeneration of tidemark between brushite and cell-seeded gel |

similar methodology with promising results when evaluating the use of a poly (ethylene glycol) hydrogel incorporating hydroxyapatite (HA) and the arginine-glycine-aspartic acid (RGD) peptide to engineer functional ligament-to-bone attachments (Paxton et al. 2009). These novel ACL graft designs represent a significant improvement over single-phased ACL grafts, and the next step is to address the challenge of biological fixation, by considering the fibrocartilage interface in the ACL scaffold design.

To this end, Spalazzi et al. pioneered the design of a tri-phasic scaffold for the regeneration of the ACL-to-bone interface (Spalazzi et al. 2006a, 2008a) (Figure 32.2b). Modeled after the native insertion, the scaffold consists of three distinct yet continuous phases, Phase A (poly (lactic-*co*-glycolic acid) [PLGA] 10:90) for fibroblast culture and ligament formation, Phase B (sintered PLGA 85:15 microspheres) is the interface region intended for fibrochondrocyte culture, and Phase C is comprised of sintered PLGA (85:15) and 45S5 bioactive glass composite microspheres for bone formation and integration (Lu et al. 2003). This design results in a "single" scaffold system with three distinct yet continuous phases, intended to support the formation of the multitissue regions observed across the ACL-bone junction. Heterotypic cellular interactions on the tri-phasic scaffold were assessed both *in vitro* (Spalazzi et al. 2006a) and *in vivo* (Spalazzi et al. 2008a). To form the ligament and bone regions, fibroblasts and osteoblasts were seeded onto Phase A and Phase C, respectively (Figure 32.2c). This controlled cell distribution resulted in the elaboration of cell type-specific matrix on each phase of the scaffold *in vitro*, with a mineralized matrix detected only on Phase C, and an extensive type I collagen matrix found on both Phases A and B. *In vivo* evaluation (Spalazzi et al. 2008a) of the co-cultured scaffold revealed extensive tissue infiltration and abundant matrix deposition on Phase A and Phase C (Figure 32.2d). Cell migration, increased matrix production, and vascularization were observed on Phase B, the interface region. Moreover, tissue continuity was maintained across all three scaffold phases. Interestingly, extracellular matrix production compensated for the decrease in mechanical properties accompanying scaffold degradation, and the phase-specific controlled matrix heterogeneity was maintained *in vivo* (Spalazzi et al. 2008a).

To form a fibrocartilage interface-like tissue at the interface phase, Spalazzi et al. extended the *in vivo* evaluation of the above scaffold system to tri-culture (Spalazzi et al. 2006a, 2008a), including chondrocytes along with fibroblasts and osteoblasts (Spalazzi et al. 2008a). Specifically, articular chondrocytes were encapsulated in a hydrogel matrix and loaded into Phase B of the scaffold, while ligament fibroblasts and osteoblasts were preseeded onto Phase A and Phase C, respectively. At 2 months postimplantation, an extensive collagen-rich matrix was prevalent in all three phases of the tri-cultured scaffolds. Moreover, a fibrocartilaginous region of chondrocyte-like cells embedded within a matrix of types I and II collagen as well as glycosaminoglycans was observed. Interestingly, both cell shape and matrix morphology of the neo-fibrocartilage resembled that of the neonatal ligament-to-bone interface (Wang et al. 2006). Moreover, the neo-fibrocartilage formed was continuous with the ligament-like tissue observed in Phase A as well as the bone-like tissue found in Phase C (Spalazzi et al. 2008a).

These promising results demonstrate that biomimetic stratified scaffold design coupled with spatial control over the distribution of interface relevant cell populations can lead to interface regeneration, and underscore the potential for continuous multitissue regeneration on a single scaffold system. In terms of clinical application, the tri-phasic scaffold can be used to guide the reestablishment of an anatomic fibrocartilage interfacial region directly on soft-tissue grafts. Specifically, the scaffold can be utilized as a graft collar during ACL reconstruction, and the feasibility of such an approach was recently demonstrated with a mechanoactive scaffold based on a composite of PLGA 85:15 nanofibers and sintered microspheres (Spalazzi et al. 2008b). It was observed that scaffold-induced compression of tendon grafts resulted in significant matrix remodeling and the upregulation of fibrocartilage interface-related markers such as type II collagen, aggrecan, and transforming growth factor-$\beta$3 (TGF-$\beta$3). These results suggest that the stratified scaffold can be used to induce the formation of an anatomic fibrocartilage interface directly on biological ACL reconstruction grafts.

In summary, current strategies in ligament-to-bone interface tissue engineering first tackles the difficult problem of soft-tissue-to-bone integration *ex vivo* by preengineering the multitissue interface through stratified scaffold design, followed by the relatively less challenging task of bone-to-bone integration *in vivo*. Functional and integrative ligament repair may be achieved by coupling both cell-based and scaffold-based approaches, as well as efforts to recapitulate the complex nanoscale to microscale organization of the native interface in scaffold design.

## 32.3 Interface Scaffold Design for Tendon-to-Bone Interface Tissue Engineering

Similar to the ligament-to-bone interface, the tendon-to-bone interface (Figure 32.1) displays a zonal distribution of extracellular matrix components (Benjamin et al. 1986; Blevins et al. 1997). As such, while tendon-to-bone and ligament-to-bone insertions are physiologically and biochemically similar, the tissue engineering strategy applied is expected to differ as the two interfaces do vary in terms of loading environment and mineral distribution with the added difference in the method of surgical repair which would also influence the subsequent healing response.

Current efforts in tendon-to-bone interface tissue engineering have centered on rotator cuff repair, motivated by the debilitating effects of this shoulder condition and the clinical need for functional solutions for integrative tendon-to-bone repair (Table 32.2). Existing cuff repair and mechanical fixation methods do not result in insertion site regeneration and are associated with high incidence of failure (Coons and Alan 2006; Derwin et al. 2006; Galatz et al. 2004; Iannotti et al. 2006), which underscore the need for functional grafting solutions that can promote interface formation and biological fixation. To address this challenge, several groups have evaluated the feasibility of integrating tendon with bone or with biomaterials through the formation of an anatomic insertion site. By surgically reattaching tendon to bone, Fujioka et al. reported that cellular reorganization occurred at the reattachment site, along with the formation of nonmineralized and mineralized fibrocartilage-like regions (Fujioka et al. 1998). Additionally, perisoteum (Chang et al. 2009) and demineralized bone matrix (DBM) (Sundar et al. 2009) have been researched for tendon-bone interface regeneration. The periosteum is known to be a source of multipotent stem cells that have the potential to differentiate into osteogenic and chondrogenic lineages. Chang et al. sutured a periosteal flap to the torn end of the rabbit infraspinatus tendon and then attached the flap to bone (Chang et al. 2009). A fibrous layer was observed at the interface between tendon and bone at 4 weeks, which later remodeled into a fibrocartilage-like matrix after 12 weeks, and failure load increased significantly over time, suggesting improved tendon-bone integration with healing. In an effort to harness the osteogenic and chondrogenic potential of DBM, Sundar et al. interposed DBM between patellar tendon and osteotomized bone in a ovine model (Sundar et al. 2009). It was found that DBM-augmented repair significantly improved functional weight bearing and the deposition of fibrocartilage and mineralized fibrocartilage at the tendon-bone interface.

**TABLE 32.2**  Scaffolds for Tendon-to-Bone Tissue Engineering

| Study | Scaffold Design | Study Model | Outcomes |
|---|---|---|---|
| Chang et al. (2009) | Periosteum attached to end of transected end of tendon | *In vivo*/Infraspinatus tendon-bone repair in rabbit model | (1) Extensive fibrocartilage and bone formation at interface<br>(2) Significant increase in failure load at interface region over time |
| Li et al. (2009) | PLGA and PCL nanofibers (unaligned) with a gradient of calcium phosphate across scaffold | *In vitro*/MC3T3 cells (mouse preosteoblasts) | (1) Gradation in mineral across scaffold produced a gradient in stiffness<br>(2) Gradient in cell density observed, higher in regions with increased mineral concentration |
| Sundar et al. (2009) | DBM interposed between tendon and bone | *In vivo*/Patella-patellar tendon-bone repair in ovine model | Augmentation with DBM increased area of fibrocartilage and mineralized fibrocartilage found at interface |
| Moffat et al. (2009a) | PLGA (85:15) nanofiber scaffolds (aligned and unaligned) | *In vitro*/human rotator cuff tendon fibroblasts | (1) Tendon fibroblasts organized and produced matrix oriented according to the underlying nanofiber organization<br>(2) Matrix deposition and scaffold mechanical properties mimicked that of human rotator cuff tendons |
| Moffat et al. (2010) | Bi-phasic nanofiber-based scaffold (aligned): Phase A: PLGA (85:15) Phase B: PLGA+ HA | *In vitro and in vivo*/bovine full-thickness articular chondrocytes in athymic rat subcutaneous model | (1) Scaffold mineral distribution mimics that of native insertion sites<br>(2) Synthesis of fibrocartilage-like matrix on Phase A and Phase B<br>(3) Regional mineral distribution maintained<br>(4) Increase in mineral density and osteointegration over time |

The delivery of osteoinductive growth factors (Rodeo et al. 2007) and the inhibition of matrix metalloproteinases (MMP) during the healing process (Bedi et al. 2010; Gulotta et al. 2010) have also been explored to improve tendon bone integration. Rodeo et al. (Rodeo et al. 2007) examined the effect of osteoinductive growth factors on tendon-bone healing in an ovine model. A mixture of osteoinductive growth factors from platelet-rich plasma were delivered via a type I collagen sponge carrier to the infraspinatus tendon–bone interface. Abundant formation of new bone, fibrocartilage, and soft tissue were observed and these changes were accompanied by an increase in tendon attachment strength. Recently, Bedi et al. (Bedi et al. 2010) and Gulotta et al. (Gulotta et al. 2010) examined the influence of MMP inhibition on tendon-bone healing and insertion site regeneration. Using a rat model, Bedi et al. applied recombinant α-2-macroglobulin (A2 M) protein (a universal MMP inhibitor) to the repaired supraspinatus tendon-bone interface, resulting in significantly greater fibrocartilage formation at 2 weeks, plus improved collagen organization accompanied by a reduction in collagen degradation.

In addition to biological grafts and cytokines, synthetic biomaterials have been investigated for tendon-to-bone integration. Implantation of a polyglycolide fiber mesh in a rat model was shown to lead to the formation of an organized fibrovascular matrix at the infraspinatus tendon-to-bone junction (Yokoya et al. 2008). Recently, nanofiber scaffolds have been explored for tendon-to-bone interface tissue engineering, largely due to their biomimetic potential and physiological relevance. These scaffolds can be tailored to match the native tendon matrix, with controlled alignment, high surface area to volume ratio, permeability, and porosity (Li et al. 2002, 2007; Ma et al. 2005; Pham et al. 2006). In order to investigate the potential of nanofiber scaffolds for tendon tissue engineering, Moffat et al. evaluated the effects of PLGA nanofiber organization (aligned vs. unaligned) on human tendon fibroblast attachment and biosynthesis (Moffat et al. 2009a). Nanofiber alignment was found to be the primary factor guiding tendon fibroblast morphology, alignment, and integrin expression. Types I and III collagen, the dominant collagen types of the supraspinatus tendon, were synthesized on the nanofiber scaffolds and it was shown that their deposition was also controlled by the underlying fiber orientation. Furthermore, scaffold mechanical properties, directly related to fiber alignment, decreased as the polymer degraded but remained within range of those reported for the native supraspinatus tendon (Itoi et al. 1995).

Building upon these promising results, Moffat et al. designed a stratified, composite nanofiber system (Figure 32.3a) consisting of distinct yet continuous noncalcified and calcified regions that mimic the organization of native tendon-to-bone insertion (Moffat et al. 2008a). The bi-phasic scaffold is produced by electrospinning, with Phase A comprised of aligned PLGA nanofibers to support the regeneration of the nonmineralized fibrocartilage region, and Phase B which is based on aligned PLGA nanofibers embedded with nanoparticles of HA (PLGA-HA) to support the regeneration of the mineralized fibrocartilage region. The bi-phasic scaffold design has been evaluated both *in vitro* (Moffat 2010) and *in vivo* (Moffat et al. 2010). It was reported that a chondrocyte-mediated fibrocartilage-like extracellular matrix

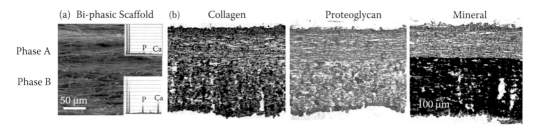

**FIGURE 32.3** (**See color insert.**) Bi-phasic nanofiber scaffold for tendon-to-bone integration. (a) Cross-section of the bi-phasic scaffold (1000×, bar = 50 μm), Insert: Elemental composition of the two phases, calcium (Ca) and phosphorous (P) present only in Phase B. (b) Matrix deposition on bi-phasic scaffold after 3 weeks of subcutaneous implantation in athymic rats (Collagen—picrosirius red, Proteoglycan—Alcian blue, Mineral—Von Kossa; 20×, bar = 100 μm). (From Moffat, K. L. et al. 2010. *Transactions of the 56th Orthopaedic Research Society.* New Orleans, LA.)

was found on each scaffold phase, while mineral distribution was maintained, with a calcified fibrocartilage formed on Phase B, through which the bi-phasic scaffold integrated with surrounding bone tissue (Figure 32.3b).

Nanofiber-based scaffolds with a gradient of mineral distribution have also been investigated for tendon-bone interface regeneration. Li et al. formed a linear gradient of calcium phosphate on PLGA and poly-ε-caprolactone (PCL) nanofiber scaffolds by varying immersion time in concentrated simulated body fluid (Li et al. 2009). The mineral gradient imparted a gradation in mechanical properties along the length of the scaffold, with lower strains and higher elastic modulus corresponding to areas of higher calcium phosphate concentration. In an alternative approach, collagen scaffolds with a compositional gradient of retroviral coating for the transcription faction RUNX2 induced fibroblasts to produce a gradient of mineralized matrix both *in vitro* and *in vivo* (Phillips et al. 2008). These systems with a linear gradient of mineral content hold significant promise for biomimetic tendon-bone interface regeneration.

Since tendon connects muscle to bone, thus for functional rotator cuff repair, the muscle-tendon interface is another critical research area that to date, has been relatively under-explored. As the tendon joins the muscle to bone, through the myotendinous junction (MTJ), which connects muscle to tendon, acts as a bridge to distribute mechanical loads (Yang and Temenoff 2009). This interface consists of a band of fibroblast-laden, interdigitating tissue that connects the dense collagen fibers of the tendon to the more elastic muscle fibers while displaying a gradient of structural properties (Tidball 1991). Current tissue engineering approaches, as demonstrated by Swasdison et al., include the culturing of myoblasts in collagen gels *in vitro* to form contractile muscle constructs with fibrils that terminate in a manner similar to the native MTJ (Swasdison and Mayne 1991, 1992). Adopting a cell-based approach, Larkin et al. evaluated a novel self-organizing system for *in vitro* MTJ formation by co-culturing skeletal muscle constructs with engineered tendon constructs. Interestingly, upregulation of paxillin was observed at the neo-interface, and the MTJ formed was able to sustain tensile loading beyond the physiological strain range (Larkin et al. 2006).

These aforementioned studies collective demonstrate the importance of the tendon-bone interface and the promise of different methodologies for facilitating tendon-bone healing, interface regeneration, and osteointegration. Functional tendon-to-bone interface tissue engineering focuses on the design of biomimetic scaffolds that are preengineered to recapitulate the inherent structural and mechanical heterogeneity of the native interface, while utilizing biomaterials combined with physiologically relevant growth factors and cytokines, in order to guide cellular differentiation and enhance tendon-to-bone integration.

## 32.4 Stratified Scaffold Design for Cartilage-to-Bone Interface Tissue Engineering

Another common interface of the musculoskeletal system is the osteochondral interface which is found between articular cartilage and subchondral bone (Figure 32.1). The articular cartilage proper can be divided into three regions: the tangential (surface) zone, the transitional (middle) zone, and the radial (deep) zone. Directly below the deep zone is the osteochondral interface (Figure 32.4a) which consists of hypertrophic chondrocytes embedded in a densely mineralized matrix (Bullough et al. 1983; Fawns and Landells 1953; Lyons et al. 2005; Oegema, Jr. and Thompson 1990). Similar to the other soft-tissue-to-bone interfaces, the osteochondral interface facilitates the pressurization and physiological loading of articular cartilage, while serving as a physical barrier for vascular invasion (Collins 1950; Mow et al. 1989; Oegema and Thompson 1992; Redler et al. 1975). Thus, regeneration of this soft-tissue-to-bone interface is a critical component of strategies for integrative and functional cartilage tissue engineering.

Stratified scaffold design has been extensively researched for osteochondral tissue engineering, with the first generation of scaffolds consisting of two distinct cartilage or bone regions joined together using

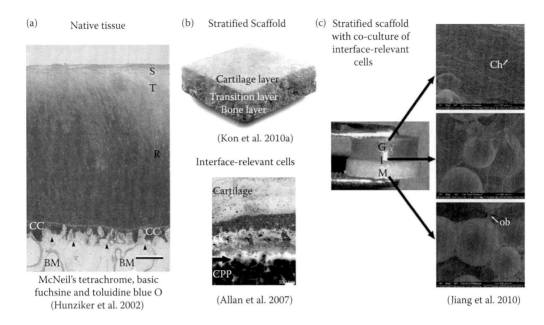

(a) Native tissue

S
T

R

CC          CC

BM          BM

McNeil's tetrachrome, basic
fuchsine and toluidine blue O
(Hunziker et al. 2002)

(b) Stratified Scaffold

Cartilage layer
Transition layer
Bone layer

(Kon et al. 2010a)

Interface-relevant cells

Cartilage

CPP

(Allan et al. 2007)

(c) Stratified scaffold
with co-culture of
interface-relevant
cells

Ch

G
I
M

ob

(Jiang et al. 2010)

**FIGURE 32.4** (**See color insert.**) Osteochondral tissue engineering. (a) Stratified organization of the human cartilage and the osteochondral junction. (b) Stratified scaffold designed to mimic zonal organization regions and cell-based approaches for cartilage-to-bone integration. (c) *In vitro* co-culture of chondrocytes and osteoblasts on a stratified scaffold. (Modified from Hunziker et al. 2002. *Osteoarthritis Cartilage.* 10(7):564–572; Kon et al. 2010a. *Injury.* 41:778–786; Allan, K. S. et al. 2007. *Tissue Eng.* 13:167–177; Jiang et al. 2010. *Ann. Biomed. Eng.* 38(6):2183–2196.)

either sutures or sealants (Table 32.3). Schaefer et al. seeded articular chondrocytes on polyglycolic acid (PGA) meshes and periosteal cells on PLGA/polyethylene glycol foams, and sutured the separate constructs together at 1 or 4 weeks post seeding (Schaefer et al. 2000). Integration between the two scaffolds was observed to be superior when brought together at week 1 instead of week 4, suggesting the importance of immediate osteoblast–chondrocyte interactions for phase-to-phase integration. Gao et al. seeded MSCs stimulated with TGF-β1 for chondrogenic differentiation on a hyaluronan sponge, and MSCs stimulated with osteogenic media on porous calcium phosphate scaffold (Gao et al. 2001). These scaffolds were then joined by a fibrin sealant and evaluated in a subcutaneous model, with continuous collagen fibers observed between the two scaffolds after 6 weeks. Utilizing sequential photo-polymerization, Alhadlaq et al. formed a bi-layered mandibular condyle-shaped osteochondral construct based on polyethylene glycol-diacrylate hydrogel. The top layer contained MSC-derived chondrocytes while the bottom layer contained MSC-derived osteoblasts (Alhadlaq and Mao 2005). After 12 weeks *in vivo*, distinct cartilaginous and osseous regions were observed, with histological integration evident between them. Similar observations have been reported for MSC cultured on biphasic scaffolds (Chen et al. 2006; Shao et al. 2006; Swieszkowski et al. 2007).

Collectively, these pioneering studies demonstrate the feasibility of engineering multiple tissues (cartilage and bone) on a multiphased scaffold; the next step is to incorporate the appropriate cell–cell and cell–material interactions found at the osteochondral interface into this scaffold design. To this end, several groups have reported on stratified scaffold designs that mimic the structural organization of the native osteochondral interface. Lu et al. and later Jiang et al. evaluated 3-D osteoblast–chondrocyte co-culture on a biomimetic, continuous multiphased osteochondral construct (Figure 32.4c) consisting of a hydrogel-based cartilage region, a polymer-ceramic composite microsphere bone region, and an interfacial region consisting of a hybrid of the hydrogel and polymer-ceramic composite (Jiang et al. 2010; Lu et al. 2005b). It was found that osteoblast and chondrocyte co-culture on this scaffold system supported the formation of

**TABLE 32.3** Scaffolds for Cartilage-to-Bone Tissue Engineering

| Study | Scaffold Design | Study Model | Outcomes |
|---|---|---|---|
| Schaefer et al. (2000) | PGA mesh sutured to PLGA-PEG foam | *In vitro*/Bovine articular chondrocytes and periosteal cells | Improved integration of cartilage and bone regions with decreased preculture time |
| Gao et al. (2001) | Hyaluronan sponge and porous calcium phosphate scaffold joined with fibrin sealant | *In vivo*/Subcutaneous rat model (MSC) | Supports MSC differentiation into continuous fibrocartilage and bone regions |
| Sherwood et al. (2002) | 90% porous d, l-PLGA/l-PLA and 55% l-PLGA/TCP composite | *In vitro*/Ovine articular chondrocytes | Gradient of material properties and porosity prevents delamination in transition region |
| Alhadlaq et al. (2005) | Bilayered PEG hydrogel | *In vivo*/Subcutaneous mouse model (MSC) | Supports MSC differentiation into stratified cartilage-and bone-like regions |
| Swieszkowski et al. (2007) | PCL and PCL/TCP composite | *In vivo*/Rabbit model (MSC) | Promotes bone healing |
| Harley et al. (2010) | Mineralized collagen I/ glycosaminoglycans (GAG) and nonmineralized collagen II/GAG with interdiffused interface region | Acellular scaffold fabrication | Biomimetic gradient of scaffold properties |
| Dormer et al. (2010) | PLGA Microsphere scaffold with opposing BMP-2 and TGF-β1 gradients | *In vitro*/Human MSC | Gradient scaffold produces regionalized matrix deposition |
| Jiang et al. (2010) | Agarose hydrogel and PLGA/ bioglass (BG) composite | *In vitro*/Bovine chondrocytes and osteoblasts | Supports region-specific co-culture of chondrocytes and osteoblasts which can lead to the production of distinct yet continuous regions of cartilage, calcified cartilage and bone-like matrices |
| Kon et al. (2010) | 100% collagen, 60% collagen/40%HA, 30% collagen/70% HA tri-layered scaffold | *In vivo*/Horse model | Regeneration of fibrocartilage and bone tissue with tidemark at interface |

distinct yet continuous cartilaginous and osseous matrices, with predesigned integration between these regions achieving a mineralized interfacial region within which direct osteoblast-chondrocyte interactions are encouraged. Taking a cell-based approach, Allan et al. seeded interface-relevant deep zone chondrocytes on a calcium polyphosphate scaffold formed a calcified cartilage-like zone atop the ceramic (Allan et al. 2007). These observations delineate the importance of both cell–cell and cell–material interactions, in addition to scaffold design, in mediating complex tissue formation.

Functional gradients have also been incorporated into scaffold design for integrative cartilage repair. Sherwood et al. designed a biphasic scaffold and evaluated chondrocyte response on the scaffold using a 3-D printing process (Sherwood et al. 2002). The upper, cartilage region is composed of PLGA/polylactic acid (PLA), with macroscopic staggered channels to facilitate cell seeding. The lower bone portion has decreased porosity and consists of PLGA and TCP. Most importantly, there is a transition region with a gradient of composition and porosity. Recently, scaffolds with either a compositional (Harley et al. 2010; Kon et al. 2010a,b) or chemical factor (Dormer et al. 2010; Singh et al. 2010a) gradient have been reported. Harley et al. designed an osteochondral scaffold with cartilage and bone regions as well as a continuous osteochondral interface-like region in between these two phases (Harley et al. 2010). While it remains to be validated *in vitro* and *in vivo*, this multiphased design is intended to promote scaffold-mediated integration within an osteochondral defect site. In a study by Dormer et al., a PLGA microsphere-based scaffold was loaded with both chondrogenic and osteogenic growth factors in opposing gradients (Dormer et al. 2010). This scaffold was then seeded with human MSCs and it was found that there was corresponding spatial distribution in matrix deposition in the scaffold. When a gradient collagen-HA scaffold was tested in an equine model (Kon et al. 2010b), distinct fibrocartilage and bone regions were observed (Figure 32.4b).

Utilizing an ethanol-based solvent evaporation technique, Singh et al. developed 3D multiphased PLGA microsphere scaffolds with continuous macroscopic gradients in stiffness. Structural gradients were produced by incorporating a high stiffness nanophase material ($CaCO_3$ or $TiO_2$) into portions of the microspheres during the scaffold fabrication process (Singh et al. 2010b). Preliminary *in vitro* studies showed that structurally homogenous scaffolds fabricated using this method can support the attachment of human umbilical cord-derived MSCs (Singh et al. 2010b). In addition to scaffolds with compositional gradient, Singh et al. have also designed microsphere scaffolds with regional growth factor release profiles (Singh et al. 2008). Both human umbilical cord MSCs and porcine chondrocytes were seeded on these scaffolds, with significant cell viability during early culturing periods.

In summary, scaffold design with multiple phases or a gradient of properties, in conjunction with the use of interface relevant cell populations and MSCs, is a promising approach to engineer the osteochondral interface. Results from the studies highlighted above underscore the importance of the cartilage-to-bone interface; thus advanced scaffold design aimed at the formation of integrated osteochondral grafts must take into consideration the regeneration of a functional and stable interface region between these distinct tissue types.

## 32.5 Summary and Future Directions

The objective of this chapter is to provide an overview of current concepts in interface tissue engineering, focusing on strategies for the design of scaffolds with a gradation of mechanical and structural properties aimed at the regeneration of the complex tissue-to-tissue interface. Specifically, stratified scaffolds have been designed to mimic the structure and function of the native soft-tissue-to-bone interface while employing spatial control over heterotypic cell interactions and supporting the formation of integrated multitissue systems. The vast potential of multiphased scaffold systems is evident from the *in vitro* and *in vivo* evaluations described here for the integrative repair of cartilage, ligament and tendon injuries. Moreover, these novel scaffolds are capable of multitissue regeneration by mediating heterotypic cellular interactions, and can be further refined by incorporating well controlled compositional and growth factor gradients, as well as the use of biochemical and biomechanical stimulation to encourage tissue growth and maturation. Furthermore, functional and integrative soft-tissue repair may be achieved by coupling both cell-based and scaffold-based approaches. Clinically, it is anticipated that stratified scaffolds would significantly improve current soft-tissue repair strategies by facilitating functional integration with host tissue, stimulating interface formation and enabling biological fixation.

It is emphasized that interface tissue engineering will be instrumental for the *ex vivo* development and *in vivo* regeneration of integrated musculoskeletal tissue systems with biomimetic functionality; however, there remain a number of challenges in this exciting area. These include the need for a greater understanding of the structure-function relationship existing at the native tissue-to-tissue interface as well as the mechanisms governing interface development and regeneration. Furthermore, the *in vivo* host environment plus the precise effects of biological, chemical, and physical stimulation on interface regeneration must be thoroughly evaluated to enable the formation and homeostasis of the neo-interface. Physiologically relevant *in vivo* models are also needed to determine the clinical potential of the designed scaffolds. Additionally, as is evident in many of the reported studies, utilization of multiple cell sources is typically necessary to ensure or enhance heterogeneous tissue formation. Ultimately, the clinical implementation of these scaffolds will require identifying an optimal cell source which is readily available, such as an adult stem cell source which can be quickly isolated and expanded.

In summary, regeneration of tissue-to-tissue junctions through interface tissue engineering represents a promising strategy for achieving biological fixation and integrative soft-tissue repair, using either biological or tissue engineering grafts. It is anticipated that these efforts will lead to the development of a new generation of functional fixation devices for soft-tissue repair as well as augment the clinical translation potential of tissue engineered grafts. Moreover, by bridging distinct types of tissue, interface tissue engineering will be instrumental for the development of integrated musculoskeletal tissue systems with biomimetic complexity and functionality.

# References

Alhadlaq, A. and Mao, J. J. 2005. Tissue-engineered osteochondral constructs in the shape of an articular condyle. *J. Bone Joint Surg. Am.* 87:936–944.

Allan, K. S., Pilliar, R. M., Wang, J., Grynpas, M. D., and Kandel, R. A. 2007. Formation of biphasic constructs containing cartilage with a calcified zone interface. *Tissue Eng.* 13:167–177.

Altman, G. H., Horan, R. L., Lu, H. H., Moreau, J., Martin, I., Richmond, J. C., and Kaplan, D. L. 2002. Silk matrix for tissue engineered anterior cruciate ligaments. *Biomaterials.* 23:4131–4141.

Bedi, A., Kovacevic, D., Hettrich, C., Gulotta, L. V., Ehteshami, J. R., Warren, R. F., and Rodeo, S. A. 2010. The effect of matrix metalloproteinase inhibition on tendon-to-bone healing in a rotator cuff repair model. *J. Shoulder. Elbow. Surg.* 19:384–391.

Benjamin, M., Evans, E. J., and Copp, L. 1986. The histology of tendon attachments to bone in man. *J. Anat.* 149:89–100.

Bitar, M. C., Knowles, J., Lewis, M. P., and Salih, V. 2005. Soluble phosphate glass fibers for repair of bone-ligament interface. *J. Mater. Sci. Mater.* Med. 16(12):1131–1136.

Blevins, F. T., Djurasovic, M., Flatow, E. L., and Vogel, K. G. 1997. Biology of the rotator cuff tendon. *Orthop. Clin. North Am.* 28:1–16.

Bullough, P. G. and Jagannath, A. 1983. The morphology of the calcification front in articular cartilage. Its significance in joint function. *J. Bone Joint Surg. Br.* 65:72–78.

Butler, D. L., Goldstein, S. A., and Guilak, F. 2000. Functional tissue engineering: The role of biomechanics. *J. Biomech. Eng.* 122:570–575.

Chang, C. H., Chen, C. H., Su, C. Y., Liu, H. T., and Yu, C. M. 2009. Rotator cuff repair with periosteum for enhancing tendon-bone healing: A biomechanical and histological study in rabbits. *Knee. Surg. Sports Traumatol. Arthrosc.* 17:1447–1453.

Chen, C. H., Chen, W. J., Shih, C. H., Yang, C. Y., Liu, S. J., and Lin, P. Y. 2003. Enveloping the tendon graft with periosteum to enhance tendon-bone healing in a bone tunnel: A biomechanical and histologic study in rabbits. *Arthroscopy.* 19:290–296.

Chen, C. H., Liu, H. W., Tsai, C. L., Yu, C. M., Lin, I. H., and Hsiue, G. H. 2008. Photoencapsulation of bone morphogenetic protein-2 and periosteal progenitor cells improve tendon graft healing in a bone tunnel. *Am. J. Sports Med.* 36:461–473.

Chen, G., Sato, T., Tanaka, J., and Tateishi, T. 2006. Preparation of a biphasic scaffold for osteochondral tissue engineering. *Mater. Sci. Eng.: C.* 26:118–123.

Collins, D. H. 1950. *The Pathology of Articular and Spinal Diseases.* Baltimore, MD: William & Wilkins.

Coons, D. A. and Alan, B. F. 2006. Tendon graft substitutes-rotator cuff patches. *Sports Med. Arthrosc.* 14:185–190.

Cooper, J. A., Lu, H. H., Ko, F. K., Freeman, J. W., and Laurencin, C. T. 2005. Fiber-based tissue-engineered scaffold for ligament replacement: Design considerations and *in vitro* evaluation. *Biomaterials.* 26:1523–1532.

Cooper, J. A., Jr., Sahota, J. S., Gorum, W. J., Carter, J., Doty, S. B., and Laurencin, C. T. 2007. Biomimetic tissue-engineered anterior cruciate ligament replacement. *Proc. Natl. Acad. Sci. USA.* 104:3049–3054.

Cooper, R. R. and Misol, S. 1970. Tendon and ligament insertion. A light and electron microscopic study. *J. Bone Joint Surg. Am.* 52:1–20.

Derwin, K. A., Baker, A. R., Spragg, R. K., Leigh, D. R., and Iannotti, J. P. 2006. Commercial extracellular matrix scaffolds for rotator cuff tendon repair. Biomechanical, biochemical, and cellular properties. *J. Bone Joint Surg. Am.* 88:2665–2672.

Dormer, N. H., Singh, M., Wang, L., Berkland, C. J., and Detamore, M. S. 2010. Osteochondral interface tissue engineering using macroscopic gradients of bioactive signals. *Ann. Biomed. Eng.* 38:2167–2182.

Dunn, M. G., Liesch, J. B., Tiku, M. L., and Zawadsky, J. P. 1995. Development of fibroblast-seeded ligament analogs for ACL reconstruction. *J. Biomed. Mater. Res.* 29:1363–1371.

Dunn, M. G., Tria, A. J., Kato, Y. P., Bechler, J. R., Ochner, R. S., Zawadsky, J. P., and Silver, F. H. 1992. Anterior cruciate ligament reconstruction using a composite collagenous prosthesis. A biomechanical and histologic study in rabbits. *Am. J. Sports Med.* 20:507–515.

Fawns, H. T. and Landells, J. W. 1953. Histochemical studies of rheumatic conditions. I. Observations on the fine structures of the matrix of normal bone and cartilage. *Ann. Rheum. Dis.* 12:105–113.

Friedman, M. J., Sherman, O. H., Fox, J. M., Del Pizzo, W., Snyder, S. J., and Ferkel, R. J. 1985. Autogeneic anterior cruciate ligament (ACL) anterior reconstruction of the knee. A review. *Clin. Orthop.* 196:9–14.

Fujioka, H., Thakur, R., Wang, G. J., Mizuno, K., Balian, G., and Hurwitz, S. R. 1998. Comparison of surgically attached and non-attached repair of the rat Achilles tendon-bone interface. Cellular organization and type X collagen expression. *Connect. Tissue Res.* 37:205–218.

Galatz, L. M., Ball, C. M., Teefey, S. A., Middleton, W. D., and Yamaguchi, K. 2004. The outcome and repair integrity of completely arthroscopically repaired large and massive rotator cuff tears. *J. Bone Joint Surg. Am.* 86-A:219–224.

Gao, J., Dennis, J. E., Solchaga, L. A., Awadallah, A. S., Goldberg, V. M., and Caplan, A. I. 2001. Tissue-engineered fabrication of an osteochondral composite graft using rat bone marrow-derived mesenchymal stem cells. *Tissue Eng.* 7:363–371.

Gulotta, L. V., Kovacevic, D., Montgomery, S., Ehteshami, J. R., Packer, J. D., and Rodeo, S. A. 2010. Stem cells genetically modified with the developmental gene MT1-MMP improve regeneration of the supraspinatus tendon-to-bone insertion site. *Am. J. Sports Med.* 38:1429–1437.

Gulotta, L. V., Kovacevic, D., Ying, L., Ehteshami, J. R., Montgomery, S., and Rodeo, S. A. 2008. Augmentation of tendon-to-bone healing with a magnesium-based bone adhesive. *Am. J. Sports Med.* 36:1290–1297.

Harley, B. A., Lynn, A. K., Wissner-Gross, Z., Bonfield, W., Yannas, I. V., and Gibson, L. J. 2010. Design of a multiphase osteochondral scaffold III: Fabrication of layered scaffolds with continuous interfaces. *J. Biomed. Mater. Res. A.* 92:1078–1093.

Hashimoto, Y., Yoshida, G., Toyoda, H., and Takaoka, K. 2007. Generation of tendon-to-bone interface "enthesis" with use of recombinant BMP-2 in a rabbit model. *J. Orthop. Res.* 25:1415–1424.

Huangfu, X. and Zhao, J. 2007. Tendon-bone healing enhancement using injectable tricalcium phosphate in a dog anterior cruciate ligament reconstruction model. *Arthroscopy.* 23:455–462.

Hunziker, E. B., Quinn, T. M., and Hauselmann, H. J. 2002. Quantitative structural organization of normal adult human articular cartilage. *Osteoarthritis Cartilage.* 10(7):564–572.

Iannotti, J. P., Codsi, M. J., Kwon, Y. W., Derwin, K., Ciccone, J., and Brems, J. J. 2006. Porcine small intestine submucosa augmentation of surgical repair of chronic two-tendon rotator cuff tears. A randomized, controlled trial. *J. Bone Joint Surg. Am.* 88:1238–1244.

Inoue, N., Ikeda, K., Aro, H. T., Frassica, F. J., Sim, F. H., and Chao, E. Y. 2002. Biologic tendon fixation to metallic implant augmented with autogenous cancellous bone graft and bone marrow in a canine model. *J. Orthop. Res.* 20:957–966.

Ishikawa, H., Koshino, T., Takeuchi, R., and Saito, T. 2001. Effects of collagen gel mixed with hydroxyapatite powder on interface between newly formed bone and grafted achilles tendon in rabbit femoral bone tunnel. *Biomaterials.* 22:1689–1694.

Itoi, E., Berglund, L. J., Grabowski, J. J., Schultz, F. M., Growney, E. S., Morrey, B. F., and An, K. N. 1995. Tensile properties of the supraspinatus tendon. *J. Orthop. Res.* 13:578–584.

Iwahashi, T., Shino, K., Nakata, K., Otsubo, H., Suzuki, T., Amano, H., and Nakamura, N. 2010. Direct anterior cruciate ligament insertion to the femur assessed by histology and 3-dimensional volume-rendered computed tomography. *Arthroscopy.* 26(9 Suppl):S13–s20.

Jiang, J., Tang, A., Ateshian, G. A., Guo, X. E., Hung, C. T., and Lu, H. H. 2010. Bioactive stratified polymer ceramic-hydrogel scaffold for integrative osteochondral repair. *Ann. Biomed. Eng.* 38(6):2183–2196.

Ju, Y. J., Muneta, T., Yoshimura, H., Koga, H., and Sekiya, I. 2008. Synovial mesenchymal stem cells accelerate early remodeling of tendon-bone healing. *Cell Tissue Res.* 332:469–478.

Karaoglu, S., Celik, C., and Korkusuz, P. 2009. The effects of bone marrow or periosteum on tendon-to-bone tunnel healing in a rabbit model. *Knee. Surg. Sports Traumatol. Arthrosc.* 17:170–178.

Kon, E., Delcogliano, M., Filardo, G., Pressato, D., Busacca, M., Grigolo, B., Desando, G., and Marcacci, M. 2010a. A novel nano-composite multi-layered biomaterial for treatment of osteochondral lesions: Technique note and an early stability pilot clinical trial. *Injury.* 41:778–786.

Kon, E., Mutini, A., Arcangeli, E., Delcogliano, M., Filardo, G., Nicoli, A. N., Pressato, D., Quarto, R., Zaffagnini, S., and Marcacci, M. 2010b. Novel nanostructured scaffold for osteochondral regeneration: Pilot study in horses. *J. Tissue Eng. Regen. Med.* 4:300–308.

Kyung, H. S., Kim, S. Y., Oh, C. W., and Kim, S. J. 2003. Tendon-to-bone tunnel healing in a rabbit model: The effect of periosteum augmentation at the tendon-to-bone interface. *Knee. Surg Sports Traumatol. Arthrosc.* 11:9–15.

Larkin, L. M., Calve, S., Kostrominova, T. Y., and Arruda, E. M. 2006. Structure and functional evaluation of tendon-skeletal muscle constructs engineered *in vitro. Tissue Eng.* 12:3149–3158.

Li, W. J., Laurencin, C. T., Caterson, E. J., Tuan, R. S., and Ko, F. K. 2002. Electrospun nanofibrous structure: A novel scaffold for tissue engineering. *J. Biomed. Mater. Res.* 60:613–621.

Li, W. J., Mauck, R. L., Cooper, J. A., Yuan, X., and Tuan, R. S. 2007. Engineering controllable anisotropy in electrospun biodegradable nanofibrous scaffolds for musculoskeletal tissue engineering. *J. Biomech.* 40:1686–1693.

Li, X. R., Xie, J. W., Lipner, J., Yuan, X. Y., Thomopoulos, S., and Xia, Y. N. 2009. Nanofiber scaffolds with gradations in mineral content for mimicking the tendon-to-bone insertion site. *Nano Lett.* 9:2763–2768.

Lim, J. K., Hui, J., Li, L., Thambyah, A., Goh, J., and Lee, E. H. 2004. Enhancement of tendon graft osteointegration using mesenchymal stem cells in a rabbit model of anterior cruciate ligament reconstruction. *Arthroscopy.* 20:899–910.

Liu, S. H., Panossian, V., al Shaikh, R., Tomin, E., Shepherd, E., Finerman, G. A., and Lane, J. M. 1997. Morphology and matrix composition during early tendon to bone healing. *Clin. Orthop. Relat. Res.* 339:253–260.

Lu, H. H., Cooper, J. A., Jr., Manuel, S., Freeman, J. W., Attawia, M. A., Ko, F. K., and Laurencin, C. T. 2005a. Anterior cruciate ligament regeneration using braided biodegradable scaffolds: *In vitro* optimization studies. *Biomaterials.* 26:4805–4816.

Lu, H. H., El Amin, S. F., Scott, K. D., and Laurencin, C. T. 2003. Three-dimensional, bioactive, biodegradable, polymer-bioactive glass composite scaffolds with improved mechanical properties support collagen synthesis and mineralization of human osteoblast-like cells in vitro. *J. Biomed. Mater. Res.* 64A:465–474.

Lu, H. H. and Jiang, J. 2006. Interface tissue engineering and the formulation of multiple-tissue systems. *Adv. Biochem. Eng. Biotechnol.* 102:91–111.

Lu, H. H., Jiang, J., Tang, A., Hung, C. T., and Guo, X. E. 2005b. Development of controlled heterogeneity on a polymer-ceramic hydrogel scaffold for osteochondral repair. *Bioceramics.* 17:607–610.

Lu, H. H., Subramony, S. D., Boushell, M. K., and Zhang, X. 2010. Tissue engineering strategies for the regeneration of orthopedic interfaces. *Ann. Biomed. Eng.* 38(6):2142–2154.

Lyons, T. J., Stoddart, R. W., McClure, S. F., and McClure, J. 2005. The tidemark of the chondro-osseous junction of the normal human knee joint. *J. Mol. Histol.* 36:207–215.

Ma, C. B., Kawamura, S., Deng, X. H., Ying, L., Schneidkraut, J., Hays, P., and Rodeo, S. A. 2007. Bone morphogenetic proteins-signaling plays a role in tendon-to-bone healing: A study of rhBMP-2 and noggin. *Am. J. Sports Med.* 35:597–604.

Ma, J., Goble, K., Smietana, M., Kostrominova, T., Larkin, L., and Arruda, E. M. 2009. Morphological and functional characteristics of three-dimensional engineered bone-ligament-bone constructs following implantation. *J. Biomech. Eng.* 131:101017.

Ma, Z., Kotaki, M., Inai, R., and Ramakrishna, S. 2005. Potential of nanofiber matrix as tissue-engineering scaffolds. *Tissue Eng.* 11:101–109.

Martinek, V., Latterman, C., Usas, A., Abramowitch, S., Woo, S. L., Fu, F. H., and Huard, J. 2002. Enhancement of tendon-bone integration of anterior cruciate ligament grafts with bone morphogenetic protein-2 gene transfer: A histological and biomechanical study. *J. Bone Joint Surg. Am.* 84-A:1123–1131.

Matyas, J. R., Anton, M. G., Shrive, N. G., and Frank, C. B. 1995. Stress governs tissue phenotype at the femoral insertion of the rabbit MCL. *J. Biomech.* 28:147–157.

Mihelic, R., Pecina, M., Jelic, M., Zoricic, S., Kusec, V., Simic, P., Bobinac, D., Lah, B., Legovic, D., and Vukicevic, S. 2004. Bone morphogenetic protein-7 (osteogenic protein-1) promotes tendon graft integration in anterior cruciate ligament reconstruction in sheep. *Am. J. Sports Med.* 32:1619–1625.

Moffat, K. L. 2010. *Biomimetic Nanofiber Scaffold Design for Tendon-to-bone Interface Tissue Engineering.* Thesis. Columbia University.

Moffat, K. L., Levine, W. N., and Lu, H. H. 2008a. *In vitro* evaluation of rotator cuff tendon fibroblasts on aligned composite scaffold of polymer nanofibers and hydroxyapatite nanoparticles. *Transactions of the 54th Orthopaedic Research Society.* San Francisco, CA.

Moffat, K. L., Cassilly, R. T., Subramony, S. D., Dargis, B. R., Zhang, X., Liu, X., Guo, X. E., Doty, S. B., Levine, W. N., and Lu, H. H. 2010. *In vivo* evalution of a bi-phasic nanofiber-based scaffold for integrative rotator cuff repair. *Transactions of the 56th Orthopaedic Research Society.* New Orleans, LA.

Moffat, K. L., Kwei, A. S., Spalazzi, J. P., Doty, S. B., Levine, W. N., and Lu, H. H. 2009a. Novel nanofiber-based scaffold for rotator cuff repair and augmentation. *Tissue Eng. Part A.* 15:115–126.

Moffat, K. L., Sun, W. H., Pena, P. E., Chahine, N. O., Doty, S. B., Ateshian, G. A., Hung, C. T., and Lu, H. H. 2008b. Characterization of the structure-function relationship at the ligament-to-bone interface. *Proc. Natl. Acad. Sci. U.S.A.* 105:7947–7952.

Moffat, K. L., Wang, I. N., Rodeo, S. A., and Lu, H. H. 2009b. Orthopedic interface tissue engineering for the biological fixation of soft tissue grafts. *Clin. Sports Med.* 28:157–176.

Mow, V. C., Proctor, C. S., and Kelly, M. A. 1989. Biomechanics of articular cartilage. In *Basic Biomechanics of the Musculoskeletal System*, ed. M. Nordin, H. F. Victor, and K. Forssen. Philadelphia, PA: Lea and Febiger, pp. 31–58.

Mutsuzaki, H., Sakane, M., Nakajima, H., Ito, A., Hattori, S., Miyanaga, Y., Ochiai, N., and Tanaka, J. 2004. Calcium-phosphate-hybridized tendon directly promotes regeneration of tendon-bone insertion. *J. Biomed. Mater. Res. A.* 70:319–327.

Nawata, K., Minamizaki, T., Yamashita, Y., and Teshima, R. 2002. Development of the attachment zones in the rat anterior cruciate ligament: Changes in the distributions of proliferating cells and fibrillar collagens during postnatal growth. *J. Orthop. Res.* 20:1339–1344.

Oegema, T. R., Jr. and Thompson, R. C., Jr. 1992. The zone of calcified cartilage. Its role in osteoarthritis. In *Articular Cartilage and Osteoarthritis*, ed. K. E. Kuettner, R. Schleyerbach, J. G. Peyron, and V. C. Hascall. New York, NY: Raven Press, pp. 319–331.

Oegema, T. R., Jr. and Thompson, R. C., Jr. 1990. Cartilage-bone interface (Tidemark). In *Cartilage Changes in Osteoarthritis*, ed. C.-G. K. Brandt. Indianapolis, In: Indiana School of Medicine Publ, pp. 43–52.

Ohtera, K., Yamada, Y., Aoki, M., Sasaki, T., and Yamakoshi, K. 2000. Effects of periosteum wrapped around tendon in a bone tunnel: A biomechanical and histological study in rabbits. *Crit. Rev. Biomed. Eng.* 28:115–118.

Ouyang, H. W., Goh, J. C., and Lee, E. H. 2004. Use of bone marrow stromal cells for tendon graft-to-bone healing: Histological and immunohistochemical studies in a rabbit model. *Am. J. Sports Med.* 32:321–327.

Paxton, J. Z., Donnelly, K., Keatch, R. P., and Baar, K. 2009. Engineering the bone-ligament interface using polyethylene glycol diacrylate incorporated with hydroxyapatite. *Tissue Eng. Part A.* 15:1201–1209.

Paxton, J. Z., Donnelly, K., Keatch, R. P., Baar, K., and Grover, L. M. 2010a. Factors affecting the longevity and strength in an in vitro model of the bone-ligament interface. *Ann. Biomed. Eng.* 38(6):2155–2166.

Paxton, J. Z., Grover, L. M., and Baar, K. 2010b. Engineering an in vitro model of a functional ligament form bone to bone. *Tissue Eng. Part A.* 16(11):3515–3525.

Pham, Q. P., Sharma, U., and Mikos, A. G. 2006. Electrospinning of polymeric nanofibers for tissue engineering applications: A review. *Tissue Eng.* 12:1197–1211.

Phillips, J. E., Burns, K. L., Le Doux, J. M., Guldberg, R. E., and Garcia, A. J. 2008. Engineering graded tissue interfaces. *Proc. Natl. Acad. Sci. U.S.A.* 105:12170–12175.

Ralphs, J. R., Benjamin, M., Waggett, A. D., Russell, D. C., Messner, K., and Gao, J. 1998. Regional differences in cell shape and gap junction expression in rat Achilles tendon: Relation to fibrocartilage differentiation. *J. Anat.* 193 (Pt 2):215–222.

Redler, I., Mow, V. C., Zimny, M. L., and Mansell, J. 1975. The ultrastructure and biomechanical significance of the tidemark of articular cartilage. *Clin. Orthop. Relat. Res.* 112:357–362.

Robertson, D. B., Daniel, D. M., and Biden, E. 1986. Soft tissue fixation to bone. *Am. J. Sports Med.* 14:398–403.

Robertson, W. J., Hatch, J. D., and Rodeo, S. A. 2007. Evaluation of tendon graft fixation using alpha-BSM calcium phosphate cement. *Arthroscopy.* 23:1087–1092.

Rodeo, S. A., Arnoczky, S. P., Torzilli, P. A., Hidaka, C., and Warren, R. F. 1993. Tendon-healing in a bone tunnel. A biomechanical and histological study in the dog. *J. Bone Joint Surg. Am.* 75:1795–1803.

Rodeo, S. A., Potter, H. G., Kawamura, S., Turner, A. S., Kim, H. J., and Atkinson, B. L. 2007. Biologic augmentation of rotator cuff tendon-healing with use of a mixture of osteoinductive growth factors. *J. Bone Joint Surg. Am.* 89:2485–2497.

Rodeo, S. A., Suzuki, K., Deng, X. H., Wozney, J., and Warren, R. F. 1999. Use of recombinant human bone morphogenetic protein-2 to enhance tendon healing in a bone tunnel. *Am. J. Sports Med.* 27:476–488.

Sasaki, K. et al. 2008. Enhancement of tendon-bone osteointegration of anterior cruciate ligament graft using granulocyte colony-stimulating factor. *Am. J. Sports Med.* 36:1519–1527.

Schaefer, D., Martin, I., Shastri, P., Padera, R. F., Langer, R., Freed, L. E., and Vunjak-Novakovic, G. 2000. *In vitro* generation of osteochondral composites. *Biomaterials.* 21:2599–2606.

Shao, X., Goh, J. C., Hutmacher, D. W., Lee, E. H., and Zigang, G. 2006. Repair of large articular osteochondral defects using hybrid scaffolds and bone marrow-derived mesenchymal stem cells in a rabbit model. *Tissue Eng.* 12:1539–1551.

Shen, H., Qiao, G., Cao, H., and Jiang, Y. 2010. An histological study of the influence of osteoinductive calcium phosphate ceramics on tendon healing pattern in a bone tunnel with suspensory fixation. *Int. Orthop.* 34:917–924.

Sherwood, J. K., Riley, S. L., Palazzolo, R., Brown, S. C., Monkhouse, D. C., Coates, M., Griffith, L. G., Landeen, L. K., and Ratcliffe, A. 2002. A three-dimensional osteochondral composite scaffold for articular cartilage repair. *Biomaterials.* 23:4739–4751.

Singh, M., Dormer, N., Salash, J., Christian, J., Moore, D., Berkland, C., and Detamore, M. 2010a. Three-dimensional macroscopic scaffolds with a gradient in stiffness for functional regeneration of interfacial tissues. *J. Biomed. Mat. Res. A.* 94:870–876.

Singh, M., Morris, C. P., Ellis, R. J., Detamore, M. S., and Berkland, C. 2008. Microsphere-based seamless scaffolds containing macroscopic gradients of encapsulated factors for tissue engineering. *Tissue Eng. Part C.* 14:299–309.

Singh, M., Sandhu, B., Scurto, A., Berkland, C., and Detamore, M. S. 2010b. Microsphere-based scaffolds for cartilage tissue engineering: Using subcritical $CO_2$ as a sintering agent. *Acta Biomater.* 6:137–143.

Soon, M. Y., Hassan, A., Hui, J. H., Goh, J. C., and Lee, E. H. 2007. An analysis of soft tissue allograft anterior cruciate ligament reconstruction in a rabbit model: A short-term study of the use of mesenchymal stem cells to enhance tendon osteointegration. *Am. J. Sports Med.* 35:962–971.

Spalazzi, J. P., Dagher, E., Doty, S. B., Guo, X. E., Rodeo, S. A., and Lu, H. H. 2008a. *In vivo* evaluation of a multiphased scaffold designed for orthopaedic interface tissue engineering and soft tissue-to-bone integration. *J. Biomed. Mater. Res. Part A.* 86A:1–12.

Spalazzi, J. P., Doty, S. B., Moffat, K. L., Levine, W. N., and Lu, H. H. 2006a. Development of controlled matrix heterogeneity on a triphasic scaffold for orthopedic interface tissue engineering. *Tissue Eng.* 12:3497–3508.

Spalazzi, J. P., Gallina, J., Fung-Kee-Fung, S. D., Konofagou, E. E., and Lu, H. H. 2006b. Elastographic imaging of strain distribution in the anterior cruciate ligament and the ligament-bone insertions. *J. Orthop. Res.* 24(10):2001–2010.

Spalazzi, J. P., Vyner, M. C., Jacobs, M. T., Moffat, K. L., and Lu, H. H. 2008b. Mechanoactive scaffold induces tendon remodeling and expression of fibrocartilage markers. *Clin. Orthop. Relat. Res.* 466:1938–1948.

Sundar, S., Pendegrass, C. J., and Blunn, G. W. 2009. Tendon bone healing can be enhanced by demineralized bone matrix: A functional and histological study. *J. Biomed. Mater. Res. B Appl. Biomater.* 88:115–122.

Swasdison, S. and Mayne, R. 1991. *In vitro* attachment of skeletal muscle fibers to a collagen gel duplicates the structure of the myotendinous junction. *Exp. Cell Res.* 193:227–231.

Swasdison, S. and Mayne, R. 1992. Formation of highly organized skeletal muscle fibers *in vitro*. Comparison with muscle development *in vivo*. *J. Cell Sci.* 102 (Pt 3):643–652.

Swieszkowski, W., Tuan, B. H. S., Kurzydlowski, K. J., and Hutmacher, D. W. 2007. Repair and regeneration of osteochondral defects in the articular joints. *Biomolec. Eng.* 24:489–495.

Thomopoulos, S., Williams, G. R., Gimbel J.A., Favata, M., and Soslowsky, L. J. 2003. Variations of biomechanical, structural, and compositional properties along the tendon to bone insertion site. *J. Orthop. Res.* 21:413–419.

Tidball, J. G. 1991. Myotendinous junction injury in relation to junction structure and molecular composition. *Exerc. Sport Sci. Rev.* 19:419–445.

Tien, Y. C., Chih, T. T., Lin, J. H., Ju, C. P., and Lin, S. D. 2004. Augmentation of tendon-bone healing by the use of calcium-phosphate cement. *J. Bone Joint Surg. Br.* 86:1072–1076.

Wang, I. E., Mitroo, S., Chen, F. H., Lu, H. H., and Doty, S. B. 2006. Age-dependent changes in matrix composition and organization at the ligament-to-bone insertion. *J. Orthop. Res.* 24:1745–1755.

Woo, S. L., Maynard, J., Butler, D. L., Lyon, R. M., Torzilli, P. A., Akeson, W. H., Cooper, R. R., and Oakes, B. 1988. Ligament, tendon, and joint capsule insertions to bone. In *Injury and Repair of the Musculosketal Soft Tissues,* ed. S. L. Woo and J. A. Bulkwater. Savannah, Georgia: American Academy of Orthopaedic Surgeons, pp. 133–166.

Yang, P. J. and Temenoff, J. S. 2009. Engineering orthopedic tissue interfaces. *Tissue Eng. Part B Rev.* 15:127–141.

Yokoya, S., Mochizuki, Y., Nagata, Y., Deie, M., and Ochi, M. 2008. Tendon-bone insertion repair and regeneration using polyglycolic acid sheet in the rabbit rotator cuff injury model. *Am. J. Sports Med.* 36:1298–1309.

Youn, I., Jones, D. G., Andrews, P. J., Cook, M. P., and Suh, J. K. 2004. Periosteal augmentation of a tendon graft improves tendon healing in the bone tunnel. *Clin. Orthop. Relat. Res.* 419:223–231.

# 33

# The Bioengineering of Dental Tissues

Rena N. D'Souza
*Texas A&M Health Science Center—Baylor College of Dentistry*

Katherine R. Regan
*Texas A&M Health Science Center—Baylor College of Dentistry*

Kerstin M. Galler
*University of Regensburg*

Songtao Shi
*University of Southern California School of Dentistry*

33.1 Introduction ........................................................................ 33-1
33.2 The Tooth and Its Supporting Structures ..................... 33-2
33.3 Genetic Control of Tooth Development.......................... 33-3
       Stages of Tooth Development • Molecular Mechanisms
       Determining Tooth Shape, Size, and Structure
33.4 Tooth Regenerative Strategies......................................... 33-7
       Stem Cells • Human Dental Pulp Stem Cells • Scaffolding
       Material • Fine-Tuning Scaffolds in Regenerative
       Dentistry • Dentin Tissue Regeneration • Tooth Regeneration
33.5 Conclusion ........................................................................ 33-14
Acknowledgments ....................................................................... 33-15
References..................................................................................... 33-15

## 33.1 Introduction

The proper size, shape, color, and alignment of teeth influence the nature of our smile and determine our uniqueness as individual humans. In addition to their esthetic value, teeth are important for the mastication of food and for proper speech. Despite these critical functions, the importance and uniqueness of teeth are frequently overlooked by health professionals. The loss of dentition to common diseases like caries and periodontal disease as well as to trauma imposes significant emotional and financial burdens on patients and their families. Despite the overall success of osseointegrated titanium implants, tooth forms and individual dental tissues that are bioengineered from natural tissues/cells represent the next wave of dental regenerative medicine. The calcified tooth matrices of enamel, dentin, and cementum each possess unique biomechanical, structural, and biochemical properties. The bioengineering of whole tooth forms involves several challenges relating to the restoration of specific shapes and sizes as well as the (re)generation of these highly specialized mineralized matrices. To provide an appreciation for the complexity of the tooth as a whole, this chapter will first discuss the components of a mature tooth and its surrounding structures. Next, the fundamental principles of tooth development that provide the molecular and genetic bases for modern bioengineering strategies will be presented. Important contributions from mouse and human genetic studies will also be summarized. Recent data from successful tooth engineering initiatives involving somatic and stem cell approaches along with the use of novel scaffolds and whole tooth organ strategies will be discussed. In projecting future research directions, this chapter concludes with a brief discussion of the challenges and opportunities existing for bioengineering one of the most complex of all vertebrate organ systems.

## 33.2 The Tooth and Its Supporting Structures

The crowns of teeth, which are exposed in the oral cavity, are covered by enamel. Under the enamel is a thick layer of dentin and a soft central core, enclosed by the pulp chamber (Figure 33.1). Enamel is the hardest calcified structure in the body as it is about 99.5% mineralized. It varies from 2 to 3 mm in thickness at the height of cusps and narrows to a knife-edge thickness at the cementoenamel junction. Enamel is deposited by ameloblasts, cells that are believed to undergo programmed cell death. Because enamel is acellular and nonvital, it cannot regenerate itself. Underlying enamel is dentin, a specialized mineralized matrix that shares several biochemical characteristics with bone. In contrast to enamel, dentin is a vital tissue harboring odontoblastic processes and some nerve endings. The formation of dentin follows the same principles that guide the formation of other hard connective tissues in the body, namely, cementum and bone.

As described by Linde and Goldberg [1] and Butler and Ritchie [2], the composition of the dentin matrix and the process of dentinogenesis are highly complex. The organic phase of dentin is composed of proteins, proteoglycans, lipids, various growth factors, and water. Among the proteins, collagen is the most abundant and offers a fibrous matrix for the deposition of carbonate apatite crystals. The collagens found in dentin are primarily type I collagen with trace amounts of type V collagen and some type I collagen trimer. An important class of dentin matrix proteins is the noncollagenous proteins or NCPs [2]. The dentin-specific NCPs are dentin phosphoproteins (DPP) or phosphophoryns and dentin sialoprotein (DSP). After type I collagen, DPP is the most abundant of the dentin matrix proteins and represents almost 50% of the dentin extracellular matrix. DPP is a polyionic macromolecule rich in phosphoserine and aspartic acid. Its high affinity for type I collagen as well as calcium makes it a strong candidate for the initiation of dentin mineralization. DSP accounts for 5–8% of the dentin matrix and has a relatively high sialic acid and carbohydrate content. Its role in dentin mineralization is presently unclear. For several years it was believed that DSP and DPP were two independent proteins encoded by individual genes. In fact DPP and DSP are specific cleavage products of a larger precursor protein that was translated from one large transcript [3]. This single gene encoding for DSP and DPP is named "dentin sialophosphoprotein" or Dspp [4].

A second category of NCPs with Ca-binding properties is classified as mineralized tissue specific, since they are found in all the calcified connective tissues, namely, dentin, bone, and cementum. These proteins include osteocalcin (OC) and bone sialoprotein (BSP). A serine-rich phosphoprotein called "dentin matrix protein 1" (Dmp-1), whose expression was first described as being restricted to odontoblasts [5], was later shown to be expressed by osteoblasts and cementoblasts [6]. Other NCPs include osteopontin and osteonectin [secreted protein acidic and rich in cysteine (SPARC)]. The fourth category of dentin NCPs is not expressed in odontoblasts but is primarily synthesized in the liver and released

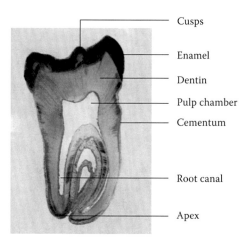

Cusps

Enamel

Dentin

Pulp chamber

Cementum

Root canal

Apex

**FIGURE 33.1** Component parts of a tooth.

into the circulation. An example of a serum-borne protein is α2HS-glycoprotein. Diffusible growth factors that appear to be sequestered within dentin matrix constitute the fifth group of dentin NCPs; this group includes the bone morphogenetic proteins (BMPs), insulin-like growth factors (IGFs), and transforming growth factor (TGF)-βs [7].

The central chamber of the tooth is occupied by a soft connective tissue called the "dental pulp," which is comprised of a heterogeneous cell population of fibroblasts, undifferentiated mesenchymal cells, nerves, blood vessels, and lymphatics. The regenerative capacity of dental pulp is well documented in the literature and best illustrated by the formation of a layer of reparative dentin beneath a carious lesion or a cavity base. As will be discussed later, somatic stem cells from the dental pulp of a deciduous molar are capable of regenerating several tissues when transplanted *in vivo*. Cementum is another calcified tissue of mesodermal origin. The cementum covering the apical third of the root is cellular (contains cementocytes), whereas that of the remaining two-thirds is acellular. Since the fibers of the periodontal ligament are anchored within the cementum, the regeneration of this complex is important when the bioengineering of whole tooth structures is considered.

## 33.3 Genetic Control of Tooth Development

### 33.3.1 Stages of Tooth Development

Teeth develop in distinct stages that are easily recognizable at the microscopic level. Hence, stages in odontogenesis are described in classic terms by the histologic appearance of the tooth organ. From early to late, these stages are described as the lamina, bud, cap, and bell (early and late) stages of tooth development [8,9]. Recent advances in the understanding of the molecular control of tooth development have led to the development of new terminology to describe tooth development as occurring in four phases: initiation, morphogenesis, cell or cytodifferentiation, and matrix apposition (Figure 33.2). The appearance of the dental lamina marks the first visible sign of tooth initiation seen at about 5 weeks of human development. The inductive influence of the dental lamina to dictate the fate of the underlying ectomesenchyme

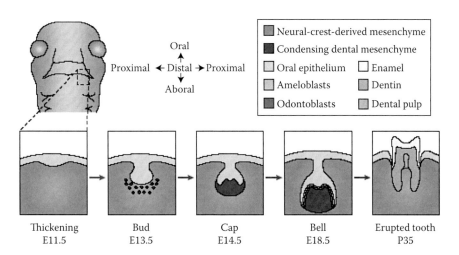

**FIGURE 33.2** Stages of tooth development. A schematic frontal view of an embryo head at embryonic day (E)11.5 is shown with a dashed box to indicate the site where the lower (mandibular) molars will form. Below, the stages of tooth development are laid out from the first signs of thickening at E11.5 to eruption of the tooth at around 5 weeks after birth. The tooth germ is formed from the oral epithelium and neural-crest-derived mesenchyme. At the bell stage of development, the ameloblasts and odontoblasts form in adjacent layers at the site of interaction between the epithelium and mesenchyme. These layers produce the enamel and dentin of the fully formed tooth. (Reproduced with permission from Tucker A and Sharpe P. 2004. *Nat Rev Genet* 5(7): 499–508.)

has been confirmed by several researchers [10]. Table 33.1 summarizes the molecules expressed in the epithelium and mesenchyme at this inductive phase. The bud stage is characterized by the continual growth of cells of the dental lamina and ectomesenchyme. The latter is condensed and termed the "dental papilla." At this point, the inductive or tooth-forming potential is transferred from the dental epithelium to the dental papilla. The transition from the bud to the cap stage is an important step in tooth development as it marks the onset of crown formation. The tooth bud assumes the shape of a cap that is surrounded by the dental papilla. The ectodermal compartment of the tooth organ is referred to as the "dental" or "enamel" organ. The enamel organ and dental papilla become encapsulated by a sac called the "dental follicle," which separates the tooth organ papilla from the other connective tissues of the jaws. A cluster of cells known as the "enamel knot" is an important organizing center within the dental organ and is important for the formation of cusps [11,12]. The enamel knot expresses a unique set of signaling molecules that influence the shape of the crown as well as the development of the dental papilla. Similar to the fate of signaling centers in other organizing tissues like the developing limb bud, the enamel knot undergoes programmed cell death, or apoptosis, after cuspal patterning is completed at the onset of the early bell stage. As the dental organ assumes the shape of a bell, several layers of cells continue to divide at different rates. A single layer of cuboidal cells called the "external" or "outer dental epithelium" lines the periphery of the dental organ, while cells that border the dental papilla and are columnar in appearance form the internal or inner dental epithelium. The latter gives rise to the ameloblasts, cells responsible for enamel formation. Cells located in the center of the dental organ produce high levels of glycosaminoglycans that are able to sequester fluids as well as growth factors leading to its expansion. This network of star-shaped cells is named the "stellate reticulum." Interposed between the stellate reticulum and the internal dental epithelium is a narrow layer of flattened cells termed the "stratum intermedium," which express high levels of alkaline phosphatase. The stratum intermedium is believed to influence the biomineralization of enamel. In the region of the apical end of the tooth organ, the internal and external dental epithelial layers meet at a junction called the "cervical loop."

At the early bell stage, each layer of the dental organ has assumed special functions and exchanges molecular information leading to cell differentiation at the late bell stage. The dental lamina, which connects the tooth organ to the oral epithelium, gradually disintegrates at the late bell stage. At the future cusp tips, cells of the internal dental epithelium stop dividing and assume a columnar shape. The most peripheral cells of the dental papilla organize along the basement membrane and differentiate into odontoblasts, the dentin-forming cells. At this time, the dental papilla is termed the "dental pulp." After the first layer of predentin matrix is deposited, the cells of the internal dental epithelium differentiate into ameloblasts or enamel-producing cells. As enamel is deposited over the dentin matrix, the ameloblasts retreat to the external surface of the crown and are believed to undergo programmed cell death. In contrast, the odontoblasts line the inner surface of dentin and remain metabolically active throughout the life of a tooth. Root formation then proceeds as epithelial cells proliferate apically and influence the differentiation of odontoblasts from the dental papilla as well as cementoblasts from the follicle mesenchyme. This process leads to the deposition of root dentin and cementum, respectively. The dental follicle that produces the components of the periodontium, namely the periodontal ligament fibroblasts, alveolar bone of the tooth socket, and the cementum, also plays a role during tooth eruption, which marks the last phase of odontogenesis.

## 33.3.2 Molecular Mechanisms Determining Tooth Shape, Size, and Structure

Similar to other organs like the limb bud, kidney, lung, and hair follicles, tooth development is regulated by temporally and spatially restricted interactions between epithelial and mesenchymal compartments. The molecular methods used in expression analyses as well as functional *in vivo* and *in vitro* tooth recombinations and bead implantation assays have greatly increased our understanding of the molecular control of tooth development. In addition, the use of genetic approaches involving transgenic mice

**TABLE 33.1** Genes Expressed during Tooth Development in Mouse[a]

| Stage of Development | Expressed in Epithelium | References | Expressed in Mesenchyme | References |
|---|---|---|---|---|
| | Up to Epithelial Thickening | | | |
| (E10–E11) | *Fgf8,9* | 21,60,63,64 | *Activin* | 70 |
| | *Bmp4* | 21,35,60,75 | *Pax9* | 21 |
| | *Shh* | 24,69 | *Barx1* | 60 |
| | *Islet1* | 65 | *Msx1 & Msx2* | 19,83,84 |
| | *Pitx2* | 66,67 | *Dlx1,2,3,5,6* | 61,62 |
| | *Wnt 10b* | 76 | *Ptc* | 24 |
| | *Follistatin* | 70 | *Gli1,2,3* | 24 |
| | *Lef1* | 20 | *Lhx6,7* | 63 |
| | *Eda, Edar* | 72 | | |
| | Bud Stage | | | |
| (E12–E13) | *Eda, Edar* | 72 | *Runx2* | 71 |
| | *Pitx2* | 66,67 | *Bmp4* | 35,75 |
| | | | *Msx1* | 35 |
| | | | *Lef1* | 20 |
| | | | *Fgf3,10* | 73 |
| | | | *Dlx1,2* | 62 |
| | | | *Lhx6,7* | 63 |
| | Cap Stage | | | |
| (E14–E15) | *Enamel knot* | | *Non-EK* epithelium | |
| | *p21* | 11 | *FgfR* | 74 |
| | *Shh* | 24 | *Eda* | 72 |
| | *Edar* | 72 | | |
| | *Edaradd* | 68 | | |
| | *Bmp 2,4,7* | 75 | | |
| | *Wnt10a* | 76 | | |
| | *Msx2* | 11,29 | | |
| | *Fgf3,4* | 10,73 | | |
| | Bell Stage | | | |
| (E16 Onwards) | *Amelogenin* | 77 | *Dspp* | 78 |
| | *Bmp5* | 75 | | |

*Source:* Reproduced with permission from About I et al. 2001. *Oper Dent* 26(4): 336–342.

[a] This list indicates the expression pattern of several genes that are thought to be important in tooth development in the mouse. A more comprehensive list of genes and their expression patterns can be found at the Gene Expression in Tooth web site (http://bite-it.helsinki.fi/). *Barx*, BarH-like homeobox; *Bmp*, bone morphogenetic protein; *Dlx*, distal-less homeobox; *Dspp*, dentin sialophosphoprotein; E, embryonic stage; *Eda*, ectodysplasin-A; *Edar*, Eda receptor; *Edaradd*, EDAR (ectodysplasin-A receptor)-associated death domain; *EK*, enamel knot; *Fgf*, fibroblast growth factor; *FgfR*, fibroblast growth factor receptor; *Gli*, GLI-Kruppel family member; *Lef*, lymphoid enhancer binding factor; *Lhx*, LIM homeodomain genes; *Msx*, homeobox, msh-like; *p21* (*CDKN1A*), cyclin-dependent kinase inhibitor 1A; *Pax*, pairedbox gene; *Pitx*, paired-related homeobox gene; *Ptc*, patched; *Runx*, *runt* homologue; *Shh*, sonic hedgehog; *Wnt*, wingless-related protein.

with targeted inactivation of various genes has provided a powerful means to delineate the *in vivo* functions of individual molecules [13,14].

*In vivo* and *in vitro* recombination studies have shown that during the formation of the epithelial bud (E12), the inductive potential shifts to the dental mesenchyme that later influences the fate of the enamel organ and its morphogenesis from the bud stage to the early bell stage (E16) [10,15–17]. Reciprocal interactions between the morphologically distinct enamel organ and papilla mesenchyme at the late bell stage (E18) then lead to the differentiation of dentin-forming odontoblasts and enamel-forming ameloblasts. As morphogenesis advances, the matrices of dentin and enamel are deposited in an organized manner, and root formation begins. Interactions between the apical extension of the enamel organ (epithelial root sheath) and papilla/follicle mesenchyme bring about the patterning of roots, the differentiation of cementoblasts and the formation of cementum. Hence, during crown and root development, morphogenesis and cytodifferentiation are controlled by epithelial–mesenchymal interactions.

As depicted in Table 33.1 [14], molecular changes in the dental mesenchyme involve proteins in the BMP, fibroblast growth factor (FGF) and wingless integration (WNT) families, including *sonic hedgehog (Shh)* as well as transcriptional molecules like the *Msx-1, -2* homeobox genes; lymphoid enhancer-binding factor 1 (Lef-1) and Pax9, a member of the paired-box-containing transcription factor gene family. The actions and interactions of these molecules are complex and described eloquently in recent reviews [13,18].

The BMPs are among the best-characterized signals in tooth development. In addition to directly influencing the morphogenesis of the enamel organ (see discussion on enamel knot below), epithelial BMP-2 and -4 are able to induce the expression of *Msx1, Msx2,* and *Lef-1* in the dental mesenchyme as shown in bead implantation assays [19–21]. The shift in *Bmp-4* expression from epithelium to mesenchyme occurs around E12 and is coincident with the transfer of inductive potential from dental epithelium to mesenchyme [19]. In the mesenchyme, *Bmp-4* in turn requires *Msx-1* to induce its own expression [20]. The FGFs are generally potent stimulators of cell proliferation and division both in the dental mesenchyme and epithelium. *Fgf-2, -4,-8,* and *-9* expression are each restricted to the dental epithelium and can stimulate *Msx-1* but not *Msx-2* expression in the underlying mesenchyme. *Fgf-8* is expressed early in odontogenesis (E10.5–E11.5), in presumptive dental epithelium, and can induce the expression of *Pax9* in the underlying mesenchyme. Interestingly, BMP-4 prevents this induction and may share an antagonistic relationship with the FGFs, similar to what is observed in limb development [22]. Recent studies by Hardcastle et al., 1998, have shown that *Shh* in beads cannot induce *Pax9, Msx-1,* or *Bmp-4* expression in dental mesenchyme but is able to stimulate other genes encoding the transmembrane protein *patched (Ptc)* and *Gli1,* a zinc finger transcription factor [23–25]. Since neither FGF-8 nor BMP-4 can stimulate *Ptc* or *Gli1,* it is assumed that the *Shh* signaling pathway is independent of the BMP and FGF pathways during tooth development [25]. Several *Wnt* genes are expressed during tooth development and may be required for the formation of the tooth bud [13]. These genes are believed to play a role in activating the intracellular pathway involving frizzled receptors, β-catenin, and the nuclear transport of Lef-1. Other signaling molecules including the Notch genes, epidermal growth factor, hepatocyte growth factor and, the platelet-derived growth factor families may also influence tooth development although the exact nature of their involvement remains to be elucidated.

The enamel knot is a transient epithelial structure that appears at the onset of cusp formation. For years it was thought that the enamel knot controlled the folding of the dental epithelium and hence cuspal morphogenesis. Recently, the morphological, cellular, and molecular events leading to the formation and disappearance of the enamel knot have been described, thus linking its role as an organizing center for tooth morphogenesis [12,26,27]. Interestingly, the cells of the enamel knot are the only cells within the enamel organ that stop proliferating [11] and undergo apoptosis [28]. Another intriguing finding linked p21, a cyclin-dependent kinase inhibitor associated with terminal differentiation events, to apoptosis of the enamel knot [12].

The enamel knot cells express several signaling molecule genes including *Bmp-2, -4, -7; Fgf-4, -9; Msx-2;* and *Shh* [23,26,29–31]. Although the precise function of each morphogen is not currently known, a model for the relationship of the inductive signaling molecules involved has been proposed by integrating morphological and molecular data [12]. Since the instructive signaling influence lies with the dental mesenchyme prior to the development of the primary enamel knot, it is likely that this tissue influences enamel knot formation. In this regard, BMP-4 in condensing dental mesenchyme functions as a paracrine molecule that can upregulate *Msx2* and *p21* expression within the enamel knot [12,27]. It is hypothesized that *p21* then prevents proliferation within the enamel knot, allowing for the growth stimulatory *Fgf-4* to be expressed exclusively in this region [11]. FGF-4 may then act singly or in concert with *Fgf-9* to influence patterning or to regulate the expression of downstream genes like *Msx1* in the underlying papilla mesenchyme [20,29]. Intriguingly, BMP-4 participates in the regulation of apoptosis later in development, perhaps in an autocrine fashion by involving genes like *Msx-2*.

Mice genetically engineered with targeted mutations in transcription factor genes like *Msx-1, Lef*-1, and *Pax9* as well as activin-βA, a member of the TGF-β superfamily, have revealed important information. Knockouts of *Bmp-2, -4,* and *Shh* have proven less informative largely due to death that occurs *in utero* prior to the onset of tooth development. In the *Msx-1, Lef*-1, *Pax9,* and activin-βA mutant strains, tooth development fails to advance beyond the bud stage. Thus, these molecules are important in directing the fate of the dental mesenchyme and its ability to influence the progress of epithelial morphogenesis to the cap stage [32–35]. Curiously, *Msx2(–/–)* knockout molars develop fully but show abnormal cuspal patterning, a poorly differentiated stellate reticulum and enamel matrix defects, suggesting that this homeobox gene is involved in the patterning and differentiation of the enamel organ [18]. As reviewed by Tucker and Sharpe, 2004 [14], molecular information on tooth development can be used to alter the shape and size of teeth. For example, when beads soaked with Bmp4 are placed on mesenchyme within the presumptive incisor region, *Msx1* expression is downregulated, and the expression of the transcription factor *Barx1* is upregulated. Since *Barx1* is normally restricted to the molar region, its misexpression within the incisor region results in the formation of a molar tooth organ instead of an incisor [36].

In addition to use of the mouse tooth organ model, the legacy of inheritable anomalies of human dentition involving the failure of teeth to develop offers a powerful system for studying the genetic pathways controlling the development of human dentition. Familial tooth agenesis is the most common dental anomaly, which affects up to 25% of the population. It is transmitted either as an autosomal-dominant, autosomal-recessive, or X-linked trait, and presents in syndromic and nonsyndromic forms. As shown by studies in the mouse, the genes involved in epithelial–mesenchymal interactions are strong candidates for human tooth agenesis. Until recently, mutations in two genes that encode for the key transcription factors *PAX9* and *MSX1* were associated with the agenesis of molars and premolars [37]. Importantly, PAX9 and MSX1 have each been excluded in other families with autosomal dominant forms of tooth agenesis. Recently, tooth agenesis has been linked to a mutation in AXIN2, a molecule known to regulate cell homeostasis [38]. Several members of this four-generation family are affected by or are at risk for colon cancer, suggesting a broader role for this molecule in cell proliferation.

Taken together, the data from mouse and human studies have provided valuable insights into the molecular and genetic control of tooth development. As illustrated below, such basic information has provided the rationale for tooth bioengineering initiatives for the regeneration of dentin matrix and whole tooth forms.

## 33.4 Tooth Regenerative Strategies

The combination of stem cells, biomolecules, and an appropriate scaffolding material is the basis of the tissue engineering paradigm and one of the keys to the success of any regenerative strategy. In general, the specifics of this paradigm vary greatly depending on the tissue targeted for regeneration. Those factors associated with dental regenerative strategies and their real-world application are more complicated and are discussed below.

### 33.4.1 Stem Cells

Over the years, the amount of research on the use of stem cells for clinical therapies has been growing, especially after researchers found that hematopoietic stem cells, a well-characterized population of postnatal stem cells, have been successfully utilized in clinics to treat hematopoietic diseases [39], autoimmune diseases [40], and solid tumors [41]. Stem cells are defined as cells that have clonogenic and self-renewing capabilities and that differentiate into multiple cell lineages. In general, there are two kinds of stem cells: embryonic and postnatal stem cells. Embryonic stem cells are derived from mammalian embryos in the blastocyst stage and have the ability to generate any terminally differentiated cell in the body; postnatal stem cells are part of tissue-specific cells of the postnatal organism into which they are committed to differentiate. Stem cell-based tissue regeneration has great clinical potential to regain physiological functions that have been damaged by various diseases.

## 33.4.2 Human Dental Pulp Stem Cells

The isolation and identification of stem cells are the first steps in studying the potential of stem cell-mediated therapy. Postnatal stem cells have been isolated from a variety of tissues including, but not limited to, skin, liver, brain, bone marrow, and peripheral blood. Recently, dental pulp stem cells (DPSCs) have been successfully isolated from adult dental pulp in extracted human teeth [42]. Similar to the other mesenchymal stem cells, DPSCs are able to generate clonogenic cell colonies *in vitro* (Figure 33.3). The majority of the individual colonies (67%) failed to proliferate beyond 20 population doublings in the culture, suggesting that only a small portion of cells maintain high proliferation potential *in vitro* [43]. Mixed multicolony DPSCs show a higher proliferation rate than bone marrow stromal stem cells (BMSSCs) in culture. cDNA microarray analysis demonstrated that highly expressed cyclin-dependent kinase 6 (cdk6) and IGF-2 in DPSCs might be, at least partially, responsible for the promoted progression of cells through G1 to the start of DNA synthesis [44–46], leading to an elevated replicative proliferation. Most postnatal stem cells reside in a specific niche microenvironment to maintain their stemness. To elucidate the DPSCs' niche environment, DPSCs were first found to express various markers associated with endothelial and/or smooth muscle cells such as STRO-1, 3G5, VCAM-1, MUC-18, and α-smooth muscle actin [42,47]. Then, immunohistochemical staining and magnetic beads sorting were applied to confirm that DPSCs, similar to BMSSCs, reside in a perivascular niche microenvironment [47]. Considering their clonogenic nature, higher proliferation rate, and specific niche microenvironment, DPSCs satisfy the three criteria characteristic of human postnatal somatic stem cells.

## 33.4.3 Scaffolding Material

The selection of an appropriate scaffolding material is critical, as it will support and direct tissue growth and allow for scaffold integration into the surrounding host tissue. While every tissue is different and requires unique growth conditions, a scaffold must meet several general criteria: (1) it must provide a nontoxic, 3-D microenvironment that offers mechanical support, (2) it must be biocompatible, and (3) it needs to be nonimmunogenic so as to avoid adverse effects in the body [48]. Controlled biodegradability, usually through the use of enzymes or by hydrolysis, is also desirable because it allows for newly formed tissue to replace the scaffolding material at a compatible rate. The ability to incorporate growth factors relevant to the specific approach and release them in a controlled manner to stimulate matrix-embedded cells or cells from the surrounding tissue is also desired. Like the story of Goldilocks, finding a material with

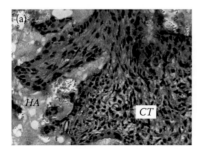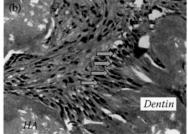

**FIGURE 33.3** (**See color insert.**) Hematoxylin and eosin staining of representative DPSC transplants. (a) After 1 week posttransplantation, DPSC transplants contain connective tissue (*CT*) around HA/TCP carrier (*HA*), without any sign of dentin formation. (b) After 6 weeks posttransplantation, DPSCs differentiate into odontoblasts (arrows) that are responsible for the dentin formation on the surface of HA/TCP (*HA*). Original magnification: 40×.

the mechanical, chemical, and biological properties that are "just right" involves some trial and error. An example of how to fine-tune a material can be found later in this chapter. A variety of constructs, namely natural and synthetic polymers, is being explored and developed to fit the criteria mentioned above. These materials can be fabricated into nanofibrous materials, porous scaffolds, and hydrogels.

### 33.4.3.1 Nanofibrous Materials

Natural materials used as tissue engineering scaffolds include collagen, fibrin, elastin alginate, silk, and glycosaminoglycans such as hyaluronan and chitosan. All of these nanofibrous materials possess many desirable properties similar to those of natural ECM, such as their mechanical strength, which can be enhanced by various chemical crosslinkers (e.g., glutaraldehyde, formaldehyde), localized biodegradability by metalloproteinases (e.g., collagenase and serine proteases) and an inherent biocompatibility [49–51]. Collagen has been particularly interesting in bone and tooth tissue engineering due to its ability to be fabricated into gels, nanofibers, porous scaffolds, and to support cell growth of human periodontal ligament cells and human dental pulp cells to form viable tissues [52–54]. However, these natural materials can be difficult to process and often risk transmitting animal-associated pathogens and inducing immunoresponses [55].

### 33.4.3.2 Porous Scaffolds

Synthetic polymers offer more control over the design of the material through manipulation of their chemical and mechanical properties (i.e., molecular weight, the configuration of polymer chains, the presence of functional groups, degradable linkages) [56]. These synthetic materials are also valued for their reproducibility and ease in controlling porosity. Synthetic polymers are also already approved for use by the Food and Drug Administration (FDA) [57]. Commonly used synthetic scaffolding materials are derived from polyester materials that readily degrade in the human body; these materials include polylactic acid (PLA), polyglycolic acid (PGA), polycaprolactone (PCL), and blends of PLA and PGA [58]. PLA in itself is a strong polymer and is useful in applications requiring structural strength; it has already been implicated as a possible scaffolding material that, when combined with stem cells from human exfoliated deciduous teeth (SHEDs), can form tissue resembling physiologic dental pulp, including microvasculature [59]. When seeded with DPSCs, PGA has been shown to form soft tissue that is similar to native pulp and is capable of forming tooth cementum-like tissue, ligament, and bone structures when used with PCL [60,61]. Polyethylene glycol (PEG) is an additional class of synthetic material showing promise as a tissue engineering scaffold [62]. Synthetic polymers also have some drawbacks, including issues associated with the fabrication of the material and chronic or acute inflammatory response.

### 33.4.3.3 Hydrogels

Hydrogels have only recently been explored for their unique properties in the field of tissue engineering. They can be fabricated from natural materials (e.g., collagen, fibrin, chitosan, hyaluronan), synthetic materials (e.g., PEG, PEG copolymers, self-assembling peptide nanofibers), or a blend of the two. Hydrogels are favored for a variety of reasons: (1) they have a high water content, (2) their viscoelastic properties mimic soft tissue, (3) they undergo degradation under mild conditions, (4) their mechanical and structural properties are similar to those of native tissue and ECM, (5) they are biocompatible, (6) they are efficient transporters of nutrients and metabolic products, (7) they allow cells to easily proliferate and differentiate within the matrix, (8) they are able to encapsulate cells uniformly, and (9) they can be delivered in a relatively noninvasive manner by injection and gelation *in situ* [51,63,64,65]. In particular, hydrogels based on self-assembling peptide nanofibers have shown great promise as a possible scaffolding material for dental tissue engineering [66,67]. Such hydrogels are favored for their easy control over material and chemical properties, bioactivity, biocompatibility, diverse functional capabilities (i.e., adhesion, degradation, mineralization, and growth factor attachment sites), and their comparable size to ECM components [68–71]. The National Institute for Dental and Craniofacial Research (NIDCR) has already implicated these materials as a possible candidate in their strategy for the regeneration of whole human teeth [72].

### 33.4.4 Fine-Tuning Scaffolds in Regenerative Dentistry

Given the complex architecture of the tooth and the presence of both soft and mineralized tissue within the oral cavity, no single scaffold can fit all the needed requirements. However, the use of one of the materials discussed (nanofibrous materials, porous scaffolds, and hydrogels) in conjunction with dental stem cells and bioactive factors presents a possible means of regenerating specific tissues within the oral cavity. Collaborative efforts by researchers in the fields of chemistry, biology, and engineering have already yielded promising results in enamel remineralization, regeneration of the dentin-pulp complex, and periodontal regeneration.

One such collaboration in the field of dentin-pulp regeneration has produced a class of self-assembling nanofiber hydrogels known as Multidomain Peptide (MDP) nanofibers. These MDPs show promise as a tunable and injectable hydrogel that could support soft tissue growth similar to dental pulp [67,73–75]. MDP nanofibers derive their name from their distinct modular domains (regions), which can be seen in Figure 33.4a. Region one represents a hydrophobic amino acid face, region two a hydrophilic amino acid face, and region three charged amino acid end groups. Each of these regions contributes to the ability of the material to self-assemble into nanofibers of controlled length (120 nm), diameter (6 nm), and height (2 nm). These nanofibers can further undergo self-assembly to form stable hydrogels by the addition of oppositely charged multivalent ions like magnesium or phosphate under physiological conditions (Figure 33.4b).

Furthermore, the modular nature of MDPs means that each region can be easily optimized independently of the other. This characteristic allows MDPs to be tailored for the specific application of regenerating dental pulp. However, the addition of phosphoserines in region three would provide sites for hydroxyapatite nucleation and encourage biomineralization deposition on the nanofibers to make this material suitable for dentin regeneration. Specific changes to the modular regions have led to improved mechanical and bioactive properties of the MDPs, illustrating how a basic scaffolding material can be fine-tuned for use as a dental tissue engineering scaffold.

Several desirable mechanical properties have resulted from the modification of the MDPs: (1) their tunable viscoelastic properties achieved by exchanging specific amino acids from regions two or three to give control over the "softness" or "hardness" of the hydrogel and (2) shear thinning behavior that allowed the material to conform to the uneven architecture before "setting" when injected into small defects in the oral cavity (Figure 33.5a). Changes in the bioactive properties resulted from several modifications: (1) the addition of cell adhesion motifs like RGD to region three, which significantly improved cell attachment, (2) insertion of an enzyme cleavable sequence that allowed for degradation of the material over

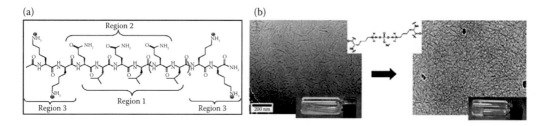

**FIGURE 33.4** Nanofibrous peptide hydrogels. (a) The three key regions that control the peptides' self-assembly into a nanostructured fiber are shown. (1) A hydrophobic face, which is the energetic driving force for self-assembly in water; (2) a hydrophilic face, which provides water solubility and opposition to region 1, creating a facial amphiphile; and (3) charged peripheral groups that limit the extent of self-assembly via electrostatic repulsion and also aid in solubility. Regions 1 and 2 are formed from a pattern of alternating hydrophobic and hydrophilic amino acids such that when the peptide is in a fully extended conformation, the amino acid side chains alternate between one side of the peptide and the other. This arrangement results in one face of the peptide being hydrophobic (region 1) while the other is hydrophilic (region 2). (b) CryoTEM images of nanofibers before and after addition of phosphate, resulting in increased fiber length and gelation.

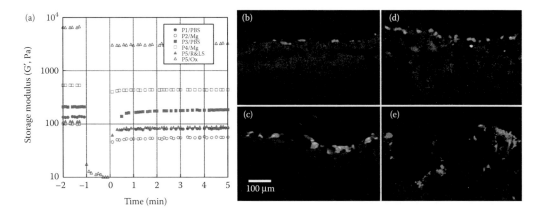

**FIGURE 33.5** **(See color insert.)** Mechanical strength of peptides prepared with different solutions. (a) A time sweep experiment showing shear recovery properties of nanofibrous scaffolds. After application of a high load, the hydrogels returned to the original storage modulus ($G'$) within 1 min. (b) Green-fluorescent cells were seeded on top of hydrogels without cleavage site (b, c) and hydrogels where the cleavage motif is present (d, e). Both peptides carry the cell adhesion motif RGD. Images show cells after 1 day (b, d) and after 5 days (c, e) in culture. Cells remain as a mono-layer on top of hydrogels without a cleavage site (c), they migrate and spread into hydrogels with a cleavage motif (e).

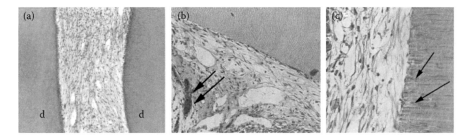

**FIGURE 33.6** **(See color insert.)** *In vivo* culture of MDP nanofibers. (a) and (b) show the formation of vascular-ized pulp-like soft connective tissue with blood formation (arrows). (c) DPSC seem to have extended their processes into the dentin tubules (arrows), which is suggestive of DPSC differentiation into odontoblasts in the presence of hydrogels containing growth factors.

time by dental stem cells (Figures 33.5b through 33.8e), and (3) incorporation of heparin molecules into the hydrogel, which bound, protected and slowly released growth factors in response to cellular activity.

Fine-tuning of the MDP nanofiber led to their testing *in vivo* in a well-known mouse model in which MPDs containing embedded DPSCs and various growth factors [vascular endothial growth factor (VEGF), TGF ß-1, and FGF2] were inserted into the pulp chamber of prepared tooth slices after removal of the original tooth tissue and treatment with ethylenediaminetetraacetic acid (EDTA) [75]. These con-structs were then subcutaneously implanted into the backs of immunodeficient mice and allowed to grow over a period of several weeks (Figure 33.6).

While more extensive research is currently underway, this approach and others similar to it are the next steps toward more viable therapies that are practical alternatives to current endodontic treatments seen in the clinic.

## 33.4.5 Dentin Tissue Regeneration

One of the most important characteristics of DPSCs is their capability to form a dentin/pulp-like com-plex upon *in vivo* transplantation in conjunction with hydroxyapatite/tricalcium phosphate as a carrier vehicle [42]. Backscatter electron microscopy (EM) analysis demonstrated that the dentin-like material formed in the transplants had a globular appearance consistent with the structure of dentin *in situ* [43]. DPSC-mediated odontogenesis is differentiable from BMSSC-mediated osteogenesis by regenerating different organ-like structures and involving different regulating molecules [76]. This capacity implies that critical factor(s) may regulate mineralized matrix-forming stem cells to generate defined mineralized tissue along with associated soft tissues. The property of multipotential differentiation of DPSCs has been demonstrated by the finding that under the proper culture conditions, DPSCs are capable of differentiating into osteo/odontogenic cells, adipocytes, and neural cells [43]. However, the assets of the multipotential differentiation of DPSCs at functional levels remain to be confirmed.

The findings on DPSCs may reveal their potential for dentin and pulp tissue regeneration. Human teeth do not undergo the type of remodeling seen in other mineralized tissues such as bone, which remodels to maintain organ integrity. Once a tooth has erupted, dentinal damage caused by mechanical trauma, exposure to chemicals or infectious processes, induces the formation of reparative dentin that serves as a protective barrier to the dental pulp with limited capacity, though structurally poorly organized [77–81]. It was reported that bone morphogenetic protein-7 is capable of stimulating tertiary dentin formation when applied to freshly cut dentin both *in vitro* and *in vivo* [82,83]. This formation probably occurs through an osteo/odontogenic induction property of BMP-7, since BMP-7-transfected human fibroblasts were able to express an osteogenic characteristic and form bone tissue *in vivo* [84]. DPSCs were also capable of forming reparative dentin structure on the surfaces of regular human dentin [76]. However, it seems that DPSCs exhibit a decreased and altered *in vivo* odontogenic capacity when loaded on the surface of human dentin. While the reason is not known, it may be associated with the microenvironment that accommodates *in vivo* differentiation of DPSCs [76]. When DPSCs were seeded onto poly-D, L-lactide-glycolide as a carrier, inserted into empty human root canals, and subsequently transplanted into immunocompromised mice subcutaneously, they generated pulp-like tissue with well-established vascularity and a continuous layer of dentin-like tissue deposited onto the canal dentinal wall. This dentin-like structure appeared to be produced by a layer of newly formed odontoblast-like cells expressing Dspp, BSP, alkaline phosphatase, and CD105. A study by Huang et al. suggested that pulp-like tissue can be regenerated *de novo* in emptied root canal space [85].

Recently, it was demonstrated that the autogenous transplantation of BMP2-treated DPSCs was able to stimulate reparative dentin formation on the amputated pulp [86]. This finding suggests that combined therapy using stem cells and growth factors may improve stem cell-mediated dentin regeneration.

### 33.4.6 Tooth Regeneration

Recently, whole tooth regeneration *in vivo* has become a popular topic in dental research. Tooth development involves a mutual signaling interaction between the epithelial and mesenchymal cells of neural ectodermal origin. It was demonstrated that tooth crown structures including dentin, odontoblasts, pulp chamber, putative Hertwig's root sheath epithelia, putative cementoblasts, and enamel organ could be regenerated using dissociated cells from pig tooth bud tissues (Figure 33.7) [87]. Further, the same research group demonstrated that cultured cells from rat tooth bud were also able to regenerate tooth structure when loaded on PGA or PLGA scaffolds [88]. These studies demonstrate for the first time that mammalian tooth structure can be regenerated in a system consisting of tooth bud progenitors and the proper scaffold. Moreover, Sharpe's group conducted a promising study to demonstrate that mice embryonic oral epithelium along with nondental stem cells can induce an odontogenic response, showing the expression of odontogenic mesenchymal cell-associated genes such as Msx1, Lhx7, and Pax9 [89]. After being transplanted into adult renal capsules, the recombination of embryonic oral epithelium with nondental stem cells (embryonic, neural, and bone marrow stem cells) gave rise to both tooth structure and bone tissue (Figure 33.8) [89]. Also, transplanted embryonic tooth primordial were able to maintain their tooth development potential within an adult environment [89]. This study clearly

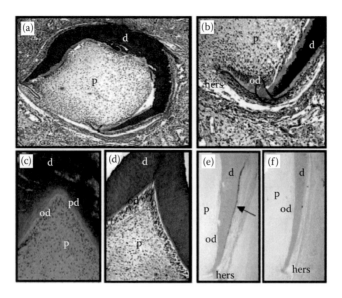

**FIGURE 33.7** **(See color insert.)** Histology and immunohistochemistry of a 20-week implant. (a) Von Kossa stain for calcified mineralization in bioengineered tooth crown (50× magnification). Dark brown stain is positive for mineralized tissues. (b) A high-magnification (400×) photomicrograph of the Hertwig's epithelial root sheath is shown, stained by the Von Kossa method to detect calcified mineralization. (c) High-magnification (200×) photomicrograph of cuspal region in bioengineered tooth crown. The tissue was stained by the Von Kossa method. (d) Hematoxylin and eosin (H&E) stain of a positive control porcine third molar cuspal region demonstrates morphology similar to that of the bioengineered tooth structure (200×). (e) BSP immunostain of 20-week-old bioengineered tooth crown (100×). Positive BSP expression is indicated by the arrow. (f) Negative preimmune control immunostain for BSP in bioengineered tooth crown (100×). Abbreviations: d, dentin; od, odontoblasts; p, pulp; pd, predentin, hers, Hertwig's epithelial root sheath. (Reproduced with permission from Young CS et al. 2002. *J Dent Res* 81(10): 695–700.)

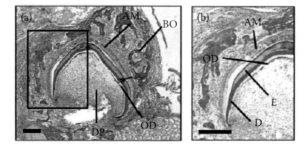

**FIGURE 33.8** **(See color insert.)** Recombinant explant between bone marrow-derived cells and oral epithelium following 12 days of development in a renal capsule. All the tissues visible are donor-derived, since the host kidney makes no cellular contribution to the tissue. Where epithelium in the recombinations was from GFP mice, *in situ* hybridization of sections of these tissues confirmed that all mesenchyme-derived cells were of wildtype origin (not shown). Scale bar: 80 μm. (a) Bioengineered tooth organ showing normal morphogenesis, cell differentiation and matrix deposition, BO: bone; DP: dental pulp. (b) High magnification view of boxed area showing functional ameloblasts (AM), odontoblasts (OD) and normal deposition of enamel (E), dentin (D) matrices. (Reproduced with permission from Ohazama A et al. 2004. *J Dent Res* 83(7): 518–522.)

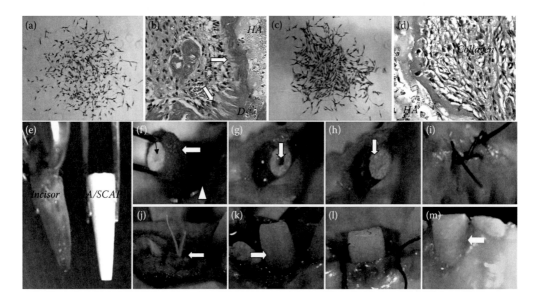

**FIGURE 33.9**   **(See color insert.)** SCAP/PDLSC-mediated root/periodontal structure as an artificial crown support for the restoration of tooth function in swine. (a) SCAP isolated from swine were capable of forming a single colony cluster when plated at a low cell density. (b) When transplanted into immunocompromised mice for 8 weeks, swine SCAP differentiate into odontoblasts (open arrows) to regenerate dentin (*D*) on the surface of the hydroxy-apatite carrier (*HA*). (c) Swine PDLSCs were capable of forming a single colony cluster. (d) After transplantation into immunocompromised mice, PDLSCs formed cementum (*C*) on the surface of hydroxyapatite carrier (*HA*). Collagen fibers were found to connect to newly formed cementum. (e) Extracted minipig lower incisor and root-shaped HA/TCP carrier loaded with SCAP. (f) Gelfoam containing $10 \times 10^6$ PDLSCs (open arrow) was used to cover the HA/SCAP (black arrow) and implanted into the lower incisor socket (open triangle). (g) HA/SCAP-Gelfoam/PDLSCs were implanted into a newly extracted incisor socket. A post channel was created inside the root shape HA carrier (open arrow). (h) The post channel was sealed with a temporary post for affixing a crown in the next step. (i) The HA/SCAP-Gelfoam/PDLSC implant was sutured for 3 months. (j) The HA/SCAP-Gelfoam/PDLSC implant (open arrow) was reexposed and the temporary post was removed to expose the post channel. (k) A premade porcelain crown was cemented to the HA/SCAP-Gelfoam/PDLSC structure. (l) The exposed section was sutured. (m) After 4 weeks' fixation, the porcelain crown was retained in the swine for exertion of masticatory function as shown by open arrows. (Reproduced with permission from Sonoyama W et al. 2006. *PLoS ONE* 20(1): e79.)

indicates that the inductive function of embryonic oral epithelium may be an important driving force for future prospects of achieving entire tooth regeneration *in vivo*.

A new population of stem cells from the root apical papilla named "SCAP" was isolated and identified as a primitive stem cell population [90]. The transplantation of SCAP along with periodontal ligament stem cells generated a root/periodontal complex capable of supporting a porcelain crown, resulting in normal tooth function in a mini pig model [90]. This work integrates a stem cell-mediated tissue regeneration strategy, engineered materials for structure, and current dental crown technologies to the recovery of tooth strength and appearance (Figure 33.9).

## 33.5 Conclusion

The last decade has witnessed an explosion of scientific and technological advances that will undoubtedly propel the field of tooth bioengineering forward. This chapter is limited in scope inasmuch as only a few tooth regenerative strategies were discussed. Therefore, readers should be mindful of several other existing dimensions of research. As presented in the current literature, there is great interest in understanding the structural, biomechanical, and bioregulatory features of dentin and bone matrices as well as the complex process of enamel biomineralization and remineralization. Such basic knowledge is essential for the development of tooth-specific biological substitutes that will best restore, maintain, or improve the functions of normal dentition. The legacy of inheritable anomalies involving tooth patterning and extracellular matrices will continue to provide a powerful means of identifying new molecular pathways that influence normal and abnormal development. Clearly, advances in the field of tooth bioengineering will depend on the clever integration of basic science knowledge from animal and human developmental and genetic studies with emerging technologies in the fields of stem cell biology, autologous cell therapy, gene therapy, materials sciences, and nanotechnology. While the clinical applications for the use of bioengineered tooth forms and matrices remain limitless, several challenges must be surmounted prior to successful therapeutic interventions. As important as the timely diagnosis, accurate prognosis and proper treatment of diseases affecting dentition will be the preparation of host sites within the oral cavity to receive bioengineered materials. In every respect, the field of tooth bioengineering encompasses broad strategies and multidisciplinary approaches directed at restoring one of the most complex organs in vertebrates.

## Acknowledgments

The authors acknowledge the support of the National Institute of Dental and Craniofacial Research (NIDCR), National Institutes of Health (NIH). The research program of RDS has been funded through NIH grants DE10517; DE07252; DE12269; DE11663 and DE13368. STS is supported by the Division of Intramural Research at the NIDCR.

## References

1. Linde A and Goldberg M. 1993. Dentinogenesis. *Crit Rev Oral Biol Med* 4(5): 679–728.
2. Butler WT and Ritchie H. 1995. The nature and functional significance of dentin extracellular matrix proteins. *Int J Dev Biol* 39(1): 169–179.
3. MacDougall M et al. 1997. Dentin phosphoprotein and dentin sialoprotein are cleavage products expressed from a single transcript coded by a gene on human chromosome 4. Dentin phosphoprotein DNA sequence determination. *J Biol Chem* 272(2): 835–842.
4. Prasad M, Butler WT, and Qin C. 2010. Dentin sialophosphoprotein in biomineralization. *Connect Tissue Res* 51(5): 404–417.
5. George A et al. 1993. Characterization of a novel dentin matrix acidic phosphoprotein. Implications for induction of biomineralization. *J Biol Chem* 268(17): 12624–12630.
6. D'Souza RN et al. 1997. Gene expression patterns of murine dentin matrix protein 1 (Dmp1) and dentin sialophosphoprotein (DSPP) suggest distinct developmental functions *in vivo*. *J Bone Miner Res* 12(12): 2040–2049.
7. Smith AJ and Lesot H. 2001. Induction and regulation of crown dentinogenesis: Embryonic events as a template for dental tissue repair? *Crit Rev Oral Biol Med.* 12(5): 425–437.
8. Ten Cate AR. 1998. *Oral Histology: Development, Structure, and Function* (5th edn.). St. Louis, MO, Mosby, Inc.
9. Avery JK. 1987. Development of teeth: Crown formation, Chapter 7. In: *Oral Development and Histology*. Pine JW, ed. Baltimore, MD, Waverly Press.
10. Mina M and Kollar EJ. 1987. The induction of odontogenesis in non-dental mesenchyme combined with early murine mandibular arch epithelium. *Arch Oral Biol* 32(2): 123–127.
11. Jernvall J et al. 1994. Evidence for the role of the enamel knot as a control center in mammalian tooth cusp formation: Non-dividing cells express growth stimulating Fgf-4 gene. *Intnl J Dev Biol* 38(3): 463–469.
12. Jernvall J et al. 1998. The life history of an embryonic signaling center: BMP-4 induces p21 and is associated with apoptosis in the mouse tooth enamel knot. *Development* 125(2): 161–169.
13. Thesleff I and Sharpe P. 1997. Signaling networks regulating dental development. *Mech Dev* 67(2): 111–123.

14. Tucker A and Sharpe P. 2004. The cutting-edge of mammalian development; how the embryo makes teeth. *Nat Rev Genet* 5(7): 499–508.

15. Lumsden AGS. 1988. Spatial organization of the epithelium and the role of neural crest cells in the initiation of the mammalian tooth. *Development* 103(Suppl); 155–169.

16. Kollar EJ and Baird GR. 1969. The influence of the dental papilla on the development of tooth shape in embryonic mouse tooth germs. *J Embryol Exp Morphol* 21(1): 131–148.

17. Kollar EJ and Baird GR. 1970. Tissue interactions in embryonic mouse tooth germs. I. Reorganization of the dental epithelium during tooth-germ reconstruction. *J Embryol Exp Morphol* 24(1): 159–171.

18. Maas R and Bei M. 1997. The genetic control of early tooth development. *Crit Rev Oral Biol Med* 8(1): 4–39.

19. Vainio S et al. 1993. Identification of BMP-4 as a signal mediating secondary induction between epithelial and mesenchymal tissues during early tooth development. *Cell* 75(1): 45–58.

20. Chen Y et al. 1996. Msx1 controls inductive signaling in mammalian tooth morphogenesis. *Development* 122(10): 3035–3044.

21. Kratochwil K et al. 1996. Lef1 expression is activated by BMP-4 and regulates inductive tissue interactions in tooth and hair development. *Genes Dev* 10(11): 1382–1394.

22. Neubüser A et al. 1997. Antagonistic interactions between FGF and BMP signaling pathways: A mechanism for positioning the sites of tooth formation. *Cell* 90(2): 247–255.

23. Bitgood MJ and McMahon AP. 1995. Hedgehog and Bmp genes are coexpressed at many diverse sites of cell-cell interaction in the mouse embryo. *Dev Biol* 172(1): 126–138.

24. Koyama E et al. 1996. Polarizing activity, sonic hedgehog, and tooth development in embryonic and postnatal mouse. *Dev Dyn* 206(1):59–72.

25. Hardcastle Z et al. 1998. The *Shh* signaling pathway in tooth development: defects in Gli2 and Gli3 mutants. *Development* 125(15): 2803–2811.

26. Vaahtokari A et al. 1996. The enamel knot as a signaling center in the developing mouse tooth. *Mech Dev* 54(1): 39–43.

27. Thesleff I and Jernvall J. 1997. The enamel knot: a putative signaling center regulating tooth development. Cold Spring: Harb Symp. *Quant Biol* 62: 257–267.

28. Vaahtokari A, Åberg T, and Thesleff I. 1996. Apoptosis in the developing tooth: association with an embryonic signaling center and suppression by EGF and FGF-4. *Development* 122(1): 121–129.

29. Kettunen P and Thesleff I. 1998. Expression and function of FGFs-4, -8, and -9 suggest functional redundancy and repetitive use as epithelial signals during tooth morphogenesis. *Dev Dyn* 211(3): 256–268.

30. MacKenzie A, Ferguson MW, and Sharpe PT. 1992. Expression patterns of the homeobox gene, Hox-8, in the mouse embryo suggest a role in specifying tooth initiation and shape. *Development* 115(2):403–420.

31. Iseki S et al. 1996. Sonic hedgehog is expressed in epithelial cells during development of whisker, hair, and tooth. *Biochem Biophys Res Comm* 218(3): 688–693.

32. Satokata I and Maas R. 1994. Msx1 deficient mice exhibit cleft palate and abnormalities of craniofacial and tooth development. *Nat Genet* 6(4): 348–356.

33. van Genderen C et al. 1994. Development of several organs that require inductive epithelial- mesenchymal interactions is impaired in LEF-1-deficient mice. *Genes Dev* 8(22): 2691–2703.

34. Peters H, Neubüser A, and Balling R. 1998. Pax genes and organogenesis: Pax9 meets tooth development. *Eur J Oral Sci* 106(Suppl 1): 38–43.

35. Matzuk MM, Kumar TR, and Bradley A. 1995. Different phenotypes for mice deficient in either activins or activin receptor type II. *Nature* 374: 356–360.

36. Tucker AS, Al Khamis A, and Sharpe PT. 1998. Interactions between Bmp-4 and Msx-1 act to restrict gene expression to odontogenic mesenchyme. *Dev Dyn* 212: 533–539.

37. Vieira AR. 2003. Oral clefts and syndromic forms of tooth agenesis as models for genetics of isolated tooth agenesis. *J Dent Res* 82(3): 162–165.

38. Lammi L et al. 2004. Mutations in AXIN2 cause familial tooth agenesis and predispose to colorectal cancer. *Am J Hum Genet* 74(5): 1043–1050.

39. Thomas ED. 1995. Bone marrow transplantation from bench to bedside. *Ann NY Acad Sci* 770: 34–41.

40. Snowden JA et al. 2004. Autologous hemopoietic stem cell transplantation in severe RA: A report from the EBMT and ABMTR. *J Rheum* 31: 482–488.

41. Rini BI et al. 2002. Allogeneic stem-cell transplantation of renal cell cancer after nonmyeloablative chemotherapy: Feasibility, engraftment, and clinical results. *J Clin Oncol* 20: 2017–2024.

42. Gronthos S et al. 2000. Postnatal human dental pulp stem cells (DPSCs) *in vitro* and *in vivo*. *Proc Natl Acad Sci U S A* 97(25): 13625–30136.

43. Gronthos S et al. 2002. Stem cell properties of human dental pulp stem cells. *J Dent Res* 81(8): 531–535.

44. Shi S, Robey PG, and Gronthos S. 2001. Comparison of gene expression profiles for human, dental pulp and bone marrow stromal stem cells by cDNA microarray analysis. *Bone* 29(6): 532–539.

45. Ekholm SV and Reed SI. 2000. Regulation of G(1) cyclin-dependent kinases in the mammalian cell cycle. *Curr Opin Cell Biol* 12(6): 676–684.

46. Grossel MJ, Baker GL, and Hinds PW. 1999. cdk6 can shorten G(1) phase dependent upon the N-terminal INK4 interaction domain. *J Biol Chem* 274(42): 29960–29967.

47. Shi S and Gronthos S. 2003. Perivascular niche of postnatal mesenchymal stem cells identified in human bone marrow and dental pulp. *J Bone Min Res* 18(4): 696–704.

48. Langer R and Vacanti JP. 1993. Tissue engineering. *Science* 260(5110): 920–926.

49. Lee CR, Grodzinsk JR, and Spector M. 2001. The effects of cross-linking of collagen-glycosaminoglycan scaffolds on compressive stiffness, chondrocyte-mediated contraction, proliferation, and biosynthesis. *Biomaterials* 22(23): 3145–3154.

50. Alberts B et al. 1994. Molecular biology of the cell (3rd edn.). Garland Publishing, Inc., New York.

51. Lee KY and Mooney DJ. 2001. Hydrogels for tissue engineering. *Chem Rev* 101(7): 1869–1879. Review.

52. Sumitaa Y et al. 2006. Performance of collagen sponge as a 3-D scaffold for tooth-tissue engineering. *Biomaterials* 27(17): 3238–3248.

53. Zhang Y et al. 2006. Novel chitosan/collagen scaffold containing transforming growth factor-beta1 DNA for periodontal tissue engineering. *Biochem Biophys Res Commun* 344(1): 362–369.

54. Kim NR, Lee DH, Chung PH, and Yang HC. 2009. Distinct differentiation properties of human dental pulp cells on collagen, gelatin, and chitosan scaffolds. *Oral Surg Oral Med Oral Pathol Oral Radiol Endod* 108(5): e94–100.

55. Friess W. 1998. Collagen-biomaterial for drug delivery. *Eur J Pharm Biopharm* 45(2): 113–136. Review.

56. Ohara T et al. 2010. Evaluation of scaffold materials for tooth tissue engineering. *J Biomed Mater Res A* 94(3): 800–805.

57. Sachlos E and Czernuszka JT. 2003. Making tissue engineering scaffolds work. Review: The application of solid freeform fabrication technology to the production of tissue engineering scaffolds. *Eur Cell Mater* 5: 29–39; discussion 39–40. Review.

58. Athanasiou KA, Niederauer GG, and Agrawal CM. 1996. Sterilization, toxicity, biocompatibility and clinical applications of polylactic acid/polyglycolic acid copolymers. *Biomaterials* (2): 93–102. Review.

59. Cordeiro MM et al. 2008. Dental pulp tissue engineering with stem cells from exfoliated deciduous teeth. *J Endod* 34(8): 962–969.

60. Mooney DJ, Powell C, Piana J, and Rutherford B. 1996. Engineering dental pulp-like tissue *in vitro*. *Biotechnol Prog* 12(6): 865–868.

61. Park CH et al. 2010. Biomimetic hybrid scaffolds for engineering human tooth-ligament interfaces. *Biomaterials* 31(23): 5945–5952.

62. Merrill EW and Salzman EW. 1995. Polyethylene oxide as a biomaterial. *ASAIO J* 6: 60–64.

63. Park JB and Lakes RS. 1992. *Biomaterials: An Introduction* (2nd edn.). Plenum Press, New York.

64. Drury JL and Mooney DJ. 2003. Hydrogels for tissue engineering: Scaffold design variables and applications. *Biomaterials* 24(24): 4337–4351. Review.

65. Lee KY, Alsberg E and Mooney DJ. 2001. Degradable and injectable poly(aldehyde guluronate) hydrogels for bone tissue engineering. *J Biomed Mater Res* 56(2): 228–233.

66. Galler KM et al. 2008. Self-assembling peptide amphiphile nanofibers as a scaffold for dental stem cells. *Tissue Eng Part A* 14(12): 2051–2058.

67. Galler KM et al. 2010. Self-assembling multidomain peptide hydrogels: Designed susceptibility to enzymatic cleavage allows enhanced cell migration and spreading. *J Am Chem Soc* 132(9): 3217–3223.

68. Shah RN et al. 2010. Supramolecular design of self-assembling nanofibers for cartilage regeneration. *Proc Natl Acad Sci USA* 107(8): 3293–3298.

69. Hartgerink JD, Beniash E, and Stupp SI. 2001. Self-assembly and mineralization of peptide-amphiphile nanofibers. *Science* 294(5547): 1684–1688.

70. Hosseinkhani H et al. 2006. Osteogenic differentiation of mesenchymal stem cells in self-assembled peptide-amphiphile nanofibers. *Biomaterials* 27(22): 4079–4086.

71. Rajangam K et al. 2006. Heparin binding nanostructures to promote growth of blood vessels. *Nano Lett* 6(9): 2086–2090.

72. Snead ML. 2008. Whole-tooth regeneration: It takes a village of scientists, clinicians, and patients. *J Dent Educ* 72(8): 903–911.

73. Dong H et al. 2007. Self-assembly of multi-domain peptides: Balancing molecular frustration controls conformation and nanostructure. *J Am Chem Soc* 129(41): 12468–12472.

74. Aulisa L, Dong H, and Hartgerink JD. 2009. Self-assembly of multidomain peptides: Sequence variation allows control over cross-linking and viscoelasticity. *Biomacromolecules* 10(9): 2694–2698.

75. Cordeiro MM et al. Dental pulp tissue engineering with stem cells from exfoliated deciduous teeth. *J Endod* 34(8): 962–969.

76. Batouli S et al. 2003. Comparison of stem cell-mediated osteogenesis and dentinogenesis. *J Dent Res* 82(12): 975–980.

77. Levin LG. 1998. Pulpal regeneration. *Pract Periodontics Aesthet Dent* 10(5): 621–624.

78. About I et al. 2001. Pulpal inflammatory responses following non-carious class V restorations. *Oper Dent* 26(4): 336–342.

79. About I et al. 2001. The effect of cavity restoration variables on odontoblast cell numbers and dental repair. *J Dent* 29(2): 109–117.

80. Murray PE et al. 2001. Restorative pulpal and repair responses. *J Am Dent Assoc* 132(4): 482–491.

81. Murray PE et al. 2000. Postoperative pulpal and repair responses. *J Am Dent Assoc* 131(3): 321–329.

82. Rutherford RB and Gu K. 2000. Treatment of inflamed ferret dental pulps with recombinant bone morphogenetic protein-7. *Eur J Oral Sci* 108(3): 202–206.

83. Sloan AJ, Rutherford RB, and Smith AJ. 2000. Stimulation of the rat dentine-pulp complex by bone morphogenetic protein-7 *in vitro*. *Arch Oral Biol* 45(2): 173–177.

84. Rutherford RB et al. 2002. Bone morphogenetic protein-transduced human fibroblasts convert to osteoblasts and form bone *in vivo*. *Tissue Eng* 8(3): 441–452.

85. Huang GT-J et al. 2010. Stem/progenitor cell-mediated *de novo* regeneration of dental pulp with newly deposited continuous layer of dentin in an *in vivo* model. *Tissue Eng.* 16(2): 605–615.

86. Iohara K et al. 2004. Dentin regeneration by dental pulp stem cell therapy with recombinant human bone morphogenetic protein 2. *J Dent Res* 83(8): 590–595.

87. Young CS et al. 2002. Tissue engineering of complex tooth structures on biodegradable polymer scaffolds. *J Dent Res* 81(10): 695–700.

88. Duailibi MT et al. 2004. Bioengineered teeth from cultured rat tooth bud cells. *J Dent Res* 83(7): 523–528.

89. Ohazama A et al. 2004. Stem-cell-based tissue engineering of murine teeth. *J Dent Res* 83(7): 518–522.

90. Sonoyama W et al. 2006. Mesenchymal stem cell-mediated functional tooth regeneration in swine. *PLoS ONE* 20(1): e79.

# 34

# Tissue Engineering of the Urogenital System

In Kap Ko
*Wake Forest University*
*School of Medicine*

Anthony Atala
*Wake Forest University*
*School of Medicine*

James J. Yoo
*Wake Forest University*
*School of Medicine*

34.1 Introduction ...................................................................................34-1
34.2 Fundamental Components of Urogenital
Tissue Engineering ........................................................................34-2
   Biomaterials • Cells • Controlling the Microenvironment
   Using Biomaterials
34.3 Engineering Specific Urogenital Structures ...........................34-6
   Bladder • Kidney • Urethra • Penis • Testis • Vagina
34.4 Perspective ....................................................................................34-12
Acknowledgment...................................................................................34-12
References................................................................................................34-12

## 34.1 Introduction

The urogenital system is made up of the urinary tract, which excretes waste, and the reproductive system. In both sexes, the urinary tract is made up of the kidneys, the ureters (which bring urine from the kidneys to the bladder), the bladder, and the urethra (the tube that connects the bladder to the outside of the body). In males, the urogenital system also includes the penis and testes, and in females it includes the vagina and uterus. Congenital disorders, cancer, trauma, infection, inflammation, iatrogenic injuries, or other conditions of the urogenital system can lead to organ damage or complete loss of organ function. If this occurs, reconstructive procedures or organ transplantation are required. Currently, urologic reconstructive procedures are usually performed with grafts composed of native nonurologic tissues, such as skin, gastrointestinal segments, or oral mucosa. However, these grafts can lead to complications after reconstruction. Often, the inherently different functional characteristics of the different tissues used in the reconstruction cause a mismatch in the urinary system. As an example, current methods of replacing bladder tissue with gastrointestinal segments can be problematic due to the opposite ways in which these two tissues handle solutes—urologic tissue normally excretes these solutes, but gastrointestinal tissue generally absorbs them, and such a mismatch can lead to metabolic complications, stone formation, infection, and even malignancy. Additionally, for patients requiring replacement of large sections of the urinary tract, donor site morbidity is likely, and in severe cases, there may be insufficient tissue available for autografting.

Owing to the limitations of current methods for reconstructing urological tissues, alternative approaches have been pursued. As such, the field of tissue engineering and regenerative medicine has emerged as a means to provide novel solutions to overcome the current challenges of medical practice. The replacement of lost or deficient urologic tissues with functionally equivalent ones created using tissue engineering techniques would improve the outcome of reconstructive surgery for urogenital organs. In this chapter, the basic components needed for successful engineering of urogenital tissues are discussed, and examples of tissue engineering techniques designed for specific urogenital structures are presented.

## 34.2 Fundamental Components of Urogenital Tissue Engineering

The main components used to engineer a functional replacement for urogenital tissue are biomaterials (scaffolds, matrices), living cells, and an appropriate microenvironment that can support cell survival and growth. A well-balanced combination of these components is crucial in fabricating engineered tissues or organs for the development of functional substitutes (Langer and Vacanti 1993). Engineering of urogenital tissue may involve matrices alone, wherein the body's natural ability to regenerate is used to orient or direct new tissue growth, or the use of matrices with cells. When cells are used, donor tissue is dissociated into individual cells which are either, implanted directly into the host or expanded in culture, attached to a support matrix and reimplanted after expansion. The implanted tissue can be autologous, allogeneic, or heterologous.

### 34.2.1 Biomaterials

Biomaterials used for urogenital tissue regeneration function as an artificial extracellular matrix (ECM) and elicit biologic and mechanical functions of native ECM found in tissues in the body. Native ECM brings cells together into tissue, controls the tissue structure, and regulates the cell phenotype (Alberts et al. 1994). Biomaterials facilitate the localization and delivery of cells and/or bioactive factors (e.g., cell adhesion peptides, growth factors) to desired sites in the body; define a 3-D space for the formation of new tissues with appropriate structure; and guide the development of new tissues with appropriate function (Kim and Mooney 1998).

The design and selection of the biomaterial is critical in the development of engineered urogenital tissues. The biomaterial must be capable of controlling the structure and function of the engineered tissue in a predesigned manner by interacting with transplanted cells and/or host cells. Generally, the ideal biomaterial should be biocompatible, promote cellular interaction and tissue development, and possess proper mechanical and physical properties. In addition, it should be biodegradable and bioresorbable to support the reconstruction of a completely normal tissue without inflammation. Such behavior of the biomaterials avoids the risk of inflammatory or foreign-body responses that may be associated with the permanent presence of a foreign material in the body. Finally, the degradation rate and the concentration of degradation products in the tissues surrounding the implant must be at a tolerable level (Bergsma et al. 1995).

The biomaterials should provide an appropriate regulation of cell behavior (e.g., adhesion, proliferation, migration, differentiation) in order to promote the development of functional new tissue. Cell behavior in engineered tissues is regulated by multiple interactions with the microenvironment, including interactions with cell-adhesion ligands (Hynes 1992) and with soluble growth factors (Deuel 1997). Cell adhesion—promoting factors (e.g., Arg-Gly-Asp [RGD] amino acid sequences) can be presented by the biomaterial itself or incorporated into the biomaterial in order to control cell behavior through ligand-induced cell receptor signaling processes (Barrera et al. 1993; Cook et al. 1997). The biomaterials provide temporary mechanical support sufficient to withstand *in vivo* forces exerted by the surrounding tissue and maintain a potential space for tissue development. The mechanical support of the biomaterials should be maintained until the engineered tissue has sufficient mechanical integrity to support itself (Atala 2007). This potentially can be achieved by an appropriate choice of mechanical and degradative properties of the biomaterials (Kim and Mooney 1998).

Generally, three classes of biomaterials have been used for engineering of urogenital tissues: naturally derived materials, such as collagen and alginate; acellular tissue matrices, such as bladder submucosa (BSM) and small-intestinal submucosa; and synthetic polymers, such as polyglycolic acid (PGA), polylactic acid (PLA), and poly(lactic-*co*-glycolic acid) (PLGA). These classes of biomaterials have been tested in regard to their biocompatibility with primary human urothelial and bladder muscle cells (Pariente et al. 2001). Naturally derived materials and acellular tissue matrices have the potential advantage of biologic recognition. Synthetic polymers can be produced reproducibly on a large scale with controlled properties of strength, degradation rate, and microstructure.

Collagen is the most abundant and ubiquitous structural protein in the body, and it may be readily purified from both animal and human tissues with an enzyme treatment and salt/acid extraction (Li 1995). Collagen has long been known to exhibit minimal inflammatory and antigenic responses (Furthmayr and Timpl 1976), and it has been approved by the U.S. Food and Drug Administration (FDA) for many types of medical applications, including wound dressings and artificial skin (Cen et al. 2008). Intermolecular cross-linking reduces the degradation rate by making the collagen molecules less susceptible to an enzymatic attack. Intermolecular cross-linking can be accomplished by various physical (e.g., ultraviolet radiation, dehydrothermal treatment) or chemical (e.g., glutaraldehyde, formaldehyde, carbodiimides) techniques (Li 1995). Collagen contains cell-adhesion domain sequences (e.g., RGD) that exhibit specific cellular interactions. This may help to retain the phenotype and activity of many types of cells, including fibroblasts (Silver and Pins 1992) and chondrocytes (Sams and Nixon 1995). This material can be processed into a wide variety of structures such as sponges, fibers, and films (Yannas and Burke 1980a; Yannas et al. 1980b; Cavallaro et al. 1994).

Alginate, a polysaccharide isolated from seaweed, has been used as an injectable cell delivery vehicle (Smidsrod and Skjak-Braek 1990) and a cell immobilization matrix (Lim and Sun 1980) owing to its gentle gelling properties in the presence of divalent ions such as calcium. Alginate is a family of copolymers of D-mannuronate and L-guluronate. The physical and mechanical properties of alginate gel are strongly correlated with the proportion and length of the polyguluronate block in the alginate chains (Smidsrod and Skjak-Braek 1990). Efforts have been made to synthesize biodegradable alginate hydrogels with mechanical properties that are controllable in a wide range by intermolecular covalent cross-linking and with cell-adhesion peptides coupled to their backbones (Rowley et al. 1999).

Polysaccharides include cellulose, alginate, hyaluronic acid, starches, dextran, heparin, chitin, and chitosan, and many of these have been used in tissue engineering and regenerative medicine (Lee et al. 2009). In particular, for urological applications, cellulose and cellulose derivatives have been used as hemostatic agents and sealants (Hong and Loughlin 2006; Msezane et al. 2008). Cellulose and cellulose derivatives are the most abundant natural polymers on the globe and they consist of (1,4)-linked β-D-glucose units. Cellulose has been of particular interest due to its abundance as a renewable resource, biodegradability, and compatibility with biological systems.

Recently, natural materials such as alginate and collagen have been used as "bio-inks" in a newly developed bioprinting technique based on inkjet technology (Boland et al. 2006; Campbell and Weiss 2007). Using this technology, these scaffold materials can be "printed" into a desired scaffold shape using a modified inkjet printer. In addition, several groups have shown that living cells can also be printed using this technology (Laflamme et al. 2005; Nakamura et al. 2005). This exciting technique can be modified so that a 3-D construct containing a precise arrangement of cells, growth factors, and ECM material can be printed (Roth et al. 2004; Ilkhanizadeh et al. 2007; Xu et al. 2009). Such constructs may eventually be implanted into a host to serve as the backbone for a new tissue or organ.

Acellular tissue matrices are collagen-rich matrices prepared by removing cellular components from tissues. The matrices are often prepared by mechanical and chemical manipulation of a segment of bladder tissue (Dahms et al. 1998; Piechota et al. 1998b; Yoo et al. 1998b; Chen et al. 1999). The matrices slowly degrade after implantation and are replaced and remodeled by ECM proteins synthesized and secreted by transplanted or ingrowing cells. Acellular tissue matrices support cell ingrowth and regeneration of urogenital tissues, including urethra and bladder, with no evidence of immunogenic rejection (Probst et al. 1997b; Chen et al. 1999). Because the structures of the proteins (e.g., collagen, elastin) in acellular matrices are well conserved and normally arranged, the mechanical properties of the acellular matrices are not significantly different from those of native BSM (Dahms et al. 1998).

Polyesters of naturally occurring α-hydroxy acids, including PGA, PLA, and PLGA, are widely used in regenerative medicine. These polymers have gained FDA approval for human use in a variety of applications, including sutures (Gilding 1981). The degradation products of PGA, PLA, and PLGA are nontoxic, natural metabolites that are eventually eliminated from the body in the form of carbon dioxide and water (Gilding 1981). Because these polymers are thermoplastics, they can easily be formed into a 3-D scaffold with a desired microstructure, gross shape, and dimension by various techniques, including molding, extrusion (Freed et al. 1994), solvent casting (Mikos et al. 1994), phase separation techniques, and gas foaming techniques (Harris et al. 1998). More recently, techniques such as electrospinning have been used to quickly create highly porous scaffolds in various conformations (Han and Gouma 2006; Choi et al. 2008; Lee et al. 2008a,b).

Many applications in urogenital tissue regeneration require a scaffold with high porosity and a high ratio of surface area to volume. This need has been addressed by processing biomaterials into configurations of fiber meshes and porous sponges using the techniques described previously. More recently, electrospinning techniques have been developed to quickly create highly porous scaffolds in various conformations including nanostructures (Han and Gouma 2006; Choi 2008; Lee et al. 2008a,b). Other biodegradable synthetic polymers, including poly(anhydrides) and poly(ortho-esters), can also be used to fabricate scaffolds for urogenital regeneration with controlled properties (Peppas and Langer 1994).

Nanotechnology, the ability to use small molecules that have distinct properties in a small scale, has been used to create "smart biomaterials for regenerative medicine" (Boccaccini and Blaker 2005; Harrison and Atala 2007). Nanoscaffolds have been manufactured specifically for bladder applications (Harrington et al. 2006). The manufacturing of biomaterials can also lead to enhanced cell alignment and tissue formation (Choi et al. 2008).

## 34.2.2 Cells

Unlike cell-free scaffold systems, cell-based techniques require cell isolation and manipulation. The general strategy for creating a cell-based scaffold is to seed cells onto the desired scaffolds, and then culture the construct *in vitro* for a short period of time. These seeded scaffolds can then be used to construct engineered tissues *in vitro*, and the engineered tissues can be implanted *in vivo* for successful integration with host tissues or organs (Langer and Vacanti 1993). Generally, the use of autologous cells is desirable because of the associated low risk of immune rejection. However, the use of adult tissue-specific autologous cells has many limitations, including difficulty in harvesting certain cell types and difficulty in culturing the cells because of their low proliferative capacity. Therefore, various types of stem cells, such as embryonic stem cells (ES cells), fetal stem cells (amniotic fluid, umbilical, placenta), induced pluripotent state cells (iPS), and tissue specific stem cells have been considered as cell sources for cell-seeded scaffold systems.

ES cells are derived from the inner cell mass of the embryo. These cells are pluripotent and possess the capacity to both self-renew and differentiate into virtually any type of cells in the body (Martin 1981). ES cells have great therapeutic potential, but their use is currently limited by ethical issues surrounding the destruction of embryos required to obtain them.

Fetal and neonatal amniotic fluid and placenta are known to contain multipotent cells, which may be useful in cell-based applications. The amniotic fluid and placental membrane contain a heterogeneous population of cell types derived from the developing fetus (Priest et al. 1978; Polgar et al. 1989). In addition, the isolation and characterization of multipotent human and mouse amniotic-fluid and placental-derived stem (AFPS) cells in 2007, indicated that AFPS cells display extensive self-renewal properties and can give rise to cells from all three germ layers (De Coppi et al. 2007a). Unlike ES cells, the AFPS cells do not form teratomas *in vivo*, strongly suggesting they could be used in future clinical applications. AFPS cell lines can be differentiated into adipogenic, osteogenic, endothelial, myogenic, neural-like, and hepatic lineages and the differentiated cells resulting from the AFPS cells are able to perform specialized tissue functions.

Adult stem cells, on the other hand, are usually isolated from tissues, organs, or bone marrow biopsies. Like ES and AFPS cells, adult stem cells have the ability to self-renew and they can differentiate into various types of cells, but their differentiation is limited to tissue-specific lineages. Many techniques for isolating and harvesting adult stem cells such as hematopoietic stem cells (Ballas et al. 2002), neural stem cells from brain (Taupin 2006; Jiao and Chen 2008), mesenchymal stem cells from bone marrow and fat (Caplan and Bruder 2001; Jiang et al. 2002; Crisan et al. 2008), liver stem cells from liver (Ikeda et al. 2008; Mimeault and Batra 2008), muscle satellite cells from skeletal muscle (Crisan, Casteilla et al. 2008), and epithelial stem cells from gut tissue (Spradling et al. 2001), have been developed over the past few decades. However, these native tissue progenitor cells are often difficult to isolate and/or maintain in culture. Despite this challenge, a number of culture techniques have been developed to increase the success of these cultures. Tissue-specific progenitor cells with unipotent capabiltiy can be derived from most tissues or organs. The advantage of these cells is that they are already programmed to become the target cell type, without any extra-lineage differentiation. By noting the location of the progenitor cells, as well as by exploring the conditions that promote differentiation and/or self-renewal, it has been possible to overcome some of the obstacles that limit cell expansion *in vitro*. One example is the urothelial cell. Urothelial cells could not be grown in the laboratory setting in the past, but only with limited success. It was believed that urothelial cells had a natural senescence that was hard to overcome. Several protocols have been developed over the last two decades that have improved urothelial growth and expansion (Cilento et al. 1994; Liebert et al. 1997; Scriven et al. 1997; Puthenveettil et al. 1999). A system of urothelial cell harvesting was developed that does not use any enzymes or serum and has a large expansion potential. Using these methods of cell culture, it is possible to expand a urothelial strain from a single specimen that initially covers a surface area of 1 cm$^2$ to one covering a surface area of 4202 m$^2$ (the equivalent area of one football field) within 8 weeks (Cilento et al. 1994).

Recently, reports of the successful transformation of adult cells into pluripotent stem cells through a type of genetic "reprogramming" have been published. Reprogramming is a technique that involves de-differentiation of adult somatic cells to produce patient-specific pluripotent stem cells, eliminating the need to create embryos. Cells generated by reprogramming would be genetically identical to the somatic cells (and thus, the patient who donated these cells) and would not be rejected. Yamanaka was the first to discover that mouse embryonic fibroblasts (MEFs) and adult mouse fibroblasts could be reprogrammed into an "iPS" (Takahashi and Yamanaka 2006). These iPS cells possessed the immortal growth characteristics of self-renewing ES cells, expressed genes specific for ES cells, and generated embryoid bodies *in vitro* and teratomas *in vivo*. When iPS cells were injected into mouse blastocysts, they contributed to a variety of cell types. However, although iPS cells selected in this way were pluripotent, they were not identical to ES cells. Unlike ES cells, chimeras made from iPS cells did not result in full-term pregnancies. Gene expression profiles of the iPS cells showed that they possessed a distinct gene expression signature that was different from that of ES cells. In addition, the epigenetic state of the iPS cells was somewhere between that found in somatic cells and that found in ES cells, suggesting that the reprogramming was incomplete.

These results were improved significantly by Wernig and Jaenisch in July 2007 (Wernig et al. 2007). In this study, DNA methylation, gene expression profiles, and the chromatin state of the reprogrammed cells were similar to those of ES cells. Teratomas induced by these cells contained differentiated cell types representing all three embryonic germ layers. Most importantly, the reprogrammed cells from this experiment were able to form viable chimeras and contribute to the germ line like ES cells, suggesting that these iPS cells were completely reprogrammed. It has recently been shown that reprogramming of human cells is possible (Takahashi et al. 2007; Yu et al. 2007). Yamanaka generated human iPS cells that are similar to human ES (hES) cells in terms of morphology, proliferation, gene expression, surface markers, and teratoma formation. Thompson's group showed that retroviral transduction of the stem cell markers *OCT4, SOX2, NANOG,* and *LIN28* could generate pluripotent stem cells. However, in both studies, the human iPS cells were similar but not identical to hES cells. Although reprogramming is an exciting phenomenon, our limited understanding of the mechanism underlying it currently limits the clinical applicability of the technique, but the future potential of reprogramming is quite exciting.

### 34.2.3 Controlling the Microenvironment Using Biomaterials

Appropriate microenvironments are also critical in the success of tissue regeneration. The roles of natural ECM and signaling molecules such as growth factors and cytokines are closely involved in cell attachment, growth, migration, differentiation, and other functions. Because the cell-free system does not require cell seeding of the scaffold, the success of tissue regeneration is closely related to its ability to recruit enough cells and reprogram these cells to form a new tissue. Thus, growth factors and cytokines play significant roles in cell-free scaffold systems, because these factors act on the target therapeutic cells or their niches *in vivo* to promote cell mobilization into scaffolds as well as growth and reprogramming of recruited cells within the scaffolds (Lee et al. 2008c; Xu et al. 2008; Zhao and Karp 2009). The release of these signaling factors should be controlled to overcome the short half-life of free growth factors. For instance, growth factors encapsulated in microspheres show a controlled-release profile using nanoscale double emulsion methods (Hanson et al. 2008) and sequential delivery of dual growth factors based on different degradation times or diffusion properties of vehicle materials is desirable for efficient tissue regeneration (Richardson et al. 2001; Sohier et al. 2006). Also, tethering growth factors to scaffolds is a very promising strategy in maximizing their effects, as this prevents internalization of growth-factor-receptor complexes by cells (Mann et al. 2001; Segers and Lee 2007; Mehta et al. 2010). For example, incorporated basic fibroblast growth factor (bFGF, FGF-2), an angiogenic factor, within a collagen scaffold was used to promote bladder regeneration in an animal study using rats (Chen et al. 2010c). Vascular endothelial growth factor (VEGF) and nerve growth factor were combined into bladder acellular matrix and synergistically regenerated functional bladder tissue in a rat model of neurogenic bladder (Kikuno et al. 2009). Several other growth factors such as hepatocyte growth factor, platelet derived growth factor-BB, insulin like growth factor-1 and heparin binding epidermal growth factor-like growth factor can be incorporated into bladder acellular matrix for urological tissue regeneration (Kanematsu et al. 2004). More promisingly, delivery of multiple growth factors at rates mimicking the *in vivo* environment has great potential in clinical applications of tissue regeneration (Chen et al. 2010a).

## 34.3 Engineering Specific Urogenital Structures

### 34.3.1 Bladder

Currently, gastrointestinal segments are commonly used in bladder repair or reconstruction procedures, but this technique has a number of limitations including infection, perforation, metabolic disturbances, urolithiasis (stone formation), and even malignancy (McDougal 1992; Atala et al. 1993; Kaefer et al. 1997). To solve these problems, physicians and scientists are turning to the field of tissue engineering. Two general strategies have been developed for bladder reconstruction using tissue engineering: a cell-free method and a cell-based scaffold system.

Cell-free scaffold systems use scaffolds without cells to create a microenvironment that is conducive to tissue regeneration. Several scaffolds and biomaterials have been used to substitute for the damaged bladder wall in bladder augmentation procedures. These biomaterials have been composed of both natural and synthetic materials including collagen, polyvinyl sponges, PGA, and Teflon. Most of these studies showed that there are limitations to using cell-free scaffolds, however. Biocompatibility issues have been reported, and this leads to biomechanical and other functional problems in the repaired bladder, including scarring, reduced reservoir volume, and graft contraction (Atala 1996, 1998).

Alternatively, small intestinal sub-mucosa (SIS) has been used for bladder regeneration. SIS was developed by the Badylak group for vascular repair (Badylak et al. 1989) and has also been used in urological applications. When SIS derived from porcine small intestine was used for bladder augmentation, it resulted in the formation of a transitional layer that was similar to that seen in the native bladder (Kropp et al. 1996a,b). More interestingly, functional cholinergic and purinergic innervation were found in both dogs (Kropp et al. 1996b) and rats (Vaught et al. 1996) that were reconstructed using SIS. However, in the dog study, SIS without cells eventually led to graft shrinkage (Zhang et al. 2006), indicating that SIS alone may not be sufficient for functional bladder reconstruction.

Other trials have been attempted using acellular bladder matrices (ABM) that were produced by mechanically and chemically removing all the cellular components from donor bladder tissue (Sutherland et al. 1996; Probst et al. 1997a; Piechota et al. 1998a; Yoo et al. 1998b; Wefer et al. 2001). Antigenicity was not evident in these studies, indicating that removal of the cellular components was successful. The matrices were able to serve as vehicles for partial bladder regeneration, but it was shown that they were not sufficient when the defect to be repaired was large. Like most cell-free scaffolds used in bladder regeneration, nonseeded ABM grafts showed promising results in terms of regenerating urothelial cell layers normally, but the muscle layer was not completely formed (Kropp et al. 1996b; Sutherland et al. 1996; Probst et al. 1997a; Yoo et al. 1998b; Zhang et al. 2006; Jayo et al. 2008b). This suggests that cell-based scaffold systems using bladder muscle cells may be critical to promote the formation of normal bladder structure and function.

Cell-based scaffold systems for bladder regeneration that are based on the use of isolated urothelial and smooth muscle cells, which are the key cellular components of the native bladder, have shown promise in early studies. In order to engineer bladder tissue *in vitro*, these cell types can be cultured and expanded *in vitro*, seeded on scaffolds, and allowed to adhere to the scaffold. They then form cellular structures on the scaffold, and this construct can be implanted into the patient. It is hypothesized that the tissue engineered 3D bladder, will exhibit fully differentiated cell populations after implantation *in vivo* and the presence of these cells will reduce the inflammatory immune response to the matrix as well as prevent graft contraction and shrinkage.

In one study, cell-seeded allogeneic ABM were used for bladder augmentation in dogs (Yoo et al. 1998b). The dog study demonstrated that matrices with autologous urothelial and smooth muscle cells produced bladder tissue that was much more similar to native bladder tissue compared to the tissue that resulted from the use of matrices without cells. The regenerated bladder tissues contained a normal cellular organization consisting of a urothelial layer surrounded by smooth muscle tissue, and urodynamic studies indicated that the bladder compliance was normal. The bladders augmented with cell-seeded matrices showed a significant increase (100%) in capacity compared with bladders augmented with cell-free matrices, which showed only a 30% increase in capacity. In addition, bladders augmented with cell-seeded matrices retained most of their diameter, while matrices implanted without cells led to graft contraction and shrinkage.

These studies were performed with biodegradable synthetic polymers and showed similar results in long-term studies (Jayo et al. 2008a,b). However, not all scaffolds perform this well if a large portion of the bladder needs replacement. Using a canine model of subtotal cystectomy, seeded and unseeded SIS were used to reconstruct the bladder. In this case, both the unseeded and seeded groups developed severely shrunken bladders and histologically, severe inflammation, fibroblast infiltration, and muscle hypertrophy could be seen (Zhang et al. 2006). Therefore, the selection of an appropriate scaffold is critical for the success of bladder tissue engineering. More recently, several studies were reported to enhance bladder regeneration through scaffold modification, such as the fabrication of modified SIS using biodegradable nanoparticles (Mondalek et al. 2010), production of a compressed collagen gel to improve mechanical properties (Engelhardt et al. 2010), and fabrication of topographically modified scaffolds with nanosurfaces (Chun et al. 2009). Various cell sources were used in these studies, including mesenchymal stem cells (Tian et al. 2010) and hair stem cells (Drewa 2008; Drewa et al. 2009). In addition, the use of bioreactors, in which mechanical stimulation can be applied to improve the cellular environment and facilitate cell–cell and cell-ECM during bladder engineering *in vitro*, has also been proposed as an important parameter for success (Farhat and Yeger 2008; Devarapalli et al. 2009).

Engineered bladder tissue for cystoplasty was used clinically in a small study starting in 1998. In this pilot study of seven patients, a cell seeded collagen scaffold either with or without omental coverage, or a combined PGA-collagen scaffold seeded with cells and covered with omentum was tested. The patients reconstructed with the engineered bladder tissue using the PGA-collagen cell-seeded scaffolds with omental coverage showed increased compliance, decreased end-filling pressures, increased capacities, and longer dry periods over time (Atala et al. 2006).

From the results above, it is evident that at this time, the use of cell-seeded matrices is superior to the use of nonseeded matrices for the reconstruction of large portions of the bladder. Although advances have been made with the engineering of bladder tissues, many challenges remain. Current research in many centers is aimed at the development of biologically active and "smart" biomaterials that may improve tissue regeneration.

## 34.3.2 Kidney

Although kidney transplantation has been successfully applied to patients with end-stage renal disease for many years, this therapy is hampered by the severe shortage of donor organs. Regenerative medicine may be able to provide solutions to this problem through the development of tissue engineered kidney structures and cell transplantation therapy (Osafune 2010, May 6 Epub ahead of print). However, due to the anatomical complexity of the kidney, which includes delicate structures such as nephrons and collecting ducts, and the need for communication between each individual cell to fulfill renal function, multidisciplinary strategies are required to organize and build a functional kidney structure in the laboratory (Yokoo and Kawamura 2009).

In most cases, trials of renal regeneration were developed using cell-based scaffold system. First of all, the development of reliable renal cell sources (Prockop 1997; Kale et al. 2003; Lin et al. 2003; Ikarashi et al. 2005; Lin et al. 2005; Yokoo et al. 2005) is the required for this. Appropriate conditions must be provided to ensure the long-term survival, differentiation, and growth of many different types of cells (Milici et al. 1985; Carley et al. 1988; Humes and Cieslinski 1992; Schena 1998). Next, appropriate synthetic biodegradable polymers to use as a template are required to provide structural support for cells. One of the first attempts at kidney regeneration using cells was performed with rabbit kidney cells. Kidney cells from distal tubules, glomeruli, and proximal tubules were expanded separately and then seeded onto PGA scaffolds. The cell seeded scaffolds were implanted subcutaneously into host athymic mice. Histological examination showed that nephron segments had formed within the polymer structures, and these cells were able to proliferate, as evidenced by BrdU staining. In another study, single renal cells were seeded onto biodegradable polymers and implanted into immune competent syngeneic hosts. These single cells appeared to proliferate, and they organized cord-like structures with host epithelial cells. These results demonstrated that single suspended cells are capable of reconstituting tubular structures, with homogeneous cell types within each tubule.

Other synthetic polymers have been used as cell scaffolds in renal tissue engineering as well. A tubular device constructed from polycarbonate was used as a scaffold for supporting mouse renal cells (Yoo et al. 1996). The tubular device was connected at one end to a silastic catheter which terminated in a reservoir, and this construct was implanted subcutaneously in athymic mice. Histological examination of the implanted device demonstrated extensive vascularization as well as formation of glomeruli and highly organized tubule-like structures. Immunocytochemical staining confirmed the presence of both proximal and distal tubular cells and cells of the thin ascending loop of Henle. Interestingly, the newly formed structures exhibited renal function by excreting high levels of solute through a yellow urine-like fluid (Yoo et al. 1996).

However, naturally derived scaffolds may have better biocompatibility and elicit fewer immune reactions than synthetic biodegradable polymers. Collagen-based scaffolds have been increasingly used in many applications (De Filippo et al. 2002; El-Kassaby et al. 2003; Falke et al. 2003; Atala et al. 2006; Murray et al. 2006). Moreover, it is thought that the use of an acellular kidney matrix would allow for transplantation of a larger number of cells due to its 3-D kidney-like architecture, resulting in greater renal tissue volumes. Thus, an acellular collagen-based kidney matrix, which is similar to the native renal architecture, was developed. In a subsequent study, it was investigated whether these collagen-based matrices could support the growth of renal cells as well as accommodate large enough volumes of renal cells to form kidney structures *in vivo* (Amiel et al. 2000).

Isolation of particular cell types that produce renal-specific factors may be a good approach for selective cell therapies to treat aspects of renal failure. For example, cells that produce erythropoietin have been isolated in culture, and these cells could eventually be used to treat the anemia that results from end-stage renal failure (Aboushwareb et al. 2008). Other more ambitious approaches are working towards the goal of total renal functional replacement. To create kidney tissue that would deliver full renal function, a culture containing all of the cell types comprising functional nephron units should be used. Optimal culture conditions to nurture renal cells have been extensively studied and cells grown under these conditions have been reported to maintain their cellular characteristics (Lanza et al. 2002).

Recent investigative efforts in the search for a reliable cell source have been expanded to stem and progenitor cells. Use of these cells for tissue regeneration is attractive due to their ability to differentiate and mature into all of the specific cell types needed. This is particularly useful in instances where primary renal cells are unavailable due to extensive tissue damage. Bone marrow-derived human mesenchymal stem cells have been shown to be a potential source due to their ability to differentiate into several cell lineages (Prockop 1997; Kale et al. 2003; Ikarashi et al. 2005). These cells have been shown to participate in kidney development when they are placed in a rat embryonic niche that allows for continued exposure to a repertoire of nephrogenic signals (Yokoo et al. 2005). These cells, however, were found to contribute mainly to regeneration of damaged glomerular endothelial cells after injury. The major cell source of kidney regeneration was found to originate from intrarenal cells in an ischemic renal injury model (Lin et al. 2005).

Another potential cell source for kidney regeneration is circulating stem cells, which have been shown to transform into tubular and glomerular epithelial cells, podocytes, mesangial cells, and interstitial cells after renal injury (Ito et al. 2001; Poulsom et al. 2001; Gupta et al. 2002; Iwano et al. 2002; Kale et al. 2003; Lin et al. 2003; Rookmaaker et al. 2003). Other stem cell types, such as human ES cells (Lin 2006), and the more recently discovered human amniotic fluid and placental stem cells can also differentiate into renal cells (Perin et al. 2007). In addition, studies have been completed to determine whether renal tissue could be formed using an alternative cell source. Nuclear transplantation (therapeutic cloning) was performed to generate histocompatible tissues, and the feasibility of engineering syngeneic renal tissues *in vivo* using these cloned cells was investigated (Lanza et al. 2002). Nuclear material from bovine dermal fibroblasts was transferred into unfertilized enucleated donor bovine eggs. Renal cells from the cloned embryos were harvested, expanded *in vitro*, and seeded onto 3-D renal devices. The devices were implanted into the back of the same steer from which the cells were cloned, and were retrieved 12 weeks later. This process produced functioning renal units. Urine production and viability were demonstrated after transplantation back into the nuclear donor animal. Chemical analysis suggested unidirectional secretion and concentration of urea nitrogen and creatinine. Microscopic analysis revealed formation of organized glomeruli and tubular structures. Immunohistochemical and real time polymerase chain reaction (RT-PCR) analysis confirmed the expression of renal mRNA and proteins. These studies demonstrated that cells derived from nuclear transfer can be successfully harvested, expanded in culture, and transplanted *in vivo* with the use of biodegradable scaffolds on which the single suspended cells can organize into tissue structures that are genetically identical to that of the host. These studies were the first demonstration of the use of therapeutic cloning for regeneration of tissues *in vivo*.

Very recently, endothelial progenitor cells encapsulated in a bioartificial niche such as hyaluronic acid gel were tested (Ratliff et al. 2010). These observations suggest that controlling stem and progenitor cell differentiation may lead to successful regeneration of kidney tissues.

### 34.3.3 Urethra

Various matrices have been developed for the purpose of urethral tissue regeneration, from biodegradable synthetic polymers such as woven meshes of PGA without cells (Bazeed et al. 1983; Olsen et al.

1992), to naturally derived collagen-based materials such bladder-derived acellular submucosa (Chen et al. 1999), and an acellular urethral submucosa (Sievert et al. 2000) in various animal models.

A relatively simple structured urethral replacement was constructed using porcine BSM (Chen et al. 1999), which proved to be a suitable substitute for repair of urethral defects in rabbits. A normal urothelial luminal lining developed, and organized muscle bundles could be seen in the scaffold matrix implanted *in vivo*. The successful outcome of this study led to clinical trials, in which some urethral defects were repaired using human bladder acellular collagen matrices (Atala et al. 1999). The neourethras were created by anastomosing the matrix in an onlay fashion to the urethral plate, and the size of the created neourethra ranged from 5 to 15 cm. After a 3-year follow-up, three of the four patients had a successful outcome in regard to cosmetic appearance and function. One patient who had a 15-cm repair developed a subglanular fistula. Similar results were obtained using acellular collagen-based matrix. Both pediatric and adult patients with primary urethral stricture disease showed successful results using this matrix (El-Kassaby et al. 2003). Another study in 30 patients with recurrent stricture disease showed that a healthy urethral bed ( two or fewer prior urethral surgeries) was needed for successful urethral reconstruction using the acellular collage-based grafts (el-Kassaby et al. 2008).

While cell-free scaffolds were successfully applied to onlay urethral repairs experimentally and clinically, it has been shown that in cases in which a tubularized repair of the urethra is needed, cell-seeding is required because when cell-free tubular scaffolds are used, inadequate urethral tissue regeneration occurs, leading to graft contracture and stricture formation (De Filippo et al. 2002). In one study, the use of collagen-based matrices seeded with autologous rabbit urothelial and smooth muscle cells (Kim et al. 2008) was shown to form new tissue that was structurally similar to native urethra. Unlike the tubularized collagen matrices without cells, these cell seeded matrices did not result in severe inflammation, fibrosis, and stricture formation. These findings were confirmed clinically. A clinical trial using tubularized nonseeded SIS for urethral stricture repair was performed in eight patients. Two patients with short inflammatory strictures maintained urethral patency. Stricture recurrence developed in the other six patients within 3 months of surgery (le Roux 2005). Other cell types such as epidermal cells and oral keratinocytes (Fu et al. 2007; Li et al. 2008a,b) have also been tried experimentally with acellular collagen matrices for urethral reconstruction. Finally, a gene transfection technique was adapted for urethral reconstruction using VEGF gene-modified urothelial cells (Guan et al. 2008).

## 34.3.4 Penis

One of the major limitations of penile reconstructive surgery is the availability of sufficient autologous tissue for use in reconstruction. Penile reconstruction was initially attempted in the late 1930s, where rib cartilage was used as a stiffener for patients with traumatic penile loss (Goodwin and Scott 1952). This material was soon discontinued due to the unsatisfactory functional and cosmetic results. Silicone rigid prostheses were developed in the 1970s and have been used widely (Small et al. 1975; Bretan 1989). However, biocompatibility issues have been a problem in selected patients (Thomalla et al. 1987; Nukui et al. 1997). Tissue transfer techniques with flaps from various nongenital sources such as the groin, dorsalis pedis, and forearm, have been used for genital reconstruction (Jordan 1999). However, operative complications such as infection, graft failure, and donor site morbidity still remained. As such, the development of a natural prosthesis composed of autologous cells was proposed. In a initial study (Yoo et al. 1998a), chondrocytes harvested from the articular surface of calf shoulders was isolated, grown, and expanded in culture. The cells were seeded onto preformed cylindrical PGA polymer rods and implanted in mice. The retrieved scaffolds seeded with cells showed milky-white, rod-shaped, solid cartilage structures. The constructs maintained their preimplantation size and shape. In a subsequent study using an autologous system, the feasibility of applying the engineered cartilage rods *in situ* was investigated (Yoo et al. 1999). Autologous chondrocytes harvested from rabbit ear were seeded onto biodegradable poly-L-lactic acid coated PGA polymer rods and implanted into the corporal spaces of rabbits. The retrieved scaffolds showed the presence of well-formed, milky-white cartilage structures within the corpora at 1 month as well mating activity. In another study using human cartilage rods, chondrocytes isolated from human ear were seeded on rod shaped biodegradable polymer scaffolds. The engineered human cartilaginous rods were flexible, elastic and able to withstand high degrees of compressive forces. The mechanical properties were comparable to those of commercially available silicone prostheses (Kim et al. 2002).

One of the major components of the penis is corporal smooth muscle, and autologous smooth muscle cells have been applied to reconstruct corporal (erectile) tissue *de novo* in several studies. Corporal smooth muscle cells were able to regenerate cavernosal tissue *de novo* when seeded onto biodegradable polymers (Kershen et al. 2002). Importantly, it has also been shown that 3-D capillary networks can be formed when endothelial cells from the corpus cavernosum are cultured on collagen. Human corporal smooth muscle cells and endothelial cells seeded on biodegradable polymer scaffolds were able to create vascularized cavernosal muscle when implanted *in vivo* (Park et al. 1999). In addition, acellular collagen matrices derived from processed donor rabbit corpora was used as a cell supportive scaffold, where human corpus cavernosal muscle and endothelial cells from donor penile tissue were expanded *in vitro*. Histological studies showed that the appropriate cell architecture formed within the collagen matrices 4 weeks after implantation (Falke et al. 2003).

In order to investigate the functional parameters of the engineered corpora, acellular corporal collagen matrices obtained from donor rabbit penis were seeded with autologous corpus cavernosal smooth muscle and endothelial cells. Histological studies demonstrated that the urethra was intact and the cells were interposed into the corporal space. Normal functional and structural parameters (cavernosography, cavernosometry, mating behavior, and sperm ejaculation) were confirmed up to 6 months after implantation, and female rabbits mated with the reconstructed males were able to conceive (Kwon et al. 2002). This technology was further confirmed when the entire rabbit corpora was removed and replaced with the engineered scaffolds seeded with autologous cell seeded collagen matrices. This neocorpora showed continuous integration into native tissue and physiologically normal in terms of contraction and relaxation in response to electric field and pharmacological stimulation. With the results of mating activity and reproductive function by the presence of sperm in engineered corpora, this strategy was proven to reconstruct structurally and functionally normal neocorpora when implanted (Chen et al. 2010b).

## 34.3.5 Testis

Patients with testicular dysfunction require androgen replacement for somatic development and maintenance. Conventional treatment for testicular dysfunction consists of periodic intramuscular injections of chemically modified testosterone or, more recently, skin patch applications. However, long-term pulsatile testosterone therapy is not optimal and can cause multiple problems, including disregulated erythropoiesis and bone density changes.

Leydig cells are the major source of testosterone production in males. An interesting controlled-release testosterone delivery system was designed using these cells. Leydig cells were microencapsulated in an alginate-poly-L-lysine solution and the encapsulated cells were injected into castrated animals to determine whether they would survive and continue producing physiologic levels of testosterone. Serum testosterone was measured serially. This experiment showed that the animals were able to maintain testosterone levels in the long term (Machluf and Atala 1998; Machluf et al. 2000), suggesting feasibility of the microencapsulation method for Leydig cells for replacement or supplementation of testosterone production (Lo et al. 2004).

Further studies showed that testicular prostheses created with chondrocytes in bioreactors could be loaded with testosterone and implanted *in vivo*. The prostheses were implanted in athymic mice with bilateral anorchia, and they released testosterone long term and maintained androgen levels in the physiologic range (Raya-Rivera et al. 2008). Recently, the Leydig cell technology was combined with these engineered prostheses for the long term functional replacement of androgen levels as well as sperm production (Nagano and Brinster 1998). In addition, fertility has been restored in mice with the transplantation of male germ line stem cells (Ogawa et al. 2000). Use of other cell types such as spermatogonial stem cells (Lo et al. 2005) and Sertoli cells, the main component of the testicular germ cell niche, can support spermatogenesis (Shinohara et al. 2003).

### 34.3.6 Vagina

Several pathological conditions, including congenital malformations and malignancy, can adversely affect normal vaginal development or anatomy. Vaginal reconstruction has traditionally been challenging due to the paucity of available native tissue. For vaginal reconstruction, acellular materials have been used experimentally in rats (Wefer et al. 2002) and cell-based scaffold systems were also investigated using vaginal derived cells (De Filippo et al. 2003). Vaginal epithelial and smooth muscle cells of female rabbits were seeded onto biodegradable polymer scaffolds, and the cell-seeded constructs were then implanted into mice. Functional studies in the tissue-engineered constructs showed similar properties to those of normal vaginal tissue. When these constructs were used for autologous total vaginal replacement in a rabbit model, patent functional vaginal structures were noted in the tissue-engineered specimens, while the noncell-seeded structures were noted to be stenotic (De Filippo et al. 2008). These studies indicated that a regenerative medicine approach to clinical vaginal reconstruction would be a realistic possibility. Clinical trials are currently being conducted.

## 34.4 Perspective

With new advances in biomaterial science, scaffold fabrication, and established cell culture methods, the fields of urogenital tissue engineering and regenerative medicine have advanced quickly within the last decade. Many experimental studies have now been performed to test new strategies for the repair or replacement of damaged or dysfunctional urologic tissues and organs, and some of these are now clinically applicable. However, the reconstruction of fully functional tissues is still challenging, and this therapy is not in widespread clinical use. In order to achieve this goal, multidisciplinary research in regenerative medicine should be conducted in a well-balanced manner. First, the combination of mechanically and structurally "smart" biomaterials and bioactive signaling can enhance efficient urological tissue regeneration by providing cells with biological cues that aid in the formation of new tissues (Azzarello et al. 2009; Yang et al. 2010). In addition, by controlling stem cell behavior with biological signaling so that the native regeneration system of the body operates properly (Roessger et al. 2009), it may be possible to enhance the efficiency of tissue formation on various scaffold materials. Finally, new techniques to manipulate and differentiate ES cells (Frimberger et al. 2006), iPS cells (De Coppi et al. 2007b), and adult stem cells into urologic lineages would allow these other cells to be used in addition to autologous cell isolation and expansion. There have been several trials to enhance the functional properties of tissue engineered products (Chen et al. 2010b), but these still need to be evaluated over the long term.

## Acknowledgment

The authors wish to thank Dr. Jennifer L. Olson for editorial assistance.

## References

Aboushwareb, T., F. Egydio, L. Straker et al. 2008. Erythropoietin producing cells for potential cell therapy. _World J Urol_ 26:295–300.

Alberts, B., D. Bray, and J. M. Lewis. 1994. The extracellular matrix of animals. In _Molecular Biology of the Cell_. B. Alberts, D. Bray and J. M. Lewis (eds.). New York, NY, Garland Publishing: 971–995.

Amiel, G. E., J. J. Yoo, and A. Atala. 2000. Renal tissue engineering using a collagen-based kidney matrix. *Tissue Eng Suppl.* 6:685.

Atala, A. 1996. This month in investigative urology: Commentary on the replacement of urologic associated mucosa. *J Urol* 156:338–339.

Atala, A. 1998. Autologous cell transplantation for urologic reconstruction. *J Urol* 159:2–3.

Atala, A. 2007. Engineering tissues, organs and cells. *J Tissue Eng Regen Med* 1:83–96.

Atala, A., S. B. Bauer, W. H. Hendren, and A. B. Retik. 1993. The effect of gastric augmentation on bladder function. *J Urol* 149:1099–1102.

Atala, A., S. B. Bauer, S. Soker, J. J. Yoo, and A. B. Retik. 2006. Tissue-engineered autologous bladders for patients needing cystoplasty. *Lancet* 367:1241–1246.

Atala, A., L. Guzman, and A. B. Retik. 1999. A novel inert collagen matrix for hypospadias repair. *J Urol* 162:1148–1151.

Azzarello, J., B. P. Kropp, K. M. Fung, and H. K. Lin. 2009. Age-dependent vascular endothelial growth factor expression and angiogenic capability of bladder smooth muscle cells: Implications for cell-seeded technology in bladder tissue engineering. *J Tissue Eng Regen Med* 3:579–589.

Badylak, S. F., G. C. Lantz, A. Coffey, and L. A. Geddes. 1989. Small intestinal submucosa as a large diameter vascular graft in the dog. *J Surg Res* 47:74–80.

Ballas, C. B., S. P. Zielske, and S. L. Gerson. 2002. Adult bone marrow stem cells for cell and gene therapies: Implications for greater use. *J Cell Biochem Suppl* 38:20–28.

Barrera, D. A., E. Zylstra, P. T. Lansbury, and R. Langer. 1993. Synthesis and RGD peptide modification of a new biodegradable copolymer poly (lactic acid-*co*-lysine). *J Am Chem Soc* 115:11010–11011.

Bazeed, M. A., J. W. Thuroff, R. A. Schmidt, and E. A. Tanagho. 1983. New treatment for urethral strictures. *Urology* 21:53–57.

Bergsma, J. E., F. R. Rozema, R. R. Bos et al. 1995. *In vivo* degradation and biocompatibility study of *in vitro* pre-degraded as-polymerized polyactide particles. *Biomaterials* 16:267–274.

Boccaccini, A. R. and J. J. Blaker. 2005. Bioactive composite materials for tissue engineering scaffolds. *Expert Rev Med Devices* 2:303–317.

Boland, T., T. Xu, B. Damon, and X. Cui. 2006. Application of inkjet printing to tissue engineering. *Biotechnol J* 1:910–917.

Bretan, P. N., Jr. 1989. History of the prosthetic treatment of impotence. *Urol Clin North Am* 16:1–5.

Campbell, P. G. and L. E. Weiss. 2007. Tissue engineering with the aid of inkjet printers. *Expert Opin Biol Ther* 7:1123–1127.

Caplan, A. I. and S. P. Bruder. 2001. Mesenchymal stem cells: Building blocks for molecular medicine in the 21st century. *Trends Mol Med* 7:259–264.

Carley, W. W., A. J. Milici, and J. A. Madri. 1988. Extracellular matrix specificity for the differentiation of capillary endothelial cells. *Exp Cell Res* 178:426–434.

Cavallaro, J. F., P. D. Kemp, and K. H. Kraus. 1994. Collagen fabrics as biomaterials. *Biotechnol Bioeng* 43:781–791.

Cen, L., W. Liu, L. Cui, W. Zhang, and Y. Cao. 2008. Collagen tissue engineering: Development of novel biomaterials and applications. *Pediatr Res* 63:492–496.

Chen, F., J. J. Yoo, and A. Atala. 1999. Acellular collagen matrix as a possible "off the shelf" biomaterial for urethral repair. *Urology* 54:407–410.

Chen, F. M., M. Zhang, and Z. F. Wu. 2010a. Toward delivery of multiple growth factors in tissue engineering. *Biomaterials* 31:6279–6308.

Chen, K. L., D. Eberli, J. J. Yoo, and A. Atala. 2010b. Bioengineered corporal tissue for structural and functional restoration of the penis. *Proc Natl Acad Sci USA* 107:3346–3350.

Chen, W., C. Shi, S. Yi et al. 2010c. Bladder regeneration by collagen scaffolds with collagen binding human basic fibroblast growth factor. *J Urol* 183:2432–2439.

Choi, J. S., S. J. Lee, G. J. Christ, A. Atala, and J. J. Yoo. 2008. The influence of electrospun aligned poly(epsilon-caprolactone)/collagen nanofiber meshes on the formation of self-aligned skeletal muscle myotubes. *Biomaterials* 29:2899–2906.

Chun, Y. W., D. Khang, K. M. Haberstroh, and T. J. Webster. 2009. The role of polymer nanosurface roughness and submicron pores in improving bladder urothelial cell density and inhibiting calcium oxalate stone formation. *Nanotechnology* 20:085104.

Cilento, B. G., M. R. Freeman, F. X. Schneck, A. B. Retik, and A. Atala. 1994. Phenotypic and cytogenetic characterization of human bladder urothelia expanded *in vitro*. *J Urol* 152:665–670.

Cook, A. D., J. S. Hrkach, N. N. Gao et al. 1997. Characterization and development of RGD-peptide-modified poly(lactic acid-co-lysine) as an interactive, resorbable biomaterial. *J Biomed Mater Res* 35:513–523.

Crisan, M., L. Casteilla, L. Lehr et al. 2008. A reservoir of brown adipocyte progenitors in human skeletal muscle. *Stem Cells* 26:2425–2433.

Dahms, S. E., H. J. Piechota, R. Dahiya, T. F. Lue, and E. A. Tanagho. 1998. Composition and biomechanical properties of the bladder acellular matrix graft: Comparative analysis in rat, pig and human. *Br J Urol* 82:411–419.

De Coppi, P., G. Bartsch, Jr., M. M. Siddiqui et al. 2007a. Isolation of amniotic stem cell lines with potential for therapy. *Nat Biotechnol* 25:100–106.

De Coppi, P., A. Callegari, A. Chiavegato et al. 2007b. Amniotic fluid and bone marrow derived mesenchymal stem cells can be converted to smooth muscle cells in the cryo-injured rat bladder and prevent compensatory hypertrophy of surviving smooth muscle cells. *J Urol* 177:369–376.

De Filippo, R. E., C. E. Bishop, L. F. Filho, J. J. Yoo, and A. Atala. 2008. Tissue engineering a complete vaginal replacement from a small biopsy of autologous tissue. *Transplantation* 86:208–214.

De Filippo, R. E., J. J. Yoo, and A. Atala. 2002. Urethral replacement using cell seeded tubularized collagen matrices. *J Urol* 168:1789–1792; discussion 1792–1783.

De Filippo, R. E., J. J. Yoo, and A. Atala. 2003. Engineering of vaginal tissue *in vivo*. *Tissue Eng* 9:301–306.

Deuel, T. F. (1997). Growth factors. *Principles of Tissue Engineering*. R. Lanza, R. Langer and W. L. Chick. New York, NY, Academic Press: 133–149.

Devarapalli, M., B. J. Lawrence, and S. V. Madihally. 2009. Modeling nutrient consumptions in large flow-through bioreactors for tissue engineering. *Biotechnol Bioeng* 103:1003–1015.

Drewa, T. 2008. Using hair-follicle stem cells for urinary bladder-wall regeneration. *Regen Med* 3:939–944.

Drewa, T., R. Joachimiak, A. Kaznica, V. Sarafian, and M. Pokrywczynska. 2009. Hair stem cells for bladder regeneration in rats: Preliminary results. *Transplant Proc* 41:4345–4351.

El-Kassaby, A., T. AbouShwareb, and A. Atala. 2008. Randomized comparative study between buccal mucosal and acellular bladder matrix grafts in complex anterior urethral strictures. *J Urol* 179:1432–1436.

El-Kassaby, A. W., A. B. Retik, J. J. Yoo, and A. Atala. 2003. Urethral stricture repair with an off-the-shelf collagen matrix. *J Urol* 169:170–173; discussion 173.

Engelhardt, E. M., E. Stegberg, R. A. Brown et al. 2010. Compressed collagen gel: A novel scaffold for human bladder cells. *J Tissue Eng Regen Med* 4:123–130.

Falke, G., J. J. Yoo, T. G. Kwon, R. Moreland, and A. Atala. 2003. Formation of corporal tissue architecture *in vivo* using human cavernosal muscle and endothelial cells seeded on collagen matrices. *Tissue Eng* 9:871–879.

Farhat, W. A. and H. Yeger. 2008. Does mechanical stimulation have any role in urinary bladder tissue engineering? *World J Urol* 26:301–305.

Freed, L. E., G. Vunjak-Novakovic, R. J. Biron et al. 1994. Biodegradable polymer scaffolds for tissue engineering. *Biotechnology (N Y)* 12:689–693.

Frimberger, D., N. Morales, J. D. Gearhart, J. P. Gearhart, and Y. Lakshmanan. 2006. Human embryoid body-derived stem cells in tissue engineering-enhanced migration in co-culture with bladder smooth muscle and urothelium. *Urology* 67:1298–1303.

Fu, Q., C. L. Deng, W. Liu, and Y. L. Cao. 2007. Urethral replacement using epidermal cell-seeded tubular acellular bladder collagen matrix. *BJU Int* 99:1162–1165.

Furthmayr, H. and R. Timpl. 1976. Immunochemistry of collagens and procollagens. *Int Rev Connect Tissue Res* 7:61–99.

Gilding, D. 1981. Biodegradable Polymers. *Biocompatibility of Clinical Implant Materials*. D. Williams. Boca Raton, FL, CRC Press: 209–232.

Goodwin, W. E. and W. W. Scott. 1952. Phalloplasty. *J Urol* 68:903–908.

Guan, Y., L. Ou, G. Hu et al. 2008. Tissue engineering of urethra using human vascular endothelial growth factor gene-modified bladder urothelial cells. *Artif Organs* 32:91–99.

Gupta, S., C. Verfaillie, D. Chmielewski, Y. Kim, and M. E. Rosenberg. 2002. A role for extrarenal cells in the regeneration following acute renal failure. *Kidney Int* 62:1285–1290.

Han, D. and P. I. Gouma. 2006. Electrospun bioscaffolds that mimic the topology of extracellular matrix. *Nanomedicine* 2:37–41.

Hanson, J. A., C. B. Chang, S. M. Graves et al. 2008. Nanoscale double emulsions stabilized by single-component block copolypeptides. *Nature* 455:85–88.

Harrington, D. A., E. Y. Cheng, M. O. Guler et al. 2006. Branched peptide-amphiphiles as self-assembling coatings for tissue engineering scaffolds. *J Biomed Mater Res A* 78:157–167.

Harris, L. D., B. S. Kim, and D. J. Mooney. 1998. Open pore biodegradable matrices formed with gas foaming. *J Biomed Mater Res* 42:396–402.

Harrison, B. S. and A. Atala. 2007. Carbon nanotube applications for tissue engineering. *Biomaterials* 28:344–353.

Hong, Y. M. and K. R. Loughlin. 2006. The use of hemostatic agents and sealants in urology. *J Urol* 176:2367–2374.

Humes, H. D. and D. A. Cieslinski. 1992. Interaction between growth factors and retinoic acid in the induction of kidney tubulogenesis in tissue culture. *Exp Cell Res* 201:8–15.

Hynes, R. O. 1992. Integrins: Versatility, modulation, and signaling in cell adhesion. *Cell* 69:11–25.

Ikarashi, K., B. Li, M. Suwa et al. 2005. Bone marrow cells contribute to regeneration of damaged glomerular endothelial cells. *Kidney Int* 67:1925–1933.

Ikeda, E., K. Yagi, M. Kojima et al. 2008. Multipotent cells from the human third molar: Feasibility of cell-based therapy for liver disease. *Differentiation* 76:495–505.

Ilkhanizadeh, S., A. I. Teixeira, and O. Hermanson. 2007. Inkjet printing of macromolecules on hydrogels to steer neural stem cell differentiation. *Biomaterials* 28:3936–3943.

Ito, T., A. Suzuki, E. Imai, M. Okabe, and M. Hori. 2001. Bone marrow is a reservoir of repopulating mesangial cells during glomerular remodeling. *J Am Soc Nephrol* 12:2625–2635.

Iwano, M., D. Plieth, T. M. Danoff et al. 2002. Evidence that fibroblasts derive from epithelium during tissue fibrosis. *J Clin Invest* 110:341–350.

Jayo, M. J., D. Jain, J. W. Ludlow et al. 2008a. Long-term durability, tissue regeneration and neo-organ growth during skeletal maturation with a neo-bladder augmentation construct. *Regen Med* 3:671–682.

Jayo, M. J., D. Jain, B. J. Wagner, and T. A. Bertram. 2008b. Early cellular and stromal responses in regeneration versus repair of a mammalian bladder using autologous cell and biodegradable scaffold technologies. *J Urol* 180:392–397.

Jiang, Y., B. N. Jahagirdar, R. L. Reinhardt et al. 2002. Pluripotency of mesenchymal stem cells derived from adult marrow. *Nature* 418:41–49.

Jiao, J. and D. F. Chen. 2008. Induction of neurogenesis in nonconventional neurogenic regions of the adult central nervous system by niche astrocyte-produced signals. *Stem Cells* 26:1221–1230.

Jordan, G. H. 1999. Penile reconstruction, phallic construction, and urethral reconstruction. *Urol Clin North Am* 26:1–13, vii.

Kaefer, M., M. S. Tobin, W. H. Hendren et al. 1997. Continent urinary diversion: The Children's Hospital experience. *J Urol* 157:1394–1399.

Kale, S., A. Karihaloo, P. R. Clark et al. 2003. Bone marrow stem cells contribute to repair of the ischemically injured renal tubule. *J Clin Invest* 112:42–49.

Kanematsu, A., S. Yamamoto, M. Ozeki et al. 2004. Collagenous matrices as release carriers of exogenous growth factors. *Biomaterials* 25:4513–4520.

Kershen, R. T., J. J. Yoo, R. B. Moreland, R. J. Krane, and A. Atala. 2002. Reconstitution of human corpus cavernosum smooth muscle *in vitro* and *in vivo*. *Tissue Eng* 8:515–524.

Kikuno, N., K. Kawamoto, H. Hirata et al. 2009. Nerve growth factor combined with vascular endothelial growth factor enhances regeneration of bladder acellular matrix graft in spinal cord injury-induced neurogenic rat bladder. *BJU Int* 103:1424–1428.

Kim, B. S., A. Atala, and J. J. Yoo. 2008. A collagen matrix derived from bladder can be used to engineer smooth muscle tissue. *World J Urol* 26:307–314.

Kim, B. S. and D. J. Mooney. 1998. Development of biocompatible synthetic extracellular matrices for tissue engineering. *Trends Biotechnol* 16:224–230.

Kim, B. S., J. J. Yoo, and A. Atala. 2002. Engineering of human cartilage rods: Potential application for penile prostheses. *J Urol* 168:1794–1797.

Kropp, B. P., M. K. Rippy, S. F. Badylak et al. 1996a. Regenerative urinary bladder augmentation using small intestinal submucosa: Urodynamic and histopathologic assessment in long-term canine bladder augmentations. *J Urol* 155:2098–2104.

Kropp, B. P., B. D. Sawyer, H. E. Shannon et al. 1996b. Characterization of small intestinal submucosa regenerated canine detrusor: Assessment of reinnervation, *in vitro* compliance and contractility. *J Urol* 156:599–607.

Kwon, T. G., J. J. Yoo, and A. Atala. 2002. Autologous penile corpora cavernosa replacement using tissue engineering techniques. *J Urol* 168:1754–1758.

Laflamme, M. A., J. Gold, C. Xu et al. 2005. Formation of human myocardium in the rat heart from human embryonic stem cells. *Am J Pathol* 167:663–671.

Langer, R. and J. P. Vacanti. 1993. Tissue engineering. *Science* 260:920–926.

Lanza, R. P., H. Y. Chung, J. J. Yoo et al. 2002. Generation of histocompatible tissues using nuclear transplantation. *Nat Biotechnol* 20:689–696.

le Roux, P. J. 2005. Endoscopic urethroplasty with unseeded small intestinal submucosa collagen matrix grafts: A pilot study. *J Urol* 173:140–143.

Lee, K. Y., L. Jeong, Y. O. Kang, S. J. Lee, and W. H. Park. 2009. Electrospinning of polysaccharides for regenerative medicine. *Adv Drug Deliv Rev* 61:1020–1032.

Lee, S. J., J. Liu, S. H. Oh et al. 2008a. Development of a composite vascular scaffolding system that withstands physiological vascular conditions. *Biomaterials* 29:2891–2898.

Lee, S. J., S. H. Oh, J. Liu et al. 2008b. The use of thermal treatments to enhance the mechanical properties of electrospun poly(epsilon-caprolactone) scaffolds. *Biomaterials* 29:1422–1430.

Lee, S. J., M. Van Dyke, A. Atala, and J. J. Yoo. 2008c. Host cell mobilization for *in situ* tissue regeneration. *Rejuvenation Res* 11:747–756.

Li, C., Y. Xu, L. Song et al. 2008a. Preliminary experimental study of tissue-engineered urethral reconstruction using oral keratinocytes seeded on BAMG. *Urol Int* 81:290–295.

Li, C., Y. M. Xu, L. J. Song et al. 2008b. Urethral reconstruction using oral keratinocyte seeded bladder acellular matrix grafts. *J Urol* 180:1538–1542.

Li, S. T. 1995. Biologic biomaterials: Tissue derived biomaterials (collagen). *The Biomedical Engineering Handbook*. J. D. Bronzino. Boca Raton, FL, CRS Press: 627–647.

Liebert, M., A. Hubbel, M. Chung et al. 1997. Expression of mal is associated with urothelial differentiation *in vitro*: Identification by differential display reverse-transcriptase polymerase chain reaction. *Differentiation* 61:177–185.

Lin, F. 2006. Stem cells in kidney regeneration following acute renal injury. *Pediatr Res* 59:74R–78R.

Lin, F., K. Cordes, L. Li et al. 2003. Hematopoietic stem cells contribute to the regeneration of renal tubules after renal ischemia-reperfusion injury in mice. *J Am Soc Nephrol* 14:1188–1199.

Lin, F., A. Moran, and P. Igarashi. 2005. Intrarenal cells, not bone marrow-derived cells, are the major source for regeneration in postischemic kidney. *J Clin Invest* 115:1756–1764.

Lim, F. and A. M. Sun. 1980. Microencapsulated islets as bioartificial endocrine pancreas. *Science* 210:908–910.

Lo, K. C., V. M. Brugh, 3rd, M. Parker, and D. J. Lamb. 2005. Isolation and enrichment of murine spermatogonial stem cells using rhodamine 123 mitochondrial dye. *Biol Reprod* 72:767–771.

Lo, K. C., Z. Lei, V. Rao Ch, J. Beck, and D. J. Lamb. 2004. *De novo* testosterone production in luteinizing hormone receptor knockout mice after transplantation of leydig stem cells. *Endocrinology* 145:4011–4015.

Machluf, M. and A. Atala. 1998. Emerging concepts for tissue and organ transplantation. *Graft* 1:31–37.

Machluf, M., A. Orsola, and A. Atala. 2000. Controlled release of therapeutic agents: Slow delivery and cell encapsulation. *World J Urol* 18:80–83.

Mann, B. K., R. H. Schmedlen, and J. L. West. 2001. Tethered-TGF-beta increases extracellular matrix production of vascular smooth muscle cells. *Biomaterials* 22:439–444.

Martin, G. R. 1981. Isolation of a pluripotent cell line from early mouse embryos cultured in medium conditioned by teratocarcinoma stem cells. *Proc Natl Acad Sci USA* 78:7634–7638.

McDougal, W. S. 1992. Metabolic complications of urinary intestinal diversion. *J Urol* 147:1199–1208.

Mehta, G., C. M. Williams, L. Alvarez et al. 2010. Synergistic effects of tethered growth factors and adhesion ligands on DNA synthesis and function of primary hepatocytes cultured on soft synthetic hydrogels. *Biomaterials* 31:4657–4671.

Mikos, A. G., M. D. Lyman, L. E. Freed, and R. Langer. 1994. Wetting of poly(L-lactic acid) and poly(DL-lactic-*co*-glycolic acid) foams for tissue culture. *Biomaterials* 15:55–58.

Milici, A. J., M. B. Furie, and W. W. Carley. 1985. The formation of fenestrations and channels by capillary endothelium *in vitro*. *Proc Natl Acad Sci USA* 82:6181–6185.

Mimeault, M. and S. K. Batra. 2008. Recent progress on tissue-resident adult stem cell biology and their therapeutic implications. *Stem Cell Rev* 4:27–49.

Mondalek, F. G., R. A. Ashley, C. C. Roth et al. 2010. Enhanced angiogenesis of modified porcine small intestinal submucosa with hyaluronic acid-poly(lactide-*co*-glycolide) nanoparticles: From fabrication to preclinical validation. *J Biomed Mater Res A.* 94:712–719.

Msezane, L. P., M. H. Katz, O. N. Gofrit, A. L. Shalhav, and K. C. Zorn. 2008. Hemostatic agents and instruments in laparoscopic renal surgery. *J Endourol* 22:403–408.

Murray, M. M., B. Forsythe, F. Chen et al. 2006. The effect of thrombin on ACL fibroblast interactions with collagen hydrogels. *J Orthop Res* 24:508–515.

Nagano, M. and R. L. Brinster. 1998. Spermatogonial transplantation and reconstitution of donor cell spermatogenesis in recipient mice. *APMIS* 106:47–55; discussion 56–47.

Nakamura, M., A. Kobayashi, F. Takagi et al. 2005. Biocompatible inkjet printing technique for designed seeding of individual living cells. *Tissue Eng* 11:1658–1666.

Nukui, F., S. Okamoto, M. Nagata, J. Kurokawa, and J. Fukui. 1997. Complications and reimplantation of penile implants. *Int J Urol* 4:52–54.

Ogawa, T., I. Dobrinski, M. R. Avarbock, and R. L. Brinster. 2000. Transplantation of male germ line stem cells restores fertility in infertile mice. *Nat Med* 6:29–34.

Olsen, L., S. Bowald, C. Busch, J. Carlsten, and I. Eriksson. 1992. Urethral reconstruction with a new synthetic absorbable device. An experimental study. *Scand J Urol Nephrol* 26:323–326.

Osafune, K. 2010. *In vitro* regeneration of kidney from pluripotent stem cells. *Exp Cell Res.* 316:2571–2577.

Pariente, J. L., B. S. Kim, and A. Atala. 2001. *In vitro* biocompatibility assessment of naturally derived and synthetic biomaterials using normal human urothelial cells. *J Biomed Mater Res* 55:33–39.

Park, H. J., J. J. Yoo, R. T. Kershen, R. Moreland, and A. Atala. 1999. Reconstitution of human corporal smooth muscle and endothelial cells *in vivo*. *J Urol* 162:1106–1109.

Peppas, N. A. and R. Langer. 1994. New challenges in biomaterials. [see comment]. *Science* 263:1715–1720.

Perin, L., S. Giuliani, D. Jin et al. 2007. Renal differentiation of amniotic fluid stem cells. *Cell Prolif* 40:936–948.

Piechota, H. J., S. E. Dahms, L. S. Nunes et al. 1998a. *In vitro* functional properties of the rat bladder regenerated by the bladder acellular matrix graft. *J Urol* 159:1717–1724.

Piechota, H. J., S. E. Dahms, L. S. Nunes et al. 1998b. *In vitro* functional properties of the rat bladder regenerated by the bladder acellular matrix graft. *J Urol* 159:1717–1724.

Polgar, K., R. Adany, G. Abel et al. 1989. Characterization of rapidly adhering amniotic fluid cells by combined immunofluorescence and phagocytosis assays. *Am J Hum Genet* 45:786–792.

Poulsom, R., S. J. Forbes, K. Hodivala-Dilke et al. 2001. Bone marrow contributes to renal parenchymal turnover and regeneration. *J Pathol* 195:229–235.

Priest, R. E., K. M. Marimuthu, and J. H. Priest. 1978. Origin of cells in human amniotic fluid cultures: Ultrastructural features. *Lab Invest* 39:106–109.

Probst, M., R. Dahiya, S. Carrier, and E. A. Tanagho. 1997a. Reproduction of functional smooth muscle tissue and partial bladder replacement. *Br J Urol* 79:505–515.

Probst, M., R. Dahiya, S. Carrier, and E. A. Tanagho. 1997b. Reproduction of functional smooth muscle tissue and partial bladder replacement. *Br J Urol* 79:505–515.

Prockop, D. J. 1997. Marrow stromal cells as stem cells for nonhematopoietic tissues. *Science* 276:71–74.

Puthenveettil, J. A., M. S. Burger, and C. A. Reznikoff. 1999. Replicative senescence in human uroepithelial cells. *Adv Exp Med Biol* 462:83–91.

Ratliff, B. B., T. Ghaly, P. Brudnicki et al. 2010. Endothelial progenitors encapsulated in bioartificial niches are insulated from systemic cytotoxicity and are angiogenesis competent. *Am J Physiol Renal Physiol* 299: F178–186.

Raya-Rivera, A. M., C. Baez, A. Atala, and J. J. Yoo. 2008. Tissue engineered testicular prostheses with prolonged testosterone release. *World J Urol* 26:351–358.

Richardson, T. P., M. C. Peters, A. B. Ennett, and D. J. Mooney. 2001. Polymeric system for dual growth factor delivery. *Nat Biotechnol* 19:1029–1034.

Roessger, A., L. Denk, and W. W. Minuth. 2009. Potential of stem/progenitor cell cultures within polyester fleeces to regenerate renal tubules. *Biomaterials* 30:3723–3732.

Rookmaaker, M. B., A. M. Smits, H. Tolboom et al. 2003. Bone-marrow-derived cells contribute to glomerular endothelial repair in experimental glomerulonephritis. *Am J Pathol* 163:553–562.

Roth, E. A., T. Xu, M. Das et al. 2004. Inkjet printing for high-throughput cell patterning. *Biomaterials* 25:3707–3715.

Rowley, J. A., G. Madlambayan, and D. J. Mooney. 1999. Alginate hydrogels as synthetic extracellular matrix materials. *Biomaterials* 20:45–53.

Sams, A. E. and A. J. Nixon. 1995. Chondrocyte-laden collagen scaffolds for resurfacing extensive articular cartilage defects. *Osteoarthritis Cartilage* 3:47–59.

Schena, F. P. 1998. Role of growth factors in acute renal failure. *Kidney Int Suppl* 66: S11–S15.

Scriven, S. D., C. Booth, D. F. Thomas, L. K. Trejdosiewicz, and J. Southgate. 1997. Reconstitution of human urothelium from monolayer cultures. *J Urol* 158:1147–1152.

Segers, V. F. and R. T. Lee. 2007. Local delivery of proteins and the use of self-assembling peptides. *Drug Discov Today* 12:561–568.

Shinohara, T., K. E. Orwig, M. R. Avarbock, and R. L. Brinster. 2003. Restoration of spermatogenesis in infertile mice by Sertoli cell transplantation. *Biol Reprod* 68:1064–1071.

Sievert, K. D., M. E. Bakircioglu, L. Nunes et al. 2000. Homologous acellular matrix graft for urethral reconstruction in the rabbit: Histological and functional evaluation. *J Urol* 163:1958–1965.

Silver, F. H. and G. Pins. 1992. Cell growth on collagen: A review of tissue engineering using scaffolds containing extracellular matrix. *J Long-Term Eff Med Implants* 2:67–80.

Small, M. P., H. M. Carrion, and J. A. Gordon. 1975. Small-Carrion penile prosthesis. New implant for management of impotence. *Urology* 5:479–486.

Smidsrod, O. and G. Skjak-Braek. 1990. Alginate as immobilization matrix for cells. *Trends Biotechnol* 8:71–78.

Sohier, J., T. J. Vlugt, N. Cabrol et al. 2006. Dual release of proteins from porous polymeric scaffolds. *J Control Release* 111:95–106.

Spradling, A., D. Drummond-Barbosa, and T. Kai. 2001. Stem cells find their niche. *Nature* 414:98–104.

Sutherland, R. S., L. S. Baskin, S. W. Hayward, and G. R. Cunha. 1996. Regeneration of bladder urothelium, smooth muscle, blood vessels and nerves into an acellular tissue matrix. *J Urol* 156:571–577.

Takahashi, K., K. Tanabe, M. Ohnuki et al. 2007. Induction of pluripotent stem cells from adult human fibroblasts by defined factors. *Cell* 131:861–872.

Takahashi, K. and S. Yamanaka. 2006. Induction of pluripotent stem cells from mouse embryonic and adult fibroblast cultures by defined factors *Cell* 126:663–676.

Taupin, P. 2006. Therapeutic potential of adult neural stem cells. *Recent Pat CNS Drug Discov* 1:299–303.

Thomalla, J. V., S. T. Thompson, R. G. Rowland, and J. J. Mulcahy. 1987. Infectious complications of penile prosthetic implants. *J Urol* 138:65–67.

Tian, H., S. Bharadwaj, Y. Liu et al. 2010. Differentiation of human bone marrow mesenchymal stem cells into bladder cells: Potential for urological tissue engineering. *Tissue Eng Part A* 16:1769–1779.

Vaught, J. D., B. P. Kropp, B. D. Sawyer et al. 1996. Detrusor regeneration in the rat using porcine small intestinal submucosal grafts: Functional innervation and receptor expression. *J Urol* 155:374–378.

Wefer, J., N. Sekido, K. D. Sievert et al. 2002. Homologous acellular matrix graft for vaginal repair in rats: A pilot study for a new reconstructive approach. *World J Urol* 20:260–263.

Wefer, J., K. D. Sievert, N. Schlote et al. 2001. Time dependent smooth muscle regeneration and maturation in a bladder acellular matrix graft: Histological studies and *in vivo* functional evaluation. *J Urol* 165:1755–1759.

Wernig, M., A. Meissner, R. Foreman et al. 2007. *In vitro* reprogramming of fibroblasts into a pluripotent ES-cell-like state *Nature* 448:318–324.

Xu, T., J. Rohozinski, W. Zhao et al. 2009. Inkjet-mediated gene transfection into living cells combined with targeted delivery. *Tissue Eng Part A* 15:95–101.

Xu, Y., Y. Shi and S. Ding. 2008. A chemical approach to stem-cell biology and regenerative medicine. *Nature* 453:338–344.

Yang, B., L. Zhou, Z. Sun et al. 2010. *In vitro* evaluation of the bioactive factors preserved in porcine small intestinal submucosa through cellular biological approaches. *J Biomed Mater Res A* 93:1100–1109.

Yannas, I. V. and J. F. Burke. 1980a. Design of an artificial skin. I. Basic design principles. *J Biomed Mater Res* 14:65–81.

Yannas, I. V., J. F. Burke, P. L. Gordon, C. Huang, and R. H. Rubenstein. 1980b. Design of an artificial skin. II. Control of chemical composition. *J Biomed Mater Res* 14:107–132.

Yokoo, T. and T. Kawamura. 2009. Xenobiotic kidney organogenesis: A new avenue for renal transplantation. *J Nephrol* 22:312–317.

Yokoo, T., T. Ohashi, J. S. Shen et al. 2005. Human mesenchymal stem cells in rodent whole-embryo culture are reprogrammed to contribute to kidney tissues. *Proc Natl Acad Sci USA* 102:3296–3300.

Yoo, J. J., S. Ashkar, and A. Atala. 1996. Creation of functional kidney structures with excretion of kidney-like fluid *in vivo*. *Pediatrics* 98 (suppl):605.

Yoo, J. J., I. Lee, and A. Atala. 1998a. Cartilage rods as a potential material for penile reconstruction. *J Urol* 160:1164–1168; discussion 1178.

Yoo, J. J., J. Meng, F. Oberpenning, and A. Atala. 1998b. Bladder augmentation using allogenic bladder submucosa seeded with cells. *Urology* 51:221–225.

Yoo, J. J., H. J. Park, I. Lee, and A. Atala. 1999. Autologous engineered cartilage rods for penile reconstruction. *J Urol* 162:1119–1121.

Yu, J., M. A. Vodyanik, K. Smuga-Otto et al. 2007. Induced pluripotent stem cell lines derived from human somatic cells. *Science* 318:1917–1920.

Zhang, Y., D. Frimberger, E. Y. Cheng, H. K. Lin, and B. P. Kropp. 2006. Challenges in a larger bladder replacement with cell-seeded and unseeded small intestinal submucosa grafts in a subtotal cystectomy model. *BJU Int* 98:1100–1105.

Zhao, W. and J. M. Karp. 2009. Controlling cell fate *in vivo*. *Chembiochem* 10:2308–2310.

# 35

# Vascular Tissue Engineering

35.1 Introduction ................................................................... 35-1
    Significance • Cardiovascular Disease
35.2 Cell Source .................................................................... 35-2
    Differentiated Cells • Endothelial Progenitors • Smooth Muscle
    Progenitors • Mesenchymal Stem Cells • Pluripotent Stem Cells
35.3 Scaffolds/Extracellular Matrix .................................... 35-5
    Synthetic Scaffolds • Natural Scaffolds • Cell Assembly • Matrix
    and Culture Effects
35.4 Growth Factor Signaling .............................................. 35-7
35.5 Vascular Grafts and Medial Equivalents ....................... 35-9
35.6 Engineered Vascular Networks .................................... 35-10
35.7 Conclusions ................................................................. 35-12
References ............................................................................. 35-12

Laura J. Suggs
*University of Texas, Austin*

## 35.1 Introduction

### 35.1.1 Significance

Cardiovascular disease is the number one cause of death in developed countries. Over 60 million Americans suffer from some type of vascular disorder [1], and disease associated with small to medium size vessels is the chief killer in the United States [2]. Over 500,000 coronary artery bypass graft (CABG) surgeries were performed in 2000 [1]. Current options for graft replacements are either autologous vessels or synthetic materials. Synthetic materials, despite being readily available and relatively inexpensive, are associated with thrombogenicity and neo-intima formation in low-flow and small-diameter vessels. Autologous vessels exhibit better patency; however, about 60% of CABG patients do not possess suitable healthy vessels to serve as a graft [3]. Vascular tissue engineering holds promise for the rescue and regeneration of tissue following ischemia, the development of small diameter blood vessel substitutes and the creation of mature blood vessel networks.

The paradigm of tissue engineering constitutes a scaffold upon which cells can adhere, proliferate, and express their differentiated function, the cells themselves and any signals, soluble or otherwise, which the cell requires. Our current understanding of the interplay between the cells and their supporting scaffold has demonstrated a reciprocal interaction where the scaffold can inform and control tissue organization and cell differentiation, and the cells are able to remodel tissue engineering matrices to better approximate natural tissue. A successful vascular tissue engineering strategy would result in a physiologically functional blood vessel or vessel network to adequately perfuse diseased or injured tissue. This strategy would necessarily be devised across various disciplines and rely on an understanding of engineering principles and the life sciences.

One approach that has been successful in tissue engineering is to enhance cell adhesion to matrices and scaffolds in order to encourage cell attachment and proliferation. This strategy becomes problematic in the presence of blood due to the ability of flowing blood to recognize foreign surfaces. Traditional, permanent cardiovascular devices have been designed to be inert to cell and platelet adhesion. As a result, many researchers have attempted to approximate the blood vessel lumen by lining constructs with a functional endothelium. The endothelium, a single layer of endothelial cells (ECs), serves as the primary regulatory for blood coagulation and transport from the blood space to the tissue space. Investigators have also looked to known angiogenic mechanisms to control EC migration, adhesion, and function in the context of forming microvascular networks. Collectively, much work has been focused on the control or seeding of terminally differentiated cells within scaffolds, however, a dramatic increase in the understanding of stem and vascular progenitor cells has driven the exploration of these cell sources for vascular tissue engineering. Furthermore, a greater understanding of how cells interact with both soluble and insoluble, or matrix, signals has resulted in novel combination strategies for regeneration of a number of vascular deficiencies.

### 35.1.2 Cardiovascular Disease

With the average age increasing, the prevalence of cardiovascular disease has continued to expand. The primary cause is atherosclerosis, a thickening of the lining of the arteries (the intima). It most commonly affects the arteries of the heart, brain, and lower limbs, and subsequent ischemia results in functional deficits and tissue damage. Antithrombotic therapy, bypass grafting and therapeutic angiogenesis are potential treatments for vascular disease. Atherosclerosis is thought to begin with some type of injury to the ECs that line blood vessels. This injury may be mechanical, such as repeated stress on the cells; or chemical, including exposure to molecules such as oxidized low-density lipoprotein (LDL). Stress on the cells that line the arterial wall may be caused by hypertension. Elevated levels of lipids and cholesterol can be due to diet, genetic disposition, or diseases such as diabetes. In response to this injury, ECs initiate the healing process. As part of healing, ECs secrete agents which recruit additional cell types. Macrophages locate themselves within the intima and accumulate lipids to form foam cells. These cells then organize to form fatty streaks which will eventually become a fibrous atherosclerotic plaque. As these lesions grow, they can become calcified which reduces distensibility and can result in thrombosis at the site of the plaque.

Ischemic heart disease is the single most common cause of death. Ischemic heart disease, or reduced blood flow to the heart, is primarily brought on by atherosclerosis in the coronary circulation. Some deaths occur suddenly as a result of acute closure on the coronary arteries while some occur because of a progressive weakening of the heart muscle. Acute coronary occlusion can be a result of thrombus formation in an atherosclerotic vessel. This thrombus can occlude the vessel resulting in a cessation of blood flow to the corresponding region of the heart. The area of muscle that has no flow and cannot function is said to be infarcted. A formed thrombus can break loose, or embolize, and occlude a downstream vessel, again resulting in myocardial infarction. Cardiac failure can also result from chronic damage. Congestive heart failure is a result of ischemic heart muscle which has reduced contractility. Back pressure, or congestion, builds up in either the pulmonary or systemic circulation depending on which side of the heart is affected. In order to compensate for this decreased output, the heart increases the volume of blood which is being pumped, and the heart muscle becomes enlarged.

## 35.2 Cell Source

### 35.2.1 Differentiated Cells

Seeding of EC populations onto synthetic device surfaces was an early tissue engineering approach to limit thrombosis. Isolation and culture of a significant population of ECs for seeding as well as their retention on a synthetic surface under blood shear is problematic. Pioneering work by Jarrell et al. proposed the isolation of microvessel endothelium from human adipose tissue from a lipo-aspirate [4]. They were able to collect a large fraction of cells that exhibited phenotypic characteristics of ECs. Subsequent high-density seeding onto synthetic graft surfaces was possible, but early clinic work did not demonstrate the necessary improvements over unseeded grafts [5]. Subsequent work with the stromal vascular fraction from adipose tissue has revealed a heterogeneous population containing ECs as well as a multipotent cell of mesenchymal lineage among others [6].

## 35.2.2 Endothelial Progenitors

Following work by Asahara and colleagues, investigators have identified endothelial progenitor cells (EPCs) from peripheral blood, bone marrow mononuclear cells, and umbilical cord blood. This early work reported the role of EPCs in enhancing postnatal vasculogenesis in a model of hind limb ischemia [7]. Subsequent preclinical work has evaluated the potential of EPCs for enhancing recovery in cardiac injury. The isolation of this cell population begins with an enrichment of CD34+ cells, which is also a marker for hematopoietic stem cells (HSCs), followed by tissue culture plastic adherence selection. Differentiation has been promoted through culture with vascular endothelial growth factor (VEGF) [8–9]. These cells share a number of other markers with HSCs including: VEGFR2/flk-1 + , Tek (Tie-2), cKit, Sca-1, CD133, and CD34 [7]. No marker to date has been definitive for the EPC. Bone marrow-derived CD34+ cells have been used to seed grafts in dogs with enhanced endothelialization, but the role of these cells is unclear as no correlation was seen between the number of cells and the degree of endothelialization [10].

Populations of EPCs with colony forming ability, endothelial colony forming cells (ECFCs) have been isolated through an extended culture process called late outgrowth. This process is also based on culture adherence and colony formation at 7–21 days. Unlike early outgrowth EPCs, ECFCs have the ability to form tubes. Markers of mature ECs have been used to characterize these cells and include: von Willebrand Factor (vWF), platelet endothelial cell adhesion molecule-1 (PECAM-1/CD31) and vascular endothelial-cadherin (VE-Cad), and by uptake of Dil-acetylated LDL and binding of lectin. ECFCs have been shown to incorporate into newly formed vasculature in animal models of ischemia. While both EPCs and ECFCs have been shown to improve neovascularization, they may have different roles in enhancing this process.

EPCs may also have the ability to mobilize toward sites of ischemia and participate in vasculogenesis [11]. The stem cell homing factor, granulocyte macrophage-colony stimulating factor has been administered systemically and enhanced the numbers of EPCs circulating in peripheral blood as well as the degree of neovascularization in a model of ischemia [12]. VEGF has also been shown to enhance the mobilization of EPCs to peripheral blood either directly in mice or via plasmid or recombinant protein in humans. Other factors that have been proposed as agents to increase the number of circulating EPCs include: Ang-1, placenta-derived growth factor (PlGF), erythropoietin and 3-hydroxy-3-methylglutaryl coenzyme A. While it is likely that increasing the number of circulating EPCs may enhance neovascularization at sites of ischemia, enhancing engraftment at the site of injury or onto a synthetic surface may also be necessary. Clinical trials with circulating EPCs (e.g., the START trial) did not show efficacy in patients with lower limb ischemia [13]. A potential engraftment factor may be stromal cell-derived factor (SDF)-1α. SDF-1α is involved in stem cell homing to the bone marrow compartment during HSC transplantation. Our group has used a polymeric delivery system to enhance stem cell homing via SDF-1α localization in a mouse model of myocardial infarction [14]. Enhancing stem cell homing in this model increased the measured functional recovery. Engraftment of EPCs onto synthetic grafts may also be enhanced via an antibody capture technique. The use of a CD34 antibody localized to graft surfaces has been evaluated in a preliminary trial, the HEALING trial [15].

## 35.2.3 Smooth Muscle Progenitors

Analogous to ECs, smooth muscle cells (SMCs) for tissue engineering have often been derived from mature tissues such as aorta in order to be evaluated in animal models. Acquiring a sufficient number of autologous cells may limit clinical translation to humans, however. In the use of SMCs and their progenitors for tissue engineered vascular graft (TEVG) fabrication; it has been proposed that early passage cells may have an enhanced ability to produce extracellular matrix components which could result in higher strengths and improved performance [16]. Smooth muscle progenitor cells have been reported to reside in peripheral blood, and express markers characteristic of mature SMCs following cytokine stimulation. SMC-positive markers include: $\alpha$-smooth muscle actin, myosin heavy chain, and calponin. It is important to note, however, that markers of angioblasts (CD34, Flk-1, Flt-1) [17]. were also seen, suggesting that they retained markers of their origin from blood. Mesenchymal stem cells (MSCs) from bone marrow, as discussed below can also exhibit SMC phenotype following stimulation with transforming growth factor (TGF)-$\beta$. Mechanical stimulation of MSCs has been shown to upregulate markers of SMCs. Specifically, uniaxial cyclic strain of 2D cultures demonstrated upregulation of smooth muscle $\alpha$-actin, calponin, as well as a number of collagen isoforms including collagen I [18].

## 35.2.4 Mesenchymal Stem Cells

MSCs are a stem cell population that are present in bone marrow, adipose tissue, or peripheral blood and can differentiate readily into terminal cells of the mesenchyme. Recent evidence suggests that MSCs can express phenotypic characteristics of endothelial, neural, smooth muscle, skeletal myoblasts, and cardiomyocytes [19–21]. Isolated, autologous bone marrow stem cells have been shown to contribute to cardiac muscle repair and formation of new blood vessels following tissue ischemia, based on the localization of genetic markers [21–22]. Cells of perivascular origin have also been isolated that share markers of both mural cells and MSCs including (CD146, NG-2, and PDGF-R$\beta$) [23,24]. These cells exhibited multilineage potential toward cells of the mesenchyme. The relationship among MSCs and mural cells including both pericytes and SMCs is still poorly understood, and it remains to be seen what cell population will be most effective for reapproximating the medial layer of TEVGs.

Clinical studies have been performed using autologous MSCs to seed the pores of synthetic grafts in an extracardiac total cavopulmonary position [25]. A 50/50 ratio of polylactic acid to polycaprolactone blend was used to construct the grafts along with other polymeric reinforcement. Safety was demonstrated at the 1 year follow-up in a total of 42 patients. It is unclear at this point what role the MSCs are playing within these constructs and whether or not they are differentiating toward the correct vascular cell type.

## 35.2.5 Pluripotent Stem Cells

Embryonic stem (ES) cells provide promise as a pluripotent cell source for vascular tissue engineering. If ES cells are to fulfill this potential, efficient, and scalable culture techniques to provide fully differentiated cell types must be developed. Clinical concerns over ES cell therapies include immunogenicity and tumorigenicity. Various strategies are currently being explored to "tailor" cells toward specific patients to circumvent problems associated with immune rejection [26,27]. Pluripotent adult stem cells have also been derived from postnatal cells using genetic manipulation. These cells are termed induced pluripotent stem cells and may provide an autologous cell source without the potential for immune rejection. They are genetically modified adult cells that behave in a similar manner to ES cells and are pluripotent [28]. Teratoma formation can still occur, however, the generation of tumors from pluripotent stem cells can be eliminated by using fully differentiated cells. Desired lineages can be enriched during differentiation using various strategies. These include induction using chemokines, co-culture with differentiated cell types, as well as genetic manipulation on the starting ES cell population. Selection based on surface markers is possible, either with or without induction, using cell sorting techniques. Cells of mesodermal origin including osteoblasts, chondrocytes, cardiomyocytes, ECs, SMCs, and hematopoetic (blood) cells have all been generated from mouse ES cells [29–33].

## 35.3 Scaffolds/Extracellular Matrix

### 35.3.1 Synthetic Scaffolds

Polyglycolic acid (PGA), a well-characterized biodegradable polymer, has been investigated for use in many tissue engineering applications. Niklason was the first to show feasibility of PGA as a scaffold for vascular tissue engineering [34]. Her group seeded a porous, degradable, tubular PGA mesh scaffold with bovine aortic SMCs and cultured the grafts in a bioreactor with pulsatile flow through the lumen of the vessel. After 8 weeks, the PGA mesh had been partially replaced by a SMC medial layer and showed increased collagen and mechanical properties. ECs were then seeded on the luminal surface. These vessels showed promising results with burst strengths over 2000 mm Hg and patency of up to 4 weeks in a porcine model. Contraction was observed in response to serotonin, endothelin-1, and prostaglandin $F_{2\alpha}$.

Poly(ethylene glycol) (PEG) possesses several advantages as a biomaterial. In addition to being hydrophilic and biocompatibile, it is resistant to protein adsorption and cell adhesion, and therefore is nonimmunogenic with very few biological interactions when rendered insoluble or chemically conjugated to proteins. It can be modified to include a variety of reactive functional groups that can be utilized to impart new properties to PEG. For example, acrylated PEG will undergo photopolymerization and can do so in the presence of cells with minimal harmful effects [35]. Additionally, PEG can be modified to include biologically-relevant molecules such as adhesion peptides [36], growth factors [37], or proteolytically degradable enzymes.

PEG hydrogel-based TEVGs have the potential to combine the advantages of a synthetic scaffold with benefits such as specific cell-material interactions, including remodeling in response to tissue genesis. Publications by West's group described photopolymerizable PEG hydrogel extracellular matrix (ECM) analogs that mimic the properties of collagen [38,39]. These hydrogels included degradable sequences, sensitive to proteases such as collagenase and elastase, in the backbone of the polymer. They also incorporated grafted adhesive peptides, such as arginine-glycine-aspartic acid (RGD), in the network. The hydrogels degraded as cells produced proteolytic enzymes. The nonimmunogenic properties and biological function of these PEG-based hydrogels present an attractive scaffold alternative. They could lead to a TEVG that, when implanted, could encourage cell growth and function and would be completely replaced over time to create totally new tissue.

### 35.3.2 Natural Scaffolds

The first TEVG was developed by Weinberg and Bell [40]. This pioneering study proved feasibility of a TEVG based on a scaffold of natural materials and vascular cells. The graft was derived from a collagen gel supported by Dacron mesh and seeded with bovine aortic SMC, EC, and fibroblasts. Initially, a collagen gel containing SMCs was cast in a tubular shape. After a 1-week culture period, Dacron mesh was wrapped around the outside of this layer to provide mechanical strength. Another layer of collagen and fibroblasts was cast over this, and the inner lumen was lined with ECs. Functional and histological staining confirmed formation of an endothelial layer and production of prostacyclin and vWF. However, this graft did not exhibit sufficient mechanical strength. Several parameters were varied, such as collagen concentration, cell density, and culture time. Nevertheless, the highest reported burst strength was approximately 325 mm Hg. This was significantly less than typical physiologic pressures of 5000 mm Hg in the coronary artery and 2000 mm Hg in the saphenous vein.

Acellular matrices have been developed as an alternative to collagen gel-based TEVGs. The major advantage of an acellular approach is the elimination of the long culture time associated with cell-seeded scaffolds. One material of interest is small intestine submucosa (SIS), a matrix that has been mechanically treated to remove cells, leaving an intact scaffold composed mainly of collagen. SIS possesses mechanical properties suitable for a vascular graft, and better compliance than current autologous vessel grafts [41]. In one case, Huynh rolled sheets of porcine SIS around a mandrel to form a TEVG [42]. The SIS matrix was cross-linked with 1-ethyl-3(3-dimethylaminopropyl) carbodiimide hydrochloride, and the inner lining was coated with bovine fibrillar collagen derivatives and treated with heparin to prevent thrombosis. These grafts were implanted into rabbits and all remained patent until harvest after 90 days. Upon examination, infiltration of SMCs and ECs from surrounding tissue was apparent. Additionally, vessels showed physiologic activity in response to vasoactive agents. Preimplant burst strengths were ~930 mm Hg. Similar work by Roeder using the carotid artery in a canine model examined burst strengths of remodeled SIS grafts after 60 days [43]. This approach produced burst strengths of ~5000 mm Hg in the explanted vessels, equivalent to the burst strength of native vessels.

Another tactic has been to use de-cellularized arterial matrices as a scaffold for TEVGs. Advantages include blood compatibility and an ECM with correctly aligned collagen and elastin fibers. Native vessels are treated with trypsin and ethylenediaminetetraacetic acid to remove cells [44]. This leaves an intact matrix that can be used for implantation. Cells may be seeded in the matrix and conditioned under pulsatile flow [45]. Fibrosis was a problem in these types of grafts, and concern remains over immune response and disease transmission with the xenogenic materials used in acellular matrices.

## 35.3.3 Cell Assembly

L'Heureux et al. created a TEVG by rolling sheets of cells around a mandrel to form a layered construct [46]. No supportive scaffold was used. Human umbilical vein SMCs and human dermal fibroblasts were grown in culture flasks to super-confluency in high ascorbic acid conditions for 1 month. The cell sheets were then rolled around a mandrel to tissue layers. After 8 weeks of culture in a bioreactor, the lumen was seeded with ECs and then cultured for another week. At the end of this period, ECs showed $\alpha$-LDL uptake and vWF and SMCs showed positive staining for $\alpha$-smooth muscle actin and desmin. Grafts showed circumferential alignment, significant ECM production, and burst strengths of about 2000 mm Hg. However, only a 50% patency rate was seen in a canine model after 1 week. Note that this was a xenograft implantation and one would expect a significant immune response. Other disadvantages included a total culture time of 3 months, and the fact that much of the graft's strength was attributed to the adventitial layer, not the medial layer as seen in native vessels.

## 35.3.4 Matrix and Culture Effects

The importance of matrix signaling has been demonstrated for both stem cells [47,48] as well as differentiated vascular cell types. Nikolovski et al. cultured SMCs on two different types of scaffolds, collagen, and PGA. They demonstrated that SMCs can sense the nature of the substrate and that SMCs proliferated to a greater degree on collagen, while SMCs exhibited greater differentiated function as measured by elastin production on PGA scaffolds. This result was confirmed not only on 2D substrates but also on 3-D scaffolds. The investigators hypothesized that the cells were "sensing" their substrate via the adsorbed protein layer and subsequently examined the composition of those proteins.

Prior work in our lab has demonstrated that an adult mesodermal progenitor cell, specifically human MSCs, seeded in a PEGylated fibrin gel within 48 h *in vitro* began to form vascular tube-like networks, in contrast to controls of unreactive PEG mixed with fibrinogen or fibrin alone [49]. These tubes stained positive for mature EC specific markers like CD31 and vWF. Real-time polymerase chain reaction

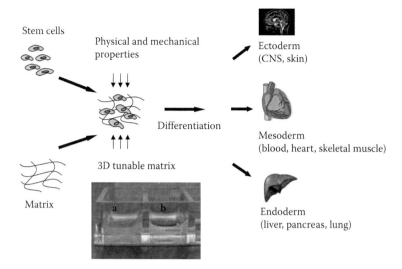

**FIGURE 35.1** Schematic of a controlled 3D matrix culture system for directing stem cell differentiation. Picture denotes 3D cell culture matrix in 4-well chamber slide. (a) Fibrin (b) PEGylated fibrin. (Reproduced with permission from Zhang, G. et al. *Acta Biomater*, 2010.)

(RT-PCR) data also demonstrated that CD31 and vWF as well as VEGF mRNA was expressed in MSCs. This demonstrates that the composition of the culture substrate or matrix can not only control the differentiated function of cells but also drive stem cell differentiation toward an EC-like phenotype. Clearly, vascular tissue engineering depends on a number of factors including media composition as well as scaffold chemistry and physical characteristics. (Figure 35.1).

## 35.4 Growth Factor Signaling

The third component of a classical tissue engineering approach is any signaling imposed on target cells to induce or maintain the desired phenotype. In particular, soluble signals have been used either as a media supplement to support maturation of TEVGs as described below, as a localized cytokine on synthetic materials in order to control cell migration and growth, or as a delivered drug from degradable matrices to encourage blood vessel network formation. A number of cytokines are involved in the stimulation of vascular cells including ECs, SMCs, and their progenitors. One of the most widely studied factors in VEGF which includes the isoforms A–F and PlGF [50]. The family of VEGF peptides is a key player in the angiogenic response [51]. VEGF can exert activity directly on ECs to stimulate migration and proliferation in the formation of neovasculature. VEGF acts to induce mobilization of EPCs into peripheral blood as well as to induce differentiation from EPCs and ECFCs. Additionally, VEGF acts as a factor to increase blood vessel permeability.

The family of fibroblast growth factors (FGFs) is another group of potent factors controlling angiogenesis [52]. Over 22 members of the FGF family have been identified and many of them act on multiple cells types. FGF1 and FGF2 have been reported to act on ECs to enhance angiogenesis. In particular FGF1 and FGF2 can promote an angiogenic phenotype in culture [53]. FGFs can exert their activity through autocrine or paracrine pathways to promote angiogenesis. Molecular cross-talk exists between the FGF and VEGF families of growth factors, and they can act synergistically to promote blood vessel formation while retaining specific activities toward ECs [54].

Platelet-derived growth factor (PDGF) has a number of activities on vascular cells including mediating collagen synthesis by fibroblasts, mediating inflammation, regulating lymph development, and recruiting stem cell mobilization [55]. PDGF has also been shown to cause dramatic effects on SMCs and their progenitors. PDGF promotes recruitment of pericytes during blood vessel development, thereby enhancing blood vessel stabilization and maturation [56]. The effects of PDGF on SMCs include enhancing proliferation, migration, and synthesis of matrix proteins. TGF-β1 is a pleiotropic growth factor that has an indirect effect on the angiogenesis cascade by upregulating production of VEGF and basic fibroblast growth factor (bFGF) from SMCs [57]. Additionally, it has been hypothesized that TGF-β1 may recruit inflammatory cells that release VEGF, bFGF, and PDGF-BB and thus further influence angiogenesis [58,59]. Furthermore, evidence has indicated that TGF-β1 may induce SMC phenotype from a population of MSCs [60–62].

Other factors involved in regulating angiogenesis and blood vessel maturation include the angiopoietins; angiopoietin-1 and -2, hepatocyte growth factor (HGF), neurotrophin nerve growth factor, erythropoietin, and insulin-like growth factor as well as members of the hedgehog (Hh) family of proteins, particularly sonic hedgehog (Shh) which has demonstrated potent angiogenic activity.

Incorporation of cytokines into synthetic materials that retain graft strength and growth factor activity is a significant challenge. The vascular growth factors VEGF and FGF-1 have been delivered from cardiovascular implants using the native affinity of these factors for natural proteins such as fibrin and heparin. Commercially available fibrin adhesive has been embedded within expanded polytetrafluoroethylene (ePTFE) grafts [63,64]. The presence of cytokine-loaded fibrin alters the drug release profile to maintain activity over a longer timecourse. Heparin has also been used in the development of affinity matrices. In particular, heparin has been covalently bound to ePTFE and to polyester grafts via charge interaction [65,66]. Heparin has been used to slow growth factor release by incorporation in fibrin and embedding in synthetic grafts. Casper et al. used a low molecular weight heparin (LMWH) grafted to PEG followed by electrospinning into poly(lactic-*co*-glycolic acid) (PLGA) grafts. Heparin and FGF retention was higher with the conjugation versus LMWH alone [67]. Other matrix proteins that have been used to mediate growth factor release include albumin to localize VEGF [68] and combinations of gelatin and heparin to localize VEGF and FGF-2 to polyurethane grafts [69].

Incorporating cytokines into cardiovascular device coatings has the potential to mediate cell growth around the device. Analogous to EC seeding on vascular conduits, enhancing signaling from a synthetic surface may encourage EC growth and migration to enhance endothelialization. In particular, VEGF has been incorporated into hydrocarbon stent coatings, EC growth was enhanced, but restenosis in animal models was not reduced [70,71]. Phosphorylcholine coatings have been used in VEGF gene delivery strategy with success [72,73]. As is the case with EC seeding, the retention of migrated ECs on device surfaces is complicated by flowing blood and the underlying stiffness of the surface.

An alternative to incorporation of growth factors either within grafts or within device coatings is to tether growth factors directly onto surfaces. In particular, the challenge with this strategy is to retain growth factor activity following tethering. Pioneering work by Ito and Imanishi reported the immobilization of insulin directly onto polymeric substrates. Enhanced cell proliferation was demonstrated relative to controls of soluble or adsorbed insulin [74]. Surface-tethering of insulin also resulted in an increase in the degree of endothelialization on vascular grafts. Cells could be maintained in tissue culture without media supplementation of serum through the use of insulin delivered via surface-tethering to microcarriers. Surface-tethering of growth factors may provide some unique advantages over soluble signals including protection against normal enzymatic inactivation as well as the highly localized action of the growth factor activity. Immobilization of growth factors using the molecularly mobile, PEG may aggregate ligand–receptor complexes on the cell surface and augment receptor-mediated functions [75]. Similar immobilization strategies have been used to encourage EC or EPC engraftment on synthetic substrates [15,76].

Mann used an acryloyl-PEG-N-hydroxy succinimide (NHS) molecule to incorporate adhesion peptides into a PEG hydrogel [77]. Tethering growth factor (GFs) such as TGF-β1 using the same acryloyl-PEG-NHS chemistry increased matrix production and elastic modulus. It is hypothesized that local presentation of the GF maintains bioactivity and promotes localized effects [37]. This same chemistry could incorporate other GFs to promote EC proliferation or activity [78]. Further, the cell adhesive domain arginine-glycine-aspartic acid-serine (RGDS) can be patterned within gels to promote EC tubulogenesis [79].

## 35.5 Vascular Grafts and Medial Equivalents

The seminal work on TEVGs by Weinberg and Bell in 1986 [80] was based on the observed contraction of a collagen by embedded fibroblasts. Contraction of 10–20-fold was possible and particular focus was directed toward the replacement of the contractile or medial layer of the TEVG. Several groups have attempted to improve upon the mechanical strength of collagen gel-based TEVGs using various methods. Tranquillo's group has investigated magnetically-oriented collagen gel fibrils and glycation cross-linking to increase mechanical strength [81,82]. They also looked at fibrin as an alternative to collagen and studied the effect of various media supplements, including ascorbic acid, TGF-B, insulin, and plasmin [83,84]. Seliktar conditioned collagen gel-based TEVGs with cyclic mechanical strain and noted increased mechanical strength through matrix metalloproteinase remodeling [85]. With the use of these methods, the burst strength of TEVGs has been increased above that of Weinberg and Bell, but is still a major concern for clinical translation.

The further refinement of TEVGs in 1999 by Niklason et al. demonstrated the increase and maintenance of burst strength of the construct. A major contributor to the success of this vessel was the pulsatile bioreactor culture system. An example of this is shown in Figure 35.2. Conditioning was performed at 165 beats/min and a radial strain of 5%. Previous work has shown that dynamic mechanical strain regulates the development of *in vitro* smooth muscle tissue [86]. The mechanical stresses imparted by the bioreactor, in addition to media supplements, contributed to vessel strength by increasing collagen synthesis *in vitro*. This idea is important for any TEVG that contains a SMC component. Further work to study the benefits of fibril alignment, cross-linking, and media supplements, as demonstrated by other groups, could lead to further improvements.

In a unique strategy, SMCs have been incorporated directly into electrospun poly(ester urethane) urea (PEUU) scaffolds [87]. Using this method, investigators could uniformly distribute a large number of cells within a material possessing the necessary strength and extensibility for use as a graft material. Using a combination of electrospinning and electrospraying maintained cell viability during processing even in the presence of organic solvents. Measured strengths were reduced by ~24%, but *in vivo* results have not yet been reported.

Media composition has been shown to be important for the bulk of cell seeding approaches described above. In particular, most rely on high concentrations of various factors in culture along with relative

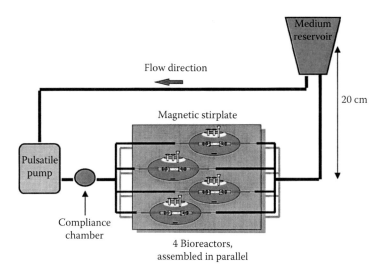

**FIGURE 35.2** Biomimetic system for vessel culture. (Reproduced with permission from Niklason, L.E. et al., *Science*, 1999. **284**(5413): 489–93.)

long periods of culture or mechanical conditioning in order to enhance burst strengths of TEVGs. For cell assembly as described by L'Heureux SMCs from human umbilical veins and fibroblasts from human dermis were cultured independently in culture supplemented with 50 µg/mL of ascorbic acid. In Nicklason's work the media was supplemented with 20% fetal bovine serum, ascorbic acid, copper, and various amino acids. Typical *in vitro* culture times range from weeks to months. It would be desirable to reduce the culture times as well as to control the cytokine composition that the cells are exposed to locally following implantation. These goals have motivated work into optimizing signaling events either in culture or following implantation. Another problem that will have to be addressed in the future is cell source if fully differentiated cells are to be used. Autologous tissue is the best cell source to prevent an immune response, yet extended culture is necessary between cell harvest and graft implantation.

The greatest challenges that TEVGs currently face are thrombosis and insufficient mechanical strength; both of these could cause catastrophic failure of a graft *in vivo*. Compliance mismatch has been implicated as a problem in previous graft failures. Close matching of mechanical properties is of importance; however, exact matching may not be necessary. Currently used autologous vessel grafts have widely varied mechanical properties, yet have been successful as replacement tissue. A successful TEVG should mimic the native artery as closely as possible, both in character and function. Ideally, the ECM should contain similar amounts of collagen and elastin to the native artery, to ensure comparable strength and recoil. The graft should also contain a confluent layer of luminal ECs to prevent thrombosis. Additionally, for a graft to be commercially feasible, it will need to be cost effective and competitive with current graft therapies. None of the previously described TEVGs meet all the requirements for a successful, implantable replacement therapy. Clearly, there is room for further research in this area.

## 35.6 Engineered Vascular Networks

There is a significant interest in neovascularization of growth of new blood vessels following ischemia. Blood vessel obstruction in various tissues such as cardiac or skeletal muscle leads to tissue hypoxia and tissue necrosis. This is particular damaging in the heart due to the postmitotic state of the mature cardiac myocyte. The restoration of blood flow through ischemic tissues may regenerate new tissue or rescue existing tissue (as in the cardiac case) leading to improved function.

Strategies for enhancing vascularization are based on the use of angiogenic agents or vascular cells that can either encourage blood vessel growth from existing vessels (angiogenesis) or participate in the assembly of blood vessels (vasculogenesis). As noted previously, a number of different stem and progenitor cell populations including: MSCs, HSCs and EPCs have demonstrated potential for vascular cell differentiation. These cells have been delivered to ischemic tissues in various animal models as well as clinical trials. The infusion of autologous MSCs following myocardial infarction and reperfusion is still ongoing to evaluate functional recovery.

The extent to which stem cells can actually participate in new blood vessels may be very dependent on the cell type and microenvironment. Very detailed fluorescent cell labeling and confocal imaging of transplanted cells into skeletal muscle revealed that while MSCs could participate in neovascularization, the extent of transdifferentiation toward vascular cell types was minimal [88]. Our laboratory has demonstrated that while MSCs could readily transdifferentiate into vascular cells including ECs *in vitro*, the extent of trandifferentiation *in vivo* in a mouse MI model was not correlated with the extent of new blood vessel formation [49,89].

Recent studies have shown the importance of the contribution of multiple cell types including vascular progenitors when engineering vascularized tissue on synthetic matrices [90]. Constructs fabricated from 50/50 poly(L-lactic acid) (PLLA)/PLGA were seeded with mouse myoblasts and human embryonic ECs. The addition of an EC population increased implant vascularization and subsequent tissue viability. Blood vessel organization, however, has only been investigated *in vivo*, and it remains unclear the relative contribution of EPC types, whether providing a purely paracrine role or differentiating and incorporating into the newly formed blood vessels [91].

Combination strategies using multiple growth factors, stem cell populations or growth factor stimulation in combination with stem cell delivery may be necessary in order to provide a robust blood vessel network. Much can be learned from vascular biology with respect to the activity of various growth factors in the development of blood vessels. The action of cytokines can be dependent on concentration, timing and the context of the target cell. It is therefore of great importance to have growth factor presentation that is tightly controlled. A major challenge in growth factory delivery is the relatively short half-life of most therapeutic peptides as well as their sensitivity to processing. Scaffold delivery systems that can deliver multiple growth factors and/or stem cells are particularly challenging. Stem cell delivery is complicated by the typically low retention of viable cells as well as the lack of understanding regarding the mechanism for enhanced blood vessel formation. Tissue engineering advances may provide solutions for combination delivery with next generation scaffolds.

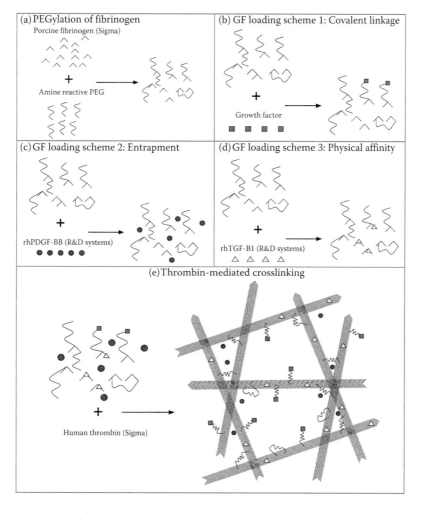

**FIGURE 35.3** Schematic of 3 mechanisms to load growth factors (GFs) into PEGylated fibrin gels. (a) Depicts PEGylation of fibrinogen with amine reactive PEG. (b) Depicts conjugation of GF through homobifunctional PEG. (Adapted from Zhang, G. et al., *Tissue Eng*, 2007. **13**(8): 2063–71; Zhang, G. et al., *Tissue Eng*, 2006. **12**(1): 9–19.) (c) Depicts admixing of GFs into PEG and fibrinogen solution. (d) Depicts physical affinity of particular GFs with fibrinogen. (e) Depicts thrombin-mediated gelation of fibrinogen into PEGylated fibrin gels loaded with multiple GFs. (Reproduced with permission from Drinnan, C.T. et al., *J Control Release*, 2010.)

Examples of matrices that have been used for combination delivery include natural proteins such as type I collagen or fibrin to treat ischemic myocardium [92,93]. The native biologic activity of structural proteins may be particularly important for maintaining cell viability and differentiated function. Designed peptides based on charged α-linked side chains have been investigated as self-assembling matrices with the ability to recruit therapeutic cell populations in a mouse myocardial model. Endothelial and SMCs were identified following delivery [94,95]. A cardiomyoctye survival factor was also delivered via self-assembling peptide with measured induction of downstream signaling [96]. Investigators have correlated the matrix physical characteristics to the organization of formed vascular networks.

Pioneering work by Mooney and colleagues demonstrated the dual delivery of growth factors with distinct kinetics. Richardson et al. incorporated VEGF and PDGF-BB into a poly(lactic-*co*-glycolic acid) (PLGA) matrix and microspheres to present a controlled dual GF release [97]. Increased blood vessel size and distribution were demonstrated with the multiple GF release compared to individual GF release. Similarly, our laboratory has demonstrated that PEGylated fibrin can be loaded with growth factors using different mechanisms with varying release profiles (Figure 35.3). Specifically, a rapid release of PDGF-BB and delayed release of TGF-β1 was demonstrated by two distinct mechanisms. These release profiles parallel vasculogenesis models for capillary tube stabilization and mural cell differentiation [98,99]. Further, differentiation of MSCs toward pericytes is predicted to require a similar GF cascade to form mature mural cells [62].

Our laboratory has also reported the combination delivery of stem cells with growth factor delivery. We looked specifically at the codelivery of HGF and MSCs in a mouse model of myocardial ischemia [89]. We demonstrated that delivery of both cells and HGF from PEGylated fibrin resulted in a 15-fold increase in cell retention with reduced fibrosis and enhanced ejection fraction as a measure of cardiac performance. An important conclusion of this study was that increases in blood vessel density could be produced through the release of the growth factor alone which was not necessarily correlated with improved cardiac output. While many growth factors are known to stimulate angiogenesis, the stabilization and maturation of newly formed vessels may be more complex and necessary for functional recovery.

## 35.7  Conclusions

Successful vascular tissue engineering strategies consider cell source, scaffold composition, as well as any additional signals that may be imposed during culture. Challenges that remain within this field are generally associated with defining the appropriate cell populations and controlling the effects of matrix composition and signaling upon the cells of interest. Cell source and the contribution of vascular progenitors in repair and blood vessel assembly are open questions. Identifying the correct cell population, scaffold characteristics and added signals for the development of blood vessels continues to be an important question within the field of vascular tissue engineering.

## References

1. Schmedlen, R.H. et al., Tissue engineered small-diameter vascular grafts. *Clin Plast Surg*, 2003. **30**(4): 507–17.
2. Tu, J.V. et al., Use of cardiac procedures and outcomes in elderly patients with myocardial infarction in the United States and Canada. *N Engl J Med*, 1997. **336**(21): 1500–5.
3. Moneta, G.L. and J.M. Porter, Arterial substitutes in peripheral vascular surgery: A review. *J Long Term Eff Med Implants*, 1995. **5**(1): 47–67.
4. Williams, S.K., D.G. Rose, and B.E. Jarrell, Microvascular endothelial cell sodding of ePTFE vascular grafts: Improved patency and stability of the cellular lining. *J Biomed Mater Res*, 1994. **28**(2): 203–12.
5. Schmidt, S.P. et al., Evaluation of expanded polytetrafluoroethylene arteriovenous access grafts onto which microvessel-derived cells were transplanted to "improve" graft performance: Preliminary results. *Ann Vasc Surg*, 1998. **12**(5): 405–11.

6. Planat-Benard, V. et al., Plasticity of human adipose lineage cells toward endothelial cells: Physiological and therapeutic perspectives. *Circulation*, 2004. **109**(5): 656–63.

7. Asahara, T. and J.M. Isner, Endothelial progenitor cells for vascular regeneration. *J Hematother Stem Cell Res*, 2002. **11**(2): 171–78.

8. Gehling, U.M. et al., *In vitro* differentiation of endothelial cells from AC133-positive progenitor cells. *Blood*, 2000. **95**(10): 3106–12.

9. Boyer, M. et al., Isolation of endothelial cells and their progenitor cells from human peripheral blood. *J Vasc Surg*, 2000. **31**(1 Pt 1): 181–89.

10. Bhattacharya, V. et al., Enhanced endothelialization and microvessel formation in polyester grafts seeded with CD34(+) bone marrow cells. *Blood*, 2000. **95**(2): 581–85.

11. Ribatti, D., The discovery of endothelial progenitor cells. An historical review. *Leuk Res*, 2007. **31**(4): 439–44.

12. Cottler-Fox, M.H. et al., Stem cell mobilization. *Hematol Am Soc Hematol Educ Program*, 2003: 419–37.

13. van Royen, N. et al., START Trial: A pilot study on STimulation of ARTeriogenesis using subcutaneous application of granulocyte-macrophage colony-stimulating factor as a new treatment for peripheral vascular disease. *Circulation*, 2005. **112**(7): 1040–46.

14. Zhang, G. et al., Controlled release of stromal cell-derived factor-1 alpha *in situ* increases c-kit+ cell homing to the infarcted heart. *Tissue Eng*, 2007. **13**(8): 2063–71.

15. Aoki, J. et al., Endothelial progenitor cell capture by stents coated with antibody against CD34: The HEALING-FIM (Healthy Endothelial Accelerated Lining Inhibits Neointimal Growth-First In Man) *Registry*. *J Am Coll Cardiol*, 2005. **45**(10): 1574–79.

16. Grassl, E.D., T.R. Oegema, and R.T. Tranquillo, Fibrin as an alternative biopolymer to type-I collagen for the fabrication of a media equivalent. *J Biomed Mater Res*, 2002. **60**(4): 607–12.

17. Simper, D. et al., Smooth muscle progenitor cells in human blood. *Circulation*, 2002. **106**(10): 1199–204.

18. Park, J.S. et al., Differential effects of equiaxial and uniaxial strain on mesenchymal stem cells. *Biotechnol Bioeng*, 2004. **88**(3): 359–68.

19. Makino, S. et al., Cardiomyocytes can be generated from marrow stromal cells *in vitro*. *J Clin Invest*, 1999. **103**(5): 697–705.

20. Pittenger, M.F. et al., Multilineage potential of adult human mesenchymal stem cells. *Science*, 1999. **284**(5411): 143–47.

21. Toma, C. et al., Human mesenchymal stem cells differentiate to a cardiomyocyte phenotype in the adult murine heart. *Circulation*, 2002. **105**(1): 93–98.

22. Strauer, B.E. et al., Repair of infarcted myocardium by autologous intracoronary mononuclear bone marrow cell transplantation in humans. *Circulation*, 2002. **106**(15): 1913–18.

23. Abedin, M., Y. Tintut, and L.L. Demer, Mesenchymal stem cells and the artery wall. *Circ Res*, 2004. **95**(7): 671–76.

24. Tintut, Y. et al., Multilineage potential of cells from the artery wall. *Circulation*, 2003. **108**(20): 2505–10.

25. Isomatsu, Y. et al., Extracardiac total cavopulmonary connection using a tissue-engineered graft. *J Thorac Cardiovasc Surg*, 2003. **126**(6): 1958–62.

26. Menasche, P., The potential of embryonic stem cells to treat heart disease. *Curr Opin Mol Ther*, 2005. **7**(4): 293–99.

27. Oh, S.K. and A.B. Choo, Human embryonic stem cells: Technological challenges towards therapy. *Clin Exp Pharmacol Physiol*, 2006. **33**(5–6): 489–95.

28. Park, I.H. et al., Reprogramming of human somatic cells to pluripotency with defined factors. *Nature*, 2008. **451**(7175): 141–46.

29. Boheler, K.R. et al., Differentiation of pluripotent embryonic stem cells into cardiomyocytes. *Circ Res*, 2002. **91**(3): 189–201.

30. Hegert, C. et al., Differentiation plasticity of chondrocytes derived from mouse embryonic stem cells. *J Cell Sci*, 2002. **115**(Pt 23): 4617–28.

31. Kramer, J., C. Hegert, and J. Rohwedel, *In vitro* differentiation of mouse ES cells: Bone and cartilage. *Methods Enzymol*, 2003. **365**: 251–68.

32. Levenberg, S. et al., Endothelial cells derived from human embryonic stem cells. *Proc Natl Acad Sci USA*, 2002. **99**(7): 4391–96.

33. Wobus, A.M. et al., Embryonic stem cells as a model to study cardiac, skeletal muscle, and vascular smooth muscle cell differentiation. *Methods Mol Biol*, 2002. **185**: 127–56.

34. Niklason, L.E. et al., Functional arteries grown *in vitro*. *Science*, 1999. **284**(5413): 489–93.

35. Hill-West, J.L. et al., Prevention of postoperative adhesions in the rat by *in situ* photopolymerization of bioresorbable hydrogel barriers. *Obstet Gynecol*, 1994. **83**(1): 59–64.

36. Hern, D.L. and J.A. Hubbell, Incorporation of adhesion peptides into nonadhesive hydrogels useful for tissue resurfacing. *J Biomed Mater Res*, 1998. **39**(2): 266–76.

37. Mann, B.K., R.H. Schmedlen, and J.L. West, Tethered-TGF-beta increases extracellular matrix production of vascular smooth muscle cells. *Biomaterials*, 2001. **22**(5): 439–44.

38. Gobin, A.S. and J.L. West, Cell migration through defined, synthetic ECM analogs. *Faseb J*, 2002. **16**(7): 751–53.

39. Mann, B.K. et al., Smooth muscle cell growth in photopolymerized hydrogels with cell adhesive and proteolytically degradable domains: Synthetic ECM analogs for tissue engineering. *Biomaterials*, 2001. **22**(22): 3045–51.

40. Weinberg, C.B. and E. Bell, A blood vessel model constructed from collagen and cultured vascular cells. *Science*, 1986. **231**(4736): 397–400.

41. Roeder, R. et al., Compliance, elastic modulus, and burst pressure of small-intestine submucosa (SIS), small-diameter vascular grafts. *J Biomed Mater Res*, 1999. **47**(1): 65–70.

42. Huynh, T. et al., Remodeling of an acellular collagen graft into a physiologically responsive neovessel. *Nat Biotechnol*, 1999. **17**(11): 1083–86.

43. Roeder, R.A., G.C. Lantz, and L.A. Geddes, Mechanical remodeling of small-intestine submucosa small-diameter vascular grafts—A preliminary report. *Biomed Instrum Technol*, 2001. **35**(2): 110–20.

44. Bader, A. et al., Engineering of human vascular aortic tissue based on a xenogeneic starter matrix. *Transplantation*, 2000. **70**(1): 7–14.

45. Teebken, O.E. et al., Tissue engineering of vascular grafts: Human cell seeding of decellularised porcine matrix. *Eur J Vasc Endovasc Surg*, 2000. **19**(4): 381–86.

46. L'Heureux, N. et al., A completely biological tissue-engineered human blood vessel. *Faseb J*, 1998. **12**(1): 47–56.

47. Engler, A.J. et al., Matrix elasticity directs stem cell lineage specification. *Cell*, 2006. **126**(4): 677–89.

48. Engler, A.J. et al., Myotubes differentiate optimally on substrates with tissue-like stiffness: Pathological implications for soft or stiff microenvironments. *J Cell Biol*, 2004. **166**(6): 877–87.

49. Zhang, G. et al., A PEGylated fibrin patch for mesenchymal stem cell delivery. *Tissue Eng*, 2006. **12**(1): 9–19.

50. Roy, H., S. Bhardwaj, and S. Yla-Herttuala, Biology of vascular endothelial growth factors. *FEBS Lett*, 2006. **580**(12): 2879–87.

51. Shibuya, M., Differential roles of vascular endothelial growth factor receptor-1 and receptor-2 in angiogenesis. *J Biochem Mol Biol*, 2006. **39**(5): 469–78.

52. Presta, M. et al., Fibroblast growth factor/fibroblast growth factor receptor system in angiogenesis. *Cytokine Growth Factor Rev*, 2005. **16**(2): 159–78.

53. Wiedlocha, A. and V. Sorensen, Signaling, internalization, and intracellular activity of fibroblast growth factor. *Curr Top Microbiol Immunol*, 2004. **286**: 45–79.

54. Distler, J.H. et al., Angiogenic and angiostatic factors in the molecular control of angiogenesis. *Q J Nucl Med*, 2003. **47**(3): 149–61.

55. Alvarez, R.H., H.M. Kantarjian, and J.E. Cortes, Biology of platelet-derived growth factor and its involvement in disease. *Mayo Clin Proc*, 2006. **81**(9): 1241–57.

56. Wang, X.T., P.Y. Liu, and J.B. Tang, PDGF gene therapy enhances expression of VEGF and bFGF genes and activates the NF-kappaB gene in signal pathways in ischemic flaps. *Plast Reconstr Surg*, 2006. **117**(1): 129–37; discussion 138–9.

57. Isner, J.M. and A. Takayuki, Therapeutic angiogenesis. *Front Biosci*, 1998. **3**: e49–69.

58. Ahrendt, G., D.E. Chickering, and J.P. Ranieri, Angiogenic growth factors: A review for tissue engineering. *Tissue Eng*, 1998. **4**(2): 117–30.

59. Li, J., Y.P. Zhang, and R.S. Kirsner, Angiogenesis in wound repair: Angiogenic growth factors and the extracellular matrix. *Microsc Res Tech*, 2003. **60**(1): 107–14.

60. Seruya, M. et al., Clonal population of adult stem cells: Life span and differentiation potential. *Cell Transplant*, 2004. **13**(2): 93–101.

61. Wang, D. et al., Proteomic profiling of bone marrow mesenchymal stem cells upon transforming growth factor beta1 stimulation. *J Biol Chem*, 2004. **279**(42): 43725–34.

62. Ross, J.J. et al., Cytokine-induced differentiation of multipotent adult progenitor cells into functional smooth muscle cells. *J. Clin. Invest*, 2006. **116**(12): 3139–49.

63. Gosselin, C. et al., ePTFE coating with fibrin glue, FGF-1, and heparin: Effect on retention of seeded endothelial cells. *J Surg Res*, 1996. **60**(2): 327–32.

64. Greisler, H.P. et al., Enhanced endothelialization of expanded polytetrafluoroethylene grafts by fibroblast growth factor type 1 pretreatment. *Surgery*, 1992. **112**(2): 244–54; discussion 254–5.

65. Mohamed, M.S., M. Mukherjee, and V.V. Kakkar, Thrombogenicity of heparin and non-heparin bound arterial prostheses: An *in vitro* evaluation. *J R Coll Surg Edinb*, 1998. **43**(3): 155–57.

66. Begovac, P.C. et al., Improvements in GORE-TEX vascular graft performance by Carmeda BioActive surface heparin immobilization. *Eur J Vasc Endovasc Surg*, 2003. **25**(5): 432–37.

67. Casper, C.L. et al., Functionalizing electrospun fibers with biologically relevant macromolecules. *Biomacromolecules*, 2005. **6**(4): 1998–2007.

68. Crombez, M. et al., Improving arterial prosthesis neo-endothelialization: Application of a proactive VEGF construct onto PTFE surfaces. *Biomaterials*, 2005. **26**(35): 7402–9.

69. Masuda, S. et al., Vascular endothelial growth factor enhances vascularization in microporous small caliber polyurethane grafts. *Asaio J*, 1997. **43**(5): M530–34.

70. Swanson, N. et al., *In vitro* evaluation of vascular endothelial growth factor (VEGF)-eluting stents. *Int J Cardiol*, 2003. **92**(2–3): 247–51.

71. Swanson, N. et al., Vascular endothelial growth factor (VEGF)-eluting stents: *In vivo* effects on thrombosis, endothelialization and intimal hyperplasia. *J Invasive Cardiol*, 2003. **15**(12): 688–92.

72. Van Belle, E. et al., Passivation of metallic stents after arterial gene transfer of phVEGF165 inhibits thrombus formation and intimal thickening. *J Am Coll Cardiol*, 1997. **29**(6): 1371–79.

73. Walter, D.H. et al., Local gene transfer of phVEGF-2 plasmid by gene-eluting stents: An alternative strategy for inhibition of restenosis. *Circulation*, 2004. **110**(1): 36–45.

74. Ito, Y., G. Chen, and Y. Imanishi, Artificial juxtacrine stimulation for tissue engineering. *J Biomater Sci Polym Ed*, 1998. **9**(8): 879–90.

75. Li, J.S. et al., Enhancement of artificial juxtacrine stimulation of insulin by co-immobilization with adhesion factors. *J Biomed Mater Res*, 1997. **37**(2): 190–97.

76. Blindt, R. et al., A novel drug-eluting stent coated with an integrin-binding cyclic Arg-Gly-Asp peptide inhibits neointimal hyperplasia by recruiting endothelial progenitor cells. *J Am Coll Cardiol*, 2006. **47**(9): 1786–95.

77. Mann, B.K. and J.L. West, Cell adhesion peptides alter smooth muscle cell adhesion, proliferation, migration, and matrix protein synthesis on modified surfaces and in polymer scaffolds. *J Biomed Mater Res*, 2002. **60**(1): 86–93.

78. Leslie-Barbick, J.E., J.J. Moon, and J.L. West, Covalently-immobilized vascular endothelial growth factor promotes endothelial cell tubulogenesis in poly(ethylene glycol) diacrylate hydrogels. *J Biomater Sci Polym Ed*, 2009. **20**(12): 1763–79.

79. Moon, J.J. et al., Micropatterning of poly(ethylene glycol) diacrylate hydrogels with biomolecules to regulate and guide endothelial morphogenesis. *Tissue Eng Part A*, 2009. **15**(3): 579–85.

80. Weinberg, C.B. and E. Bell, A blood vessel model constructed from collagen and cultured vascular cells. *Science*, 1986. **231**(4736): 397–400.

81. Girton, T.S., T.R. Oegema, and R.T. Tranquillo, Exploiting glycation to stiffen and strengthen tissue equivalents for tissue engineering. *J Biomed Mater Res*, 1999. **46**(1): 87–92.

82. Tranquillo, R.T. et al., Magnetically orientated tissue-equivalent tubes: Application to a circumferentially orientated media-equivalent. *Biomaterials*, 1996. **17**(3): 349–57.

83. Grassl, E.D., T.R. Oegema, and R.T. Tranquillo, Fibrin as an alternative biopolymer to type-I collagen for the fabrication of a media equivalent. *J Biomed Mater Res*, 2002. **60**(4): 607–12.

84. Neidert, M.R. et al., Enhanced fibrin remodeling *in vitro* with TGF-beta1, insulin and plasmin for improved tissue-equivalents. *Biomaterials*, 2002. **23**(17): 3717–31.

85. Seliktar, D., R.M. Nerem, and Z.S. Galis, The role of matrix metalloproteinase-2 in the remodeling of cell-seeded vascular constructs subjected to cyclic strain. *Ann Biomed Eng*, 2001. **29**(11): 923–34.

86. Kim, B.S. et al., Cyclic mechanical strain regulates the development of engineered smooth muscle tissue. *Nat Biotechnol*, 1999. **17**(10): 979–83.

87. Stankus, J.J. et al., Microintegrating smooth muscle cells into a biodegradable, elastomeric fiber matrix. *Biomaterials*, 2006. **27**(5): 735–44.

88. O'Neill, T.J.t. et al., Mobilization of bone marrow-derived cells enhances the angiogenic response to hypoxia without transdifferentiation into endothelial cells. *Circ Res*, 2005. **97**(10): 1027–35.

89. Zhang, G. et al., Enhancing efficacy of stem cell transplantation to the heart with a PEGylated fibrin biomatrix. *Tissue Eng Part A*, 2008. **14**(6): 1025–36.

90. Levenberg, S. et al., Engineering vascularized skeletal muscle tissue. *Nat Biotechnol*, 2005. **23**(7): 879–84.

91. Murayama, T. et al., Determination of bone marrow-derived endothelial progenitor cell significance in angiogenic growth factor-induced neovascularization *in vivo*. *Exp Hematol*, 2002. **30**(8): 967–72.

92. Liu, J. et al., Autologous stem cell transplantation for myocardial repair. *Am J Physiol Heart Circ Physiol*, 2004. **287**(2): H501–11.

93. Xiang, Z. et al., Collagen-GAG scaffolds grafted onto myocardial infarcts in a rat model: A delivery vehicle for mesenchymal stem cells. *Tissue Eng*, 2006. **12**(9): 2467–78.

94. Davis, M.E. et al., Injectable self-assembling peptide nanofibers create intramyocardial microenvironments for endothelial cells. *Circulation*, 2005. **111**(4): 442–50.

95. Narmoneva, D.A. et al., Self-assembling short oligopeptides and the promotion of angiogenesis. *Biomaterials*, 2005. **26**(23): 4837–46.

96. Davis, M.E. et al., Local myocardial insulin-like growth factor 1 (IGF-1) delivery with biotinylated peptide nanofibers improves cell therapy for myocardial infarction. *Proc Natl Acad Sci USA*, 2006. **103**(21): 8155–60.

97. Richardson, T.P. et al., Polymeric system for dual growth factor delivery. *Nat Biotechnol*, 2001. **19**(11): 1029–34.

98. Hirschi, K.K. et al., Endothelial cells modulate the proliferation of mural cell precursors via platelet-derived growth factor-BB and heterotypic cell contact. *Circ Res*, 1999. **84**(3): 298–305.

99. Hirschi, K.K., S.A. Rohovsky, and P.A. D'Amore, PDGF, TGF-B, and heterotpic cell-cell interactions mediate endothelial cell-induced recruitment of 10T1/2 cells and their differentiation to smooth muscle fate. *J Cell Biol*, 1998. **141**(3): 805–14.

100. Zhang, G., C.T. Drinnan, L.R. Geuss, and L.J. Suggs, Vascular differentiation of bone marrow stem cells is directed by a tunable three-dimensional matrix. *Acta Biomater*, 2010. **6**(9): 3395–403.

101. Drinnan, C.T., G. Zhang, M.A. Alexander, A.S. Pulido, and L.J. Suggs, Multimodal release of transforming growth factor-beta1 and the BB isoform of platelet derived growth factor from PEGylated fibrin gels. *J Control Release*, 2010. **147**(2): 180–5.

# 36

# Neural Engineering

36.1 Overview of the Anatomy of the Nervous System.....................36-1
36.2 Peripheral Nerve Repair ...............................................................36-2
    Injuries and Treatments • Biomaterials in Peripheral Nerve
    Repair • Cellular and Growth Factor–Containing Nerve
    Guides • Summary
36.3 CNS Repair .....................................................................................36-7
    Brain Injuries and Spinal Cord Injuries • Biomaterials in CNS
    Research • Cellular Therapies in Spinal Cord Repair
36.4. Animal Models of Nervous System Injury Research ..............36-12
36.5 Overall Summary of Neural Tissue Engineering...................36-12
References...................................................................................................36-12

Yen-Chih Lin
*University of Pittsburgh*

Kacey G. Marra
*University of Pittsburgh*

## 36.1 Overview of the Anatomy of the Nervous System

The nervous system can be divided into three parts: the central nervous system (CNS), the peripheral nervous system (PNS), and the autonomic nervous system (ANS) (Dawson et al. 2003). The CNS consists of the brain and spinal cord. The PNS resides outside the CNS and forms a network to collect information from sensory responses. The ANS is identified by primary ganglia of the head and neck, sympathetic chain and adrenal gland (Gabella and Larry 2009). The primary function of the nervous system is to receive input from the environment and innervate muscle tissues in response. To accomplish this task, neurons, which are the basic unit of the functional nervous system (Dawson et al. 2003), form a highly specific interconnecting network from the brain to the spinal cord. There are 12 paired cranial nerve and 31 paired spinal nerve connections between the CNS and the PNS, which result in motor/efferent, sensory/afferent, or mixed function. Furthermore, internal environments such as cardiorespiratory activities, glandular secretions, vasodilatation and genital erectile tissue responses are monitored by an array of visceral receptors, chemoreceptors, and stretch receptors via autonomic nerves from the CNS (Keller et al. 2009).

The morphology of a neuron is characterized by a prominent round nucleus cell body, an axon (a long cell process), and dendrites (numerous short cell processes). The nervous system contains a network of neurons that communicate with each other by means of the synapse. The cell bodies of peripheral neurons originate in the spinal cord, specifically the dorsal root ganglion and autonomic ganglion, while the axons extend from the centrally located cell bodies and terminate in neuromuscular endings (motor neurons), end organs, or receptors (sensory or sympathetic fibers).

Astrocytes, oligodendrocytes, ependyma, and microglial cells are four major support cells in the mammalian CNS. Astrocytes provide a structural scaffold for other elements of the CNS and regulate the exchange of fluid. Fibrous and protoplasmic astrocytes are two types of astrocytes. Oligodendrocytes coat the axons in the CNS with myelin. The primary function of the ependyma is to interact with astrocytes to form a barrier separating the ventricles of the brain and cerebrospinal fluid (CSF) from the CNS neurons. Microglia are the specialized macrophage in the CNS (Streit 2001). All of these four different cells are known as glial or neuroglial cells (Dawson et al. 2003).

The spinal cord is a long cylinder of gray and white nerve tissue which support cells located in the upper two-thirds of the vertebral canal extending from the brain. In a cross-sectional view, the center region of the spinal cord, which contains cell bodies, dendrites, axons, and glial cells, is gray and butterfly shaped. Outside this region resides white tissue matter composed of axons and glial cells associated with sensory and motor neurons. The following nerves connect the connecting spinal cord to receive incoming signals from the body receptor and sends signals to the body reactors: 8 pairs of cervical nerves, 12 pairs of thoracic, 5 pairs of lumbar, 5 of pairs sacral, and 1 coccygeal nerve.

The PNS is composed of axons, Schwann cells, fibroblast support cells, and blood vessels. Schwann cells are the glial components of the PNS. A Schwann cell is characterized by their variably shaped nucleus and a coarse chromatin pattern surrounded by a thin rim of cytoplasm. Within the PNS, Schwann cells are located around the axons (myelinated axons) or are related to several axons (nonmyelinated axons) and aid in axon function. The ratio of unmyelinated and myelinated axons among sensory and motor nerves receptor is 4:1 (Maggi et al. 2003). The primary function of a Schwann cell is similar to the oligodendrocytes in the CNS (Gallo et al. 2009). The Schwann cells align longitudinally along the length of an axon and concentrically envelope the axons with tightly compressed lipid membranes were referred to as the neurilemma. Large myelinated nerve fibers (10–20 μm) are associated with fast conduction rates, and mainly respond to sensory input and motor outflow to skeletal muscles; intermediate myelinated nerve fibers (3–8 μm) usually conduct messages in response to light touches, pressure, temperature, and pain sensation; small unmyelinated nerve fibers (0.2–1.5 μm) have the slowest conduction rate.

A peripheral nerve consists of axons covered by protective support tissue. Beginning with the basic unit of nerve trunk organization is myelinated or unmyelinated axons embedded in collagen-rich connective tissue termed the endoneurium. The endoneurium, which divides nerve fibers into small undulating groupings which allows nerves to resist elongation under tension, is comprised of glycosaminoglycan and collagen (Sunderland 1968). Furthermore, fibroblast support cells, mast cells and macrophages reside within the endoneurium (Terzis and Smith 1990). A number of nerve fibers are further embedded by an endoneurium layer termed the perineurium, known as a fascicle. The epineurium surrounds and binds groups of fascicles and blood vessel into an anatomical nerve trunk.

Overall, neurons are the highly differentiated elemental cell unit that the entire nervous system is composed of, but the components of support cells differ in CNS, PNS, and ANS. Moreover, it is well known that the nervous system, especially CNS, cannot be easily regenerated on its own due to its specific differentiation. Therefore, nerve tissue repair is a relevant treatment concept in human health care as it directly impacts the quality of life (Yang et al. 2004).

## 36.2 Peripheral Nerve Repair

### 36.2.1 Injuries and Treatments

Nervous system injuries are most commonly caused by trauma (Ichihara et al. 2008), bone fractures or joint dislocations (Millesi 1998). Injuries to the peripheral nerves result in partial or total loss of motor, sensory and autonomic functions conveyed by the lesioned nerves to the denervated segments of the body, due to the interruption of axonal continuity, degeneration of nerve fibers distal to the lesion and eventual death of axotomized neurons (Navarro et al. 2007). Additionally, neurons are comprised of specific shapes and are highly metabolically active resulting in the handicap of nerve regeneration (Dawson et al. 2003; Toth 2009). Therefore, the potential for nerve regeneration based on the severity of nerve damage that does not disrupt the connective tissue macrostructure is extremely poor when large segments of nerve trunks are lost.

There has been more than a century of experience in surgical management, yet repair of a nerve gap remains a challenge in microsurgery (Johnson et al. 2005). The major strategy of current treatments for clinical peripheral nerve surgery is autograft as a replacement. However, only about 50% of patients significantly regain useful functions after post operation (Lee and Wolfe 2000). As a result, many researchers have investigated the use of synthetic or biological guidance channels, muscle, vein grafts, and acellular graft materials as nerve conduits (Glasby et al. 1986; Fansa et al. 2001; Meek and Coert 2002; Walsh et al. 2009). However, the comorbidity of harvesting donor grafts, acute immunization, and weak axonal reconnections are major deterrents. Nerve anastamosis and regeneration remains limited by gap length (Pabari et al. 2010). The challenge of designing nerve guides that meet all of these requirements has rendered the clinical success of a peripheral nerve substitute for gaps surpassing 3 cm thus far elusive.

Tissue engineering has seen an increase in potential nerve repair treatments in the past decade (Battiston et al. 2009). Tubes to repair nerve trunks have been used experimentally to study the regeneration process (Dahlin 2008). Nerve guides (also referenced as guidance channels or conduits) are cylindrical conduits of either biologic-based or synthetic materials that have been used since the beginning of the late 1970s to bridge nerve defects. (Lundborg 2000) Many reports demonstrate that nerve guides can conserve neurotrophic factors from endogenous cells within the site of injury, and support fibrin clot formation between the injured nerve stumps, preventing neuroma and fibrosis and mitigating mechanical force across a nerve gap (Lundborg 2000; Meek et al. 2002; Taras and Jacoby 2008). The successful nerve guide must provide an adequate scaffold for axon regeneration, be semi-permeable, and degrade at an appropriate rate as the nerve regenerates (Ichihara et al. 2008). For the development of artificial nerve grafts, a desirable biomaterial must be biocompatible, have a negligible inflammatory response, and promote axonal elongation.

## 36.2.2 Biomaterials in Peripheral Nerve Repair

There are many required characteristics for biomaterials suitable for tissue engineering applications. First, the material must be easily formed into a similar configuration of target tissue (Hudson et al. 2000). Second, an implanted scaffold should be biocompatible and noncytotoxic as to avoid degradable products affecting adjacent cells (Schlosshauer et al. 2006). Third, the biomaterial must have a controlled degrading rate so as to provide support for the entire tissue regeneration period (Kokai et al. 2009). Finally, the biomaterial should have an appropriate swelling ratio to maintain the wound moistness and also avoid compression of the tissue injury (Lin et al. 2009).

### 36.2.2.1 Native Materials

Collagen, an essential protein of the extracellular matrix in mammals, is a suitable material for generating artificial substitutes for diseased or damaged tissue and organs as collagen can aid in the proliferation of cells (Wang et al. 2003; Zhang et al. 2006). Approximately 49% of the total protein in nerves is composed of collagen types I and III (Bunge et al. 1989). As such, collagen has been widely assessed as a biomaterial for nerve guide fabrication (Valentini et al. 1987; Archibald et al. 1991; Li et al. 1992; Stocum 1998; Ceballos et al. 1999; Hutmacher 2001; Verdu et al. 2002; Whitlock et al. 2009). When compared to synthetic materials for conduits, literature suggests that a natural material, such as collagen, can enhance axonal regeneration, myelination and vascularization in a 10 mm rat sciatic nerve defect (Kemp et al. 2009). Using a rat sciatic nerve crush injury model, a collagen conduit was found to be retained and concentrated at the nerve injury site to enhance the functional restoration following nerve damage (Sun et al. 2009). The increase in nerve area and a dramatic increase in myelinated nerve fiber numbers were attributed to previous work demonstrating that collagen rapidly revascularizes and integrates into the host tissue following implantation (Felix et al. 2005). Moreover, Alluin et al. reported a 1 cm segment of the peroneal nerve innervating the tibialis anterior muscle was removed and immediately replaced by a biodegradable nerve guide fabricated from highly purified type I and III collagen derived from porcine skin. The data indicate that motor axonal regeneration and locomotor recovery can be obtained with the insertion of this collagen tube (Alluin et al. 2009). Gibby et al. also demonstrated the potential of collagen as a nerve guide in cat radial and sural nerve defect models (Gibby et al. 1983). Yoshitani et al.

examined a collagen-based guide coating with synthetic material can induce functional recovery of the injured phrenic nerve and was aided by coverage with a pedicled pericardial fat pad in dog animal model. Archibald et al. examined collagen-based nerve guides in both rat and nonhuman primate models and demonstrated that the collagen nerve guides were as efficient as autografts (Archibald et al. 1991). More recently, Tyner et al. reported that a collagen nerve guide enhanced linear nerve outgrowth and reduced neuroma formation after peripheral nerve injury in a rat model (Tyner et al. 2007).

There are additional studies supporting the use of collagen as a nerve guide. Bushnell et al. reported that collagen tubes might offer a clinically effective option for restoration of sensory function in the early follow-up period (Bushnell et al. 2008). Furthermore, modification of collagen tubes with peptide sequence resulted in an improved interaction between Schwann cells and the nerve guide biomaterial (Bozkurt et al. 2007). Waitayawinyu et al. determined that type I collagen conduits and autografts produced comparable results, which were significantly better than PGA conduits, for gaps up to 10 mm in length in rat animal model (Waitayawinyu et al. 2007). Though collagen guides have demonstrated success in animal models of peripheral nerve regeneration, the rapid degradation rate of the material requires that the collagen be cross-linked in order to provide mechanical stability for the regenerative period required for critical size defects (Harley et al. 2004; Alluin et al. 2009). This limits the use of collagen in long peripheral nerve gaps.

Alginate, extracted from brown seaweed, is composed of linearly unbranched polymers $\beta$-$(1 \rightarrow 4)$-linked D-mannuronic acid ($M$) and $\alpha$-$(1 \rightarrow 4)$-linked L-guluronic acid (G) residues. Alginate sponge is suitable for cell attachment, proliferation, and differentiation due to its biocompatibility and hydrophilicity (Shapiro and Cohen 1997). Suzuki et al. examined an alginate-based scaffold using a 50-mm gap in a cat sciatic nerve model. Many newly developed nerve fasciculi were found, and the implanted nerve guidance material had completely degraded with little inflammation. This freeze-dried alginate scaffold allows the nerve to regenerate across longer gaps than described in previous literature (Suzuki et al. 1999). Matsuura et al. also fabricated a novel biodegradable alginate gel sponge sheet and demonstrated that an alginate sponge can enhance nerve repair (Matsuura et al. 2006).

Chitosan is a linear polysaccharide comprised of $\beta$1- to $\beta$4-linked D-glucosamine residues, and its potential as a biomaterial is based on its cationic nature and high charge density in solution (Kuo et al. 2009; Lin et al. 2009). Moreover, chitosan membranes and fibers have excellent neuroglial cell affinity, especially Schwann cell (Yuan et al. 2004). Jiao et al. examined a chitosan-based artificial nerve graft to bridge a long-term delayed 10-mm defect in SD rats, and the results showed that Schwann cells survived and sustained their ability to myelinate axons at least 6 months. In addition, the atrophic denervated muscle could be reinnervated by regenerated axons through new muscle–nerve connections (Jiao et al. 2009). Lin et al. reported that modification of a chitosan matrix by gold nanoparticles not only provides the mechanical strength necessary, but also enhances the cellular response (Lin et al. 2008).

Silk fibroin is another native biomaterial studied in nerve repair, and is characterized by its slow degradation rate, strong mechanical strength and neuro-biocompatibility (Uebersax et al. 2007; Yang et al. 2009; Madduri et al. 2010). Yang et al. reported that silk fibroin has good biocompatibility with dorsal root ganglia and is also beneficial to the survival of Schwann cells without exerting any significant cytotoxic effects on their phenotype or function in *in vitro* experiments (Yang et al. 2007). They further investigated the degradation behavior of nerve guidance conduits comprised of silk fibroin. These results collectively indicated that silk fibroin-based conduits were able to degrade at a significantly increasing rate as compared to silk fibroin fibers, thus meeting the requirements of peripheral nerve regeneration (Yang et al. 2009). Researchers have also developed silk fibroin conduits loaded with glial cell line-derived neurotrophic factor (GDNF) and nerve growth factor (NGF) to strengthen functional recovery of injured peripheral nerves (Yang et al. 2007; Madduri et al. 2010).

Hyaluronic acid, (HA), also referred to as hyaluronan, is an important constituent of extracellular matrix, and has been used as a viscoelastic biomaterial for medical purposes, such as injectable fillers, and in drug delivery systems. The hyaluronan-based nerve conduit is not cytotoxic and shows good biocompatibility *in vitro*, indicative of a suitable material for peripheral nerve repair (Jansen et al. 2004). Ikeda et al. reported that coating the nerve tissue with IIA was the most effective method of reducing extraneural and intraneural scarring after neurolysis (Ikeda et al. 2003). In general, however, HA hydrogels lack sufficient mechanical and degradative properties on its own to be particularly useful in long gap peripheral nerve repair. Small intestinal submucosa (SIS), is another native polymeric material that has been examined as a tissue-engineered substrate for a variety of applications, including nerve regeneration (Voytik-Harbin et al. 1997; Badylak et al. 1998; Hadlock et al. 2001; Lindberg and Badylak 2001). In addition to SIS, purified natural extracellular matrix (ECM) components such as laminin and fibronectin participate in axonal development (Schmidt and Leach 2003). Laminin is the first ECM protein expressed during embryogenesis and has been shown to both promote axonal outgrowth and guide developing neurites (Ciardelli and Chiono 2006).

### 36.2.2.2 Synthetic Materials

In general, synthetic materials are attractive candidates for nerve tissue engineering applications due to their chemical and physical properties (e.g., stiffness, degradation rate, and porosity) can in theory be optimized to the specific needs of the application. Axonal regeneration is based on varying parameters of the conduit such as porosity, wall thickness, and Schwann cell seeding density, has been examined (Rutkowski and Heath 2002). This section describes polymers that have FDA approval, such as poly(lactic acid) (PLA), poly(glycolic acid) (PGA), poly(caprolactone) (PCL), and copolymers (Hadlock et al. 1999; Rodriguez et al. 1999; Maquet et al. 2000). PLA conduits have been modified with various of polymers, such as poly(vinyl alcohol), PCL, or plasticizers and implanted into nerve gap models with promising results (den Dunnen et al. 1996; Heath and Rutkowski 1998; Luciano et al. 2000; Rutkowski and Heath 2002). PCL/PLA copolymer tubes are highly permeable, which permits the necessary exchange of nutrients and molecules in the wound site (den Dunnen and Meek 2001). Caprolactone has been mixed with trimethylene carbonate to produce flexibility and tailored degradation rates for nerve guides (Pego et al. 2001). All mechanical properties and degradation rates can be controlled by altering the monomer ratio or addition of cross-linking reagent during the fabrication of nerve guides.

The use of nondegradable synthetic polymers such as silicone (Lundborg et al. 1982; Kakinoki et al. 1995), polyethylene (Madison et al. 1987), polyurethanes (Robinson et al. 1991), Teflon (Lanzetta et al. 2003), and polysulfone (Navarro et al. 1996) is another strategy that has been examined in nerve tissue engineering. For example, Johansson et al. reported that porous silicone tubes, due to its large surface area, diminished inflammatory response and firm adhesion to the tissue, and may be an appropriate material for the development of new implantable electronic nerve devices (Johansson et al. 2009). Polyethylene tubes have been implanted in a 4-mm mouse sciatic nerve defect and demonstrated similar results to unmodified PLA tubes. These tubes were further modified by the inclusion of a laminin gel within the conduits, which enhanced axonal outgrowth (Madison et al. 1987). Teflon, polysulfone (Navarro et al. 1996), poly(pyrrole) and poly(pyrrole)/hyaluronic acid (Schmidt et al. 1997; Collier et al. 2000) composites have also been examined as nerve guides, with satisfactory results. However, nondegradable synthetic polymers are not ideal for tissue engineering applications due to nondigestion, immune response, and fibrous adhesion.

## 36.2.3 Cellular and Growth Factor–Containing Nerve Guides

Although tubular nerve guides can promote axonal elongation over relatively short gaps, the inclusion of cells and/or growth factors within a guide can significantly improve nerve regeneration. Schwann cells are a significant cell phenotype participating in peripheral nerve regeneration (Dezawa 2002; Court et al. 2006). Schwann cells are the myelinating cells of the PNS, and can secrete extracellular matrix, cell adhesion molecules, integrins and neurotrophins (Dawson et al. 2003). Therefore, Schwann cells seeded in artificial conduits would is a promising strategy to repair peripheral nerve injuries (Guenard et al. 1992; Rutkowski et al. 2004; Kim et al. 2007). Schwann cells have been seeded in

SIS (Hadlock et al. 2001), acellular autologous matrices (Fansa and Keilhoff 2004), poly(caprolactone) (Galla et al. 2004), PLGA (Hadlock et al. 2000), and collagen tubes (Ansselin et al. 1997, 1998) and have resulted in improved recovery of animal models in long-term experiments. Schwann cells incorporation can enhance regeneration of peripheral axons over a distance normally prohibitive in the early stages of regeneration (1–3 months). Although additional Schwann cells can significantly help nerve repair, a challenge for using autologous Schwann cells is the donor site morbidity. In order to obtain autologous Schwann cells, a peripheral nerve must be resected, and time for expansion of Schwann cells is necessary. As an alternative, adult mesenchymal stem cells (MSCs) are present in various adult tissues, such as bone marrow and can potentially be transfected into Schwann cells. Adipose tissue is an attractive source of MSCs and can be harvested from a patient in a minimally invasive manner, producing a large quantity of autologous cells (Lin et al. 2009). Kingham et al. demonstrated that adipose stem cells (ASC) differentiated into a Schwann cell phenotype can promote neurite outgrowth *in vitro* (Kingham et al. 2007). Summa et al. further tested fibrin nerve conduits seeded with ASCs which differentiated to a Schwann cell-like phenotype for sciatic nerve injury repair and observed that ASCs enhanced axon regeneration, without the limitations of the donor-site morbidity associated with isolation of Schwann cells, and could be a clinically translatable route towards new methods to enhance peripheral nerve repair (di Summa et al. 2010). Bone marrow stem cells (BMSCs) also have demonstrated the capability of differentiation into Schwann cells. BMSCs have been shown to promote peripheral nerve regeneration not only via their direct release of neurotrophic factors, but through indirect modulation of cellular behaviors of Schwann cells (Wang et al. 2009). Tohill et al. reported rat BMSCs trans-differentiated into neuronal phenotypes can express glial markers and stimulate nerve regeneration (Tohill et al. 2004).

In addition to cellular incorporation, the delivery of neurotrophic factors has been studied. Scaffolds were modified with growth factors such as acidic and basic fibroblast growth factors, (aFGF and bFGF), vascular endothelial growth factor (VEGF), endothelial growth factor (EGF), leukemia inhibitory factor (LIF), and insulin-like growth factor (IGF), and have been investigated as potential additives for *r* improved nerve regeneration (Tan et al. 1996; Yaginuma et al. 1996; Terenghi 1999; Loh et al. 2001; Fine et al. 2002; Galla et al. 2004).

Neurotrophins are a family of growth factors which specifically target neuronal behavior. Nerve growth factor (NGF), brain-derived neurotrophic factor (BDNF), neurotrophin-3 (NT-3), neurotrophin-4/5 (NT-4/5), ciliary neurotrophic factor (CNTF), and glial cell line-derived growth factor (GDNF) are neurotrophic factors (Schmidt and Leach 2003), Terenghi 1999) a known promoter of neuron outgrowth and branching (Eppley et al. 1991; Whitworth et al. 1996). However, the short half-life of NGF limits clinical application. Xu et al. reported NGF embedded in polyphosphoester microspheres can extend biological activity (Xu et al. 2002). NGF has also been encapsulated within biodegradable microspheres or lipid microtubules (Dodla and Bellamkonda 2008), adsorbed onto the polymer surface of a nerve guide or coated on the inside of the nerve guides with centrifugal casting (Piotrowicz and Shoichet 2006). BDNF has been demonstrated to support motor neuron survival (Sendtner et al. 1992) and promote both motor neuron (Braun et al. 1996) and sensory neuron axonal outgrowth (Oudega and Hagg 1999). Osmotic mini-pumps (Moir et al. 2000; Boyd and Gordon 2002), calcium alginate spheres (Vögelin et al. 2006), or directly modified collagen nerve guide matrices (Utley et al. 1996, Böstrom and Camacho 1998) are various delivery systems which are used in peripheral nerve regeneration. GDNF, which is one of the dopaminergic factors derived from neurons of the midbrain (Iwase et al. 2005) promotes proliferation, migration and differentiation of Schwann cells and promotes the survival of motor and sensory neurons (Henderson et al. 1994; Airaksinen and Saarma 2002; Paratcha and Ledda 2008). Chitosan (Patel et al. 2007), collagen/PLGA (Piquilloud et al. 2007), collagen/PVA (Barras et al. 2002; Fine et al. 2002), or PCL (Kokai et al. 2010) nerve guides modified with GDNF has resulted in enhanced nerve regeneration in preclinical models. Recently, Kokai has shown that double-walled PLGA/PLA microspheres encapsulating GDNF embedded into the walls of PCL guides can improve axonal regeneration. (Kokai et al. 2009, 2010).

## 36.2.4 Summary

Polymeric nerve guides can be used in treating nerve lesions instead of autologous nerves. However, polymer nerve guides have not been shown to repair peripheral nerve defects in humans >3 cm. To improve on existing nerve guide designs, many are studying the essential tissue engineering paradigm: scaffolds, cells and growth factors.

# 36.3 CNS Repair

## 36.3.1 Brain Injuries and Spinal Cord Injuries

The incidence of spinal cord injuries (SCI) in the United States has reached 12,000 new cases per year (Center 2004); approximately 255,702 individuals already live with spinal cord injury (SCI) in the United States. Motor vehicle accidents are the main cause of SCI (42%), followed by falls (27.1%), knife and gunshot injuries (15.3%), and recreational activities (7.4%) (Becker et al. 2003). In all, 77.8% of the cases occur in males (Becker et al. 2003; Talac et al. 2004) with most cases occurring at ages between 16 and 30 years old (Center 2004).

Multiple health problems, such as recurrent kidney stones, urinary tract infection, pressure sores, and cardiac and respiratory dysfunction, arise as a result of the loss of sensory and motor functions in regions below the level of the injury (Talac et al. 2004). Pneumonia, pulmonary emboli, and septicemia are the leading causes of death in individuals that survive the initial SCI (Becker et al. 2003). Treatments that reduce autonomic dysfunction and neuropathic pain will significantly improve the quality of life of individuals living with a SCI (Anderson et al. 2002, 2007; Vogel et al. 2002).

### 36.3.1.1 Pathophysiology of CNS and Clinical Treatment

A SCI is characterized by the progressive destruction of spinal cord tissue (Norenberg et al. 2004; Talac et al. 2004). In the initial impact, which most commonly occurs in the form of a compression or contusion of the spinal cord tissue, fragments of bone, vertebral disk, or ligament affect axons, neurons, glial cells, and blood vessels (Becker et al. 2003). The initial damage triggers focal hemorrhage, local edema, vasospasm, and the loss of microcirculation (Becker et al. 2003; Norenberg et al. 2004). The ischemia expands to the surrounding tissue, leading to additional neuronal death (Becker et al. 2003). Cells far beyond the original lesion are affected in both antegrade and retrograde directions. The apoptotic death of oligodendrocytes occurs as white matter tracts degenerates. An inflammatory response that includes the infiltration of neutrophils, monocytes, and lymphocytes to the site of the injury is observed 24 h after the initial insult (Norenberg et al. 2004; Talac et al. 2004). Cytotoxic extracellular levels of excitatory amino acids such as glutamate and free radicals are also reached after the impact (Norenberg et al. 2004; Talac et al. 2004). In humans, large cystic regions surrounded by scar tissue are formed (Profyris et al. 2004).

### 36.3.1.2 Nonpermissive Environment for Nerve Regeneration

Unlike the peripheral nervous system, the CNS has a limited capacity of regeneration following injury. As regenerating axons reaches the proximity of the injury, axons cease to grow. The inability for axons to regenerate and cross the site of injury has been attributed to the formation of a glial scar which contains inhibitory substrates (Fawcett and Asher 1999; Hermanns et al. 2001; McKerracher 2001; Jacobs and Fehlings 2003; Lee et al. 2003). Inhibitory molecules present in the injured spinal cord include myelin-associated inhibitors such as Nogo-A, myelin-associated glycoprotein (MAG), and oligodendrocyte myelin glycoprotein (OMgp), all of which are known to cause growth cone collapse (McKerracher 2001; Jacobs and Fehlings 2003; Lee et al. 2003). Fortunately, growth cones are dynamic structures and can be "reawakened into a regenerative state" as demonstrated by Tom and colleagues using an *in vitro* system of adult dorsal root ganglion (DRG) in a gradient of aggrecan (Tom et al. 2004).

In lesions that open the meninges, the glial scar is composed mainly of reactive astrocytes mixed with meningeal fibroblasts (Fawcett and Asher 1999; McKerracher 2001; Jacobs and Fehlings 2003). Oligodendrocyte precursor cells and inflammatory cells have also been identified in the glial scar (Fawcett and Asher 1999; McKerracher 2001; Jacobs and Fehlings 2003). The inability of axons to regenerate through the glial scar was attributed for many years to the physical barrier presented by the scar (Fitch and Silver 1997; Stichel and Muller 1998,2004). However, proteoglycans present in the glial scar (e.g., chondroitin sulfate proteoglycans: CSPGs) are highly inhibitory of axonal growth (Fitch and Silver 1997; Jacobs and Fehlings 2003; Talac et al. 2004). Astrocytes in the glial scar are known to produce four types of proteoglycans: heparan sulfate proteoglycan (HSPG), dermatan sulfate proteoglycan (DSPG), keratan sulfate proteoglycan (KSPG), and chondroitin sulfate proteoglycan (CSPG) (Silver and Miller 2004). CSPGs, in particular, are produced within 24 hours after injury and remain at the injury site for months (Silver and Miller 2004). An important role of the glial scar involves the stabilization of the spinal cord tissue after injury. For instance, astrocytes limit cellular degeneration, ameliorate the inflammatory response, and assist in the repair of the blood brain barrier.

## 36.3.2 Biomaterials in CNS Research

Similar to research in peripheral nerve tissue engineering, native or synthetic biomaterials have been extensively investigated. Tubular conduits aimed to guide regeneration across the transected spinal cord, and as sponges or gels that could potentially reduce glial scar formation (Cheng et al. 2007). Cells and signal factors have been incorporated into these biomaterials to further improve axonal regrowth.

### 36.3.2.1 Native Materials

Collagen is a suitable material for generating artificial substitutes for diseased or damaged tissue and organs. Petter-Punchner et al. tested a scaffold fabricated from fibrin sealant and equine collagen. The results demonstrated that the fibrin sealant–collagen scaffold treatment has significantly affected axonal regrowth, especially regrowth of myelination and vascularization (Petter-Puchner et al. 2007). Liu and colleagues observed axonal regrowth through a collagen guidance channel used to bridge the rat spinal cord and the nerve root (Liu et al. 1997, 2001). Miyazaki et al. demonstrated that a porcine collagen-derived matrix that delivered growth factors can enhance spinal fusion in rats (Miyazaki et al. 2009).

Alginate gel is widely used in drug delivery systems, and alginate sponges can significantly reduce connective tissue scar formation after a completely transected rat SCI model (Kataoka et al. 2004; Ciofani et al. 2008). Peter et al. implanted alginate-based highly anisotropic capillary hydrogels (ACH) into acute cervical spinal cord lesions in adult rats and showed that alginate-based ACH integrates into the spinal cord parenchyma without major inflammatory responses while maintaining their anisotropic structure (Prang et al. 2006). The advantages of agarose as a biomaterial are its low immune or inflammatory response, which effectively delineate pathways for regenerating axons to follow, and it is easy to shape. Shula et al. reported uniaxial channels within agarose scaffolds stimulate and guide linear axonal growth (Stokols and Tuszynski 2006). Thomas et al. reported neurotrophin-3 expressing autologous bone marrow stromal cells that were seeded in templated agarose scaffolds can enhance regeneration of long-tract axons through sites of SCI (Gros et al. 2010).

The proteoglycans derived from activated glial cells inhibit neuronal regeneration. Hyatt et al. reported that fibrin gel embedded with chondroitinase can reduce glial cell secretion of glycosaminoglycans after spinal cord lesion (Hyatt et al. 2010). King et al. demonstrated that a fibrin and fibronectin injected mixture supported robust growth of axons (King et al. 2010). Taylor et al. fabricated a fibrin scaffold modified with neurotrophin-3. This fibrin scaffold combined with growth factor enhanced the spinal cord repair in rats (Taylor and Sakiyama-Elbert 2006). Both fibrin gel and fibrin scaffold shows promise as a suitable biomaterial for filling cavities at SCI sites.

Fibers of poly-β-hydroxybutyrate (PHB) (a biodegradable polymer of bacterial and algae origin (Hazari et al. 1999)) coated with an alginate hydrogel containing fibronectin were implanted in a cervical

SCI in adult rats (Novikov et al. 2002). PHB fibers demonstrated improved neuronal survival in comparison with the implantation of only alginate hydrogel or fibronectin. Novikova et al. demonstrated PHB scaffold seeded with Schwann cells significantly promote spinal cord repair (Novikova et al. 2008). Silk (Uebersax et al. 2007), chitosan (Nomura et al. 2008; Li et al. 2009), self-assembling peptide nanofibers (Guo et al. 2009), and hyaluronic acid (Wang and Spector 2009) are more examples of natural materials that have been examined in spinal cord research.

### 36.3.2.2 Synthetic Polymers

Polyethylene glycol (PEG) is a hydrophilic polymer and membrane fusogen that has been examined in spinal cord repair (Luo et al. 2002). PEG has been shown to immediately repair physically damaged of spinal cord cell membrane, restore electrical impulse conduction, and reverse the permeabilization produced by the injury (Murakami et al. 1999; Borgens and Shi 2000; Borgens and Bohnert 2002; Donaldson et al. 2002). *In vivo* studies using adult guinea-pig spinal cords model demonstrated an increase in nerve impulse conduction after treating the injured spinal cord membranes for two minutes with a 50% PEG solution prepared in distilled water (Shi and Borgens 2000). Furthermore, PEG was shown to inhibit necrosis and apoptotic cell death following SCI through two pathways: repair of plasma membranes and protection of mitochondria (Luo and Shi 2007). Kang et al. investigated conjugation of PEG to FGF2 and compared its distribution relative to unmodified FGF2 in injured spinal cord tissue. PEGylation of FGF2 enhanced tissue penetration by reducing its rate of elimination (Kang et al. 2010). Moreover, PEG-complexes are promising as multifunctional injectable scaffolds for the treatment of CNS injuries (Comolli et al. 2009).

Poly-(lactide-*co*-glycolide) (PLGA) is also a potential neural tissue engineering material due to the ease of fabrication, mechanical strength, and biodegradability. Gautier et al. investigated a series of characterizations of PLGA and PLA guidance channels both *in vitro* and *in vivo* (Gautier et al. 1998). These guidance channel structures minimized scar tissue formation and contributed to the accumulation of growth promoting molecules in the site of injury (Oudega et al. 2001). These guidance channels could also be incorporated into the spinal cord tracts (Friedman et al. 2002). However, the authors concluded that PLGA is not suitable for spinal cord applications due to the fast resorption of this polymer and the high degree of swelling that could potentially lead to the compression of the spinal cord stumps (Gautier et al. 1998). To overcome this disadvantage, different configurations of PLGA were fabricated (Li et al. 2009; Xiong et al. 2009; Yao et al. 2009). Recently, PLGA particles have been shown to be an excellent cell/drug-delivery candidate in stroke-induced brain cavities (Bible et al. 2009). Wang et al. constructed trimethylated chitosan surface-modified PLGA nanoparticles to deliver drugs to the brain (Wang et al. 2010).

Guidance channels comprised of poly (D,L-lactic acid) have demonstrated slower degradation rates and less water absorption than PLGA (Gautier et al. 1998). The guidance channels prepared using poly(D,L-lactic acid) and a mixture of poly(L-lactic acid) and 10% poly(L-lactic acid) oligomers were implanted into a 3–4 mm long gap created at the T8–T9 level of a rat spinal cord (Oudega et al. 2001). Axons were observed to grow into the channel during the first 2 months (postsurgery), and retracted or died in a later time point due to collapse of the guidance channel walls. Patist and colleagues studied the suitability of a freeze-dried poly(D,L-lactic acid) foam containing BDNF in promoting regeneration in the transected adult rat thoracic spinal cord (Patist et al. 2004). Hurtado et al. developed Schwann cells seeded onto macroporous scaffolds to effectively promote axonal regeneration in the injured spinal cord (Hurtado et al. 2006). Finally, Li et al. devised patterned multiwalled PLA conduits (Li et al. 2007).

Poly(2-hydroxyethyl methacrylate) (pHEMA) is a nonbiodegradable material. One of pHEMA's physical characteristics is that it is easily tailorable, and been used extensively in medical applications. Tsai et al. implanted poly(2-hydroxyethyl methacrylate-*co*-methyl methacrylate) (pHEMA-MMA) hydrogel guidance channels into a T8 transected spinal cord in adult Sprague-Dawley rats; the hydrogel guidance channel improved specific supraspinal and local axonal regeneration after complete spinal cord transection (Tsai et al. 2004). In another study, modifications of pHEMA with cholesterol and laminin have been developed to design scaffolds that promote cell–surface interactions (Kubinov et al. 2009). Poly[*N*-(2-hydroxypropyl)methacrylamide] (pHPMA) (NeuroGel™) is another biocompatible commercial hydrogel. Woerly et al. reported pHPMA conjugated RGD peptides when implanted into a completely transected spinal cord reduces the necrosis and cavitation in the site of lesion (Woerly et al. 2001). The authors also implanted the same hydrogel into the completely transected cat spinal cord, and demonstrated reduction of cavitation and enhanced angiogenesis (Woerly et al. 2004).

### 36.3.2.3 Neurotrophic Factors

Although guidance channels can direct axon growth in a specific direction and reduce scar tissue formation, molecular cues such as those provided by neurotrophic factors can significantly enhance axonal guidance to their targets in the injured spinal cord. Neurotrophic factors are able to promote the growth or survival of neurons during development (Jones et al. 2001). Sayer et al. reported that treatment with neurotrophic factors reduced ascending sensory and corticospinal motor axons in adult rat spinal cord (Sayer et al. 2002). Oudega et al. demonstrated that neurotrophins promoted regeneration of sensory axons in the adult rat spinal cord (Oudega and Hagg 1999; Sayer et al. 2002). There are many reports demonstrating that neurotrophic factors delivered by continuous infusion (Oudega and Hagg 1999; Novikov et al. 2002), direct injection (Sayer et al. 2002), and incorporation into a gel or scaffold (Oudega and Hagg 1999; Patist et al. 2004; Taylor et al. 2004) can direct the growth of axons into the site of injury. As neurotrophins have been reported to be helpful for the lesion-induced recovery of spinal cord, studies on endogenous neurotrophins, particularly nerve growth factor (NGF) (Oudega and Hagg 1999; Sayer et al. 2002), brain-derived neurotrophic factor (BDNF) (Oudega and Hagg 1999; Sayer et al. 2002) and neurotrophin-3 (NT-3) (Oudega and Hagg 1999; Sayer et al. 2002) in injured spinal cords might provide important advances in clinical treatment (Li et al. 2007). For example, the infusion of NGF during the first 2 weeks into a SCI promoted sensory axon regrowth (Oudega and Hagg 1999). Rodrigues et al. grafted mesenchymal stem cells (MSCs), which continuously produced BDNF, into a rat spinal cord ventral horn, and reported promising spinal cord regeneration (Rodrigues Hell et al. 2009). Delivery of NT-3 elicited the growth of corticospinal axons after injection into a rat SCI (Oudega and Hagg 1999). Zhang et al. reported evaluation of temporal changes in the levels of NGF, BDNF, NT-3, and NT-4 in adult rhesus monkeys subjected to T8 spinal hemisection. They demonstrated that intrinsic NGF, BDNF, and NT-3 may play a local role in the responses to the SCI in primates (Zhang et al. 2008).

## 36.3.3 Cellular Therapies in Spinal Cord Repair

Cell transplantation therapies examined for SCI repair include the use of olfactory ensheathing cells, Schwann cells, neural and embryonic stem cells, as described in the next several sections.

### 36.3.3.1 Olfactory Ensheathing Cells

Olfactory ensheathing cells (OECs) are the main glial cell type that populate mammalian olfactory nerves (Pastrana et al. 2007) and have been shown to myelinate peripheral nerves in the presence of meningeal cells (Franklin 2003). OECs promoted the regeneration of axons when implanted into the injured adult mammalian CNS (Barnett 2004; Barnett and Riddell 2004). Pastrana et al. showed that BDNF production by OECs plays a direct role in the promotion of axon regeneration of adult CNS neurons (Pastrana et al. 2007). In order to monitor the migratory ability of OECs, Lee and colleagues concluded that the OECs were not able to cross the host–graft interface in a completely transected spinal cord of female Sprague–Dawley rats (Lee et al. 2004). OECs have been shown to alter the morphology of sympathetic preganglionic neurons, and hence modify their activity in the neuronal networks responsible for the dysreflexic reaction (Kalincík et al. 2010). Srivastava et al. reported neural progenitor cell co-transplantation with OECs for neurotrophic factor support may be a better approach for functional restoration in kainic acid-induced rat model of cognitive dysfunction (Srivastava et al. 2009). Shi et al.

demonstrated that OECs can protect the white matter from ischemic injury, but the potential mechanisms of transplanted OEC-mediated recovery need further studies (Shi et al. 2010)

### 36.3.3.2 Schwann Cells (SCs)

Schwann cells (SCs) produce growth factors, cell adhesion molecules, and extracellular matrix components contribute to the supportive environment present in peripheral nerves, and can become a substitute for the axon bridge (Jones et al. 2003). Although SCs are not present in the spinal cord, reports have shown that SC transplantation can augment repair in the injured spinal cord (Firouzi et al. 2006). When SCs were implanted into the injured rat spinal cord, axonal regeneration and myelination within the region of implantation was improved (Jones et al. 2003). Hurtado et al. reported that SC-seeded PLA scaffolds effectively promoted axonal regeneration in the injured spinal cord (Hurtado et al. 2006). Tabesh et al. has published a review of biodegradable polymer scaffolds seeded with SCs for SCI (Tabesh et al. 2009). SCs genetically modified to express neurotrophin is another strategy to improve spinal cord repair. Pettingill et al. transplanted the neurotrophin overexpressing SCs into early postnatal rats and showed significantly enhanced neuronal survival (Pettingill et al. 2008). Transplantation of cell adhesion molecule L1 gene overexpressing SCs enhances early events in spinal cord repair after injury in an adult mouse model (Lavdas et al. 2010). In extensive research, translation of SCs, which were rapid and efficiently induced by spheroid-forming cells from subcutaneous fat tissue shows therapeutic promise for repair of damage to the CNS (Chi et al. 2010). While promising, none of the current strategies have demonstrated full functional recovery after SCI, and further research is necessary.

### 36.3.3.3 Stem Cells

Both adult stem cells and embryonic stem cells have been proposed and examined as possible cellular therapies for SCI (Cummings et al. 2005, 2006). Embryonic stem cells are pluripotent cells able to differentiate into the various cell types of the body. McDonald et al. demonstrated that implanting embryonic stem cells into a contusion of rat spinal cord can differentiate into astrocytes, oligodendrocytes, and neurons (McDonald et al. 2004). Adipose-derived stem cells, which are believed to be mesenchymal stem cells, family have been examined in SCI. Xu et al., has produced SC-like cells from ASCs. These cells may benefit the treatment of both peripheral and central nerve injuries (Xu et al. 2008). Kim et al. reported human ASCs significantly improved motor recovery and enhanced morphometric change when implanted in a contusive SCI in rats (Kim and Kwak 2007). Oh et al. also reported that a hypoxic preconditioning treatment for adipose tissue-derived mesenchymal stem cells co-cultured with DsRed-engineered neural stem cells can improve both the cell survival and the gene expression of the engineered NSCs, indicating combined stem cell and gene therapies for SCI as a potential therapy (Oh et al. 2010).

Bone marrow-derived stem cells have been widely examined for nerve regeneration in the spinal cord. The transplantation of bone marrow stem cells into the injured cord promoted axonal sprouting and in some instances, improvements in behavioral tests were observed (Lee et al. 2003; Ankeny et al. 2004; Zhao et al. 2004; Lu et al. 2005; Kang et al. 2006; Ohta et al. 2008; Wright et al. 2008; Cao and Feng 2009; Furuya et al. 2009; Jung et al. 2009; Matsuda et al. 2009; Paul et al. 2009). Jung et al. compared the therapeutic effects between autologous and allogeneic bone-marrow-derived mesenchymal stem cell transplantation in experimentally induced SCI of dogs. They demonstrated that both autologous and allogeneic MSC transplantation could be clinically useful therapeutic approaches for treating SCI (Jung et al. 2009). Ide and colleagues examined the effects of BMSCs in subacute SCI (2 weeks postinjury) by transplanting the cells directly into the lesion. The results showed BMSC transplantation had markedly beneficial effects on tissue repair and axonal outgrowth in the rat model (Ide et al. 2010).

In summary, there are multiple promising strategies to promote axon regrowth or eliminate the inhibitory molecules to improve the repair of the injured spinal cord. In cases of extensive neural tissue loss, the implantation of stem cells or neural progenitor cells offers a strategy to replenish the glia and/or neurons lost. The inability of the regenerating axons to emerge from the graft and the polymer scaffold are two important issues which require additional studies.

## 36.4 Animal Models of Nervous System Injury Research

Animal models play important roles in the preclinical screening and assessment of potential nerve tissue engineering therapies, and, can be used to determine whether a specific construct can regenerate axons. Applicable animal model selection requires close resemblance of the target human organ. Nevertheless, it is generally well accepted to choose a small animal model for preliminary investigations. A final preclinical animal model for nerve system repair should be performed on a non-human primate model such as a rhesus monkey (Zhang et al. 2009). Another issue that should be addressed when choosing an animal model is the age of the animal. Immature animals can more easily repair defects compared to skeletally mature animals. Furuya et al. (2009) and Sun et al. (2009) have all investigated biopolymer conduits containing stem cells or NGF on the promotion of sciatic nerve regeneration in a rat sciatic nerve crush injury model. Suzuki et al. chose a cat animal model to investigate peripheral nerve regeneration across long gap (Suzuki et al. 1999). Jung et al. reported the evaluation of autologous or allogeneic bone marrow-derived mesenchymal stem cell transplantation in canine SCI (Jung et al. 2009). Polymer conduits treated with autologous stem cells were implanted in a rhesus monkey model (Hu et al. 2007; Zhang et al. 2009).

## 36.5 Overall Summary of Neural Tissue Engineering

Tissue engineering applies the principles of engineering and life sciences toward the development of biological substitutes that restore tissue. This field is a rapidly growing and exciting field, especially neural tissue engineering. Extensive research is being conducted in this area. Axon re-growth in long gaps is still a challenge in both PNS and CNS repair. The principle aim of a novel scaffold design should be to mimic the target tissue as much as possible, which includes tailored mechanical properties and suitable degradation rates. Stem cell therapy is another strategy in this field. The design of novel hydrogels that can encapsulate cells or deliver drugs to the injury are among the most promising treatments. The future trends of nervous system repair are cell therapy, gene therapy, drug delivery, and tissue engineering therapy.

## References

http://www.spinalinjury.net/html/_spinal_cord_101.html.

Airaksinen, MS and Saarma, M. 2002. The GDNF family: Signalling, biological functions and therapeutic value. *Nat Rev Neurosci* 3(5):383–394.

Alluin, O, Wittmann, C, Marqueste, T et al. 2009. Functional recovery after peripheral nerve injury and implantation of a collagen guide. *Biomaterials* 30(3):363–373.

Anderson, CJ, Krajci, KA, and Vogel, LC. 2002. Life satisfaction in adults with pediatric-onset spinal cord injuries. *J Spinal Cord Med* 25(3):184–190.

Anderson, KD, Borisoff, JF, Johnson, RD, Stiens, SA, and Elliott, SL. 2007. The impact of spinal cord injury on sexual function: Concerns of the general population. *Spinal Cord* 45(5):328–337.

Ankeny, DP, McTigue, DM, and Jakeman, LB. 2004. Bone marrow transplants provide tissue protection and directional guidance for axons after contusive spinal cord injury in rats. *Exp Neurol* 190(1):17–31.

Ansselin, AD, Fink, T, and Davey, DF. 1997. Peripheral nerve regeneration through nerve guides seeded with adult Schwann cells. *Neuropathol Appl Neurobiol* 23(5):387–398.

Ansselin, AD, Fink, T, and Davey, DF. 1998. An alternative to nerve grafts in peripheral nerve repair: Nerve guides seeded with adult Schwann cells. *Acta Chur Aust* 30(S147):19–24.

Archibald, S, Krarup, C, Shefner, J, Li, S, and Madison, R. 1991. A collagen-based nerve guide conduit for peripheral nerve repair: An electrophysiological study of nerve regeneration in rodents and nonhuman primates. *J Comp Neurol* 306(4):685–696.

Badylak, SF, Record, R, Lindberg, K, Hodde, J, and Park, K. 1998. Small intestinal submucosa: A substrate for *in vitro* cell growth. *J Biomater Sci Polym Ed* 9(8):863–878.

Barnett, SC. 2004. Olfactor ensheathing cells: Unique glial cell types? *J Neurotrauma* 21(4):375–382.

Barnett, SC and Riddell, JS. 2004. Olfactory ensheathing cells (OECs) and the treatment of CNS injury: Advantages and possible caveats. *J Anat* 204:57–67.

Barras, F, Pasche, P, Bouche, N, Aebischer, P, and Zurn, AD. 2002. Glial cell line-derived neurotrophic factor released by synthetic guidance channels promotes facial nerve regeneration in the rat. *J Neurosci Res* 70(6):746–755.

Battiston, B, Raimondo, S, Tos, P, Gaidano, V, Audisio, C, Scevola, A, Perroteau, I, and Geuna, S. 2009. Chapter 11: Tissue engineering of peripheral nerves. *Int Rev Neurobiol* 87:227–249.

Becker, D, Sadowsky, CL, and McDonald, JW. 2003. Restoring function after spinal cord injury. *The Neurologist* 9:1–15.

Bible, E, Chau, DYS, Alexander, MR et al. 2009. The support of neural stem cells transplanted into stroke-induced brain cavities by PLGA particles. *Biomaterials* 30(16):2985–2994.

Borgens, RB and Shi, R. 2000. Immediate recovery from spinal cord injury through molecular repair of nerve membranes with polyethylene glycol. *FASEB* 14:27–35.

Borgens, R, Shi, R, and Bohnert, D. 2002. Behavioral recovery from spinal cord injury following delayed application of polyethylene glycol. *J Exp Biol* 205:1–12.

Böstrom, M and Camacho, N. 1998. Potential role of bone morphogenetic proteins in fracure healing. *Clin Orthop Rel Res* 355S:S274-S282.

Boyd, JG and Gordon, T. 2002. A dose-dependent facilitation and inhibition of peripheral nerve regeneration by brain-derived neurotrophic factor. *Eur J Neurosc* 15(4):613–626.

Bozkurt, A, Lassner, F, Tank, J et al. 2007. A bioartifical nerve guide using a resorbable collagen matrix. *J Plastic, Reconstr Aesthetic Surg* 60(4):S4–S4.

Braun, S, Croizat, B, Lagrange, M, Warter, J, and Poindron, P. 1996. Neurotrophins increase motoneurons' ability to innervate skeletal muscle fibers in rat spinal cord—human muscle cocultures. *J Neurol Sci* 136(1–2):17–23.

Bunge, M, Bunge, R, Kleitman, N, and Dean, A. 1989. Role of peripheral nerve extracellular matrix in Schwann cell function and in neurite regeneration. *Dev Neurosci* 11(4–5):348–360.

Bushnell, BD, McWilliams, AD, Whitener, GB, and Messer, TM. 2008. Early clinical experience with collagen nerve tubes in digital nerve repair. *J Hand Surg* 33(7):1081–1087.

Cao, FJ, and Feng, SQ. 2009. Human umbilical cord mesenchymal stem cells and the treatment of spinal cord injury. *Chin Med J (Engl)* 122(2):225–231.

Ceballos, D, Navarro, X, Dubey, N et al. 1999. Magnetically aligned collagen gel filling a collagen nerve guide improves peripheral nerve regeneration. *Exp Neurol* 158(2):290–300.

Center, NSCIS. 2004. Spinal cord injury: Fact and figures at a glance. *J Spinal Cord Med* 27(2).

Cheng, H, Huang, YC, Chang, PT, and Huang, YY. 2007. Laminin-incorporated nerve conduits made by plasma treatment for repairing spinal cord injury. *Biochem Biophys Res Commun* 357(4):938–944.

Chi, GF, Kim, M-r, Kim, D-W, Jiang, MH, and Son, Y. 2010. Schwann cells differentiated from spheroid-forming cells of rat subcutaneous fat tissue myelinate axons in the spinal cord injury. *Exp Neurol* 222(2):304–317.

Ciardelli, G, and Chiono, V. 2006. Materials for peripheral nerve regeneration. *Macromol Biosci* 6(1):13–26.

Ciofani, G, Raffa, V, Pizzorusso, T, Menciassi, A, and Dario, P. 2008. Characterization of an alginate-based drug delivery system for neurological applications. *Med Eng Phys* 30(7):848–855.

Collier, JH, Camp, JP., Hudson, TW., and Schmidt, CE. 2000. Synthesis and characterization of polypyrrole-hyaluronic acid composite biomaterials for tissue engineering applications. *J Biomed Mater Res* 50(4):574–584.

Comolli, N, Neuhuber, B, Fischer, I, and Lowman, A. 2009. *in vitro* analysis of PNIPAAm-PEG, a novel, injectable scaffold for spinal cord repair. *Acta Biomater* 5(4):1046–1055.

Court, FA, Wrabetz, L, and Feltri, ML. 2006. Basal lamina: Schwann cells wrap to the rhythm of space–time. *Curr Opin Neurobiol* 16(5):501–507.

Cummings, BJ, Uchida, N, Tamaki, SJ et al. 2005. Human neural stem cells differentiate and promote loco-motor recovery in spinal cord-injured mice. *Proc Natl Acad Sci USA* 102(39):14069–14074.

Cummings, BJ, Uchida, N, Tamaki, SJ, and Anderson, AJ. 2006. Human neural stem cell differentiation following transplantation into spinal cord injured mice: Association with recovery of locomotor function. *Neurol Res* 28(5):474–481.

Dahlin, LB. 2008. Techniques of peripheral nerve repair. Scandinavian. *J Surg* 97:310–316.

Dawson, TP, Neal, JW, Llewellyn, L, and Thomas, C. 2003. *Neuropathology Techniques*. London, Arnold, pp. 135–138.

den Dunnen, WF and Meek, MF. 2001. Sensory nerve function and auto-mutilation after reconstruction of various gap lengths with nerve guides and autologous nerve grafts. *Biomaterials* 22(10):1171–1176.

den Dunnen, WF, Stokroos, I, Blaauw, EH et al. 1996. Light-microscopic and electron-microscopic evalu-ation of short-term nerve regeneration using a biodegradable poly(DL-lactide-epsilon-caprolacton) nerve guide. *J Biomed Mater Res* 31(1):105–115.

Dezawa, M. 2002. Central and peripheral nerve regeneration by transplantation of Schwann cells and transdifferentiated bone marrow stromal cells. *Anat Sci Int* 77(1):12–25.

di Summa, PG, Kingham, PJ, Raffoul, W, Wiberg, M, Terenghi, G, and Kalbermatten, DF. 2010. Adipose-derived stem cells enhance peripheral nerve regeneration. *J Plastic, Reconstr Aesthetic Surg* 63:1544–1552.

Dodla, MC and Bellamkonda, RV. 2008. Differences between the effect of anisotropic and isotropic lam-inin and nerve growth factor presenting scaffolds on nerve regeneration across long peripheral nerve gaps. *Biomaterials* 29(1):33–46.

Donaldson, J, Shi, R, and Borgens, R. 2002. Polyethylene glycol rapidly restores physiological functions in damaged sciatic nerves of guinea pigs. *Neurosurgery* 50:147–157.

Eppley, BL, Snyders, RV, Winkelmann, TM, and Roufa, DG. 1991. Efficacy of nerve growth factor in regeneration of the mandibular nerve: A preliminary report. *J Oral Maxillofacial Surg* 49(1):61–68.

Fansa, H and Keilhoff, G. 2004. Comparison of different biogenic matrices seeded with cultured Schwann cells for bridging peripheral nerve defects. *Neurol Res* 26(2):167–173.

Fansa, H, Keilhoff, G, Wolf, G, and Schneider, W. 2001. Tissue engineering of peripheral nerves: A comparison of venous and acellular muscle grafts with cultured *Schwann cells Plast Reconstr Surg* 107(2):485–494.

Fawcett, JW and Asher, RA. 1999. The glial scar and central nervous system repair. *Brain Res Bull* 49(6):377–391.

Felix, S, Hisham, F, Gerald, W, and Gerburg, K. 2005. Collagen nerve conduits—Assessment of biocom-patibility and axonal regeneration. *Bio-Med Mater Eng* 15(1):3–12.

Fine, EG, Decosterd, I, Papaloizos, M, Zurn, AD, and Aebischer, P. 2002. GDNF and NGF released by synthetic guidance channels support sciatic nerve regeneration across a long gap. *Eur J Neurosci* 15(4):589–601.

Firouzi, M, Moshayedi, P, Saberi, H et al. 2006. Transplantation of Schwann cells to subarachnoid space induces repair in contused rat spinal cord. *Neurosci Lett* 402(1–2):66–70.

Fitch, MT and Silver, J. 1997. Glial cell extracellular matrix: Boundaries for axon growth in development and regeneration. *Cell Tissue Res* 290:379–384.

Franklin, RJM. 2003. Remyelination by transplanted olfactory ensheathing cells. *Anatom Record* 271B:71–76.

Friedman, JA, Windebank, AJ, Moore, MJ et al. 2002. Biodegradable polymer grafts for surgical repair of the injured spinal cord. *Neurosurgery* 51:742–752.

Furuya, T, Hashimoto, M, Koda, M, Okawa, A, Murata, A, Takahashi, K, Yamashita, T, and Yamazaki, M. 2009. Treatment of rat spinal cord injury with a Rho-kinase inhibitor and bone marrow stromal cell transplantation. *Brain Res* 1295:192–202.

Gabella, G and Larry, RS 2009. Autonomic nervous system: Neuroanatomy. *Encyclopedia of Neuroscience*. Oxford, Academic Press: pp. 961–966.

Galla, TJ, Vedecnik, SV, Halbgewachs, J et al. 2004. Fibrin/Schwann cell matrix in poly-epsilon-caprolactone conduits enhancing guided nerve regeneration. *Int J Artif Organs* 27:127–136.

Gallo, V, Chew, LJ, and Larry, RS (2009). Neurotransmitter and hormone receptors on oligodendrocytes and schwann cells. *Encyclopedia of Neuroscience*. Oxford, Academic Press: pp. 1051–1059.

Gautier, SE, Oudega, M, Fragoso, M et al. 1998. Poly(alpha-hydroxyacids) for application in the spinal cord: Resorbability and biocompatibility with adult rat Schwann cells and spinal cord. *J Biomed Mater Res* 42:642–654.

Gibby, WA, Koerber, HR, and Horch, KW. 1983. A quantitative evaluation of suture and tubulization nerve repair techniques. *J Neurosurg* 58(4):574–579.

Glasby, MA, Gschmeissner, S, Hitchcock, RJ, and Huang, CL. 1986. Regeneration of the sciatic nerve in rats. The effect of muscle basement membrane. *J Bone Jt Surg Br* 68(5):829–833.

Glasby, MA, Gschmeissner, SE, Huang, CL, and De Souza, BA. 1986. Degenerated muscle grafts used for peripheral nerve repair in primates. *J Hand Surg* [Br] 11(3):347–351.

Gros, T, Sakamoto, JS, Blesch, A, Havton, LA, and Tuszynski, MH. 2010. Regeneration of long-tract axons through sites of spinal cord injury using templated agarose scaffolds. *Biomaterials* 31(26):6719–6729.

Guenard, V, Kleitman, N, Morrissey, TK, Bunge, RP, and Aebischer, P. 1992. Syngeneic Schwann cells derived from adult nerves seeded in semipermeable guidance channels enhance peripheral nerve regeneration. *J Neurosci* 12(9):3310–3320.

Guo, J, Leung, KKG, Su, H et al. 2009. Self-assembling peptide nanofiber scaffold promotes the reconstruction of acutely injured brain. *Nanomed: Nanotechnol, Biol Med* 5(3):345–351.

Hadlock, T, Sundback, C, Hunter, D, Cheney, M, and Vacanti, JP. 2000. A polymer foam conduit seeded with Schwann cells promotes guided peripheral nerve regeneration. *Tissue Eng* 6(2):119–127.

Hadlock, TA, Sundback, CA, Hunter, DA, Vacanti, JP, and Cheney, ML. 2001. A new artificial nerve graft containing rolled Schwann cell monolayers. *Microsurgery* 21(3):96–101.

Hadlock, T, Sundback, C, Koka, R et al. 1999. A novel, biodegradable polymer conduit delivers neurotrophins and promotes nerve regeneration. *Laryngoscope* 109(9):1412–1416.

Harley, B, Spilker, M, Wu, J et al. 2004. Optimal degradation rate for collagen chambers used for regeneration of peripheral nerves over long gaps. *Cells Tissues Organs* 176(1–3):153–165.

Hazari, A, Johansson-Ruden, G, Junemo-Bostrom, K et al. 1999. A new resorbable wrap-around implant as an alternative nerve repair technique. *J Hand Surg (British and European Volume)* 24B(3):291–295.

Heath, CA and Rutkowski, GE. 1998. The development of bioartificial nerve grafts for peripheral-nerve regeneration. *Trends Biotechnol* 16(4):163–168.

Henderson, CE, Phillips, HS, Pollock, RA, Davies, AM, Lemeulle, C, Armanini, M, Simmons, L, Moffet, B, Vandlen, RA, and Simpson, LC. 1994. GDNF: A potent survival factor for motoneurons present in peripheral nerve and muscle. *Science* 266(5187):1062–1064.

Hermanns, S, Klapka, N, and Muller, HW. 2001. The collagenous lesion scar—An obstacle for axonal regeneration in brain and spinal cord injury. *Restor Neurol Neurosci* 19:139–148.

Hu, J, Zhu, Q-T, Liu, X-L, Xu, Y-b, and Zhu, J-K. 2007. Repair of extended peripheral nerve lesions in rhesus monkeys using acellular allogenic nerve grafts implanted with autologous mesenchymal stem cells. *Exp Neurol* 204(2):658–666.

Hudson, TW, Evans, GRD, and Schmidt., CE. 2000. Engineering strategies for peripheral nerve repair. *Orthop Clin North Am* 31(3):NA.

Hurtado, A, Moon, LDF, Maquet, V et al. 2006. Poly (D,L-lactic acid) macroporous guidance scaffolds seeded with Schwann cells genetically modified to secrete a bi-functional neurotrophin implanted in the completely transected adult rat thoracic spinal cord. *Biomaterials* 27(3):430–442.

Hutmacher, DW. 2001. Scaffold design and fabrication technologies for engineering tissues-state of the art and future perspectives. *J Biomater Sci Polym Ed* 12(1):107–124.

Hyatt, AJT, Wang, D, Kwok, JC, Fawcett, JW, and Martin, KR. 2010. Controlled release of chondroitinase ABC from fibrin gel reduces the level of inhibitory glycosaminoglycan chains in lesioned spinal cord. *J Control Release* 147(1):24–29.

Ichihara, S, Inada, Y, and Nakamura, T. 2008. Artificial nerve tubes and their application for repair of peripheral nerve injury: An update of current concepts. *Injury* 39(Supplement 4):29–39.

Ide, C, Nakai, Y, Nakano, N et al. 2010. Bone marrow stromal cell transplantation for treatment of subacute spinal cord injury in the rat. *Brain Res* 1332:32–47.

Ikeda, K, Yamauchi, D, Osamura, N, Hagiwara, N, and Tomita, K. 2003. Hyaluronic acid prevents peripheral nerve adhesion. *Br J Plastic Surg* 56(4):342–347.

Iwase, T, Jung, C, Bae, H, Zhang, M, and Solivan, B. 2005. Glial cell line derived neurotrophic factor-induced signaling in Schwann cells. *J Neurochem* 94:1488–1499.

Jacobs, WB and Fehlings, MG. 2003. The molecular basis of neural regeneration. *Neurosurgery* 53:943–949.

Jansen, K, van der Werff, JFA, van Wachem, PB et al. 2004. A hyaluronan-based nerve guide: *In vitro* cytotoxicity, subcutaneous tissue reactions, and degradation in the rat. *Biomaterials* 25(3):483–489.

Jiao, H, Yao, J, Yang, Y et al. 2009. Chitosan/polyglycolic acid nerve grafts for axon regeneration from prolonged axotomized neurons to chronically denervated segments. *Biomaterials* 30(28):5004–5018.

Johansson, F, Wallman, L, Danielsen, N, Schouenborg, J, and Kanje, M. 2009. Porous silicon as a potential electrode material in a nerve repair setting: Tissue reactions. *Acta Biomaterialia* 5(6):2230–2237.

Johnson, EO, Zoubos, AB, and Soucacos, PN. 2005. Regeneration and repair of peripheral nerves. *Injury* 36(4, Suppl 1):S24-S29.

Jones, DG, Anderson, ER, and Galvin, KA. 2003. Spinal cord regeneration: Moving tentatively towards new perspectives. *NeuroRehabilitation* 18:339–351.

Jones, LL, Oudega, M, Bunge, MB, and Tuszynski, MH. 2001. Neurotrophic factors, cellular bridges and gene therapy for spinal cord injury. *J Physiol* 533:83–89.

Jung, D-I, Ha, J, Kang, B-T et al. 2009. A comparison of autologous and allogenic bone marrow-derived mesenchymal stem cell transplantation in canine spinal cord injury. *J Neurol Sci* 285(1–2):67–77.

Kakinoki, R, Nishijima, N, Ueba, Y, Oka, M, and Yamamuro, T. 1995. Relationship between axonal regeneration and vascularity in tubulation—an experimental study in rats. *Neurosci Res* 23(1):35–45.

Kalincík, T, Choi, EA, Féron, F, Bianco, J, Sutharsan, R, Hayward, I, Mackay-Sim, A, Carrive, P, and Waite, PM. 2010. Olfactory ensheathing cells reduce duration of autonomic dysreflexia in rats with high spinal cord injury. *Autonom Neurosci* 154(1–2):20–29.

Kang, CE, Tator, CH, and Shoichet, MS. 2010. Poly(ethylene glycol) modification enhances penetration of fibroblast growth factor 2 to injured spinal cord tissue from an intrathecal delivery system. *J Control Release* 144(1):25–31.

Kang, SK, Shin, MJ, Jung, JS, Kim, YG, and Kim, CH. 2006. Autologous adipose tissue-derived stromal cells for treatment of spinal cord injury. *Stem Cells Dev* 15(4):583–594.

Kataoka, K, Suzuki, Y, Kitada, M et al. 2004. Alginate enhances elongation of early regenerating axons in spinal cord of young rats. *Tissue Eng* 10(3/4):493–504.

Keller, NR, Robertson, D, and Larry, RS (2009). Autonomic nervous system: General overview. *Encyclopedia of Neuroscience*. Oxford, Academic Press: pp. 941–949.

Kemp, SWP, Syed, S, Walsh, SK, Zochodne, DW, and Midha, R. 2009. Collagen nerve conduits promote enhanced axonal regeneration, Schwann cell association, and neovascularization compared to silicone conduits. *Tissue Eng Part* 15(8):1975–1988.

Kim, SB and Kwak, H. 2007. Poster 278: The effects of human adipose tissue-derived mesenchymal stem cells transplantation on neurologic recovery in rats with spinal cord injury. *Arch Phys Med Rehab* 88(9):E91-E91.

Kim, S-M, Lee, S-K, and Lee, J-H. 2007. Peripheral nerve regeneration using a three dimensionally cultured Schwann cell conduit. *J Craniofacial Surg* 18(3):475–488. 10.1097/01.scs.0000249362.41170.f3.

King, VR, Alovskaya, A, Wei, DYT, Brown, RA, and Priestley, JV. 2010. The use of injectable forms of fibrin and fibronectin to support axonal ingrowth after spinal cord injury. *Biomaterials* 31(15):4447–4456.

Kingham, PJ, Kalbermatten, DF, Mahay, D et al. 2007. Adipose-derived stem cells differentiate into a Schwann cell phenotype and promote neurite outgrowth in vitro. *Exp Neurol* 207(2):267–274.

Kokai, LE, Ghaznavi, AM, Marra, KG. 2010. Incorporation of double-walled microspheres into polymer nerve guides for the sustained delivery of glial cell line-derived neurotrophic factor. *Biomaterials* 31(8):2313–2322.

Kokai, LE, Lin, Y-C, Oyster, NM, Marra, KG. 2009. Diffusion of soluble factors through degradable polymer nerve guides: Controlling manufacturing parameters. *Acta Biomaterial* 5(7):2540–2550.

Kokai, LE, Tan, H, Jhunjhunwala, S et al. 2010. Protein bioactivity and polymer orientation is affected by stabilizer incorporation for double-walled microspheres. *J Control Release* 141(2):168–176.

Kubinová, S, Horák, D, Syková, E. 2009. Cholesterol-modified superporous poly(2-hydroxyethyl methacrylate) scaffolds for tissue engineering. *Biomaterials* 30(27):4601–4609.

Kuo, Y-C, Yeh, C-F, and Yang, J-T. 2009. Differentiation of bone marrow stromal cells in poly(lactide-*co*-glycolide)/chitosan scaffolds. *Biomaterials* 30(34):6604–6613.

Lanzetta, M, Gal, A, Wright, B, and Owen, E. 2003. Effect of FK506 and basic fibroblast growth factor on nerve regeneration using a polytetrafluoroethylene chamber for nerve repair. *Int Surg* 88(1):47–51.

Lavdas, AA, Chen, J, Papastefanaki, F et al. 2010. Schwann cells engineered to express the cell adhesion molecule L1 accelerate myelination and motor recovery after spinal cord injury. *Exp Neurol* 221(1):206–216.

Lee, DHS, Strittmatter, SM, and Sah, DWY. 2003. Targeting the nogo receptor to treat central nervous system injuries. *Nature* 2:1–7.

Lee, I-H, Bulte, JWM, Schweinhardt, P et al. 2004. *in vivo* magnetic resonance tracking of olfactory ensheathing glia grafted into the rat spinal cord. *Exp Neurol* 187:509–516.

Lee, SK and Wolfe, SW. 2000. Peripheral nerve injury and repair. *J Am Acad Orthop Surg* 8(4):243–252.

Li, S, Archibald, S, Krarup, C, and Madison, R. 1992. Peripheral nerve repair with collagen conduits. *Clin Mater* 9(3–4):195–200.

Li, X, Hou, S, Feng, X et al. 2009. Patterning of neural stem cells on poly(lactic-*co*-glycolic acid) film modified by hydrophobin. *Colloids Surf B: Biointerfaces* 74(1):370–374.

Li, X, Yang, Z, Zhang, A, Wang, T, and Chen, W. 2009. Repair of thoracic spinal cord injury by chitosan tube implantation in adult rats. *Biomaterials* 30(6):1121–1132.

Li, X-L, Zhang, W, Zhou, X et al. 2007. Temporal changes in the expression of some neurotrophins in spinal cord transected adult rats. *Neuropeptides* 41(3):135–143.

Lin, Y-C, Brayfield, CA, Gerlach, JC, Peter Rubin, J, and Marra, KG. 2009. Peptide modification of polyethersulfone surfaces to improve adipose-derived stem cell adhesion. *Acta Biomater* 5(5):1416–1424.

Lin, Y-C, Tan, F-j, Marra, KG, Jan, S-S, and Liu, D-C. 2009. Synthesis and characterization of collagen/hyaluronan/chitosan composite sponges for potential biomedical applications. *Acta Biomater* 5(7):2591–2600.

Lin, Y-L, Jen, J-C, Hsu, S-h, and Chiu, I-M. 2008. Sciatic nerve repair by microgrooved nerve conduits made of chitosan-gold nanocomposites. *Surg Neurol* 70(Suppl 1):S9–S18.

Lindberg, K, and Badylak, SF. 2001. Porcine small intestinal submucosa (SIS): A bioscaffold supporting *in vitro* primary human epidermal cell differentiation and synthesis of basement membrane proteins. *Burns* 27(3):254–266.

Liu, S, Peulve, P, Jin, O et al. 1997. Axonal regrowth through collagen tubes bridging the spinal cord to nerve roots. *J Neurosci Res* 49:425–432.

Liu, S, Said, G, and Tadie, M. 2001. Regrowth of the rostral spinal axons into the caudal ventral roots through a collagen tube implanted into hemisected adult rat spinal cord. *Neurosurgery* 49(1):143–151.

Loh, NK, Woerly, S, Bunt, SM, Wilton, SD, and Harvey, AR. 2001. The regrowth of axons within tissue defects in the CNS is promoted by implanted hydrogel matrices that contain BDNF and CNTF producing fibroblasts. *Exp Neurol* 170(1):72–84.

Lu, P, Jones, LL, and Tuszynski, MH. 2005. BDNF-expressing marrow stromal cells support extensive axonal growth at sites of spinal cord injury. *Exp Neurol* 191(2):344–360.

Luciano, RM, de Carvalho Zavaglia, CA, and de Rezende Duek, EA. 2000. Preparation of bioabsorbable nerve guide tubes. *Artif Organs* 24(3):206–208.

Lundborg, G. 2000. A 25-year perspective of peripheral nerve surgery: Evolving neuroscientific concepts and clinical significance. _J Hand Surg_ 25(3):391–414.

Lundborg, G, Dahlin, LB, Danielsen, N et al. 1982. Nerve regeneration in silicone chambers: Influence of gap length and of distal stump components. _Exp Neurol_ 76(2):361–375.

Luo, J, Borgens, R, and Shi, R. 2002. Polyethylene glycol immediately repairs neuronal membranes and inhibits free radical production after acute spinal cord injury. _J Neurochem_ 83:471–480.

Luo, J and Shi, R. 2007. Polyethylene glycol inhibits apoptotic cell death following traumatic spinal cord injury. _Brain Res_ 1155:10–16.

Madduri, S, Papaloizos, M, and Gander, B. 2010. Trophically and topographically functionalized silk fibroin nerve conduits for guided peripheral nerve regeneration. _Biomaterials_ 31(8):2323–2334.

Madison, RD, da Silva, C, Dikkes, P, Sidman, RL, and Chiu, T-H. 1987. Peripheral nerve regeneration with entubulation repair: Comparison of biodegradeable nerve guides versus polyethylene tubes and the effects of a laminin-containing gel. _Exp Neurol_ 95(2):378–390.

Madison, RD, Da Silva, CF, Dikkes, P, Sidman, RL, and Chio, T-H. 1987. Peripheral nerve regeneration with entubulation repair: Comparison of biodegradeable nerve guides versus polyethylene tubes and the effects of a laminin-containing gel. _Exp Neurol_ 95(2):378–390.

Maggi, S, Lowe, J, and Mackinnon, S. 2003. Pathophysiology of nerve injury. _Clin Plastic Surg_ 30(2):109–126.

Maquet, V, Martin, D, Malgrange, B et al. 2000. Peripheral nerve regeneration using bioresorbable macroporous scaffolds. _J Biomed Mater Res_ 52(4):639–651.

Matsuda, R, Yoshikawa, M, Kimura, H et al. 2009. Cotransplantation of mouse embryonic stem cells and bone marrow stromal cells following spinal cord injury suppresses tumor development. _Cell Transplant_ 18(1):39–54.

Matsuura, S, Obara, T, Tsuchiya, N, Suzuki, Y, and Habuchi, T. 2006. Cavernous nerve regeneration by biodegradable alginate gel sponge sheet placement without sutures. _Urology_ 68(6):1366–1371.

McDonald, JW, Becker, D, Holekamp, TF et al. 2004. Repair of the injured spinal cord and the potential of embryonic stem cell transplantation. _J Neurotrauma_ 21(4):383–393.

McKerracher, L. 2001. Spinal cord repair: Strategies to promote axon regeneration. _Neurobiol Dis_ 8:11–18.

Meek, MF, Coert, JH. 2002. Clinical use of nerve conduits in peripheral-nerve repair: Review of the literature. _J Reconstr Microsurg_ 18(02):097–110.

Meek, MF, Varejao, AS, and Geuna, S. 2002. Muscle grafts and alternatives for nerve repair. _J Oral Maxillofac Surg_ 60(9):1095–1096.

Millesi, H 1998. Trauma involving the brachial plexus. Management of peripheral nerve problems. G. E. Omer, M. Spinner and A. L. Van Beek (Eds) Philadelphia, PA, W.B. Saunders Company.

Miyazaki, M, Morishita, Y, He, W et al. 2009. A porcine collagen-derived matrix as a carrier for recombinant human bone morphogenetic protein-2 enhances spinal fusion in rats. _Spine J_ 9(1):22–30.

Moir, M, Wang, M, To, M, Lum, J, and Terris, D. 2000. Delayed repair of transected nerves: Effect of brain-derived neurotrophic factor. _Arch Otolaryngol-Head Neck Surg_ 126(4):501–505.

Murakami, H, Kobayashi, M., Takeuchi, H. and Kawashima, Y. 1999. Preparation of poly(DL-lactide-_co_-glycolide) nanoparticles by modified spontaneous emulsification solvent diffusion method. Int. _J Pharm_ 187(2):143–152.

Navarro, X, Rodríguez, F, Labrador, R et al. 1996. Peripheral nerve regeneration through bioresorbable and durable nerve guides. _J Peripheral Nervous System_ 1(1):53–64.

Navarro, X, Viv, M, and Valero-Cabr, A. 2007. Neural plasticity after peripheral nerve injury and regeneration. _Progr Neurobiol_ 82(4):163–201.

Nomura, H, Zahir, T, Kim, H et al. 2008. Extramedullary chitosan channels promote survival of transplanted neural stem and progenitor cells and create a tissue bridge after complete spinal cord transection. _Tissue Eng Part A_ 14(5):649–65.

Norenberg, MD, Smith, J, and Marcillo, A. 2004. The pathology of human spinal cord injury: Defining the problems. _J Neurotrauma_ 21(4):429–440.

Novikov, LN, Novikona, LN, Mosahebi, A et al. 2002. A novel biodegradable implant for neuronal rescue and regeneration after spinal cord injury. *Biomaterials* 23:3369–3376.

Novikova, LN, Pettersson, J, Brohlin, M, Wiberg, M, and Novikov, LN. 2008. Biodegradable poly-[beta]-hydroxybutyrate scaffold seeded with Schwann cells to promote spinal cord repair. *Biomaterials* 29(9):1198–1206.

Oh, JS, Ha, Y, An, SS, Khan, M, Pennant, WA, Kim, HJ, Yoon do, H, Lee, M, and Kim, KN. 2010. Hypoxia-preconditioned adipose tissue-derived mesenchymal stem cell increase the survival and gene expression of engineered neural stem cells in a spinal cord injury model. *Neuroscience Letters* 472(3):215–219.

Ohta, Y, Takenaga, M, Tokura, Y et al. 2008. Mature adipocyte-derived cells, dedifferentiated fat cells (DFAT), promoted functional recovery from spinal cord injury-induced motor dysfunction in rats. *Cell Transplant* 17(8):877–886.

Oudega, M, Gautier, SE, Chapon, P et al. 2001. Axonal regeneration into Schwann cell grafts within resorbable poly(alpha-hydroxyacid) guidance channels in the adult rat spinal cord. *Biomaterials* 22:1125–1136.

Oudega, M, and Hagg, T. 1999. Neurotrophins promote regeneration of sensory axons in the adult rat spinal cord. *Brain Res* 818(2):431–438.

Pabari, A, Yang, SY, Seifalian, AM, and Mosahebi, A. 2010. Modern surgical management of peripheral nerve gap. *J Plastic, Reconstr Aesthetic Surg* 63(12):1941–1948.

Paratcha, G, Ledda, F. 2008. GDNF and GFR[alpha]: A versatile molecular complex for developing neurons. *Trends Neurosci* 31(8):384–391.

Pastrana, E, Moreno-Flores, MT, Avila, J et al. 2007. BDNF production by olfactory ensheathing cells contributes to axonal regeneration of cultured adult CNS neurons. *Neurochem Int* 50(3):491–498.

Patel, M, Mao, L, Wu, B, and VandeVord, PJ. 2007. GDNF-chitosan blended nerve guides: A functional study. *J Tissue Eng Regenerative Med* 1(5):360–367.

Patist, CM, Mulder, MB, Gautier, SE et al. 2004. Freeze-dried poly(D,L-lactic acid) macroporous guidance scaffolds impregnated with brain-derived neurotrophic factor in the transected adult rat thoracic spinal cord. *Biomaterials* 25:1569–1582.

Paul, C, Samdani, AF, Betz, RR, Fischer, I, and Neuhuber, B. 2009. Grafting of human bone marrow stromal cells into spinal cord injury: A comparison of delivery methods. *Spine (Phila Pa 1976)* 34(4):328–34.

Pego, AP, Poot, AA, Grijpma, DW, and Feijen, J. 2001. Copolymers of trimethylene carbonate and epsilon-caprolactone for porous nerve guides: Synthesis and properties. *J Biomater Sci Polym Ed* 12(1):35–53.

Petter-Puchner, AH, Froetscher, W, Krametter-Froetscher, R et al. 2007. The long-term neurocompatibility of human fibrin sealant and equine collagen as biomatrices in experimental spinal cord injury. *Exp Toxicol Pathol* 58(4):237–245.

Pettingill, LN, Minter, RL, and Shepherd, RK. 2008. Schwann cells genetically modified to express neurotrophins promote spiral ganglion neuron survival in vitro. *Neuroscience* 152(3):821–828.

Piotrowicz, A and Shoichet, MS. 2006. Nerve guidance channels as drug delivery vehicles. *Biomaterials* 27(9):2018–2027.

Piquilloud, G, Christen, T, Pfister, LA, Gander, B, and Papaloïzos, MY. 2007. Variations in glial cell line-derived neurotrophic factor release from biodegradable nerve conduits modify the rate of functional motor recovery after rat primary nerve repairs. *Eur J Neurosci* 26(5):1109–1117.

Prang, P, Müller, R, Eljaouhari, A et al. 2006. The promotion of oriented axonal regrowth in the injured spinal cord by alginate-based anisotropic capillary hydrogels. *Biomaterials* 27(19):3560–3569.

Profyris, C, Cheema, SS, Zang, D et al. 2004. Degenerative and regenerative mechanisms governing spinal cord injury. *Neurobiol Dis* 15:415–436.

Robinson, P, van der Lei, B, Hoppen, H et al. 1991. Nerve regeneration through a two-ply biodegradable nerve guide in the rat and the influence of ACTH4–9 nerve growth factor. *Microsurgery* 12(6):412–419.

Rodrigues Hell, RC, Silva Costa, MM, Goes, AM, and Oliveira, ALR. 2009. Local injection of BDNF producing mesenchymal stem cells increases neuronal survival and synaptic stability following ventral root avulsion. *Neurobiol Dis* 33(2):290–300.

Rodriguez, FJ, Gomez, N., Perego, G., and Navarro, X. 1999. Highly permeable polylactide-capro-lactone nerve guides enhance peripheral nerve regeneration through long gaps. *Biomaterials* 20(16):1489–1500.

Rutkowski, GE and Heath, CA. 2002. Development of a bioartificial nerve graft. I. Design based on a reaction-diffusion model. *Biotechnol Progr* 18(2):362–372.

Rutkowski, GE and Heath, CA. 2002. Development of a bioartificial nerve graft. II. Nerve regeneration in vitro. *Biotechnol Progr* 18(2):373–379.

Rutkowski, GE, Miller, CA, Jeftinija, S, and Mallapragada, SK. 2004. Synergistic effects of micropatterned biodegradable conduits and Schwann cells on sciatic nerve regeneration. *J Neural Eng* 1(3):151–157.

Sayer, FT, Oudega, M, and Hagg, T. 2002. Neurotrophins reduce degeneration of injured ascending sensory and corticospinal motor axons in adult rat spinal cord. *Exp Neurol* 175:282–296.

Schlosshauer, B, Dreesmann, L, Schaller, H-E, and Sinis, N. 2006. Synthetic nerve guide implants in humans: A comprehensive survey. [Review]. *Neurosurgery* 59(4):740–748.

Schmidt, CE and Leach, JB. 2003. Neural tissue engineering: Strategies for repair and regeneration. *Ann Rev Biomed Eng* 5(1):293–347.

Schmidt, CE, Shastri, VR, Vacanti, JP, and Langer, R. 1997. Stimulation of neurite outgrowth using an electrically conducting polymer. *Proc Natl Acad Sci USA* 94:8948–8953.

Sendtner, M, Holtmann, B, Kolbeck, R, Thoenen, H, and Barde, Y. 1992. Brain-derived neurotrophic factor prevents the death of motoneurons in newborn rats after nerve section. *Nature* 360(6406):757–759.

Shapiro, L and Cohen, S. 1997. Novel alginate sponges for cell culture and transplantation. *Biomaterials* 18(8):583–590.

Shi, R and Borgens, R. 2000. Anatomical repair of nerve membranes in crushed mammalian spinal cord with polyethylene glycol. *J Neurocytol* 29:633–643.

Shi, X, Kang, Y, Hu, Q, Chen, C, Yang, L, Wang, K, Chen, L, Huang, H, and Zhou, C. 2010. A long-term observation of olfactory ensheathing cells transplantation to repair white matter and functional recovery in a focal ischemia model in rat. *Brain Res* 1317:257–267.

Silver, J and Miller, JH. 2004. Regeneration beyond the glial scar. *Nature* 5:146–156.

Srivastava, N, Seth, K, Khanna, VK, Ansari, RW, and Agrawal, AK. 2009. Long-term functional restoration by neural progenitor cell transplantation in rat model of cognitive dysfunction: Co-transplantation with olfactory ensheathing cells for neurotrophic factor support. *Int J Dev Neurosci* 27(1):103–110.

Stichel, CC and Muller, HW. 1998. The CNS lesion scar: New vistas on an old regeneration barrier. *Cell Tissue Res* 294:1–9.

Stocum, DL. 1998. Regenerative biology and engineering: Strategies for tissue restoration. *Wound Repair Regen* 6(4):276–290.

Stokols, S and Tuszynski, MH. 2006. Freeze-dried agarose scaffolds with uniaxial channels stimulate and guide linear axonal growth following spinal cord injury. *Biomaterials* 27(3):443–451.

Streit, WJ. 2001. Microglia and Macrophages in the Developing CNS. *NeuroToxicology* 22(5):619–624.

Sun, W, Sun, C, Lin, H et al. 2009. The effect of collagen-binding NGF-[beta] on the promotion of sciatic nerve regeneration in a rat sciatic nerve crush injury model. *Biomaterials* 30(27):4649–4656.

Sunderland, S (1968). *Nerves and Nerve Injuries*. Baltimore, The Williams & Wilkins Company.

Suzuki, Y, Tanihara, M, Ohnishi, K et al. 1999. Cat peripheral nerve regeneration across 50 mm gap repaired with a novel nerve guide composed of freeze-dried alginate gel. *Neurosci Lett* 259(2):75–78.

Tabesh, H, Amoabediny, G, Nik, NS et al. 2009. The role of biodegradable engineered scaffolds seeded with Schwann cells for spinal cord regeneration. *Neurochem Int* 54(2):73–83.

Talac, R, Friedman, JA, Moore, MJ et al. 2004. Animal models of spinal cord injury for evaluation of tissue engineering treatment strategies. *Biomaterials* 25:1505–1510.

Tan, SA, Deglon, N, Zurn, AD et al. 1996. Rescue of motoneurons from axotomy induced cell death by polymer encapsulated cells genetically engineered to release CNTF. *Cell Trans* 5:577–587.

Taras, JS, and Jacoby, SM. 2008. Repair of lacerated peripheral nerves with nerve conduits. *Tech Hand Upper Extremity Surg* 12(2):100–106.

Taylor, S, McDonald, J, and Sakiyama-Elbert, S. 2004. Controlled release of neurotrophin-3 from fibrin gels for spinal cord injury. *J Control Release* 98:281–294.

Taylor, SJ, and Sakiyama-Elbert, SE. 2006. Effect of controlled delivery of neurotrophin-3 from fibrin on spinal cord injury in a long term model. *J Control Release* 116(2):204–210.

Terenghi, G. 1999. Peripheral nerve regeneration and neurotrophic factors. *J Anat.* 194:1–14.

Terzis, JK and Smith, KL (1990). The peripheral nerve. *Structure, Function and Reconstruction.* New York, NY, Hampton Press.

Tohill, M, Mantovani, C, Wiberg, M, and Terenghi, G. 2004. Rat bone marrow mesenchymal stem cells express glial markers and stimulate nerve regeneration. *Neurosci Lett* 362(3):200–203.

Tom, VJ, Steinmetz, MP, Miller, JH, Doller, CM, and Silver, J. 2004. Studies on the development and behavior of the dystrophic growth cone, the hallmark of regeneration failure, in an *in vitro* model of the glial scar and after spinal cord injury. *J Neurosci* 24:6531–6539.

Toth, C. 2009. Peripheral nerve injuries attributable to sport and recreation. *Phys Med Rehab Clin North Am* 20(1):77–100.

Tsai, EC, Dalton, PD, Shoichet, MS, and Tator, CH. 2004. Synthetic hydrogel guidance channels facilitate regeneration of adult rat brainstem motor axons after complete spinal cord transection. *J Neurotrauma* 21(6):789–804.

Tyner, TR, Parks, N, Faria, S et al. 2007. Effects of collagen nerve guide on neuroma formation and neuropathic pain in a rat model. *Am J Surg* 193(1):e1–e6.

Uebersax, L, Mattotti, M, Papaloizos, M et al. 2007. Silk fibroin matrices for the controlled release of nerve growth factor (NGF). *Biomaterials* 28(30):4449–4460.

Utley, D, Lewin, S, Cheng, E et al. 1996. Brain-derived neurotrophic factor and collagen tubulization enhance functional recovery after peripheral nerve transection and repair. *Arch Otolaryngol-Head Neck Surg* 122(4):407–413.

Valentini, RF, Aebischer, P, Winn, SR, and Galletti, PM. 1987. Collagen- and laminin-containing gels impede peripheral nerve regeneration through semipermeable nerve guidance channels. *Exp Neurol* 98(2):350–356.

Verdu, E, Labrador, RO, Rodriguez, FJ et al. 2002. Alignment of collagen and laminin-containing gels improve nerve regeneration within silicone tubes. *Restor Neurol Neurosci* 20(5):169–179.

Vogel, LC, Krajci, KA, and Anderson, CJ. 2002. Adults with pediatric-onset spinal cord injury: Part 1: Prevalence of medical complications. *J Spinal Cord Med* 25(2):106–116.

Vögelin, E, Baker, JM, Gates, J et al. 2006. Effects of local continuous release of brain derived neurotrophic factor (BDNF) on peripheral nerve regeneration in a rat model. *Exp Neurol* 199(2):348–353.

Voytik-Harbin, SL, Brightman, AO, Kraine, MR, Waisner, B, and Badylak, SF. 1997. Identification of extractractable growth factors from small intestinal submucosa. *J Cell Biochem* 67:478–491.

Waitayawinyu, T, Parisi, DM, Miller, B et al. 2007. A comparison of polyglycolic acid versus type 1 collagen bioabsorbable nerve conduits in a rat model: An alternative to autografting. *J Hand Surg* 32(10):1521–1529.

Walsh, S, Biernaskie, J, Kemp, SWP, and Midha, R. 2009. Supplementation of acellular nerve grafts with skin derived precursor cells promotes peripheral nerve regeneration. *Neuroscience* 164(3):1097–1107.

Wang, J, Ding, F, Gu, Y, Liu, J, and Gu, X. 2009. Bone marrow mesenchymal stem cells promote cell proliferation and neurotrophic function of Schwann cells *in vitro* and in vivo. *Brain Res* 1262:7–15.

Wang, T-W and Spector, M. 2009. Development of hyaluronic acid-based scaffolds for brain tissue engineering. *Acta Biomaterialia* 5(7):2371–2384.

Wang, XH, Li, DP, Wang, WJ et al. 2003. Crosslinked collagen/chitosan matrix for artificial livers. *Biomaterials* 24(19):3213–3220.

Wang, ZH, Wang, ZY, Sun, CS et al. 2010. Trimethylated chitosan-conjugated PLGA nanoparticles for the delivery of drugs to the brain. *Biomaterials* 31(5):908–915.

Whitlock, EL, Tuffaha, SH, Luciano, JP et al. 2009. Processed allografts and type I collagen conduits for repair of peripheral nerve gaps. *Muscle Nerve* 39(6):787–799.

Whitworth, I, Brown, R, Doré, C et al. 1996. Nerve growth factor enhances nerve regeneration through fibronectin grafts. *J Hand Surg* 21(4):514–522.

Woerly, S, Doan, VD, Sosa, N, Vellis, JD, and Espinosa-Jeffrey, A. 2004. Prevention of gliotic scar formation by NeuroGel allows partial endogenous repair of transected cat spinal cord. *J Neurosci Res* 75:262–272.

Woerly, S, Pinet, E, Robertis, LD, Diep, DV, and Bousmina, M. 2001. Spinal cord repair with PHPMA hydrogel containing RGD peptides (NeuroGel™). *Biomaterials* 22:1095–1111.

Wright, KT, Masri, WE, Osman, A et al. 2008. The cell culture expansion of bone marrow stromal cells from humans with spinal cord injury: Implications for future cell transplantation therapy. *Spinal Cord* 46(12):811–7.

Xiong, Y, Zeng, Y-S, Zeng, C-G et al. 2009. Synaptic transmission of neural stem cells seeded in 3-dimensional PLGA scaffolds. *Biomaterials* 30(22):3711–3722.

Xu, X, Yu, H, Gao, S et al. 2002. Polyphosphoester microspheres for sustained release of biologically active nerve growth factor. *Biomaterials* 23(17):3765–3772.

Xu, Y, Liu, L, Li, Y et al. 2008. Myelin-forming ability of Schwann cell-like cells induced from rat adipose-derived stem cells in vitro. *Brain Res* 1239:49–55.

Yaginuma, H, Tomita, M, Takashita, N et al. 1996. A novel type of programmed neuronal death in the cervical spinal cord of the chick embryo. *J Neurosci* 16(11):3685–703.

Yang, F, Murugan, R, Ramakrishna, S et al. 2004. Fabrication of nano-structured porous PLLA scaffold intended for nerve tissue engineering. *Biomaterials* 25(10):1891–1900.

Yang, Y, Chen, X, Ding, F et al. 2007. Biocompatibility evaluation of silk fibroin with peripheral nerve tissues and cells in vitro. *Biomaterials* 28(9):1643–1652.

Yang, Y, Ding, F, Wu, J et al. 2007. Development and evaluation of silk fibroin-based nerve grafts used for peripheral nerve regeneration. *Biomaterials* 28(36):5526–5535.

Yang, Y, Zhao, Y, Gu, Y et al. 2009. Degradation behaviors of nerve guidance conduits made up of silk fibroin *in vitro* and in vivo. *Polymer Degrad Stability* 94(12):2213–2220.

Yao, L, Wang, S, Cui, W et al. 2009. Effect of functionalized micropatterned PLGA on guided neurite growth. *Acta Biomater* 5(2):580–588.

Yuan, Y, Zhang, P, Yang, Y, Wang, X, and Gu, X. 2004. The interaction of Schwann cells with chitosan membranes and fibers in vitro. *Biomaterials* 25(18):4273–4278.

Zhang, H-T, Gao, Z-Y, Chen, Y-Z, and Wang, T-H. 2008. Temporal changes in the level of neurotrophins in the spinal cord and associated precentral gyrus following spinal hemisection in adult Rhesus monkeys. *J Chem Neuroanatomy* 36(3–4):138–143.

Zhang, P, Zhang, C, Kou, Y et al. 2009. The histological analysis of biological conduit sleeve bridging rhesus monkey median nerve injury with small gap. *Artificial Cells, Blood Substitutes, and Biotechnol: An Int J* 37(2):101–104.

Zhang, Y, Cheng, X, Wang, J et al. 2006. Novel chitosan/collagen scaffold containing transforming growth factor-[beta]1 DNA for periodontal tissue engineering. *Biochem Biophys Res Commun* 344(1):362–369.

Zhao, ZM, Li, HJ, Liu, HY et al. 2004. Intraspinal transplantation of CD34+ human umbilical cord blood cells after spinal cord hemisection injury improves functional recovery in adult rats. *Cell Transplant* 13(2):113–122.

# 37

# Tumor Engineering: Applications for Cancer Biology and Drug Development

37.1 Introduction ............................................................ 37-1
37.2 Cancer Fundamentals and Relationship to Tissue Engineering ............................................................ 37-2
37.3 Preclinical Drug Evaluation ................................... 37-4
Monolayer Cell Culture • Animal Models • Tumor Explants
37.4 Advanced 3D Models of Cancer ............................. 37-6
Spheroids • Bioengineered Tumors
37.5 Tools for Creation of a Bioengineered Tumor Model .............. 37-8
ECM Gels • Polymer Scaffolds • Signaling Molecules • Cocultures • Bioreactors
37.6 Applications of Advanced 3D Cancer Models ......................... 37-12
Improve Evaluation of New Cancer Drugs • Study the Impact of a 3D Microenvironment upon Angiogenesis • Create More Advanced Animal Models
37.7 Conclusions ........................................................... 37-14
References ................................................................. 37-14

Joseph A. Ludwig
*University of Texas, Houston*
*MD Anderson Cancer Center*

Emily Burdett
*BioScience Research Collaborative*

## 37.1 Introduction

Though considerable progress has been made since the advent of the modern chemotherapy era, cancer remains a leading cause of death throughout the developed world. Within the United States alone, more than half a million people die of their malignancies each year, often despite receiving treatment that, unfortunately, fails to provide long-term control of tumor growth secondary to *de novo* or acquired drug resistance. While concerted efforts by academic institutions, the pharmaceutical industry, and governmental agencies such as the Food and Drug Administration (FDA) strive to rapidly transition promising therapies along the drug development pipeline from the lab bench to the bedside, a number of hurdles exist both preclinically and clinically.

A major one, which contributes to the drug development costs averaging more than 1.7 billion dollars per year for each FDA-approved drug,[1] is the inability to accurately predict in advance which preclinical drug candidates will ultimately prove beneficial in time-consuming and costly late-stage clinical trials. As oncologists and cancer biologists can attest to, though it is relatively easy to eradicate cancer within cell lines and animals, potential drug candidates tested with these model systems often show little or no efficacy when tested in humans. To close this void, preclinical models of cancer must improve to the fullest extent possible to better replicate, *ex vivo,* the complexity that occurs naturally. Toward that end, applications previously intended for regenerative tissue engineering are finding new uses for the creation of bioengineered tumor models, that is, multicellular three-dimensional (3D) tumor-like constructs that rely upon nonnative biomimetic microenvironments or scaffolds to recapitulate defining cancer characteristics such as malignant transformation, invasion, or growth.

As described in the previous chapters, a diverse range of tissue engineering applications have emerged or are on the near horizon that promise to improve survival and/or quality of life either by supplanting worn out or defective human tissues or augmenting poorly functioning ones. Examples include biological substitutes for damaged joints, biosynthetic bone grafts or skin grafts, and many others. Unlike those applications however, which by and large are intended for regenerative purposes for eventual *in vivo* transplantation, bioengineered tumors serve an altogether different purpose—to provide a high fidelity *ex vivo* model of human tumor biology that cannot otherwise be studied as readily in patients (or animal models) for myriad reasons, including practical limitations in biopsy frequency, limited patient numbers (especially for rare tumor types), uncontrollable conditions (serum growth factors, immune surveillance, etc.) and restricted evaluation in humans to those drugs which are either FDA-approved or in clinical trials.

To obviate some of those inherent challenges, the nascent field of tumor bioengineering offers a multidisciplinary approach that draws upon lessons learned for regenerative bioengineering applications and applies them to the field of cancer biology. The result of this convergence is a greater capacity to define the precise contributions that 3D geometry, cell–cell interaction, tumor stroma, and drug diffusion have upon tumor growth, metastatic potential, and chemosensitivity that would not otherwise be possible using traditional two-dimensional (2D) monolayer cell growth. Ultimately, of course, the knowledge gained from 3D bioengineered tumor models should serve to improve the lives of cancer patients by explaining divergent preclinical and clinical drug responses.

Paralleling the overarching structure of this book, this chapter first discusses the fundamentals (with sections that focus on the relationship between cancer biology and tissue engineering as well as the current paradigm of preclinical drug testing), next describes advanced 3D models and enabling technologies used for bioengineered tumors, and finally highlights potential applications by which bioengineered tumors may contribute to our understanding of cancer biology. Though all models, including recent bioengineered tumor models used to understand cancer biology, will undoubtedly fall short of the goal of exactly mimicking the complex *in vivo* biology, considerable progress toward that goal has been made since traditional 2D culture was first used. Just as ancient Greeks philosophers realized a spherical Earth better fit their experimental observations than the planar one originally conceptualized, cancer biologists have understood for some time that cancer cells grown in 3D culture often mimic *in vivo* conditions better than 2D monolayer cell culture upon plastic substratum. As the effects that spatial and temporal cues have upon the cancer phenotype are better comprehended, we anticipate the field of tissue engineering will play an ever-greater role in identifying novel targets amenable to biologically targeted cancer treatment.

## 37.2  Cancer Fundamentals and Relationship to Tissue Engineering

Though a comprehensive discussion of cancer biology is beyond the scope of this text, a brief introduction is in order, with particular attention to the remarkable overlap that exists between normal cellular processes that occur physiologically (and within tissue-engineered models) and anomalous ones, which are subverted by malignant cells during their malignant transformation. At its simplest, malignant tumors (as opposed to benign neoplasms) may be defined generically as an accumulation of dysfunctional cells, originally derived from a single corrupted normal cell, that gain the ability to invade and metastasize—often to the detriment of the host. A fuller understanding for those macroscopic events of tumor growth and metastasis, however, can be attributed by and large to either somatic or spontaneous genetic errors that lead to amplification and/or upregulation of cancer-promoting genes (oncogenes) or loss of function mutations in tumor suppressor genes. This multistep process of tumorigenesis imbues malignant cells with several molecular hallmarks of cancer.

As described succinctly by Hanahan and Weinberg more than a decade ago, those hallmarks include the ability to evade apoptosis, self-sufficiency in growth signals, insensitivity to antigrowth signals, an unlimited replicative potential, as well as interactions at the tumor–stroma interface that promote angiogenesis, invasion, and metastasis.[2] Although such capabilities are invariably required for cancer formation, growth, and invasion, not all are unique to cancer and, given the appropriate setting, normal cells may transiently exhibit some of those same cancer-like features (Table 37.1).

For example, during embryogenesis human stem cells and their more differentiated progenitors expand at an incredible rate, forming organs and complex anatomical structures at a pace rivaling tumor formation. The capacity for brisk neoplasia can be similarly observed during hepatic regeneration following partial hepatectomy. Like their malignant counterparts, noncancerous human stems cells have

**TABLE 37.1** Comparisons of Malignant Neoplasms, Wounds, and Bioengineered Tissues

| | Cancers | Wounds | Bioengineered Tissues |
|---|---|---|---|
| Growth signals | Tumors often grow without reliance upon growth factors secondary to activating mutations in cognate receptors, receptor amplification, or upregulation of downstream pathways | Initial clot contains fibrin, fibronectin, and platelets as well as mitogens and chemoattractants that recruit the cells needed for wound healing | Growth factors can be used with synthetic scaffolds or hydrogels in an attempt to mimic the wound healing process and improve growth and survival of the cells of interest |
| Antigrowth signals | Can become insensitive to antigrowth signals and proliferate unhindered | Responsive, such that wounds normally avoid overgrowth (keloids being an exception) | Responsive to antigrowth signals |
| Tissue invasion | Can invade into and beyond natural tissue borders | Wounds are transiently invaded by a host of inflammatory cells (lymphocytes, macrophages, etc.) to form "granulation tissue" | Bioengineered tissues can be embedded *in vivo* for regenerative purposes. Though invasion does not occur, interaction with the host tissue can be helpful in maintaining implant viability, growth, and function |
| Distant spread | The ability to metastasize is a fundamental trait of cancers (as opposed to benign neoplasms) | Does not occur | Does not occur |
| Replication potential | Unlimited secondary to altered telomeres | Stem cells possess unlimited replication potential | Limited, although human mesenchymal stem cells have been used for regenerative purposes |
| Angiogenesis | Tumor cells and recruited cancer-associated fibroblasts often secrete VEGF and other growth factors to stimulate angiogenesis | Angiogenesis is a critical early physiological process necessary for wound healing | Bioengineered tissues have been designed to promote angiogenesis through addition of exogenous angiogenic factors. Required for long-term viability of *in vivo* tissue implants |
| Apoptosis | Can evade apoptosis through a process called anoikis | Occurs normally. Apoptosis plays an especially important role during embryogenesis | Occurs normally. Biomimetic scaffolds and ECMs can be provided in an attempt to avoid programmed cell death |

the capacity for unlimited self-renewal, can often migrate to foreign locations with the body as needed, and can elicit physiological angiogenesis. Finally, as Dovorak highlighted more than two decades ago, numerous parallels exist between tumor formation and wound healing such that tumors can, in some sense, be described as "wounds that do not heal."[3] Both tumors and wounds lay a foundation of fibrin–fibronectin matrix and growth factors that serve as chemoattractants for inflammatory cells; mainly fibroblasts, lymphocytes, and endothelial cells. In the initial phases of both wound healing and tumor formation, angiogenesis is required to supply nutrients, exchange oxygen, and remove waste and, just as a wound's fibrin-clot evolves to form highly cellular and vascularized granulation tissue, tumors coerce their surrounding stroma to further their capacity to grow and invade.

Perhaps what most distinguishes neoplasms (both malignant and benign) from normal physiological phenomena such as wound healing, embryogenesis, and tissue regeneration is that cancer's cells have lost their homeostatic cues between the surrounding stroma and themselves, and therefore, continue to propagate without respect for their surrounding environment. Malignant neoplasms go one step further and not only fail to recognize normal cellular or tissue boundaries but can also grow within foreign environments such lymph nodes or bone (for carcinomas) or lung tissue (for sarcomas) through a process of anoikis (the ability for anchorage-independent cell growth). Analogous to the "seed and soil" example, it is now recognized that the intrinsic properties of the cancer cell ("seed") and surrounding stroma ("soil") are critical for tumor metastasis.

Given this dysfunctional bidirectional signaling that occurs between tumor and stroma, one might be tempted to mistakenly discount the impact that spatial and temporal cues have upon a cancer's phenotype. However, most cancer cells grown *in vitro* still require a minimal supplement of growth factors, most often provided with the addition of fetal calf serum, and many cell types require plates specially coated with collagen or other matrix components to grow. Also, splitting cells too sparsely can limit cell growth by depriving them of required paracrine signaling. Thus, even cancer cells cannot entirely forgo their reliance upon stroma and extracellular matrix (ECM) for survival.

As has readily become apparent, a cancer's phenotype is also critically dependent upon the presence or absence of adherent culture surfaces, the extracellular matrix, and the design and chemical makeup of extracellular scaffolding material, which together can promote 3D *in vitro* cancer growth that better replicates *in vivo* conditions. Tissue engineers have, of course, known of the marked impact the surrounding stroma and extracellular environment has upon cell and tissue growth from the very beginning of their collective effort to create *ex vivo* tissue. As a prelude to discussing how lessons learned from the tissue engineering field can be applied to the science of cancer biology to create improved higher fidelity 3D *ex vivo* tumor models, the limitations of current 2D monolayer culture and xenograft models are noted with special attention to their use for evaluation of potential antineoplastic agents.

## 37.3 Preclinical Drug Evaluation

### 37.3.1 Monolayer Cell Culture

Since the advent of *in vitro* immortalized cancer growth on traditional 2D monolayers, individual cell lines and diverse cancer panels have been widely used for evaluation of antineoplastic drug candidates.[4] For example, more than two decades ago the National Cancer Institute established a panel of 60 unique cancer cell lines used to screen more than 100,000 compounds; many other cancer cell lines have been used with similar intent.[4–7] Via a number of high-throughput technologies measuring the expression at the gene and protein level, correlations between expression and drug efficacy have been used to identify drugs with unique mechanisms of action and elucidated resistance mechanisms.[4–6]

However, despite the undeniable scientific advances, 2D monolayer culture has generally failed to serve as a reliable predictor of clinical benefit for promising drugs that transition into the clinical arena.[8,9] The reasons for this are myriad but the artificial growth environment itself is considered to be a likely culprit.[4] The immortalization process tends to enrich for the most rapidly proliferating cancer cells capable surviving on uncoated tissue culture plastic as opposed to ones that would naturally grow at a more subdued rates in the native 3D environment *in vivo*.[7] Furthermore, although fetal calf serum is usually added to culture medium as a surrogate for missing growth factors, 2D monolayer culture lacks other critical features such as an ECM, human soluble signaling molecules, and a 3D architecture composed of stromal cells and irregular microvasculature.[10] The influence of those factors on cancer cells have been thoroughly discussed elsewhere.[10–15]

For the reason that the vast majority of anticancer drugs work by indiscriminant targeting the processes responsible for cell division, rather than specific proteins or pathways responsible for other cancer traits (e.g., resistance to apoptosis, immortality, metastatic potential, growth factor independence), the recent trend in preclinical *in vitro* drug testing has been to move beyond traditional 2D culture models and rely more heavily upon emerging 3D ones or to animal models, though animal models have their own limitations noted below.

## 37.3.2 Animal Models

Of course an alternative to *in vitro* models that better reproduce the biological complexity of human tumors is to use tumor xenografts within an animal model. That strategy allows several of the 3D microenvironmental cues missing during monolayer growth to be replaced, albeit incompletely since major differences exist between human and animal tissues.[16] By far the most widespread xenograft model employed for preclinical drug evaluation is the subcutaneous human tumor xenograft.[17] Briefly summarized, human tumor cells are implanted subcutaneously in immunodeficient mice and allowed to grow sufficiently to be detectible by physical calipers or luminescent measures. Then experimental therapeutics are compared to placebo controls for potential efficacy and molecular pathways within responding or resistant xenografts can be interrogated to monitor if the drug effect occurred through the hypothesized mechanism of action.[16] By evaluating drug pharmacokinetics and toxicity, animal models additionally serve as a necessary step prior to phase I human clinical trials.

Unfortunately, as with *in vitro* testing, the majority of drugs that appear promising in xenograft models fail to display equal efficacy in those early phase I/II trials.[8,9,18] Again, this might be expected given the subtle differences that exist between the human and mouse 3D tumor microenvironment; such differences are likely to be especially pronounced using a foreign subcutaneous tumor placement rather than orthotopic site.[16,17] Sophisticated animal models can be used to overcome some of these shortcomings, either by orthotopic xenograft placement or autochthonous tumor models whereby tumors arise within their expected locations induced by genetic manipulation and carcinogen exposure.[19–21] Though biological data from those models are likely to be relevant to the human clinical experience, their added complexity and technical difficulty often precludes their extensive use. Moreover, not all cancer types can be adapted for orthotopic or autochthonous study. In summary, a critical role for animal models persists but they are not yet reliable enough to predict human drug response.

## 37.3.3 Tumor Explants

Tumor explants, typically millimeter size pieces tumor specimens directly transplanted in animals without transient *in vitro* culture, offers a third alternative for preclinical drug evaluation. Whereas standard *in vitro* culture often results in dedifferentiated cells that stray far from the original *in vivo* phenotype, tumor explants have the distinct advantage of maintaining cell differentiation in a near native state. This is especially helpful, as many of the signaling cascades targeted by biologically oriented therapies are likely to remain essentially unaltered within the explants and, thereby, provide a truer reflection of how the original tumors may have responded. In the rare instances when patients and their respective tumor explants were exposed to the same drug, strong correlations in drug efficacy have been reported.

Though explants probably offer the highest fidelity to native human tumors, they are also the most technically demanding and least commonly employed for cancer research. Since tumor explants are derived from patients' tumors, there are obviously finite amounts available, all the limitations of animal models exist, and the cost of surgical tissue acquisition can be prohibitive unless the surgical resection is planned as part of routine clinical care.

# 37.4 Advanced 3D Models of Cancer

## 37.4.1 Spheroids

Advanced 3D cancer models have been developed with the intent of overcoming many of the challenges inherent in 2D monolayer culture, xenografts, and tumor explants. Since its invention in the early 1970s, the most commonly studied 3D cancer model has been the human tumor spheroid, defined as a small (<1 mm diameter), tightly bound spherical aggregate of cancer cells derived from a cancer cell line. Similar to the embryoid bodies often used in stem cell research, spheroids tend to form when transformed cells are maintained under nonadherent conditions. Most healthy adherent cell types will undergo a process called anoikis, or apoptosis triggered by lack of adherence to a surface, but cancer cells have developed mechanisms to resist this, and can therefore survive while suspended long term in cell culture media. The individual cells in suspension will then aggregate together and over time these loosely bound cell masses will develop into the more tightly bound spheroids. Because spheroids provide cancer cells with both a 3D architecture and extensive cell–cell contacts, they model the *in vivo* cellular environment much more effectively than 2D monolayers and exhibit many of the biological properties of solid tumors, including cell morphology,[22,23] growth kinetics,[22] gene expression,[22] and drug response.[23,24]

### 37.4.1.1 Spheroid Formation Techniques

Various methods can be used to induce spheroid formation. One method used by cancer biologists involves subjecting a cell suspension to constant mixing.[25,26] This is most commonly done using a spinner flask, where a small rotor continually stirs the solution. The resulting sheer stress at the walls of the flask prevents cells from attaching or settling to the bottom, ultimately resulting in spheroid formation.[25,26] The size and number of spheroids produced by this method is relatively consistent, and can be controlled by varying factors like cell density or stirring speed.[27,28] The spinner flask is not appropriate for all applications, however, because the high sheer stresses encountered by the cells can damage them.[27] The rotary wall vessel reactor uses a similar method to produce spheroids, but is gentler on the cells because of lower sheer stress. In that system, a cell suspension is placed between an outer cylinder that rotates and an inner one held stationary, resulting in constant liquid motion around the inner cylinder. This was originally developed as a method to mimic microgravity but can successfully produce spheroids as well. Despite its advantages, the rotary wall vessel reactor requires expensive and cumbersome specialized equipment that confine its general use.[27,28]

A simpler and more commonly used spheroid formation technique is liquid overlay, which involves plating a cell solution on a nonadherent surface. Because this method avoids shear stress problems and eliminates the need for specialized equipment, it is more accessible to the general oncological research community. Briefly, nonadherent tissue culture surfaces can be easily achieved by coating tissue culture plates with thin films of agar.[29] The agar prevents cells from adhering to the plate surface which leads to cell aggregation and eventual spheroid formation. Though other types of nonadherent coatings are available, agar remains popular because it is easy to use and inexpensive. Commercially available nonbinding and low adhesion tissue culture plates are becoming widespread and produce similar results when used for spheroid culture. A disadvantage of the liquid overlay technique is that the resulting spheroids can be highly varied in size and number, a challenge to ensuring uniformity among experimental samples.[27] One way to avoid this problem is to produce individual spheroids within agar-coated 96 well plates; the concavity of the agar surface yields a single spheroid per well of consistent size and cell composition. Scaling up for high-throughput applications can be difficult using this method because each spheroid is produced one at a time, yet the simplicity inherent in the liquid overlay culture method has made it extremely popular with cancer researchers.[22–24,30]

Other techniques developed in recent years have sought to improve the consistency of spheroids even further though none of these have obtained mainstream popularity. One method, that grows spheroids within hanging drops of liquid, has been very successful in the creation of single spheroids of consistent size and cell number.[27,31] As with other methods, this process is also difficult to scale up. Additionally, extra handling steps are required because cells can only be maintained in hanging drops for short time periods.[28] Other groups have created microfluidic chips where very small spheroids of defined geometry are formed within prefabricate microwells. This technique, along with various others, has only seen limited use due to the precise equipment requirements.[32]

### 37.4.1.2 Spheroids as a Model of Tumor Microregions and Micrometastases

As with other 3D tissue models, diffusional gradients are present within the structure of tumor spheroids. But unlike models of healthy tissues, these gradients can often be beneficial in mimicking certain aspects of tumor biology. One of the hallmarks of cancer is the ability of a growing tumor to recruit a vasculature. However, this vasculature is not present during the early stages of formation of a nascent tumor or micrometastasis, and angiogenesis is only triggered when the tumor reaches a large enough size where hypoxia and lack of nutrients become detrimental to cells. Additionally, the angiogenesis that occurs during tumor formation is not the same carefully orchestrated process involved in the growth and healing of healthy tissues. Instead, the vasculature that forms within a tumor is often highly irregular. This results in an uneven blood supply throughout the tumor, and microregions often exist where the blood supply is not adequate to meet the cells' metabolic needs. Tumors therefore become heterogeneous tissues with marked variations in cell metabolic activity and even the presence of secondary necroses where the blood supply becomes too low. Because of this heterogeneity, many researchers consider tumor spheroids to be a good model of *in vivo* cancer biology because its 3D structure results in a similar metabolic distribution. In order for cells on the interior of a spheroid to remain viable, oxygen and nutrients must diffuse in while waste products diffuse out. The result is a stratified structure where cell viability decreases as distance from the spheroid surface increases.[27,28] The outer rim of the spheroid is made up of rapidly proliferating cells where nutrients and oxygen are quickly supplied and waste products are just as quickly removed. The inner cell layers, conversely, are relatively quiescent and under higher metabolic stress due to hypoxia and accumulation of waste by-products. Since the limit of diffusion of small molecules like oxygen through the cell mass is only about 150–200 μm, spheroids with a diameter over about 500 μm will also contain a necrotic core.[27,28] A spheroid system, therefore, effectively mimics the variation in physiological stress and oxygenation experienced by cells within nascent tumors, micrometastases, and avascular tumor microregions, which makes them a good model of the growth kinetics and heterogeneity found in some areas of solid tumors.[28,33]

## 37.4.2 Bioengineered Tumors

Although they more effectively mimic the native state inherent in the host, tumor spheroids still suffer from several of the limitations present within 2D monolayer culture. They are devoid of their extracellular surroundings and lack environmental cues provided by an ECM, other cell types (such as fibroblasts, endothelial cells, etc.), and 3D scaffolding that would exist *in vivo*. In an attempt to overcome those limitations, the nascent scientific discipline of tumor bioengineering has emerged largely through cross-disciplinary collaboration between tissue engineers and cancer biologists who recognize the complementary strengths each discipline brings to the other.

As with any emerging scientific discipline, it remains difficult to precisely define the scope of research implied under the rubric of bioengineered tumors. Some prominent scientists have reasonably defined tumor engineering as "the construction of complex culture models that recapitulate aspects of the *in vivo* tumor microenvironment to study the dynamics of tumor development, progression, and therapy on multiple scales."[34] While that definition is certainly true, and accurately describes the end goal, it is a little ambiguous with respect to the requirement for "complexity," as nonbioengineered tumor models may be equally complex. We propose a slightly different definition and suggest that bioengineered tumors require three fundamental traits:

1. Formation of 3D cellular structures that are more complex than would naturally occur in the absence of tissue-engineered conditions (i.e., beyond 2D culture and self-forming spheroids)
2. Reliance upon tissue engineering processes that enables the interaction between the cancer cells to be measured and precisely controlled
3. Recreation of aspects of tumor behavior (e.g., tumor growth kinetics, invasion, metastasis, angiogenesis, and drug sensitivity) that occurs *in vivo* with high fidelity

All three traits are required, as the presence of just one or two traits can be found within traditional cancer models. For example, tumor spheroids have higher 3D order and better mimic the *in vivo* tumor phenotype but form through innate biological programming independent of tissue engineering processes. Since 3D spheroids form spontaneously without the aid of external tissue engineering control, they obviously cannot be said to be "bioengineered." Equally true, exotic tissue-engineered surfaces exist for 2D cell culture but lack any higher 3D cell architecture; in such cases, despite a clear reliance upon tissue engineering, the criteria are unmet because monolayer cultures lack tumor-like properties.[35]

Within the definition proposed above, a number of enabling technologies formerly used in tissue engineering applications are being adapted for use in bioengineered tumors. Several key applications will be discussed herein after briefly describing the core technologies used within those applications.

## 37.5 Tools for Creation of a Bioengineered Tumor Model

### 37.5.1 ECM Gels

ECM gel culture is a widely used technique in the cancer biology field that has been used to study the effect of 3D growth on cancer cell behavior. In this scenario, tumor cells are suspended in a gel-like matrix. Over time, the individual cells will migrate toward one another and form spheroid-like structures within the gel. These spheroids are similar to traditional spheroids; however, they experience both cell–cell and cell–matrix interactions, which in many cases is a better mimic of their natural *in vivo* microenvironment.

Various materials have been used as a basis for gel culture, including collagen and alginate; however, recent research commonly employs Matrigel or similar crude ECM extracts. Matrigel is a biologically complex undefined mixture of ECM molecules and growth factors derived from the ESH mouse sarcoma cell line, which has proven to be a good platform for the growth of both cancerous and healthy cell types because of its diverse signaling and attachment capabilities. Numerous methods can be used for Matrigel embedding, including suspending cells within the matrix itself, as well as floating cells on top of a preformed matrix gel.

Gel embedding offers a variety of advantages over traditional spheroid culture. For one, the signaling environment offered by the Matrigel is much more similar to the complex signaling milieu encountered by tumor cells *in vivo*. Although more invasive cancers usually form disorganized cell masses within the gel, less invasive cancers (typically lower-grade ones which still resemble their cell type of origin) usually form complex structures reminiscent of the *in vivo* host tumor. For example, when breast carcinoma cells are placed within ECM gel culture, less invasive tumor types form ductal structures similar to those seen in native breast tissue. This demonstrates that signaling molecules and 3D structural environments act to encourage the cells to organize into their native structure; it also gives a system whereby the invasiveness of a given cancer cell line can be evaluated and compared to other cell lines. Additionally, for many tissue types, it offers the chance to compare the growth of cancerous cells to their cell type of origin.

Most adherent cell types will undergo anoikis, or apoptosis due to lack of adhesion, when placed in a nonadherent environment required for traditional spheroid formation. Gel embedding, however, offers adhesion sights to these healthy cells within the matrix. Like their cancerous counterparts, they will subsequently migrate together and often form tissue-like structures within the gel. Mina Bissel's laboratory at U.C. Berkley, which has pioneered much of the work in Matrigel embedding, has used these advantages to study various breast carcinoma cell lines and to compare them to native breast tissue.[36–38]

One disadvantage of using naturally derived sources, such as Matrigel, is the ill-defined and irreproducible nature of the mixture. Because the composition of Matrigel and other EHS-derived ECM gels is unknown, it can be hard to ensure that the signaling environment is a good mimic of the particular tumor type under study. In recent years, ECM extracts from a variety of specific tissue types have become available, so it is now possible to study select cancer types within their native ECM. To date, this has yet to be used extensively for 3D cancer cell culture. Some research is underway to develop artificial ECM gels that have a well-defined and tailored molecular makeup, and this may offer a viable alternative for 3D models when studying the particular effects of various biological molecules or inhibitors.

## 37.5.2 Polymer Scaffolds

As the tissue engineering field has made greater contributions toward the development of 3D cancer models, researchers have begun to use many of the polymer matrices developed for tissue culture as an alternative method to provide cancer cells with a 3D architecture. These polymer scaffolds offer the advantage of superior mechanical properties and more tunable characteristics such as porosity, degradation properties, mechanical strength, and surface functionality.

The majority of published work relating to bioengineered tumor models has focused on the interaction between cancer cells and polymer scaffolds. Polymers that have been investigated include porous chitosan,[39,40] surface-modified poly(lactic acid) and poly(lactic-*co*-glycolic acid) (PLGA) microparticles,[41,42] porous PLGA discs,[43] and alginate-l-lysine-alginate hydrogels.[44] Cancer cell lines were found to attach and proliferate on these materials and to form 3D structures that were histologically and morphologically similar to *in vivo* tumors. These models have been evaluated preliminarily as a platform to study cancer drug response and the creation of angiogenic factors under hypoxic conditions, and results suggest significant changes in comparison to 2D controls and greater similarity to the *in vivo* phenotype.

The polymer scaffold that is used in the creation of a bioengineered tumor serves many of the same roles as in traditional tissue engineering pursuits. First, it should provide a basic architecture for 3D cell growth and attachment. A 3D architecture, including both cell–cell and cell–matrix attachments, plays an important role in dictating cell behavior, including cell migration, proliferation rates, response to signaling molecules, and resistance to apoptosis. Second, researchers can use the polymer matrix as a means to mimic the mechanical strength and signaling capabilities provided by the ECM molecules *in vivo*. Signaling provided by ECM molecules has been investigated extensively in cancer biology and has been shown to modify both cancer cell signaling and drug response. Signaling through the β1-integrin has been particularly well known for the effect it has on the phenotype of a wide variety of cancers. Although not as extensively studied, substrate stiffness has also been shown to exert an effect on cancer cell growth, especially as it pertains to cancer cell migration rates. A polymer matrix with mechanical properties tuned to match the *in vivo* tumor tissue and modified to mimic natural ECM signaling is therefore preferred when creating a bioengineered tumor model. Finally, a polymer scaffold must be biocompatible and maintain adequate porosity to allow for cancer cell migration and oxygen and nutrient transfer within the construct without sacrificing mechanical integrity. Some factors with less relevance when used to model cancer include scaffold immunogenicity and degradation rate, since patient implantation will not occur.

Although only a small number of materials have been investigated thus far in tumor models, many others could be adapted for that purpose or, at the very least, serve as an ideal starting place. As mentioned in the introduction, malignant cells rely upon their surrounding tissue environment or "soil" for growth signals and often metastasize to specific locations conducive to tumor survival and growth. Therefore, to the extent bioengineered tissues replicate those environments, they may serve as an easily controlled model of tumor invasion and metastasis. As the science of bioengineered tumors evolves in parallel with the field of tissue engineering, new polymer scaffold materials used for tissue regeneration may be adapted to the specific needs of cancer-type-specific tumor models.

### 37.5.3 Signaling Molecules

In common with tissue regeneration/engineering, wound healing, and tumor growth, is the reliance upon various signaling molecules (proteins, peptides, or glycoprotein-related growth factors and cytokines) for a host of cellular effects, including chemotaxis, mitogenesis, morphogenesis, metabolism, and apoptosis.[45] As occurs physiologically, those effects are impacted by systemic exposures of hormones and circulating growth factors (growth hormone, insulin, insulin-like growth factor, etc.) as well as by localized, autocrine- and paracrine-induced, time and spatially dependent concentrations unique to a particular microenvironment. Malignant cells, to a certain extent, rely upon the same signaling cascades as do healing wounds and regenerating tissues but, as discussed previously, often acquire independence from specific growth factors through amplification or activating mutations of their cognate growth factor receptors, which clearly obviates the need for receptor–ligand binding for downstream pathway activation. In addition to heterotypic signaling (i.e., signaling by one cell type to affect another), cancer cells may acquire the capacity to manufacture growth factors directly and, thereby induce an autocrine positive feedback loop that reinforces tumor growth and invasion.[46–48] A number of excellent reviews exist which thoroughly describe this phenomenon.

As discussed previously, ECM gels like Matrigel may serve as a biologically derived, albeit poorly defined, source for many of the growth factors needed for the purposes of tissue engineering or bioengineered tumors. Such gel-based systems, while adequate for providing uniform growth factor concentrations and even some temporal control over release parameters, are not as ideally suited for mimicking the local tumor microenvironment as are tunable, biocompatible polymer scaffolds. A number of modern approaches have sought to better orchestrate spatially dependent signaling by integrating signaling molecules within polymer scaffolds through covalent immobilization (using chemical crosslinking) or noncovalent methods such as growth factor-encapsulated, crosslinked microspheres[49] or nanoparticles.[50] Other methods of growth factor delivery include localized bolus injection,[51] release from coated scaffolds,[52,53] and release from within biodegradable polymer scaffolds.[54–57]

Using "wound healing" as the paradigm for future development, a number of tissue-engineered models have naturally sought to replicate the temporal release of sequential growth factors. By extension to tumor bioengineering, cancer biologists may adapt such models as new tools in their arsenal to interrogate the tumor–ECM microenvironment. As this occurs, one would anticipate that biologically targeted therapies will evolve beyond antiangiogenic therapy to include ones aimed at disrupting the ECM–tumor interrelationship as well.

### 37.5.4 Cocultures

Just as in healthy tissues, tumors do not exist is isolation but are composed of an amalgamation of diverse cell types, including nonmalignant ones. In fact, cancer-associated fibroblasts (CAF), lymphocytes, endothelial cells, and macrophages together can routinely account for up to 90% of the tumor volume; presumably stimulated by the cancer-associated inflammatory state and a vigorous but ineffective immune response.

CAFs, the most prominent nonmalignant intratumoral cell type (especially within breast and pancreatic carcinomas),[1,58] play a critical tumorigenic role by contributing superfluous signaling molecules, including hepatocyte growth factor (HGF), fibroblast growth factor (FGF), interleukin-6 (IL-6), and others.[59] In certain epithelial cancer types, they have been shown to produce insulin-like growth factor

1 (IGF-1), a potent stimulant of mitogenesis and tumorigenesis.[60,61] CAFs may work in concert with endothelial cells by promoting angiogenic factors such as vascular endothelial growth factor (VEGF), platelet-derived growth factor (PDGF), and SDF-1α.[62,63] Even tissue invasion and metastasis can be encouraged by CAFs by contributing to the transforming growth factor-β (TGF-β)-mediated epithelial-to-mesenchymal transition, a process characterized by reduced cell adhesion, repressed expression of E-cadherin, and enhanced cell motility.[64,65] Finally, proinvasion proteases such as matrix metalloproteases and plasminogen activators can be supplemented by CAFs to directly aid tumor invasion.[66]

Other cell types with that have a multifaceted role in the tumor–host relationship include endothelial cells, tumor-infiltrating lymphocytes (TIL), pericytes, and others. Endothelial cells are required in order to produce enough vascularity within the tumor necessary to reach a significant size. Paradoxically, immune cells can simultaneously serve both to reinforce and suppress tumor growth and maintenance; some immune cells are responsible for detecting and eliminating irregular cells, such as those that have undergone a malignant transformation whereas others can be signaled to produce inflammatory molecules that can both aid in vascularization as well as increasing the rate of genetic changes that occur within the cells, thus aiding in tumor progression. The role that macrophages play in tumor progression has been studied extensively, and in some cases, they appear to be required in order for tumor progression to occur.

On account of the importance of stromal cells, some researchers have investigated 3D cocultures that combine cancer cells with one or more other cell types within their environment. These have taken many forms but the majority is spheroid cocultures (i.e., a cancer spheroid combined with a fibroblast spheroid or a cancer spheroid combined with a monolayer or suspension of stromal cells). As an example of one such approach, prostate cancer spheroids have been combined with osteoblasts to aid in understanding the effect of the bone microenvironment on prostate cancer metastases.

Although stromal cells play a vital role in dictating cancer cell behavior, incorporating them into a general tissue engineering strategy will be challenging. Culture conditions that can accommodate both cell types must be optimized, the scaffold/signaling environment must be compatible with both malignant and normal cell types, and the models systems must be able to account for differences in cell proliferation rates. With the complexity inherent in such a culture scheme, many tissue engineers simply try to mimic the signaling molecules expressed by stromal cells directly without attempting to achieve the real-world molecular cross-talk that occurs within patients' tissues and/or tumors.

## 37.5.5 Bioreactors

A fifth tool that may be invariably used in the development of a bioengineered tumor are bioreactors, which allow for careful monitoring of cell and tissue culture growth under highly controlled, reproducible, and sometimes automated conditions. Given the ability to precisely control pH, temperature, fluid pressure, shear stress, nutrient concentrations, waste removal, and diffusion of oxygen, it is not surprising that bioreactors have found a valuable functional niche both within industry and academia.[67] Depending upon the bioreactor type, some offer unique advantages over another. For example, the spinner-flask bioreactors may improve surface deposition of cells onto 3D scaffolds; rotating-wall vessel (RWV) bioreactors can mimic conditions of microgravity; and specialized reactors can provide mechanical stress under physiological conditions that mimic tissues exposed to repetitive weight bearing (e.g., cartilage and bones). Furthermore, unlike static culture methods, direct perfusion bioreactors (whereby culture medium flows steadily through porous scaffolds) excel in achieving both uniform cell seeding throughout the interior and exterior 3D compartments and homogeneous nutrient- and oxygen-gradients free of hypoxic and/or nutrient deficient regions typical of spheroids.

As experts in tissue engineering are aware for the reasons mentioned above, bioreactors are especially adept at producing 3D tissues that more closely resemble their normal or cancerous tissue counterparts. Specifically with respect to cancer, RWV bioreactors using prostate[68] or melanoma[69] cell lines can elicit 3D structures bearing close resemblance to *in vivo* tumor morphology. That bioreactors promise to maintain certain cancer types in their native, differentiated state is perhaps the most important and potentially useful rationale for their use as preclinical models as opposed to comparatively inferior approaches such as monolayer, spheroid, or static 3D culture. This supposition stems from the fact that many of the recently FDA-approved anticancer therapeutics are aimed at specific molecular targets and/or pathways known to vary considerably depending upon the differentiation state; by extension, if the bioreactor-enabled preclinical 3D models are nearly equivalent to human tumors with respect to differentiation, then preclinical models should serve as better predictors of subsequent clinical efficacy.

## 37.6 Applications of Advanced 3D Cancer Models

### 37.6.1 Improve Evaluation of New Cancer Drugs

Though pharmacokinetic evaluation of drug absorption, metabolism, excretion, and toxicity in animals remains a mandatory step that precedes introduction into human clinical trials, a peristent Achilles' heel of animal and *in vitro* cancer models alike has been the general lack of predictive value with respect to drug efficacy.[8,9,18,70–72] For lack of a better strategy, those traditional preclinical models have remained the most popular. Yet, mirroring a trend toward multidisciplinary "team" science, it has become increasingly common for cancer biologists and tissue engineers to work collaboratively, blending valuable aspects of 3D tissue engineering into well-established *in vitro* cancer models. By doing so, there has been some early success in achieving several principle goals of *ex vivo* cancer models: (1) better prediction in advance of human trials, which drugs will succeed in combating cancer, (2) help define the mechanism(s) by which drug resistance develops, and (3) investigate the impact the tumor–ECM interaction has upon drug sensitivity, cell differentiation, invasion, and metastasis.

As described earlier in this chapter, monolayer cultures have been woefully inadequate in meeting those goals. By mimicking some of the features of *in vivo* tumors (e.g., regions of local hypoxia or nutrient deprivation, slower cell proliferation, reliance upon spatial cues, and cell–cell interaction) tumor spheroids have had more success and paved the way for more advanced drug testing models.

Just as most *in vivo* tumors are considerably more chemoresistant than *in vitro* models of the same cancer type, so too are most cancer spheroids for several reasons.[27,30] First, most drugs are limited by their diffusion when they are placed in static culture with a 3D tumor construct. Therefore, drugs in the interior of the construct are exposed to a lower drug concentration than drugs on the periphery, which can contribute to lower cell death. This has actually been exploited in several studies that examined large molecule and antibody therapies in order to understand how well they can diffuse into a tissue. Second, cell–cell attachments provided by the 3D structure and E-cadherin-mediated pathways can help to protect the cell against cell death and to avoid anoikis. Third, cell matrix attachments and the resulting 3D cell morphology can also play a role in altering the cell's phenotype and protect it from drug-induced apoptosis. Finally, cells within a 3D structure will often proliferate at a much lower rate than cells grown in monolayers. Because most cytotoxic drugs target the cell cycle, a lower proliferative rate results in lower overall cell death. A thorough description of the malignant cell lines tested in spheroid culture and a detailed assessment of the challenges associated in moving from monolayer to spheroid culture for purposes of drug testing are reviewed elsewhere.[28]

Cell aggregates embedded within natural or synthetic ECM have proven particularly useful for teasing apart the impact cell–ECM interactions have upon differentiation and invasion.[73] One prominent example developed by Bissell and colleagues found that breast cells embedded within a laminin-rich ECM formed either organized polarized acinus-like structures or bizarre highly proliferative colonies when normal or malignant cells were, respectively, used as the source.[74] Since the effects of biologically targeted drugs are highly dependent upon their respective gene or protein targets, maintaining the differentiation status and expression profile of tumor models in a pattern closer to their *in vivo* counterpart would be expected to more accurately assess a drug candidate's clinical potential. This was conclusively demonstrated by Fischbach et al. using a 3D model of human oral squamous carcinoma cells that were maintained on poly(lactide-*co*-glycolide) scaffolds; in that system, the oral cancer cells grown in 2D were sensitive to LY294002, a PI3-kinase inhibitor, whereas the same cells grown in 3D were resistant.[43,75]

## 37.6.2 Study the Impact of a 3D Microenvironment upon Angiogenesis

In recognition that tumors must fully rely upon angiogenesis to grow beyond a microscopic size, anti-angiogenic small molecules and antibodies targeting VEGF and other endothelial growth factors have received intense scrutiny as a promising cancer therapy.[76,77] Though such therapies have proven moderately successful, there remains considerable room for improvement and much remains to be learned to optimize antiangiogenic treatment. As nicely reviewed by Verbridge et al., bioengineered tumor models overcome many of the potential limitations of *in vitro*- and animal-based models of angiogenesis and are particularly useful for studying the impact that the cell–cell, cell–ECM, and 3D architecture have upon the angiogenic process.[78]

To examine spatiotemporal control of angiogenesis, lithographic techniques have been used to build 3D microfluidic structures within a calcium alginate hydrogel seeded with cells.[79] The effect of cell–cell interaction upon blood vessel formation has been modeled by micropatterning techniques[80,81] and the role of the ECM matrix has been extensively studied using a number of natural and synthetic biodegradable scaffolds that allow time-variable release of growth factors.[82,83] Some, designed with covalently linked VEGF within the synthetic matrix, have even been used to assess the effect of cell-mediated growth factor release that occurs as endothelial cells invade and locally remodel the ECM.[84] Though less often considered, mechanical forces that increase cytoskeletal tension may favor capillary network formation by human endothelial cells.[85] Advanced 3D models using photo-cross-linked RGD-modified polyacrylamide[86] or ionic-cross-linked alginate hydrogels[87] can provide a novel means to alter the surrounding elasticity in ways not previously possible with traditional 2D monolayer culture.[88] Altered pH and temperature may also be used to change ECM stiffness but those parameters must of course remain within physiological ranges safe for cell survival.

## 37.6.3 Create More Advanced Animal Models

The most widely used animal model for studying cancer remains the subcutaneous human tumor xenograft and although this model has provided scientists with an incredible wealth of preclinical data, the foreign location of tumor growth also confounds the conclusions that can be drawn. Orthotopic models overcome this shortcoming by placing a given tumor within its tissue type of origin in the mouse but have their own challenges, as they are more technically demanding and have not been developed for all tissue types.

Given the clinical raison d'être for tissue engineering and regenerative medicine, and vast experience using implanted noncancerous tissues for that purpose, it should be no surprise that *ex vivo* tissue-engineered tumor models meant for xenograft use are better tumor biomimetics than human subcutaneous or orthotopic models. Cancer cells that are first grown on 3D structures prior to later *in vivo* implantation often maintain a more differentiated state; plus, the biodegradable polymer matrix offers a more reliable delivery vehicle for tumor cells than just media alone. Furthermore, the field of tissue engineering has also devoted considerable attention to resolving the issues of perfusion and hypoxia in an effort to avoid the substantial cell death that often occurs within days of *in vivo* tissue implantation.

In the oral squamous cell model described earlier, larger tumor sizes were observed when cells were grown initially in 3D culture, as opposed to 2D, prior to *in vivo* implantation.[43] Tissue-engineered human tumors could also theoretically be used to study cancers that metastasize to bone, such as prostate, colon, or breast cancer among others. As an example, in the first model, to integrate engineered bone into a murine model for the purpose of studying breast cancer metastasis, Rosenblatt et al. used silk scaffolds coated with bone morphogenetic protein-2 (BMP-2) and seeded with bone marrow stromal cells as an implanted surrogate of human bone.[89,90] As the fields of tissue engineering and cancer biology forge an even stronger alliance, tissue-engineered scaffolds and ECMs are likely to find widespread utility for improved *in vivo* models.

## 37.7 Conclusions

Given the substantial scientific overlap that exists between the scientific disciplines of tissue engineering and cancer biology, and exponential progress that both fields have made in the high-throughput postgenomic era, the stage has been set for potential convergence of the fields. That has, of course, already occurred before for other engineering disciplines, as concepts from electrical engineering have been applied to cancer biology in describing the aberrant cancer signaling cascades as dysfunctional "circuits" amenable to measurement and control. Similarly, the field of systems biology is rooted, in part, on concepts relating to control process engineering (i.e., stability, fragility, and feedback loops that can either blunt or magnify the input signals of mechanical systems), which from a biological perspective can be useful in deciphering how normal and malignant cells maintain homeostasis and evade apoptosis. Improved control and measurement of the cell–cell and cell–ECM relationship, a distinct advantage inherent in tissue engineering, will almost certainly enable the creation of better cancer models, which should serve to more reliably assess preclinical drug effectiveness, enable a better understanding of cancer biology, and allow a better glimpse of the role ECM plays in tumorigenesis.

## References

1. Kalluri R, Zeisberg M. Fibroblasts in cancer. *Nat Rev Cancer* 2006; 6:392–401.
2. Hanahan D, Weinberg RA. The hallmarks of cancer. *Cell* 2000; 100:57–70.
3. Dvorak HF. Tumors: Wounds that do not heal. Similarities between tumor stroma generation and wound healing. *N Engl J Med* 1986; 315:1650–9.
4. Shoemaker RH. The NCI60 human tumour cell line anticancer drug screen. *Nat Rev Cancer* 2006; 6:813–23.
5. Holbeck SL. Update on NCI *in vitro* drug screen utilities. *Eur J Cancer* 2004; 40:785–93.
6. Monga M, Sausville EA. Developmental therapeutics program at the NCI: Molecular target and drug discovery process. *Leukemia* 2002; 16:520–6.
7. Ertel A, Verghese A, Byers SW, Ochs M, Tozeren A. Pathway-specific differences between tumor cell lines and normal and tumor tissue cells. *Mol Cancer* 2006; 5:55.
8. Johnson JI, Decker S, Zaharevitz D et al. Relationships between drug activity in NCI preclinical *in vitro* and *in vivo* models and early clinical trials. *Br J Cancer* 2001; 84:1424–31.
9. Voskoglou-Nomikos T, Pater JL, Seymour L. Clinical predictive value of the *in vitro* cell line, human xenograft, and mouse allograft preclinical cancer models. *Clin Cancer Res* 2003; 9:4227–39.
10. Mueller MM, Fusenig NE. Friends or foes—Bipolar effects of the tumour stroma in cancer. *Nat Rev Cancer* 2004; 4:839–49.
11. Bissell MJ, Radisky D. Putting tumours in context. *Nat Rev Cancer* 2001; 1:46–54.
12. Jacks T, Weinberg RA. Taking the study of cancer cell survival to a new dimension. *Cell* 2002; 111:923–5.
13. Wernert N. The multiple roles of tumour stroma. *Virchows Arch* 1997; 430:433–43.
14. Liotta LA, Kohn EC. The microenvironment of the tumour-host interface. *Nature* 2001; 411:375–9.
15. Zahir N, Weaver VM. Death in the third dimension: Apoptosis regulation and tissue architecture. *Curr Opin Genet Dev* 2004; 14:71–80.
16. Kung AL. Practices and pitfalls of mouse cancer models in drug discovery. *Adv Cancer Res* 2007; 96:191–212.
17. Teicher BA. Tumor models for efficacy determination. *Mol Cancer Ther* 2006; 5:2435–43.
18. Kelland LR. Of mice and men: Values and liabilities of the athymic nude mouse model in anticancer drug development. *Eur J Cancer* 2004; 40:827–36.

19. Killion JJ, Radinsky R, Fidler IJ. Orthotopic models are necessary to predict therapy of transplantable tumors in mice. *Cancer Metastasis Rev* 1998; 17:279–84.

20. Sharpless NE, Depinho RA. The mighty mouse: Genetically engineered mouse models in cancer drug development. *Nat Rev Drug Discov* 2006; 5:741–54.

21. Talmadge JE, Lenz BF, Klabansky R et al. Therapy of autochthonous skin cancers in mice with intravenously injected liposomes containing muramyltripeptide. *Cancer Res* 1986; 46:1160–3.

22. Lawlor ER, Scheel C, Irving J, Sorensen PH. Anchorage-independent multi-cellular spheroids as an *in vitro* model of growth signaling in Ewing tumors. *Oncogene* 2002; 21:307–18.

23. Myatt SS, Redfern CP, Burchill SA. p38MAPK-Dependent sensitivity of Ewing's sarcoma family of tumors to fenretinide-induced cell death. *Clin Cancer Res* 2005; 11:3136–48.

24. Kang HG, Jenabi JM, Zhang J et al. E-cadherin cell-cell adhesion in ewing tumor cells mediates suppression of anoikis through activation of the ErbB4 tyrosine kinase. *Cancer Res* 2007; 67:3094–105.

25. Sutherland RM, Inch WR, McCredie JA, Kruuv J. A multi-component radiation survival curve using an *in vitro* tumour model. *Int J Radiat Biol Relat Stud Phys Chem Med* 1970; 18:491–5.

26. Durand RE, Sutherland RM. Effects of intercellular contact on repair of radiation damage. *Exp Cell Res* 1972; 71:75–80.

27. Lin RZ, Chang HY. Recent advances in three-dimensional multicellular spheroid culture for biomedical research. *Biotechnol J* 2008; 3:1172–84.

28. Friedrich J, Ebner R, Kunz-Schughart LA. Experimental anti-tumor therapy in 3-D: Spheroids— old hat or new challenge? *Int J Radiat Biol* 2007; 83:849–71.

29. Yuhas JM, Li AP, Martinez AO, Ladman AJ. A simplified method for production and growth of multicellular tumor spheroids. *Cancer Res* 1977; 37:3639–43.

30. Friedrich J, Seidel C, Ebner R, Kunz-Schughart LA. Spheroid-based drug screen: Considerations and practical approach. *Nat Protoc* 2009; 4:309–24.

31. Timmins NE, Nielsen LK. Generation of multicellular tumor spheroids by the hanging-drop method. *Methods Mol Med* 2007; 140:141–51.

32. Wu LY, Di Carlo D, Lee LP. Microfluidic self-assembly of tumor spheroids for anticancer drug discovery. *Biomed Microdevices* 2008; 10:197–202.

33. Kunz-Schughart LA. Multicellular tumor spheroids: Intermediates between monolayer culture and *in vivo* tumor. *Cell Biol Int* 1999; 23:157–61.

34. Ghajar CM, Bissell MJ. Tumor engineering: The other face of tissue engineering. *Tissue Eng Part A*; 16:2153–6.

35. Burdett E, Kasper FK, Mikos AG, Ludwig JA. Engineering tumors: A tissue engineering perspective in cancer biology. *Tissue Eng Part B Rev* 2010; 16:351–9.

36. Lee GY, Kenny PA, Lee EH, Bissell MJ. Three-dimensional culture models of normal and malignant breast epithelial cells. *Nat Methods* 2007; 4:359–65.

37. Petersen OW, Ronnov-Jessen L, Howlett AR, Bissell MJ. Interaction with basement membrane serves to rapidly distinguish growth and differentiation pattern of normal and malignant human breast epithelial cells. *Proc Natl Acad Sci USA* 1992; 89:9064–8.

38. Wang F, Weaver VM, Petersen OW et al. Reciprocal interactions between beta1-integrin and epidermal growth factor receptor in three-dimensional basement membrane breast cultures: A different perspective in epithelial biology. *Proc Natl Acad Sci USA* 1998; 95:14821–6.

39. Dhiman HK, Ray AR, Panda AK. Characterization and evaluation of chitosan matrix for *in vitro* growth of MCF-7 breast cancer cell lines. *Biomaterials* 2004; 25:5147–54.

40. Dhiman HK, Ray AR, Panda AK. Three-dimensional chitosan scaffold-based MCF-7 cell culture for the determination of the cytotoxicity of tamoxifen. *Biomaterials* 2005; 26:979–86.

41. Sahoo SK, Panda AK, Labhasetwar V. Characterization of porous PLGA/PLA microparticles as a scaffold for three dimensional growth of breast cancer cells. *Biomacromolecules* 2005; 6:1132–9.

42. Horning JL, Sahoo SK, Vijayaraghavalu S et al. 3-D tumor model for *in vitro* evaluation of anticancer drugs. *Mol Pharm* 2008; 5:849–62.

43. Fischbach C, Chen R, Matsumoto T et al. Engineering tumors with 3D scaffolds. *Nat Methods* 2007; 4:855–60.

44. Coutu DL, Yousefi AM, Galipeau J. Three-dimensional porous scaffolds at the crossroads of tissue engineering and cell-based gene therapy. *J Cell Biochem* 2009; 108:537–46.

45. Chen FM, Zhang M, Wu ZF. Toward delivery of multiple growth factors in tissue engineering. *Biomaterials*; 31:6279–308.

46. Marek L, Ware KE, Fritzsche A et al. Fibroblast growth factor (FGF) and FGF receptor-mediated autocrine signaling in non-small-cell lung cancer cells. *Mol Pharmacol* 2009; 75:196–207.

47. Park M, Park H, Kim WH, Cho H, Lee JH. Presence of autocrine hepatocyte growth factor-Met signaling and its role in proliferation and migration of SNU-484 gastric cancer cell line. *Exp Mol Med* 2005; 37:213–9.

48. Sawhney RS, Cookson MM, Sharma B, Hauser J, Brattain MG. Autocrine transforming growth factor alpha regulates cell adhesion by multiple signaling via specific phosphorylation sites of p70S6 kinase in colon cancer cells. *J Biol Chem* 2004; 279:47379–90.

49. Chen F, Wu Z, Wang Q et al. Preparation and biological characteristics of recombinant human bone morphogenetic protein-2-loaded dextran-co-gelatin hydrogel microspheres, *in vitro* and *in vivo* studies. *Pharmacology* 2005; 75:133–44.

50. Chen FM, Ma ZW, Dong GY, Wu ZF. Composite glycidyl methacrylated dextran (Dex-GMA)/gelatin nanoparticles for localized protein delivery. Acta *Pharmacol Sin* 2009; 30:485–93.

51. Kawaguchi H, Nakamura K, Tabata Y et al. Acceleration of fracture healing in nonhuman primates by fibroblast growth factor-2. *J Clin Endocrinol Metab* 2001; 86:875–80.

52. Lind M, Overgaard S, Nguyen T, Ongpipattanakul B, Bunger C, Soballe K. Transforming growth factor-beta stimulates bone ongrowth. Hydroxyapatite-coated implants studied in dogs. *Acta Orthop Scand* 1996; 67:611–6.

53. Liu Y, Huse RO, de Groot K, Buser D, Hunziker EB. Delivery mode and efficacy of BMP-2 in association with implants. *J Dent Res* 2007; 86:84–9.

54. Uebersax L, Merkle HP, Meinel L. Biopolymer-based growth factor delivery for tissue repair: From natural concepts to engineered systems. *Tissue Eng Part B Rev* 2009; 15:263–89.

55. Sohier J, Vlugt TJ, Cabrol N, Van Blitterswijk C, de Groot K, Bezemer JM. Dual release of proteins from porous polymeric scaffolds. *J Control Release* 2006; 111:95–106.

56. Ginty PJ, Barry JJ, White LJ, Howdle SM, Shakesheff KM. Controlling protein release from scaffolds using polymer blends and composites. *Eur J Pharm Biopharm* 2008; 68:82–9.

57. Woo BH, Fink BF, Page R et al. Enhancement of bone growth by sustained delivery of recombinant human bone morphogenetic protein-2 in a polymeric matrix. *Pharm Res* 2001; 18:1747–53.

58. Ostman A, Augsten M. Cancer-associated fibroblasts and tumor growth— bystanders turning into key players. *Curr Opin Genet Dev* 2009; 19:67–73.

59. Pietras K, Ostman A. Hallmarks of cancer: Interactions with the tumor stroma. *Exp Cell Res* 2010; 316:1324–31.

60. Strnad H, Lacina L, Kolar M et al. Head and neck squamous cancer stromal fibroblasts produce growth factors influencing phenotype of normal human keratinocytes. *Histochem Cell Biol*; 133:201–11.

61. LeBedis C, Chen K, Fallavollita L, Boutros T, Brodt P. Peripheral lymph node stromal cells can promote growth and tumorigenicity of breast carcinoma cells through the release of IGF-I and EGF. *Int J Cancer* 2002; 100:2–8.

62. Orimo A, Weinberg RA. Stromal fibroblasts in cancer: A novel tumor-promoting cell type. *Cell Cycle* 2006; 5:1597–601.

63. Orimo A, Gupta PB, Sgroi DC et al. Stromal fibroblasts present in invasive human breast carcinomas promote tumor growth and angiogenesis through elevated SDF-1/CXCL12 secretion. *Cell* 2005; 121:335–48.

64. Bhowmick NA, Moses HL. Tumor-stroma interactions. *Curr Opin Genet Dev* 2005; 15:97–101.

65. Bhowmick NA, Neilson EG, Moses HL. Stromal fibroblasts in cancer initiation and progression. *Nature* 2004; 432:332–7.

66. Joyce JA, Pollard JW. Microenvironmental regulation of metastasis. *Nat Rev Cancer* 2009; 9:239–52.

67. Martin I, Wendt D, Heberer M. The role of bioreactors in tissue engineering. *Trends Biotechnol* 2004; 22:80–6.

68. Rhee HW, Zhau HE, Pathak S et al. Permanent phenotypic and genotypic changes of prostate cancer cells cultured in a three-dimensional rotating-wall vessel. *In Vitro Cell Dev Biol Anim* 2001; 37:127–40.

69. Licato LL, Prieto VG, Grimm EA. A novel preclinical model of human malignant melanoma utilizing bioreactor rotating-wall vessels. *In Vitro Cell Dev Biol Anim* 2001; 37:121–6.

70. Balis FM. Evolution of anticancer drug discovery and the role of cell-based screening. *J Natl Cancer Inst* 2002; 94:78–9.

71. Kerbel RS. Human tumor xenografts as predictive preclinical models for anticancer drug activity in humans: Better than commonly perceived-but they can be improved. *Cancer Biol Ther* 2003; 2:S134–9.

72. Sausville EA. Overview. Cancer drug discovery: Pathway promise or covalent certainty for drug effect— quo vadis? *Curr Opin Investig Drugs* 2000; 1:511–3.

73. Debnath J, Brugge JS. Modelling glandular epithelial cancers in three-dimensional cultures. *Nat Rev Cancer* 2005; 5:675–88.

74. Nelson CM, Bissell MJ. Modeling dynamic reciprocity: Engineering three-dimensional culture models of breast architecture, function, and neoplastic transformation. *Semin Cancer Biol* 2005; 15:342–52.

75. Fischbach C, Kong HJ, Hsiong SX, Evangelista MB, Yuen W, Mooney DJ. Cancer cell angiogenic capability is regulated by 3D culture and integrin engagement. *Proc Natl Acad Sci USA* 2009; 106:399–404.

76. Folkman J. Tumor angiogenesis: Therapeutic implications. *N Engl J Med* 1971; 285:1182–6.

77. Jain RK. Normalization of tumor vasculature: An emerging concept in antiangiogenic therapy. *Science* 2005; 307:58–62.

78. Verbridge SS, Chandler EM, Fischbach C. Tissue-engineered three-dimensional tumor models to study tumor angiogenesis. *Tissue Eng Part A*; 16:2147–52.

79. Choi NW, Cabodi M, Held B, Gleghorn JP, Bonassar LJ, Stroock AD. Microfluidic scaffolds for tissue engineering. *Nat Mater* 2007; 6:908–15.

80. Tan CP, Cipriany BR, Lin DM, Craighead HG. Nanoscale resolution, multicomponent biomolecular arrays generated by aligned printing with parylene peel-off. *Nano Lett* 2010; 10:719–25.

81. Tan CP, Seo BR, Brooks DJ, Chandler EM, Craighead HG, Fischbach C. Parylene peel-off arrays to probe the role of cell-cell interactions in tumour angiogenesis. *Integr Biol (Camb)* 2009; 1:587–94.

82. Hern DL, Hubbell JA. Incorporation of adhesion peptides into nonadhesive hydrogels useful for tissue resurfacing. *J Biomed Mater Res* 1998; 39:266–76.

83. Zisch AH, Lutolf MP, Hubbell JA. Biopolymeric delivery matrices for angiogenic growth factors. *Cardiovasc Pathol* 2003; 12:295–310.

84. Zisch AH, Lutolf MP, Ehrbar M et al. Cell-demanded release of VEGF from synthetic, biointeractive cell ingrowth matrices for vascularized tissue growth. *FASEB J* 2003; 17:2260–2.

85. Mammoto A, Connor KM, Mammoto T et al. A mechanosensitive transcriptional mechanism that controls angiogenesis. *Nature* 2009; 457:1103–8.

86. Ulrich TA, de Juan Pardo EM, Kumar S. The mechanical rigidity of the extracellular matrix regulates the structure, motility, and proliferation of glioma cells. *Cancer Res* 2009; 69:4167–74.

87. Genes NG, Rowley JA, Mooney DJ, Bonassar LJ. Effect of substrate mechanics on chondrocyte adhesion to modified alginate surfaces. *Arch Biochem Biophys* 2004; 422:161–7.

88. Mammoto T, Ingber DE. Mechanical control of tissue and organ development. *Development* 2010; 137:1407–20.

89. Moreau JE, Anderson K, Mauney JR, Nguyen T, Kaplan DL, Rosenblatt M. Tissue-engineered bone serves as a target for metastasis of human breast cancer in a mouse model. *Cancer Res* 2007; 67:10304–8.

90. Kuperwasser C, Dessain S, Bierbaum BE et al. A mouse model of human breast cancer metastasis to human bone. *Cancer Res* 2005; 65:6130–8.

# Index

## A

AAc, *see* Acrylic acid (AAc)
AAV, *see* Adeno-associated virus (AAV)
Abbreviations list, 7-2 to 7-3, **11**-13 to **11**-15
ABM, *see* Acellular bladder matrices (ABM)
ABS, *see* Acrylonitrile butadiene styrene (ABS)
Accordion-like honeycomb (ALH), **11**-13
Acellular bladder matrices (ABM), **34**-7
Acellular collagen-based kidney matrix, **34**-8
ACH, *see* Anisotropic capillary hydrogels (ACH)
ACI, *see* Autologous chondrocyte implantation (ACI)
Acidic fibroblast growth factors, **36**-6
ACL, *see* Anterior cruciate ligament (ACL)
ACP, *see* Amorphous calcium phosphate (ACP)
Acrylates, **20**-6
Acrylic acid (AAc), **12**-4
Acrylonitrile butadiene styrene (ABS), **31**-5
Activated leukocyte cell adhesion molecule
    (ALCAM), **10**-3
ADAS cells, *see* Adipose-derived adult stromal cells
    (ADAS cells)
ADCC, *see* Antibody-dependent cellular cytotoxicity
    (ADCC)
Adeno-associated virus (AAV), **18**-2, **18**-3
Adenoviruses, **18**-2 to **18**-3
AdhD, *see* Aldo–keto reductase activity (AdhD)
Adhesion factors, **17**-7
    in ECM, **17**-8
Adhesion peptides, **21**-4
Adiponectin, **7**-13
Adipose-derived adult stromal cells (ADAS cells),
    **28**-2, **30**-12, **30**-14
    limitation, **30**-16
    scaffold materials, **30**-16
Adipose derived stem cells (ADSC), **12**-9
Adipose stem cells (ASCs), **27**-8, **36**-6, **36**-11
Adipose tissue, **36**-6
Adipose tissue-derived MSCs (ATSCs), **27**-8
ADSC, *see* Adipose derived stem cells (ADSC)
Adult chondrocytes, **30**-17
Adult stem cells, **34**-4 to **34**-5
AFPS cells, *see* Amniotic-fluid and placental-derived
    stem cells (AFPS cells)

Agarose, **13**-5
Agarose gel electrophoresis, **13**-5; *see also* Gel
        electrophoresis
    agarose concentration, **13**-5
    applied voltage, **13**-5 to **13**-6
    band visualization, **13**-6
    DNA loading buffer, **13**-6
    technical considerations, **13**-5
Agarose layered culture system, **30**-6
Aggrecan, **30**-2
ALCAM, *see* Activated leukocyte cell adhesion
        molecule (ALCAM)
Aldehyde dehydrogenase (ALDH), **9**-8
ALDH, *see* Aldehyde dehydrogenase (ALDH)
Aldo–keto reductase activity (AdhD), **4**-6
Alginate, **27**-6
ALH, *see* Accordion-like honeycomb (ALH)
Aliphatic diacids, **5**-10
Alkaline phosphatase (ALP), **7**-3, **11**-13
    assay, **13**-4
    as bone formation marker, **6**-2
    as conjugated enzymes, **13**-23
    in hypertrophic chondrocytes, **21**-5
$\alpha$-2-Macroglobulin (A2 M), **32**-9
$\alpha$-TCP, see Alpha-tricalcium phosphate ($\alpha$-TCP)
Alpha-tricalcium phosphate ($\alpha$-TCP), **3**-2, **3**-3; *see also*
        Tricalcium phosphates (TCPs)
A2 M, *see* $\alpha$-2-Macroglobulin (A2 M)
Ameloblasts, **33**-4
Amine-terminated methoxy poly(ethylene glycol)
        (AMPEG), **11**-13
Amniotic-fluid and placental-derived stem cells
        (AFPS cells), **34**-4; *see also* Embryonic
        stem cells (ESCs)
Amorphous calcium phosphate (ACP), **3**-5
AMPEG, *see* Amine-terminated methoxy
        poly(ethylene glycol) (AMPEG)
Ang-1, *see* Angiopoietin-1 (Ang-1)
Angiogenesis, **24**-2 to **24**-3; *see also*
        Neovascularization
    cell–cell interaction on, **37**-13
Angiopoietin-1 (Ang-1), **24**-3
Animal models, **37**-5
Anisotropic capillary hydrogels (ACH), **36**-8

Anisotropy, **15**-5
Anoikis, *see* Apoptosis
ANS, *see* Autonomic nervous system (ANS)
Anterior cruciate ligament (ACL), **12**-10, **29**-1
  neotissue formation, **32**-3
  silk-fiber matrix as, **2**-10
Anterior visceral endoderm (AVE), **8**-11
Antibody-dependent cellular cytotoxicity (ADCC),
    **9**-7
Anti-differentiation factors, **8**-11
Antigen, **9**-6
Antigen-presenting cells (APCs), **9**-6
  professional, **9**-6
Apatite, **3**-3; *see also* Calcium phosphate (CaP);
      Hydroxyapatite (HA)
  CHA, **3**-4
  chemical and crystallographic characteristics,
      **3**-4
  coral-derived, **3**-10
  fluorapatite, **3**-4
  HA, **3**-3
  nonstoichiometric, **3**-4
  silicon-substituted, **3**-5
  stoichiometric, **3**-3
APCs, *see* Antigen-presenting cells (APCs)
Apoptosis, **37**-6
Apt, *see* A10 RNA aptamer (Apt)
Arg–Glu–Asp–Val peptide (REDV peptide), **12**-5
Arginine-glycine-aspartic acid (RGD), **12**-7
  adhesive peptides, **35**-5
  as cell-adhesion domain sequences, **34**-2
  cell attachment stimulation, **19**-7
  domain, **12**-2
  for functional ligament-to-bone attachments,
      **32**-6
  in MSC culturing, **23**-6
A10 RNA aptamer (Apt), **11**-13
Aromatic diacids, **5**-10
Arteriogenesis, **24**-4; *see also* Neovascularization
Articular cartilage, **7**-4, **22**-22
Astrocytes, **36**-1
Asymmetric divisions, **8**-5
Atherosclerosis, **14**-4, **35**-2; *see also*
      Mechanotransduction abnormalities
Atherosclerotic plaque, **35**-2
Atom transfer radical polymerization, **5**-14
ATSCs, *see* Adipose tissue-derived MSCs (ATSCs)
Autocrine signaling, **7**-5
Autologous chondrocyte implantation (ACI),
    **30**-3
  advantages, **30**-7
Autologous grafts, **2**-11
Autonomic nervous system (ANS), **36**-1
AVE, *see* Anterior visceral endoderm (AVE)
Axial force, **15**-6
Axons, **36**-2
  guidance channels, **36**-10

**B**

BAD, *see* BCL2-associated agonist of cell death (BAD)
Basement membrane (BM), **24**-3
Basic fibroblast growth factor (bFGF), **28**-12, **30**-5,
      **34**-6, **36**-6
BAX, *see* BCL2-associated X protein (BAX)
B cells, **9**-5
  expression, **9**-6
  negative selection, **9**-6
  V-D-J rearrangement, **9**-5
BCEs, *see* Bovine adrenal capillary endothelial cells
      (BCEs)
BCL2-associated agonist of cell death (BAD), **7**-6
BCL2-associated X protein (BAX), **7**-7
BDNF, *see* Brain-derived neurotrophic factor (BDNF)
  clinical applications, **3**-10
  whitlockite, **3**-3
β-mercaptoethanol, **13**-9
Beta sheets, **2**-4; *see also* Silk
β-TCP, *see* Beta-tricalcium phosphate (β-TCP)
Beta-Tricalcium phosphate (β-TCP), **3**-2; *see also*
      Tricalcium phosphates (TCPs)
BFU-E (Burst-forming units erythroid), **9**-4
Biaxial force, **15**-6
Biglycan, **29**-2 to **29**-3
Bioactive agents, **17**-1, **17**-7; *see also* Drug delivery
Bioactive factors, **27**-5
Bioactive glass, **27**-5
Bioactive glass ceramic nanoparticles (nBGC), **11**-14
Bioartificial tissues
  cultivation, **26**-2
  dynamic tissue culture method, **26**-9
Bioceramics, **27**-5
Biochemical influences, **21**-2
Biodegradation, **17**-4
Bioengineered tumor, **37**-7 to **37**-8
Bioengineered tumor model
  bioreactors, **37**-11 to **37**-12
  cocultures, **37**-10 to **37**-11
  ECM gels, **37**-8 to **37**-9
  polymer scaffolds, **37**-9 to **37**-10
  signaling molecules, **37**-10
  tools, **37**-8
Bioerosion, **17**-4
  bioerodible drug delivery systems, **17**-5
  mechanism of, **17**-4
  surface erosion, **17**-4
Biological barriers, **19**-1, **19**-3
Biological spatial scales, **26**-2
Biomaterial, **2**-5; *see also* Micropatterned biomaterial;
      Peripheral nerve repair
  acellular tissue matrices, **34**-3
  alginate, **34**-3
  biodegradable synthetic polymer, **34**-4
  cell-based scaffold, **34**-4
  cellulose, **34**-3

characteristics, **34**-2
classes of, **34**-2
collagen, **34**-3
functions, **34**-2
induced pluripotent state cells, **34**-4
mechanical properties, **14**-12
nanoscaffolds, **34**-4
natural, **4**-1
polysaccharides, **34**-3
protein-engineered, **4**-1
Biomaterial mechanics, **14**-6; *see also* Cellular
    mechanotransduction
cancerous tumor suppression, **14**-11
cardiovascular engineering, **14**-11
cell–substrate interactions, **14**-6 to **14**-9
cellular behavior regulation, **14**-9 to **14**-10
engineering with stem cells, **14**-12
neural engineering, **14**-10 to **14**-11
potential target and applications, **14**-10
Biomedical imaging, **25**-1, **25**-12
infrared imaging, **25**-6
nuclear magnetic resonance, **25**-6 to **25**-12
optical imaging, **25**-2 to **25**-4
radiation-based imaging, **25**-4 to **25**-5
ultrasound, **25**-5
Biomimetic approaches, **12**-1, **13**-1; *see also*
    Biomimetic surface modifications; Scaffold;
    Tissue engineering
composite scaffolds, **12**-8 to **12**-10
growth factor-presenting materials, **12**-5 to **12**-6
hydrogels, **12**-6 to **12**-8
principle, **22**-2
scaffolds mimicking ECM structure, **12**-10 to
    **12**-11
for vessel culture, **35**-9
Biomimetic surface modifications, **12**-3, **12**-4
functional groups, **12**-4
protein immobilization, **12**-5
Bioreactor, **22**-2, **30**-16, **37**-11 to **37**-12; *see also*
    Micro-bioreactor; Perfusion bioreactors;
    Tissue engineering bioreactors; Vascular
    bioreactors
biochemical and mechanical cues, **22**-7 to **22**-8
first-generation, **22**-2
general requirements, **22**-6 to **22**-7
issues in, **22**-8 to **22**-9
mammalian cells and, **22**-3
mass transport considerations, **22**-7
principle, **22**-6
as shipping containers, **22**-8 to **22**-9
spinner flask, **22**-19
for tissue culture, **22**-2
types, **22**-8
Bioresorption, **3**-8
CaP blocks, **3**-8
CaP cements, **3**-14
Biot number, **26**-8

on growth rates, **26**-11
Biphasic calcium phosphate (BCP), **3**-10 to **3**-11, **12**-9
Bladder submucosa (BSM), **34**-2
Bladder tissue engineering, **25**-11
Blastocyst, **8**-4; *see also* Embryonic stem cells (ESCs)
Blood cell differentiation, **9**-2
Blood vessel, **22**-5
functional engineered, **22**-17
network's job, **23**-9
wall, **22**-17
Blotting, **13**-20; *see also* Molecular biology techniques
eastern blot, **13**-23 to **13**-24
northern blot, **13**-21 to **13**-22
southern blot, **13**-20 to **13**-21
western blot, **13**-22 to **13**-23
Bluing, **13**-2
Blunting enzymes, **13**-11
Klenow fragment, **13**-11 to **13**-12
technical considerations, **13**-13
BM, *see* Basement membrane (BM)
BMSC, *see* Bone marrow mesenchymal stem cells
    (BMSC); Bone marrow stromal cells
    (BMSCs)
BMSSCs, *see* Bone marrow stromal stem cells
    (BMSSCs)
Bone, **2**-8, **22**-19; *see also* Bone tissue engineering
    bioreactor
bioreactors, **22**-21
cells, **7**-3
components for tissue engineering, **22**-21
functional bone engineering, **22**-19
gene therapy, **18**-8 to **18**-9
grafts, **6**-2
implants, **2**-8 to **2**-9
induction, **6**-2
inorganic phase of, **3**-1
loading and shear stresses, **7**-15
marrow, **9**-11
shear forces effect on, **23**-4 to **23**-6
therapeutic trials, **18**-9
types of, **22**-19
Bone biology; *see also* Bone engineering
bone-lining cells, **27**-2
cancellous bone, **27**-2
composition of, **27**-2
cortical bone, **27**-2
dynamics of, **27**-3 to **27**-4
endochondral bone formation, **27**-4
hormone effect, **27**-3
lamellar bone, **27**-2
periosteum, **27**-2
shape, **27**-1
structure, **27**-1 to **27**-2
Bone engineering, **22**-19, **27**-1, **27**-13
alginate, **27**-6
bioactive factors, **27**-5
bioactive glass, **27**-5

Bone engineering (*Continued*)
  bioceramics, **27**-5
  BMPs, **27**-9 to **27**-10
  chitosan, **27**-6
  chondroitin sulfate, **27**-6, **27**-7
  clinical translation, **27**-12 to **27**-13
  collagen type I, **27**-6
  effect of delivering combinations, **27**-10
  ESCs, **27**-8
  fibrin, **27**-6
  fibroblast growth factors, **27**-10
  gelatin hydrogels, **27**-6
  glass ceramics, **27**-5
  hyaluronan, **27**-6
  insulin-like growth factor, **27**-10
  material characteristics, **27**-5
  MDSCs, **27**-9
  MSCs, **27**-8
  multiple growth factor delivery, **27**-11
  nanoscale features, **27**-11 to **27**-12
  osteoblasts, **27**-7 to **27**-8
  periosteal-derived progenitor cells, **27**-8
  platelet-derived growth factors, **27**-10
  silk fibroin, **27**-6
  transforming growth factors, **27**-9
Bone-lining cells, **27**-2 to **27**-3
Bone marrow
  pluripotent cells, **10**-1
  stem cells, **36**-11
Bone marrow mesenchymal stem cells (BMSC), **11**-13
Bone marrow stromal cells (BMSCs), **10**-1, **28**-2,
      **36**-6; *see also* Mesenchymal stem cells
      (MSCs)
  differentiation, **10**-4
  mesenchymal stromal cells, **21**-6, **28**-13, **30**-11
  research on, **10**-1
Bone marrow stromal stem cells (BMSSCs), **33**-8
Bone morphogenetic protein (BMP), **7**-9, **11**-13
  ATSCs, **27**-8
  bind to extracellular matrix, **6**-3
  for bone tunnel osteointegration, **32**-4
  on cartilage homeostasis, **7**-10
  challenges and opportunities, **6**-4
  clinical applications, **6**-4
  as diffusible growth factors, **33**-3
  family in mammals, **6**-3
  isolation from, **6**-1, **6**-2
  matrix production stimulation, **30**-5
  in osteogenic differentiation, **21**-2
  as osteoinductive protein, **28**-8
  receptors, **6**-2
  with silk scaffolds, **2**-9
  structure, **7**-9
Bone-patellar-bone graft, **29**-4
Bone sialoprotein (BSP), **33**-2
  osteoblasts differentiation mark, **21**-6
BoneSource®, **3**-15; *see also* CaP cements

Bone tissue engineering bioreactor, **22**-5, **22**-19;
      *see also* Bone tissue engineering; Tissue
      engineering bioreactors
  bone bioreactors, **22**-21
  challenges, **22**-22
  features, **22**-4
  limitations, **22**-22
  osteoblast in, **23**-4
  perfusion bioreactors, **22**-19 to **22**-21
  schematics of, **22**-20
  spinner flask bioreactor, **22**-19
Bone volume over total tissue volume (BV/TV), **28**-7
Bovine adrenal capillary endothelial cells (BCEs),
      **16**-11
Bovine serum albumin (BSA), **11**-13, **16**-11
Brain-derived neurotrophic factor (BDNF), **36**-6,
      **36**-10
Brownian motion, **17**-3
BSA, *see* Bovine serum albumin (BSA)
BSM, *see* Bladder submucosa (BSM)
BSP, *see* Bone sialoprotein (BSP)
Bursa of fabricius, **9**-5
Burst-forming units erythroid, *see* BFU-E (Burst-
      forming units erythroid)
BV/TV, *see* Bone volume over total tissue volume (BV/
      TV)

# C

CA, *see* Cellular automata (CA)
CABG, *see* Coronary artery bypass graft (CABG)
CAF, *see* Cancer-associated fibroblasts (CAF)
Calcium deficient hydroxyapatite (CDHA or s-HA),
      **3**-3
Calcium phosphate (CaP), **3**-1; *see also* Apatite
  abbreviations of, **3**-2
  apatites, **3**-3
  dicalcium phosphate, **3**-2
  drawback of, **3**-8
  octacalcium phosphate, **3**-3
  osteoinductivity, **3**-15
  physicochemical properties, **3**-1
  porous, **3**-8
  remodeling, **3**-8
  tetracalcium phosphate, **3**-3
  tricalcium phosphate, **3**-2 to **3**-3
Calcium phosphate cement (CPC), **11**-14
Calcium sources, **3**-12
Calf intestinal alkaline phosphatase (CIP), **13**-13 to
      **13**-14
Calmodulin-binding domains (CBDs), **4**-6
cAMP, *see* Cyclic adenosine monophosphate (cAMP)
Cancellous bone, **27**-2
Cancer, **14**-5, **37**-1; *see also* Cancer 3D models;
      Mechanotransduction abnormalities
  adherent culture surfaces, **37**-4
  animal model for, **37**-13

cancerous tumor suppression, **14**-11
cancer-promoting genes, **37**-3
cell metastasis, **14**-11
characteristics, **37**-3, **37**-4
drug development hurdles, **37**-1
drug resistance of, **37**-1
and engineering applications, **37**-2
gene therapy, **18**-17 to **18**-18
malignant tumors, **37**-2
Cancer 3D models, **37**-6; *see also* Spheroids
   3D microenvironment impact on angiogenesis,
      **37**-13
   animal models creation, **37**-13 to **37**-14
   bioengineered tumors, **37**-7 to **37**-8
   cancer drugs evaluation, **37**-12 to **37**-13
Cancer-associated fibroblasts (CAF), **37**-10
   tissue invasion and metastasis, **37**-11
CaP, *see* Calcium phosphate (CaP)
CaP blocks/granules, **3**-5, **3**-15; *see also* Calcium
      phosphate (CaP)
   biological properties, **3**-8
   bioresorption, **3**-8
   clinical applications, **3**-9 to **3**-11
   commercial, **3**-6 to **3**-7
   *in vivo* animal studies, **3**-8
   mechanical properties, **3**-8
   precipitation route, **3**-5
   production methods, **3**-5
   sol–gel method, **3**-5
   structure–property relationships, **3**-8
   tissue response of, **3**-9
CaP cements, **3**-11; *see also* Calcium phosphate (CaP)
   biological properties, **3**-14
   bioresorption, **3**-14
   clinical applications, **3**-15
   commercially available, **3**-11
   injection of, **3**-12
   *in vivo* animal studies, **3**-14
   mechanical properties, **3**-13
   setting of cement, **3**-12
   structure–property relationships, **3**-13
   transversal section of, **3**-14
CaP ceramics, **3**-1; *see also* Calcium phosphate (CaP)
Caprolactone, **36**-5
Carbon nanofibers (CNFs), **11**-14
Carbonated apatite (CHA), **3**-4; *see also* Apatite
Carboxymethylchitosan (CMCht), **19**-4
Cardiac gene therapy, **18**-14
   cell injection, **18**-16
   cell-mediated delivery, **18**-16, **18**-17
   clinical trials, **18**-15
   genes studied in preclinical cardiac trials, **18**-16
   *in vivo* cardiac studies, **18**-15, **18**-16
   scaffold-based cell therapy, **18**-16 to **18**-17
Cardiac myopathy, **14**-4; *see also*
      Mechanotransduction abnormalities
Cardiac tissue, **22**-14

Cardiac tissue engineering bioreactors, **22**-3, **22**-14;
      *see also* Tissue engineering bioreactors
   biomimetic paradigm for, **22**-15
   cardiac tissue requirements, **22**-14
   challenges, **22**-17
   design strategies, **22**-14
   electrical stimulation bioreactors, **22**-16
   features, **22**-4
   limitations, **22**-17
   mechanical stimulation bioreactors, **22**-16
   perfusion bioreactor, **22**-14 to **22**-15
Cardiotoxin (CDTX), **28**-14
Cardiovascular disease, **35**-1, **35**-2
Cardiovascular engineering, **14**-11
Cartilage, **2**-9, **22**-22, **22**-25
   shear forces effect on, **23**-3 to **23**-4
Cartilage derived morphogenetic proteins (CDMPs),
      **6**-1
Cartilage engineering, **30**-16
   adult chondrocytes, **30**-17
   limitations, **30**-18 to **30**-19
   stem cell differentiation, **30**-17, **30**-18
Cartilage engineering, zonal, **30**-4
   growth factor delivery, **30**-5 to **30**-6
   layered culture systems, **30**-6 to **30**-7
   monolayer cell studies, **30**-4 to **30**-5
   scaffold-supported culture, **30**-5
Cartilage regeneration, articular, **28**-17
Cartilage tissue, **22**-22, **30**-1; *see also* Chondrogenesis
   age and disease, **30**-3
   composition, **30**-1 to **30**-2
   hypoxic condition, **30**-14
   structure, **30**-2 to **30**-3
   treatment, **30**-3
Cartilage tissue engineering, **30**-4
   limitations, **30**-4
   model, **30**-4
   tissue growth model, **26**-5
Cartilage tissue engineering bioreactors, **22**-5, **22**-22;
      *see also* Tissue engineering bioreactors
   challenges, **22**-25
   design strategies, **22**-22
   features, **22**-4
   limitations, **22**-25
   mechanical loading bioreactors, **22**-24
   performance of, **22**-22 to **22**-23
   perfusion bioreactors, **22**-23 to **22**-24
   surface shear bioreactor, **22**-24 to **22**-25
CBDs, *see* Calmodulin-binding domains (CBDs)
CDHA or s-HA, *see* Calcium deficient hydroxyapatite
      (CDHA or s-HA)
CD45 isoforms, **9**-10
cdk6, *see* Cyclin-dependent kinase 6 (cdk6)
CDMPs, *see* Cartilage derived morphogenetic proteins
      (CDMPs)
CD33 myeloid marker, **9**-5
CDTX, *see* Cardiotoxin (CDTX)

Cdx2, **8**-4
    for cell phenotypes, **8**-5
Cell, **23**-1
    adhesion control, **14**-11
    adhesion via integrins, **23**-2
    assembly, **24**-4 to **24**-5, **35**-36
    binding domain IKVAV, **4**-9
    FA-mediated mechanotransduction, **23**-2
    free scaffold systems, **34**-6
    function modulation, **23**-1
    generated responses, **15**-2
    homeostasis, **7**-5
    hydrogels, **16**-13
    injection, **18**-16
    mediated delivery, **18**-16 to **18**-17
    mediated gene therapy, **18**-6
    metastasis, **14**-11
    migration, **26**-3 to **26**-4, **26**-13
    patterning, **16**-14; *see also* Micropatterned
        biomaterials
    population dynamics, **26**-4
    proliferation, **26**-3
    types, **14**-8, **14**-12, **19**-2
Cell adhesion, **35**-2
    control, **14**-11
    proteins, **4**-9, **12**-2
Cell encapsulation, **20**-1, **20**-11; *see also* Gelation
        mechanisms
    advantages, **20**-1
    gelation mechanisms in, **20**-2
    hydrogels, **20**-1 to **20**-2
    hydrogel structure and degradation, **20**-8
    scaffold, **20**-1
Cell engineering, **19**-1, **19**-2
    differentiated cells, **19**-2
    genetic vaccination, **19**-6
    intracellular delivery, **19**-3 to **19**-4
    liposomal formulations, **19**-7
    MNPs, **19**-7
    nanoparticles, **19**-4 to **19**-7
    nanoparticles' intracellular reservoir, **19**-4
    PCI-mediated gene delivery, **19**-6
    PEG-liposome formulations, **19**-7
    QDs, **19**-6
    siRNA, **19**-5
    stem cells, **19**-2
    stimuli-sensitive nanocarriers, **19**-6
Cell–substrate interactions, **14**-6; *see also* Biomaterial
        mechanics
    parameters affecting, **14**-6
    porosity, **14**-8 to **14**-9
    stiffness, **14**-6 to **14**-8
    topography, **14**-9
Cellular automata (CA), **26**-4
Cellular behavior regulation, **14**-9
    combinatorial designs, **14**-10
    heterogeneous materials/gradients, **14**-10

Cellular behaviors, **12**-7, **16**-1
Cellular functions, **11**-5, **20**-1
Cellular internalization mechanism, **19**-3
Cellular mechanotransduction, **14**-1; *see*
        *also* Biomaterial mechanics;
        Mechanotransduction
    cell migratory behavior, **14**-2
    in disease, **14**-3
    mechanical changes and cellular behavior, **14**-2
        to **14**-3
    mechanobiology, **14**-2
    mediators of, **14**-2
    overview, **14**-1 to **14**-2
    referenced models of, **14**-3
Cellular microenvironment, **16**-1
    components in, **12**-2, **12**-3
    control, **16**-1
Cellular Potts model (CPM), **26**-4 to **26**-5
Cementum, **33**-4
Central nervous system (CNS), **36**-1
    biomaterials in CNS research, **36**-8
    pathophysiology of, **36**-7
    repair, **36**-7
    support cells in, **36**-2
Central nervous system repair, **36**-7
    alginate gel, **36**-8
    brain and spinal cord injuries, **36**-7
    collagen, **36**-8
    cytotoxic amino acids, **36**-7
    glial scar, **36**-8
    olfactory ensheathing cells, **36**-10
    PHB fibers, **36**-8
    poptotic death of oligodendrocytes, **36**-7
    progressive destruction, **36**-7
    proteoglycans, **36**-8
    regeneration capacity, **36**-7
    Schwann cells, **36**-11
    stem cells, **36**-11
Cerebrospinal fluid (CSF), **36**-1
CFC, *see* Colony-forming cells (CFC)
CFU, *see* Colony-forming unit (CFU)
CG, *see* Chitosan–gelatin (CG)
CH, *see* Chitosan scaffolds (CH)
CH1, *see* nHA-chitosan scaffold (CH1)
CHA, *see* Carbonated apatite (CHA)
Chain extender, **5**-11
Chemical patterning, **16**-2
Chemical patterning techniques, **16**-2; *see also*
        Micropatterned biomaterials
    capillary force lithography, **16**-6
    layer-by-layer deposition, **16**-6
    microcontact printing, **16**-4 to **16**-5
    micromolding, **16**-5 to **16**-6
    photolithography, **16**-3 to **16**-4
    processing steps, **16**-4
    SAMs, **16**-2 to **16**-3
Chemisorption, **16**-2

Chitosan, **27**-6
Chitosan–gelatin (CG), **11**-13
Chitosan–nanohydroxyapatite (nHA), **11**-14
Chitosan scaffolds (CH), **11**-14
Chondrocytes, **7**-4, **30**-2
  BMP-2, **7**-10
  cartilage ECM, **7**-4
  coculture, **21**-4 to **21**-6
  dedifferentiation of, **21**-5
  ECM, **7**-4
  FGF-2, **7**-10
  hypertrophic, **21**-5
  IGF in, **7**-7
  interleukin, **7**-12
  markers, **21**-6
  mechanotransduction, **7**-14, **7**-16
  PDGF effect on, **7**-10
  TGF-β1 impact on ECM production, **7**-9
  VEGF interaction, **7**-10
Chondrogenesis, **30**-8; *see also* Growth factor (GF);
      Chondrogenic culture conditions for stem
      cell
  limitations in ESC, **30**-9, **30**-11, **30**-12
  *in vitro* ESC, **30**-8
  *in vitro* MSCs, **30**-11
Chondrogenic culture conditions for stem cell, **30**-18
  ADAS, **30**-15
  ESC, **30**-10
  MSCs, **30**-13
Chondroitin sulfate, **27**-6, **27**-7
Chondroitin sulfate proteoglycan (CSPG), **36**-8
Ciliary neurotrophic factor (CNTF), **36**-6
CIP, *see* Calf intestinal alkaline phosphatase (CIP)
c-Jun N-terminal kinases (JNK), **7**-7
CL, *see* Colloidal lithography (CL)
Cleavages, **8**-3
CLI, *see* Critical limb ischemia (CLI)
Click reactions, **20**-7 to **20**-8
CLP, *see* Common lymphoid progenitors (CLP)
CMCht, *see* Carboxymethylchitosan (CMCht)
CMP, *see* Common myeloid progenitors (CMP)
CNFs, *see* Carbon nanofibers (CNFs)
CNS, *see* Central nervous system (CNS)
CNTF, *see* Ciliary neurotrophic factor (CNTF)
Coculture, **21**-1, **37**-10 to **37**-11; *see also* Mesenchymal
      stem cells (MSCs)
  cells of interest, **21**-2
  with chondrocytes, **21**-4
  conditioned media systems, **21**-4
  future outlook, **21**-9 to **21**-10
  mesenchymal and endothelial lineages, **21**-8 to
      **21**-9
  mesenchymal stem cells, **21**-2 to **21**-3
  methods, **21**-3
  three-dimensional, **21**-4
  for two cell populations, **21**-3
  two-dimensional, **21**-3 to **21**-4

Cohesion, **3**-13
Cohesive Technology Opportunity Stratification
      (CTOS), **1**-4 to **1**-5, **1**-6; *see also* Generally
      Critical Concepts (GCC)
Collagen, **20**-9, **33**-2
  content, **30**-2
  type I, **27**-6, **29**-2
  type III, **29**-2
Collateralization, *see* Arteriogenesis
Colloidal lithography (CL), **16**-7, **16**-8 to **16**-10
Colony-forming cells (CFC), **9**-2
Colony-forming unit (CFU), **9**-2, **10**-2
Common lymphoid progenitors (CLP), **9**-5
  B cells, **9**-5 to **9**-6
  dendritic cells, **9**-6 to **9**-7
  NK cells, **9**-7
  T cell, **9**-6
Common myeloid progenitors (CMP), **9**-3
  granulocytes, **9**-5
  monocytes, **9**-5
  platelets, **9**-4 to **9**-5
  red blood cells, **9**-4
Compliance, **15**-6; *see also* Stiffness
Compression, **15**-4
  stresses, **15**-5
Compressive loading systems, **15**-15; *see also*
      Mechanical conditioning
  hydrostatic pressure systems, **15**-16
  using plate, **15**-17
Computed tomography (CT), **11**-14
  MicroCT, **25**-5
  for noninvasive *in vivo* imaging, **11**-9
  three-dimensional, **28**-2
Conjugated enzymes, **13**-23
Connective tissue (CT), **33**-8
Connexin 43, **21**-7
Contractile proteins, **15**-2
Contrast agent, **25**-8
Coral apatites, **3**-10; *see also* Apatite
Cornea, **2**-10
Corneal transparency, **2**-10
Coronary artery bypass graft (CABG), **35**-1
Cortical bone, **27**-2
CPC, *see* Calcium phosphate cement (CPC)
CPM, *see* Cellular Potts model (CPM)
Cranial nerves, **36**-1
Craniofacial bioengineering; *see also* Soft-tissue
      regeneration; Tooth regeneration
  articular cartilage regeneration, **28**-17
  bone regeneration, **28**-2
  after bone replacement, **28**-3
  calvarial-derived osteoblasts, **28**-4
  calvarial healing, **28**-5 to **28**-6
  challenges, **28**-1 to **28**-2
  controlled release technology, **28**-7
  gene therapy, **28**-8
  *in vivo* transduction of hMSCs, **28**-9

Craniofacial bioengineering (*Continued*)
    mandibular transplant, **28**-3
    postsurgical synostosis regulation, **28**-7
    viral delivery of the therapeutic gene, **28**-8
Critical limb ischemia (CLI), **18**-10
    angiogenic gene therapy, **18**-14
Crystallizable fragment (Fc), **4**-9
Crystal violet, **13**-3
    technical considerations, **13**-3 to **13**-4
CSF, *see* Cerebrospinal fluid (CSF)
CSPG, *see* Chondroitin sulfate proteoglycan (CSPG)
CT, *see* Computed tomography (CT); Connective
    tissue (CT)
CTC, *see* Cytotoxic T cells (CTC)
CTOS, *see* Cohesive Technology Opportunity
    Stratification (CTOS)
Culture conditions, **4**-4
Cycle threshold, **13**-16
Cyclic adenosine monophosphate (cAMP), **23**-5
Cyclin-dependent kinase 6 (cdk6), **33**-8
Cytokine gene therapy, **18**-17 to **18**-18
Cytokines, **7**-5, **18**-10, **7**-17; *see also* Interleukin-1
    (IL-1); Interleukin-6 (IL-6); Tumor necrosis
    factor
Cytotoxic amino acids, **36**-7
Cytotoxic T cells (CTC), **18**-18

# D

DBM, *see* Demineralized bone matrix (DBM)
DCP, *see* Dicalcium phosphates (DCP)
DCPD, *see* Dicalcium phosphate dihydrate (DCPD)
DCs, *see* Dendritic cells (DCs)
Decorin, **29**-2 to **29**-3
De-differentiation, **10**-4
Default pathway, *see* Neuroectoderm specification
Del1, *see* Developmental endothelial locus-1 (Del1)
Demineralized bone matrix (DBM), **32**-8
Dendritic cells (DCs), **9**-6 to **9**-7
Dental follicle, **33**-4
Dental lamina, **33**-4
Dental organ, *see* Enamel—organ
Dental pulp, **33**-4
Dental pulp stem cells (DPSCs), **33**-8
Dental stem cells (DSC), **28**-16
Dental tissue bioengineering, **33**-1
    fine-tuning scaffolds in, **33**-10 to **33**-11
    histology and immunohistochemistry of implant,
        **33**-13
    human dental pulp stem cells, **33**-8
    hydrogels, **33**-9
    nanofibrous materials, **33**-9
    porous scaffolds, **33**-9
    recombinant explant, **33**-13
    regeneration, **33**-12 to **33**-14
    regenerative strategies, **33**-7
    scaffolding material, **33**-8 to **33**-9

    whole tooth regeneration, **33**-12
Dentin, **33**-2
    tissue regeneration, **33**-11 to **33**-12
Dentin matrix protein 1 (Dmp-1), **33**-2
Dentin phosphoproteins (DPP), **33**-2
Dentin sialoprotein (DSP), **33**-2
Deoxyribonucleotide triphosphates (dNTPs), **13**-15
Dermatan sulfate proteoglycan (DSPG), **36**-8
Desaminotyrosyl-tyrosine alkyl esters, **5**-12
Developmental endothelial locus-1 (Del1), **30**-3
Dex, *see* Dexamethasone (Dex)
Dexamethasone (Dex), **19**-4, **21**-7
Diabetes, **18**-10
    therapeutic trials, **18**-11 to **18**-13
    wound healing, **18**-9 to **18**-10
Dicalcium phosphate dihydrate (DCPD), **3**-2; *see also*
    Calcium phosphate (CaP)
Dicalcium phosphates (DCP), **3**-2; *see also* Calcium
    phosphate (CaP)
*Dictyostelium discoideum*, **26**-4
Differentiated cells, **35**-2 to **35**-3
Diffusion, **17**-2; *see also* Drug delivery
    driven drug release, **17**-3
    Fick's second law, **17**-3
    from swellable polymers, **17**-3 to **17**-4
Diffusion tensor imaging, **25**-9
Diffusion-weighted imaging, **25**-9
Digestive enzymes, **18**-7
Divalent metal ions, **13**-6
Dmp-1, *see* Dentin matrix protein 1 (Dmp-1)
DNA ligase, **13**-10
    ligation reaction, **13**-11
    mechanism of, **13**-12
    T4 DNA ligase, **13**-10
DNA modification enzymes, **13**-10; *see also* Molecular
    biology techniques
    blunting enzymes, **13**-11 to **13**-13
    calf intestinal phosphatase, **13**-13
    DNA ligase, **13**-10 to **13**-11
DNA polymerase, **13**-15
DN stage, *see* Double negative stage (DN stage)
dNTPs, *see* Deoxyribonucleotide triphosphates
    (dNTPs)
Dorsal root ganglion (DRG), **36**-7
DOTA, *see* 1,4,7,10-Tetraazacyclododecane-
    N,N′,N″,N‴-tetraacetic acid (DOTA)
Double negative stage (DN stage), **9**-6
Double positive stage (DP stage), **9**-6
Double-stranded DNA (dsDNA), **13**-6
DPP, *see* Dentin phosphoproteins (DPP)
DPSCs, *see* Dental pulp stem cells (DPSCs)
DP stage, *see* Double positive stage (DP stage)
DRG, *see* Dorsal root ganglion (DRG)
Drug
    limitation due to diffusion, **37**-12
    resistance of cancer, **37**-1
Drug delivery, **17**-1; *see also* Diffusion

affinity binding, **17**-12 to **17**-13
applications of, **17**-1
bioerosion, **17**-4 to **17**-5
classical drug delivery systems, **17**-2, **17**-8
controlled drug delivery, **17**-1, **17**-2
covalent binding, **17**-12
diffusion, **17**-2
drug admixing with cell substrate, **17**-10 to **17**-11
drugs entrapped within cell substrate, **17**-11 to **17**-12
gel-based and gel-like systems, **17**-10
goals of, **17**-1
mechanisms of, **17**-2
microparticulate systems, **17**-9 to **17**-10
monolithic polymer systems, **17**-9
overall release profiles, **17**-6
particulate systems within cell substrate, **7**-13
PEGylation, **17**-8
protein degradation, **17**-7 to **17**-8
stimuli-responsive systems, **17**-5
in tissue engineering, **17**-6 to **17**-7, **17**-8
from tissue engineering scaffolds and matrices, **17**-10 to **17**-13
Drug evaluation, preclinical, **37**-4
animal models, **37**-5
monolayer cell culture, **37**-4 to **37**-5
tumor explants, **37**-5 to **37**-6
DSC, *see* Dental stem cells (DSC)
dsDNA, *see* Double-stranded DNA (dsDNA)
DSP, *see* Dentin sialoprotein (DSP)
DSPG, *see* Dermatan sulfate proteoglycan (DSPG)
Dynamic loads, **15**-6
Dynamic seeding method, **26**-9
Dynamic tissue culture, **26**-9
Dystrophin, **14**-5

# E

Early thymic progenitors (ETP), **9**-6
Eastern blot, **13**-23; *see also* Blotting
EB, *see* Ethidium bromide (EB)
EBL, *see* Electron-beam lithography (EBL)
EBs, *see* Embryoid bodies (EBs)
E-cadherin, **4**-9 to **4**-10, **8**-13
binding partners, **8**-4
EC cells, *see* Embryonic carcinoma cells (EC cells)
ECFCs, *see* Endothelial colony forming cells (ECFCs)
ECM, *see* Extracellular matrix (ECM)
*E. coli, see Escherichia coli (E. coli)*
EDA, *see* N-(2-aminoethyl-3-aminopropyl) trimethoxysilane (EDA)
EDTA, *see* Ethylenediaminetetraacetic acid (EDTA)
EGF, *see* Endothelial growth factor (EGF); Epidermal growth factor (EGF)
Elasticity imaging, **25**-5
Elastic modulus, **4**-5
Elastin, **11**-2, **29**-2

like sequences, **4**-5
Elastin-like-polypeptide (ELP), **20**-4
Electrical stimulation bioreactors, **22**-16; *see also* Cardiac tissue engineering bioreactors
Electron-beam lithography (EBL), **12**-7
Electron microscopy (EM), **33**-12
Electron rich catalysts, **5**-7
Electroporation, **18**-4
Electrospinning, **12**-11
ELP, *see* Elastin-like-polypeptide (ELP)
EM, *see* Electron microscopy (EM)
Embryoid bodies (EBs), **8**-3
differentiation, **8**-12
formation, **8**-13 to **8**-15, **15**-11
Embryonic carcinoma cells (EC cells), **8**-1; *see also* Embryonic stem cells (ESCs)
differentiation in *in vitro* culture, **8**-3
Embryonic development, **8**-3
blastocyst, **8**-4
Cdx2, **8**-5
cell specification, **8**-4
cleavages, **8**-3
compaction processes, **8**-3 to **8**-4
morula, **8**-3
trophoblast, **8**-4
zygote, **8**-3
Embryonic stem cells (ESCs), **8**-1, **8**-15, **19**-2, **33**-7, **34**-4; *see also* Embryonic carcinoma cells (EC cells); Mesenchymal stem cells (MSCs); Stem cells
alternate derivation methods, **8**-7
blastomere derivation, **8**-7 to **8**-8
characteristics, **8**-5
clinical outlook, **8**-14
culture conditions for undifferentiated, **8**-9 to **8**-10
derivation of, **8**-3
differentiation, **8**-11 to **8**-12, **36**-11
early embryonic development, **8**-3 to **8**-5
embryoid body differentiation, **8**-12 to **8**-14
epiblast stem cells, **8**-10 to **8**-11
induced pluripotent stem cells, **8**-9
*in vivo* differentiation capacity, **8**-6
late embryonic development, **8**-11
legal issues, **8**-1 to **8**-2
origin and derivation of, **8**-1
phase images, **8**-10
pluripotency, **8**-5 to **8**-6, **8**-7, **10**-5, **30**-7; *see also* Mammalian development
propagation, **8**-9
publication records, **8**-2
research history, **8**-1
self-renewal, **8**-5, **10**-3
somatic cell nuclear transfer, **8**-8
spontaneous aggregation of, **8**-13
teratoma formation, **8**-6
tetraploid complementation, **8**-6
Emergent behavior, **26**-13

EMT, *see* Epithelial mesenchymal transition (EMT)
Enamel, **33**-2
    knot, **33**-4, **33**-5 to **33**-6
    organ, **33**-4
Encapsulation conditions, **17**-7
Endochondral bone formation, **27**-4
Endocrine signal, **7**-5
Endocrine signaling, **7**-13
Endocytosis, **19**-3
Endoneurium, **36**-2
Endothelial cells (ECs)
    and angiogenesis, **24**-3
    in blood coagulation and transport, **35**-2
    in blood vessels, **22**-17
    in cardiovascular engineering, **14**-11
    effect of hemodynamic shear forces, **23**-9
    migration, **14**-2
    self-assembly of, **24**-4 to **24**-5
    for vascularization strategies, **24**-10
Endothelial colony forming cells (ECFCs), **35**-3
Endothelial growth factor (EGF), **36**-6
Endothelial precursor cells (EPCs), **24**-3
Endothelial progenitor cells (EPCs), **35**-3
Endotoxin, **4**-3
Engineered protein biomaterials, *see* Protein-
    engineered biomaterials
Engineered vascular networks, **35**-10 to **35**-12
Engineering specific urogenital structures, **34**-6
    bladder, **34**-6 to **34**-8
    kidney, **34**-8 to **34**-9
    penis, **34**-10 to **34**-11
    testis, **34**-11 to **34**-12
    urethra, **34**-9 to **34**-10
    vagina, **34**-12
Enhanced contrast, **25**-8
EO, *see* Ethylene oxide (EO)
Eosin, **13**-2; *see also* Hematoxylin and eosin (H&E)
EPCs, *see* Endothelial precursor cells (EPCs);
    Endothelial progenitor cells (EPCs)
Ependyma, **36**-1
Epiblast stem cells (EpiSCs), **8**-10 to **8**-11
Epidermal growth factor (EGF), **2**-10, **12**-6
Epigenetic promoters, **18**-1
EpiSCs, *see* Epiblast stem cells (EpiSCs)
Epithelial mesenchymal transition (EMT), **30**-7
Epithelial stem cells, **34**-5
EPO, *see* Erythropoietin (EPO)
Equibiaxial, **15**-6
ERK, *see* Extracellular signal-regulated kinase (ERK)
Erythrocytes, **9**-1; *see also* Hematopoietic system; Red
    blood cells
Erythropoietin (EPO), **9**-4
*Escherichia coli* (*E. coli*), **2**-5
ESCs, *see* Embryonic stem cells (ESCs)
Ethidium bromide (EB), **13**-6
Ethylenediaminetetraacetic acid (EDTA), **33**-11
Ethylene oxide (EO), **28**-7

ETP, *see* Early thymic progenitors (ETP)
Eukaryotic yeast, **4**-3
European garden spider (*Araneus diadematus*), **2**-2;
    *see also* Spider silks
Extracellular matrix (ECM), **11**-14
    adhesion factors in, **17**-8
    in axonal development, **36**-5
    biomacromolecules in, **12**-2
    BMPs bind to, **6**-3
    cancer cell reliance on, **37**-4
    in cartilage, **30**-1
    cell-binding domains, **4**-8
    cell function modulation, **23**-1
    cell migratory behavior and mechanical
      properties of, **14**-2
    chondrocyte, **7**-4
    components, **16**-5
    environment construction and proteins involved,
      **12**-5
    fibrin, **24**-8
    of fibrous connective tissue, **29**-2
    $\gamma$-carboxyglutamic acid-containing proteins in, **7**-3
    gel culture, **37**-8 to **37**-9
    growth factors and, **17**-8
    heparin, **12**-6
    in mechanoregulation, **14**-2
    in morphogenesis, **6**-3
    noncollagenous components of, **7**-3
    osteoblasts, **7**-3 to **7**-4
    peptide domains, **4**-1
    proteins, **7**-10
    role of, **4**-8
    scaffolding, **6**-3
    scaffolds mimicking structure of, **12**-10 to **12**-11
    specific molecules, **23**-1
    zones, **7**-4
Extracellular signal, **7**-4
Extracellular signal-regulated kinase (ERK), **7**-7, **23**-2

## F

FA, *see* Focal adhesion (FA)
FAC, *see* Focal adhesion complex (FAC)
FACS, *see* Fluorescence-activated cell sorting (FACS)
FAK, *see* Focal adhesion kinase (FAK)
Fascicle, **36**-2
FB, *see* Fluorobenzoyl (FB)
FBS, *see* Fetal bovine serum (FBS)
Fc, *see* Crystallizable fragment (Fc)
FDA, *see* U.S. Food and Drug Administration (FDA)
Feeder-free culture methods, **8**-9
Fetal bovine serum (FBS), **10**-6
    substitutes for, **10**-7
FGF, *see* Fibroblast growth factor (FGF)
Fibrin, **17**-13
    analogs, **17**-13
    based scaffolds, **27**-12

in bone engineering, **27**-6
cytokine-loaded, **35**-8
in gene therapy, **18**-17
heparin-conjugated fibrin gel, **12**-6
sealant–collagen scaffold treatment, **36**-8
Fibrinogen, **17**-13
Fibroblast, **23**-7, **29**-3; *see also* Fibrous connective
    tissues
    cellular alignment, **29**-9
    ECM synthesis and remodeling, **29**-9 to **29**-10
    mechanical stimulation, **29**-8 to **29**-9
    mechanosensation in dermal, **23**-8
    proliferation and differentiation, **29**-9
    strain magnitude and rate, **29**-10
Fibroblast growth factor (FGF), **4**-10, **6**-3, **27**-10
    in angiogenesis, **35**-7
    from cardiovascular implants, **35**-8
    in FGFtreated parietal defects, **28**-5
    molecular changes in dental mesenchyme, **33**-5
    tumorigenic role, **37**-10
Fibroins, **2**-2; *see also* Silk fibers
    production, **2**-5
    silk fibroin-based conduits, **2**-11
    spidroins, **2**-2
Fibronectin (FN), **16**-5, **29**-3
Fibronectin-derived peptide ligands, **4**-8
Fibrous connective tissues, **29**-2 to **29**-3; *see also*
    Tendon and ligament engineering
    enzymes and growth factors, **29**-3
    structure-property relationships, **29**-3 to **29**-4
Fick's second law, **17**-3
Filopodia, **16**-7
FITC, *see* Fluorescein isothiocyanate (FITC)
Flexcell tension system, **15**-15; *see also* Tensile loading
    systems
Fluid shear systems, **15**-9; *see also* Mechanical
    conditioning
    cone-and-plate, **15**-10
    parallel plate system, **15**-9
    Reynolds number, **15**-10
Fluorapatite, **3**-4; *see also* Apatite
Fluorescein isothiocyanate (FITC), **19**-5
Fluorescence-activated cell sorting (FACS), **9**-3
Fluorescence-labeled primers, **13**-17
Fluorescence resonance energy transfer (FRET), **13**-17
Fluorobenzoyl (FB), **11**-14
FN, *see* Fibronectin (FN)
Focal adhesion (FA), **23**-2
Focal adhesion complex (FAC), **7**-14
Focal adhesion kinase (FAK), **7**-7, **23**-2
Force, **15**-1, **15**-4
Fourier transform infrared (FT-IR), **25**-6
Four-point bending systems, **15**-14; *see also* Tensile
    loading systems
FRET, *see* Fluorescence resonance energy transfer
    (FRET)
FT-IR, *see* Fourier transform infrared (FT-IR)

Fumarate, **20**-6
Fumarate-based macromers, **20**-6
Functional tissue engineering, **22**-2; *see also* Tissue
    engineering

## G

GAGs, *see* Glycosaminoglycan (GAGs)
GAM, *see* Gene Activated Matrix (GAM)
γ-carboxyglutamic acid-containing proteins, **7**-3
GAPD, *see* Glyceraldehyde-3-phosphate
    dehydrogenase (GAPD)
Gastrointestinal tissue functionality, **34**-1
Gastrulation, **8**-11, **30**-7
GCC, *see* Generally Critical Concepts (GCC)
G-CSF (Granulocyte colony-stimulating factor), **9**-11
    mobilized peripheral blood, **9**-11 to **9**-12
GDF-5, *see* Growth/differentiation factors (GDF-5)
GDNF, *see* Glial cell line-derived neurotrophic factor
    (GDNF)
Gelatin hydrogels, **27**-6
Gelation mechanisms, **20**-2; *see also* Cell
    encapsulation; Radical chain
    polymerizations; Step growth
    polymerization
    via covalent crosslinking, **20**-5 to **20**-8
    examples of, **20**-3
    via noncovalent interactions, **20**-3 to **20**-5
    Pluronic F-127, **20**-4
    pNiPAAm, **20**-4
    self-assembling polypeptides, **20**-4 to **20**-5
    stimuli responsive hydrogel, **20**-3
Gel-based and gel-like systems, **17**-10
Gel electrophoresis, **13**-4; *see also* Molecular biology
    techniques
    agarose, **13**-5 to **13**-6
    polyacrylamide, **13**-6 to **13**-7
    SDS-PAGE, **13**-8 to **13**-9
Gel embedding, **37**-8
Gendicine, **18**-2 to **18**-3
Gene Activated Matrix (GAM), **18**-8
Generally Critical Concepts (GCC), **1**-4; *see also*
    Cohesive Technology Opportunity
    Stratification (CTOS)
    assignment of weights to, **1**-7
Gene therapy, **18**-1, **18**-18, **28**-8; *see also* Vectors
    bone regeneration, **18**-8
    cancer, **18**-17 to **18**-18
    delivery technique, **18**-2 to **18**-6
    diabetic wound healing, **18**-9 to **18**-10
    epigenetic promoters, **18**-1
    *ex vivo* gene delivery, **18**-6
    liposomal complex internalization, **18**-3
    lower-limb ischemia, **18**-10
    myocardial infarction, **18**-14 to **18**-17
    naked plasmid DNA, **18**-7
    oncolytic virus therapy, **18**-18

Gene therapy (*Continued*)
    systemic and local gene delivery, **18**-6 to **18**-7
    therapeutic agent dose, **18**-7 to **18**-8
    therapeutic clinical trials, **18**-8
    vectors of, **18**-2
Genetic vaccination, **19**-6
Germ cell, **19**-2
    tumors, *see* Teratocarcinomas
Germ layers, **19**-2; *see also* Stem cells
GF, *see* Growth factor (GF)
GFOGER, *see* Gly–Phe–Hyp–Gly–Glu–Arg
       (GFOGER)
GFP, *see* Green fluorescent protein (GFP)
GH, *see* Growth hormone (GH)
Glass ceramics, **27**-5
Glial cell, **36**-2
Glial cell line-derived neurotrophic factor (GDNF),
       **36**-4, **36**-6
Glial scar, **36**-8
Glyceraldehyde-3-phosphate dehydrogenase (GAPD),
       **19**-5
Glycophorin A, **9**-4
Glycoproteins, **29**-3
Glycosaminoglycan (GAGs), **7**-4, **17**-12, **27**-6, **30**-2
Gly–Phe–Hyp–Gly–Glu–Arg (GFOGER), **21**-4
GMP, *see* Granulocyte–monocyte progenitor (GMP)
Gradients, **25**-8
Granulocyte–monocyte progenitor (GMP), **9**-3
Gray matter, **36**-2
Grb2, *see* Growth factor receptor-binding protein 2
       (Grb2)
Green fluorescent protein (GFP), **19**-5
Growth/differentiation factors (GDF-5), **6**-2
Growth factor (GF), **11**-14, **17**-6 to **17**-7, **27**-11; *see also*
       Fibroblast growth factor (FGF)
    for ADAS chondrogenesis, **30**-14
    anabolic, **7**-5
    catabolic growth factors, **7**-10
    delivery of, **17**-9
    dual growth factor studies, **7**-16
    encapsulation, **12**-5 to **12**-6
    for ESC chondrogenesis, **30**-8 to **30**-9
    fibroblastic growth factor, **7**-10
    heparin binding, **17**-13
    insulin-like growth factor, **7**-5 to **7**-6
    interleukin-1, **7**-11
    interleukin-6, **7**-12
    for MSCs chondrogenesis, **30**-11 to **30**-12
    physical entrapment of, **12**-6
    platelet-derived growth factor, **7**-10
    role of, **12**-5
    signaling, **35**-7 to **35**-8
    TGF-β superfamily, **7**-7 to **7**-10
    tumor necrosis factor, **7**-13
    VEGF, **7**-10
    in vessel formation, **24**-7 to **24**-9
Growth factor receptor-binding protein 2 (Grb2), **7**-15

Growth hormone (GH), **7**-5, **7**-13
Guidance channels, **36**-9

## H

H&E, *see* Hematoxylin and eosin (H&E)
HA, *see* Hydroxyapatite (HA)
HA-coll, *see* Hyaluronic acid–collagen (HA-coll)
Hamstring tendon graft, **29**-4
HARV, *see* High-aspect ratio vessel (HARV)
HBDC, *see* Human bone-derived cells (HBDC)
HBGFs, *see* Heparin binding growth factors (HBGFs)
HCA, *see* Hydroxylcarbonate apatite (HCA)
hCHs, *see* Human chondrocytes (hCHs)
HCN channels, *see* Hyperpolarization-activated cyclic
       nucleotide-gated channels (HCN channels)
Head group, **16**-2
Heart, **22**-14
Heart tissue engineering, **23**-8
Hematopoietic cell surface antigens, **10**-3
Hematopoietic lineage commitment process, **9**-3
    lymphoid progenitors and progeny, **9**-5 to **9**-7
    multipotent cells, **9**-7
    myeloid progenitors and progeny, **9**-3 to **9**-5
Hematopoietic stem cells (HSC), **9**-3, **9**-7, **27**-2; *see also*
       Hematopoietic system
    bone marrow, **9**-11
    CD34+ cells, **35**-3
    CD45 isoforms, **9**-10
    *ex vivo* expansion of, **9**-12
    fate decisions, **9**-9
    G-CSF mobilized peripheral blood, **9**-11 to **9**-12
    hematopoietic niche, **9**-10 to **9**-11
    identification strategies, **9**-7 to **9**-9
    immunodeficient animal models, **9**-10
    quiescence and cell fate decisions, **9**-9 to **9**-10
    self-renewal, **9**-9
    sources for clinical transplantation, **9**-11
    in subendochondral niche, **21**-6
    transplant assays, **9**-10
    umbilical cord blood, **9**-12
Hematopoietic stem cells identification strategies, **9**-7
    aldefluor, **9**-8
    day 2 homing assay, **9**-9
    functional characteristics, **9**-8
    human HSPCs, **9**-8
    immunophenotype, **9**-8
    mouse HSCs, **9**-8
    side population, **9**-8
Hematopoietic stem or progenitor cell (HSPC), **9**-3,
       **9**-8
Hematopoietic system, **9**-1, **9**-12; *see also*
       Hematopoietic stem cells (HSC)
    blood cell differentiation, **9**-2
    hematopoietic hierarchy, **9**-1, **9**-4
    hematopoietic stem cells, **9**-3
    mature blood cells, **9**-1 to **9**-2

precursor cells, **9**-2
primitive hematopoietic cells, **9**-7
progenitor cells, **9**-2 to **9**-3
Hematoxylin, **13**-2
Hematoxylin and eosin (H&E), **13**-2
    staining, **28**-11
Heparan sulfate, **17**-12, **17**-13
Heparan sulfate proteoglycan (HSPG), **36**-8
Heparin, **12**-5, **17**-12
    in ECM, **12**-6
Heparin binding growth factors (HBGFs), **17**-13
Hepatocyte growth factor (HGF), **12**-7, **37**-10
hESCs, *see* Human ESCs (hESCs)
Hexafluoro-isopropanol (HFIP), **2**-5
HFF, *see* Human foreskin fibroblasts (HFF)
HFIP, *see* Hexafluoro-isopropanol (HFIP)
HGF, *see* Hepatocyte growth factor (HGF)
hGH, *see* Human growth hormone (hGH)
hHGF, *see* Human hepatocyte growth factor (hHGF)
HIFs, *see* Hypoxia-inducible transcription factors
        (HIFs)
High-aspect ratio vessel (HARV), **22**-2
Histochemistry, **13**-1; *see also* Molecular biology
        techniques
    alkaline phosphatase assay, **13**-4
    crystal violet, **13**-3
    hematoxylin and eosin, **13**-2
    Oil Red O, **13**-4
    stains, **13**-3
    toluidine blue, **13**-3
Histology, **11**-9
HIV, *see* Human immunodeficiency virus (HIV)
HLA, *see* Human leukocyte antigen (HLA)
hMSC, *see* Human mesenchymal stem cell (hMSC)
Honorary stem cells, **9**-1
Hormones, **7**-13
    adiponectin, **7**-13
    on bone cells, **27**-3
    in bone engineering, **27**-9
    on cell differentiation, **17**-7
    as cell-directive domains, **4**-10
    growth hormone, **7**-13
    on osteoblasts and chondrocytes, **7**-17
    parathyroid hormone, **7**-13
    as signaling molecules, **7**-1, **7**-5
Horseradish peroxidase (HRP), **12**-7, **13**-23
Housekeeping gene, **13**-19
HPA, *see* 3-(4-Hydroxyphenyl) propionic acid (HPA)
hPTH, *see* Human parathyroid hormone (hPTH)
HRP, *see* Horseradish peroxidase (HRP)
HSC, *see* Hematopoietic stem cells (HSC)
HSPC, *see* Hematopoietic stem or progenitor cell
        (HSPC)
HSPG, *see* Heparan sulfate proteoglycan (HSPG)
Human bone-derived cells (HBDC), **11**-14
Human chondrocytes (hCHs), **2**-9
Human dental pulp stem cells, **33**-8

Human ESCs (hESCs), **27**-8
Human foreskin fibroblasts (HFF), **12**-8
Human growth hormone (hGH), **17**-11
Human hepatocyte growth factor (hHGF), **18**-14
Human immunodeficiency virus (HIV), **19**-6
Human leukocyte antigen (HLA), **10**-2
Human mesenchymal stem cell (hMSC), **11**-14, **12**-5,
        **14**-9, **28**-7
    osteogenesis and scaffold degradability, **2**-8
Human neuroblastoma cells, **14**-9
Human parathyroid hormone (hPTH), **18**-9
Human umbilical vein endothelial cells (HUVEC),
        **12**-5, **19**-5
HUVEC, *see* Human umbilical vein endothelial cells
        (HUVEC)
Hyaluronan, **27**-6, *see* Hyaluronic acid (HA)
Hyaluronic acid (HA), **16**-5, **36**-4
    in microfluidic system, **16**-10
    nanogels internalization, **19**-5
Hyaluronic acid–collagen (HA-coll), **11**-14
Hybrid multiscale model, **26**-6, **26**-13; *see also* Tissue
        cultivation multiscale modeling
    dynamic seeding method, **26**-9
    dynamic tissue culture, **26**-9
    for mass transport dynamics, **26**-6 to **26**-8
    mass transport dynamics and cellular functions,
        **26**-8 to **26**-9
    for population dynamic, **26**-6
Hydrogel, **12**-6, **33**-9; *see also* Gelation mechanisms
    cell encapsulation, **20**-1 to **20**-2
    and controlled cell interactions, **12**-6
    degradation modes, **20**-10 to **20**-11
    degrading enzymes, **12**-8
    features of, **12**-7
    growth factor encapsulation, **12**-5 to **12**-6
    hydrophilic polymers as, **5**-2
    in microfluidic system, **16**-10
    microparticles, **17**-10
    natural, **12**-8
    PEG, **12**-7
    PEG-based, **17**-11, **30**-5
    PEG-MA, **16**-13
    self-assembling, **20**-3
    structure and degradation, **20**-8
    structure in tissue development, **20**-8 to **20**-10
    impact of temporal changes in, **20**-9
    thermoresponsive, **20**-3
    two-dimensional culture hydrogel system, **12**-8
Hydrophilic polymers, **5**-2
Hydrophobic polymers, **5**-2
Hydrostatic pressure systems, **15**-16; *see also*
        Compressive loading systems
Hydroxyapatite (HA), **3**-2, **3**-3, **11**-14; *see also* Apatite
    acicular microcrystalline, **3**-13
    categories, **3**-3
    clinical applications, **3**-9 to **3**-10
    HA/TCP carrier, **33**-8

Hydroxyapatite (HA) (*Continued*)
  in ligament-to-bone attachments, **32**-6
  in tooth composite, **28**-10
Hydroxylcarbonate apatite (HCA), **11**-14
3-(4-Hydroxyphenyl) propionic acid (HPA), **12**-7
Hyperpolarization-activated cyclic nucleotide-gated
      channels (HCN channels), **18**-16
Hypertrophic chondrocytes, **30**-8
Hypertrophy, **14**-4, **15**-2
Hypoxia-inducible transcription factors (HIFs), **27**-10

# I

IACUC, *see* Institutional Animal Care and Use
      Committee (IACUC)
ICAM, *see* Intercellular adhesion molecule (ICAM)
ICM, *see* Inner cell mass (ICM)
IDE, *see* Investigational Device Exemption (IDE)
IF, *see* Interstitial fibrous (IF)
Ig, *see* Immunoglobulin (Ig)
IGF-1R, *see* Insulin-like growth factor-1 receptor
      (IGF-1R)
IGFBP, *see* Insulin-like growth factor binding protein
      (IGFBP)
IKLLI, *see* Ile–Lys–Leu–Leu–Ile (IKLLI)
IKVAV, *see* Ile–Lys–Val–Ala–Val (IKVAV)
IL, *see* Imprint lithography (IL)
IL-6, *see* Interleukin-6 (IL-6)
IL-6R, *see* Interleukin-6 receptor (IL-6R)
IL-1Ra, *see* Interleukin-1 receptor antagonist (IL-1Ra)
Ile–Lys–Leu–Leu–Ile (IKLLI), **12**-7
Ile–Lys–Val–Ala–Val (IKVAV), **12**-7
Imaging agents, **11**-10, **11**-12
Imaging techniques, **25**-1; *see also* Biomedical imaging
Immune cell
    as anti-tumor, **37**-11
    types, **9**-2
Immunoblot, *see* Western blot
Immunoglobulin (Ig), **4**-9
    IgG, **13**-23
    superfamily, **4**-10
Imprint lithography (IL), **16**-7 to **16**-8
Induced pluripotent stem cell (iPS cell), **8**-9, **10**-6,
      **34**-4; *see also* Embryonic stem cells (ESCs)
Infrared imaging, **25**-6; *see also* Biomedical imaging
Inner cell mass (ICM), **8**-3
Inositol 1,4,5-trisphosphate receptors (InsP3Rs),
      **23**-6
In-plane displacement systems, **15**-15, **15**-16; *see also*
      Tensile loading systems
InsP3Rs, *see* Inositol 1,4,5-trisphosphate receptors
      (InsP3Rs)
Institutional Animal Care and Use Committee
      (IACUC), **28**-11
Institutional review board (IRB), **28**-10
Insulin-like growth factor (IGF), **6**-3, **7**-5 to **7**-6; *see*
      *also* Growth factor (GF)

  in chondrocytes, **7**-7
  in dentin matrix, **33**-3
  IGF-1, **27**-10, **30**-5, **37**-10 to **37**-11
  IGFBPs, **7**-6
  in osteoblast, **7**-7
  in scaffold modification, **36**-6
  signaling pathway, **7**-6 to **7**-7
Insulin-like growth factor-1 receptor (IGF-1R), **7**-6
Insulin-like growth factor binding protein (IGFBP),
      **7**-6
Insulin receptor substrate (IRS), **7**-6
Insulin, transferrin, selenium (ITS), **30**-9
Integrated microdevices, **22**-11
Integrin–ligand binding, **4**-8
Integrin, **12**-2, **23**-2
    cell adhesion via, **23**-2
    domain, **7**-14
    functions, **23**-2
    hypertrophy and, **14**-4
    mechanotransduction signaling, **7**-15
    signal pathways, **7**-14
    signaling, **14**-2
    as transmembrane cell surface receptors, **15**-4
Intercellular adhesion molecule (ICAM), **10**-3, **11**-14
Interface tissue engineering, **32**-1
    bi-phasic nanofiber scaffold, **32**-9
    cartilage-to-bone, **32**-10 to **32**-13
    fibrocartilage interface, **32**-3, **32**-7
    functional gradients, **32**-12
    future directions, **32**-13 to **32**-14
    interface regeneration, **32**-7
    ligament-to-bone, **32**-4 to **32**-7
    multiple tissues engineering, **32**-11
    myotendinous junction, **32**-10
    nanofiber alignment, **32**-9
    osteochondral tissue engineering, **32**-11
    periosteum, **32**-8
    PLGA/polyethylene glycol foams, **32**-11
    rotator cuff repair, **32**-8
    scaffolds, **32**-5, **32**-12
    soft-to-hard tissue interfaces, **32**-2 to **32**-3
    tendon-to-bone interfaces, **32**-7 to **32**-10
    3D multiphased PLGA microsphere scaffolds,
      **32**-13
Interleukin-1 (IL-1), **7**-5, **7**-11
    in chondrocytes, **7**-12
    in osteoblasts, **7**-12
    signaling pathway, **7**-11
Interleukin-6 (IL-6), **7**-12, **37**-10
Interleukin-6 receptor (IL-6R), **7**-12
Interleukin-1 receptor activate kinase (IRAK), **7**-11
Interleukin-1 receptor antagonist (IL-1Ra), **7**-11
Interpenetrating polymer networks (IPNs), **11**-14
Interstitial fibrous (IF), **28**-12
Intervertebral disc (IVD), **21**-4
Intima, **35**-2
Investigational Device Exemption (IDE), **4**-11

*In vitro* fertilization (IVF), **8**-1
IPNs, *see* Interpenetrating polymer networks (IPNs)
iPS cell, *see* Induced pluripotent stem cell (iPS cell)
IRAK, *see* Interleukin-1 receptor activate kinase (IRAK)
IRB, *see* Institutional review board (IRB)
Irgacure® 2959, **20**-6
IRS, *see* Insulin receptor substrate (IRS)
Ischemic heart disease, **35**-2
Isoleucine-lysine-valine-alanine-valine (IKVAV), **11**-14, **20**-4
Isotropy, **15**-5
Ito cells, *see* Pericytes
ITS, *see* Insulin, transferrin, selenium (ITS)
IVD, *see* Intervertebral disc (IVD)
IVF, *see* In vitro fertilization (IVF)

# J

JNK, *see* c-Jun N-terminal kinases (JNK)
Joint alteration procedures, **30**-3
JunB, *see* jun B proto-oncogene (JunB)
jun B proto-oncogene (JunB), **7**-12

# K

Keratan sulfate proteoglycan (KSPG), **36**-8
Kevlar 49, **2**-3
Kit⁺Sca⁺Lin⁻ (KSL), **9**-8
KLDL, *see* Lysine-leucine-aspartic acid-leucine (KLDL)
Klenow fragment, **13**-11 to **13**-12
KSL, *see* Kit⁺Sca⁺Lin⁻ (KSL)
KSPG, *see* Keratan sulfate proteoglycan (KSPG)

# L

Lactic acid, **5**-8; *see also* Poly(esters)
Lamellar bone, **27**-2
Laminin peptides, **5**-15
LCST, *see* Lower critical solution temperature (LCST)
LDL, *see* Low-density lipoprotein (LDL)
Lentivirus, **18**-4
Leucine zippers, **4**-6
Leukaphaeresis, **9**-11
Leukemia inhibitory factor (LIF), **8**-9, **36**-6
Leukocyte adhesion receptors, **14**-4
Leukocyte function-associated antigen-1 (LFA-1), **10**-3
LFA-1, *see* Leukocyte function-associated antigen-1 (LFA-1)
LIF, *see* Leukemia inhibitory factor (LIF)
Ligament, **2**-9 to **2**-10, **32**-1; *see also* Tendon and ligament engineering
    allografts, **29**-2
    reconstruction, **29**-2
Lipid-raft endocytic internalization, **19**-3

Lipoplexes, **18**-5
Lipoprotein receptor-related protein 5 (Lrp-5), **7**-4
Liposomal complex internalization, **18**-3
Liposomal formulations, **19**-7
Liquid/powder ratio (L/P ratio), **3**-12
Lithographic techniques, **16**-7
Liver stem cells, **34**-5
Living cell, **15**-1
    arrays, **22**-9
Living polymerizations, **5**-3
    radical, **5**-14
ʟ-lactide, **5**-8; *see also* Poly(esters)
LMWH, *see* Low molecular weight heparin (LMWH)
Longitudinal tensile loading systems, **15**-11, **15**-12; *see also* Tensile loading systems
Long-term HSC (LT-HSC), **9**-3, **9**-7
Low molecular weight heparin (LMWH), **35**-8
Low-density lipoprotein (LDL), **14**-4, **35**-2
Lower critical solution temperature (LCST), **20**-4
L/P ratio, *see* Liquid/powder ratio (L/P ratio)
Lrp-5, *see* Lipoprotein receptor-related protein 5 (Lrp-5)
LT-HSC, *see* Long-term HSC (LT-HSC)
Lymphocytes, **9**-1; *see also* Hematopoietic system
Lympho-hematopoietic system, **9**-3
Lysine-leucine-aspartic acid-leucine (KLDL), **20**-4
Lysosomal degradation, **19**-3

# M

Macrophage colony-stimulating factor (M-CSF), **7**-12
MAG, *see* Myelin-associated glycoprotein (MAG)
Magnetic nanoparticles (MNPs), **19**-6
Magnetic resonance imaging (MRI), **11**-9, **25**-7 to **25**-8; *see also* Nuclear magnetic resonance (NMR)
    of nanocomposites, **11**-12
Magnetic resonance microscopy (MRM), **25**-11
Magnetite cationic liposomes (MCLs), **19**-7
Magnetization transfer, **25**-9
Major histocompatibility class (MHC), **10**-5
    proteins, **9**-6
Mammalian development, **30**-7; *see also* Chondrogenesis
Mandibular condyle, **31**-2
    tissue engineering, **31**-6 to **31**-7
MAP, *see* Mitogen-activated protein (MAP)
Map erk kinase (MEK), **7**-16
MAPK, *see* Mitogen-activated protein kinase (MAPK)
Marrow stem cells, *see* Mesenchymal stem cells (MSCs)
Mass transport
    dynamic continuous model, **26**-6 to **26**-8
    limitations, **26**-4
    on tissue growth and structure, **26**-9 to **26**-11
Material morphologies, **2**-6
Matrices, **17**-10

Matrigel, **4**-1, **37**-8; *see also* Extracellular matrix—gel
    culture
    disadvantage of, **37**-9
    as growth factor source, **37**-10
Matrix and culture effects, **35**-6 to **35**-7
Matrix Gla protein (MGP), **7**-3
Matrix metalloproteinases (MMP), **4**-7 to **4**-8, **5**-5,
    **20**-7
    disrupting physical barrier, **12**-8
    ECM digetion by, **7**-3
    during healing process, **32**-9
    MMP-1, **29**-3
Matrix-contracting systems, **15**-15; *see also* Tensile
    loading systems
MBGs, *see* Mesoporous bioactive glass (MBGs)
MCL, *see* Medial collateral ligament (MCL)
MCLs, *see* Magnetite cationic liposomes (MCLs)
MCP-1, *see* Monocyte chemotactic protein-1 (MCP-1)
M-CSF, *see* Macrophage colony-stimulating factor
    (M-CSF)
MDP, *see* Monocyte-DC progenitor (MDP);
    Multidomain peptide (MDP)
MDSCs, *see* Muscle-derived stem cells (MDSCs)
Mechanical conditioning, **15**-1
    cell-generated responses, **15**-2
    compressive loading systems, **15**-15 to **15**-17
    current technologies, **15**-6
    devices used to study physical force effects, **15**-7
        to **15**-8
    fluid shear systems, **15**-9 to **15**-11
    living cell, **15**-1
    mechanical stimulation and cell responses, **15**-2
    micromechanical cell response, **15**-3 to **15**-4
    tensegrity model, **15**-3 to **15**-4
    tensile loading systems, **15**-11 to **15**-15
    upcoming technologies, **15**-18
Mechanical loading bioreactors, **22**-24; *see also*
    Cartilage tissue engineering bioreactors
Mechanical stimulation bioreactors, **22**-16; *see also*
    Cardiac tissue engineering bioreactors
Mechanical therapies, **14**-5 to **14**-6; *see also*
    Mechanotransduction abnormalities
Mechanosensors, **14**-2
Mechanotransduction, **7**-14, **15**-4, **29**-8; *see also*
    Cellular mechanotransduction; Shear forces
    chondrocytes, **7**-16
    FA-mediated, **23**-2
    integrins, **7**-14 to **7**-15
    osteoblasts, **7**-15 to **7**-16
Mechanotransduction abnormalities, **14**-3; *see also*
    Cellular mechanotransduction
    atherosclerosis, **14**-4
    cancer, **14**-5
    cardiac myopathy, **14**-4
    mechanical therapies, **14**-5 to **14**-6
    muscular dystrophies, **14**-4 to **14**-5
Medial collateral ligament (MCL), **29**-9

MEFs, *see* Mouse embryonic fibroblasts (MEFs)
Megakaryocyte—erythroid progenitor (MEP), **9**-3
MEK, *see* Map erk kinase (MEK)
Membrane molecules, **21**-4
Membrane receptors, **23**-2
MEP, *see* Megakaryocyte—erythroid progenitor
    (MEP)
Mesangial cells, *see* Pericytes
Mesenchymal stem cells (MSCs), **10**-1, **11**-14, **21**-2 to
    **21**-3, **27**-2; *see also* Coculture; Embryonic
    stem cells (ESCs)
    BDNF production, **36**-10
    bioreactors for, **22**-8
    characteristics, **10**-2
    chondrocyte coculture with, **21**-5 to **21**-6
    colony forming unit assay, **10**-2
    concerns, **10**-6 to **10**-7
    differentiation capacity, **10**-3 to **10**-4
    differentiation into hypertrophic chondrocytes,
        **21**-5
    direct osteoblast coculture with, **21**-7
    human, **10**-2
    indirect osteoblast coculture with, **21**-7
    isolation, **10**-2
    multipotent, **32**-4
    myoblast coculture with, **21**-8
    niche, **10**-4 to **10**-5
    osteoblast coculture with, **21**-6 to **21**-7
    plasticity of, **10**-3, **10**-4
    self-renewal capacity, **10**-3
    source, **36**-6
    surface marker and flow cytometry, **10**-3
    surgical trauma reduction, **28**-7
    therapeutic applications, **10**-5 to **10**-6
    tumorigenesis potential of, **10**-7
Mesenchymal stem cells (MSe), **35**-4
Mesoporous bioactive glass (MBGs), **11**-14
Methacrylates, **5**-13, **20**-6
    2-nitrobenzyl, **5**-13 to **5**-14
    responsive, **5**-13
Methoxy poly(ethylene glycol) (MPEG), **11**-14
Methylcellulose, **8**-14
Methylene blue, **13**-3
Methylmethacrylate (MMA), **11**-14
MGP, *see* Matrix Gla protein (MGP)
MHC, *see* Major histocompatibility class (MHC)
MI, *see* Myocardial infarction (MI)
Michael addition, **5**-10, **20**-7
Micro-bioreactor, **22**-3, **22**-9; *see also* Tissue
    engineering bioreactors
    advantage of, **22**-9
    applications, **22**-11
    cellular microenvironment, **22**-9 to **22**-10
    flow conditions, **22**-10 to **22**-11
    hematopoietic stem cell expansion, **22**-12 to **22**-14
    human liver cell, **22**-11 to **22**-12
    integrated microdevices, **22**-11

key features, **22**-4
micropatterned cell co-culture, **22**-12
perfusion bioreactor, **22**-13
substrate geometry and stiffness, **22**-10
Microcomputed tomography (μCT), **28**-7
Microcontact printing (μCP), **16**-3, **16**-4
processing steps, **16**-5
MicroCT, **25**-5; *see also* Computed tomography (CT);
Radiation-based imaging
Microfluidic device, **22**-9
flow, **22**-10 to **22**-11
Microfluidics, **22**-9
cardiomyocyte organoid fabrication, **16**-11
techniques, **16**-10
Microglia, **36**-2
Micromolding, **16**-5
Microparticulate systems, **17**-9
hydrogel microparticles, **17**-10
poly(phosphoester) microspheres, **17**-9 to **17**-10
surface functionalization, **17**-10
Micropatterned biomaterials, **16**-1, **16**-14
chemical patterning, **16**-2 to **16**-6
patterning, **16**-2
surface modification, **16**-2
three-dimensional patterning, **16**-10
topographical patterning, **16**-6 to **16**-10
Micro positron emission tomography (microPET),
**11**-14, **25**-5; *see also* Radiation-based
imaging
Migration speed on seed distribution, **26**-11 to **26**-13
Mitogen-activated protein (MAP), **7**-7
Mitogen-activated protein kinase (MAPK), **7**-7, **14**-3,
**23**-4
MMA, *see* Methylmethacrylate (MMA)
MNPs, *see* Magnetic nanoparticles (MNPs)
Molecular beacon technique, **13**-17
Molecular biology techniques, **13**-1
blotting, **13**-20 to **13**-24
DNA modification enzymes, **13**-10
gel electrophoresis, **13**-4 to **13**-9
histochemistry, **13**-1 to **13**-4
polymerase chain reaction, **13**-14 to **13**-20
restriction enzymes, **13**-9 to **13**-10
Monocyte chemotactic protein-1 (MCP-1), **24**-9
Monocyte-DC progenitor (MDP), **9**-7
Monolayer cell culture, **37**-4 to **37**-5
Monolithic polymer systems, **17**-9
Morphogenesis, **6**-1, **6**-2
bone, **6**-1
and tissue engineering, **6**-1
Morphogens, **21**-6
Morula, **8**-3
Mouse embryonic fibroblasts (MEFs), **8**-8, **34**-5
MPEG, *see* Methoxy poly(ethylene glycol) (MPEG)
MPPs, *see* Multipotent progenitors (MPPs)
MRI, *see* Magnetic resonance imaging (MRI)
MRM, *see* Magnetic resonance microscopy (MRM)

MSCs, *see* Mesenchymal stem cells (MSCs)
MSe, *see* Mesenchymal stem cells (MSe)
MTJ, *see* Myotendinous junction (MTJ)
Multidomain peptide (MDP), **33**-10
Multipotent, **19**-2; *see also* Stem cells
cells, **9**-7
Multipotent progenitors (MPPs), **9**-7
Mural cells, *see* Pericytes
Muscle satellite cells, **34**-5
Muscle-derived stem cells (MDSCs), **27**-9
Muscular dystrophy, **14**-3, **14**-4 to **14**-5; *see also*
Mechanotransduction abnormalities
μCP, see Microcontact printing (μCP)
μCT, see Microcomputed tomography (μCT)
Myelin-associated glycoprotein (MAG), **36**-7
Myocardial infarction (MI), **18**-14
Myocardium, native, **22**-14
Myotendinous junction (MTJ), **32**-10

# N

*N*-(2-aminoethyl-3-aminopropyl) trimethoxysilane
(EDA), **16**-4
Nanobiomaterials, **11**-1; *see also* Tissue engineering
(TE)
drug delivery system, **11**-10 to **11**-11
future developments, **11**-13
imaging, **11**-12 to **11**-13
incorporated polymer scaffolds, **11**-4 to **11**-5
nanofibrous scaffolds, **11**-2
nano-HA-PLGA-peptide drug delivery
system, **11**-9
polymer/composite scaffolds, **11**-6 to **11**-8
SEM images of, **11**-5
for therapeutic delivery, **11**-5
tissue engineering scaffold properties, **11**-2
tissue formation process imaging, **11**-9
Nanofibers, **11**-2; *see also* Extracellular matrix (ECM)
Nanofibrous peptide hydrogels, **33**-10
mechanical strength of, **33**-11
Nanofibrous scaffolds, **11**-3 to **11**-4; *see also* Scaffold
fabrication, **11**-2
SEM imaging of, **11**-3
starting materials for, **11**-2
Nano-HA-PLGA-peptide drug delivery system, **11**-9
Nano-hydroxyapatite/polyamide (n-HA/PA), **11**-14
Nanoparticles (NP), **11**-14
Nanotechnology, **11**-1
Nanotechnology-based cell engineering strategies,
**19**-1; *see also* Cell engineering
National Institute for Dental and Craniofacial
Research (NIDCR), **33**-9, **33**-15
National Institutes of Health (NIH), **33**-15
Natural Killer cells (NK cells), **9**-7
Natural scaffolds, **35**-5 to **35**-6; *see also* Scaffold
nBGC, *see* Bioactive glass ceramic nanoparticles
(nBGC)

NCAM, *see* Neural Cell Adhesion Molecule (NCAM)
NCPs, *see* Noncollagenous proteins (NCPs)
Near infrared (NIR), **11**-14
Negative selection, **9**-6
Neoplasia, **37**-3
Neovascularization, **24**-1; *see also* Vascularizing
    engineered tissues
 angiogenesis, **24**-2 to **24**-3
 arteriogenesis, **24**-4
 limitations in tissue engineering, **24**-1
 mechanisms, **24**-1, **24**-2
 vasculogenesis, **24**-3
Nerve growth factor (NGF), **12**-6
 for cellular therapy, **17**-9
 for lesion-induced recovery, **36**-10
 silk fibroin conduits with, **36**-4
Nerve guide, **36**-3
 axonal elongation, **36**-5
Nervous system, **36**-1
 injury models, **36**-12
 neuron, **36**-1
 parts, **36**-1
 peripheral nervous system, **36**-2
 spinal cord, **36**-2
 support cells of CNS, **36**-1
Neural Cell Adhesion Molecule (NCAM), **4**-10
Neural engineering, **14**-10 to **14**-11
Neural stem cells (NSC), **11**-14, **34**-5
Neural tissue engineering, **36**-12; *see also* Central
    nervous system repair; Peripheral nerve
    repair; Spinal cord injuries (SCI); Vascular
    tissue engineering
Neurilemma, **36**-2
Neuroectoderm specification, **8**-11
NeuroGel™, **36**-10
Neuroglial cells, *see* Glial cell
Neuron, **36**-1
Neurotrophins, **36**-6
 NT-3, **11**-14, **36**-6, **36**-10
 NT-4/5, **36**-6
Neutrophils, **9**-5
Newton's third law, **15**-2
NF-κB, see Nuclear transcription factor—kappaB
    (NF-κB)
NGF, *see* Nerve growth factor (NGF)
nHA, *see* Chitosan–nanohydroxyapatite (nHA)
nHA-chitosan scaffold (CH1), **11**-14
n-HA/PA, *see* Nano-hydroxyapatite/polyamide
    (n-HA/PA)
Niche, **10**-4
NIDCR, *see* National Institute for Dental and
    Craniofacial Research (NIDCR)
NIH, *see* National Institutes of Health (NIH)
NIPAAm, *see* N-isopropylacrylamide (NIPAAm)
NIR, *see* Near infrared (NIR)
N-isopropylacrylamide (NIPAAm), **15**-18
Nitric oxide synthase type II (NOS2), **7**-12

2-Nitrobenzyl (meth)acrylate, **5**-13 to **5**-14
Nitrocellulose membranes, **13**-20, **13**-23
Nitroxide-mediated polymerizations (NMP), **5**-14
NK cells, *see* Natural Killer cells (NK cells)
NMP, *see* Nitroxide-mediated polymerizations (NMP)
NMR, *see* Nuclear magnetic resonance (NMR)
NOD-*scid* IL-2Rγ $^{-/-}$ mice (NSG), **9**-10
Noncollagenous proteins (NCPs), **33**-2
Noncovalent interactions, **20**-2
Nonintegrin-mediated sequences, **12**-5
Non-naturally occurring peptides, **5**-15
Nonspecific binding, **13**-14
Nonviral vectors, **18**-4
 lipids, **18**-5
 naked DNA, **18**-4
 polymers, **18**-5
Norian Skeletal, **3**-15; *see also* CaP cements
Northern blot, **13**-21; *see also* Blotting
 advantages, **13**-21
 drawbacks, **13**-22
 technical considerations, **13**-22
NOS2, *see* Nitric oxide synthase type II (NOS2)
NP, *see* Nanoparticles (NP)
NSC, *see* Neural stem cells (NSC)
NSG, *see* NOD-*scid* IL-2Rγ $^{-/-}$ mice (NSG)
Nuclear envelope proteins, **14**-5
Nuclear magnetic resonance (NMR), **25**-6; *see also*
    Biomedical imaging
 advantages, **25**-8
 contrast agents and techniques, **25**-8 to **25**-9
 diffusion tensor imaging, **25**-9
 diffusion-weighted imaging, **25**-9
 disadvantage of, **25**-8
 examples, **25**-10 to **25**-12
 experiment, **25**-6 to **25**-7
 implantable coils, **25**-9 to **25**-10
 magnetization transfer, **25**-9
 MRI and spectroscopy, **25**-7 to **25**-8
 native contrast, **25**-8
 principles of, **25**-6 to **25**-7
 proton-density weighted images, **25**-8
 17.6-Tesla vertical bore magnet, **25**-7
 transverse relaxation, **25**-8
Nuclear transcription factor—kappaB (NF-κB), **7**-11,
    **7**-12
Nucleic acids, **17**-7
NuCore® Injectable Nucleus, **4**-11; *see also* Protein-
    engineered biomaterials
Nylon membrane, **13**-20

# O

OA, *see* Osteoarthritis (OA)
OC, *see* Osteocalcin (OC)
OCN, *see* Osteonectin (OCN)
OCP, *see* Octacalcium phosphate (OCP)
Oct4, *see* Octamer-binding transcription factor 4 (Oct4)

Octacalcium phosphate (OCP), **3**-3; *see also* Calcium phosphate (CaP)
Octamer-binding transcription factor 4 (Oct4), **8**-5
Odontoblasts, **33**-4
OECs, *see* Olfactory ensheathing cells (OECs)
Oil Red O, **13**-4
Olfactory ensheathing cells (OECs), **36**-10
Oligodendrocyte myelin glycoprotein (OMgp), **36**-7
Oligodendrocytes, **36**-1
    apoptotic death, **36**-7
Oligomeric matrix protein, **30**-3
OMgp, *see* Oligodendrocyte myelin glycoprotein (OMgp)
Oncolytic virus therapy, **18**-18
Optical imaging, **25**-2; *see also* Biomedical imaging
    application of, **25**-2
    bioluminescence, **25**-2, **25**-3
    fluorescence, **25**-2, **25**-3
    imaging setup, **25**-2
    *in vivo*, **25**-2
    QDs, **25**-4
    for structural studies, **25**-4
    transgenes expression tracking, **25**-4
Oral squamous cell model, **37**-13
Orthopedic tissues, **21**-1; *see also* Coculture
    replacement of injured, **21**-2
Osteoarthritis (OA), **30**-1
Osteoblasts, **7**-3, **27**-7 to **27**-8; *see also* Mesenchymal stem cells (MSCs)
    BMP-2, **7**-9
    bone extracellular matrix, **7**-1 to **7**-4
    coculture with MSCs, **21**-6, **21**-7
    FGF-2, **7**-10
    IGF in, **7**-7
    IL-1 in, **7**-12
    mechanotransduction, **7**-14, **7**-15 to **7**-16
    seeding, **31**-5
    TGF-β1 in, **7**-9
    VEGF interaction, **7**-10
Osteocalcin (OC), **33**-2
Osteoclasts, **7**-3
Osteocytes, **7**-3
Osteogenic markers, **2**-8 to **2**-9, **21**-9
Osteonectin (OCN), **7**-3
Out-of-plane circular substrate systems, **15**-14; *see also* Tensile loading systems
Outer dental epithelium, **33**-4

**P**

PAD, *see* Peripheral arterial disease (PAD)
PAGE, *see* Polyacrylamide gel electrophoresis (PAGE)
PAMAM, *see* Polyamidoamine (PAMAM)
Paracrine signaling, **7**-5
Parathyroid hormone (PTH), **7**-3, **7**-13, **27**-3
PBAEs, *see* Poly(β-amino esters) (PBAEs)
PBT, *see* Poly(butylene terephthalate) (PBT)

PCI-mediated gene delivery, *see* Photochemical internalization-mediated gene delivery (PCI-mediated gene delivery)
PCL, *see* Poly(ε-caprolactone) (PCL)
PCL/PLA copolymer tubes, **36**-5
PCR, *see* Polymerase chain reaction (PCR)
PD liposomes, *see* pH-dependent liposomes (PD liposomes)
PDGF, *see* Platelet derived growth factor (PDGF)
PDGFR, *see* Platelet-derived growth factor receptor (PDGFR)
PDL, *see* Periodontal ligament (PDL)
PDMS, *see* Polydimethylsiloxane (PDMS)
PDN, *see* Poly(dioxanone) (PDN)
pDNA, *see* Plasmid DNA (pDNA)
PDSGR, *see* Pro–Asp–Ser–Gly–Arg (PDSGR)
PECAM, *see* Platelet endothelial cell adhesion molecule (PECAM)
Peclet number, **26**-8
PEG, *see* Polyethylene glycol (PEG)
PEGDA, *see* Poly(ethylene glycol) diacrylate (PEGDA)
PEG-liposome formulations, **19**-7
PEG-MA hydrogels, *see* Polyethylene glycol methacrylate hydrogels (PEG-MA hydrogels)
PEGylated fibrinogen (PF), **11**-14
PEGylation, **17**-8
    for gene therapy, **18**-7
PEI-HA, *see* Poly(ethylenimine)-hyaluronic acid (PEI-HA)
PEO, *see* Poly(ethylene oxide) (PEO)
PEODA, *see* Poly(ethylene oxide) diacrylate (PEODA)
Peptide amphiphile (PA), **5**-15, **12**-6
Peptides, **20**-4
Perfusion bioreactors; *see also* Bone tissue engineering bioreactor; Micro-bioreactors
    for anatomically shaped grafts, **22**-20 to **22**-21
    in cartilage tissue engineering, **22**-23 to **22**-24
    culture bioreactors, **22**-15 to **22**-16
    for cylindrical constructs, **22**-19 to **22**-20
    for hematopoietic stem cell expansion, **22**-13
    seeding bioreactors, **22**-14 to **22**-15
Pericytes, **10**-4
Periodontal ligament (PDL), **28**-2
Periosteal-derived progenitor cells, **27**-8
Periosteum, **27**-2, **32**-8
Peripheral arterial disease (PAD), **18**-10
Peripheral nerve repair, **36**-2, **36**-7; *see also* Biomaterial
    BMSCs in, **36**-6
    cellular and growth factor–containing nerve guides, **36**-5
    delivery systems in, **36**-6
    injuries, **36**-2
    MSCs, **36**-6
    Schwann cells, **36**-5 to **36**-6
    surgical management, **36**-2 to **36**-3

Peripheral nerve repair (*Continued*)
  synthetic materials in, 36-5
  tissue engineering, 36-3
Peripheral nervous system (PNS), **2**-11, **36**-1; *see also* Peripheral nerve repair
  Schwann cells, **36**-2
PET, *see* Polyethylene terephthalate (PET)
Petri dish, **22**-2
PF, *see* PEGylated fibrinogen (PF)
PG, *see* Polycaprolactone-gelatin (PG)
PGA, *see* Polyglycolic acid (PGA)
PGE2, *see* Prostaglandin E2 (PGE2)
PGS, *see* Poly(glycerol-co-sebacate) (PGS)
Phagocytosis, **19**-3
Pharmacologically active agents, *see* Bioactive agents
Phase separation, **16**-7
PHB, *see* Poly-β-hydroxybutyrate (PHB)
PHB, *see* Poly(3-hydroxybutyrate) (P3HB or PHB)
P3HB, *see* Poly(3-hydroxybutyrate) (P3HB or PHB)
PHBV, *see* Poly(3-hydroxybutyrate-*co*-3-hydroxyvalerate) (PHBV); Poly(3-hydroxybutyrate-*co*-hydroxyvalerate) (PHBV)
pH-dependent liposomes (PD liposomes), **19**-5
PHEMA, *see* Poly(2-hydroxyethyl methacrylate) (PHEMA)
Photochemical internalization-mediated gene delivery (PCI-mediated gene delivery), **19**-6
Photoinitiating systems, **20**-5
Photolithography, **16**-3 to **16**-4
Photomask, **16**-3
Photoresist, **16**-3
Photpolymerizable polymers, **24**-7
pHPMA, *see* Poly[*N*-(2-hydroxypropyl) methacrylamide] (pHPMA)
PHSRN, **4**-9
Physical protein adsorption, **12**-4
Physisorption, **16**-2 to **16**-3
PicoGreen, **13**-6
Pinocytosis, **19**-3
PLA, *see* Polylactic acid (PLA)
Placenta, **9**-12
Placental growth factor (PlGF), **18**-14, **35**-3
Plasmid DNA (pDNA), **11**-14
Plasticity, **10**-3
Platelet, **9**-4 to **9**-5
Platelet derived growth factor (PDGF), **3**-14
Platelet endothelial cell adhesion molecule (PECAM), **11**-14
Platelet-derived growth factor receptor (PDGFR), **7**-10
  anastomosis of vasculature, **28**-12
  for ECFCs haracterization, **35**-3
PLCL, *see* Poly[(L-lactide)-*co*-(e-caprolactone)] (PLCL)
PLGA, *see* Poly(lactic-*co*-glycolic acid) (PLGA)
PlGF, *see* Placental growth factor (PlGF)
PLLA, *see* Poly(L-lactic acid) (PLLA)

Pluripotent, **19**-2; *see also* Stem cells
Pluripotent stem cells, *see* Embryonic stem cells
Pluronic F-127, **20**-4
Pluronics®, **20**-3
PMMA, *see* Poly(methyl methacrylate) (PMMA)
pNiPAAm, *see* Poly(*N*-isopropylacrylamide) (pNiPAAm)
POC, *see* Poly(1,8-octanediol-*co*-citric acid) (POC)
POE, *see* Poly(ortho esters) (POE)
Polyacrylamide gel electrophoresis (PAGE), **13**-6, **13**-7; *see also* Gel electrophoresis
Poly(acrylates), **5**-13
  synthesis, **5**-14
Poly(α-hydroxy)esters, **12**-3, **27**-7
Polyamidoamine (PAMAM), **11**-14, **19**-4
  CMCht/PAMAM dendrimer nanoparticles, **19**-4
Poly(anhydrides), **5**-10
  application, **5**-11
  methacrylated, **5**-11
  synthesis, **5**-10
Poly(β-amino esters) (PBAEs), **5**-9
  formation, **5**-10
Poly-β-hydroxybutyrate (PHB), **36**-8
Poly(butylene terephthalate) (PBT), **11**-14
Polycaprolactone-gelatin (PG), **12**-11
Polydimethylsiloxane (PDMS), **11**-14, **14**-6
Poly(D-L-lactic-*co*-glycolic acid) (PLGA), **11**-14
  scaffolds, **28**-3
Poly(dioxanone) (PDN), **5**-8
Poly(ε-caprolactone) (PCL), **11**-2, **12**-10, **32**-10
  AAc–PCL films, **12**-4
  for bone engineering, **27**-7
  glass transition temperatures, **5**-8
  melting temperature of, **5**-8
  nanofibers in SBF solution, **12**-9
  PCL/PLA copolymer tubes, **36**-5
Poly(esters), **5**-7
  condensation reactions, **5**-9
  degradation, **5**-8
  glycolide monomer, **5**-7
  poly(α-esters), **5**-7 to **5**-8
  poly(β-amino esters), **5**-9
  poly(propylene fumarate), **5**-8
  ring-opening polymerization, **5**-7
Polyethersulfone nonwoven fibers, **12**-11
Polyethylene, **36**-5
Polyethylene glycol (PEG), **4**-3, **11**-2, **11**-14, **27**-7
  advantages, **35**-5
  based hydrogels x, **5**-5
  cellular interactions, **5**-6
  in spinal cord repair, **36**-9
  synthesis, **5**-6
  as tissue engineering scaffold, **33**-9
Poly(ethylene glycol) diacrylate (PEGDA), **30**-6, **28**-12, **31**-5
Polyethylene glycol methacrylate hydrogels (PEG-MA hydrogels), **16**-13

Poly(ethylene oxide) (PEO), **11**-14, *see* Polyethylene glycol (PEG)
Poly(ethylene oxide) diacrylate (PEODA), **30**-6
Polyethylene terephthalate (PET), **11**-14
Poly(ethylenimine)-hyaluronic acid (PEI-HA), **11**-14
Poly(glycerol-co-sebacate) (PGS), **5**-9, **11**-14
Polyglycolic acid (PGA), **5**-7, **32**-11, **33**-9, **36**-5; *see also* Poly(esters)
    hybrid scaffolds, **12**-10
    in bone engineering, **27**-7
    in tooth dentin–ligament–bone complexes formation, **28**-10
Poly(3-hydroxybutyrate) (P3HB or PHB), **11**-14, **27**-7
Poly(3-hydroxybutyrate-*co*-hydroxyvalerate) (PHBV), **11**-14
Poly(3-hydroxybutyrate-*co*-3-hydroxyvalerate) (PHBV), **27**-10
Poly(2-hydroxyethyl methacrylate) (PHEMA), **4**-3, **12**-10, **36**-9
Polylactic acid (PLA), **11**-2, **11**-14, **27**-7, **33**-9
    enantiomers, **27**-7
    in nerve tissue engineering, **36**-5
Poly(lactic acid-*co*-glycolic acid) (PLGA), **5**-8, **32**-6
    in drug delivery, **17**-9
Poly(lactic-*co*-glycolic acid) (PLGA), **4**-3, **11**-2
    amorphous nature, **27**-7
    in neural tissue engineering, **36**-9
    in tumor engineering, **37**-9
Poly(ʟ-lactic acid) (PLLA), **5**-8, **11**-14
Poly[(ʟ-lactide)-*co*-(e-caprolactone)] (PLCL), **12**-8 to **12**-9
Polymer
    with FDA approval, **36**-5
    natural, **12**-8
    scaffolds, **37**-9 to **37**-10
    thermoresponsive, **20**-3
Polymerase chain reaction (PCR), **13**-14; *see also* Molecular biology techniques
    annealing, **13**-14 to **13**-15
    cycle parameters, **13**-14
    denaturing, **13**-14
    primer design, **13**-15 to **13**-16
    real-time quantitative PCR, **13**-16 to **13**-20
    technical considerations, **13**-14
    traditional, **13**-14
Polymeric diols, **5**-11
Polymerization mechanisms, **5**-2
    chain growth polymerizations, **5**-3
    monomer conversion progression, **5**-4
    polymer molecular weight progression, **5**-4
    step growth mechanism, **5**-2 to **5**-3
Poly(methacrylates), **5**-13
    synthesis, **5**-14
Poly(methyl methacrylate) (PMMA), **4**-3, **11**-2, **11**-14
    imprint lithography, **16**-7 to **16**-8
    in teeth regeneration, **28**-11

Poly[*N*-(2-hydroxypropyl)methacrylamide] (pHPMA), **36**-10
Poly(*N*-isopropylacrylamide) (pNiPAAm), **20**-3, **20**-4
Poly(1,8-octanediol-*co*-citric acid) (POC), **11**-14
Poly(ortho esters) (POE), **5**-11
Poly(peptides), **5**-14
Poly(peptoids), **5**-15
    structure of, **5**-16
Polyplexes, **18**-5
Poly(propylene fumarate) (PPF), **5**-8, **11**-2, **11**-15
    advantages, **5**-8
    in bone engineering, **27**-7
    structure of, **5**-9
Poly(propylene fumarate)/propylene fumarate-diacrylate (PPF/PF-DA), **11**-15
Polypyrrole (Ppy), **11**-15
Polysulfone, **36**-5
Poly(trimethylene carbonate) (PTMC), **5**-8
Polyurethanes, **5**-11, **36**-5
    limitation, **5**-12
    structure of, **5**-12
Poly(vinyl alcohol) (PVA), **11**-2
Poly(vinyl alcohol)/poly(acrylic acid) (PVA/PAA), **11**-15
Poly(vinylidene fluoride) (PVDF), **13**-24
Population dynamic discrete model, **26**-6
Porous 3D silk fibroin scaffolds, **2**-8
Positron emission tomography (PET), **11**-9, **25**-1, **25**-4; *see also* Radiation-based imaging
Postnatal stem cells, **10**-1, **33**-7; *see also* Mesenchymal stem cells (MSCs)
p21 peptide, **4**-10
PPF, *see* Poly(propylene fumarate) (PPF)
PPF/PF-DA, *see* Poly(propylene fumarate)/propylene fumarate-diacrylate (PPF/PF-DA)
Ppy, *see* Polypyrrole (Ppy)
Pressure, **15**-4
PRG4, *see* Proteoglycan 4 gene (PRG4)
Primer-dimers, **13**-15
Primitive streak (PS), **8**-11, **30**-7
    induction, **8**-12
Printing, *see* Stamping
Pro–Asp–Ser–Gly–Arg (PDSGR), **12**-7
Progenitor cells, **8**-22 to **8**-25
Progressive destruction, **36**-7
Proinvasion proteases, **37**-11
Proline-rich domains, **4**-6
Prostaglandin E2 (PGE2), **7**-12
Prostate specific membrane antigen (PSMA), **11**-15
Protein-engineered biomaterials, **4**-1
    as alternative to traditional biomaterials, **4**-1
    applications of, **4**-11
    cell–cell adhesion domains, **4**-9 to **4**-10
    cell-directive domains, **4**-10
    challenges, **4**-3
    crosslinking domains, **4**-5 to **4**-7
    degradation domains, **4**-7 to **4**-8

Protein-engineered biomaterials (*Continued*)
  design and synthesis of, 4-4 to 4-5
  ECM cell-binding domains, 4-8 to 4-9
  host selection, 4-3 to 4-4
  modular protein engineering design strategy, 4-2
  peptide domain categories, 4-10
  purification, 4-4
  solid-phase synthesis, 4-3
  structural domains, 4-7
  synthesis of, 4-3 to 4-5
  target proteins, 4-4
Protein engineering, 4-1
Proteoglycan 4 gene (PRG4), 30-4
Proteoglycans (PGs), **6**-3
  function in ECM, **29**-2
Proteolytic enzymes, 5-5
Proton-density weighted images, 25-8
PS, *see* Primitive streak (PS)
Pseudo poly(amino acids), **5**-12 to **5**-13
PSMA, *see* Prostate specific membrane antigen
    (PSMA)
PTH, *see* Parathyroid hormone (PTH)
PTMC, *see* Poly(trimethylene carbonate) (PTMC)
PVA, *see* Poly(vinyl alcohol) (PVA)
PVA/PAA, *see* Poly(vinyl alcohol)/poly(acrylic acid)
    (PVA/PAA)
PVDF, *see* Poly(vinylidene fluoride) (PVDF)

# Q

QDs, *see* Quantum dots (QDs)
qPCR, *see* Real-time quantitative PCR (qPCR)
Quantum dots (QDs), **19**-6, **25**-4; *see also* Optical
    imaging
Quiescence, 9-9

# R

Rabbit anti-mouse XYZ, **13**-23
Radiation-based imaging, **25**-4; *see also* Biomedical
    imaging
  microCT, **25**-5
  microPET systems, **25**-5
  PET, **25**-4
  sections in, **25**-4
Radical chain polymerizations, **20**-5; *see also* Gelation
    mechanisms
  acrylates, **20**-6
  fumarate-based macromers, **20**-6
  methacrylates, **20**-6
  photoinitiating systems, **20**-5
  redox initiating systems, **20**-5
  UV photoinitiators, **20**-6
Radiofrequency (RF), **25**-7
Radio-frequency glow discharge (RFGD), **28**-7
RAFT, *see* Reversible addition-fragmentation chain
    transfer (RAFT)

Ras/MAPK, *see* Rat sarcoma guanine triphosphatase/
    mitogen-activated protein kinases (Ras/
    MAPK)
Rat sarcoma guanine triphosphatase/mitogen-
    activated protein kinases (Ras/MAPK), **7**-6
Reactive oxygen species (ROS), **9**-5
Real time polymerase chain reaction (RT-PCR), **34**-9
Real-time quantitative PCR (qPCR), **13**-16; *see also*
    Polymerase chain reaction (PCR)
  advantage, **13**-17
  baseline fluorescence, **13**-16
  cycle threshold, **13**-16
  DNA concentration vs. cycle number curve, **13**-16
  fluorescence chemistries, **13**-17
  fluorescence-labeled primers, **13**-17
  molecular beacon technique, **13**-17
  quantification, **13**-19 to **13**-20
  technical considerations, **13**-19
Receptor proteins, **7**-5
Recombinant human (rh), **11**-15
Red blood cells, **9**-4
Redox initiating systems, **20**-5
REDV peptide, *see* Arg–Glu–Asp–Val peptide (REDV
    peptide)
Reprogramming, **34**-5
Resilin, **4**-7
Responsive (meth)acrylates, **5**-13
Resting osteoblasts, *see* Bone-lining cells
Restriction enzymes, **13**-9; *see also* Molecular biology
    techniques
  application of, **13**-9
  blunt cut, **13**-10
  enzyme activity, **13**-10
  sticky cut, **13**-9
  technical considerations, **13**-10
  types, **13**-9
Retroviruses, **18**-2, **18**-3
Reversible addition-fragmentation chain transfer
    (RAFT), **5**-14
Reynolds number, **15**-10
RF, *see* Radiofrequency (RF)
RFGD, *see* Radio-frequency glow discharge (RFGD)
RGD (arginine-glycine-aspartic acid), **4**-5, **5**-14
  cell adhesion, **4**-9
rh, *see* Recombinant human (rh)
Rho-associated kinase (ROCK), **8**-10, **23**-6
Rho-generated cytoskeletal tension, **14**-5
ROCK, *see* Rho-associated kinase (ROCK)
Root dentin, **33**-4
ROS, *see* Reactive oxygen species (ROS)
Rotating wall vessels (RWV), **22**-2
  bioreactors, **37**-11
Rotator cuff repair, **32**-8
Rouget, *see* Pericytes
RT-PCR, *see* Real time polymerase chain reaction
    (RT-PCR)
Runt related transcription factor 2 (Runx2), **7**-3

Runx2, *see* Runt related transcription factor 2
        (Runx2)
RWV, *see* Rotating wall vessels (RWV)

# S

SAEs, *see* Serious adverse events (SAEs)
SAMs, *see* Self-assembled monolayers (SAMs)
Sarcomeric proteins, **14**-4
SBF, *see* Simulated body fluid (SBF)
Scaffold, **2**-8, **11**-2, **12**-2, **17**-10, **30**-8; *see also*
        Biomimetic approaches
    adhesion-related protein immobilization, **12**-5
    anchored VEGF, **24**-8
    based cell therapy, **18**-16 to **18**-17
    biomimetic, **12**-2, **12**-4
    biphasic, **12**-9 to **12**-10
    bi-phasic nanofiber scaffold, **32**-9
    cell encapsulation, **20**-1
    cell-based scaffold, **34**-4
    collagen-modified PLLA, **12**-5
    composite, **12**-8 to **12**-10
    in dentistry, **33**-8 to **33**-9
    fine-tuning in sentistry, **33**-10 to **33**-11
    functionalized with bioactive molecules, **12**-5
    functions, **32**-5
    for gene therapy, **18**-5
    ligament-to-bone scaffolds, **32**-5, **32**-6
    matrix, **35**-5
    mediated gene therapy, **18**-5
    microvascular patterns within, **24**-5 to **24**-7
    mimicking ECM structure, **12**-10 to **12**-11
    nanofibrous, **11**-2, **11**-3 to **11**-4
    nanoscaffolds, **34**-4
    natural, **35**-5 to **35**-6
    osteoblasts seeding, **31**-5
    PCL-PGA fabrication, **12**-10
    physical protein adsorption, **12**-4
    poly(α-hydroxy)esters used as, **12**-3
    porous, **14**-8 to **14**-9, **33**-9
    spatial distribution in, **26**-12
    tendon-to-bone interface scaffolds, **32**-8
    3D multiphased PLGA microsphere scaffolds,
        **32**-13
    tissue growth in, **26**-2
    tissue-engineered, **18**-7
    topographic control of, **14**-9
    vascularization of, **24**-4 to **24**-5
    vascularized, **24**-10 to **24**-11
Scanning electron microscope (SEM), **11**-15
Schwann cells (SCs), **36**-11
    in peripheral nerve regeneration, **36**-5 to **36**-6
SCI, *see* Spinal cord injuries (SCI)
SCNT, *see* Somatic cell nuclear transfer (SCNT)
Scorpion primers, **13**-17, **13**-18
SCs, *see* Schwann cells (SCs)
SDF, *see* Stromal cell-derived factor (SDF)

SDS, *see* Sodium dodecyl sulfate (SDS)
SDS-PAGE, *see* Sodium dodecyl sulfate
        polyacrylamide gel electrophoresis
        (SDS-PAGE)
sECM, *see* Synthetic extracellular matrix (sECM)
Second messengers, **7**-5
Secondary lymphoid organs, **9**-6
Secreted protein acidic and rich in cysteine (SPARC),
        **33**-2
Seeding method, dynamic, **26**-9
Self-assembled monolayers (SAMs), **16**-2 to **16**-3
Self-assembling polypeptides, **20**-4 to **20**-5
Self-assembly, **16**-13
    advantages, **16**-14
    microgel, **16**-13
    of nanostructures, **12**-11
    of peptides, **20**-4
Self-renewal, **9**-9
    MSCs, **10**-3
SEM, *see* Scanning electron microscope (SEM)
Serious adverse events (SAEs), **18**-7
SF, *see* Silk fibroin (SF)
SFF, *see* Solid free-form fabrication (SFF)
Shear forces, **15**-5; *see also* Cellular
        mechanotransduction
    bone, **23**-4 to **23**-6
    cardiac, **23**-8
    cartilage, **23**-3 to **23**-4
    effect on tissue-specific cells, **23**-2
    skeletal muscle, **23**-9 to **23**-10
    skin, **23**-7 to **23**-8
    tendons, **23**-6 to **23**-7
    vascular grafts, **23**-9
Shear stress, **15**-5
    wall, **15**-9
SHEDs, *see* Stem cells from human exfoliated
        deciduous teeth (SHEDs)
Short-term HSCs (ST-HSCs), **9**-7
Sialoproteins osteopontin, **7**-3
Side-population (SP), **9**-8
Signal expression in engineered tissues, **7**-1
    anabolic growth factors, **7**-5
    catabolic growth factors, **7**-10
    chondrocytes, **7**-4
    dual growth factor studies, **7**-16
    hormones, **7**-13
    mechanotransduction, **7**-14
    osteoblasts, **7**-1
    signaling pathway overview, **7**-4
Signal transducer and activator of transcription
        (STAT), **7**-12
Signaling molecules, **4**-10, **23**-2, **37**-10
Signaling pathway, **7**-4
    autocrine signaling, **7**-5
    endocrine signal, **7**-5
    extracellular signal, **7**-4
    paracrine signaling, **7**-5

Silicone, **36**-5
Silk, **2**-1, **2**-11; *see also* Silk fibers; Silk moth;
      Spider silks
  biocompatibility, **2**-3 to **2**-4
  biodegradability of, **2**-4
  blends, **2**-7 to **2**-8
  in bone implants, **2**-8 to **2**-9
  in cartilage regeneration, **2**-9
  chemically modified, **2**-7
  chimeric recombinant systems, **2**-6
  in corneal tissue engineering, **2**-10 to **2**-11
  expression hosts for recombinant silk expression,
    **2**-6
  genetically engineered, **2**-5 to **2**-7
  insect, **2**-3
  *in vivo* degradation of, **2**-4
  length range of recombinant constructs obtained,
    **2**-6
  mechanical properties of, **2**-3
  native, **2**-5
  origin, **2**-1
  overview, **2**-2
  porous 3D silk fibroin scaffolds, **2**-8
  silk fibroin-based conduits, **2**-11
  silk-based biomaterials, **2**-5
  skin regeneration, **2**-10
  structure, **2**-2
  sulfonation of, **2**-7
  target tissue engineering applications, **2**-8
  in tendon and ligament repair, **2**-9 to **2**-10
  tissue engineering applications, **2**-5
Silk fibers, **2**-2; *see also* Fibroins
  mechanical properties of, **2**-3
Silk fibroin (SF), **11**-15
  advantage, **27**-6
Silk-elastin-like protein polymers, **2**-7
Silk-keratin blends, **2**-7
Silk moth
  fibroin, **2**-2
  inbred, **2**-1
  repetitive amino acid sequences found in, **2**-2
  wild, **2**-1
Simulated body fluid (SBF), **11**-15
  carbonated hydroxyapatite crystal formation, **12**-9
Single-stranded chains (ssDNA), **13**-14
Single-walled carbon nanotubes (SWCNT), **11**-15
SIS, *see* Small intestinal submucosa (SIS)
Skeletal development, *see* Chondrogenesis
Skeletal muscle, **23**-9 to **23**-10
Skeletal muscle precursors (SMPs), **28**-14
Skeletal Repair System (SRS), **3**-15
Skeleton, **7**-1
Skin, **23**-7
  fibroblasts, **23**-7 to **23**-8
  regeneration, **2**-10
  shear forces, **23**-8
  stretching of epidermis, **23**-7

Slow turning lateral vessels (STLV), **22**-2
Smad pathway, **7**-8
Smads function, **6**-2
Small intestinal submucosa (SIS), **36**-5
  for bladder regeneration, **34**-6
  in vascular tissue engineering, **35**-6
SMC, *see* Smooth muscle cells (SMC)
Smooth muscle cells (SMC), **16**-8, **22**-17
  F-actin stained, **16**-9
  for tissue engineering, **35**-4
Smooth muscle progenitors, **35**-4
SMPs, *see* Skeletal muscle precursors (SMPs)
Sodium dodecyl sulfate (SDS), **13**-8
  action on proteins, **13**-8
Sodium dodecyl sulfate polyacrylamide gel
    electrophoresis (SDS-PAGE), **13**-8 to **13**-9
Soft-tissue regeneration, **28**-11; *see also* Craniofacial
    bioengineering
  adipose tissue grafts, **28**-12 to **28**-13
  barrier in, **28**-12
  cell homing, **28**-15
  ectopic stem cell in damaged muscle, **28**-16
  hybrid implant fabrication, **28**-12
  *in vivo* implantation of bFGF and microchanneled
    PEG hydrogel, **28**-13
  nonmuscle stem cells, **28**-15
  satellite cells, **28**-13
  skeletal muscle engraft, **28**-14
Solid free-form fabrication (SFF), **31**-4
Solid-phase synthesis, **4**-3
Somatic cell nuclear transfer (SCNT), **8**-8
Somatic cells, **19**-2
Sonic hedgehog (Shh), **33**-5, **35**-8
Sonoporation, **18**-4
Southern blot, **13**-20; *see also* Blotting
Sox9, **30**-11
SP, *see* Side-population (SP)
SPARC, *see* Secreted protein acidic and rich in
    cysteine (SPARC)
Spatial distribution in scaffold, **26**-12
Spectroscopy, **25**-7 to **25**-8; *see also* Nuclear magnetic
    resonance (NMR)
Spheroids, **37**-6
  characteristics, **37**-12
  hanging drops of liquid, **37**-7
  liquid overlay, **37**-6
  microfluidic chips, **37**-7
  as model of tumor microregions, **37**-7
  reason for chemoresistance, **37**-13
Spider silks, **2**-1; *see also* Silk
  biocompatibility of, **2**-3
  European garden spider, **2**-2
  mechanical properties of, **2**-3
Spidroins, **2**-2
  isolation, **2**-5
  repetitive amino acid sequences found in, **2**-2
Spinal cord, **36**-2

Spinal cord injuries (SCI), **36**-7
Spinal cord repair, **36**-10
  olfactory ensheathing cells, **36**-10 to **36**-11
Spinal nerve, **36**-1
Spinner flask bioreactor, **22**-19; *see also* Bone tissue
      engineering bioreactor
Spin–spin relaxation, **25**-8
SPION, *see* Super paramagnetic iron oxide
      nanoparticles (SPION)
SPM, *see* Sulfopropylmethacrylate (SPM)
SRS, *see* Skeletal Repair System (SRS)
ssDNA, *see* Single-stranded chains (ssDNA)
SSEAs, *see* Stage-specific embryonic antigens
      (SSEAs)
SS-ILP, *see* Super small–insulin-loaded polymer
      microparticle (SS-ILP)
Stage-specific embryonic antigens (SSEAs), **8**-7
Stains, **13**-3
Stamping, **16**-11 to **16**-13
STAT, *see* Signal transducer and activator of
      transcription (STAT)
Static loads, **15**-6
Stellate reticulum, **33**-4
Stem cells, **19**-2
  amniotic fluid-derived, **19**-2
  classification, **19**-2
  differentiation, **30**-17, **30**-18
  division, **10**-3
  engineering with, **14**-12
  periosteum, **32**-8
  subtype of, **19**-2
  tooth regeneration, **33**-7
  for vascularization strategies, **24**-9 to **24**-10
Stem cells from human exfoliated deciduous teeth
      (SHEDs), **33**-9
Stem cells in cartilage engineering, **30**-7; *see also*
      Chondrogenesis
  adipose-derived adult stem cells, **30**-12
  bone marrow MSCs, **30**-11
  ESC, **30**-7
Step growth polymerization, **20**-7; *see also* Gelation
      mechanisms
  advantages of, **20**-7
  click reactions, **20**-7 to **20**-8
  Michael-type addition, **20**-7
ST-HSCs, *see* Short-term HSCs (ST-HSCs)
Stiffness, **15**-5
Stimuli-responsive systems, **17**-5
  enzyme-responsive systems, **17**-5
  pH-responsive systems, **17**-5
STLV, *see* Slow turning lateral vessels (STLV)
Strain, **15**-5
  relationship between stress and, **15**-6
  hardens, **15**-6
Stratified scaffold design, **32**-10 to **32**-13
Stratum intermedium, **33**-4
Strength, **15**-6

Stress, **15**-5
Stress-strain curve, **15**-6
Stromal cell-derived factor (SDF), **35**-3
  1α, **24**-3
Subcutaneous human tumor xenograft, **37**-13
Substrate stiffness, **14**-6; *see also* Cell–substrate
      interactions
  cell migration and, **14**-8
  diseased vs. healthy tissues, **14**-7
  effects of, **14**-6
  human neutrophil morphology and, **14**-7
Sulfopropylmethacrylate (SPM), **11**-15
Superficial zone protein (SZP), **30**-3
Super paramagnetic iron oxide nanoparticles
      (SPION), **11**-15
Super small–insulin-loaded polymer microparticle
      (SS-ILP), **11**-15
Surface erosion, **17**-4; *see also* Bioerosion
Surface modification, **16**-2
  technique, **12**-4
Surface osteocytes, *see* Bone-lining cells
Surface patterning, **16**-2
Surface seeding mode, **26**-9
Surface shear bioreactor, **22**-24 to **22**-25; *see
      also* Cartilage tissue engineering
      bioreactors
SWCNT, *see* Single-walled carbon nanotubes
      (SWCNT)
SYBR green, **13**-17
Symmetric divisions, **8**-5
Synthetic biomaterials, **5**-1 to **5**-2
  degradation, **5**-4
  degradation byproducts, **5**-5
  enzymatic degradation, **5**-4 to **5**-5
  hydrolytic degradation, **5**-4
  mass loss profile, **5**-5
  monomer choice, **5**-2
  non-polymeric, **5**-14 to **5**-16
  poly(acrylates), **5**-13 to **5**-14
  poly(anhydrides), **5**-10 to **5**-11
  poly(esters), **5**-7 to **5**-10
  poly(ethylene glycol), **5**-6
  poly(methacrylates), **5**-13 to **5**-14
  poly(ortho esters), **5**-11
  poly(urethanes), **5**-11 to **5**-12
  polymerization mechanisms, **5**-2
  pseudo poly(amino acids), **5**-12 to **5**-13
  stimuli-responsive degradation, **5**-5
Synthetic extracellular matrix (sECM), **20**-7
  grafts, **29**-5
  materials, **11**-2
Synthetic polymers, **4**-3
  PEG, **36**-9
  PLGA, **36**-9
  symmetric divisions, 19
Synthetic scaffolds, **35**-5
SZP, *see* Superficial zone protein (SZP)

# T

TA, *see* Tibialis anterior (TA)
TAAs, *see* Tumor-associated antigens (TAAs)
TAE, *see* Tris-acetate-EDTA (TAE)
Tail group, **16**-2
TAMCPP, *see* 5,10,15-Tri(4-acetamidophenyl)-20-mono(4-carboxyl-phenyl) porphyrin (TAMCPP)
T cell, **9**-6
TCPs, *see* Tricalcium phosphates (TCPs)
T4 DNA ligase, **13**-10
Technology development strategic directions, **1**-1, **1**-8
Teflon, **36**-5
Telomerase, **10**-7
Temporomandibular joint (TMJ), **31**-1
   bioengineering conference, **31**-6
   condyle, **22**-21
   disc tissue engineering, **31**-3 to **31**-4
   future of, **31**-6 to **31**-7
   human skull, **31**-2
   mandibular condyle, **31**-2, **31**-6 to **31**-7
   osteoblasts seeding, **31**-5
   tibial condyle-shaped scaffold, **31**-4
   tissue structure and function, **31**-2 to **31**-3
Tenascin, **29**-3
Tendon, **22**-25
   cyclical stretching, **23**-6
   shear forces effect on, **23**-6 to **23**-7
Tendon and ligament engineering, **29**-1; *see also* Fibroblast; Fibrous connective tissues
   advantages of, **29**-2
   allografts, **29**-2, **29**-4 to **29**-5
   animal models, **29**-12
   autograft, **29**-2
   biomaterial scaffold, **29**-7 to **29**-8
   bioreactor systems, **29**-8
   cell source, **29**-6 to **29**-7
   challenges and issues, **29**-11, **29**-13
   collagen ratio, **29**-3
   failures in, **29**-5 to **29**-6
   glycosaminoglycans, **29**-3
   injuries, **29**-1
   *in vivo* models to demonstrate efficacy, **29**-11
   synthetic prosthesis, **29**-5
   tendon autograft, **29**-2
   tissue engineering paradigm, **29**-6
Tendon/ligament tissue engineering bioreactors, **22**-5, **22**-25; *see also* Tissue engineering bioreactors
   challenges, **22**-26
   design principles, **22**-25 to **22**-26
   key features, **22**-4
   limitations, **22**-26
   traction mechanisms, **22**-25
Tendon markers, **23**-6
Tendons, **2**-9 to **2**-10, **32**-1

Tensegrity model, **15**-3
Tensile loading systems, **15**-11; *see also* Mechanical conditioning
   flexcell tension system, **15**-15
   four-point bending systems, **15**-14
   groups, **15**-11
   in-plane displacement systems, **15**-15, **15**-16
   longitudinal tensile loading systems, **15**-11, **15**-12
   matrix-contracting systems, **15**-15
   out-of-plane circular substrate systems, **15**-14
   stress causing factors, **15**-15
   tension application methods, **15**-12 to **15**-13
Tensile stresses, **15**-5
Tension, **15**-4
Teratocarcinomas, **8**-3
Teratoma, **8**-6
TERM, *see* Tissue engineering and regenerative medicine (TERM)
TERMIS-NA, *see* Tissue Engineering and Regenerative Medicine Society, North American chapter (TERMIS-NA)
Tetanus toxin C (TTC), **11**-15
Tethered growth factors, **4**-8
1,4,7,10-Tetraazacyclododecane-N,N',N'',N'''-tetraacetic acid (DOTA), **11**-14
Tetracalcium phosphate (TTCP), **3**-3; *see also* Calcium phosphate (CaP)
Tetraploid complementation, **8**-6
TEVG, *see* Tissue engineered vascular graft (TEVG)
TGase, *see* Transglutaminase (TGase)
TGF, *see* Transforming growth factor (TGF)
TGF-beta3, *see* Transforming growth factor-beta3 (TGF-beta3)
TGF-β superfamily, **7**-7; see also Growth factor (GF)
   bone morphogenic protein, **7**-9
   signaling pathway, **7**-7 to **7**-8
   smad pathway, **7**-8
   TGF-β1, **7**-8 to **7**-9
Thiele modulus, **26**-8
   effect on growth rates, **26**-10
Thin layer chromatography (TLC), **13**-24
Three-dimensional patterning techniques, **16**-10; *see also* Micropatterned biomaterials
   microfluidics, **16**-10 to **16**-11
   self-assembly, **16**-13 to **16**-14
   stamping/printing, **16**-11 to **16**-13
Thrombopoietin (TPO), **9**-5
Tibial condyle-shaped scaffold, **31**-4
Tibialis anterior (TA), **28**-15
TIL, *see* Tumor-infiltrating lymphocytes (TIL)
TIMP-1, *see* Tissue inhibitor of metalloproteinase-1 (TIMP-1)
Tissue cultivation multiscale modeling, **26**-1; *see also* Hybrid multiscale model
   bioartificial tissue cultivation, **26**-2
   biological spatial scales, **26**-2
   biot number effect on growth rates, **26**-11

cell migration, 26-3 to 26-4
cell population dynamics, 26-4
cell proliferation, 26-3
cellular Potts model, 26-4 to 26-5
emergent behavior, 26-13
factors in, 26-3
*in vitro* growth of cartilage tissues model, 26-5
mass transport limitations, 26-4
mass transport on, 26-9 to 26-11
migration speed on seed distribution, 26-11 to 26-13
modeling framework for, 26-5 to 26-6
spatial distribution in scaffold, 26-12
Thiele modulus effect on growth rates, 26-10
tissue growth in 3D scaffold, 26-2
tissue growth model, 26-5
Tissue culture
  dynamic, 26-9
  plates, 37-6
Tissue engineered vascular graft (TEVG), 35-4
Tissue-engineered human tumors, 37-13
Tissue engineering (TE), 6-1, 11-1; *see also* Bone engineering; Cell engineering; Dental tissue bioengineering; Nanobiomaterials
  basis of, 6-1
  biomaterial roles in, 12-1, 12-2
  biomimetic approaches in, 12-1
  bladder, 25-11
  cell stiffness, 14-8
  cellular behavior regulation, 14-9
  challenge component, 1-2
  components for, 22-21
  control process engineering, 37-14
  controlled drug delivery, 17-1
  critical concepts for, 1-4
  drug delivery in, 17-1, 17-8
  drug properties and design considerations, 17-7 to 17-8
  drugs of interest in, 17-6 to 17-7
  goal of, 3-1
  heart, 23-8
  mandibular condyle, 31-6 to 31-7
  modulators of strategy, 1-5, 1-8
  and morphogenesis, 6-1
  nanobiomaterial-based drug delivery system in, 11-10 to 11-11
  nanobiomaterials based imaging in, 11-12 to 11-13
  nanotechnology-based approaches, 11-1
  neoplasm and wound comparison, 37-3
  neovascularization limitations in, 24-1
  neural, 36-12
  on perfusion and hypoxia, 37-13
  products, 1-9, 12-1
  products for bone regeneration, 18-8
  publication records, 8-2
  stakeholders, 1-2
  strategic directions in, 1-2, 1-5, 1-8

strategic steps, 1-3
structures, 11-2
tissue regeneration, 12-10
tissue vascularization, 21-8
Tissue engineering and regenerative medicine (TERM), 19-1
Tissue Engineering and Regenerative Medicine Society, North American chapter (TERMIS-NA), 1-8
Tissue engineering bioreactors, 22-2; *see also* Bioreactor; Bone tissue engineering bioreactor; Cardiac tissue engineering bioreactors; Cartilage tissue engineering bioreactors; Micro-bioreactor; Tendon/ligament tissue engineering bioreactors; Vascular bioreactors
  bioreactors, 22-5
  cardiac tissue engineering bioreactors, 22-3
  cartilage tissue engineering bioreactors, 22-5
  challenges, 22-26 to 22-27
  current trends, 22-5 to 22-6
  features, 22-4
  micro-bioreactors, 22-3
  overview, 22-3
  tendon tissue-engineering bioreactors, 22-5
  vascular bioreactors, 22-5
Tissue grafting, 28-1
  growth model, 26-5
  inhibitor of metalloproteinase, 7-12
Tissue inhibitor of metalloproteinase-1 (TIMP-1), 29-3
Tissue interface, 12-9
Tissue necrosis factor-α (TNF-α), 7-5
Tissue plasminogen activator (tPA), 4-8
Tissue progenitor cells, 34-5
Tissue regeneration; *see also* Craniofacial bioengineering
Tissue scaffold, 7-1
Tissue structure and function, 31-2 to 31-3
TLC, *see* Thin layer chromatography (TLC)
TMJ, *see* Temporomandibular joint (TMJ)
TNF-α, see Tissue necrosis factor-α (TNF-α)
Toluidine blue, 13-3
Tooth, 33-2; *see also* Dental tissue bioengineering
  agenesis, 33-7
  dental papilla, 33-4
  dental pulp, 33-3
  development stages, 33-3 to 33-4
  genes expression, 33-6
  molecular mechanisms of, 33-4 to 33-7
  parts of, 33-2
Tooth regeneration, 28-9; *see also* Craniofacial bioengineering; Soft-tissue regeneration
  procedure, 28-10 to 28-11
  *in vivo* orthotopic and ectopic implantation, 28-10

Topographical patterning, **16**-6; *see also*
     Micropatterned biomaterials
   colloidal lithography, **16**-8 to **16**-10
   F-actin stained SMC, **16**-9
   imprint lithography, **16**-7 to **16**-8
   substrate's topography, **16**-7
Totipotent, **19**-2; *see also* Stem cells
tPA, *see* Tissue plasminogen activator (tPA)
TPO, *see* Thrombopoietin (TPO)
Traction mechanisms, **22**-25
TRADD, *see* Tumor necrosis factor receptor-
     associated death domain protein (TRADD)
TRAF, *see* Tumor necrosis factor receptor-associated
     factor (TRAF)
Transdifferentiation, **10**-4
Transforming growth factor (TGF), **2**-9, **7**-4, **27**-9,
     **30**-5, **33**-3
Transforming growth factor-beta3 (TGF-beta3), **2**-9,
     **8**-11, **27**-9, **28**-15, **29**-3, **32**-7
Transglutaminase (TGase), **4**-6
Transmembrane cell surface receptors, **15**-4
5,10,15-Tri(4-acetamidophenyl)-20-mono(4-carboxyl-
     phenyl) porphyrin (TAMCPP), **19**-6
Tricalcium phosphates (TCPs), **3**-2 to **3**-3, **32**-4;
     *see also* Calcium phosphate (CaP)
Tris-acetate-EDTA (TAE), **13**-5
Trophoblast, **8**-4; *see also* Embryonic stem cells (ESCs)
TTC, *see* Tetanus toxin C (TTC)
TTCP, *see* Tetracalcium phosphate (TTCP)
Tumor; *see also* Cancer
   biomimetics, **37**-13
   and host relationship, **37**-11
   necrosis factor, **7**-13
   and stroma, **37**-4
   and wound healing, **37**-4
Tumor engineering, **37**-1; *see also* Drug evaluation,
     preclinical; Spheroids
   polymers, **37**-9
   spatially dependent signaling, **37**-10
Tumor necrosis factor receptor-associated death
     domain protein (TRADD), **7**-13
Tumor necrosis factor receptor-associated factor
     (TRAF), **7**-11
Tumor-associated antigens (TAAs), **18**-18
Tumor-infiltrating lymphocytes (TIL), **37**-11
Tyr–Ile–Gly–Ser–Arg (YIGSR), **12**-7

## U

UCB, *see* Umbilical cord blood (UCB)
Ultimate strength, **15**-6
Ultrasonography, *see* Ultrasound imaging
Ultrasound imaging, **25**-5; *see also* Biomedical imaging
   disadvantage, **25**-5
   elasticity imaging, **25**-5
Ultraviolet (UV), **16**-3, **28**-7
   photoinitiators, **20**-6

Umbilical cord blood (UCB), **22**-13
Uniaxial force, *see* Axial force
Unipotent, **9**-1, **19**-2; *see also* Stem cells
uPA, *see* Urokinase plasminogin activator (uPA)
Urogenital system, **34**-1; *see also* Urogenital system
     tissue engineering
   reconstruction limitation, **34**-1
   tissue functionality, **34**-1
Urogenital system tissue engineering, **34**-1; *see also*
     Engineering specific urogenital structures
   acellular tissue matrices, **34**-3
   alginate, **34**-3
   biodegradable synthetic polymer, **34**-4
   biomaterial characteristics, **34**-2
   cell-based scaffold, **34**-4
   cellulose, **34**-3
   collagen, **34**-3
   extracellular matrix, **34**-2
   microenvironment control, **34**-6 to **34**-8
   nanoscaffolds, **34**-4
   pluripotent state cells, **34**-4
   polyesters of $\alpha$-hydroxy acids, **34**-3
Urokinase plasminogin activator (uPA), **4**-8
Urothelial cells, **34**-5
U.S. Food and Drug Administration (FDA), **34**-3
UV, *see* Ultraviolet (UV)

## V

Variable regions, **9**-5
Vascular bioreactors, **22**-5, **22**-17; *see also* Tissue
     engineering bioreactors
   challenges, **22**-19
   design, **22**-18 to **22**-19
   features, **22**-4
   requirements, **22**-17 to **22**-18
   for tissue-engineered artery cultivation, **22**-18
Vascular cell adhesion molecule (VCAM), **10**-3
Vascular endothelial-cadherin (VE-Cad), **35**-3
Vascular endothelial growth factor (VEGF), **3**-14
   in bladder regeneration, **34**-6
   BMP-2 on, **7**-10
   CAFs on, **37**-11
   host tissue against, **28**/12
   periosteal cells and, **27**-8
   in postnatal vasculogenesis, **35**-3
   proteolytic degradation sites on, **4**-8
Vascular grafts, **23**-9
   and medial equivalents, **35**-9
Vascular tissue engineering, **35**-1
   cell adhesion enhancement, **35**-2
   cell assembly, **35**-36
   differentiated cells, **35**-2 to **35**-3
   endothelial progenitors, **35**-3
   engineered vascular networks, **35**-10 to **35**-12
   growth factor signaling, **35**-7 to **35**-8
   matrix and culture effects, **35**-6 to **35**-7

mesenchymal stem cells, **35**-4
natural scaffolds, **35**-5 to **35**-6
pluripotent stem cells
    scaffolds/extracellular matrix, **35**-5
smooth muscle progenitors, **35**-4
synthetic scaffolds, **35**-5
vascular grafts and medial equivalents, **35**-9
Vascularizing engineered tissues, **24**-4; *see also*
        Neovascularization
approaches for promoting, **24**-2
cell self-assembly, **24**-4 to **24**-5
cell-based strategies, **24**-9 to **24**-10
growth factors, **24**-7 to **24**-9
inducing vascularization, **24**-7 to **24**-10
micromolding, **24**-6
patterned structures, **24**-5 to **24**-7
prefabrication approaches, **24**-10
prevascularized constructs, **24**-4 to **24**-7
surgical approaches, **24**-10 to **24**-11
three-dimensional confocal microscopy image,
        **24**-5
Vasculogenesis, **24**-3; *see also* Neovascularization
VCAM, *see* Vascular cell adhesion molecule (VCAM)
V-D-J rearrangement, **9**-5
VE-Cad, *see* Vascular endothelial-cadherin
        (VE-Cad)
Vectors, **18**-2; *see also* Gene therapy
cell-mediated gene therapy, **18**-6
of gene delivery, **18**-2
nonviral, **18**-4 to **18**-5
scaffolds, **18**-5
viral, **18**-2 to **18**-4
Vegetalisingfactor-1 (Vg1), **7**-7
VEGF, *see* Vascular endothelial growth factor (VEGF)
Vessel maturation, **24**-3
Vessel patterning, **24**-6
Vg1, *see* Vegetalisingfactor-1 (Vg1)
Viral gene delivery, **18**-2
    AAV, **18**-3
    adenoviruses, **18**-2 to **18**-3

DNA viruses, **18**-2
retroviruses, **18**-2, **18**-3
VK staining, *see* von-Kossa staining (VK staining)
von-Kossa staining (VK staining), **28**-11
von Willebrand Factor (vWF), **35**-3
Voxel, **25**-8
vWF, *see* von Willebrand Factor (vWF)

**W**

Weak interactions, **12**-11
Western blot, **13**-22; *see also* Blotting
basic steps, **13**-22
technical considerations, **13**-23
White tissue matter, **36**-2
Whitlockite, **3**-3; *see also* Beta-Tricalcium phosphate
        (β-TCP)
Whole tooth regeneration, **33**-12
Wingless integration (WNT), **33**-5
WNT, *see* Wingless integration (WNT)
Wnt repressors, **8**-11
Wound healing, **18**-9
WW domains, **4**-6

**X**

Xenografts, **18**-8
Xylene, **13**-2

**Y**

Yamanaka factors, **8**-9
YIGSR, *see* Tyr–Ile–Gly–Ser–Arg (YIGSR)
Young's modulus, **15**-5

**Z**

Zonal cartilage engineering, *see* Cartilage
        engineering, zonal
Zonal release, **17**-10 to **17**-11